HANDBUCH DER MEDIZINISCHEN RADIOLOGIE

ENCYCLOPEDIA OF MEDICAL RADIOLOGY

HERAUSGEGEBEN VON · EDITED BY

L. DIETHELM F. HEUCK O. OLSSON K. RANNIGER F. STRNAD
MAINZ STUTTGART LUND RICHMOND/VA. FRANKFURT/M.

H. VIETEN A. ZUPPINGER
DÜSSELDORF BERN

BAND / VOLUME XIII
TEIL / PART 1

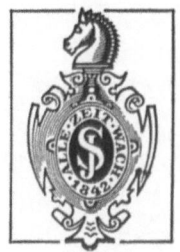

SPRINGER-VERLAG BERLIN · HEIDELBERG · NEW YORK 1973

RÖNTGENDIAGNOSTIK DES UROGENITALSYSTEMS
TEIL 1

ROENTGEN DIAGNOSIS OF THE UROGENITAL SYSTEM
PART 1

VON · BY

O. OLSSON

REDIGIERT VON · EDITED BY

O. OLSSON
LUND

MIT 448 ABBILDUNGEN (810 EINZELDARSTELLUNGEN)
WITH 448 FIGURES (810 SEPARATE ILLUSTRATIONS)

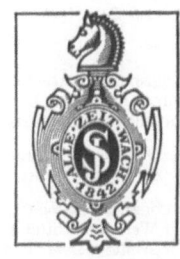

SPRINGER-VERLAG   BERLIN · HEIDELBERG · NEW YORK   1973

Professor Olle Olsson, M. D.
Department of Diagnostic Radiology
University Hospital
S-22185 Lund 5
Sweden

ISBN 978-3-642-95251-7   ISBN 978-3-642-95249-4 (eBook)
DOI 10.1007/978-3-642-95249-4

Gesamtherstellung: Sellier GmbH Freising

Softcover reprint of the hardcover 1st edition 1973

Preface

In 1962 in the series Handbuch der Urologie — Encyclopedia of Urology — Encyclopédie d'Urologie the roentgen examination of the kidney and ureter was extensively presented by the present author in collaboration with Gösta Jönsson. The roentgen examination of the distal genital tract and the male genital organs was presented by Lindblom and Romanus.

In the corresponding series Handbuch der Medizinischen Radiologie — Encyclopedia of Medical Radiology ten years later, we have arrived at the publication of the *roentgenology of the kidney and the urinary tract*. It was felt expedient that the entire chapter on urologic roentgenology be revised by the present author on the basis of a greatly enlarged current material from the Department of Diagnostic Radiology, University Hospital, Lund, Sweden. This hospital is a regional university hospital for a population of approximately 1,200,000 inhabitants in southern Sweden. Patients with specific problems for qualified diagnostic and therapeutic procedures are referred to Lund from other hospitals within the region, both central and local hospitals, and consulting cases are sent from very wide distances.

The present edition represents a complete revision of the earlier work, with the addition of several new chapters. Reference will nevertheless often be made in this work to the corresponding part of the Encyclopedia of Urology. To make possible the incorporation of a suitable number of illustrations — so important in roentgen-diagnostic publications — a very large number of new illustrations are added to a number included from the previous work.

The author wishes to extend warm appreciation and thanks to all members of his excellent staff in the Department of Diagnostic Radiology in Lund. He also wishes to express his gratitude to the heads and staffs of the clinical departments referring patients for roentgen examination for their close daily, fruitful cooperation. This gratitude is directed particularly to Professor Gösta Jönsson, Chairman of the Department of Urology.

Lund, November 1973   OLLE OLSSON

Inhaltsverzeichnis — Contents

XII

Part I:
Roentgendiagnosis of the kidney and the ureter

By

Olle Olsson

A. Introduction

Perusal of the urologic literature and current journals will convince any critical reader of the need for a comprehensive presentation of urologic diagnostic radiology in which the examination techniques and evaluation of the findings are based on fundamental roentgen-diagnostic principles. It is apparent from the literature that diagnostic radiology is widely practised without sufficient fundamental knowledge of physics, of the different examinations methods, of radiation protection, pharmacology of the contrast media, physiologic principles of dynamics, etc., all factors to be considered in the planning and performance of the examinations and in the interpretation of the findings.

Diagnostic radiology requires special training. Such training should first span the entire field before specialization is attempted in any particular branch of it. It is not possible to master any sector of diagnostic radiology without wide knowledge of the subject as a whole. Diagnostic radiology of the urinary tract occupies a central position in general diagnostic radiology. Roentgen-diagnostics of the urinary tract places great demands on the examiner's knowledge of diagnostic radiology in general because the original urologic disease may manifest itself outside the urinary tract, e. g. in the skeleton, lungs, vascular system, etc., just as the urologic disease may be only one component of a more or less generalized disease. In addition, the methods used in urologic roentgen examinations are in wide use in general diagnostic radiology.

Several fundamental technical details such as film, processing units, roentgen machines, high voltage technique, automatization, radiation protection, pharmacology and side effects of contrast media, etc. must be studied and tested in various branches of diagnostic radiology and evaluated on the basis of as wide experience as possible.

Technical skill in the performance of certain details of the examination such as arterial puncture and catheterization can be acquired and maintained only if the daily work includes a number of angiographic examinations. All technical variations as well as measures to avoid complications require cumulative experience.

The technical equipment, particularly for angiography, is specialized and expensive and thus cannot be procured for only occasional examinations.

Technical advances and clinical research have given diagnostic radiology a solid value of its own; therefore it is wrong to regard it or use it simply as a gratuitous supplement to the clinical investigation of any disease. Diagnostic radiology yields information on anatomic, pathologic and, to no small extent, on physiologic conditions. The method is based on a refined technique permitting wide variation and on detailed roentgen anatomy, which is ordinary normal anatomy with special attention to the many normal variants and presented in detailed densograms known as roentgen pictures.

Normal and pathologic conditions should be studied as closely as possible, with all necessary variations of the examination technique, and the results of the examination should be described in anatomic and pathologic nomenclature and not in photographic terms.

Only findings made in complete examinations should be considered, and then in full detail. If a roentgen examination is performed only half-heartedly or it is interrupted simply because preliminary findings happen to fit in with a preconceived opinion, or if technically poor examinations are accepted, the result may be a serious misdiagnosis.

Principles of examinations. The indications for the examination should be well founded, problems to be solved well defined, and the examination planned accordingly. The written referral for the roentgen examination must contain all information necessary for its planning.

The doctor requesting the examination must know what knowledge may be gained from the examination and should be able to assess the strain the examination implies for his patient.

The examiner should be competent and be able to perform the examination in the most rational manner. The examination should therefore always be performed by, or under the supervision of, a roentgenologist. Examinations by amateurs are condemnable.

The equipment should be of good quality. The roentgen machines must give the necessary output. The tubes, film, cassette material, etc., must be of good quality and continuously checked.

The patient should be properly prepared for the examination.

Every examination should be performed in such a way as to yield as much information as possible. This implies that the examination should include all necessary technical variations.

No examination should be performed in a standardized manner but varied according to the information desired regarding the specific patient and to problems arising in the course of the examination.

During an examination planned in a certain way, new problems may arise. The procedure should then be modified in a manner providing the best possibilities of solving such new problems.

Utilization of all possible modifications of a method is necessary to obtain the information desired. The roentgenologist must therefore perform or supervise the examination and study the films continuously while the patient is still available for further study, if necessary.

The films should document the results of a competent examination. Diagnostic radiology consisting of examination of films produced under standarized conditions is likely to lead to guesswork and is therefore condemnable.

If properly performed, the examination usually leads to a clearcut diagnosis. Often, however, the result of a basic examination may lead to a more specialized procedure to define diagnostic criteria. Occasionally the end result nevertheless offers more than one diagnostic possibility. In such cases findings at other clinical examinations and laboratory studies may help in arriving at the diagnosis. This process of the diagnostic combination of roentgen findings and other findings calls for team work between the roentgenologist and the referring colleague. Therefore regular daily staff discussions in the roentgendiagnostic department between roentgenologists and referring colleagues, with demonstration of examination results, are of great importance.

Reports. The result of the examination is described in a report. This report should be as short and distinct as possible. It should be based on studies at examination and of the resulting films, with anatomy, physiology and pathology as the basis. Photographic terms should not be used. No expression relating to visual impression should be included if not related to basic medical understanding. Reports on localization, etc., should be given in anatomically defined terms.

In a competent examination the films represent the end result of the examination and not the examination itself. Therefore the films need interpretation by the roentgenologist responsible for the examination. I have seen departments of diagnostic radiology in which films are given to the referring physician directly, without first being checked and studied by the roentgenologist. This practice is not compatible with serious roentgenology.

B. Examination fundamentals

I. Equipment

The following presentation is limited to a few points of general interest concerning the equipment necessary for urologic roentgen-diagnosis.

The roentgen apparatus should have a high output to permit performance of examinations with high voltage technique and with short exposure time. The apparatus should satisfy the highest requirements of routine work, i. e. renal angiography. This examination thus dictates the capacity of the apparatus. The frequency of exposures necessary for routine work, 5—10/sec. representing the various phases of the renal circulation, can be secured with a 6-valve machine which is also preferable to a large 4-valve machine from the point of view of radiation dose.

All types of roentgen examinations require strict consideration of the radiation dose. This holds especially for urologic roentgen examinations.

Pyelography must be performed under fluoroscopic control. Any examination table for pyelography not permitting fluoroscopy is unsatisfactory. It must offer the possibility of taking films under fluoroscopy and with a Potter-Bucky grid. Fluoroscopy should be performed under optimal conditions, preferably with the use of an image intensifier with television.

Angiography requires satisfactory equipment. To perform this type of examination with make-shift apparatus is no longer defensible. A film changer for film sheets or rolls should be available, although only one-plane films are necessary. The changer should be equipped with a program selector. It is better not to perform renal angiography at all than to perform it incompletely or in a *laissez-faire* manner.

For cine-radiography some sort of image intensifying technique should be used, with an image intensifier and television. Other methods give far too large a radiation dose. Electron-beam recording (EBR) will soon be available for cine-radiography.

The films should be examined under optimal conditions. This implies, among other things, that the viewing box space should be large enough to permit simultaneous examination of all the films during a urographic examination and permit comparison with previous examinations.

All work should be done with the right tools. Special work may require special tools. If such tools are not available, the work should not be done.

II. Radiation protection

In a situation in which a great number of chemical agents with possible serious somatic and genetic effects create enormous risks to populations, the sense of responsibility exhibited by the radiological profession should always be a model of the highest standards. Responsible radiologists in their daily work continuously observe the radiation problem with the aim of reducing radiation wherever possible to the smallest possible patient dose. Reference should here be made to the important work done by the the affiliation of the International Commission on Radiation Protection and the International Commission on Radiation Units and Measurements with the International Society of Radiology and the World Health Organization.

Many conclusions as to the proportion between radiation for diagnostic purposes and the total radiation of the population and as to genetic as well as general effects of roentgen radiation are based on loose grounds. Reliable research has shown that there is every reason to secure maximum protection against radiation, particularly of the gonads. A fair proportion of the radiation received by the reproductive organs is due to urologic diagnostic radiology. A reduction of the dose in this field is thus highly desirable.

In highly civilized countries the cumulative dose received in association with roentgen examinations is said to be less than 25% of the background radiation. It should be noted, however, that in background radiation the dose rate is very low. There is experimental evidence to support the opinion that radiation given at low dose rate produces mutation in a lower frequency than the same amount given at high dose rate. In their third report on radiation hazards the World Health Organization Expert Committee on Radiation concludes that under certain provisions for the population at large, exposure of a large number of individuals to small doses of radiation may produce the same number of mutations as exposure of a small group to larger doses. The production of chromosomal aberrations is indicated to be dose-rate dependent and irradiation of mature sperm seems to give a higher frequency of chromosomal aberration than does radiation of spermatogonia.

Although there is no reason to believe that ionizing radiation is the only, or even the principle environmental factor that can produce an increased number of mutations in man, exposure to radiation should be kept as low as possible.

Of all the sources of artificial radiation, roentgen examination is the most important. In a survey of conditions in Denmark, HAMMER-JACOBSEN (1963) found an equal distribution of roentgen examinations in males and females and the frequency of examination highest in patients above 40 years of age. He found further that 20—25% of examinations had a radiation distribution close to the gonads and that 13—14% of examinations included fluoroscopy. In a specific study on gonad doses, the very important fact is illustrated that there are very great variations in dose at the same type of examination at different hospitals, thus making mandatory a close scrutiny of the techniques for urologic roentgen examinations. A reduction is desirable, basically because the genetically significant dose per person per year has been found to be as high as 22 mR.

In Sweden urography including plain roentgenograms represents about 20% of the genetically significant dose produced by roentgen examinations (LARSSON, 1958). A marked reduction in the radiation dose during urography thus markedly influences the dosage received by the entire population.

The most important point for reducing population radiation is to keep to strict indications for every examination of the urinary tract. No examination should be performed unless the indication is rational, which means that the reason for the examination must be perfectly defined. The requisition for a roentgen examination must include all the facts necessary for choosing examination conditions which satisfy the need for the greatest possible information at the lowest possible radiation dose.

Roentgen examination of pregnant women should be kept low. In the earliest phases of pregnancy no examination requiring radiation at or close to the uterus should be performed. It is in some centers advocated that examination in this field of female patients of fertile age should be performed only during menstruation periods, thus assuring that the patient is not pregnant.

The second point to be stressed is that every examination should be performed with proper skill and that the technique selected should be such as to give the best possible information. It is necessary that the number of competent radiologists and assisting personnel should be sufficient. Medical students should be trained to respect radiation. Roentgen diagnostics should be performed only by competent roentgenologists and all roentgendiagnostic facilities in large hospitals should preferably be centralized, including personnel.

Keeping the radiation dose as low as possible can be aided by not using fluoroscopy, or, in spite of well-trimmed technique, by using it as seldom and for as short periods as possible and in recording by using the minimal number of exposures with the smallest possible field and the highest possible voltage. Such a small increase in voltage as from 60 to 90 kV can bring down the MaS-product from 250 to 30 with a corresponding reduction of the radiation dose.

Each roentgen tube must be provided with collimating cones or diaphragms preferably with light-beam localisers to limit the useful beam to the minimum size required for the examination. This will also enhance film quality. The examination tables for fluoroscopy should be equipped with well designed protective arrangements and the examiner should wear a lead rubber apron and gloves. The fluoroscopic equipment should preferably be an image intensifier-TV set-up. Correctly used, such equipment reduces radiation markedly.

Reduction of the radiation dose to which the patient is exposed during urologic roentgen examination can also be secured by covering the gonads of the patient with lead rubber. This is simple as far as males are concerned, and although more difficult, can also be secured to a fair degree in females. It is important that this precaution be strictly observed. We have found that during urography without protection of the gonads the testes will receive an average dose of 1,900 mR as against only 140 mR with lead protection and 20 mR with all proper radiation measures. At plain radiography including a film of the bladder, the dose could be reduced to 5 mR. In females proper protection will reduce the gonadal dose received in association with roentgenography of the kidneys by 30—40 %. In examinations in which the films must include the bladder, such as in complete urography, the reduction in the dose for females is small because some of the films must include the ovaries. The number of such films should therefore be kept as low as possible.

Regulations for radiation protection of the personnel should be meticulously observed. During the exposure no member of the staff should be in the examination room. Should it be necessary for the roentgenologist to be in the examination room during pyelography, for example, effective screening must be available. This is best secured by hanging up a suitably designed lead rubber curtain. The curtain may be placed and shaped according to specific requirements.

Strict attention should be given to radiation protection of both patients and personnel, especially in angiographic procedures. The most precise collimation possible during fluoroscopy and exposure will diminish radiation of the patients' gonads. At fluoroscopy — with image intensification, television and brightness control — the fluoroscopy time should be as low as possible. This rule must be observed particularly when fluoroscopy of the pelvic area may occasionally be necessary during catheterization from the femoral artery.

SVAHN et al. (1971) made a thorough study of radiation dosage in procedures carried out in the angiographic section of our department. They have concluded, on the basis of this study, that: 1. the gonads should be shielded, 2. the beam should be carefully collimated and the smallest possible field size be used for filming and fluoroscopy, 3. full-scale radiography should be replaced by 70 mm fluorography in certain examinations or by video-tape recording, 4. correctly adjusted automatic exposure and brightness control should be used. A general recommendation can be added: the examinations should be performed only by experienced roentgenologists.

The personnel should be checked continuously for radiation dosage. The film method is to be recommended. All members of our staff wear a film readily visible on lapel or blouse. Half of the film is completely protected. The film is developed after it has been worn for one week. If the wearer is found to have been exposed to radiation, he is given necessary instructions to avoid further exposure.

Continuous control and checking of radiation dosage and instruction on radiation protection are necessary and should be part and parcel of the daily routine.

III. Preparation of the patient for roentgen examination

For a roentgen examination to yield a maximum amount of information, the patient must be properly prepared.

A self-evident but unfortunately often neglected part of the preparation is to inform the patient as to what is to be done, and why. This is all the more important if the examination is likely to cause discomfort or pain or otherwise imply a strain on the patient. Such information promotes cooperation with the patient and thereby facilitates the examination. True and proper information should also be given the patient as to possible hazards included in the examination procedure.

Additional special preparation is often necessary. Since the kidneys and the urinary tract are situated in the retroperitoneal space behind the peritoneal organs, the contents of the digestive tract can be projected onto the urinary tract. The digestive tract should therefore be as empty as possible at examination of the kidneys and ureters. This can be secured by ordering the patient not to eat on the morning of the examination and by cleansing the tract. Usually a purgative is given the day before examination and two enemas, one the evening before and one the morning of the examination. The purgative is usually castor oil, which should be given early on the day before the examination because if given late in the day it will disturb the patient's sleep. If the patient cannot tolerate such a strong purgative as castor oil, a milder laxative may be used, but in such case, on two successive days.

For drastic purgation, tannic acid or Clysodrast has been used. The reports of several deaths in connection with multiple tannic acid enemas and toxicity studies in animal experiments (RAMBO et al., 1966) have resulted in the possibly somewhat hasty prohibition of these media in preparation for colon examinations. There was no detectable difference between the colonic or other toxic effects of Clysodrast and tannic acid.

Experience has shown that preparation with purgatives is time-consuming for personnel when practiced on hospital patients and that out-patients cannot always follow the rules completely. This results in poor preparation and, accordingly, risk of unsatisfactory examination. Therefore methods are continuously being tried to simplify the preparation while maintaining the highest quality. So-called contact laxatives do not influence the small bowel, have a selective effect on the colon, and are easy to administer. In our department we are using such a preparation (Bisacodil) given in dragée form, with a final cleansing with a ready-packed micro-enema. In order to minimize side effects it has been recommended (HEGEDÜS, 1971) to restrict fluid intake to maximum three liters per 24 hours. Coffee and tea are restricted, as are fat and slag-forming food. The patient follows a simple diet list during one day of preparation. With lunch on that day the patient takes two pills of the contact laxative and with dinner another two pills. The morning of the examination day the micro-enema is applied for emptying the rectum. For children this type of preparation is applicable with slight modifications.

This simple preparation has given better results than the former purgatives in a large comparative material. In 8—10 % the patients have a slight feeling of nausea, epigastric pain or dizziness. More serious side effects can be seen in exceptional cases, with exhaustion and fainting. Undoubtedly the results can be bettered and new media will be introduced.

The most important factor in all preparation is to get rid of intestinal gas, particularly in the colon. The gas is often abundant because of swallowed air or impaired absorption of gas. The major part of intestinal gas is swallowed air, which can pass rapidly into the colon. It has thus been shown (MAGNUSSON, 1931) that air introduced into the stomach by means of a stomach tube passes to the caecum within 6—15 minutes. Swallowed air is usually removed by eructation. In a bedridden patient, however, swallowed air passes through the pylorus, particularly if he is lying on the left side, i.e. when the pylorus is the highest part of the stomach. This is one of the reasons bedridden patients usually have more intestinal gas than others. The patient should therefore, if possible, be up and about before the examination, or sitting or lying on the right side, not on the left.

According to LILJA and WAHREN (1934) meteorism in pyelography is to a large extent due to impaired absorption of gas as a consequence of cystoscopy and trauma of catheterization, which causes a reflexogenic circulatory disturbance in the splenic area. These authors claim that meteorism is less marked if cystoscopy is performed under good anesthesia.

Various drugs have been used to diminish the intestinal gas, such as absorbents, atropine, pitressin, etc. The simplest and most important procedure, however, is to cleanse the intestine of gas and fecal matter in the manner described above. The examination should be performed early in the morning and without undue delay after the last enema and the patient should, if possible, be up and about before the examination. If disturbing meteorism or fecal contents persist, the patient may be prepared again for examination the following day.

Subcutaneous injections of posterior pituitary lobe extracts have been employed as a more direct means of getting rid of intestinal gas (COLLIN and ROOT, JUTRAS and CANTERO, SCHEIBEL, 1936). The preparations used were not pure enough to guarantee constant results. Deaths reported in connection with the use of pituitary extracts seem to have been due to impurities.

Since the availability of synthetic Vasopressin with its contracting effect on the smooth muscles, our department has taken up this type of preparation (GÖTHLIN, 1971). The patient is given 10—20 international units of 8 Lysine Vasopressin, Postacton (Ferring AB, Sweden). The preparation has been used in adult patients of all age groups (with the exception of pregnant women and patients with recent myocardial infarctions), with usually good or excellent results, best in the age group approximating 40 years. Poor results were seen in only 5 % of the cases. The best results are obtained when the Vasopressin is administered 30—45 minutes before the examination. The patients grow pale soon after the injection and in about one-third of the cases slight discomfort is experienced of the type epigastric pain and nausea. This discomfort is very seldom marked.

Opinions differ on the use of enema, particularly in the preparation of the patient for urography. It is claimed that the fluid infused can be absorbed from the bowel and cause diuresis, with consequent dilution of the contrast excreted and decrease in density. It has been shown, however (STEINERT, 1952) that absorption of the water is so slow as to be negligible if urography is performed soon after the enema. Our experience definitely endorses this opinion.

It has been discussed whether or not dehydration is necessary for patients who are to undergo urography, in order to increase concentration of contrast medium in the kidney pelvis. DUNBAR et al. (1960) made a very thorough study and an extensive list of pertinent literature is to be found in their paper. The authors found a slight and consistent improvement in quality of the urogram following dehydration in their study of 21 normal male adults subjected to urography. The improvement was minimal in the early stages of the examination and greater in the latter half of the first hour but was not of a degree warranting the inclusion of dehydration as a necessary part of the preparation for urography. Experiments in rabbits gave strikingly similar results.

Meteorism is more common in children than in adults. WYATT (1941) recommends the same measures to control meteorism in children as in adults, i.e. before the examination the child should be erect, prone with the head slightly raised or lying on the right side, but never on the left. A detailed rationale for managing meteorism has been devised by GYLLENSVÄRD et al. (1953). They recommend sedatives, the postures described above, and that the child be given a milk meal, with the addition of a viscosing agent.

The most important thing is to remove gas likely to be projected over the kidneys. A simple measure for this purpose has been suggested by KOSENOW (1955). He gives children 100—250 cm³ fluid in the form of milk, tea or juice before urography. The stomach thus filled with gas and fluid pushes aside intestinal gas so that with the patient supine the kidneys will be projected over the homogenous stomach. One can also fill the stomach with gas and thus secure a large homogenous gas bubble over the kidneys. This can be accomplished by the use of a carbonated fruit salt or carbonated beverage (BERG and ALLEN 1952, BERG and DUFRESNE, 1956).

Experience has shown that in small children up to an age of 1 to 2 years preparation has little effect and is thus unnecessary. After that age contact laxatives as described above can be used with suitable modifications.

Examination of a patient during an acute attack of a disease requires no preparation. More specific means of preparation are discussed in connection with the various examination methods.

C. Examination methods

I. Plain radiography[1]

Plain radiography of the urinary tract constitutes the basis of all other roentgen examinations of the kidney and the urinary tract.

The patient must be well prepared for the examination and the examination technique must be satisfactory as the difference in density permitting distinction between the kidneys and the surrounding tissue is small.

Plain radiography of the urinary tract in adults should include preferably two exposures: one of the kidneys and the major part of the ureters with the region of the suprarenals in the upper margin of the film (with a film 12 × 17 inches), and one of the lower part of the ureters and the bladder (usually with a film 18 × 10 inches). The two films should of course overlap each other in order to ensure that they cover the entire urinary tract. The focus-film distance should preferably be 1 m. The exposure of a separate film of the lower urinary tract and bladder has the advantage that the beam can then be directed roughly in line with the longitudinal axis of the pelvic canal. In such a film the contents of the small pelvis are projected free from the skeleton. Moreover, the method also permits suitable adjustment of the voltage and exposure time in the examination of patients above the age of fertility. The kidneys are influenced by the respiration and by the heart beat; therefore the exposure time must be fairly short and the voltage high, with consequent loss of contrast. The urinary bladder which is not influenced by respiration and heart beat, tolerates a longer exposure time, so that films may be taken with lower voltage and consequently better contrast. This is of importance in the evaluation of the thickness of the wall of the bladder, for example, and for demonstrating small, less opaque ureteric or vesical concrements.

The kidneys are of the same density as the surrounding tissue. However, as a rule the kidney can be outlined because of its fatty capsule. It is also possible to demonstrate the hilum and part of the sinus because of their content of fat. The medial outline of the kidney pelvis can sometimes be recognized, particularly if the pelvis is dilated. Normal ureters, on the other hand, will not be visible in plain roentgenograms. In the fatty capsule, local accumulation of fat laterally may indicate presence of lobulation or of a double kidney. In reduction of the volume of a kidney, the fatty capsule may be thickened correspondingly. Thus in a slight general reduction in size, a slight thickening of the fatty capsule may be seen on the side involved. In local scar formation a local fat pad may be seen. In marked shrinkage the fat may be abundant and occasionally the fat may be seen on both sides of the renal capsule: outside the capsule, fat padding increases; inside the capsule, fatty replacement of destroyed renal tissue occurs.

It is difficult to recognize the outline of normal kidneys if the fatty capsule is thin. In early infancy and in old age the capsule is normally thin. The so called oblique views (turning of the patient about 45° to the right on examination of the right kidney, and to

---

1 "Survey films" and "scout films" are other terms for these films. "Plain films" is an expression not always adequate but most commonly used.

the left for the left kidney) will enhance definition because a much larger area of the fatty capsule will then coincide with the direction of the roentgen rays. The upper part of the urinary bladder is well outlined because of the surrounding layer of fat; in women patients a clear border is usually seen between the bladder and the uterus.

1. Position of kidneys

The position of the kidneys varies within a fairly wide range. The right kidney is usually somewhat lower than the left. In one third of all persons both kidneys are at the same level. In children the kidneys are relatively lower than in adults and it is claimed (PETRÉN, 1943) on the basis of anatomic studies that the right kidney assumes its definitive position at the age of 5—7 years, the left at 8—10 years.

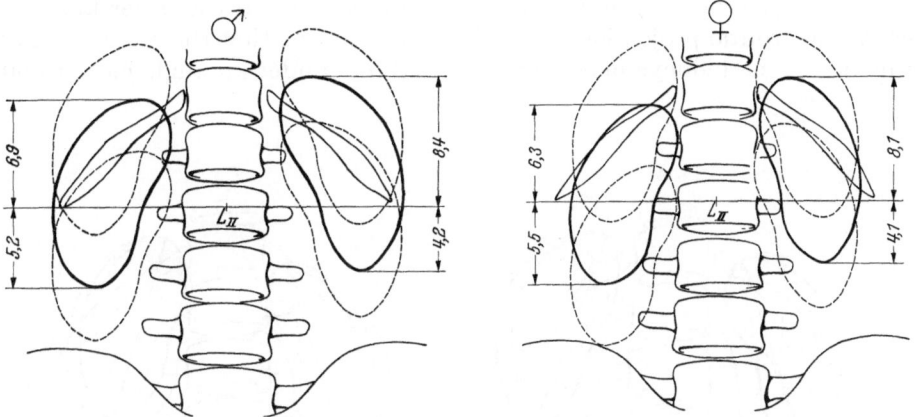

Fig. 1. Distances in cm, cranially and caudally from the middle of vertebra LII, of the poles of normal adult kidneys in plain roentgenograms. Dotted lines indicate ± 2 s (After MOËLL)

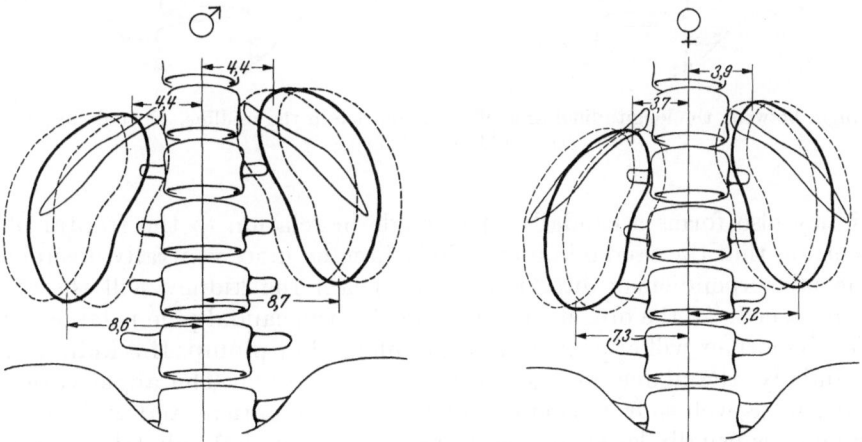

Fig. 2. Distances in cm of the cranial and caudal poles of normal adult kidneys from the midline in plain roentgenograms. Dotted lines indicate ± 2 s (After MOËLL)

The posterior surface of the kidney is usually situated 5—9 cm ventral to the surface of the skin of the back. The kidneys are usually related to the twelfth rib. As a rule, the level is such that the middle of the kidney is projected at the level of the upper half of the second lumbar vertebra. Sometimes, however, the poles of the kidneys may be situated the height of a vertebral body above or below the ordinary level (Fig. 1a, b). The most medial part of the kidney is usually projected onto or close to the tip of a transverse process, usually that of the first lumbar vertebra (Fig. 2a, b). The longitudinal axis of the kidneys forms an angle of up to about 20° with the midline of the body (Fig. 3 a, b). The medial outline of the kidney usually runs parallel to, and at a distance from, the psoas muscle varying with the thickness of the fatty capsule. The position of the kidneys in relation to the midline (distance and angle) and to the middle of the second lumbar vertebra was determined in 100 normal men and 100 women, aged 20 to 40 years, with apparently healthy kidneys. Statistical analysis showed that in males both kidneys are situated more laterally and that the angle between the longitudinal axis of the kidney and the midline is greater than in females. In both sexes the right kidney was lower than the left. The results are given graphically in the diagrams (MOËLL).

The kidneys lying on the angulated plane provided by the iliopsoas muscles are rotated with the medial parts anteriorly. The angle is fairly marked, which can be illustrated in a projection close to the lateral projection of the body. In such a projection the kidney pelvis on one side will be seen in a true lateral projection and the other kidney pelvis in a practically true frontal projection in the film. This means that the angulation is so great that the planes of the kidneys meet in the medial line under an angle close to 90°.

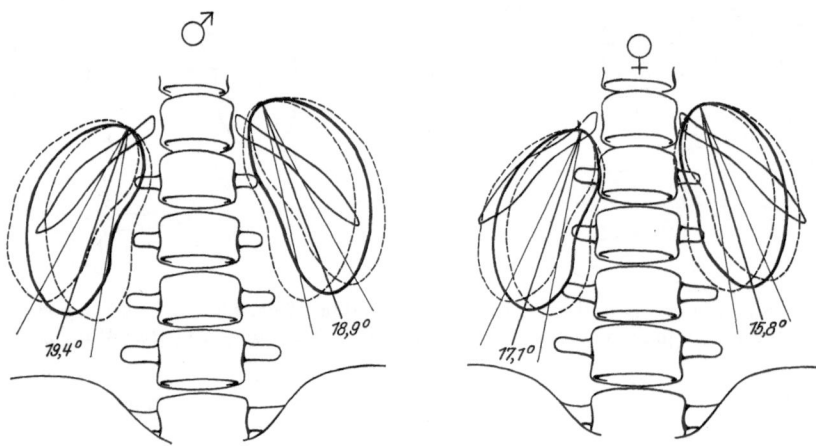

Fig. 3. The angle between the longitudinal axis of the kidneys and the midline. Dotted lines indicate ± 2 s. (After MOËLL)

The kidney also forms a caudally open angle in relation to the frontal plane of the body. This means that the caudal kidney pole is directed more ventrally in supine position. With the usual perpendicular direction of the beam the kidney will therefore appear somewhat shortened. As the object film distance for the caudal pole is larger than for the cranial pole, the former will appear somewhat enlarged or plump. If a kidney is markedly displaced caudally, the above changes will be very marked. The angle varies widely in different patients as well as from side to side in the same patient and with the respiratory phase. The angle is usually larger on the right than on the left side (HEGEDÜS, 1972).

The angle between the long axis of the kidney and the sagittal plane of the body may differ with body build: a short, stout person can have a greater angle. This angle may change if the kidney pelvis dilates or if an expansive lesion presses the kidney. Note, however, that a difference in the angle between the two sides is very common. This depends to a great extent upon the position of the kidneys: a higher position makes the angle smaller and a lower position increases the angle since the lower kidney pole is then more influenced by the psoas muscle.

The mobility of the kidneys in cranio-caudal direction is not insignificant. Respiratory excursions, which are well known from anatomic and roentgenologic studies, are made possible by the fact that the renal fascia encloses a space, closed cranially up to the diaphragm and laterally but open caudally (Fig. 4). The posterior leaf of the renal fascia is the muscle fascia of the psoas muscle. This posterior leaf is more or less fixed while the anterior leaf is fairly slack. Since this cranially closed sac is attached to the diaphragm, the upper part of the sac and the kidney follow the excursions of respiration. Since the perirenal fascia is a direct extension from the diaphragm, the movable diaphragm is a *sine qua non* for normal renal mobility. The range of mobility is limited by the vascular pedicle, by the attachment of the kidney to the suprarenal and by the fact that connective tissue runs from the renal fascia through the fatty capsule to unite with the fibrous capsule of the kidney. But even then the kidney is still fairly movable. Normally the range of movement is about 3 cm, somewhat less on the right side than on the left and somewhat larger for women than for men. On deep respiration, however, excursions of up to 10 cm may be recorded. These respiratory excursions of the kidneys have long been utilized for dia-

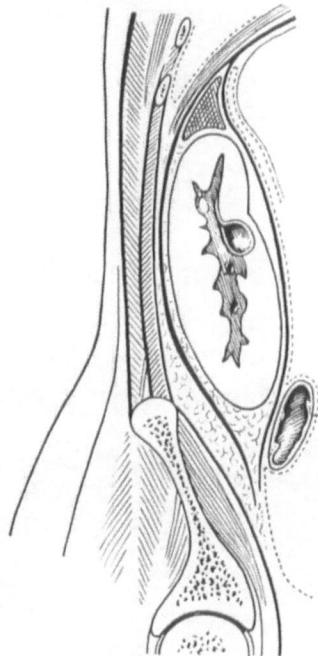

Fig. 4. Schematic drawing (after GEROTA) demonstrating relation of renal fascia to kidney and adrenal and to diaphragm

gnostic purposes and have been systematically charted to form the basis of a supplementary examination method (HILGENFELDT, 1936; HESS, 1939; BACON, 1940). It may be useful for locating calculi and metal fragments, for example, within or outside the kidney. It can also be used in the diagnosis of processes preventing excursions, *e.g.* edema, perinephritis etc. It is, however, of value only as a supplement to other examination methods.

The best demonstration of renal mobility is obtained by examining the patient in supine and in erect position and comparing the position of the kidneys in the two resulting films in relation to landmarks in the lumbar spine (Fig. 5).

KEATS (1931) in a large material found increased mobility of the kidneys in 18 % of women and 1 % of men and CAMPBELL (1967) stated that 90 % of mobile kidneys occurred in women. It is generally a condition of adult life and is much more common on the right side than on the left (80 % versus 15 %, 5 % bilateral) (THOMPSON and WALKER, 1948). (Fig. 5). It has been suggested that decreased renal blood flow could be the cause of pain in some of these patients. GÖTHLIN (1972) of our department has studied patients with mobile kidneys in supine and erect positions with a dye-dilution technique and found that the renal blood flow is unaffected and that there is no increase in vascular resistance in the erect position.

Extrarenal processes can displace the kidney. Enlargement of the liver, for example, can displace the right kidney distally, while shrinkage of the liver, as in cirrhosis, may be accompanied by cranial displacement of the right kidney. An enlarged spleen may displace the left kidney caudally and medially and flatten it, and so on.

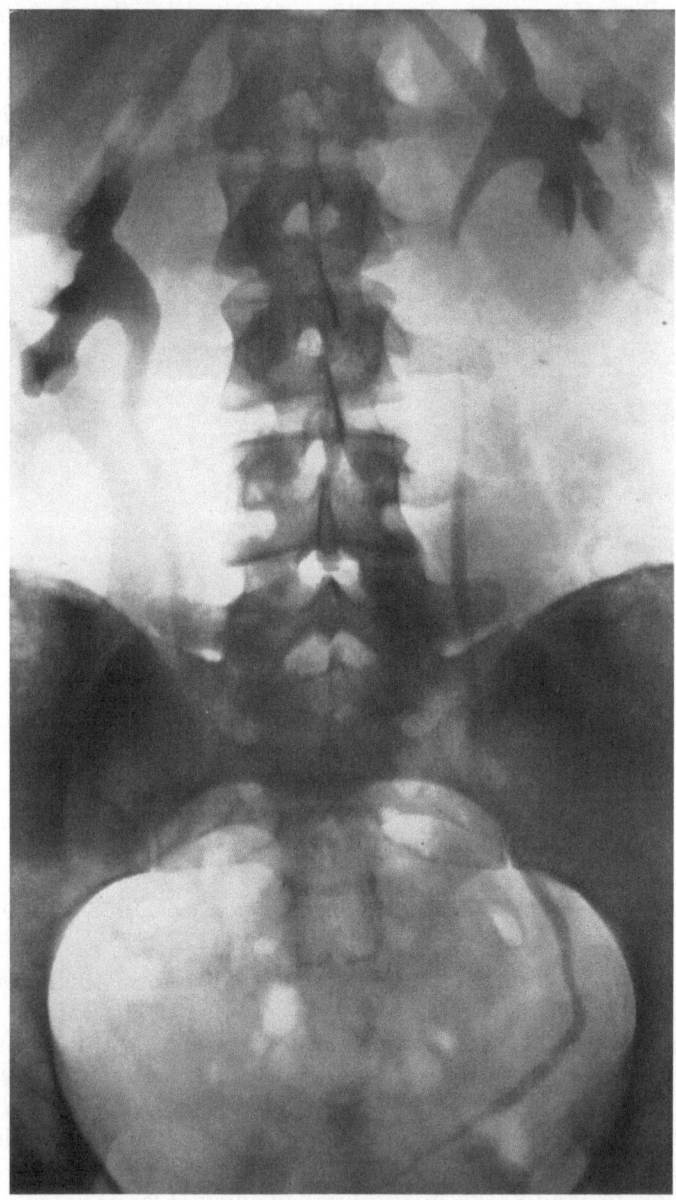

Fig. 5. Mobile kidneys. Urography. a) Prone position, b) Upright position. Both kidneys, especially the right kidney, move markedly downwards. Left kidney rotates slightly, the right kidney markedly

A certain range of movement of the kidney in ventrodorsal direction is demonstrable. The position of the kidney in supine position is sometimes different from that in prone position. In the supine position the upper pole can fall ventrally and sometimes laterally (see Fig. 23).

The range of movement of the kidney in mediolateral direction is very small. Definitely pathologic are cases where the kidney can be shifted manually across the midline

(ISAACS, 1971). This is due to a defect in the fascial attachment medially (SANDERS, 1957). A moderate range of movement towards the midline is sometimes demonstrable on examination of the patient in the lateral position and with the beam horizontal (PRATHER, 1948).

In ptosis approaching a pathologic condition the kidney is displaced, usually with the right kidney in caudal direction. As the kidney is also displaced forwards along the psoas muscle, it rotates with the lower pole directed ventrally. Therefore in plain roentgenograms in supine position the caudally displaced kidney will appear shorter than usual, and the increase in object-film distance will result in geometric enlargement of the lower

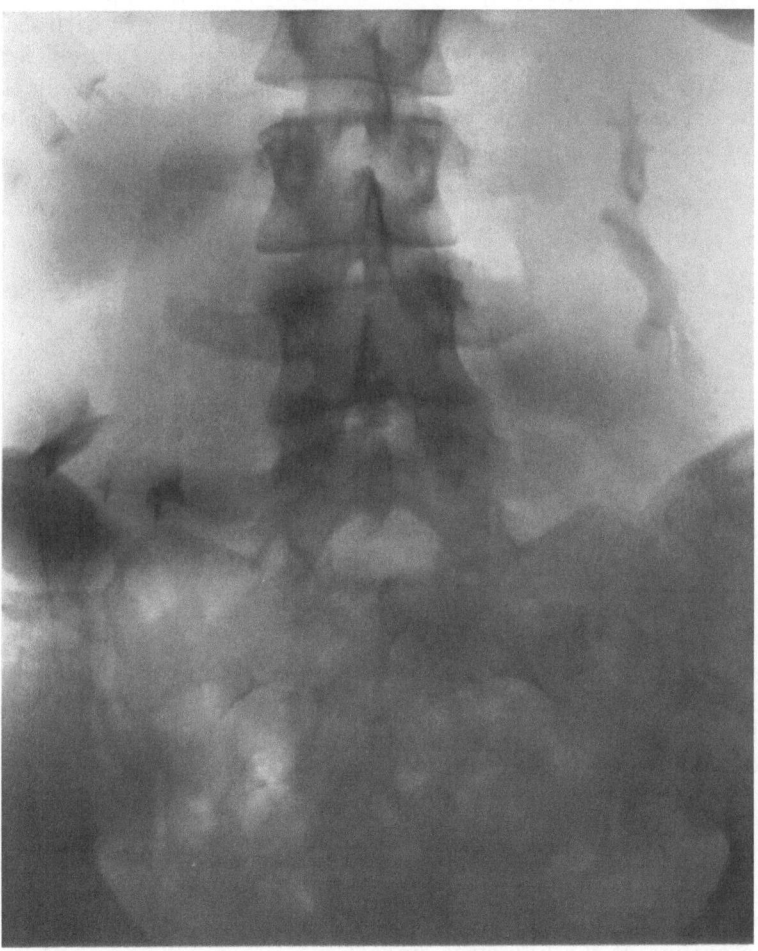

Fig. 5b

renal pole, which will then appear plump. The ptotic kidney is also situated more laterally than normally.

It is clear from the remarks set forth above that it is sometimes difficult to decide whether the position and mobility of the kidney in a given case is normal or pathologic.

It is stressed by COOK et al. (1971) that the upper urinary tract is the structure most commonly displaced by a retroperitoneal mass. It can be displaced in any direction except posteriorly. Forward displacement cannot be caused by an intraperitoneal mass. The lateral projection during urography is therefore helpful in determining whether an extrarenal mass is intra- or extraperitoneal. In a lateral projection obtained with a horizontal beam the renal pelvis normally lies posterior to the anterior border of the adjacent vertebral bodies. If the pelvis is located at the levels Th 12 to L 3, as is usually the case, the ureters lie posterior to the anterior margin of the vertebral bodies of L 1 and L 2 and do not usually cross anteriorly to the spine until they reach L 4 or L 5.

2. Shape of kidneys

The normal range of variation in the shape of the kidneys is wide. Occasionally the kidneys are long and narrow, occasionally short and thick. The upper pole of the left kidney is often very narrow because of modelling of the kidney by the spleen. The lower pole on that side then appears plump or its lateral outline will bulge. The relationship between the kidney and the liver produces a corresponding shape on the right side. The kidneys are most frequently bean-shaped although long kidneys with scarcely any rolling of the hilum are sometimes seen. Occasionally, however, the kidney is markedly rolled and angular and its lateral outline will then bulge. The distance between the surface of the kidney and the pelvis may be large, sometimes so large that it is not possible to exclude the presence of a space-occupying lesion in the kidney.

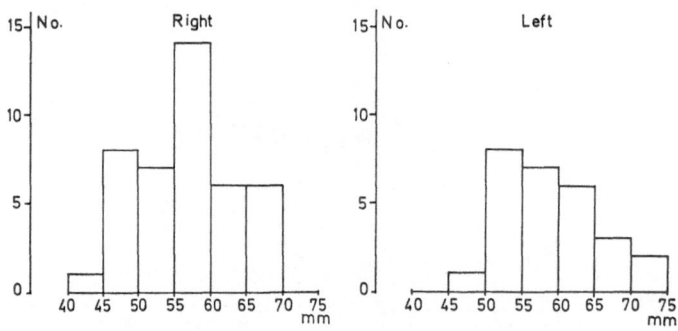

Fig. 6. Classification of the kidneys according to thickness. Average thickness of right kidney = 57.3 mm, of left kidney = 59.9 mm (Hegedüs 1972)

The outline of the kidney is smooth as a rule, with the exception of the medial part where it may be interrupted or a recess may be seen due to the renal hilum. The width of the hilum varies and it is often possible to delimit only the cranial or caudal border distinctly. In double renal pelvis an unusually wide hilum or double hilum may be seen. Below the hilum the medial outline of the kidney bulges more than cranially to the hilum. This medial outline usually runs parallel to the edge of the psoas muscle, alongside it or, if the fatty capsule is thick, some distance from it.

The surface of the kidney may be uneven because of persistent fetal lobulation. Such lobulation corresponds to the pyramids and occurs regularly before 4 years of age but may persist later. Usually only the deep furrows persist, namely those bordering on the pars cranialis, pars intermedia, and pars caudalis of the kidney (Löfgren, 1949). Otherwise the outline of the kidney is smooth.

The different shapes of the kidneys are also a reflection of the renal thickness, which differs between the two sides (Fig. 6).

3. Size of kidneys

The size of the kidneys is important *per se* and for estimating the amount of kidney parenchyma, especially in cases of generalized parenchymal diseases (see chapter L). The kidneys vary widely in length and breadth. In roentgenograms taken at a focus-film distance of 1 metre and without correction for ordinary variation in the object-film distance the length and breadth of the kidneys has been measured by Moëll (1956). Pertinent references are given in his paper of 1961.

The determinations were made on plain roentgenograms of the abdomen of 100 males and 100 females 20—49 years of age with apparently healthy kidneys. The total area (sum of products of length × width of right and left kidney) and kidney weights found

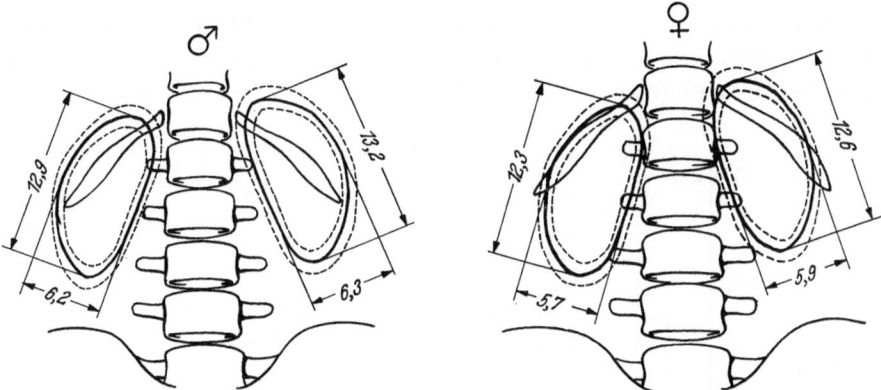

Fig. 7. Size of normal kidneys in males and females (After MoËLL)

post mortem were also correlated to form an opinion of the mass of the renal parenchyma. In males both the right and the left kidney were significantly larger than in females, also the total area. The left kidney was also significantly larger than the right in males and females. The results are given in the figures (Fig. 7a, b).

The sizes of normal kidneys in adults are as follows with the standard deviation within brackets:

males $\left\{\begin{array}{l}\text{right } 12.9 \ (0.80) \times 6.3 \ (0.45) \\ \text{left } \quad 13.2 \ (0.49) \times 6.3 \ (0.49)\end{array}\right.$ females $\left\{\begin{array}{l}\text{right } 12.3 \ (0.79) \times 5.7 \ (0.46) \\ \text{left } \quad 12.6 \ (0.77) \times 5.9 \ (0.42)\end{array}\right.$

The kidney-weight can be predicted from the diagram (Fig. 8) representing a material of over one hundred pairs of kidneys. The figures are treated logarithmically. The thin lines indicate a range of 2s.

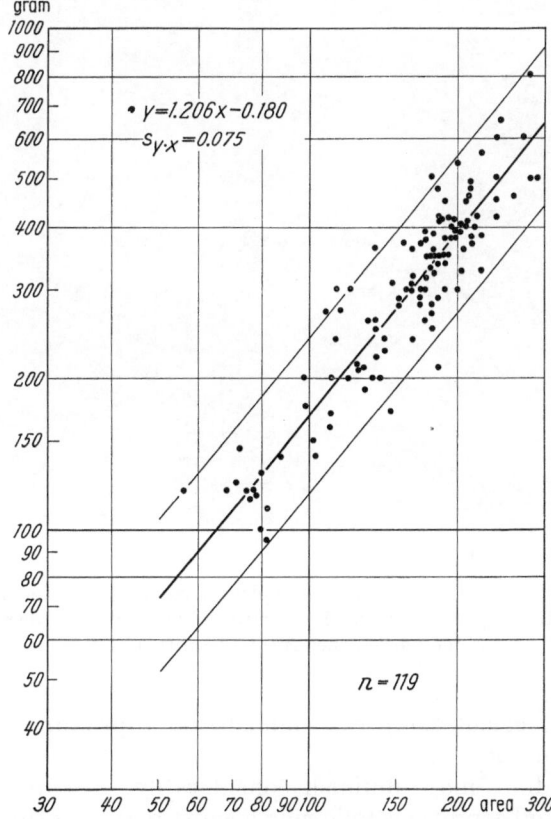

Fig. 8. Diagram for estimation of kidney weight from area of kidney in roentgenogram. Thin borderlines represent 2 s (After MoËLL)

The size of the kidneys was not found to vary appreciably with body build (stature, body weight, m² body surface, and area of vertebra L_{II}, as measured in the roentgenogram). On the basis of angiographic studies HEGEDÜS (1971) has made an investigation of

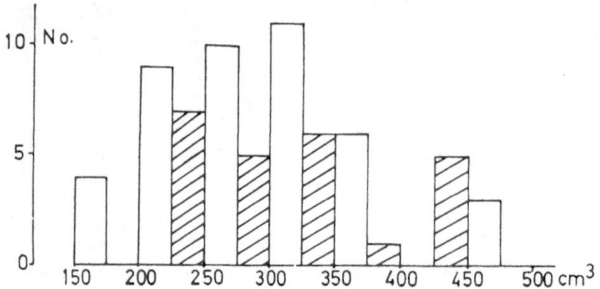

Fig. 9. Classification of the kidneys according to the roentgenologic volume. Average value of right kidney = 295 cm³ (open fields), of left kidney = 311 cm³ (hatched fields) (HEGEDÜS 1972)

kidney volume (Fig. 9). The roentgenologic volume was related to volume of autopsy kidneys, with the post mortem skrinkage of the kidney specimens taken into account. The average decrease was found to be 24 %. The roentgenologic volume (using the true

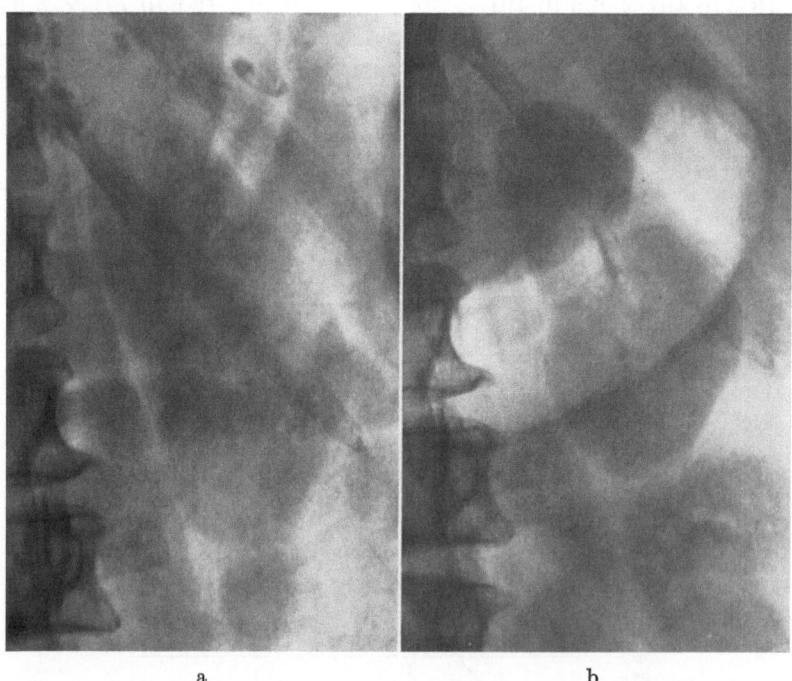

a   b

Fig. 10. Rapid fall in blood pressure in connection with splenoportography: a) left kidney at beginning of examination; b) same kidney after rapid fall in blood pressure. Kidney size has decreased markedly; length of kidney diminished from 12 cm to 10 cm

lateral projection in the calculation) was found to be approximately 50 volume percent higher than the true volume.

The size of the kidney may diminish considerably in connection with shock and after restoration of normal conditions following a short period of shock the size may return to normal (Fig. 10).

4. Calcifications projected onto the urinary tract

Calcifications are often seen at plain roentgenography of the urinary tract. They may be situated within or outside the urinary tract. Calcifications in the kidneys may be of many types and will be discussed in association with various diseases. Calcifications projected onto the urinary tract but situated outside the urinary pathways are, for example, calcified lymph nodes, gallstones, extrarenal vascular calcifications, fecal matter, etc. It is necessary, of course, to decide whether they are intra-or extrarenal. This may be determined readily by changing the projection and taking oblique views in the manner described above. Calcifications situated within the kidney, thus in the renal parenchyma or renal pelvis, are then projected onto the kidney, regardless of the angle of projection. Calcifications lying outside the kidney will, in suitable projection, be projected outside the kidney. The more distant a calcification is from the anterior or posterior surface of the kidney, the less the angle of projection need be changed to project it outside the kidney. The closer an extrarenal calcification is situated to the kidney, the more the angle of projection must be changed to show that it really lies outside the kidney. Judging from certain urologic handbooks, various elaborate and unnecessary procedures are sometimes used for ascertaining whether calcifications are situated within or outside the kidney. Such procedures can be replaced by the simple measures described above.

Change in projection is of importance also in the examination of calcifications in or beneath the ureter.

It may be well in this connection to mention a source of error which, although not common, is very embarrassing if it leads to erroneous interpretation. A fibroma or atheroma in the skin of the back and raised above the surface of the skin may cause a local increase in density which may be projected onto the kidney and simulate a stone. The source of error is well known from chest examinations but should be borne in mind even in the examination of kidneys. Oblique views will show that it is a question of a finding dorsal to the kidney and a glance at the patient's back will explain it.

Calcifications in the veins, phlebolites, are very common. They may be unilateral or bilateral, solitary or multiple, and of various sizes an shapes. They are often very dense and laminated. Occasionally they occur exclusively on one side. They are important in differentiation from ureteric stones. It may be difficult in some cases to decide whether a calcification or one of many calcifications is a phlebolite or a ureteric stone. Urography or pyelography will solve the problem (see chapter E).

Prostatic calcifications are often seen. They vary widely in size, number and distribution. They are usually symmetrical but occasionally occur almost exclusively on one side.

The suprarenals are fairly often seen as triangular, soft tissue densities surrounded by fat and situated cranially to the kidneys.

In plain roentgenograms a rounded soft tissue formation is often seen above the left kidney. This has been misinterpreted as suprarenal tumor. In reality it is the contracted fornix part of the stomach which, because of its backward tilt, lies with its axis in line with the beam, with the result that the organ tends to appear as a density in the roentgenogram.

Plain roentgenography is important per se and as a guide to planning of subsequent examination with contrast medium. *It is wrong to undertake roentgen examination of the urinary tract with contrast medium without previous, careful plain roentgenography.*

II. Additional methods

1. Zonography and tomography

If it is difficult to outline the kidneys because of lack of perirenal fat, zonography or tomography may be resorted to. These methods, by enhancing the contrast, can facilitate recognition of the outline of the kidney. If for some reason the intestine cannot be cleansed satisfactorily, it may be difficult to study the kidney. In such cases zonography is valuable. The method should not, however, be used routinely as a substitute for plain roentgenography. Neither should it be used simply to avoid proper preparation of the patient.

Another indication for tomography is in outlining the kidneys in association with retroperitoneal pneumography. It may occasionally be used to advantage in connection with nephrography, for example, but it should not be resorted to for purposes served equally well by simpler ordinary methods.

On the basis of antero-posterior plain roentgenograms of the abdomen, Dure-Smith and McArdle (1972) have constructed a diagram to facilitate the choice of level for tomography of the kidneys. Using the predicted level of cut with one cut 2 cm above and another 2 cm below this level, the kidney could be shown in the great majority of cases with an optimal angle of swing for routine use of 25°. Zonography was found not to eliminate overlying bowel gas adequately and multi-leaf cassettes were found to give an unacceptable loss of detail.

Transversal tomography may be of value on occasion in association with retroperitoneal pneumography.

2. Retroperitoneal pneumography

If it is difficult to demonstrate the kidneys and suprarenals by plain roentgenography, gas may be injected into the retroperitoneal space to increase the contrast between these organs and the surrounding tissue. The gas may be injected directly around the kidney. The examination is usually known as perirenal gas insufflation or pneumoren (Rosenstein, 1921; Carelli, 1921). This method has been used to some extent and has been discussed in the literature (Sinner, 1955). However, it has been more or less superseded by the method described by Ruiz Rivas in 1947, in a preliminary report, and in 1950, in further detail. This method is simple and more reliable. It has been described under various names such as retropneumoperitoneum, pneumoretroperitoneum, retroperitoneal emphysema, retroperitoneal gas insufflation, perirenal gas contrast, extraperitoneal pneumography. It will be referred to here as retroperitoneal pneumography. This method has received much attention in the literature (see Cocchi, 1957).

Anatomy. The method is based on the fact that retroperitoneal organs, in this case the kidneys and suprarenals, are embedded in more or less fatty connective tissue continuous with connective tissue in other regions. The pelvic connective tissue thus continues directly upwards *inter alia* into the retroperitoneum and further through and above the diaphragm. The retroperitoneal connective tissue is voluminous in those spaces situated on either side of the lumbar spine and containing the kidneys and suprarenals enclosed in the renal fascia. This fascia is described as surrounding the kidneys and suprarenals like a veil closed laterally and cranially but more or less wide open caudally (Fig. 11). Gas injected into the connective tissue space retrorectally can pass up into this retroperitoneal space and, via the caudal opening, enter the renal fascia and surround the kidney and suprarenal and find its way into the interstices in the connective tissue between these two organs. The fatter the connective tissue the quicker the gas will enter the loose tissue, while denser connective tissue will offer more resistance to the passage of the gas. Sometimes the connection between the kidney and the suprarenal may be so dense as not to permit the passage of gas between the two organs.

Technique. The patient is prepared for the examination in the same way as for urography. Some authors recommend premedication of one sort or another, mainly sedatives, but this is, as a rule, unnecessary.

Contrast media: Various types of gas such as nitrogen, carbon dioxide, nitrous oxide and helium have been used. Attempts have been made to use pentane, the boiling point of which is lower than normal body temperature and which thus volatilizes in the tissues.

Oxygen is most commonly used because it is rapidly absorbed, usually within 24 hours, and because it involves scarcely any risk of embolism. This gas, if it enters the vascular system, may be bound by the blood pigments (see under "Hazards" below). The gas most readily soluble in the blood, however, is carbon dioxid, whereas air is absorbed only slowly. The use of helium has been suggested by LEVINE (1952) and SENGER *et al.* (1953). This gas should *not* be used, however, because it is the least soluble and therefore the most dangerous. Statements that helium "casts a somewhat darker shadow than the air" and that it gives a "slightly sharper contrast than air" only reveal astonishing lack of knowledge of the fundamentals of diagnostic radiology.

The amount of gas used varies between $^1/_2$—$1^1/_2$ liters. In children the dose may be reduced down to 100 ml.

Many authors have expressed the view that tomography is necessary in association with retroperitoneal pneumography (GANDINI and GIBBA, 1954; GIRAUD *et al.*, 1956, etc). It is not necessary but may on occasion be helpful. Transverse-section tomography

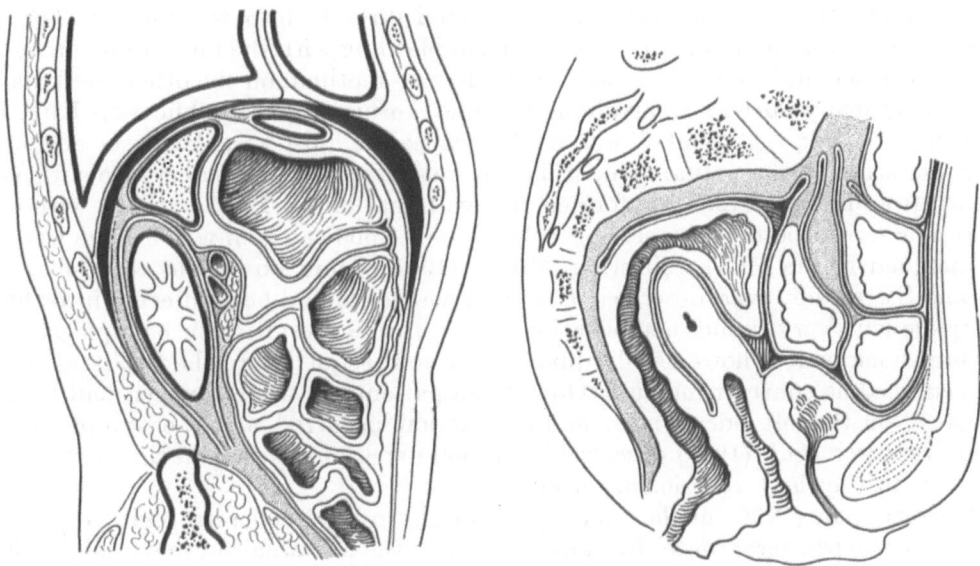

Fig. 11. Schematic drawing (after RUIZ RIVAS) illustrating relation between retrorectal-retroperitoneal connective tissue space and renal fascia

may also be used. Abdominal angiography has been performed in association with this examination method (GOODWIN *et al.*, 1955, etc.). To judge from illustrations in the literature, the method is used in connection with many other procedures, mostly unjustifiably.

The use of high voltage technique, about 200 kV, rational in methods where gas is used as contrast agent, is advocated by ENGELKAMP (1960).

Puncture technique. The coccyx is identified and puncture is made with an ordinary lumbar needle immediately adjacent to this bone. The tip of the needle is directed medially and cranially and towards the sacrum. Penetration of the rectal mucosa can be avoided by palpation with a finger in the rectum. A modification with the introduction of the needle through one of the coccygeal intervertebral spaces has been suggested (PALUBINSKAS and HODSON, 1958). The advantage of this procedure is that the needle is held more firmly in position. Another modification is presented by LANDES and RANSOM (1959). They place two thin vinyl catheters in the retro-rectal space.

To be sure that the tip of the needle is not situated within a blood vessel, aspiration is tried and, to secure a free injection space, a small amount of physiologie saline can be injected. Via a sterile pipette with a layer of cotton wool for sterilising the gas, the needle is then connected with a gas container of the type used for therapeutic pneumothorax or gas myelography, for example. During puncture and injection of the gas the patient may be in the knee-elbow position or lying on his side, preferably with the side of greater diagnostic interest uppermost. The gas is injected fairly slowly. Some authors check the position of the gas under fluoroscopy after a few hundred millimetres have been injected. This is, as a rule, not neccessary. After the gas has been injected films are exposed, usually plain films and possibly with the patient in different positions, including the erect position to secure passage of the gas to those areas of greatest diagnostic interest. During and after the injection of gas the patient has a feeling of fullness or abdominal tension and occasionally slight pain in the diaphragm, sometimes radiating up to the shoulders.

The equipment necessary for the procedure is simple. The items are listed by BLAND (1958).

Hazards. Deaths, mostly from gas embolism, have been known to occur in association with pneumoren. This is not surprising since the gas is injected quite close to the kidney and might therefore be accidentally injected directly into the kidney. The lesion caused by the actual puncture may also result in bleeding with the formation of a perirenal hematoma (COPE and SCHATZKI, 1939). RUIZ RIVAS' method, on the other hand, has been described by many authors as involving no risks. In his original publication RUIZ RIVAS stated that the risk of gas emboli was small because the most vascular tissue encountered during puncture is the actual skin, while the retor-rectal tsisue is very poor in vessels. STEINBACH and SMITH (1955) performed the examination on 1,995 patients without any fatalities or serious complications. In a collection of 1,500 cases, of which some were probably included in the above collection, MOSCA (1951) found no serious reactions. STEINBACH and SMITH, however, described 4 cases in which gas had been injected into the presacral tissue with very serious complications, 2 fatal, one resulting in hemiplegia and one in severe shock which, however, disappeared without sequelae. In the two fatal cases, air had been used as contrast medium. One of the patients in whom oxygen had been used was placed on the left side as soon as the reaction occurred and the symptoms disappeared. DURANT et al. (1947) observed in animal experiments that in this posture no air trap arose in the right ventricular outflow tract.

RANSOM et al. (1956) made a survey including over 9,000 retroperitoneal pneumographies by the presacral route. In 24 of these cases the examination was fatal and in 33 it caused severe non-fatal reactions (over 2,000 examinations of the pneumoren type caused 34 deaths and 31 severe non-fatal reactions). The investigation showed that the frequency of fatalities was equal when air or oxygen was used and the authors concluded that oxygen is not safer than air to any significant degree and recommended the use of carbon dioxide, which is 20 times more soluble in blood than is oxygen. (STAUFFER et al. in 1957 and GROSSE-BROCKHOFF et al. in 1959 used this gas as a contrast medium for angiocardiography and injected large amounts directly into the vascular system without undesirable reactions.)

Since the above dates, further cases of general reactions have been described without, however, contributing to our knowledge of the risks involved in the use of the method. A strange case of gas embolism in association with the use of oxygen, 600 ml, described by SCHULTE (1959) must be mentioned however. The examination was accompanied not only by shock, but also by the simultaneous appearance of cherry-sized livid spots on the skin of the back at the level of the low ribs. The general reactions disappeared as soon as the patient was placed on the left side.

METZLET et al. (1972) report on retroperitoneal pneumography in 98 patients through the use of carbon dioxide. All of the patients had marked pain in the back and abdomen. Marked rise in blood pressure occurred in three of five patients with pheochromocytoma.

It is obvious that all precautions must be taken. It must be checked, for example, that the tip of the needle is not situated within the lumen of a vessel. This check must be repeated on observation of any change in the position of the needle during the examination. The gas must be injected slowly, and gas soluble in blood should be used.

Other complications are emphysema of the scrotum, of the mediastinum and of the neck. In addition, cases of pneumothorax and pneumoperitoneum have been described. Poor asepsis will, of course, favor infection.

In the evaluation of the risks it may be convenient first to consider the indications. Retroperitoneal pneumography should not be used unless other roentgen methods have first been tried without success. The large series of retroperitoneal pneumography reported by some authors only show that the method is undoubtedly often used on very loose indications or quite unnecessarily.

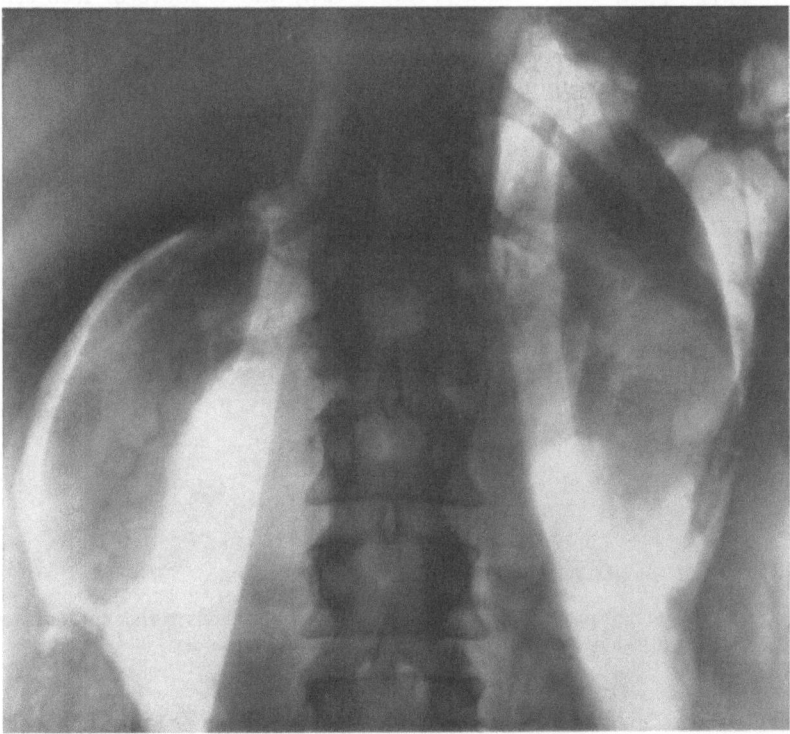

Fig. 12. Retroperitoneal pneumography

The method is contraindicated by any local inflammatory process at the intended site of injection and by poor general condition, particularly when due to cardiac insufficiency.

Normal anatomy. Normally it is not difficult for the gas to enter the renal fascia and surround the kidneys (Fig. 12). Since the gas may flow into the renal fascia and partly accumulate outside the latter, the fascia is sometimes seen as a thin membrane along part of the lateral outline of the kidney (Fig. 13). As previously mentioned, the kidney is held in position by a large number of connective tissue bands running from the fascia to the surface of the kidney, which can be loosened by the gas when it forces its way into the connective tissue. The kidney may then be mobilized. COONEY et al. (1955) described a case of complete tilting of the kidney, which rotated 90° without causing any symptoms whatsoever. As a rule the mobility of the kidney in this type of examination appears to be limited, as judged by a comparative examination of seven cases by POLVAR and BRAGGION (1952). The fat forming the capsule of the kidney, a thick layer on the posterior surface of the kidney and thinner ventrally, often has a reticular or areolar appearance because of the division of the connective tissue, which can vary from one individual to another and with the examination technique, such as with varying thickness of the layers at tomography and with the amount of gas (VESPIGNANI and ZENNARO, 1951). It will sometimes give the outline of the kidney an irregular appearance which must not be interpreted as pathologic.

On occasion, only a small amount of gas or no gas at all will enter the interstices between the kidney and the suprarenal if the connective tissue is dense, and the upper pole of the kidney cannot then be defined.

The suprarenals vary in size, position and shape. Judging from the literature, demonstration of suprarenals by this method appears to be both simple and reliable. But this is by no means always the case. The right suprarenal is usually situated adjacent to the upper pole of the kidney, like a cap, and is more or less triangular with an elongated cranial tip. The depths in sagittal direction may vary widely, for which reason many advocate not only frontal tomography, but also lateral tomography. The shape of the left suprarenal is more irregular and has been described as semilunar. It is situated more medially and lower in relation to the renal pole. It may sometimes be difficult to define the outline of the suprarenals exactly because they vary in consistency

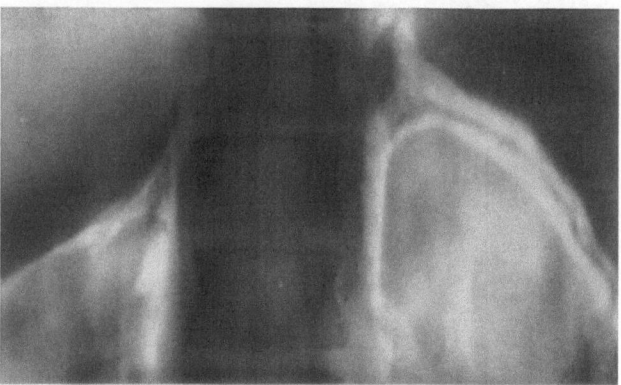

Fig. 13. Retroperitoneal pneumography. Tomogram (film from simultaneous serial multisection tomography) showing renal fascia on left side and adrenals

with the amount of fat in the parenchyma or because of the thickness and reticulation of the fatty capsule. They also vary in size. Thus on the basis of frontal films, STEINBACH and SMITH (1955) gave the following planimetric values: for the right suprarenal 2—7,8 cm, with a mean of 4.2 cm², and for the left suprarenal 2—8.7 cm², with an average of 4.3 cm². This wide range, which does not take into account the above-mentioned wide variation in sagittal diameter, makes it difficult to diagnose hyper- and hypoplasia. In the evaluation of the appearance of the suprarenal by this method the examiner must rely largely on his experience.

3. Roentgen examination of the surgically exposed kidney

Roentgen examination of the kidney during operation has been used particularly for locating calculi and for checking that no stones have been left at operation.

On examination of the kidney during operation a cassette is placed over the operative field (SUTHERLAND, 1935; ASTRALDI and URIBURU, 1937) or a film is placed in the actual wound. The latter method is the more important. The procedure is briefly as follows: The kidney is exposed, a film is inserted and placed against the kidney, the roentgen tube is adjusted and the beam coned to cover the kidney. As a rule a suitably sized film is wrapped in black paper and then packed in a sheet of rubber, a sterilized operation sleeve or the like. Special cases have also been designed for this purpose. ÅKERLUND (1937) had ready-packed films made similar to those employed in dentistry. A ready-packed film of this type is placed in a sterilized rubber glove. In order to prevent infection when the packed film is being introduced into the glove, use is made of a loading guide, consisting of a metal sleeve. The whole package is held against the exposed kidney by means of elastic ribbons. The disadvantage of a package of this type is the lack of intensifying screens, which reduces contrast and makes a longer exposure time necessary and may thus cause poor definition, and small stone fragments may not be demonstrable.

In an attempt to eliminate these disadvantages, ordinary cassettes have been used (Jaches; Francois, 1932) or thin cassettes made particularly for the purpose (Benjamin, 1931; Puigvert Gorro, 1943). Such stiff cassettes are, however, difficult to insert into the operative wound.

In order to secure a flexible, small, suitable packed film with intensifying screens, Olle Olsson (1948) designed a rubber cassette similar to that employed in industry for

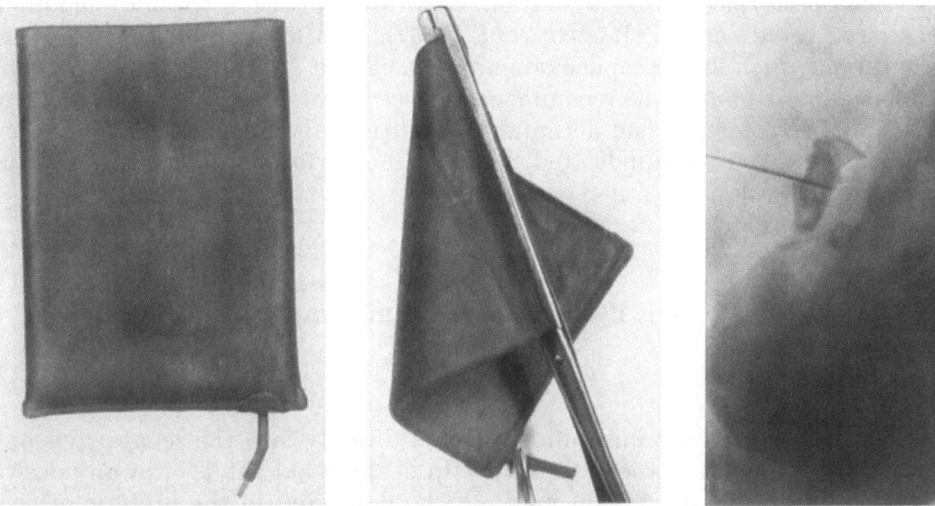

Fig. 14. Flexible, easily sterilized rubber cassette with flexible intensifying screens for roentgen examination of operatively exposed kidney. Film obtained with cassette

the roentgen inspection of material (Fig. 14). The cassette consists simply of a flat rubber bag 10 × 15 cm. The film and two intensifying screens are dropped into the bag. The mouth of the bag is closed by means of a clamp. The bottom of the bag is provided with a spout through which the air content of the closed bag may be withdrawn by means of a syringe. This decreases the thickness of the cassette and at the same time presses the screens tight against the film, which is important for obtaining sharp pictures.

The screens are of the type used for industrial purposes. They are supplied in standard sizes such as 9 × 12 cm. In these screens the fluorescent coating has been applied to a flexible material.

Thanks both to the material of which the cassette is made and the construction of the screens, the loaded cassette is very flexible. In other words it is an easily sterilizable, convenient and flexible cassette with intensifying screens. The cassette has been dimensioned to suit a standard-sized film 9 × 12 cm (4 × 5 inches). As mentioned, standard screens, coarse and fine-grained, are available for this size of film.

The rubber cassette is sterilized in the same manner as the rest of the rubber articles used at operation. An assistant with sterilized gloves holds up the sterilized cassette in the dark room of the operation department, where it is loaded with the aid of a guide consisting of a metal sleeve. The mouth of the cassette is closed by the assistant with a single pair of resection tongs or with two, one on each side. The mouth may also be closed in any other suitable manner. If tongs are used, such types should be chosen as may be used as handles when the cassette is being introduced into the operative wound. When loaded, the cassette is placed on the assistant's table and the air is withdrawn. Every time the syringe is removed from the spout, the latter is closed by means of a clip. As a rule about 60 cc of air can be sucked out of the cassette. When the air has been withdrawn, the spout is sealed by means of a small stopper. The cassette is then ready for use. It is immaterial which of the two screens is placed next to the organ to be examined. To render possible the double-sided use of this cassette the practice of making one of the sides of the cassette of lead rubber, for example, to prevent secondary radiation from the underlayer, has been discarded.

Roentgen examination for stones in the surgically exposed kidney has been used mainly for locating concrements in the renal pelvis (see section on Renal Calculi). Pyelography (FRANCOIS, 1932; HEUSSER, 1937) and renal angiography (ALKEN, 1951; GRAVES, 1956) have also been performed during operation. Fluoroscopy with a specially modified apparatus has also been described (BASKIN et al., 1957). Apart from the difficulty in securing sterile conditions, such fluoroscopic examinations, like all other fluoroscopic examinations during operation, are not to be recommended because of the difficulty in securing satisfactory radiation protection and acceptable conditions for fluoroscopy. If fluoroscopy is nevertheless considered to be indicated, it should be performed with the use of an image intensifier and television.

III. Pyelography and urography

1. Pyelography

In pyelography, contrast medium is injected directly into the renal pelvis or via the ureter, as a rule through a catheter with the tip in the renal pelvis or at any desired level of the ureter. The contrast medium may also be deposited in the ureteric orifice or the urinary bladder and the ureter then filled by gravity or by reflux by high pressure in the bladder. Particularly in children with an incompetent ureteric orifice it is usually easy to obtain a filling of the renal pelvis by lowering the head and allowing the contrast medium to flow from the bladder into the ureter and further into the renal pelvis. A filling can also be obtained by percutaneous puncture of the renal pelvis or the ureter and injection via a needle or cannula, or via an opening after pyelostomy or via a fistula, so-called antegrade pyelography.

a) Contrast media

Originally silver was used as a contrast element in the form of Collargol (Ag has the atomic number 47, atomic weight 107,88; the corresponding figures for iodine are 53 and 126,92, for barium 56 and 137,37 and for thorium 90 and 232,15). Collargol was often attended by serious side reactions, however. It was soon superseded by halogen salts such as sodium and potassium bromide or iodide and lithium iodide. These contrast media are also sometimes attended by clinical reactions and experimentally they have been proved to cause damage to the epithelium of the renal pelvis and the ureter with desquamation, edema, hyperemia and hemorrhage.

Later a colloidal thorium dioxide was used as a contrast medium. It was believed to be ideal because it was almost non-irritable. It was soon realized, however, that if this insoluble and non-absorbable contrast medium escaped into the tissues in association with reflux, for example, it would remain there and give rise to granuloma. That the radioactive effect of thorium can lead to malignant metaplasia is well known. Therefore thorium should be completely abandoned as a contrast agent. Judging from the literature, it is still in use in some quarters for special purposes, but even then it is not acceptable. Thorotrast is still of clinical interest because rests of the medium persistent after pyelography performed many years previously with thorotrast and with the medium lodged in the tissues, possibly in granulomatous masses, are still occasionally observed (Fig. 15).

Later the contrast media which we now use for urography became available. They are the only media that should be used for pyelography.

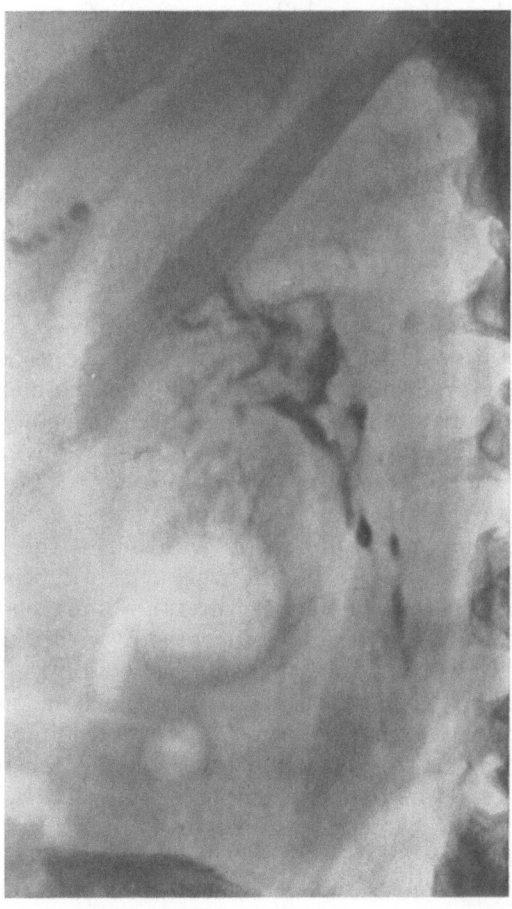

Fig. 15. Patient who several years previously underwent pyelography with thorium dioxide. Remainder of contrast medium lodged in tissues intrarenally and along double ureters after extravasation by backflow during procedure

Judging from illustrations in papers and textbooks, there seems to be a tendency to use contrast media of too high a density. High concentration of the contrast media will produce sharp outlines of the hollow organs examined, but too high a density is likely to mask changes within the renal pelvis, even fairly marked changes such as polyps or stones. Therefore the examiner should use the contrast medium in a concentration that, in relation to kilo-voltage used, can give well detailed pyelograms.

Possibly as a reaction against too high a density of contrast medium with its above-mentioned disadvantages, gas, particularly oxygen, has been used as a contrast medium. Gas can undoubtedly be indicated in certain investigations, *e.g.* so-called double-contrast examinations. A mixture of hydrogen superoxide solution with ordinary contrast medium has been suggested (KLAMI, 1954) to induce the formation of gas bubbles in pathologic processes in the renal pelvis which liberate oxygen from hydrogen peroxide. The advantage, if any, of this method appears to be very small.

b) Method

Pyelography can be performed in two essentially different ways, namely with and without fluoroscopic control.

Usually it is performed without such control. Contrast medium warmed to body temperature is injected via the catheter, and films are taken after a certain amount of contrast medium has been injected or when the patient complains of a feeling of tension or pain. Attempts have been made to calculate the amount of contrast medium that should preferably be injected by measuring the volume of the contents of the normal renal pelvis. This volume varies normally from 4 to 12 cc. In addition, some of the contrast medium may flow back, or, upon malposition of the catheter, it may be deposited in a single calyx. This method is therefore not reliable. The contrast medium was injected until the patient reported discomfort in the region of the kidneys, which was taken as a sign that the renal pelvis was filled. The pain threshold varies considerably from patient to patient, however; therefore this method has severe inherent sources of error. The difficulty in obtaining a suitable degree of filling of the renal pelvis is great and reflux often occurs, which inter alia may make interpretation of the films difficult (see chapter on backflow).

The other and better procedure is to carry out the examination under fluoroscopic control. It can be improved by the use of an image intensifier and television. This variation of pyelography has been called pyeloscopy, which name is obviously not correct. A more correct designation is pyeloradioscopy or pyelofluoroscopy.

In the performance of fluoroscopy the field must be coned, the voltage relatively high, and the current as low as possible. The duration of the fluoroscopic examination should be reduced to a minimum. This holds for every type of fluoroscopy, also when an image intensifier is used. Advertisements of manufacturers and the technique of less conscientious roentgenologists often neglect the fact that fluoroscopy with the use of image intensifiers calls for the same restrictions regarding radiation protection as does all other fluoroscopic work. An image intensifier working with 3 mA gives the same output as does an ordinary fluoroscope working with the same current, other data being equal. In an investigation of radiation hazards attending the use of transportable image intensifiers, KOCKUM et al. (1958) conclude that roentgen units of this type require additional radiation safety standards, especially when placed in the hands of radiologically unskilled workers. This also holds when a TV system is used.

During fluoroscopy well coned films can be obtained in suitable projection and with a suitable degree of compression.

The position of the catheter must be checked in pyelography. The tip of the catheter should be situated in the confluence of the renal pelvis or in the upper part of the ureter. If it is not checked it may be too high, e. g. in a calyx, and a filling may be obtained of that calyx only, which may then be inflated and cause risk of misinterpretation. The tip of the catheter may occasionally be pushed inadvertently into the renal parenchyma and the contrast medium deposited there, or be inserted through the renal parenchyma with deposition of the contrast medium subcapsularly. A gentle technique must be used in inserting the catheter up into the ureter in order to prevent lesions in the ureteral mucosa or deeper in the ureter.

If the ureter is to be examined, the catheter is withdrawn a suitable distance. The entire ureter can be examined by using a catheter with an olive-shaped tip or an acorn bulb, metal bulb, or cone tip. These catheters block the ureteric orifice. Films may be taken also during the actual injection of the contrast medium, (when protective measures against radiation hazards should, of course, be strictly observed.)

If the renal pelvis is dilated and its drainage obstructed, attempts may be made to aspirate the contrast medium after the examination; otherwise the catheter may be left *in situ* for some hours in order to facilitate drainage.

During pyelography the movements of the kidney will be studied under application of manual pressure or during the respiratory cycle (SCHEELE, 1930; ALFERMANN, 1950).

Fluoroscopy and spot-film radiography are valuable particularly during pyelography and urography (JUNKER, 1936; PREVÔT, 1939), not only for the reasons given above but also in the study of the motility of the renal pelvis and the ureter. Kymography has also been used for this purpose, also cine-radiography. The latter method should be used only with an image intensifier.

It is possible clearly to distinguish systole and diastole in the renal pelvis (NARATH, 1951) and to study the course of certain contractions. The two renal pelves contract independently of one another with regard to rhythm and frequency, with pressure fluctuations of 3—4 mm/Hg (KIIL, 1957).

The literature on the motility of the renal pelvis is considerable. It must be stressed, however, that it is to a large extent of limited value. Examination with a catheter which partly obstructs the flow and influences the motility, together with retrograde injection of a contrast medium which, in addition, is not quite inert, interferes with physiology. An experimental situation in which pyelography is used does not provide a sound basis for investigation of true physiologic conditions in the urinary pathways. Reference may here be made to PREVÔT and BERNING (1950), DAVIS (1950), NARATH (1951) and KIIL (1957), for example, who have presented extensive surveys of pertinent literature.

As mentioned, the kidney is tilted so that the cranial pole of the kidney is situated more dorsally than the caudal pole, and the medial part is higher *i.e.* more ventral than the lateral (Fig. 16). The confluence is therefore situated further ventrally than the rest of the renal pelvis. This is of importance in the performance of urography and pyelography.

The specific gravity of ordinary contrast media is higher than that of body fluids such as urine, blood etc. This gives rise to a *layer formation* between contrast medium and the rest of the contents of a cavity (the phenomenon is sometimes incorrectly called sedimentation). Ignorance of this phenomenon has often resulted in misinterpretation and erroneous evaluation of the actual findings in examinations of different kinds with contrast media, particularly in urologic radiology. The phenomenon was first described by LAURELL (1924) and has since been studied in further detail by RIBBING (1933) in retrograde pyelography and by ETTINGER (1943) in urography. Formerly it was believed that only Thorotrast was capable of causing this phenomenon, because of its poor miscibility with urine, but it has since been shown that water soluble contrast media infused into the renal pelvis via the catheter for retrograde pyelography or contrast urine coming from the papillae during urography can produce the same phenomenon, which is also confirmed by daily experience. This is why the dorsal and cranial calyces are filled first and most completely, since, because of the position of the kidney, they are situated lowest when the patient is in the supine position.

Layer formation is of importance in the evaluation of the pelviureteric junction. A narrow junction in the film or a band-like transverse filling defect at the site of the junction may be caused only by incomplete filling of this most ventrally located anatomic part. What looks like narrowing of the junction may thus mean just incomplete filling of a lumen of ordinary diameter. This also holds for "narrowing" of the ureter, which may be caused by a bend of the ureter in the ventral-dorsal plane and incomplete filling of the bend. Suitable and complete filling of all parts of the renal pelvis and the ureter therefore requires examination of the patient in different positions. This is also necessary for free projections and suitable filling of single calyces and for obtaining a three-dimensional impression of the renal pelvis, and therefore provides further support for the view that the examination should be carried out under fluoroscopic control. In certain conditions

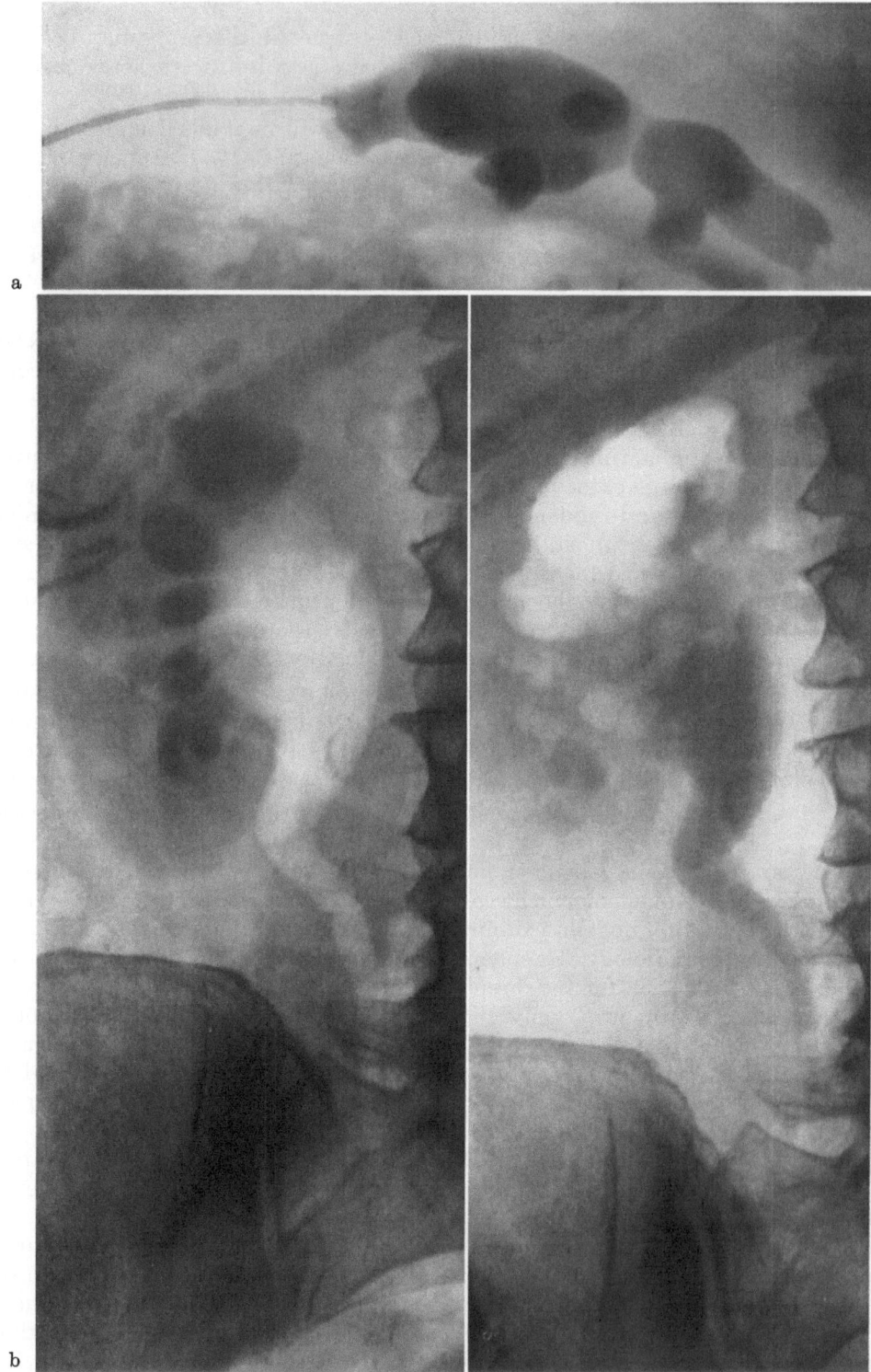

Fig. 16. a) Position of calyces, confluence and ureter when patient is examined in supine position. Cranial ualyces lowest, confluence highest. b) Roentgenograms illustrating position of calyces and kidney pelvis and creter in antero-posterior direction. Urography in patient with operative fistula between ureters and small bowel with gas passing from bowel to urinary pathways. Left part of picture supine position: calyces with dorsal position filled with urographic contrast medium whereas confluence part of kidney pelvis and ureter are filled with gas which has lower specific gravity than urographic contrast medium. Right hand picture prone position: distribution of gas and urographic contrast medium reversed.

the layer formation plays a special rôle and dictates several steps in the method (see chapter on dilatation).

In association with pyelography, contractions of the renal pelvis are sometimes seen, especially on less gentle catheterization. Cases have been described (HENDRIOCK, 1934) in which marked contractions of the entire renal pelvis have been observed during catheterization. The examination should therefore be performed as carefully as possible.

Pyelography is undoubtedly in abundant use in the study of the kidney pelvis. In a great majority of cases urography would be a better and less traumatic method of examination.

c) Roentgen anatomy

The discussion of the anatomy of the renal pelvis requires an acceptable nomenclature. The nomenclature used by anatomists differs from that used by clinicians. In addition

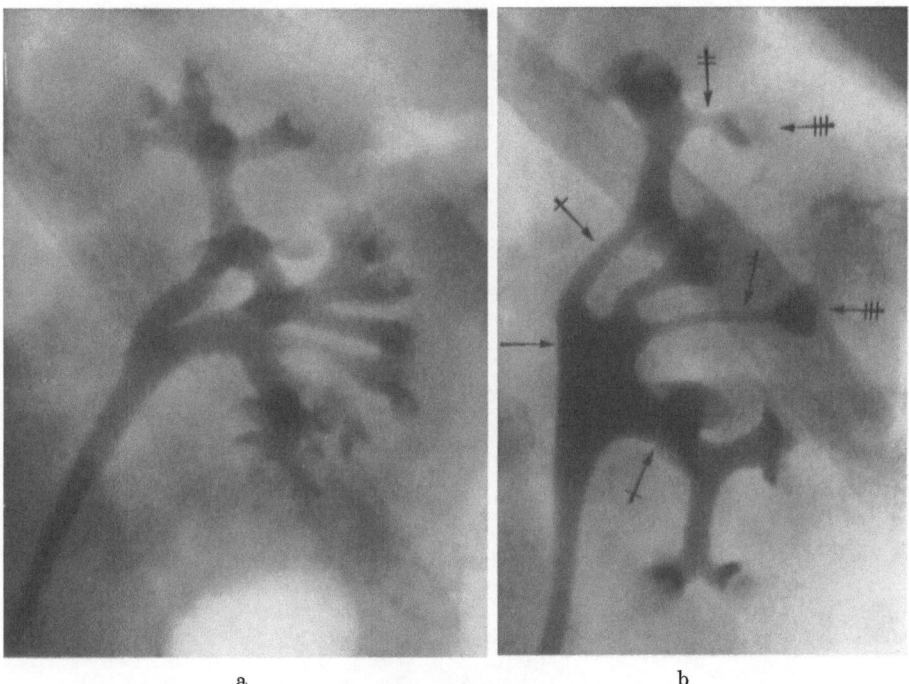

a   b

Fig. 17. Varying primary anatomy of kidney pelvis. Nomenclature of kidney pelvis demonstrated in b. → confluence → branch ⊹→ stem of calyx ⫴→ calyx

the nomenclature in the clinical literature is by no means uniform. Thus, some authors use the term renal pelvis to designate the entire renal pelvis, while others mean only that part of it formed after the confluence of the individual calyces. Some authors call this part the saccus or ampulla, which are sometimes very inappropriate names. The term calyx is used with the epithet minor to describe a single calyx, but also used with the epithet major to designate a group of calyces. Important parts, as far as nomenclature is concerned, are the stems of the calyces minores and majores. We use a nomenclature presented in 1946 by JOHNSSON of our department. According to this, that part of the renal pelvis where the different calyces meet is called the confluence; the calyces majores, the branches; after which come the stems of the calyces and the calyces.

Wide variations occur in the shape, width and branching of the renal pelvis, in the number of calyces, in the size and length of the stems, and in the important region of the pelviureteric junction (Fig. 17—25). These variations in shape are based on embryologic

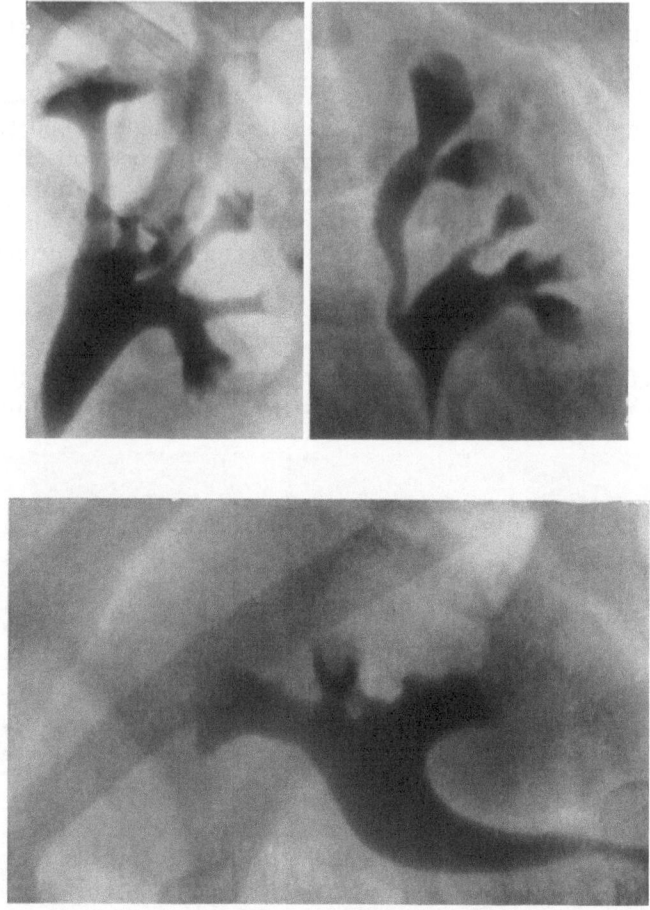

Fig. 18. Other examples of infinite variation in morphology of kidney pelvis

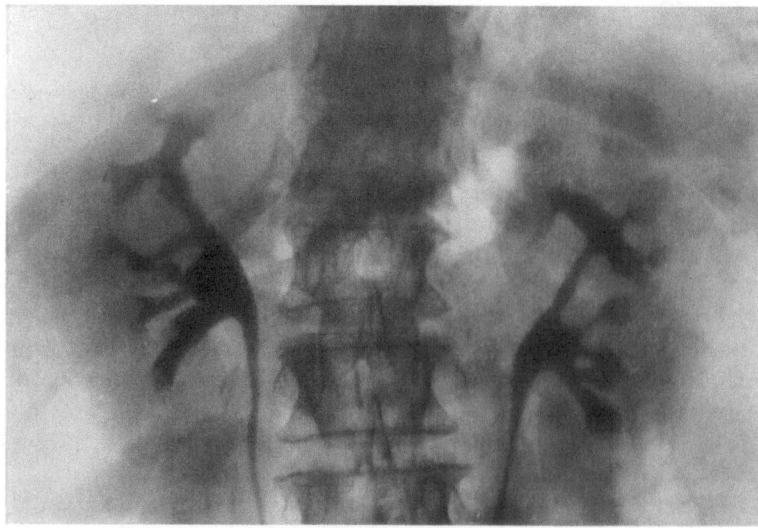

Fig. 19. Both upper kidney poles dominant with large upper branches

conditions and are related to great differences in the time at which production of urine in the fetal kidney causes the breakthrough of the septa outlining the adjoining ureteral "anlage". At an early breakthrough a dendritic kidney pelvis results. If there is a lag in the breakthrough, an ampullary kidney pelvis is found, with short calyces (LUDWIG, 1971).

The kidney is built up of 14 papillae with 6 in the cranial part, 4 in the intermediate part, and 4 in the caudal part. These papillae are arranged in a ventral row and a dorsal row. Often several papillae fuse, always in the tips of the papillae, so that the number found in a normal kidney is usually 8 or 9 (LÖFGREN, 1949). This fusion of the papillae has a strong moulding effect on the calyces, with the result that calyces of widely different shapes occur. The shape varies also with the degree of filling. At urography and pyelography it is necessary to take films at suitable angles, usually by turning the patient, in order to obtain true lateral projections of the individual calyces of particular interest in a given case.

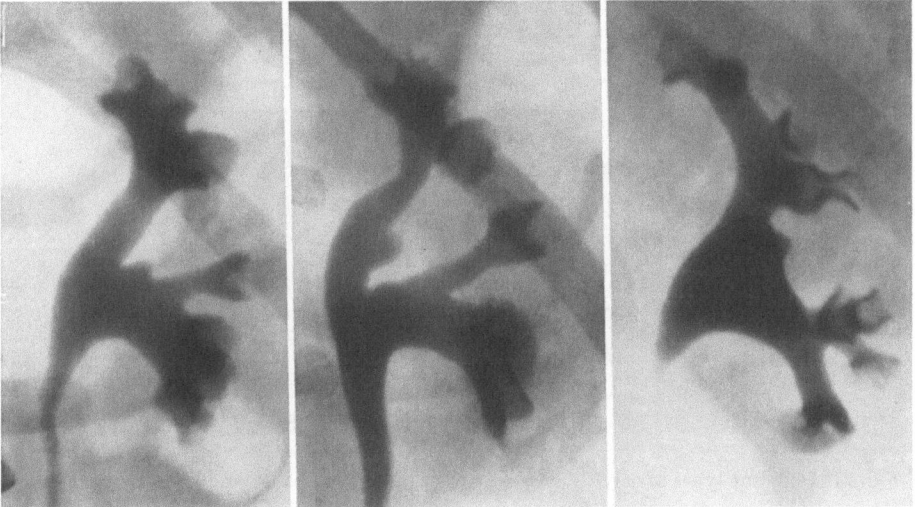

Fig. 20. Small sprout from caudal branch, cranial branch and confluence without a calyx. This anatomic variant is not uncommon

The renal pelvis is often divided into two parts, the division coinciding with the primary bifurcation angle. The upper branch is then of the same shape as the upper part of a double kidney (see chapter on anomalies) and the upper pole may be large and the lower pole smaller than ordinarily is the case.

A not uncommon variant of the renal pelvis is a small sprout usually from the base of the upper branch (Fig. 20). It has the appearance of a calyx that has been blocked and is probably due to some slight disorder during embryologic development. A microcalyx or otherwise unsually shaped calyx is sometimes seen at this site, which corresponds to the primary bifurcation angle in embryonal life (Fig. 21).

The calyces vary widely in shape, even when they are completely filled with contrast medium. The stem may be very long or short, wide or very narrow. Several calyces may lie close together with a common stem. The actual calyx can vary widely in diameter and deviate from its normally round shape. The edge of the calyx may be angular or rounded and vary in different parts of the circumference of one and the same calyx and may be of different height. Detailed examination of the anatomy may require several well coned films in different projections secured by turning the patient or angulating the beam. During urography under ureteric compression, pictures should be made routinely with the patient turned to the right and to the left, in order to have each calyx in a suitable projection. Occasionally very small calyces with long or short stems, so-called micro-calyces, are seen (Fig. 22).

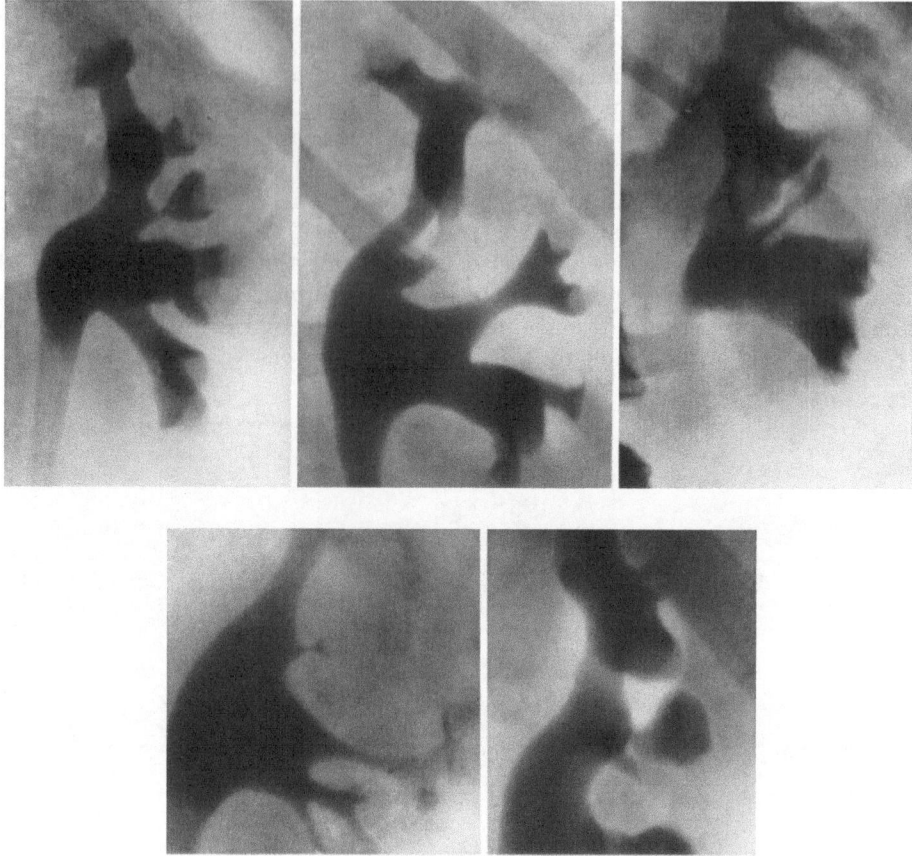

Fig. 21. Different types of calyces at same site as of sprout formation illustrated in Fig. 20

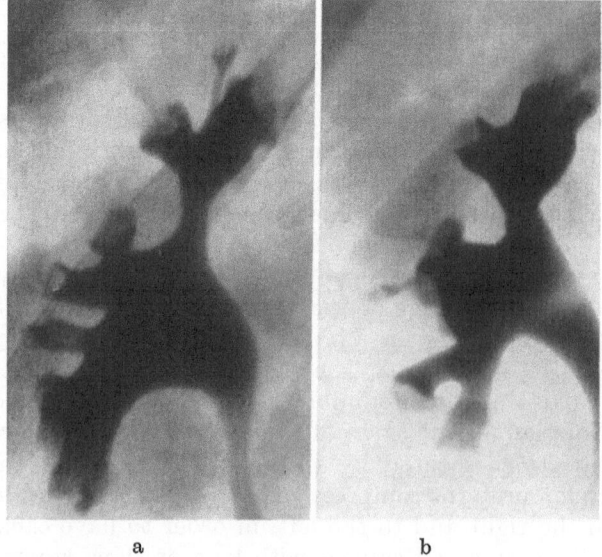

a   b

Fig. 22. Microcalyces in a) cranial and b) middle part of kidney pelvis

Not only the size and shape of the papillae influence the form of the calyces, but also the form of the sinus and the amount of sinus fat. The branches and stems may form different-sized angles with one another, usually acute. If the sinus fat is abundant, however, the branches may be pushed apart and one or more of the angles between them may then be rounded to such an extent as to simulate a space-occupying lesion.

A certain similarity is often, although not always, seen between the shapes of the renal pelves on either side.

In a renal pelvis with many and long branches pathologic changes are easier to recognize than in renal pelves in which the calyces are, so to say, situated directly on the confluence.

The confluence may have the shape of a sac or ampulla, but it may also be very narrow. If the confluence is wide, it may, of course, be difficult to draw a line of distinction between normal width and pathologic widening.

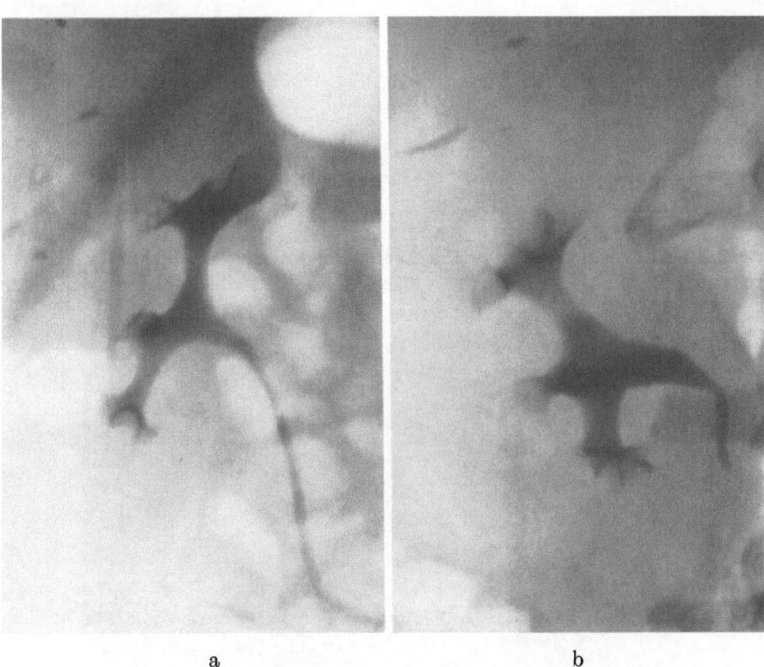

a   b

Fig. 23. Roentgen anatomy: Position of kidney in a) supine position and b) prone position of patient with mobile kidney

Change of position of the patient may cause an apparent change in the shape of the kidney pelvis (Fig. 23).

At urography, contrast urine in the ducts of the papillae often causes a blush of the papillae.

The pelviureteric junction varies widely, from a confluence gradually tapering and merging with the ureter to a distinctly outlined confluence merging abruptly with the ureter. The actual pelviureteric junction in such cases varies considerably in width. The level of the pelviureteric junction also varies and the ureter may be described as having a high or low point of departure from the renal pelvis. In the evaluation of the width, films must be taken in different planes and it is important that the region under examination be completely filled with contrast medium (Fig. 24, 25).

The anatomic background of the variation is the arrangement of muscle fibers in the kidney pelvis. At the base of the calyces the circular direction dominates; at the pelviureteric junction there is one circular and one more longitudinal layer with continuity

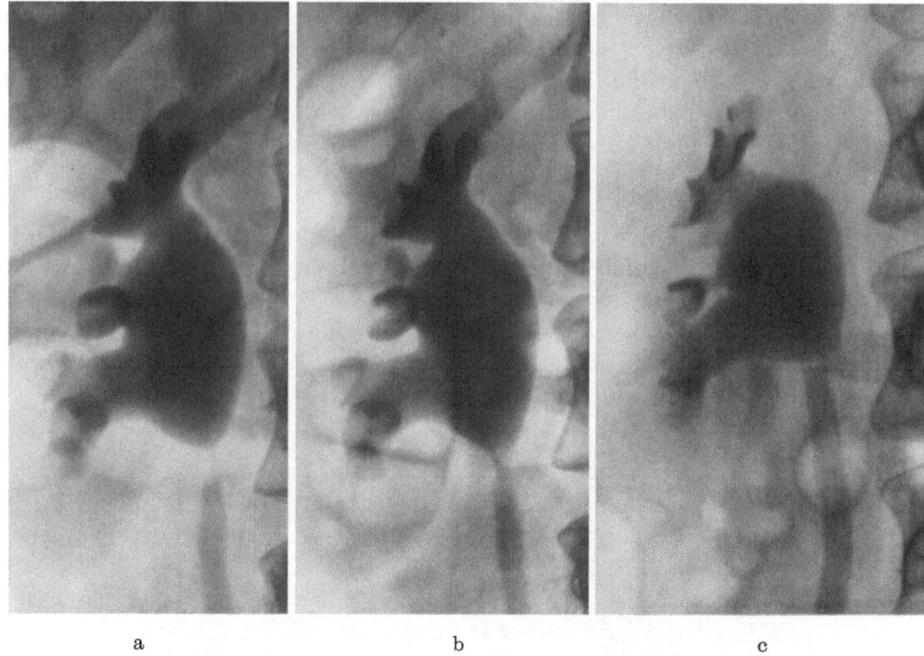

a   b   c

Fig. 24. Pelviureteric junction. Urography: a) diastole, pelviureteric junction not filled; b) systole, junction filled and of ordinary width; c) ureteric compression released. Slight ptosis of kidney causes fold at junction.

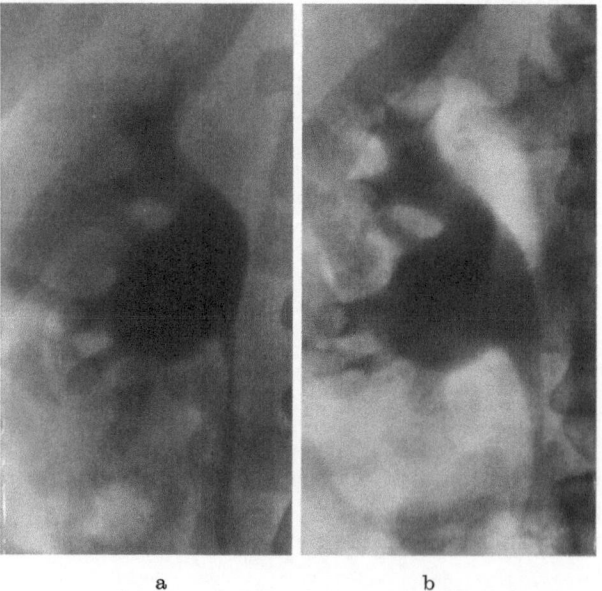

a   b

Fig. 25. Pelviureteric junction. Urography: a) frontal and b) oblique projection. Junction is flat and therefore of narrow appearance in a) but of ordinary width in b)

over into the layers in the ureter. There is no anatomic sphincter in the pelviureteric junction (Ludwig, 1971).

Pyelography provides good possibilities for studying the ureter in the manner described above. At urography (see below) films taken immediately after release of ureteric compression provide a good basis for the study of the ureters. Normally the filling obtained of the ureter during urography is not continuous. If it is so, this is due to the examination

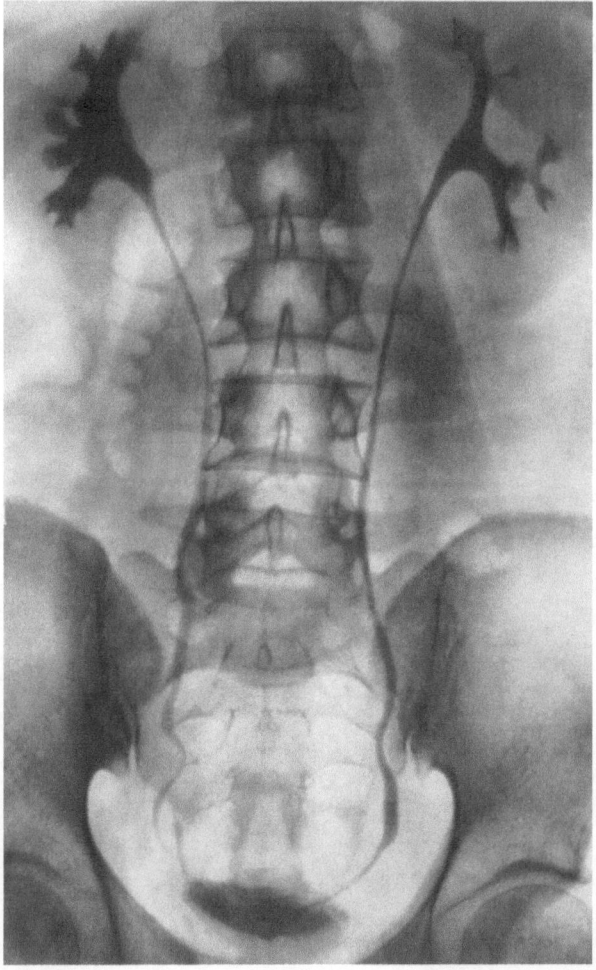

a

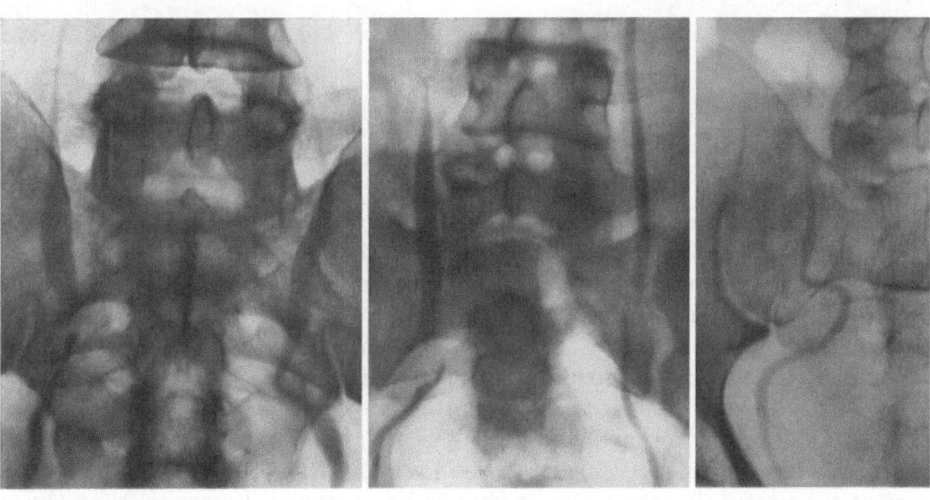

b

Fig. 26. a) Course of ureters; b) variation in roentgen anatomy of ureters at point of intersection between
ureter — iliac artery

3*

technique or to some pathologic condition, usually a more or less marked stasis in the ureteric orifice or distal thereto.

The ureters run from the kidneys medially, often in a slight curve up along the psoas muscle and then more or less parallel with and fairly close to the spine, to the lower part of the ileosacral joints. There they bend laterally, occasionally markedly, at other times less markedly, making an extra bend over the iliac artery and then again run medially to the ureteric orifice in the bladder (Fig. 27). At the same time the ureters pass from a dorsal to a more ventral position in relation to the promontory, at which level the ureters

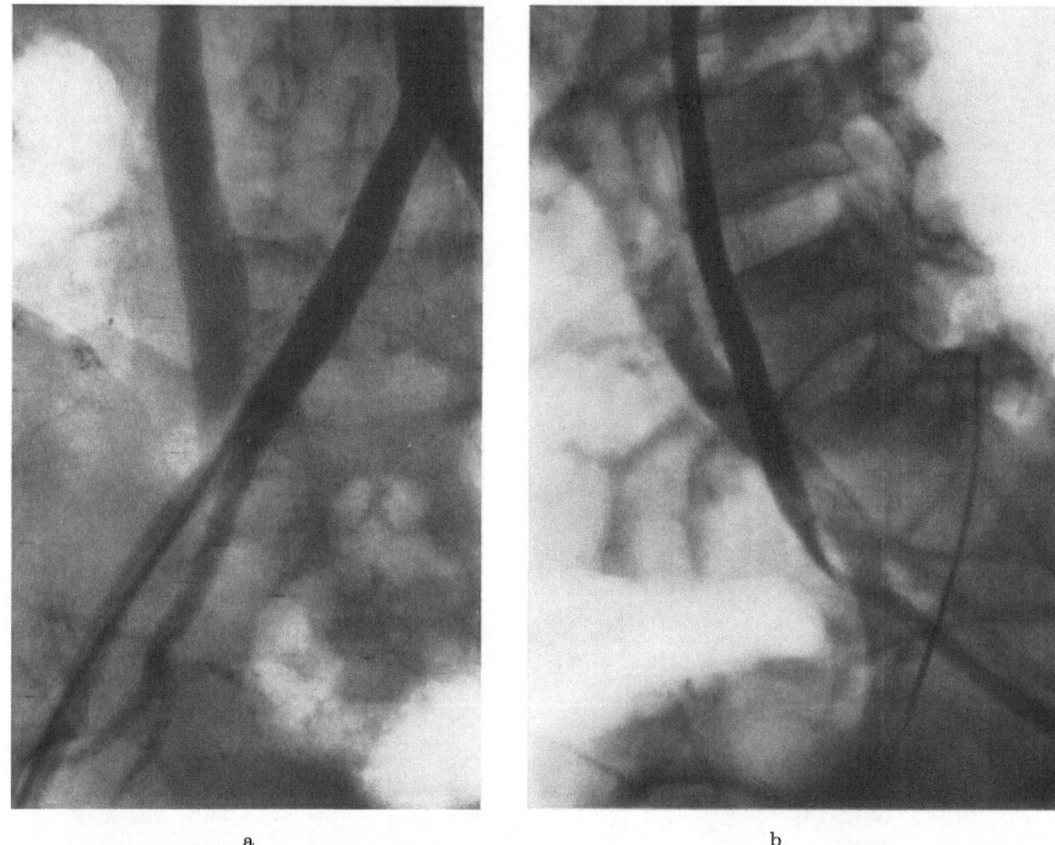

a   b

Fig. 27. Relationship ureter — iliac artery. Contrast medium and catheter in right femoral artery. Narrowing by impression of ureter at level crossed by artery. a) frontal view; b) lateral view

have their most ventral position during the entire course from the kidney pelvis to the bladder. The last section extends in a fairly sharp angle medially and ventrally (Fig. 26). This part can best be shown with the patient sitting leaning forward and the beam directed obliquely downwards, from behind. This projection is usually not necessary, however.

The ureteric orifice is often distinct when a small amount of contrast medium is in the bladder and the interureteric ridge can be seen (as a result of layer formation). If a normal-sized uterus is not situated in the midline, it can dislocate the ureter. If the floor of the bladder is high, the lowest segment or the distal part of the ureters may be lifted.

The spina ischiadica is often used as a landmark in the description of stones in the distal part of the ureter, for example. It should be observed, however, that the ureter is situated approximately $1^1/_2$ inches from the spina ischiadica both cranially and ventrally, and that the ureter nowhere in its course comes near the spine (Wadsworth and Uhlen-huth, 1956). Occasionally the ureter may be very tortuous during ureteric compression, which need not imply disease. Often the ureter is slightly widened, particularly on the right side, immediately above the level where the ureter crosses the iliac artery. In fact, the ureter is almost always somewhat wider above this level than below it.

The ureter may be influenced in its course by adjacent tissue. Thus osteophytes in connection with spondylosis deformans may influence and make an impression on the ureter (Fig. 28). A widened and tortuous aorta may also impress and displace the ureter, especially when an aortic aneurysm is present (Fig. 29). Retroperitoneal tumors and enlarged lymph glands may also displace and/or infiltrate the ureter (Fig. 30). Super-

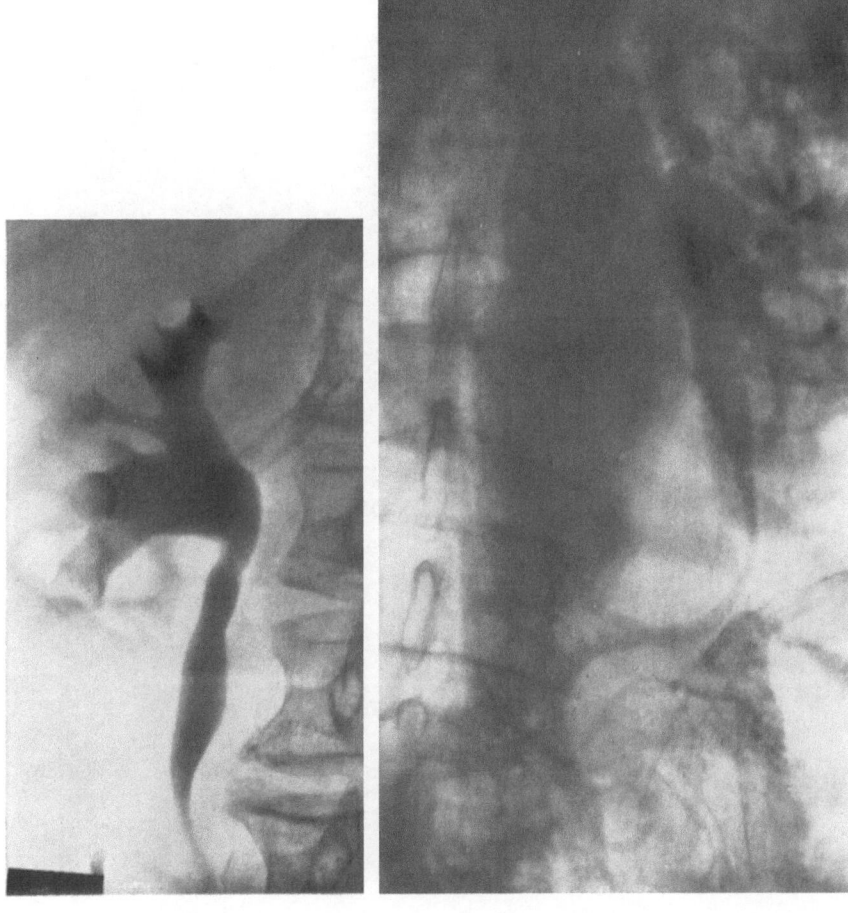

Fig. 28   Fig. 29

Fig. 28. Impression and slight displacement of right ureter by osteophytes in spondylosis deformans

Fig. 29. Displacement of left ureter by aortic aneurysm

numerary and anomalous arteries and veins can cause displacement and make an impression, as can, for example (see below), a large diverticulum of the bladder.

Ureteric peristalsis can be studied cinematographically or kymographically. Ureteric contractions always travel to the end of the ureter, with no relationship between pressure amplitude and speed of travel. Retrograde contractions occasionally occur (KIIL, 1957). JULIAN and GIBBA (1957) state that the average speed of the peristaltic wave varies between two and six cm per second and that the renal excretory rate determines the frequency of the contractile waves, usually three or four per minute.

The peristalsis in the ureter is influenced by several intra- and extraureteral factors and the adaptability is great. Adhesion of the ureter and changes in the ureteral wall markedly influence peristalsis (Melchior and Rathert, 1971).

The renal pelvis often shows filling defects in the form of indentations in various parts of the edge of the renal pelvis or band-shaped defects across a branch, the stem of a calyx, or across the confluence. The changes responsible for some of these defects have long been known. Thus Wolke (1936) showed that a rigid artery may cause such a defect. These phenomena have, however, also been the subject of much discussion in which spastic conditions have been supposed, but not proved. Such spastic conditions have also

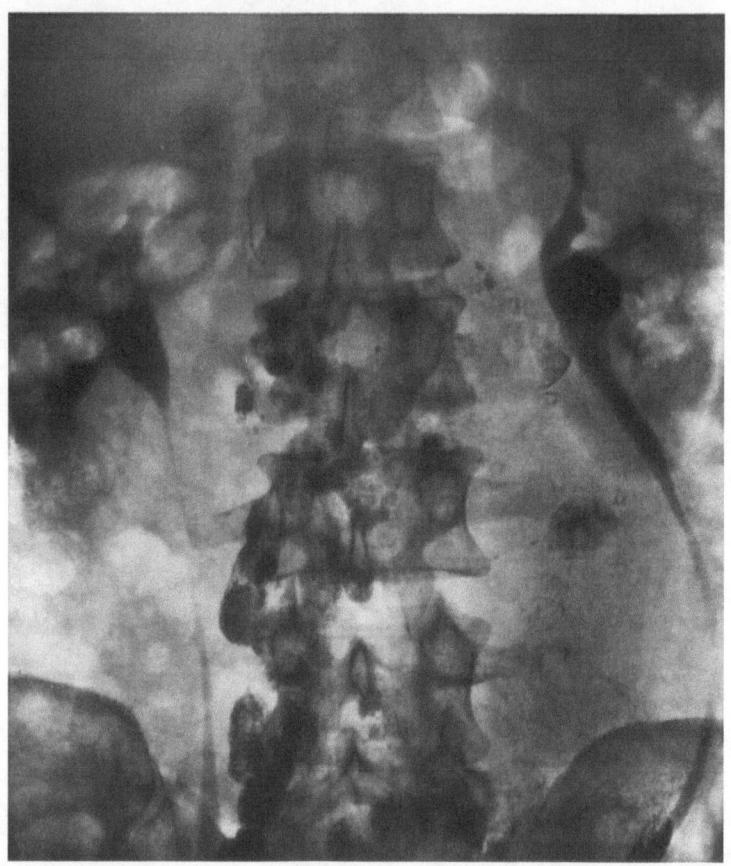

Fig. 30. Displacement of left ureter by enlarged glands — metastases from malignant teratoma of testes, lymphography

been supposed to occur locally in sphincters, the existence of which has not always been proved. Borgard (1944, 1948) compared pyelograms with the vascular anatomy as seen at operation, and in some cases he believed that normal vessels were observed to produce stasis in the calyces with pyelitis as a consequence. Günther (1950) tried to explain the defects as spasms due to pyelitis and described (1952) the cause as "Unruhe, Spasmophilie" etc. but presented no evidence in support of his claim.

On the basis of angiographic studies in from early arteriographic to late phases when contrast medium is present in the kidney pelvis, it can be shown that normal arteries and also veins can cause slight impressions in the kidney pelvis varying with differences in the position of the patient and degree of filling of the kidney pelvis (Fig. 32). The linear filling defects can thus be explained by vessels, usually arteries, sometimes veins,

ometimes a combination of the edge of the parenchyma and vessels. Common to most
f these changes is the fact that they can be observed when the renal pelvis is not completely
lled, i.e. before application of ureteric compression, and that they disappear as soon
s the renal pelvis has been filled during compression. They can also appear distinctly
uring diastole, while they will disappear upon increase in tonus during systole. Decrease
ι tonus of the renal pelvis favors demonstration.

The anatomy of the kidney pelvis and the ureter may also be influenced by anomalies
ι the vasculature, both arteries and veins. Fig. 31 represents a patient with two renal
rteries on the right side. The caudal artery, starting from a low segment of the lumbar
orta, crosses the ureter close to the pelviureteric junction and causes a slight impression

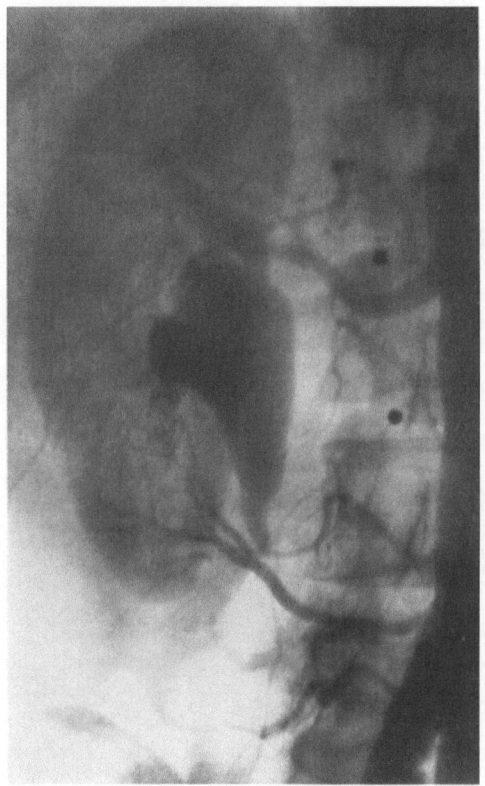

Fig. 31. Multiple renal arteries: slight compression of ureter by artery to caudal kidney pole stemming from
aorta at bifurcation in iliac arteries

in the ureter. The influence on the ureter with slight displacement and impression by an
anomalous vein from the caudal part of the left kidney is illustrated in Fig. 32.

The anatomy of the hilum can usually be studied completely in the nephrogram.
Large anatomic variations can be seen, and in the nephrogram it will also be shown
distinctly that certain defects in the renal pelvis, especially in its edges, correspond to
and are thus due to, the edge of the parenchyma.

The distance between the renal pelvis and the outer border of the parenchyma is of
diagnostic interest because it decreases with scar formation in the parenchyma and increases in the presence of a space-occupying lesion. In normal kidneys the measurement at
a focus-film distance of 100 cm was found to be 2—2.7 cm and in only one instance did
it reach 3 cm (BILLING, 1954). The distance between the renal pelvis and the outer margin
of the parenchyma in the poles of the kidney may, however, exceed 3 cm.

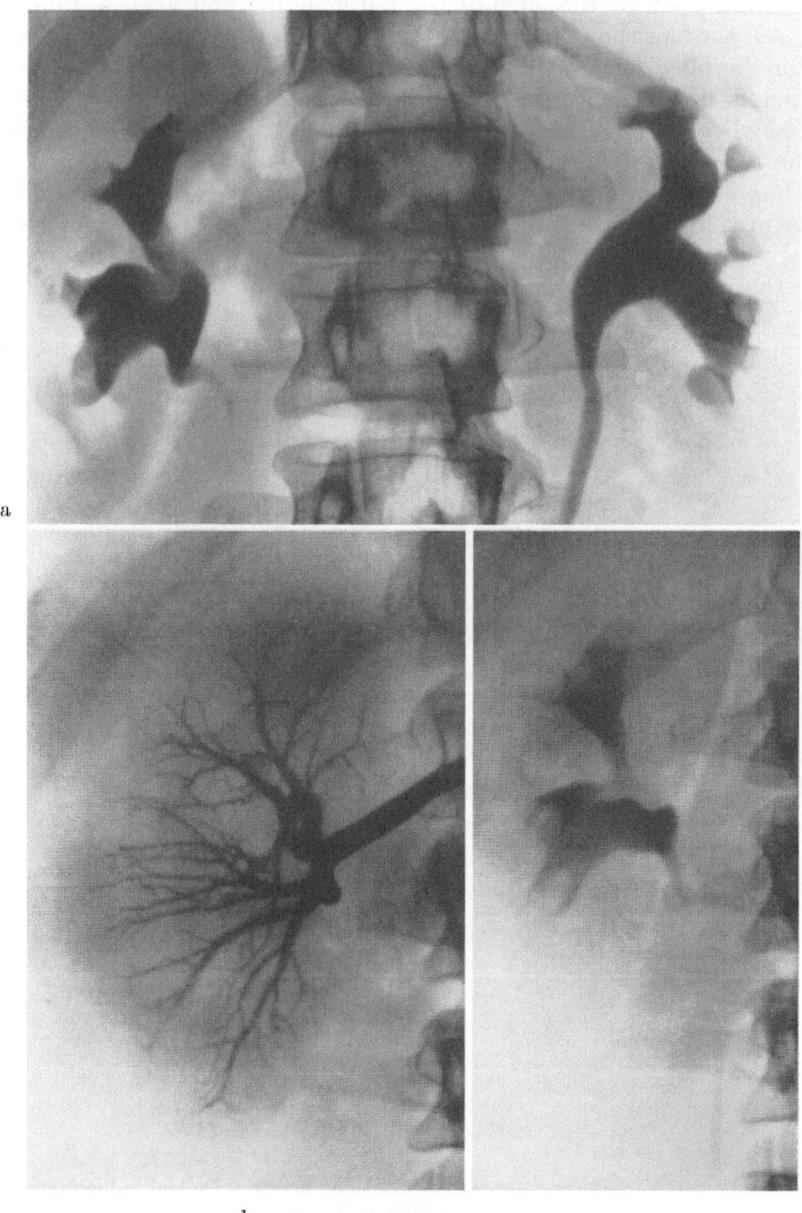

Fig. 32. Filling defect in right kidney pelvis caused by artery. Comparison with arteriogram shows complete agreement between defect in urogram shown in end phase of angiography and ventral branch, which impresses kidney pelvis b) renal angiography, c) urography in end phase of angiography.
Influence on ureter of anomalous veins from caudal part of left kidney. d) Urography, e) angiography venous phase

d) Antegrade pyelography (Fig. 33)

In certain cases in which the renal pelvis is dilated and in which no excretion is obtained at urography, in which retrograde pyelography cannot be resorted to because it is not possible to pass the catheter, for example, and in which angiography does not yield sufficient information, the renal pelvis may be punctured percutaneously and contrast medium be deposited directly into it (Weens and Florence, 1947; Wickbom, 1954; Floyd and Guy, 1956). The method has been called antegrade pyelography. A

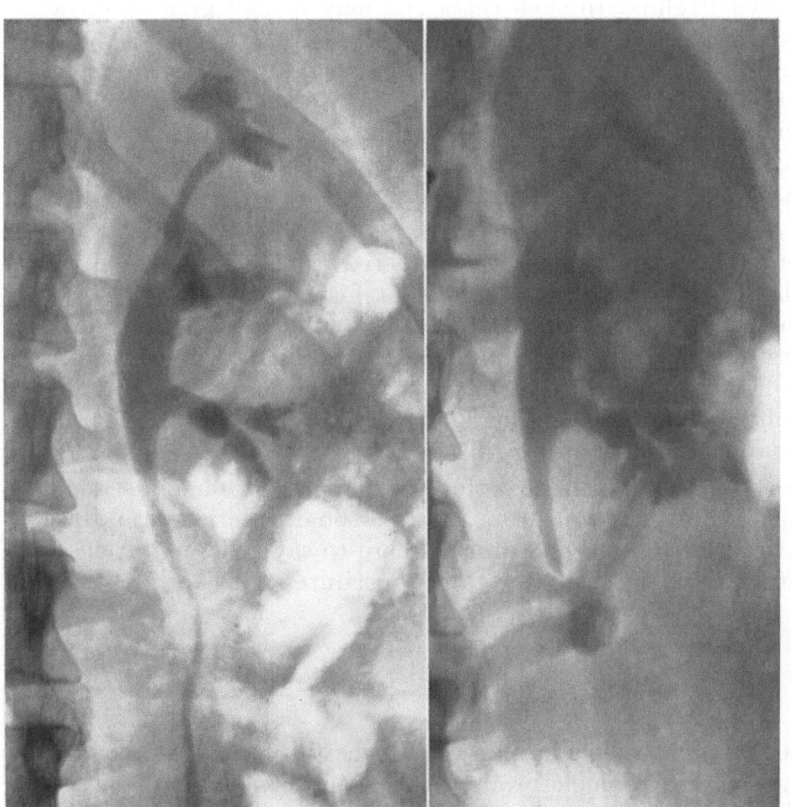 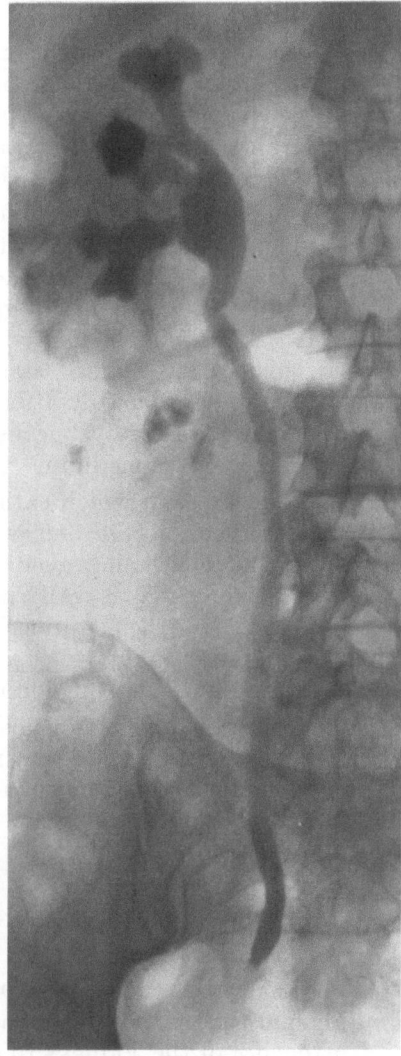

Fig. 32. d, e   Fig. 33

Fig. 33. Antegrade pyelography. Long-standing pain on right side; no excretion on right side at urography. At antegrade pyelography after percutaneous puncture of right kidney pelvis: moderate dilatation of right ureter down to complete block. At operation: coagulum in ureter

special type of antegrade pyelography is that in which the contrast medium is deposited directly into the renal pelvis via a catheter inserted for pyelostomy or via a fistula out to the skin.

e) Contraindications

As a rule, pyelography should not be performed if urography will yield the desired information. Broadly speaking, in these cases pyelography is a supplementary method to urography. The more the examiner is familiar with urography, the less will he resort to pyelography. The most important risk of pyelography is infection, and rise in temperature is not uncommon after pyelography. Attempts have been made to control or eliminate this risk by incorporation of an antibacterial agent in the contrast medium (BLOOM and RICHARDSON, 1959). The problem is complicated, however, and is made still more difficult by the nosocomial infections with resistant bacteria which regularly occur in large hospitals.

According to many experienced urologists, pyelography should not as a rule be used in the investigation of patients with tuberculosis and co-existent cystitis or of patients with obstructed drainage of the renal pelvis, thus in many cases of hydronephrosis. In cases in which the renal pelvis contains stagnant urine, the risk of infection is great. Other risks are instrumental lesions (see chapter on renal tuberculosis) and perforation (see chapter on injury to the kidney and the urinary tract).

If pyelography is performed instead of urography, because of renal insufficiency, measures should be taken to avoid reflux. In such cases one may in fact give an intravenous injection via the backflow (see chapter on backflow). Pyelography is occasionally performed instead of urography because of hypersensitivity to the contrast medium. The risk of reflux should be observed especially in such cases. Symptoms of hypersensitivity may also occur in association with retrograde pyelography without backflow. One case was described by BURROS et al. (1958) in which bilateral pyelography was followed by anuria, probably because of edema of the ureteric mucosa due to hypersensitivity to the contrast medium.

For cases in which catheterization is nevertheless considered to be indicated and the risk of infection regarded as slight, pyelography is, of course, preferred by many urologists. The tendency is, however, to start the investigation with urography and continue with pyelography only if really necessary. The better the urographic examination is performed and the more the examiner is familiar with the diagnostic possibilities of the method and the more he is able to use suitable modifications for all aspects of problems presenting themselves during the examination, the less often will pyelography be necessary.

As to the question whether pyelography can be performed on both sides in one session experienced urologists and roentgenologists can, from their personal experience, produce evidence both for and against either alternative. Suffice it here to say that limitation of the procedure to one side at a time is naturally the safer procedure and this is the technique we use.

2. Urography

Since the end of the 1920's urography has had an established place as an important diagnostic tool in the management of urologic problems. The method is based on the capacity of the kidneys to clear the blood of certain crystalline substances in which, for the purpose of urography, two or three iodine atoms have been incorporated in the molecule, and which are concentrated in the kidneys because of their reabsorption of water.

a) Contrast media

Most contrast media for urography contain two or three iodine atoms per molecule bound to a pyridine or benzene ring. All of the media contain a carboxyl group to make them water-soluble. As a rule, the carboxyl group is attached directly to the ring, but a CH_2-group may be inserted between the ring and the carboxyl group. If a larger hydrocarbon group radical is inserted, less will be excreted in the urine and more in the bile. If the amino-groups are acylated with lower fatty acid radicals (acetyl, propionyl) it will make the salts more soluble and less toxic. If higher fatty acids are used for acylation less will be excreted in the urine and more in the bile. A keto-group or an amino-group facilitates the introduction of iodine in the pyridine benzene ring. Only 2 iodine atoms can be introduced into the pyridine ring or 3 in the benzene ring, if the amino group is attached in the meta position in relation to the carboxyl groups.

Below is given a list of common contrast media together with the chemical formulas molecular weights, iodine content, official and commercial names (trade marks):

Table 1. *Contrast media used for urography*

    I. *N-Methyl-3,5-diiodo-4-pyridone-2,6-dicarbon in acid* is used in the form of the di-sodium salt.

       Structural formula

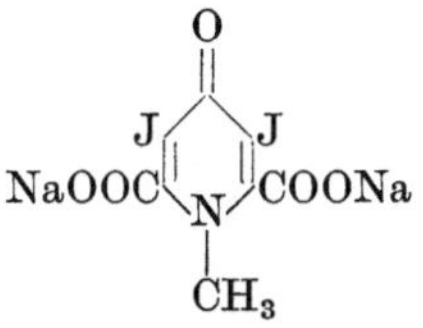

Molecular weight	*Iodine content*
492.9	51.5 %

Official names:
Sodium Iodomethamate USP
Iodoxyl BP

Trade marks:
Uroselectan B, Schering AG,
Neo-Iopax, Schering Corp.,
Uropac, May & Baker,
Urombrine, Dagran,
Urumbrine, Boots
Pyelectan, Glaxo

  II. *3,5-diiodo-4-pyridone-N-acetic acid* is used in the form of the salt of diethanolamine-(a), diethylamino-(b), morfoline-(c) or methylglucamine-(d).

      Structural formulas:

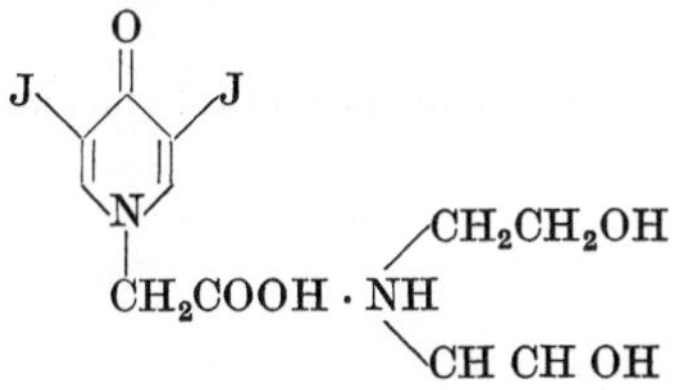

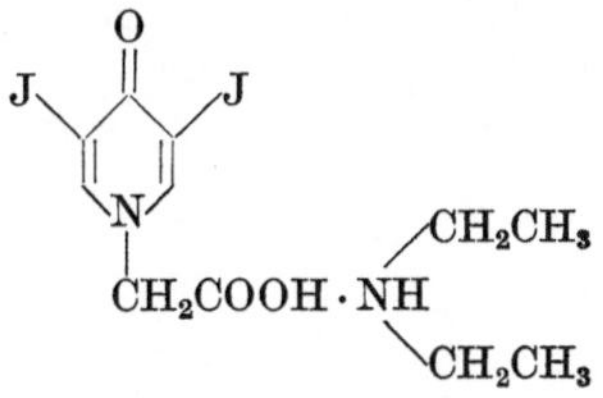

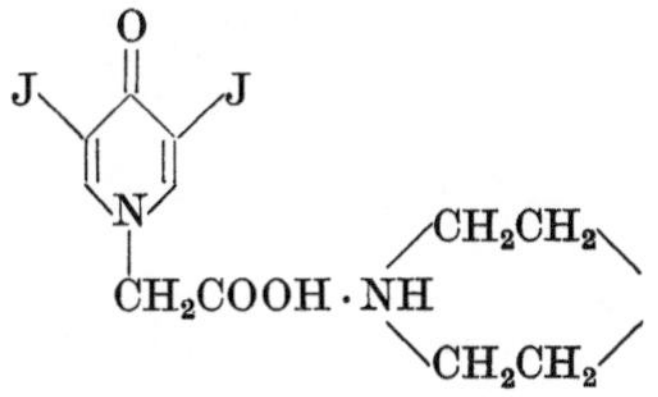

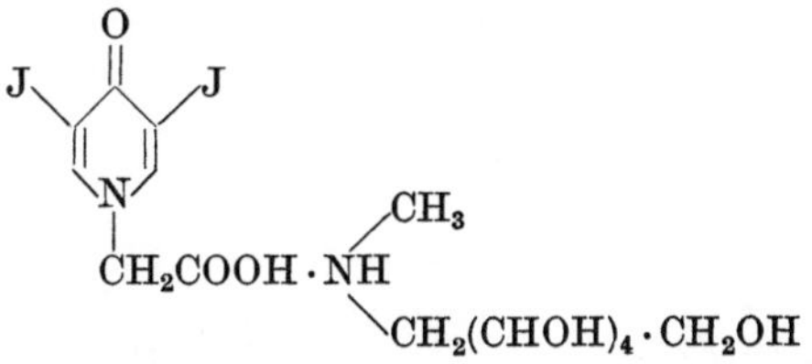

Molecular weight	*Iodine content*
a) 510.1	49.8%
b) 478.1	53.1%
c) 492.1	51.6%
d) 600.2	42.3%

Official names:
Iodopyracet USP
Diodone BP
Diodonum NFN

Trade marks:
a) Perabrodil, Bayer,
   Arteriodone, May & Baker,
   Dijodon, Leo,
   Diodrast, Winthrop-Stearns,
   Leodrast, Loven,
   Neo-Ténébryl, Guerbet,
   Nosydrast, Winthrop-Stearns
   Nosylan, Winthrop-Stearns,
   Perjodal, Pharmacia,
   Pyelombrine, Dagra,
   Pyelosil, Glaxo
   Pylumbrin, Boots,
   Umbradil, Astra,
   Uriodone, May & Baker,
   Vasiodone, May & Baker,
a + b) Iodopyracet compound solution, USP,
       Diodrast compound solution, Winthrop-Stearns,
       Falitrast U, Fahlberg-List,
c) Joduron, Cilag,
d) Perabrodil M, Bayer,
   Glucadiodone, Guerbet,
   Hydrombrine, Dagra,
   Pyelombrine M, Dagra.

III. *3-Acetylamino-2,4,6-tri-iodobenzoic acid* is used in the form of the sodium salt or the methyl glucamine salt.

Structural formulas:

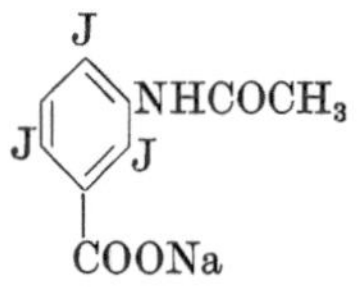

a)

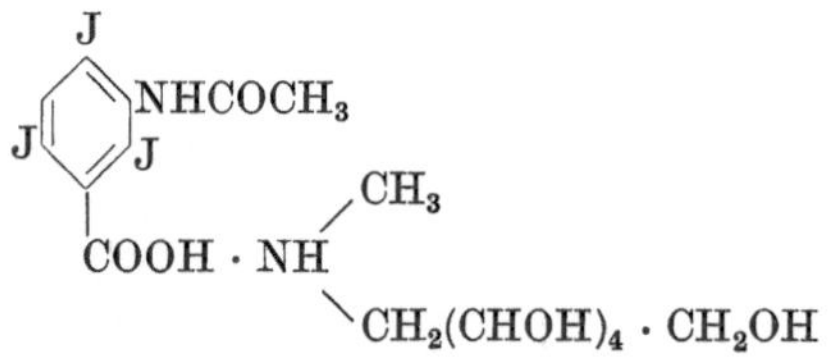

b)

Molecular weight	*Iodine content*
a) 578.9	65.8 %
b) 752.1	50.6 %

Official names:
Sodium Acetrizoate NND
Acidum acetrizoicum NFN

Trade marks:
a) Urokon Sodium, Mallinckrodt,
   Acetiodone, Guerbet,
   Diaginol, May & Baker,
   Iodopaque, Labaz,
   Rheopak, Astra,
   Triabrodil, Bayer,
   Trijodyl, Lundbeck,
   Triopac, Cilag,
   Triurol, Leo,
   Urokon, Pharmacia,
   Vesamin, Byk-Gulden,
b) Fortombrine M, Dagra.

IV. *3,5-Diacetylamino-2,4,6-triiodobenzoic acid* is used in the form of the sodium and methyl glucamine salt.

Structural formulas:

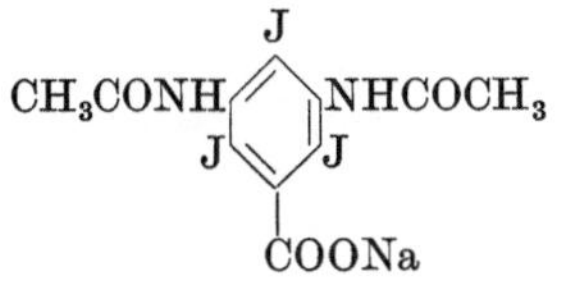

a)

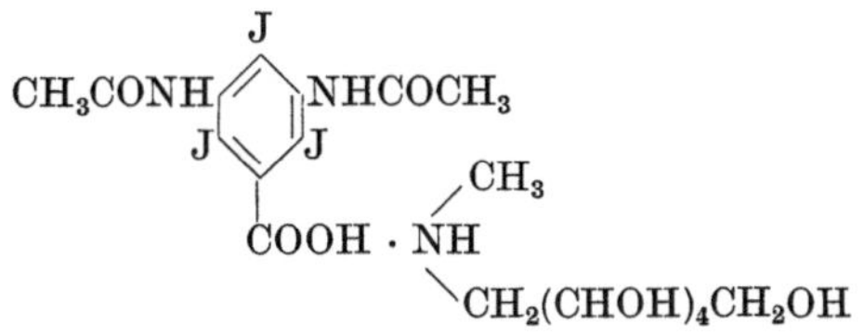

b)

Molecular weight	*Iodine content*
a) 635.9	59.9 %
b) 809.2	47.1 %

Official names:
Diatrizoate Sodium NND
Acidum amidotrizoicum NFN

Trade marks:

a) Hypaque Sodium, Winthrop-Stearns,
    Hypaque, Winthrop
a + b) Urografin (10 a + 66 b), Schering AG,
    Renografin (10 a + 66 b), Squibb,
        Hypaque M (1 a + 2 b), Winthrop.
    Angiografin, Schering AG.

V. *3,5-Dipropionylamino-2,4,6-tri-iodo-benzoic acid* is used in the form of sodium salt.
Structural formula:

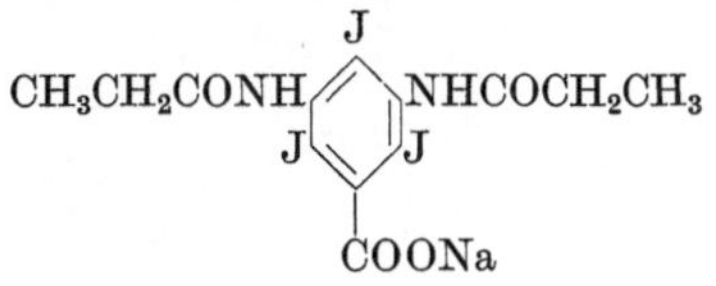

Molecular weight	*Iodine content*
663.9	57.4 %

Official name:
Sodium diprotrizoate NNR

Trade mark:
Miokon Sodium, Mallinckrodt.

VI. *5-Acetamido-2,4,6-triiodo-N-methylisophthalamic acid* is used in the form of the sodium salt or the meglumine (methylglucamine) salt or the meglumine (methylglucamine) and sodium salt)[2].
Structural formulas:

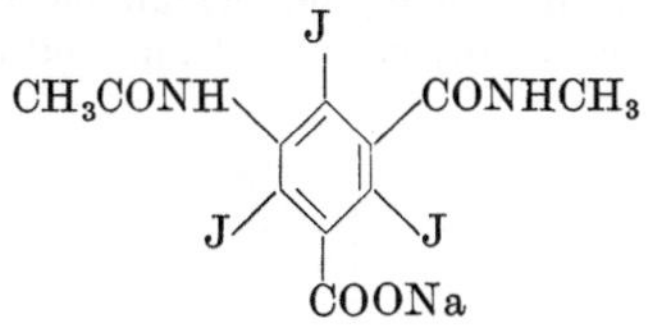

a)

---

[2] Reference is made to STRAIN (1970): "Chemical composition and names of some principal water-soluble and cholecystographic contrast media."

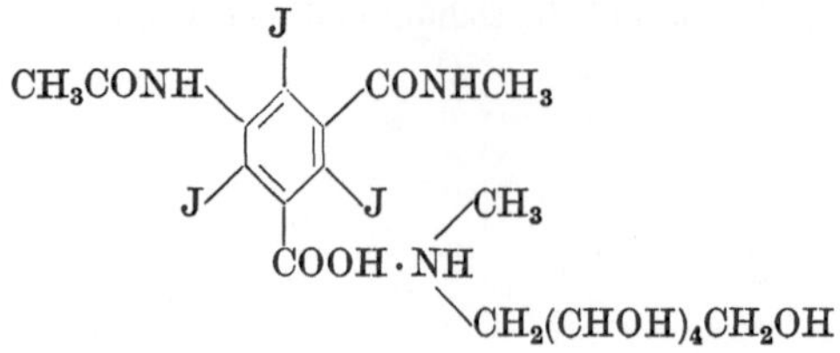

$$CH_3CONH \underset{J}{\overset{J}{\bigcirc}} CONHCH_3$$
COOH · NH — CH₃
CH₂(CHOH)₄CH₂OH

b)

Molecular weight   *Iodine content*
a) 635.9   59.9%
b) 809.2   47.1%

Official names:
Acidum iotalamicum rJNN
Jodtalaminum NFN

Trade marks:
a) Conray   Mallinckrodt
   Angio-Conray
b) Conray Meglumin

VII. *3-Acetamido-5-acetamidomethyl-2,4,6-triiodobenzoic acid* is used in the form of the meglumine (methyl-glucamine) salt or the meglumine (methylglucamine) and sodium salt.
Structural formulas:

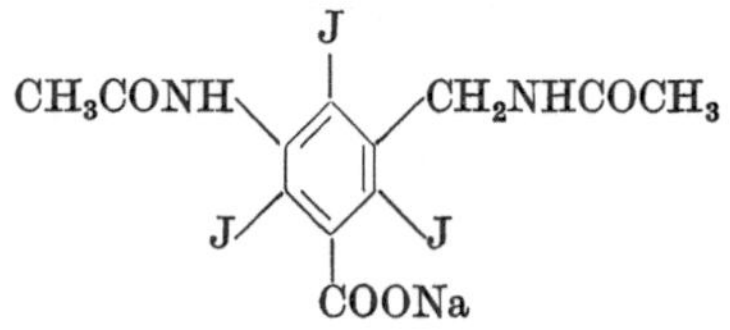

$$CH_3CONH \underset{J}{\overset{J}{\bigcirc}} CH_2NHCOCH_3$$
COONa

a)

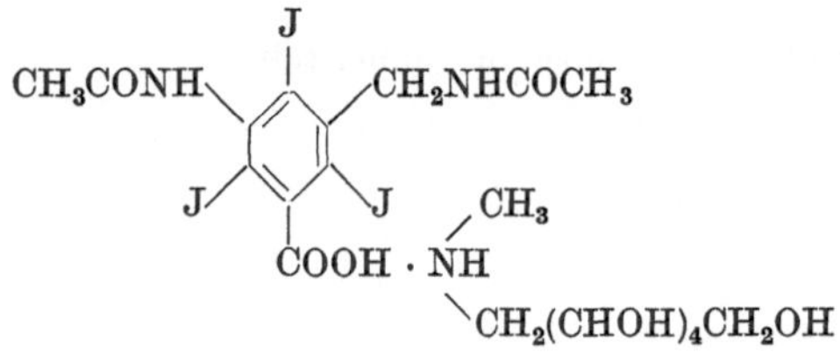

$$CH_3CONH \underset{J}{\overset{J}{\bigcirc}} CH_2NHCOCH_3$$
COOH · NH — CH₃
CH₂(CHOH)₄CH₂OH

b)

Molecular weight   *Iodine content*
a) 649.9   58.6 %
b) 823.2   46.3 %

Official names:
Jodamidum rJNN

Trade marks:
a) Uromiro 300, Bracco
a + b) Uromiro 380 (10a + 61b)

VIII. *3-Acetamido-2,4,6-triiodo-5 (N-methyl acetamido) benzoic acid* is used in the form of the sodium, calcium and magnesium salt or the meglumine (methylglucamine) and calcium salt or the meglumine (methylglucamine), sodium and calcium salt or the meglumine (methylglucamine), sodium, calcium and magnesium salt.

Structural formulas:

$$CH_3CONH \underset{J}{\overset{J}{\bigcirc}} \overset{CH_3}{\underset{}{N}}COCH_3$$
COONa

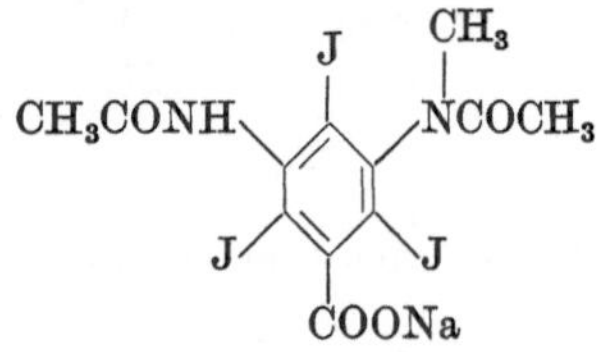

a)

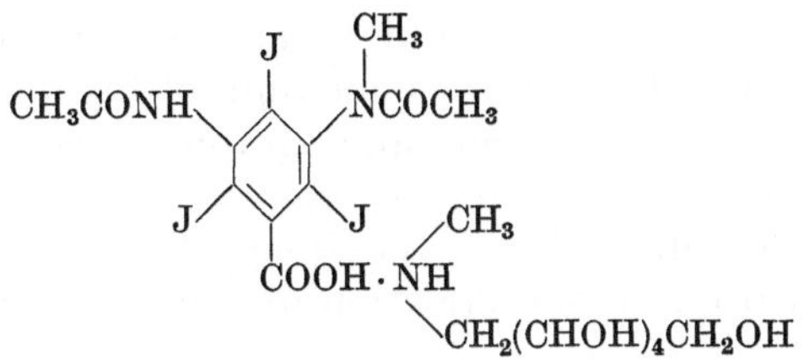

b)

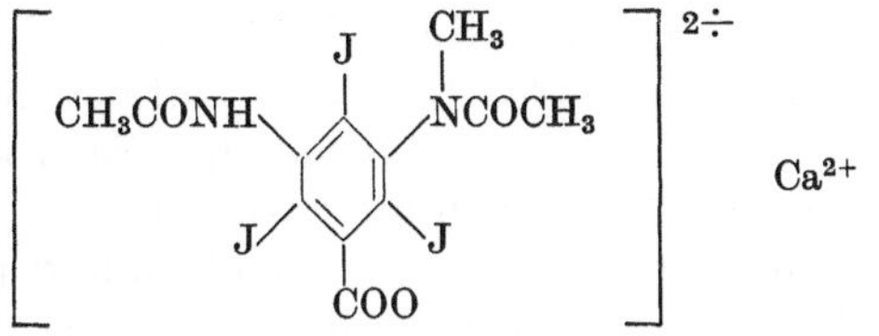

c)

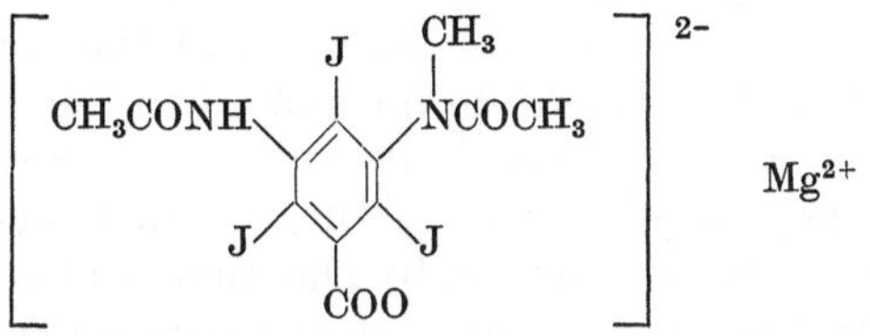

d)

Molecular weight		Iodine content
a)	649.9	58.6 %
b)	823.2	46.3 %
c)	1 293.9	58.8 %
d)	1 278.1	59.6 %

Official names:
Acidum metrizoicum NFN
Natrii metrizoas p INN

Trade marks:

a + c + d)	Isopaque (27.6 a + 1.4 c + 1 d), Nyegaard & CO. A/S
	Ronpacon (27.6 a + 1.4 c + 1 d), Cilag-Chemie AG
	Triosil (27.6 a + 1.4 c + 1 d), Glaxo
b + c)	Isopaque Cerebral (52.3 b + 1 c), Nyegaard & CO. A/S
	Ronpacon 280 (52.3 b + 1 c), Cilag-Chemie AG
a + b + c)	Isopaque Coronar 9 a + 58 b + 1 c) Nyegaard & CO. A/S
a + b + c + d)	Ronpacon 370 (28 a + 38.8 b + 1,4 c + 1 d), Cilag-Chemie AG
	ev. (10 a + 65 b + 1,1 c)

For brevity and clarity these groups of contrast media will hereafter be referred to as the di-iodine group and the tri-iodine group (with 2 and 3 iodine atoms, respectively, in the molecule). The contrast media within each of these groups differ considerably in quality.

To be acceptable for such a common examination method as urography, the contrast medium must naturally be of low toxicity and must be well tolerated by the organism. Contrast media of the di-iodine and tri-iodine groups are of low toxicity. The LD 50 for the di-iodine group is, for example, about 3.5 g per kg body weight when used intravenously while the LD 50 of the tri-iodine group is still lower, namely 10—15 g per kg body weight.

All contrast media have a certain generalized effect on the respiration and blood vessels. Contrast media belonging to the di-iodine group and some of those belonging to the tri-iodine group produce a fairly protracted dilatation of the vessels and sometimes contraction, while others such as diatrizoate sodium belonging to the tri-iodine group have hardly any demonstrable effect on the circulation.

The local tolerance of the tissues to the contrast media is high. This is of imortance in the diagnosis of diseases requiring a large amount of contrast medium of high concentration in an organ to be studied, *e.g.* in the kidneys for renal angiography. The specific local tolerance of the kidneys will be discussed in the chapter on renal angiography.

Contrast media are capable of causing hypersensitivity reactions. This side effect will be discussed in association with the description of the injection of contrast medium.

b) Excretion of contrast medium during urography

Contrast media used for urography are excreted in the urine. About $^1/_2$—1 liter of urine is produced per day, which implies that each kidney excretes $^1/_4$—$^1/_2$ ml per minute. The excretion may increase somewhat during urography because of the diuresis produced by the contrast medium. This diuretic effect is different with different media.

The contrast medium is excreted partly by ultrafiltration in the glomeruli and partly by excretion from the tubular epithelium. The amount excreted in either way varies from one medium to another. The principal excretion is by glomerular filtration however. The amount filtrated is directly proportional to the concentration of the contrast medium in the plasma. A high concentration of contrast medium not bound to the plasma protein will thus result in high ultrafiltration. This increased ultrafiltration, however, is accompanied by an increase in diuresis by the diuretic effect of the contrast medium. The increased excretion is thus balanced, partially or completely, by the increased amount of urine, so that the concentration of the contrast medium in the excreted urine will remain unchanged. This regulation of the concentration of the contrast medium in the urine is known from experience with other diuretics such as para-amino-hippuric acid, which is excreted in the same way as diodrast (Rapoport *et al.*, 1949). From a practical point of view, a higher iodine content in the excreted urine may give superior contrast conditions for studying the calyces and other details. On the other hand, an increase in diuresis may help fill the calyces more completetely and thus enhance the study of details. There is some difference in the molecular concentration of different media. It has thus been shown by Bennes and by Cattell (1970) that sodium diatrizoate is excreted in higher concentration in the urine than methylglucamine diatrizoate. This interesting physiological observation does not mean any remarkable difference in the contrast concentration in the kidney pelvis and the quality of the urogram, however.

Upon dehydration, the reabsorption of water is so marked that the concentration of the contrast medium in the urine will be higher than is normal. Thus if the osmotic pressure — if this term should still be used — on the tissue side is high, as it is in a dehydrated person, the reabsorption of water in the distal convolute tubuli will be increased to such an extent that the concentration of the contrast medium excreted will be higher than otherwise would be the case. A high osmotic pressure on the tissue side will thus permit a higher osmotic pressure on the tubular side, which in turn will result in the possibility that the kidneys will excrete a urine richer in contrast medium.

The contrast medium excreted by the tubules is proportional to the blood concentration only if this is low, but since the tubular excretion easily reaches a maximum with the ordinary doses used for urography (this maximum is 25 to 50 mg/min of diodrast iodine/ 100 ml) the concentration is said not to increase further with increasing dose. Thus a further increase in the dose will, as a rule, not increase the density of the contrast urine in the kidney pelvis because, firstly, the increase in concentration by filtration is lowered through dilution by the increased diuresis and, secondly, the concentration by tubular excretion depends on the low excretion maximum of the tubules.

This thus implies that the actual maximum molecular concentration of the various contrast media — independently of differences in the way they are excreted — is fairly equal for ordinary doses used for urography. An increased dose leads only to a prolongation of the constant level, which in human beings can be shown during urography simply by determining the specific gravity of the urine (Harrow, 1955). Contrast density of the urogram, as mentioned, can be improved to a certain extent by restriction of fluid intake. KEATES (1953) thus found an increase in di-iodine concentration inpatients who had been deprived of fluid for 18 hours when compared with those deprived for 7 hours.

In children below one year of age the concentration is often low due to their large fluid intake (WYATT, 1941). It should also be observed that during the first 2 weeks of life clearances in infants show low values, which afterwards increase, but with a wide individual variation (VESTERDAL and TUDVAD, 1949). It has been pointed out by NOGRADY and SCOTT-DUNBAR (1968) that in infants in the first month of life, excretion of intravenously injected urographic contrast media is prolonged. The maximum concentration appears to be achieved at approximately 1—3 hours after injection. Therefore the number of films during the early part of the examination of infants should be restricted and the total examination period prolonged.

HARROW (1955) suggested the use of a mixture of different contrast media because of the difference in the way contrast media are excreted, some being excreted mainly by glomerular filtration, others mainly by tubular excretion. Tubular secretion is negligible in modern contrast media, however; therefore this proposal no longer has validity.

An important possibility of improving the contrast density of the urogram is to increase the amount of radiopaque component of the contrast medium without increasing the osmotic pressure. This can be done by using contrast molecules containing several iodine atoms. The tri-iodine media represent examples of this. A solution of tri-iodine of given tonicity contains more iodine than a di-iodine solution of the same tonicity (see below).

As to the contrast density, the literature contains numerous reports of trials with, and the relative value of, new contrast media in comparison with other media. Such comparisons are often of little or no value because the authors appear to have limited knowledge of the way in which the contrast medium is excreted and have not considered the sources of error in the evaluation of the results. MADSEN (1957) has pointed out that subjects to be examined represent such heterogenous conditions for excretion and technique of exposures that these factors alone make any evaluation illusory. It is better, but probably not sufficient, to submit the same patient to urography on two occasions within a short period. The only reliable basis is afforded by precise clinical and laboratory studies. Such investigations have shown that if the patient is dehydrated the amount of iodine excreted, i.e. the factor of importance, is larger if contrast media of the di-iodine group are used, while in non-dehydrated patients contrast media of the tri-iodine group are superior.

The excretion of contrast media, however, also depends on the secretory pressure of the kidney and on the intrapelvic pressure. If the secretory pressure is lowered because of a fall in the arterial blood pressure, urinary secretion ceases. WICKBOM (1950) has shown this in urography of human beings in whom excretion ceased when the blood pressure was lowered down to 70 mm Hg. I have seen cases in which excretion ceased on fall of the blood pressure to 80 mm/Hg. This has been investigated experimentally by EDLING et al. (1954). An increase in the intrapelvic pressure can also increase or impair the excretion of contrast medium. This is discussed in the chapter on urography during renal colic.

It is difficult to judge the density of contrast medium. This depends not only on the density of the contrast urine excreted but also on the amount of urine in the renal pelvis with which the contrast urine is diluted. In addition, the width of the renal pelvis must be considered, the thickness of the layer of contrast urine increasing with the width of the renal pelvis. In the beginning of excretion the contrast density of the urine in the renal pelvis will be lower because the excreted contrast medium will be diluted by the urine in the dead space in the tubules and renal pelvis. Not until this urine has been removed by contrast urine will the density in the renal pelvis increase. If the renal pelvis is contracted or unusually small, the thickness of the layer will be less and the density of the contrast will therefore accordingly be low at a late stage of the examination, while if the renal pelvis is wide, there will be a thick layer and therefore high contrast density. After application of ureteric compression the renal pelvis will increase in width and the contrast density thereby increase. In fact the width is of decisive importance in judging density. This obvious and important point has been clearly illustrated schematically by MINDER (1936).

"An X-ray beam does not measure concentration but rather the total number of iodine atoms in its pathway. Hence radiographic density may be increased not only by increasing the concentration but also by simply increasing the volume while keeping the concentration constant" (DURE-SMITH et al., 1971). This is a good expression of an important fact. The authors believe, however, that this fact has not been taken into consideration by earlier workers in the field, which is a wrong assumption, as seen above.

In addition, excretion of contrast medium is also judged by such a crude method as estimating the differences in the density as seen in the film. Despite standardization of the method of preparation of the patient, of the contrast injection, of the type and amount of contrast medium used, of exposure, development and viewing and even if it be assumed that the thickness of the layer of contrast medium in the renal pelvis is always the same, there still remains the fact that the film reproduces contrast densities poorly, and the power of the eye to perceive differences in intensity of contrast is low.

As mentioned, modern contrast media have such a high iodine content that often a good contrast density can be secured in the renal pelvis even if a fair portion of the renal parenchyma is no longer functioning. This is demonstrated by the term selective pyelography (OLLE OLSSON, 1943), which implies that small portions of the kidney can excrete contrast urine of ordinary density, while other parts excrete urine of low density or no urine at all. This phenomenon can be demonstrated in films taken immediately after a kidney with local lesions has begun to excrete contrast urine. Later on in the examination this difference disappears and the renal pelvis can be filled with dense contrast urine coming from only a small portion of the kidney. Even in generalized kidney disease with decreasing capacity of the kidney to concentrate urine, the contrast density may be fairly high for a long time. This explains why the excretion of contrast urine may sometimes be good even in the presence of fairly severe renal damage. With a decrease in capacity of clearance by more than 50 % the contrast density in urography may still be good enough for diagnostic purposes.

On the other hand, if the contrast excretion is low, this decrease may vary widely without its being demonstrable in the film or detectable by the examiner as reduced contrast density. Finally, the absence of demonstrable excretion of contrast urine in urography may mean anything between impaired excretion and no excretion at all. The above remarks elucidate the possibility of judging renal function from the density of the contrast urine. It is obvious that this method for judging renal function is very crude. Neither is anything else to be expected, since urography aims at securing an excretion of contrast urine as dense as possible in as short a time as possible, and it must be said to have filled this requirement very well.

Another method for judging the excretion of contrast medium has been suggested by RAVASINI (1935). He determines the time between the injection of contrast medium intravenously and the appearance of the contrast medium in the renal pelvis. According to this method, several films are taken soon after the injection of the contrast medium. In such an evaluation of the excretion the blood pressure must be taken into account. It the blood pressure falls on injection of contrast medium, excretion will be delayed. The amount of contrast medium injected and the concentration of the medium are also important. In my opinion, function can be better evaluated by determining the interval between the time of injection of a small amount of contrast medium and the appearance in the renal pelvis. Such a method, which might be called mini-urography, permits fine assessment of excretion.

Heterotopic excretion of contrast media. The nature of an intravenous cholegraphic or urographic agent is based on the structure of the contrast medium molecule. The 5-position in the aromatic ring seems to be the decisive factor as to the lipophilic or hydrophilic nature of the medium, the former constituting a cholegraphic, the latter a urographic agent. This may also be expressed as the protein-binding capacity of a contrast medium.

As pointed out by LASSER *et al.* (1962), the more strongly protein-bound contrast media appear to be excreted preferentially in the bile. In the triiodobenzoate acid compounds, the absence of a prosthetic group at the 5-position in the benzene ring seems to determine the strong binding to albumin. This is the case with Urokon, and specifically with Cholegrafin. The latter is therefore a cholegraphic medium, and on the same but slightly weaker grounds Urokon (sodium acetrizoate) also often leads to gallbladder filling at urography. WOLLEY *et al.* (1957) after intravenous administration of Urokon-sodium 70 % for urography in 'standard doses', could demonstrate gallbladder filling in 12 out of 25 patients two hours after its injection. Media such as Hypaque and Urografin (sodium diatrizoate), on the other hand, exhibit weak protein binding and seldom fill the gallbladder. SEGALL (1969), in reporting on contrast filling of the gallbladder at urography in five subjects, pointed out the rarity of this phenomenon.

Sodium metrizoate (Isopaque), consisting of a balanced mixture of sodium, calcium, magnesium and methyl-glucamine salts and metrizoate acid, is closely related to sodium diatrizoate. When using this contrast medium for urography we have found that filling of the gallbladder is fairly often obtained in connection with the injection of the contrast medium. Filling of the gallbladder may be seen already during the actual examination but it seldom occurs under ordinary conditions.

In a few patients who had been subjected to urography or angiography demonstrating ordinary conditions in the urinary pathways, considerable filling of the gallbladder was observed on examination of the bowel later the same day. The interval between the injection and the time of filling was about four hours. In a series of 25 patients, in whom ordinary conditions had been demonstrated at urography, no filling of the gallbladder could be observed in any one of the patients in examinations performed five hours and 24 hours, respectively, after urography, specifically to see if such filling occurred. Filling of the gallbladder in connection with normal urography using Isopaque as contrast medium is thus a rare phenomenon.

On the other hand, the gallbladder is often contrast-filled at urography or angiography if stasis in the urinary pathways is present. This occurs more often with sodium metrizoate than with the diatrizoate media. We have encountered several cases in which during urography in connection with an attack of pain (sometimes persisting throughout the examination) a marked or only slight stasis was present on one side only and at the same time filling of the gallbladder was observable during the actual examination. When this happens it may be used as an extra sign of diagnostic importance when the acute examination is performed for the purpose of a clinical differential diagnosis between an attack of cholelithiasis and urolithiasis, and if signs of stasis at urography are slight or absent when the examination is performed after the subsidence of pain.

Filling of the gallbladder during the actual examination can be slight but may sometimes be quite marked. If minimal, an increase in concentration will usually occur during the following hours and good filling may persist and be seen on the next day.

We also have noticed filling of the gallbladder in a patient who immediately after injection of the contrast medium had a marked fall in blood pressure. No excretion could be seen through the kidneys until the blood pressure had risen.

Filling of the gallbladder occurred in a patient with polycystic renal disease; this represents a borderline case of heterotopic excretion of contrast medium, as in uremia. This type of excretion thus seems to be the same with sodium metrizoate as with other contrast media.

The difference in excretion in the bile between the salts of metrizoate and diatrizoate acids is not related to a great difference in the chemical composition, the only difference in this respect being the addition of a methyl group in the 3-position in the metrizoate

4*

compound. This may affect excretion under certain conditions. Another factor seems more plausible, however, in relation to the excretion of the contrast medium through the liver in patients with acutely impaired renal excretion in renal colic. Dawson et al. (1968) in experiments with rabbits and cats reported a half-life of intravenously injected sodium metrizoate (100 mg/kg) of 55 minutes, with an excretion of 88.4 and 86.6 % respectively in the urine, and 2.2 and 4.8 % respectively in the bile. In man, disappearance of the contrast medium Isopaque 350 from the blood was found to be a two-rate process, with half-lives of about 15 minutes and 2 hours. As compared with the corresponding figures for sodium diatrizoate in the first of the two-rate processes related to available water space, sodium metrizoate was found to have a considerably shorter half-life, i.e. 15 minutes as compared with 52 minutes (Stokes and Ter-Pergossian, 1964). It is probably this difference that explains the excretion of the sodium metrizoate through the liver, with filling of the gallbladder more rapidly if acute, unbalanced stasis is present in the urinary pathways. The choice by the organism of the liver route for eliminating a contrast medium, which under ordinary conditions offers specifically rapid excretion through the kidneys, may be looked upon as a conditional safety resort (Olle Olsson, 1971).

In renal insufficiency contrast medium injected for renal angiography, for example, is often seen to be excreted also through the bowel mucosa with a marked collection of the excreted medium in the colon (Fig. 34).

Occasionally contrast excretion is seen in the stomach (Scholtz, 1941).

Siemensen and Augustin (1972) in experiments on rabbits with terminal renal insufficiency and with and without blockage of the flow of bile from the liver, studied the excretion of Jodipamide and Diatrizoate under hemodialysis. With regard to the high degree of protein binding of Jodipamide and corresponding limited possibility of dialysis, the authors recommend caution in the use of this contrast medium in uremic patients with concomitant disease in the liver and/or gallbladder.

During cholegraphy some of the contrast medium is always excreted via the kidneys. In hepatic cellular failure the renal excretion of the medium may be increased and thereby convert cholegraphy into urography. A case has been described by Theander (1956) in which such an unintentional urogram revealed a space-occupying lesion in the right kidney, the kidney on the right side always being included in gallbladder survey films.

c) Injection and dose of contrast medium

The patient is prepared for the examination in the same way as for plain roentgenography of the urinary tract. In view of the smallness of many of the pathologic changes that can be seen during urography, proper preparation of the patient is important (see chapter B). Some authors recommend dehydration by restriction of fluid intake prior to the examination. This may be useful when di-iodines are used as a contrast medium, but is hardly necessary when tri-iodines are employed, except for patients with a large fluid intake. Withdrawal of fluids should, according to many authors, also imply that water enema should not be given because water can be absorbed from the large intestine. Since such water absorption is slow, a water enema is not contraindicated if given shortly before urography (Steinert, 1952), regardless of the type of contrast medium used.

As a rule, about 20 ml of contrast medium is injected for urography. We generally use 30—40 % solutions for the tri-iodine. Investigations of the tolerance to contrast media in association with angiocardiography have shown that large amounts can be used and therefore if, for some technical reason, the filling of the renal pelvis during ureteric compression is not satisfactory, the compression may be adjusted and a further dose of 20—40 ml, for example, injected. For children, the dose of contrast medium need not be so large, but should not be too small, 12—20 ml usually being suitable. If the dose is too small, contrast may be poor because of the relatively low tubular secretion in infants.

If desirable, the examiner may try a small dose of contrast medium for urography. In adults, good urography is sometimes possible with such a small dose as 3 ml of a contrast medium in ordinary concentration.

The medium is usually administered intravenously but may be given intra-arterially, intra-muscularly, or subcutaneously. On extravascular injection we usually dilute the contrast medium with one or two parts of distilled water and, before injecting it, we

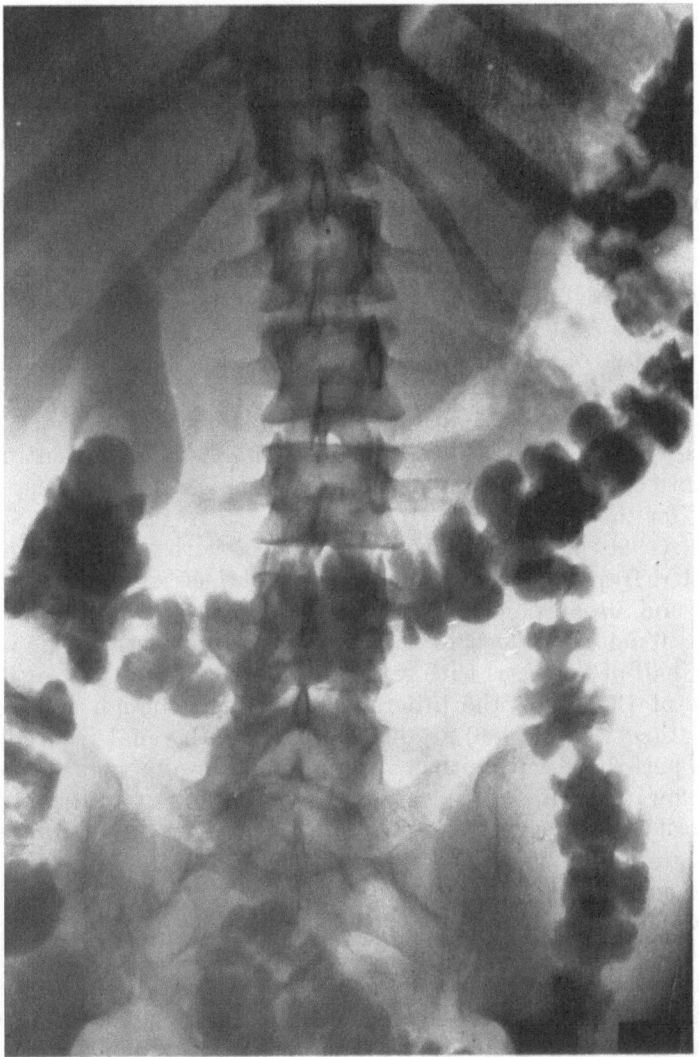

Fig. 34. Heterotopic excretion of contrast medium: filling of bowel and of gall bladder after angiography in patient with uremia

prepare the site of injection with hyaluronidase to increase the rate of absorption (OLLE OLSSON and LÖFGREN, 1949).

Any extravasation following the intravenous injection of modern contrast media will cause only a reddening and tenderness and requires no special treatment.

Oral and rectal administration of contrast media have been tried but as yet without success.

Contrast medium has also been injected into the medulla of bones, e.g. in the tibia or the sternum. In such case the contrast medium must be diluted considerably, although large amounts may be injected within a fairly short time (WALLDÉN, 1944). This method is not widely used, however.

Before the injection of contrast medium, the patient should empty the bladder, as a full bladder interferes with the excretion and transport of urine. As is known, filling of the bladder with oil was once used for urography instead of ureteric compression. It has been observed (NOGRADY et al., 1963) that at urography in infants and children during physiologic retention of bladder urine, stasis is produced in the upper urinary tract. This may occasionally simulate hydronephrosis and can be used to improve filling of the pelvic calyceal system.

d) Urography in renal insufficiency

With the contrast media formerly available, injection of contrast medium in marked renal insufficiency was counterindicated. With media now available, renal insufficiency is usually no absolute counterindication for urography. The relative counterindication lies in the fact that with low clearance values the excretion of contrast medium is so poor that it is of no diagnostic value.

In evaluation of renal function by means of plasma creatinine concentration, SCHWARTZ et al. (1963) found little evidence of nephrotoxicity after injection of three-iodinated contrast media. In only five of 90 patients was an unexplained rise in plasma creatinine concentration found after urographic examination, and in four of these cases the change was transient. With a plasma creatinine concentration between 1.5 and 5.0 mg per 100 ml, the anatomy of the kidney pelvis could be studied and with concentration above 5 mg per 100 ml, a faint concentration in the kidney pelvis was found in half of the patients, usually sufficient for morphologic study.

BARTLEY et al. (1968) presented a study of 161 cases with serum creatinine ranging from 0.9 to 5.5 mg %. Urography was performed with the injection of 40 ml of Urografin 60 %. Diagnostically useful urographic examinations were obtained in all cases with serum creatinine below 1.6 mg %, in 90 % of the cases with serum creatinine of 1.7—2.6 mg %, and in more than half of the cases with serum creatinine of 2.7—3.3 mg %. In one patient with a creatinine of 13.6 mg % the urography was good enough to exclude obstruction on both sides. FULTON et al. (1969) studied 55 cases with renal insufficiency where urography had been performed with either a large injection of contrast medium or infusion urography (see below) and found the urographic examinations to be diagnostically sufficient in the great majority of the cases. STAGE et al. (1971) in 225 cases with serum creatinine over 1.6 mg % at urography using Urografin 76 % in a large dose of 80—150 ml, found the examinations sufficient for diagnosis in all cases with creatinine below 6 mg % but also in several cases with creatine values above this level. In only 12 patients was the contrast filling of the ureters insufficient for diagnosis of a possible obstacle.

KELSEY and CATTELL (1971) studied the value of urography in 48 cases with severe non-oliguric renal failure with a blood urea of more than 200 ml per 100 ml creatinine clearance of less than 10 ml per minute, and found that the kidneys could be well outlined in all but four patients. In each of 10 patients with extrarenal obstruction this could be diagnosed and in only two patients without obstruction was no pyelogram seen. No ill effects were observed. The authors stress the necessity of the availability of dialysis.

OWMAN (1972) in a survey of the literature on the toxic effect on the kidneys of contrast media points out the important indication for urography in renal insufficiency in the differentiation between cases with and without obstruction of the urinary pathways as cause of the insufficiency. On the basis of this survey the author concludes that urography should be performed in the examination of patients with acute or chronic renal insufficiency, particularly if there is a problem of excluding obstacle to urinary drainage. It is important, however, that the patient undergoing such an examination is not dehydrated. The examination must be performed with a large dose of contrast medium, one single dose to be preferred to infusion urography. The duration of the examination should in certain cases be prolonged and films taken on the second day may reveal excretion. Tomography or zonography is often useful or necessary. Counter-indications are a marked state of dehydration, concomitant insufficiency of the liver, and the presence of myeloma.

It may be mentioned in this connection that acute renal failure has been seen to occur shortly after urography in patients with long-standing diabetes and azotemia (PILLAY et al., 1970).

e) Urography in patients with myeloma

Patients with myeloma have received particular attention from the point of view of possible damage to the kidneys by the urographic procedure. Renal lesions are very common in myelomatosis. This type of lesion includes acute glomerulonephritis, nephrotic syndrome, water-losing nephritis, Fanconi's syndrome, renal tubular acidosis, acute tubular necrosis, and acute and chronic pyelonephritis, as related by SANCHEZ and DOMS (1960) who underlined the fact that renal disease is a common guise under which myeloma may masquerade and elude detection. Patients with this disease are therefore often referred for urography, which is performed on the basis of the objective urinary findings, e. g. proteinuria. Urography may then be followed by acute or gradually increasing anuria (HOLMAN, 1939; BARTELS et al., 1954; KILMANN et al., 1957; PERILLE and CONN, 1958). For additional literature see SVOBODA, 1967. The latter author also reports on urography in 14 patients with myeloma without reactions but stresses the necessity of the strongest possible indications for urography in myelomatous patients.

MYERS and WITTEN (1971) stress that dehydration from vomiting or associated with the preparation for urography has been the common denominator that has preceded acute renal failure in myeloma. This may be an important factor but cannot be solely responsible for the acute renal failure.

In 40 patients with myeloma in whom 52 urographies were performed mainly before establishment of the diagnosis of myeloma, VIX (1966) found no evidence of renal damage by urography and the author concluded that indications for urography in myeloma should be restricted in the same way as for other cases with decrease in renal function. In an editorial (1961) LEUCUTIA summarizes precautions in this way: "Urography should not be performed in cases of multiple myeloma. In occult cases of multiple myeloma, a diligent search should be made for protein abnormalities by electrophoretic studies of the blood serum and urine, and if they are present urography should be omitted. In cases of proteinuria the possibility of multiple myeloma masquerading under the guise of a nephropathy should be kept in mind and urography performed only after the elimination of this possibility." This would exclude every patient with myeloma from examination by urography. To me the solution of the problem of urography in relation to myelomatosis lies in the fact that myeloma forces upon the clinician and the roentgenologist the necessity of having the strongest indications before urography is performed. It should be mentioned here that multiple myeloma in itself may cause acute renal failure. KJELDSBERG and HOLMAN (1971) report a case where a patient with unsuspected multiple myeloma had acute renal failure three weeks after documentation of normal renal function. No urography was performed and there was no evidence of dehydration.

f) Reactions[3]

General reactions to contrast media fall into two groups, namely those due mainly to hypertonicity and specific toxicity of the contrast medium as described above and, secondly, reactions caused by hypersensitivity to the media. The severity of the latter varies from very slight to fatal.

---

[3] The reader is referred to the report on a symposium on contrast media toxicity published in Investigative Radiology, Nov.-Dec., 1970.

The injection of the contrast medium is sometimes followed by a feeling of burning, reddening, nausea or vomiting, but the reaction is usually transient. Sometimes reactions of another type appear, namely urticaria in the form of single wheals or more widespread changes coalescing to form large regions of edema. Such edema may be serious if it involves the larynx and causes respiratory difficulties. A special type of reaction has been described by SUSSMAN & MILLER (1956) and IMBUR and BOURNE (1972). This is iodide mumps and consists of a swelling of the salivary glands occurring some days after the injection of contrast medium. The contrast medium for urography is not excreted in the urine in the form of mineralized iodine but leaves the body without undergoing any chemical change (HECHT, 1938).

Shock occasionally develops, with the usual signs: imperceptible pulse, pallor, and severe drop in blood pressure. Such shock may be fatal but is rarely so. PENDERGRASS et al. (1958) made two large-scale inquiries in the United States into deaths occurring during urography. The first inquiry, which covered four million urographies, revealed 31 deaths, of which 25 were classified as immediate. The second inquiry revealed 8.6 deaths per one million examinations. WOLFROMM (1966) reported 15 deaths and 166 severe reactions in nearly one million urographies performed between 1955 and 1965, representing one death per approximately 70,000 examinations and one severe reaction in approximately 3,000. TONIOLO (1966) found a mortality rate of one in 85.000 examinations.

Little difference was found in the incidence of reaction among various contrast media, and no advantage was found in the use of methyl-glucamine, from which a certain protective action was expected (ANSELL, 1970).

No decrease in mortality rate has been shown with the use of any new contrast medium, which may be due partly to increasing dosage and partly to less restrictive selection of patients.

It may be well to point out here that urography should not always be held responsible for any serious condition which may arise soon after examination. This is illustrated by a case described by COUNTS et al. (1957) in which fatal intra-abdominal bleeding was erroneously interpreted as shock caused by the contrast medium used in urography.

Because of the risk of severe reactions to the injection of contrast medium the examination room should always be equipped with an emergency tray with analeptics and antihistaminics and with instruments for artificial respiration, thoracotomy, and heart massage. It may be mentioned that hydrocortisone has been successfully used in the treatment of severe reactions (WRIGHT, 1959). Adrenaline should not be used because it may cause ventricular fibrillation.

All steps should be taken, of course, to prevent such reactions such as testing the patient before the examination for any hypersensitivity to the contrast medium in contemplated urography and, secondly, simultaneous administration of anti-histaminics to try to counteract such reactions. Attempts have also been made to desensibilize hypersensitive patients.

Injections of 1—2 ml intravenously as a provocation test, intracutaneous injection of a small amount of contrast medium or a drop of the medium into the conjunctiva bulbi have been used as a test. Care should be taken that such a test dose and the examination dose should be of the same type and preferably from the same batch. Since side reactions may occur several hours after the injection, the test injection should preferably be given the day before the actual examination.

ALYEA and HAINES (1947) have compared the results of such test injections with those of injections for the examination proper. Their study confirmed clinical experience that there is no parallel between the results of the injections and reactions to the contrast medium nor between the incidence of allergic symptoms such as asthma and reactions to contrast media. If there is a personal history of asthma, hay fever or drug sensitivity and the skin test is positive, there is a definite possibility that the patient will have a general reaction to the drug, according to these authors. In such cases the performance or non-performance of the examination depends on the indication. On contrast injection of the same type but for definitely different purposes e. g. cerebral angiography, we have often found that patients hypersensitive to the test dose showed no untoward reactions to subsequent angiography, which had to be performed on vital indications, and this despite the use of repeated injections.

On the basis of a questionnaire to a large number of teaching hospitals in the United States, FISCHER and DOUST (1971) analyzed data regarding the difference in the death rate between hospitals where a pre-test was made before urography and hospitals where no test was made. There was no significant statistical difference in the data from the two sources. It is therefore concluded that the pre-test is of no value in avoiding death or major complications in urography.

PENDERGRASS et al. have described a case of death following injection of a test dose. Another case of death following intravenous injection of 1 ml contrast medium has been described by PAYNE et al. (1956). I have also observed a case of sudden death following intravenous injection of 2 ml of contrast medium as a test injection. Death was due to bronchospasm which could not be controlled. Emergency therapy including immediate heart massage after thoracotomy was unsuccessful.

Although fatal reactions are rare, the frequency of mild reactions is not insignificant. It is true, however, that they have become much less common since the introduction of tri-iodine contrast media. Attempts have been made to prevent reactions by using anti-histaminics in association with the contrast injection (CREPEA et al., 1949) or by adding a small amount of antihistamine to the contrast medium injected (OLLE OLSSON, 1951). Such an admixture has been found to reduce the frequency of reactions but not to prevent them altogether. GETZOFF (1951), INMAN (1952) and MOORE and SANDERS (1953) also reported a certain effect of anti-histaminics in association with the injection of contrast medium. Other authors, however, have found such drugs to have no effect. Here it may be pointed out that it has been demonstrated experimentally (ROCKOFF et al., 1971) that the contrast media of the methyl-glucamine type are capable of liberating histamine, as was previously found regarding sodium salts. WINTER (1955) and DOYLE (1959) have found reactions to Miokon significantly to diminish when chlor-trimetone was incorporated with the contrast medium (diprotrizoate 30 cc 50% + chlortrimetone malcate 1 cc mixed).

Attempts to desensibilize patients according to allergologic principles have been performed by ARNER (1959) and we have seen patients who first reacted markedly to the contrast medium but after such desensibilization showed no reaction at all. The sensibility may be specific for a certain contrast medium. We have had a patient who could not be desensibilized to Hypaque, while desensibilization to Miokon was successful. The whole question of desensibilization is difficult to evaluate, however, because of the — fortunately — very low incidence of serious reactions. To sum up: reactions of this type can occur, the roentgenologist must deem them possible at every contrast injection, and in choosing the indications for examination this fact must be kept in mind.

g) Examination technique

Urography may be used for studying renal function or renal anatomy, or both. The evaluation of function should include not only the capacity of the kidneys to excrete contrast medium, but also the capacity of the urinary tract to receive and to transport it. The morphologic examination is possible only in a functioning kidney and is therefore in reality a combination of functional and morphologic examination. If only function is to be studied, excretion is assessed on the basis of films taken at suitable intervals from the commencement of the excretion of contrast urine: its excretion from different parts of the renal parenchyma, the concentration of the contrast medium, the filling of the renal pelvis and the ureter, and further transport of contrast urine.

It has been found (Wolpert, 1965) that the rapid injection of 50 cc of contrast medium of high concentration could cause an increase in the kidney size of approximately 0.5 cm at maximum, the first five minutes after injection, due possibly to the diuretic effect of the contrast medium. In almost $1/3$ of the cases a slight size reduction was found instead.

Usually a single dose of 20 cc of contrast medium is sufficient for a complete urography. An increases in the dose to 40 cc or 60 cc will enhance filling of the kidney pelvis with branches. If after the first dose the filling is found not to be good, another injection may be made. Large single-dose injections with a modern contrast medium give better results than the infusion technique (see below).

The first excretory urogram should be taken 1 to 3 minutes after the injection of contrast medium. Excretion of the contrast medium will be seen with collection of contrast urine in the periphery of the renal pelvis, thus in the calyces. The most dorsal calyces will be filled first because of the high specific gravity of the contrast urine. The program of the rest of the examinations will vary with the information desired and the findings made in the films as they are developed and studied (Fig. 35).

If drainage of the kidney is not obstructed, the renal pelves and ureters will never be completely filled. Owing to the rhythmic contractions of the renal pelvis, certain parts will be filled, while others will be contracted. Since diastole is much longer than systole, the set of films will be dominated by those taken during diastole, with relatively good filling of most of the calyces. The cranial calyces are filled first and then the dorsal, as mentioned, because of the position of the kidney and the high specific gravity of the contrast urine. The caudal and ventral calyces are often not filled, or filled only incompletely. Normally the filling of the ureter is never continuous; usually the upper and lower thirds are filled, while the middle third is void of contrast medium, or a filling may be obtained of other segments of the ureter.

Detailed examination of the anatomy therefore requires the accumulation of contrast urine in the renal pelvis by ureteric compression and examination of the entire ureter requires films taken when the contrast urine, on release of ureteric compression, flows from the renal pelvis down through the ureter.

As mentioned, examination of the anatomy of the kidney requires acceptable renal function. Compression should therefore not be applied until satisfactory excretion has been demonstrated. This can usually be done in a single film, well coned for the kidneys only, and taken 3 minutes after the contrast injection. This is definitely in opposition to methods for urography in which compression is applied before injection of contrast medium, particularly types of media where compression is recommended to be applied several minutes before the injection (Servadio, 1965). It is also in opposition to methods where application of ureteral compression is recommended to follow directly after injection of the contrast medium.

In experiments on rabbits, Olin and Reese (1973) in studying renal perfusion and minute volume of the heart in connection with abdominal compression, found increase in blood pressure and pulse and in the pressure in the inferior caval vein. The authors conclude that the ureteric compression should be applied, at the earliest, five minutes after the injection of the contrast medium.

Different methods have been described for ureteric compression. The best results are obtained by the use of a couple of rubber bags placed over each ureter and inflated to a pressure of 0.3—0.4 kg/cm² (Steinert, 1952). The pressure should be increased only slowly. A large single balloon placed over the middle of the abdomen often dislocates the ureters laterally and results in poor compression and also increases the intra-abdominal pressure, with consequent impairment of renal function (Bradley and Bradley, 1947). Some examination tables are equipped with an appliance for the application of compression, but such accessories fixed to the examination table prevent change in the posture of the patient during the examination. Change in posture is important, particularly for taking

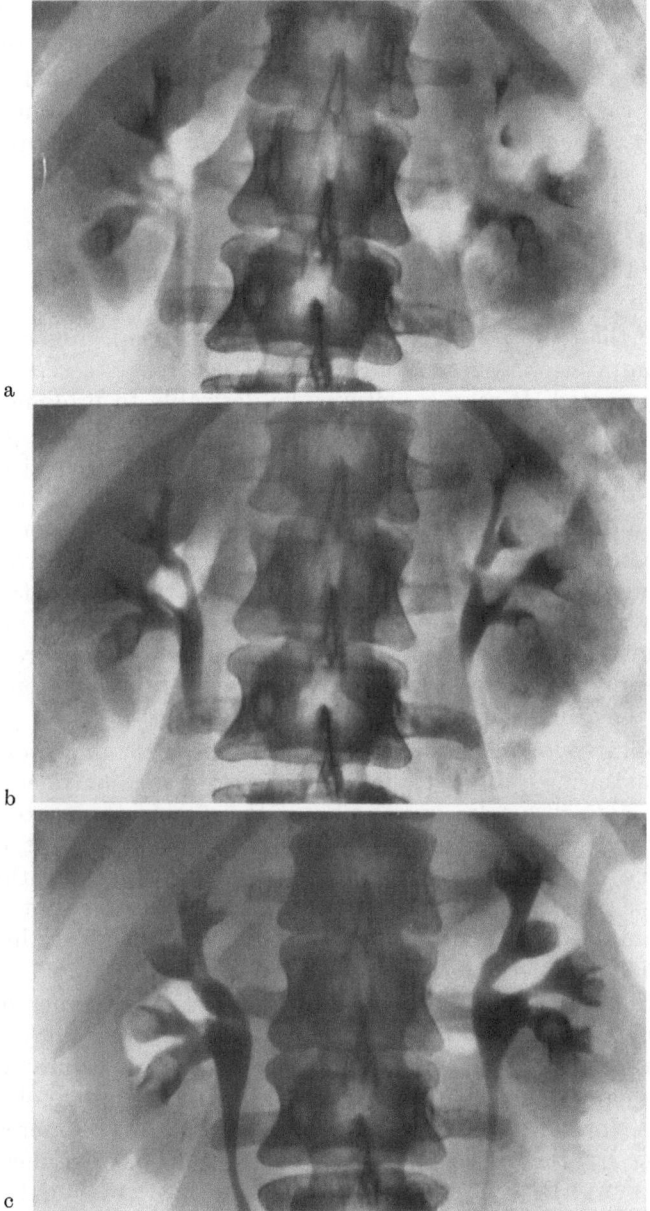

Fig. 35. Urography: a) excretion starting, b) maximal filling with free flow, c) after ureteric compression lasting 5 min. Note filling defects caused by arteries in b) in two branches on left side. These disappear upon slight distention of pelvis by compression

oblique films for demonstrating details of the renal pelvis. Compression appliances of this type are constructed in such a way that they cause a rapid increase in the pressure, which makes their use still less desirable.

It has been questioned whether ureteric compression does really obstruct flow through the ureters (CARLSON, 1946). Such an opinion only serves to demonstrate lack of knowledge of the technique of ureteric compression and of interpretation of the findings when compression is used. In fact, flow through the ureter can be completely obstructed, and prolonged compression can produce such an increase in intrapelvic pressure as to cause renal colic. It is also possible in this way to cause distention of the renal pelvis with rupture of the fornix and sinus reflux. The effect of compression of the ureter is best seen in comparison of the flow in the two ureters on compression of one of these.

Occasionally when it is difficult to obtain a filling of the renal pelves because of their being markedly contracted, it may be advisable to inject an antispasmodic drug (SINGER, 1947; MÖCKEL, 1954). Such antispasmodics should be used only exceptionally as they do not always produce the desired effect.

Occasionally the injection of the contrast medium or the compression causes a fall in the blood pressure, with decreased secretory pressure and cessation of excretion as a result. Injection of ephedrine with consequent increase in the blood pressure will be followed immediately by excretion.

A good filling of the renal pelvis usually requires 5—10 minutes of ureteric compression. Sometimes compression must be adjusted. If necessary, a second dose of contrast medium should be injected. It may sometimes be desirable to prolong compression for a considerable time. It may also be necessary to take films with the patient in different postures possibly including the erect position. In the examination of individual calyces, well coned films in different projections are always necessary.

The examination is concluded with films of the ureter and bladder taken on release of compression. The contrast urine then rushes through the ureters which are then filled along their entire length (see Fig. 26). It is important that the films of the ureters be sharp. Experience has shown that on release of the compression the patient moves and therefore must be properly instructed not to do so. Sharp roentgenograms are necessary because examination of the ureters is important for the detection of papilloma, cystic ureteritis etc., the changes often being very slight.

On release of compression with flow of contrast urine through the ureter into the bladder, where the contrast urine is diluted, a jet of ureter urine is sometimes seen in the bladder (Fig. 36). This may convey a false impression of the site of the ureteric orifice. The jet phenomenon is physiologic and should be regarded as a normal roentgenographic finding (GÖTHLIN, 1964). The direction of the jet may vary with the position of the ureteric orifice and its shape. The jet is often directed cranially in a patient with prostatic hyperplasia, for example. Deformation of the orifice by tumor or by inflammatory lesion may also cause unusual directions of the jet (Fig. 36c).

After injection of contrast medium the renal parenchyma becomes denser because the contrast medium is condensed in the excretory system of the kidney. This phenomenon is called the nephrographic effect. It is most striking in a kidney with normal renal parenchyma, which cannot be drained because of increased intrapelvic pressure or low secretory pressure. Normally the nephrographic effect can be increased markedly by loading the kidneys by the injection of a large dose of contrast medium (WEENS and FLORENCE, 1947; VESEY, DOTTER and STEINBERG, 1950. WALL and ROSE, 1951; DETAR and HARRIS, 1954). VESEY, DOTTER and STEINBERG (1950) injected 50 ml 70 % diodrast within 2 seconds and took films of the kidneys 16—28 seconds later. Satisfactory nephrograms were obtained in 18 of 25 cases by this technique.

The papillae often increase in contrast density because of stoppage of flow of contrast urine of high concentration in the papillary ducts. This is thus a sign of stasis. This increase in contrast may be extensive or limited to a few papillae and should not be confused with papillary ulcerations. On the other hand, papillary ulceration should not be missed by mistaking it for this phenomenon. If it is very marked, it can simulate medullary sponge kidney.

It is well known that substances secreted by the tubules can block the excretion of other substances such as phenol red, para-amino-hippuric acid (PAH) and penicillin. In animal experiments EDLING, HELANDER and SELDINGER (1957) showed that the nephrographic effect is reduced if the injection of the contrast medium is preceded by injection of any of these agents.

In the many comparisons of the value of urography and pyelography it is widely believed that urography cannot yield desired information on morphologic problems. In view
of what is said above it should be borne in mind that urography is often, if not most
often, performed in such a way that the amount of information it gives on the morphology

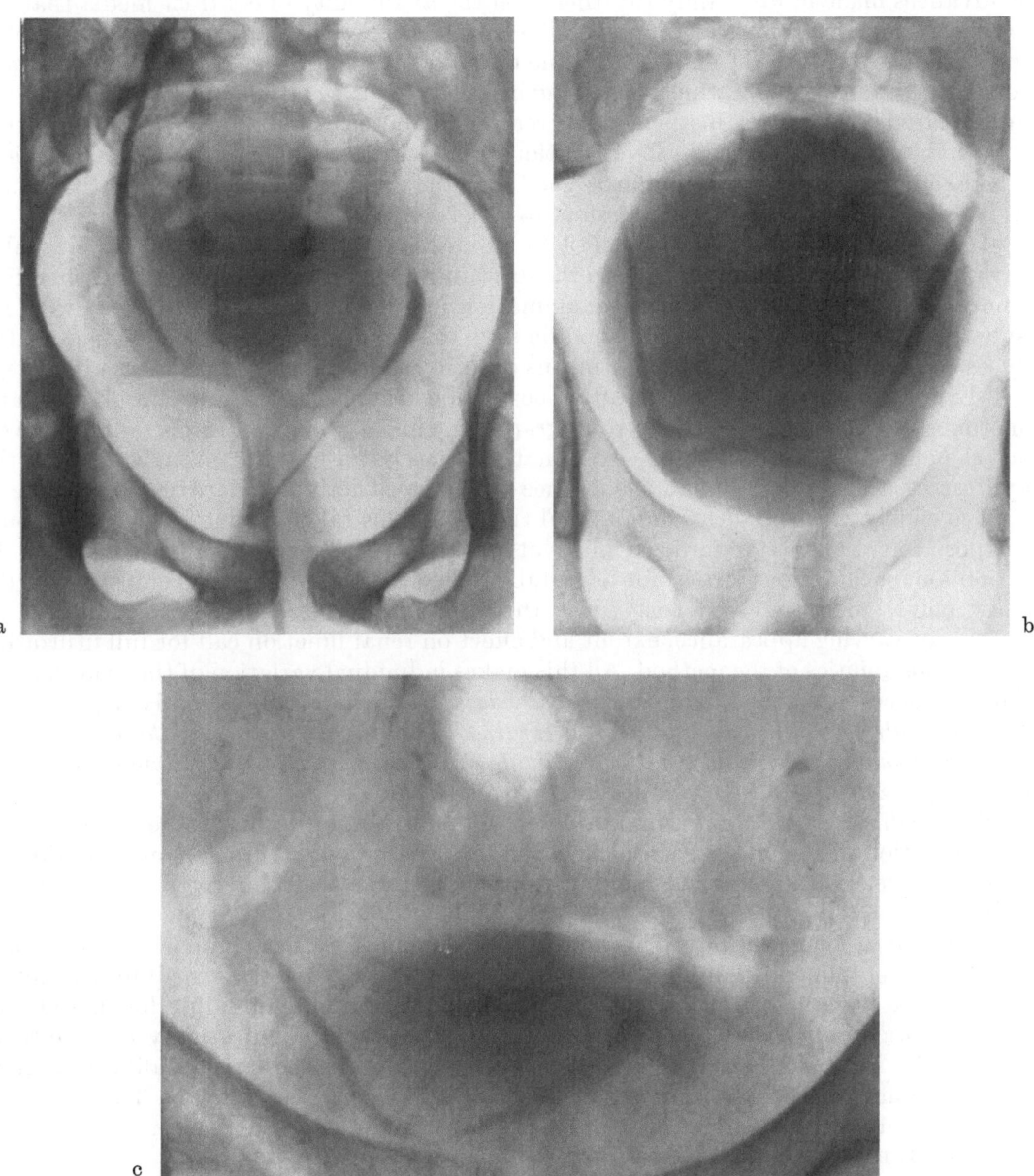

Fig. 36. a) Ureteric jet. A stream of contrast urine is ejected from left ureteric orifice through the bladder to
base at right of midline; b) Bilateral ureteric jet. c) Jet from a right ureteric orifice directed to the left cranially
in patient with cystitis affecting the ureteric orifice

of the kidneys will depend almost entirely on chance. If *properly* performed, urography
can, however, as a rule, give satisfactory information on the anatomy in addition to the
information it yields about the function of the kidney and the urinary pathways.

Some authors disapprove of the use of urography in the investigation of morphologic
changes in general or for certain purposes. Thus v. LICHTENBERG and BOEMINGHAUS are

often referred to. As a matter of principle, ureteric compression should not be used in an examination of function, which has, of course, been emphasized by pioneers in this field. I would here once more stress that in the examination of physiologic conditions, *e. g.* in the investigation of stasis, compression should not be applied. In other cases and with the advances made in urography together with the availability of contrast media that are excreted in high concentration, it is possible to make combined functional and morphologic examinations with the emphasis on the morphology. This often also makes retrograde pyelography unnecessary, which is an important advantage if check examinations are contemplated that do not in themselves require catheterization. Such a combined examination often also simplifies investigation and gives more richly faceted information. If the excretion of contrast medium is good and the examination technique satisfactory, it is possible, with the use of compression, to judge even details of the morphology.

An investigation by Dihlmann (1958) produced statistical evidence of the value of compression, but in his investigation the examinations were standardized and therefore do not show the true value of the examination method. I can therefore agree with his results but not with his conclusion when he says that incipient pathologic changes of the calyces can still be recognized best by means of retrograde pyelography. This is not always true. Even incipient changes can often be demonstrated distinctly by urography, and sometimes urography is superior to pyelography in this respect. It is important, however, that, as pointed out previously, the examination steps be adjusted to circumstances in the way described above and not in accordance with any strictly standardized procedure.

It is widely accepted as a fundamental rule that films taken during urography should be exposed at certain standardized intervals after injection of the contrast medium. In my opinion, such a procedure is not acceptable; the excretion, filling and emptying of the kidney pelvis and flow of contrast urine through the ureters as well as the pathologic processes of varying appearance, extent and effect on renal function call for full utilization of all the possibilities of the method. All this makes individual variation of the examination technique necessary. All standardization and *laissez-faire* procedures imply a poor technique. *The films should never be taken according to hard-and-fast rules. The examination procedure should instead be adjusted according to the requirements of the individual case and with full utilization of all the possibilities of the method.*

Modifications of urographic methodology. Modification according to needs instead of standardization of technique should be a rule in urography rather than an exception, as stressed above. Certain marked modifications have been used, however, under specific conditions:

1. Drip-infusion urography. This implies infusion of contrast medium in a large volume of fluid. The recommended dosage (Schenker, 1964) is 1 cc of contrast medium per pound mixed with 1 cc per pound of 5% dextrose in water. The minimum adult dose is 150 cc of each or a total volume of 300 cc. The infusion is made rapidly and usually takes 6 to 10 minutes. The indications are mainly a second procedure to increase the quality of a study which was found to be unsatisfactory when made in the conventional way. The literature illustrates different views on the value of drip-infusion urography (see, for example, Vitt and Burgher, 1966; Lenson *et al.*, 1971).

2. Rapid sequence and washout urography. As these modifications are used mainly as screening tests in renal hypertension to find patients with unilateral renal artery stenosis, they are mentioned together. Rapid-sequence urography (Maxwell *et al.*, 1962) means that after the injection of contrast medium films are taken at intervals of approximately 20 seconds for approximately 1 to 2 minutes, in order to demonstrate any difference in nephrographic effect or excretion into the renal pelvis between the two sides. Washout urography (Amplatz, 1962, 1964) implies an infusion of 500 cc saline and 40 grams of urea to wash out excreted contrast medium from the kidney pelvis. The washout procedure takes a longer time in a kidney with low urine production because of stenosis of the renal artery.

h) Urography at health-check examinations

A large number of important renal lesions have very discreet clinical symptomatology or none at all. Therefore urography must be used in many instances with fairly wide indications. In one situation we use urography in health-check examinations: in our department every angiographic procedure ends with a film of the kidneys. The often fairly large amount of contrast medium injected for the angiographic procedure, be it angiocardiography, celiac angiography, phlebography of the legs, or other types of examinations, causes good filling of the renal pelvis, usually good enough to study not-too-small details in the morphology of the kidneys. Therefore at the end of the angiographic examination or, in certain cases, during the actual examination, a single film including both kidneys can be taken and studied. In this way we have detected a considerable number of cases of anomalies of the kidneys, chronic pyelonephritis, hydronephrosis, and a few cases of renal expansivity which, at renal angiography, have been found to represent carcinoma or cyst. The additional time, cost and radiation involved in taking this single film of the kidneys is negligible in relation to the full angiographic procedure. When, during the actual angiographic procedure, the kidneys are included in the examination, at for example celiac angiography or superior mesenteric angiography, we study the resulting urogram while the catheter is still inserted. If changes are found in the kidney, at the end of the procedure the catheter is removed from, for instance, the celiac artery and introduced into the renal artery, and renal angiography is performed in the same session (for examples see OLLE OLSSON, 1973).

IV. Renal angiography

The kidney is an organ very well suited to angiography. It is a hilar organ with — usually — only one artery. This artery is fairly wide, since $\frac{1}{4}$ of the heart volume per minute passes through the kidneys. Actually the width of the renal artery is greater than that of any other artery to an organ of corresponding size. The kidney itself is a vascular sponge, the architecture of the organ being based on vasculature. Because of this great vascularity, pathologic processes in the kidney express themselves to a very great extent as vascular changes.

Angiography is thus highly suitable for the study of the anatomy and pathoanatomy of the kidney and for the study of important physiologic parameters.

Abdominal angiography with its important subdivision, renal angiography, presents an object lesson of the importance of basic knowledge for realization and full utilization of the latent possibilities of an examination method. The method, devised in 1929 by DOS SANTOS, LAMAS and CALDAS was ahead of its time. Its clinical application was heroic but premature. The results were informative and intriguing, but the risks were great. In many quarters the method fell into disgrace, and strong objections were justly raised against its use. Subsequent advances in the entire field of angiography, however, provided a much safer basis for renal angiography. Improvements in examination techniques and in the chemistry of the contrast media, more precise knowledge of the tolerance of the organism as a whole and of individual organs to contrast media, advances in normal and pathologic roentgen anatomy, and cumulative clinical experience have given renal angiography a well-established position in diagnostic radiology.

Nevertheless, the literature still reveals divergence of opinion on the value of renal angiography. Unduly enthusiastic or deprecatory opinions only too often demonstrate lack of experience in many important sections of angiography. The controversy is largely subjective and may abate with increasing knowledge and experience.

In renal angiography all the vessels of the kidney can be studied, thus not only the arteries. An examination performed to study the ateries only, should be referred to as arteriography. The veins in the kidney are, however, often of diagnostic importance.

They can be studied in the late phase of angiography or in association with cavography or by renal phlebography. The capillary phase is usually of still greater importance. Renal angiography should therefore be performed in such a way as to yield as detailed information as possible on the different phases, which should be considered together in the final interpretation of the findings. Renal angiography should always be properly planned and performed; nothing should be left to chance.

Renal angiography can be performed as aortic renal angiography, when the contrast medium is injected into the abdominal aorta, or as selective renal angiography, when the medium is injected directly into the renal artery. A method in which the contrast medium is injected mainly into the aorta through a catheter with side holes and a tip hole in a drawn-out tip which is anchored in one renal artery is called semi-selective renal angiography (BOIJSEN, 1959).

Abdominal angiography encompasses an extensive vascular region, of which the renal circulation is an important part. If renal angiography is to justify its name, selective filling of the renal arteries is highly desirable. The value of a given technique for renal angiography is thus largely dependent on the possibility of obtaining a selective filling of the renal vessels. The various techniques available will accordingly be evaluated from this point of view.

A filling of the renal arteries can be obtained by different measures such as direct (percutaneous) aortic puncture, catheterization of the aorta, or selective catheterization of a renal artery.

1. Aortic puncture

With the patient supine and with a needle 1.2 mm in outer diameter with a stylet, the lumbar aorta is punctured laterally from the left side immediately below the twelfth rib, with the needle directed ventrally, medially, and cranially in an attempt to puncture the aorta above the origin of the renal arteries. If puncture is successful, arterial blood will flow from the tip of the needle on removal of the stylet. This flow of arterial blood indicates that the tip of the needle lies free in an artery, but does not indicate with certainty that it is in the aorta. This is an important point because a dose of contrast medium adjusted with due allowance for dilution, with the relatively large volume of blood in the aorta, can be injected directly into a mesenteric or a lumbar artery, or into a renal artery, for example, if the tip of the needle happens to have pierced that artery instead of the aorta. DOS SANTOS (1937) tried to avoid injection of contrast medium directly into a renal artery by avoiding puncture of that part of the aorta from which the renal arteries usually arise. He called that section *la zone dangereuse*. In renal angiography, however, it is desirable to deposit the contrast medium as close to the renal arteries as possible. To avoid injection of contrast medium directly into an artery branching from the aorta, BAZY *et al.* (1948) modified the method: they fitted the puncture needle with a silver stylet a few centimeters longer than the needle so that they could palpate the opposite side of the vessel wall. If the stylet can be advanced more than 2 cm beyond the tip of the needle, the needle must lie free in a branch of the aorta. A needle was constructed on these principles (LINDGREN, 1953) with a movable stop-screw to prevent displacement of the needle during the injection.

2. Catheterization

Another method is catheterization with its many modifications, These fall into two groups, namely open and percutaneous catheterization. The former method was introduced by FARINAS (1946) who exposed the femoral artery, inserted a catheter up into the aorta and injected the contrast medium through the catheter. The percutaneous method was described by PEIRCE in 1953. He punctured the femoral artery with a wider needle and passed a catheter via the lumen of the needle. Needles used for this purpose must have a large bore, as the lumen of the catheter should be as wide as possible.

To avoid having to pass the catheter through a cannula and thereby to permit the introduction of a catheter of the same outer diameter or of even larger diameter than that of the needle used for puncture SELDINGER (1953) devised his excellent modification. Poisseuille's law states that when pressure and viscosity are constant, the rate of flow through narrow tubes is inversely proportional to the length of the tube and directly proportional to the 4th power of the radius of the tube. The cross section of the catheter therefore has a dominant influence on the flow of the injected contrast medium. This is utilized in the construction in the following way: a flexible guide reinforced with a central wire is introduced into the cannula with which the vessel is punctured, after which the cannula is withdrawn completely and a polyethylene catheter is threaded over the guide and fed up into the vessel.

The catheterization method permits examination of the patient in supine position. This is of importance from the point of view of selectivity. The heavy contrast medium flows along the dorsal part of the aorta, and since the renal arteries spring from the aorta more dorsally than the mesenteric artery, it is possible, with the use of a suitable injection pressure, to obtain a filling of the renal arteries without any disturbing filling of the otherwise superimposed mesenteric artery. By placing the tip of the catheter in proper relation to the origin of the renal arteries it is also possible to a certain extent to avoid a filling of the splenic artery and hepatic artery. If the tip of the catheter is not in proper position, the bulk of the contrast medium may flow into one side, e. g. if the tip of the catheter faces the orifice of a renal artery or if the contrast medium is injected against the wall of the aorta and flows along it.

A combination of translumbar and catheterization methods has been described by CUÉLLAR (1956). This method has no advantages.

The advantages of the catheterization method over aortic puncture are that the contrast medium can be deposited more correctly, the contrast dose can be kept low, the patient can be examined in the supine position, the object-film distance can accordingly be kept short, and the patient may be turned and tilted during the examination. The only advantage of direct aortic puncture over catheterization is that it usually requires less time.

Further refinement of the catheterization method to secure greater selectivity can be achieved by *selective catheterization* of either renal artery. Methods for performing selective catherization by exposure or by percutaneous puncture have been suggested. The first method of selective catheterization was devised at our department by TILLANDER (1951). He used a special catheter, the tip of which consisted of small steel links. This flexible steel tip was manipulated by a strong magnetic field so that the tip of the catheter could be passed into the renal artery under fluoroscopic control. BIERMAN et al. (1951) used a radiopaque cardiac catheter with a fixed curve at the tip. The catheter was inserted into the arterial system by exposure of a suitable artery of sufficient caliber and could be advanced into any one of the branches of the aorta.

The percutaneous method is to be preferred. ÖDMAN (1956) proposed the use of a polyethylene catheter, the tip of which can be moulded into suitable shape by immersion in hot water and by dipping into cold water immediately after. The catheter is radiopaque, which is a great advantage when feeding it into the renal artery under fluoroscopic control. It is introduced percutaneously, e. g. into the femoral artery by the SELDINGER technique.

EDHOLM and SELDINGER (1956) use an ordinary catheter which is bent by warming it cautiously above a match flame. The metal guide is introduced into the lumen of the catheter until it projects beyond its tip, and the curvature of the catheter is then straightened. The catheter is introduced into the aorta. When the guide is withdrawn, the catheter will again bend and can be manipulated into the renal artery.

GOLLMANN (1957) modified this method, using a suitably bent wire instead of the reinforcing, straight wire. Another modification by the same author was giving the wire a flexible tip to permit passage of the wire also through tortuous arteries (GOLLMANN, 1958).

The catheter for renal angiography should be thin and thin-walled. During the procedure the catheter should be rinsed well with physiologic saline in order to prevent clotting.

In puncturing the artery the anterior arterial wall can easily be felt with the needle. The tip of the needle should then rapidly penetrate this anterior wall and, if possible, not touch the posterior wall. Techniques recommended to pierce both the anterior and posterior walls and then withdraw the catheter until blood comes out, are not advisable. The risk of hematoma is greater with such a procedure. The introduction of the catheter should be done with great care and the catheter should not be forced up the iliac artery of the aorta. Difficulties may arise if the arteries are very tortuous and if great atherosclerotic plaques are present.

We have a motto in all of our angiographic procedures: "Never force but never give up."

If conditions in the iliac artery on one side do not permit introduction of the catheter, the other side may be used. In exceptional cases the catheter can be introduced from above after puncture of the brachial artery.

When the catheter has been introduced into the renal artery, the return flow through the catheter is checked to make sure that the tip is free in the artery and that the catheter does not occlude the vessel. We therefore seldom use catheters with side-holes for selective studies but use instead those with a hole at the tip. The tip of catheters with side holes is likely to be introduced too far into the vessel, whereas if a catheter with a hole only at the tip is introduced too far into the artery, no return flow will occur. If the return flow stops, the catheter is immediately withdrawn into the aorta. In addition, care should be taken that the catheter is introduced only a short distance into the mouth of the renal artery. This is important because in 7 % of our material the dorsal branch of the renal artery has an early departure. If, in such a case. the catheter is fed past the origin of a dorsal branch departing early, it will enter directly into the ventral artery and give a filling only of the region supplied by this branch, which in addition receives the entire dose of contrast medium that is diluted only slightly by the blood. The catheter may also be pushed directly into the dorsal branch.

Technical problems, catheter devices, fluid dynamics, and other aspects have been studied widely. Reference is made to monographs by OLIN (1963), LUDIN (1966) and ALMÉN (1966).

Instruments of different kinds have been proposed for the catheterization procedure. In my opinion, the safest method of performing angiography is the manual method because thereby the examiner continuously feels with his fingers any obstacles met by the tip of the catheter. For renal angiography instruments are therefore not recommended.

The catheter should be properly curved according to the course of the renal artery. The artery constantly arises from the aorta at the level of the first lumbar vertebra. If at plain roentgenography it has been shown that the kidney is low, it may be concluded that the renal artery springs at an acute angle from the aorta. The catheter should then be bent accordingly. Secondly, the catheter should be formed so as not to be fed too far into the renal artery because in that case only the ventral branch or the dorsal branch may be catheterized. When studying the films it is important to note where the contrast medium has been deposited.

If a kidney is supplied by more than one renal artery, selective angiography of each of the arteries should be performed, with due precaution not to block the flow in a thin, supplementary artery. Finding of, or suspicion of, multiple arterial supply may also make necessary continuation of the study with the aortic, non-selective technique. In such a case the guidewire is again introduced into the catheter for this selective study, the catheter is withdrawn, and on the guidewire a catheter for a non-selective study is introduced.

To avoid misinterpretation, the examiner must be familiar with the normal anatomy and check that all intrarenal arteries are filled and that all parts of the kidney show an accumulation of contrast medium in the nephrographic phase. Reproductions of angiograms in the literature reveal that this source of error has occasionally escaped attention. The selective technique should therefore not be used alone in most cases where there is reason to suspect multiple arteries, such as in double kidney, fused kidney, dystopia, or hydronephrosis.

The catheterization should be performed with fluoroscopy, using image intensifier and television. This technique is valuable particularly in angiographic work since the illumination of the examination room facilitates maintainance of sterility. The observation capacity of the examiner is also greatly enhanced. Test injections can easily be checked fluoroscopically, but occasionally it is advisable to freeze the test injection on a video tape recorder or on film.

Difficulties in finding the renal artery for selective catheterization are overcome with training. It may be necessary occasionally to withdraw the catheter and change its bending. A special method has been designed (DREVVATNE, 1969) to facilitate catheterization: an arotic injection is made, the stage with filling of the aorta and the renal arteries is frozen on a disc recorder and reversed. This reversed picture is shown to the examiner on his TV screen. With this picture on his monitor during fluoroscopy, he can perform the catheterization using the picture as a map and thus easily find the origin of the renal artery.

In non-selective renal angiography the dose of contrast medium should usually be 25—40 ml and the injection pressure approximately 6 kg per cm^2. At selective technique the dose can be kept very low, from 3—8 cc, and injection pressure at 2—2$\frac{1}{2}$ kg per cm^2. Several injections can be made in order to secure the correct timing, filling, and projection.

Some authors believe stereo-roentgenography to be useful. The procedure usually requires two injections, which is not advisable with contrast media of the di-iodine type but may be performed with the best tri-iodine contrast media. It is preferable in such cases, however, to use simultaneous stereography according to FERNSTRÖM and LINDBLOM (1955). We do not use stereography as we consider it unnecessary if the examiner is familiar with the normal anatomy of the renal arteries (see below). Instead, selective angiography with its low contrast dose for each injection can be used and suitable projections chosen to completely elucidate the problem at hand. One important projection is the true lateral projection of the kidney, as proposed by HEGEDÜS (1971).

At the end of the examination the catheter is withdrawn and pressure is applied to the puncture site to avoid formation of a hematoma. This pressure should be moderate and prolonged and the patient must be carefully observed.

3. Comparison between selective and aortic renal angiography

Of the methods available for renal angiography, the examiner may choose between the aortic and the selective methods. For some cases in which it is desirable to examine the aorta and both of the renal arteries, such as in atherosclerosis, or other types of renal artery stenosis, or if both renal arteries are to be compared, such as for assessment of potential renal function, the aortic method is to be preferred. This also holds for some patients with multiple renal arteries. Otherwise the selective method is the method of choice. This method has the following disadvantages, however: risk of blood clot formation may be incurred, although rarely; there is the theoretical possibility of infarction of some vessel region if it should be obstructed by the passing of the catheter too far without being observed; it requires more time than the other method; it may be necessary to supplement

5*

the examination or repeat it, using the aortic method if multiple arteries are found or suspected.

The selective technique fits in directly with basic roentgen-diagnostic principles: it makes possible avoidance of superimposition; it gives free choice of correct projections; it allows low doses of contrast medium, repeated injections, and correct timing.

We have had wide experience with both aortic and selective renal angiography. The selective technique, in our opinion, is far superior to the aortic but for the exceptions described above. This opinion is strengthened particularly in those cases in which the information needed would make the selective method the method of choice, but in which for some reason the method could not be used, also in those cases examined first by the aortic method and later by the selective. *In renal angiography, then, as in all types of angiography, the technique should be as selective as possible.*

4. Angiography of operatively exposed kidney

A special type of examination is angiography of the surgically exposed kidney, described by ALKEN (1950). The contrast medium is injected directly into the renal artery or one of its branches at operation. GRAVES (1956) described a special injection needle for this purpose. Films are taken of the exposed kidney (for technique see page 17) and provide a good basis for detailed study of parenchymal changes. It is believed to be of value when explorative surgery, for example, reveals changes possibly indicating partial nephrectomy.

5. Injection of contrast medium

In aortic angiography the contrast medium may be injected by hand. If a catheter is used, greater pressure is required and a mechanical injector should be used, The injector described by DOS SANTOS is unsuitable because gas is then in direct contact with the contrast fluid. Modifications eliminating this risk have been described by CHRISTOPHE and HONORÉ (1947) and LINDGREN (1953). More elaborate injectors have been devised for angiography. They are designed for more complicated angiographic procedures than renal angiography.

It should be pointed out that renal angiography can be performed very simply by manual injection and manual cassette changing. Refinement of technique is necessary, however, in a heavy program of angiographic procedures, and should be applicable also to renal angiography.

Timing of the exposures is important. Well-timed exposures are easily obtained by taking films in rapid succession. The timing problem can be solved in a simple way by a method devised by OLIN (1958) with E. C. G. control. It consists of a simple device plugged into the circuit: film changer — electrocardiograph — electric pressure syringe — roentgen apparatus with program selector. Signals from the electrocardiograph pass through a transistorized amplifier to a relay, which releases the program. It is apparent that this requires an apparatus permitting exposures in relatively rapid succession. Various types of such an apparatus with program selector are available. When the film changer is started, injection from the pressure syringe is started in association with the next QRS-complex. The flow in the arteries varies rhythmically with the heart beat; the rate of flow is highest in systole and drops rapidly immediately afterwards. Thus, to obtain the best possible filling of the arterial branches of the kidney with the smallest possible amount of contrast medium, the latter should be injected in the beginning of diastole when the blood flow to the kidney is lowest.

Many authors state the examination should be carried out under general anaesthesia. Apnea can be readily secured under anaesthesia, but it can also be achieved without anaesthesia by good co-operation with the patient. We therefore find general anaesthesia unnecessary, like WEYDE (1952) and MALUF and McCOY (1955). A method using reduction of the blood pressure to secure the important nephrographic phase based on WICKBOM's observations referred to above has been described by LINDGREN (1953). With good timing of the pictures it is not necessary to use this method, which may imply a risk by prolonging the time the vessels are exposed to the contrast medium.

6. Contrast media

For many years the use of renal angiography was severely limited by the toxicity of the contrast media. The method therefore fell into disgrace. The contrast media used were halogen salts, particularly sodium iodide.

More complex water-soluble contrast media superseded the iodides; this implied a considerable advance. Though di-iodine contrast media are going out of use in angiography, they are still used to such an extent as to require a brief comment. Renal angiography is often performed without the examiner's having any opinion of the tolerance of the kidney to the contrast media, and many authors go so far as to say that the method involves no risks at all. Perusal of the literature will reveal, however, that the use of contrast media of the di-iodine type has been followed by severe renal injury, occasionally with a fatal issue (OLLE OLSSON, 1955). Further cases have been described (LANDELIUS, 1955; BERG, 1956; EDLING and HELANDER, 1957, altogether 320 cases with 5 serious reactions). A collection has been published by McAFEE (1957) based on a survey of 13,207 abdominal aortograms of all kinds with only 375 by the catheterization method, with an overall complication rate of 1.02 % and a mortality rate of 0.28%. In 1,732 cases more than 40 cc of contrast medium had been injected.

In a systematic investigation of the NPN, albuminuria, cylindruria and size of kidney after renal angiography with di-iodine contrast medium injected directly into the aorta in a 60 per cent solution, IDBOHRN (1956) found signs of slight renal injury in 11 cases out of 39, and in 2 out of 15 in which a 50% solution had been used under otherwise identical conditions. In an experimental investigation IDBOHRN and BERG (1954) using a refined technique well adapted for investigation of the tolerance of the kidneys to contrast media found that injury can occur at concentrations of di-iodine contrast media above a critical level lying somewhere between 10 % and 17.5 % concentration in the actual renal artery. The tolerance appears to vary from one individual to another. By studies on renal function and experimental renal angiography on dogs WIDÉN (1958) verified the patho-anatomic findings of IDBOHRN and Berg.

The tri-iodine contrast media have been studied in the same way (BERG, IDBOHRN and WENDEBERG, 1958). It was shown that Urografin and Hypaque produce no histologically demonstrable renal damage. Triurol, however, in a concentration of 25% and more, usually caused histologic changes. Miokon in 50 % concentration was also followed by renal injury. Control experiments with Umbradil in 17.5 % concentration produced toxic changes in half of the animals studied (see Fig. 37). It should be observed that these concentrations refer to the actual concentration in the renal artery, which can be assessed if the experimental design is suitable. In an investigation by IDBOHRN and NORGREN it was shown that renal blood flow was not affected by the best tri-iodine media (see OLLE OLSSON, 1961).

In an investigation by EDLING et al. (1958) with 60 per cent Urografin and 50 per cent Miokon in large doses injected through a catheter inserted in the aorta of dogs, no renal injury was demonstrable despite the use of very large doses. It should be remembered that contrast medium injected in this way is diluted with aortic blood and does not correspond to the actual concentration in the renal arteries. One can, however, agree with the authors when they conclude that properly performed aortographies, preferably by transfemoral catheterization, will not damage healthy kidneys, although it should perhaps be added: with the use of the best tri-iodine contrast media. It is thus obvious that certain tri-iodine contrast media are the best media hitherto available for renal angiography and that there is no reason to use the di-iodine media. The last-mentioned authors also performed an investigation on dogs with selective renal angiography using di-iodine media as well as one of the less good tri-iodine media. This contrast medium produced renal damage when used in a large dose, while a small dose produced no change. This implies that the risks of renal damage are small, but may be somewhat greater in selective angiography than in aortic angiography.

There are many contributions to the study of the effects of contrast media on the organism. In a paper from 1962 (LASSER et al.) it is concluded that the contrast media bind with albumen and that for the three iodobenzoic acid compounds the presence or absence of a prosthetic group at the 5-position appears to determine the relative weakness or strength of binding with albumen. There is a relation between this binding and the crenation effect of red blood cells. Evidence was also found that local and systemic toxicity

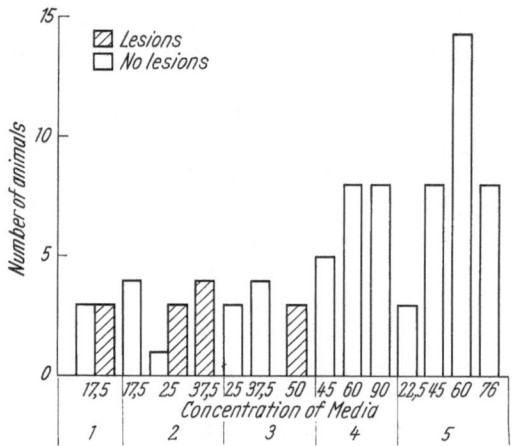

Fig. 37. Diagram. 1. Umbradil, 2. Triurol, 3. Miokon, 4. Hypaque, 5. Urografin. (Modified after BERG, IDBOHRN & WENDEBERG)

from contrast material is mediated by derangements of the blood elements and blood vessels also in relation to contrast binding albumen. In another study from 1962 LASSER et al. found in experiments on dogs that injection of the basic non-halogenated molecule of the contrast medium constructed with prosthetic groups in odd positions of the benzene ring appears to be without visible histologic effects. James et al. (1965) found, also in experiments on dogs, indications that histologic changes were correlated with stasis and that the absence of stasis was associated with irregular occurrence of morphologic changes. In experiments on dogs LÉLEK (1965) found that selective catheterization of the renal artery could lead to a reduction in renal function only if the procedure was carried out traumatically.

With finer methodology of registering damage to the renal parenchyma we can expect registration of very slight, rapidly disappearing effects on certain renal functions caused by the catheterization procedure and the injection of the contrast medium, which is indicated by clinical experiments performed by KAUDE and NORDENDFELT (1971).

Using a very sensitive kinetostatic method, the Colcemid method, EVENSEN and SKALPE (1971) with sodium metrizoate (Isopaque 260) found that smaller doses corresponding to approximately 50 ml injected twice into the renal artery of a patient weighing 70 kg would kill between 3—4 % of the tubular cells and a dose of 100 ml would kill 9 % of the cells. Regeneration is rapid. The authors conclude that the amount of sodium metrizoate used in clinical selective renal angiography represents no risk to kidneys with normal blood supply.

Dose of contrast medium. For aortic renal angiography we use 25—30 ml of Urografin; for selective angiography with injection directly into a renal artery, 5 ml. For lean patients we use 60% solution, for obese patients, 76%.

We keep the exposure time as short as possible with a voltage of approximately 100 kV. We take films in series related to the diagnostic problems to be solved.

7. Risks

On direct puncture, some or all of the contrast medium may be deposited extra-vascularly. As a rule, this will produce slight discomfort, at the most. Pleural effusion may occur on the injected side, however. Pneumothorax may also develop due to puncture of the pleural cavity if the lung extends far down, such as in emphysema.

Contrast medium may also be accidentally deposited subintimally in the aorta as in the carotid artery in carotid angiography, for example (IDBOHRN, 1951), i. e. a fairly well defined accumulation of contrast medium will be seen which does not mix with the blood (GAYLIS and LAWS, 1956; BOBLITT et al., 1959). The amount of contrast medium deposited subintimally may be small or large. If the amount thus deposited is small, complications will not occur. If the amount is large, symptoms of the type seen in dissecting aneurysms may occur with a fatal issue.

Haemorrhage may occur at the site of puncture on catheterization, as well as on direct puncture. Such haemorrhage in association with aortography is usually very slight. It is also slight if the femoral artery is punctured. Care should be taken, however, to puncture the artery well below the inguinal ligament, so that any subsequent haematoma may be readily discovered. If the artery is punctured higher up, haematoma may develop retro-peritoneally and remain concealed for a considerable time.

A case report is given by ANTONI and LINDGREN (1949) of an aged, arteriosclerotic man in whom abdominal aortography (prone position, pillow under upper part of abdomen, percutaneous puncture) was followed by a flaccid paraplegia. Without discussing the contrast medium used they believe the lesion to have been caused by the compression of the aorta, thus constituting in reality a Steno's experiment in man.

If the contrast medium intended to be injected into the aorta is injected directly into the renal artery, the concentration may exceed the tolerance of the renal parenchyma, with renal damage as a consequence. This may also occur if the flow in the distal part of the aorta is obstructed (BARNES et al., 1959). Upon accidental injection into a lumbar artery, the contrast medium may damage the spinal cord (ABESHOUSE and TIONGSON, 1956; McCORMACK, 1956; BAURYS, 1956; CONGER et al., 1957; HARE, 1957). The tolerance of the spinal cord to contrast medium has been studied by HOL and SKJERVEN (1954). They claim that examination of animals in supine position favors damage to the spine because the contrast medium is heavy and will therefore flow dorsally. TARAZI et al. (1956) state that the large volume of contrast media injected through a site near a major radicular artery and the use of the supine position have increased the frequency and extent of damage to the spinal cord. With the use of the catheterization technique with a small amount of a suitable contrast medium, this risk is very small indeed.

A case of a marked lesion of the renal artery in connection with selective angiography is described by GILL et al. (1972). The authors report a production of marked stenosis of the renal artery and subsequent diastolic hypertension. A corresponding complication with a stenosis in one of multiple renal arteries causing hypertensive disease has been reported by BERGENTZ and HEGEDÜS (1971). In this case the kidney was removed, reparational surgery was performed and the kidney was again introduced, with excellent results.

Sometimes spasm is seen (Fig. 38). The pathologic nephrogram due to spasm produced by traumatization of the arterial wall by the catheter, by occlusion of the vessel by the catheter, and by too large a dose of contrast medium has been described by EDSMAN (1957) and studied experimentally by EDLING and HELANDER (1959). One or more intrarenal branches show no contrast filling and ischemia occurs peripherally in a circumscribed region or around the whole kidney. This gives the nephrogram a characteristic appearance with irregular parts of increased density intermingled with mostly cortical, irregular filling defects.

Spasm may also occur in a kidney with multiple arteries if the entire dose of contrast medium is injected into a thin supplementary artery which is occluded by the catheter. LODIN and THORÉN (1955) suggested that the examination might be performed under

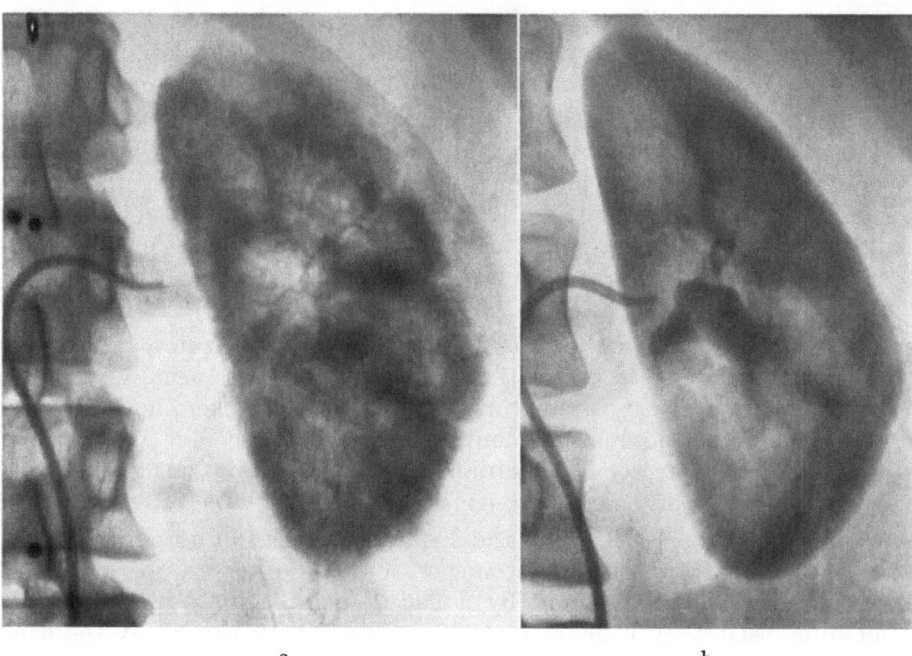

a   b

Fig. 38. Spasm at renal angiography: a) during actual spasm, b) after spasm has subsided (nephrographic phase)

ganglionic block to counteract the risk of spasm. Under anaesthesia the vessels are occasionally wider than otherwise. In my opinion, neither ganglionic block nor anaesthesia is necessary. Spasm is best avoided by using a small dose of a good contrast medium and proper catheterization technique.

AMPLATZ in 1968 drew attention to the possibility of catheter embolisation from clots formed on the outside of cardiac catheters. A thorough study of this phenomenon was made by JACOBSON (1969). Among other things, he found that oscillography before and after arterial catheterization for angiography enabled the early detection of the site of asymptomatic thrombo-emboli and that the frequency of thrombo-embolism varied with the total area of the outer wall of the inserted part of the catheter. When a long catheter was kept in the blood stream, a generalized platelet reaction occurred consisting of an increase in platelet adhesiveness. Fortunately these results have application to renal angiography only to a limited extent. Great care should nevertheless be taken to avoid thrombo-embolism locally by exact technique, short examination time and continuous rinsing of the catheter.

Thrombogenicity of vascular catheters can be markedly minimized by heparinization of the catheters (JACOBSSON and SCHLOSSMAN, 1972).

Attention is here drawn to a paper by STEIN and HILLGARTNER (1968) on alteration of coagulation mechanism of blood by contrast media. The authors found transient depression of levels of variable blood coagulation factors in more than half of the patients examined with angiographic procedures and they consider it conceivable that binding or inactivation of the coagulation factors alpha and beta globulins is the cause of the depressed assays found in both in vivo and in vitro studies.

We have performed studies of the puncture site in a number of patients in whom catheterization was performed from the other femoral artery on an earlier occasion (WINTZELL, 1969) and we found no marked changes.

In 1968 FOLIN of our department made a review of complications of percutaneous femoral catheterization in renal angiography wherein 1,818 renal angiographies with catheterization of the femoral artery in 1,319 adults were studied. The complications were as follows:

Table 2. *Complications*

Renal angiography 1817 $\Big\langle$ 711 LA
1106 Sel. a.

1. Hematoma at puncture site of considerable size (1 operation necessary)	5
2. More than 1° rise in temperature	6
3. Intimalesion	5
4. Thrombosis in femoral vein	2
5. Embolia pulm.	1
6. Perforation of artery wall	1
7. Broken guide wire	2
8. Coagulum in renal artery	1
9. Thrombosis in femoral artery	1

It is seen from the figures in the table that there is a certain risk. This risk is fairly small but indicates the need for a technique which is as exact as possible and for correct indications for the examination.

It may be well to stress here that certain authors claim that renal angiography is of little or no value in the investigation of urologic problems and should therefore not be performed (NESBITT, 1955); CONGER *et al.*, 1957). Such a view represents an unproductive, conservative attitude and is not acceptable, but is undoubtedly a healthy counter-weight to the postulation by many uncritical authors that renal angiography is a perfectly safe procedure regardless of how it is performed. From reports and illustrations on record, it is apparent that the technique employed often leaves much to be desired. In my opinion, renal angiography is an indispensable diagnostic method when performed properly and upon good indications. The entire examination must therefore be performed by a trained roentgenologist.

8. Anatomy and roentgen anatomy

a) Arteries

The two renal arteries arise from the aorta in the sectional mid-plane and usually at the same level, *i. e.* at the lower third of the first lumbar vertebra or at the disk between the first and second lumbar vertebrae (Fig. 39). The superior mesenteric artery arises somewhat cranial thereto and from a more ventral aspect. The origin of the right renal artery is, as a rule, somewhat more cranial than that of the left. The right renal artery most frequently runs a horizontal or descending course; the left, a horizontal or ascending course. The renal artery always enters the upper part of the hilum cranial to the renal pelvis and here the artery has its center of divergence. In 68 % of all cases the artery divides after it has entered the hilum (HOU-JENSEN, 1929). It may, however, divide earlier and in 20—40 % two renal arteries occur on either side (POIRIER and CHARPY, 1923). The renal artery is of end-artery type down to the interlobar branches, so that each

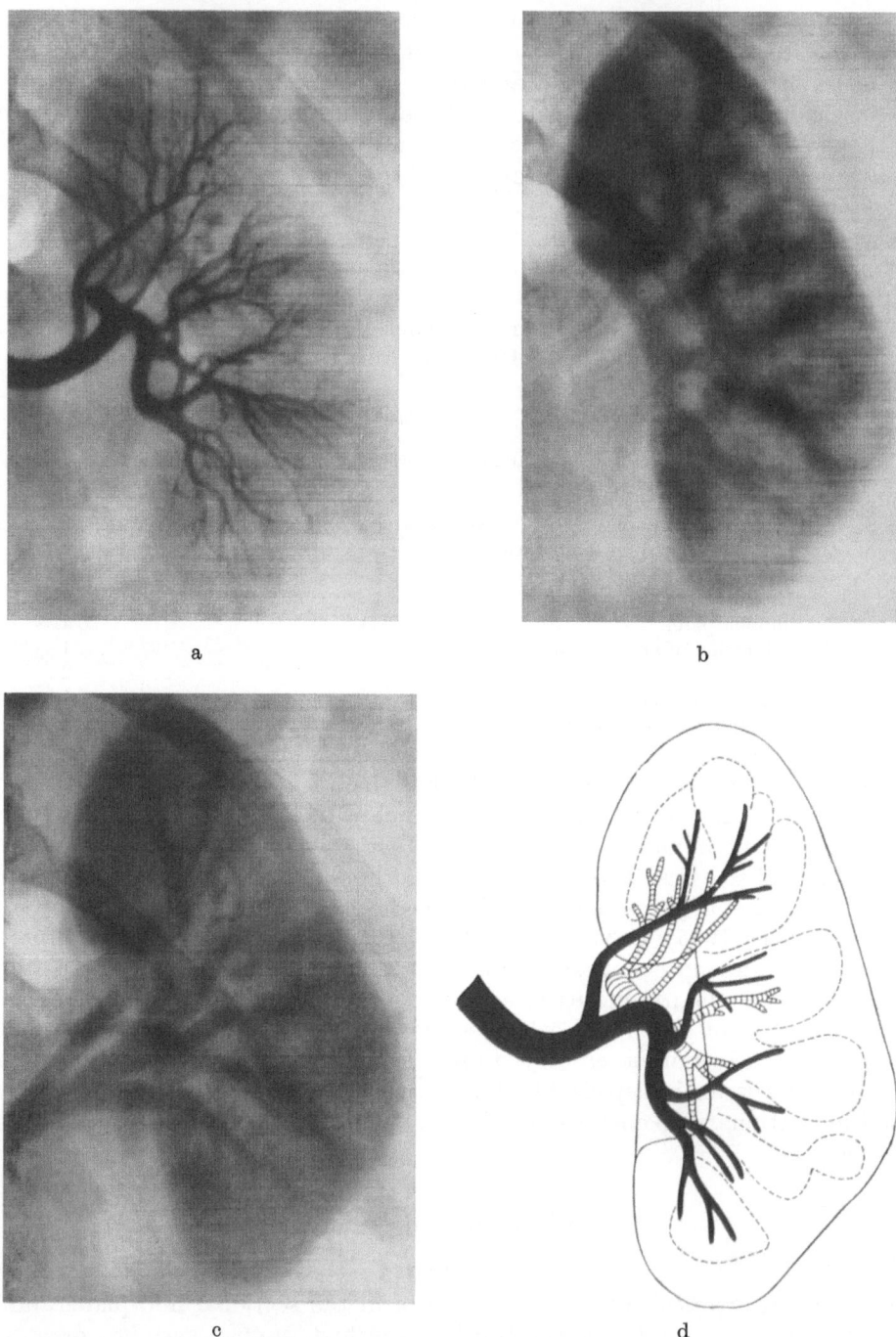

Fig. 39. Renal angiogram and renal artery skiagram: a)—d) frontal view, e)—g) oblique view (ventral arterial
branch shown in black, dorsal branch, hatched)

branch has its own field of supply and does not anastomose with the other territories at
that level. The kidney has an anterior territory and a posterior territory divided by an
intermediate region fairly poor in vessels somewhat posterior to the longitudinal plane
of the kidney. There is a segmental arrangement of the intrarenal arteries, which is said
to be constant. The region of supply of the renal artery has been described as being divided into 5 segments, apical, upper, middle, lower, posterior, each of which is supplied

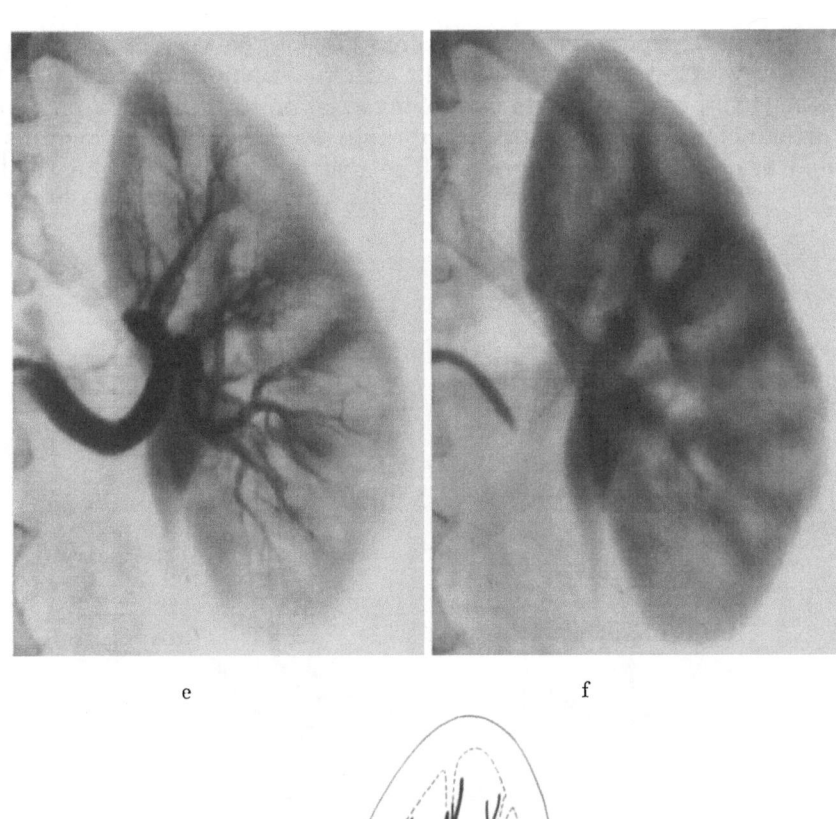

e   f

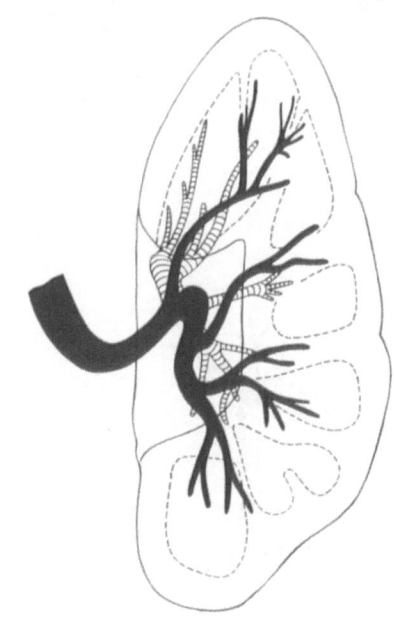

g

by its own artery without collateral circulation (GRAVES, 1954). The artery to the apical segment had the most varying origin. Some kidneys have, as normal variants, branches running directly to the upper and the lower pole (almost 20 % and 1 % respectively (HELLSTRÖM, 1928, BERGENDAL, 1936). It should be observed that the arborization does not coincide with the lobation of the kidney (SMITHUIS, 1956). It may be very irregular, one branch, for example, dividing within the hilum and running to both poles (CHIAUDANO, 1955). (See chapter on anomalies).

Selective angiography will give a clear impression of the anatomy of the vessels, knowledge of which is necessary for proper interpretation of the films. Knowledge of the course of the vessels is likewise of importance prior to any operation on the kidney, particularly if resection is contemplated. The anatomy of the vessels and their segmental distribution should therefore be founded on the angiographic findings. From this starting point BOIJSEN (1959) made an exhaustive investigation of the anatomy of the renal artery and its branches. The segmental distribution was studied in angiograms of autopsy specimens and in our clinical angiograms. The distribution is based on the localization

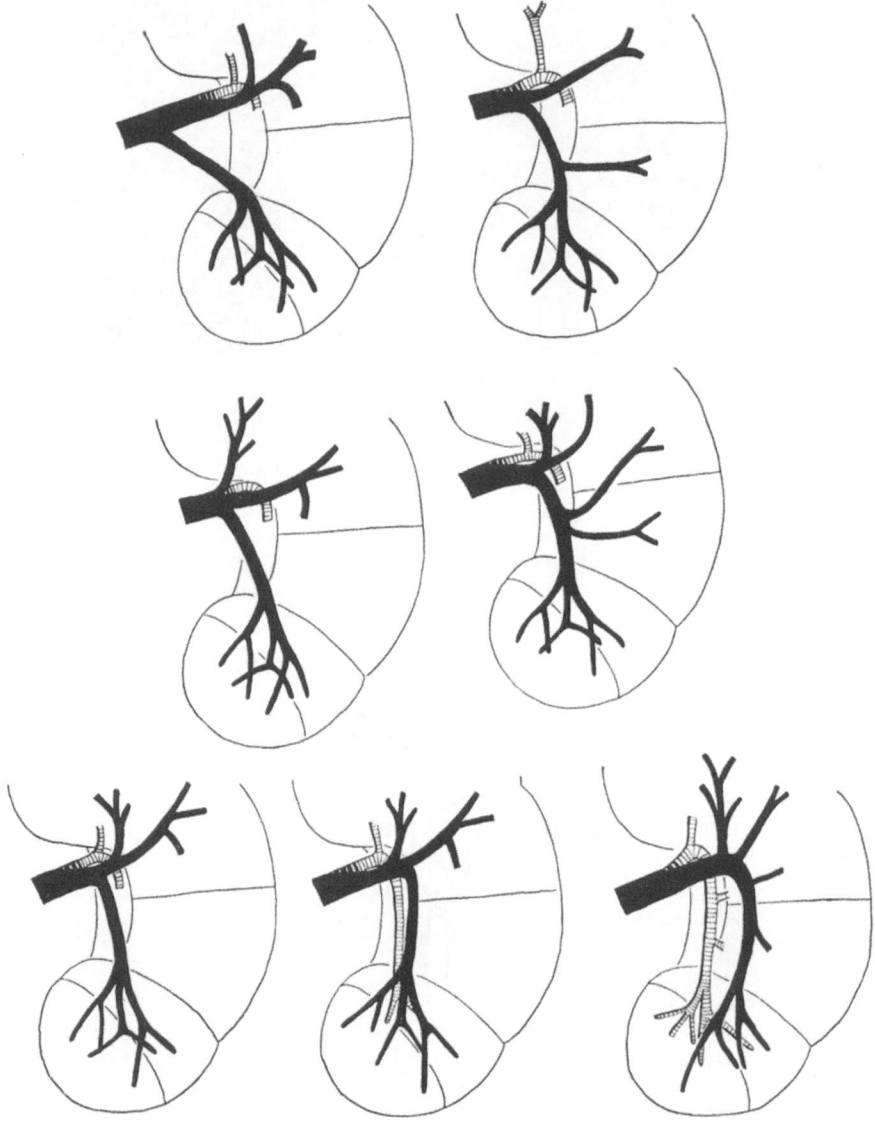

Fig. 40. Diagram of left caudal renal pole showing common variations of arterial supply

of seven pairs of pyramids described by LÖFGREN (1949). In principle, there is a ventral field and a dorsal field supplied by arteries arising from the renal artery. These arteries run ventrally and dorsally, respectively, to the renal pelvis and always supply the inter-mediate parts of the kidney, namely the fourth and fifth ventral and dorsal pyramids respectively. They often extend cranially and caudally so far as to include all the ventral and dorsal pyramids. More commonly, however, the ventral arteries supply not only the ventral area of the intermediate part, but also the ventral and dorsal pyramids in the inferior part and the dorsal artery, the two uppermost pairs of pyramids in the superior part and the dorsal intermediate part.

Owing to the tilted position of the kidney and the characteristic appearance of the dorsal and ventral branches of the renal artery, a single projection is often sufficient to chart the course and field of supply of these branches. Sometimes oblique views are helpful (Figs. 39, 42). As a rule, the dorsal branch gives the impression of being the first branch from the renal artery, in most cases it is much narrower than the ventral branch, and, owing to the position of the kidney, it runs more medially than the ventral branch and its field of supply is also situated more medially. Separate arteries from the renal artery sometimes run to the two poles before division into dorsal and ventral branches, though, as a rule, the poles are supplied by the ventral and dorsal branch respectively.

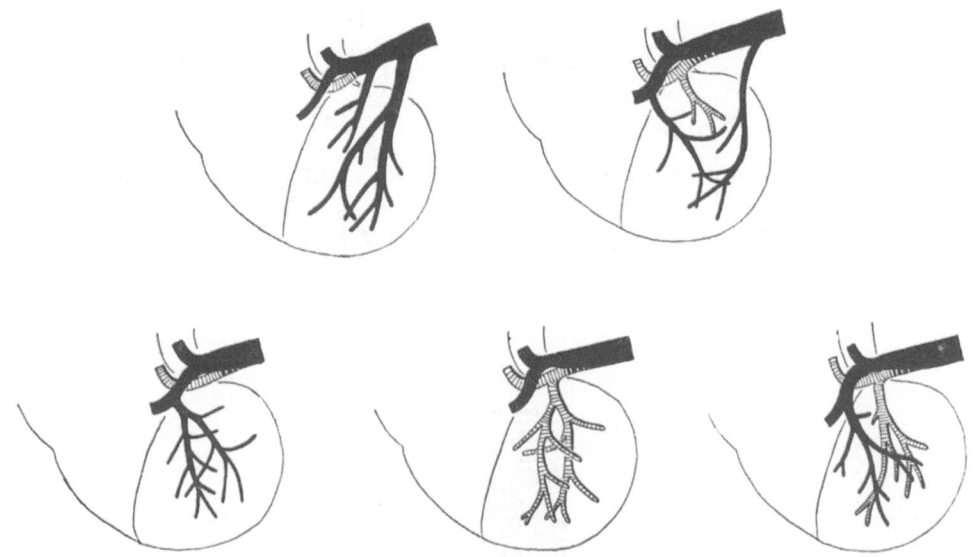

Fig. 41. Diagram showing common variations in origin, course, and field of supply of arterial branches to caudal pole (after BOIJSEN)

The nutrition of the first two pairs of pyramids varies widely; they are often supplied by several arteries (Fig. 40). The supply to the pars inferior, on the other hand, is more regular, usually with only one artery running to the lower pole (Fig. 41). In 30 % of the cases in our material the dorsal branch supplied the dorsal pyramids; the ventral branch, only the ventral pyramids in the lower pole. In 60 % of the cases the entire inferior part was supplied by a lower polar artery arising from the renal artery or its ventral branch (Fig. 42). In these cases the vessels to the lower pole can be ligated in the hilum so that an almost horizontal incision can be made through the lower part of the kidney on resection of the lower renal pole.

The renal arteries are end-arteries, so that examination by the selective technique will be incomplete if the kidney is supplied by more than one renal artery. Of our series of "normal" kidneys, we found supplementary arteries in 20 %. We did not find the number of renal arteries to vary with the normal variation in the shape of the renal pelvis. On the other hand, we did find that double kidneys and kidneys with hydronephrosis due to obstruction of the pelviureteric junction were supplied by multiple arteries in 50 % of the cases. Almost all kidneys with a congenital malformation had multiple renal arteries. Multiple arteries will be discussed in association with anomalies and hydronephrosis.

The problems of the arterial supply and the nutritional areas of the different arterial branches has been the object of further studies by Hegedüs (1971) of our department. Hegedüs made the following findings on the basis of a three-dimensional concept of the kidney arrived at at roentgenologic examination through the use of a true lateral projection together with a frontal projection:

In more than 50 % of cases the renal arteries and their primary branches run a sometimes markedly tortuous course around the kidney pelvis. Two primary branches were

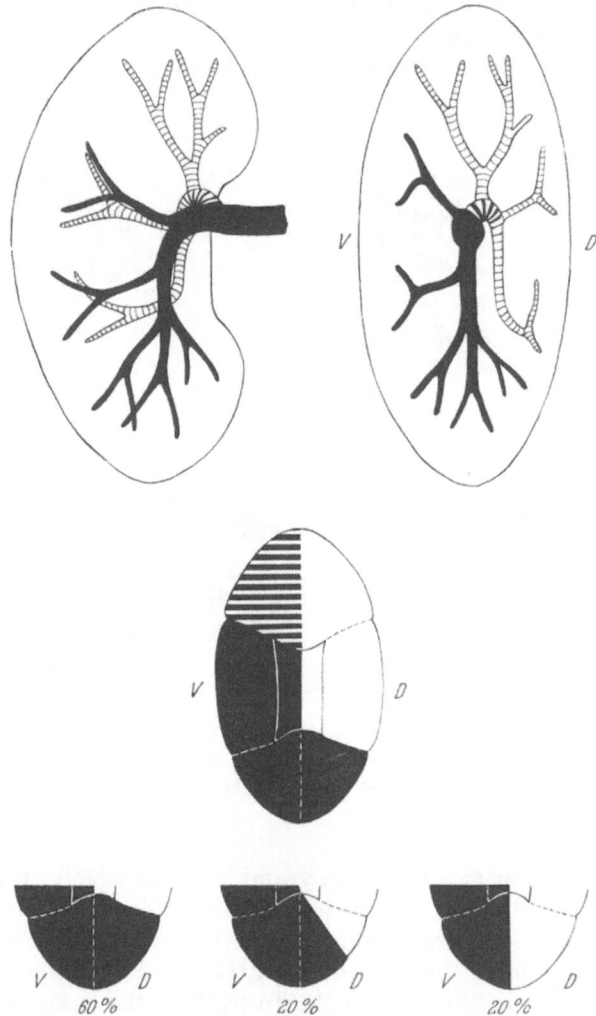

Fig. 42. Schematic illustration of segmental distribution of ventral and dorsal branch of renal artery

found in approximately 70 % of the kidneys examined, three primary branches in 20 %, and four primary branches in 10 %. In less than 50 % of the cases the plane dividing the nutritive zones between the ventral and dorsal arteries was mainly longitudinal, indicating a ventral-dorsal division of supply. In more than 50 % of the cases, however, the plane dividing the nutritive zones was mainly transversely oriented, indicating a cranio-caudal division of the zones of supply, whereas in a small percentage of cases the division was of a mixed type.

Hegedüs found, further, that in kidneys supplied by multiple arteries the following groups could be differentiated:

Group I — the two arteries behaved like two primary branches.

Group II — the larger of the arteries behaved like a main renal artery with primary branches, while the smaller artery replaced a secondary branch.

Group III — the larger of the arteries represented a main artery with all the primary and secondary branches, whereas the smaller renal artery was a tertiary branch dividing into a few interlobar arteries. In a small group the larger arteries supplied the whole kidney, with the exception of the supply from one small interlobar artery, which had a separate aortic origin.

The caliber of the artery is of importance from certain diagnostic points of view. It is described in the anatomic literature as being 6 mm wide. We have found a considerable range of variation of the caliber of the renal artery in normals and a general tendency of

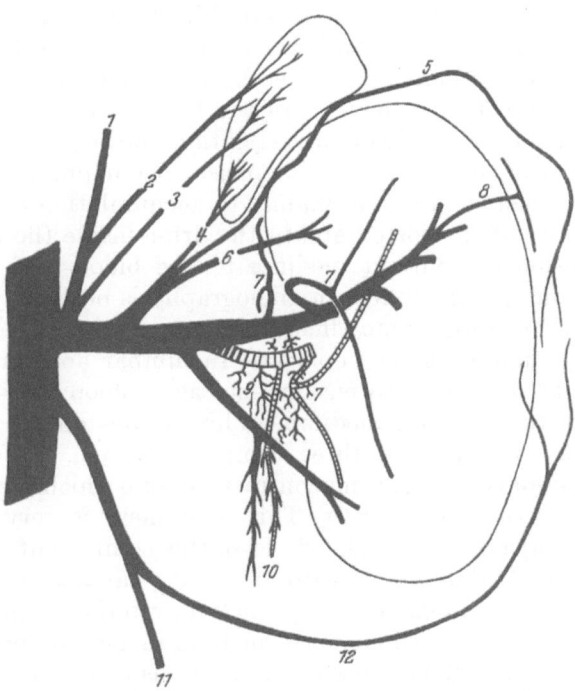

Fig. 43. Diagram of arteries arising from renal artery or its intrarenal branches and supplying extrarenal parts. 1. Inferior phrenic artery. 2—4. Arteries to adrenal. 5. Superior capsular artery. 6. R. sup. pyr. IV. 7—8. Middle capsular arteries: recurrent (7) and perforating (8) arteries. 9. Pelvic arteries. 10. Ureteric arteries (ventral and dorsal). 11. Internal spermatic artery. 12. Inferior capsular artery, which together with the superior capsular artery forms "l' arcade exorénale" (SCHMERBER). Occasionally, although rarely, the inferior capsular artery departs from the renal artery. (After BOIJSEN)

the caliber to decrease with increasing age. In a clinical material EDSMAN (1957) found the renal artery, as measured on angiograms, to range between 6.1 and 9.7 mm in the majority of cases in males, the corresponding figures for women being 4.6—8.2 mm. There was no difference in the luminal diameter of the single renal artery on the right side and on the left side in his material.

The capsular arteries, arteria capsularis superior and arteria capsularis media and inferior, will often be filled in selective angiography (Fig. 43). They stand out distinctly because of the relatively slow rate of flow and they appear filled with contrast medium longer than the renal artery. These arteries can be displaced by tumors. They may also contribute to the supply of renal carcinoma and occasionally be the main supply, and are of interest as collaterals in blockage of the main renal artery.

Renal pelvic arteries can also be observed. They are so narrow, however, that they can as a rule scarcely be discerned except in pathologic processes in the renal pelvis, e. g. pyelonephritis. This is also the case with the ureteric arteries (Boijsen, 1959).

Magnification radiography should be mentioned in this connection. With the use of tubes of very fine focus, it is possible to obtain renal angiograms with a definition making it possible to observe glomeruli closely.

Mention should be made here of photographic and electronic substraction methods and methods for direct and indirect color fluorography and radiography.

b) Nephrographic phase

It has been suggested that the nephrographic phase be called instead the capillary phase. This is not a correct designation, however, because the phase represents not only the contrast medium in the capillaries but also that in the excretory system of the kidney. This has been investigated by Edling and Helander (1959) in well designed experiments in which Thorotrast which cannot be excreted by the kidney was injected into one renal artery, and water soluble contrast medium of the type excreted by the kidney was injected into the other renal artery. Their investigation showed that the capillary filling is only a minor component of the nephrographic phase. The nephrographic effect is initially due to a very slight vascular phase, and mainly to accumulation of the contrast medium in the tubular epithelium of the cortex and in the urine inside the tubuli. If excretion is obstructed, back-diffusion of contrast medium to the blood may occur. Bolin (1966) points out that the nephrographic effect in angiography is not always distinguished from that in urography. The nephrographic effect in urography is due to an accumulation of contrast medium in the lumina of the nephrons. In lumbar aortography with low blood pressure (Lindgren, 1953) the hypotension decreases blood flow and thus decreases admixture of blood to the contrast medium. In his studies on the nephrographic phase Bolin finds this to be comprised of three components: one, the cortical vascular bed together with the intra-renal veins contains contrast medium which leaves the kidney at a rate corresponding to that of the cortical flow. This component is very small and short and specifically short if the injection time is short. Two, this component represents the volume of contrast medium in the tubular cells with an uptake capacity of approximately 8 ml. The washout of half of this tubular contrast medium requires approximately 6 seconds. Three, this component is the filtered contrast medium in the lumina of the nephrons and the small amount in the medullary vessels. On the basis of these and other data, Bolin has presented a method for measuring the contrast medium in the kidney during angiography by densitometry. With certain modifications of ordinary selective angiography but without sacrificing any of the information usually obtained through that method, the new method can give information on the passage of the contrast medium through the kidney and on flow, filtration and tubular cell activity in the kidney.

About 10 seconds after the injection of the contrast medium, the nephrographic phase usually begins to reach a maximum at which it persists for a period varying with the blood pressure. If the blood pressure is lowered, it may persist for several seconds. In this phase a dense accumulation of contrast medium is first seen in the cortex and columnae Bertini, while the pyramids appear as contrast defects against the rest of the kidney. The density of contrast then increases in the pyramids and thereby in the entire renal parenchyma. Because of the different directions of these pyramids in relation to the hilum, the density of the kidney will be irregular and vary greatly with the rate of injection of the contrast medium. If the amount of contrast medium injected is small or if the contrast medium is injected at a slow rate, these differences in the nephrographic phase will be blurred.

The outline of the kidney appears distinctly in the nephrogram and the hilum and sinus are as a rule readily recognized. Any persisting foetal lobation can also be seen. The hilum varies considerably in shape.

HEGEDÜS (1971), using frontal and true lateral views of the kidney, has been able to study in the nephrographic phase the regions of the renal parenchyma fed by the different branches of the main renal artery. This technique allows a thorough study of the shape, size and volume of the kidneys. There are great variations in the shape of the kidney: the ovoid type, for example, with a smooth surface, the ovoid type with a lobulated surface, kidneys with impressions from the liver or spleen, and kidneys with large hilar lips. The thickness of the kidneys varies greatly, as does the volume. It has been pointed out by KING et al. (1968) that as a normal anatomic variation a large cortical mass can project into the renal sinus. Such a mass appears as an expansive lesion at urography. At angiography the arteries deviate around the mass and in the nephrographic phase the mass increases in density, as does the remainder of the cortex. HEGEDÜS and FAARUP (1972) have designed a simple and reliable technique for quantitative estimation of the volume of the total kidney and of the superficial cortex of the kidney (Fig. 44). ("Superficial cortex" means the cortex volume excluding the columnae Bertini.) In their analysis of total cortical volume and superficial cortical volume these authors found the most stable parameter in normal kidneys to be the ratio between the volume of the superficial cortex and that of the total kidney.

c) Venous phase

The veins, which are wide (about twice as wide as the arteries), lie ventral to the latter and follow them in their course. Like the arteries, they may be duplicated, although less often than arteries (HELLSTRÖM, 1928). They are formed from 1—4 trunks in the hilum. In contradistinction to the intrarenal arteries, the veins present no segmental arrangement, there being a free anastomosis of venous channels throughout the kidneys (GRAVES, 1956).

The veins become visible usually about 10 seconds after the injection of the contrast medium, occasionally earlier, and the filling usually reaches a maximum approximately 20 seconds after the end of injection. The use of a highly concentrated contrast medium will increase the visibility of the veins because the contrast blood is not cleared completely from contrast medium. This also appears to be the case if renal function is impaired. If the examination is carried out with the patient holding his breath in different respiratory phases, considerable differences can be seen in the course of the veins. In many instances it is important to study the veins, for example in venous thrombosis, hydronephrosis, tumor, etc.

d) Flow studies during angiography

The general principle at each roentgen-diagnostic procedure is to extract as much useful information as possible. In renal angiography, as in many other angiographic procedures, the study, in addition to obtaining initial morphologic information, can be extended to include physiologic parameters of great diagnostic value, directly or by modification of technique at recording, or by adding a new supplementary technique. Flow studies of the kidney during angiographic procedures represent such an addition.

A crude appreciation of the flow in the renal artery can be made from serial films by studying the caliber of the renal artery, the size of the kidney and, to some extent, the dilution of the contrast medium injected. Greater accuracy and objectivity result from the use of densitometry of serial films or TV recordings (SILVERMAN, 1969).

The best method at angiography in morphologic studies was found by OLIN and GÖTHLIN (1971) to be the dye-dilution technique. After a single injection of Indocyanine 3 into the renal artery, blood samples were automatically and continuously sucked from the renal vein through a catheter in the vein to a spectrometer and automatically reinfused into the vein. The spectrometer recording allows calculation of renal blood flow.

Normal kidneys, anomalous kidneys and kidneys with different types and degrees of pathology have been studied, and are continuously being studied, by a standardized,

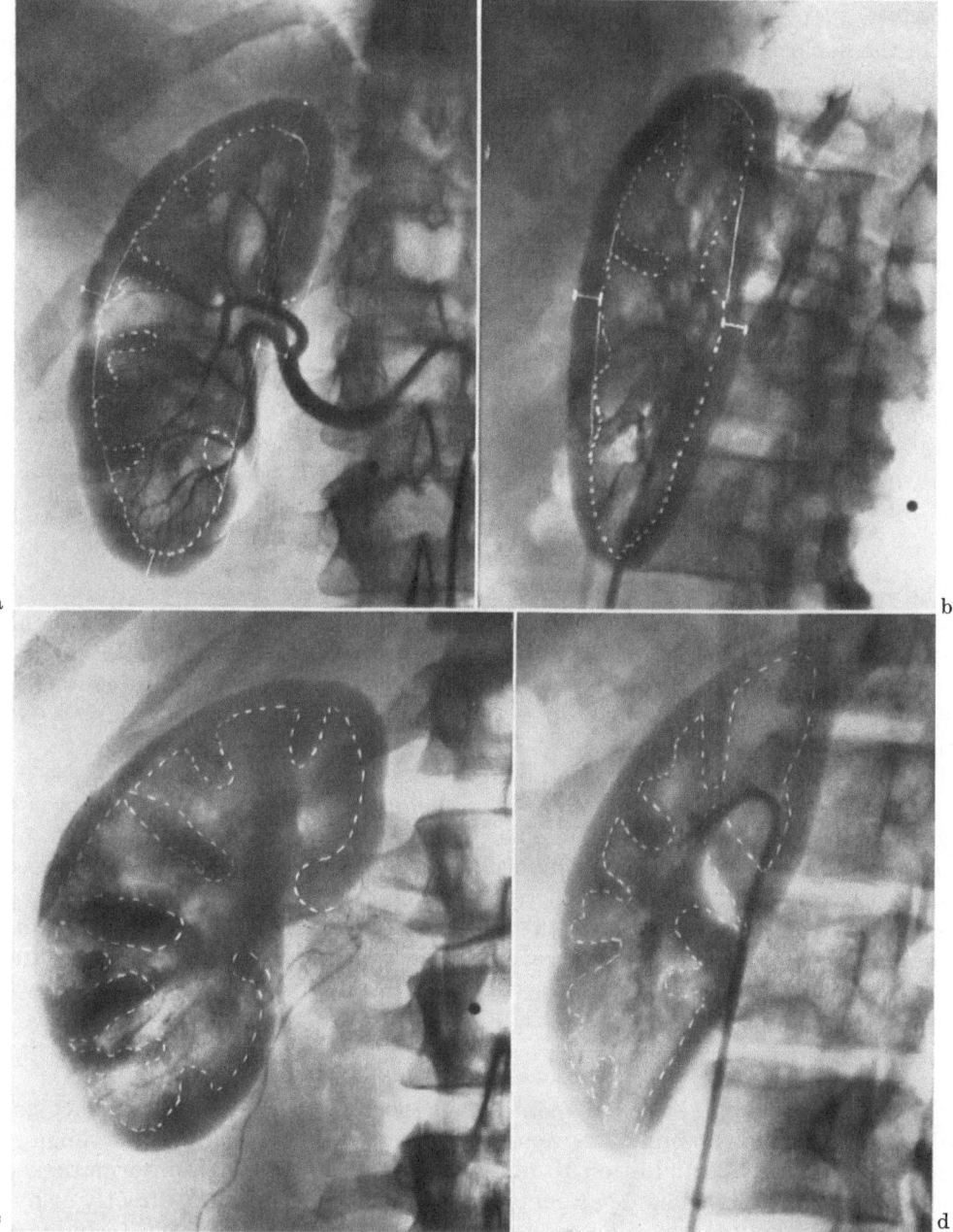

Fig. 44. Estimation of superficiae cortex according to HEGEDÜS & FAARUP. a) and b) few columnae Bertini,
c) and d) large columnae Bertini

easily practicable technique. Values for different pathologic lesions are collected and
compared at the same time as the range of normal variations is established. At this early
stage of this extensive project, information of decisive importance in diagnosis has already
been obtained, and no doubt this additional technique will very soon have routine application in selected diagnostic situations.

The technique can be developed to make possible determination of glomerular filtration and tubular secretion simultaneously and will allow refined diagnostic determination
and a certain degree of prognostic evaluation, and may influence decision on certain indications for surgery.

e) Pharmacoangiography

In connection with angiography, enhancement of findings may be achieved and subliminal symptomatology may be transferred into well detectable signs by use of certains drugs in connection with the angiographic procedure. Thus in our department ABRAMS, BOIJSEN and BORGSTRÖM (1962) started animal experiments to study the effects of epinephrine on the renal circulation. This drug was later used to cause contraction of normal vasculature in the kidney, resulting in better demonstration of pathologic vasculature, which did not react to epinephrine (ABRAMS, 1964).

For details of the pharmacologic effects of epinephrine and other drugs generally and specifically, the reader is referred to reviews by, for instance, ABRAMS (1964), ELKIN and MENG (1965), CHVOJKA and DOLEZEL (1971) and to the very thorough study by ABRAMS and OBREZ (1971). It must be pointed out that the reaction of tumor vessels to epinephrine is not specific. The vessels in inflammatory lesions may also be unresponsive to epinephrine, which makes the use of this drug less important in the sometimes difficult differential diagnosis between renal tumor and inflammatory lesions (KAHN and WISE, 1967; BECKER et al., 1967).

EKELUND et al. (1972) advocate the use of angiotensin, dose 0.5 micrograms, to enhance the demonstration of pathologic vasculature in the kidney. This drug had been used by ELKIN and MENG (1966) in experiments on dogs, where it had been shown to have a more peripheral vasoconstrictive effect than epinephrine. The results with epinephrine were somewhat unpredictable. As angiotensin is supposed to act more peripherally in the blood vessels than catecholamines this drug may have better effect, especially in the differential diagnosis between tumor with low vascularity and cyst. This diagnostic addition seems to offer definite advantages.

The use of acetylcholine is advocated by ABRAMS (1972) and by VESIN (1973). This drug causes vasodilatation and thus enhances filling of arteries and veins, and in this connection is supposed to provide better possibilities for demonstration of pathologic vasculature.

Drugs can also be used to improve the venous phase at angiography. Here, as in other angiographic regions, the injection of a vaso-dilatative drug may cause improvement. Thus FREED et al. (1968) in experimental studies on dogs, demonstrated improvement of venous filling after injection of bradykinin into the renal artery. HELETÄ and VIRTAMA (1970) have demonstrated the same effect in homo. The injection into the renal artery of 20 Mg bradykinin thus gives a better demonstration of the renal vein.

A survey of pharmaco-angiography of the kidney is given by EKELUND (1973).

V. Renal phlebography

In certain conditions such as suspected thrombosis of the renal vein or of the inferior caval vein by an ordinary thrombus or tumor thrombus, phlebography may be informative. This examination can be performed in association with cavography. Both femoral veins are then punctured and contrast medium injected at the same time on both sides. A catheter may also be passed via an arm vein (exposed or percutaneously), the catheter then being fed through the right auricle of the heart down into the inferior caval vein. It is also possible to perform selective catheterization of the renal vein and selective renal phlebography (Fig. 45). GOSPODINOW and TOPALOW (1959) catheterized via the left spermatic vein, which is an unnecessarily complicated procedure.

Cavography is performed with the patient supine and preferably turned slightly to the side to be studied, with the head end somewhat raised. This position facilitates the filling of the renal vein because of the high specific gravity of the contrast medium. After manual injection of 15—20 cm³ contrast medium (best tri-iodine medium) into each femoral vein, exposures are made, preferably with a cassette changer. During the injection the patient

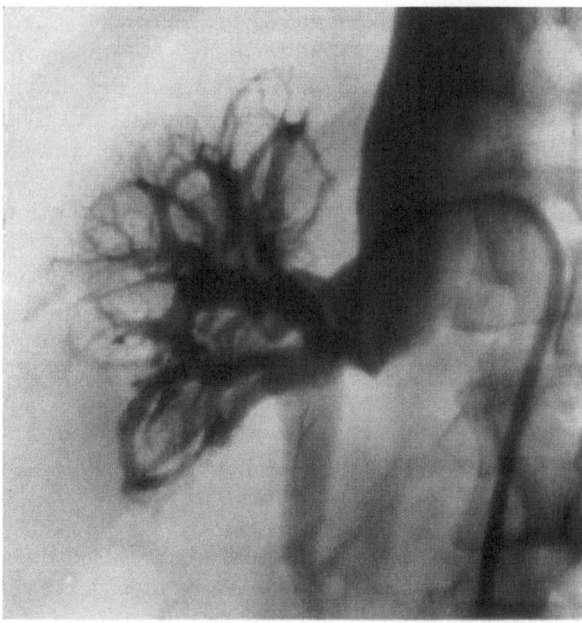

Fig. 45. Renal phlebography: selective catheterization of renal vein; filling of renal vein and intrarenal tributaries and of inferior caval vein

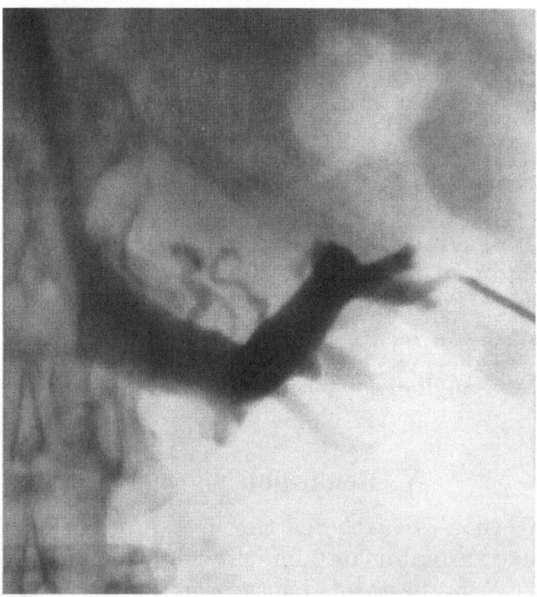

Fig. 46. Accidental puncture of kidney and injection into intrarenal venous branch; filling of renal vein and of lateral part of inferior caval vein. (Puncture made for splenoportography)

may be instructed to strain when the head of the column of contrast medium has passed the origin of the renal vein. This facilitates the filling of the vein. If the flow in the renal vein is unobstructed, streamlining in the caval vein will be seen. At selective catheterization 10—20 ml is injected into the renal vein.

The best method of performing renal phlebography is to inject contrast medium through a catheter into the renal vein with simultaneous blockage of the arterial back pressure. This can be secured by injecting into the renal artery a small dose of epinephrine or angiotensin, thus decreasing the renal blood flow. During the period of reduced flow the contrast medium is injected through the catheter into the renal vein, giving a filling of the veins in retrograde direction as peripherally as the arcuate veins (OLIN and REUTER, 1965). Another method is to block arterial flow through a balloon in the renal artery (JENSEN and OLIN, 1971).

In animal experiments BRAEDEL and HERAVI (1972) have used a non-renotropic contrast medium, Biligrafin forte, for phlebography. As only about 10% of this contrast medium is excreted by the kidney, an intra-arterial injection of the medium into the renal artery produced good demonstration of the veins.

A special type of renal phlebography with catheterization is that performed on patients in whom an anastomosis has been surgically established between the splenic and renal vein because of portal hypertension. In such cases we have been able to catheterize both the renal vein and the anastomosis and to pass the catheter into the stump of the splenic vein.

A special form of phlebography with a filling of veins in the direction of flow., i. e. from the side of the kidney, has occasionally occurred accidentally in association with direct puncture of the kidney and injection of contrast medium directly into the renal parenchyma (Fig. 46). This has occurred in connection with splenoportography in which the needle has accidentally been inserted into the kidney instead of into the spleen. Excellent renal phlebograms were obtained without any side effects of the puncture. Two such cases have been described by LEGER et al., 1957). We have also had two such cases in our department.

Normal anatomy

The inferior caval vein crosses the right part of the spine. It is fairly straight and has a caliber of 1.5—3 cm. It anastomoses richly with the spinal and other veins, which can be observed if the vein is compressed by a pathologic process or artificially. On performance of the Valsava maneuver, contrast medium injected will enter the renal vein in retrograde direction.

On catheterization of the renal vein and injection of contrast medium directly into that vein, a considerable retrograde filling will be obtained of venous radicles as well as of the main trunks (see above). Filling of all renal veins will be possible through the use of the method of decreasing or blocking arterial flow.

It is usually said in the anatomic literature that multiplicity of renal veins is a rare occurrence. Multiplicity is found fairly often at renal phlebography, however.

D. Anomalies

Those anomalies which are of greatest importance and most easily accessible to diagnostic roentgenology will here be dealt with first, in contrast to most descriptions of the anomalies. No attempt will be made here to include all anomalies which are due to embryologic disturbances. Some will be described in appropriate chapters, e. g. polycystic disease in association with renal cyst, stenosis of the pelviureteric junction in association with dilatation of the urinary pathways, etc. It must be pointed out that renal abnormalities are often found in combination with other developmental abberations. Thus, in multiple congenital anomalies, renal ectopia and other types of renal malformations are often present. The finding of renal ectopia, for example, is an indication for thorough investigation of other abnormalities such as skeletal, cardiovascular and gastro-intestinal anomalies. When certain anomalies are recognized, it is imperative to investigate the possibility of renal ectopia (MALEK et al., 1971).

In a report on seven cases involving severe fetal urologic malformation with dilatation of the kidney pelvis and ureters, pulmonary hyperplasia was severe and in all the patients pneumothorax and/or pneumomediastinum was present (RENERT *et al.*, 1972). The authors recommend early urologic evaluation when unexplained respiratory problems are noted at birth.

PARKER in 1895 described a malformation syndrome with absence of abdominal muscles in an infant with undescended testicles and anomaly of the urinary tract. ANDRÉN *et al.* (1964) and CREMIN (1971) have described this symptom in the radiologic literature. The triad of lesions usually noted in this syndrome, according to CREMIN, are:

1. absence of abdominal muscles, the degree of involvement varying from severe to mild, but with low erecti usually involved,

2. undescended testicles,

3. anomalies of the urinary tract. These are: varying degree of dysplasia, dilatation of the kidney pelvis and ureters due to absence of muscle fibers, dilatation of the bladder, often with a urachal diverticulum, and dilatation of the posterior part of the urethra.

I. Anomalies of the renal pelvis and associated anomalies of the ureter

As mentioned in the description of the normal anatomy, the shape of the renal pelvis varies so widely that it is often difficult to decide whether or not the organ should be regarded as normal. Not infrequently the kidney pelvis has a shape which makes it impossible to exclude a slight impression in it by a small expansive process in the kidney parenchyma. This makes it necessary to perform renal angiography in certain cases in order to exclude tumor.

A small process from the confluence or upper or lower branch, for example, is described in connection with the anatomy. This probably represents a slight inhibitory malformation. A definite but rare congenital anomaly of the renal pelvis is illustrated in Fig. 47 The most common of all anomalies is the double renal pelvis with forked ureter or complete double ureter.

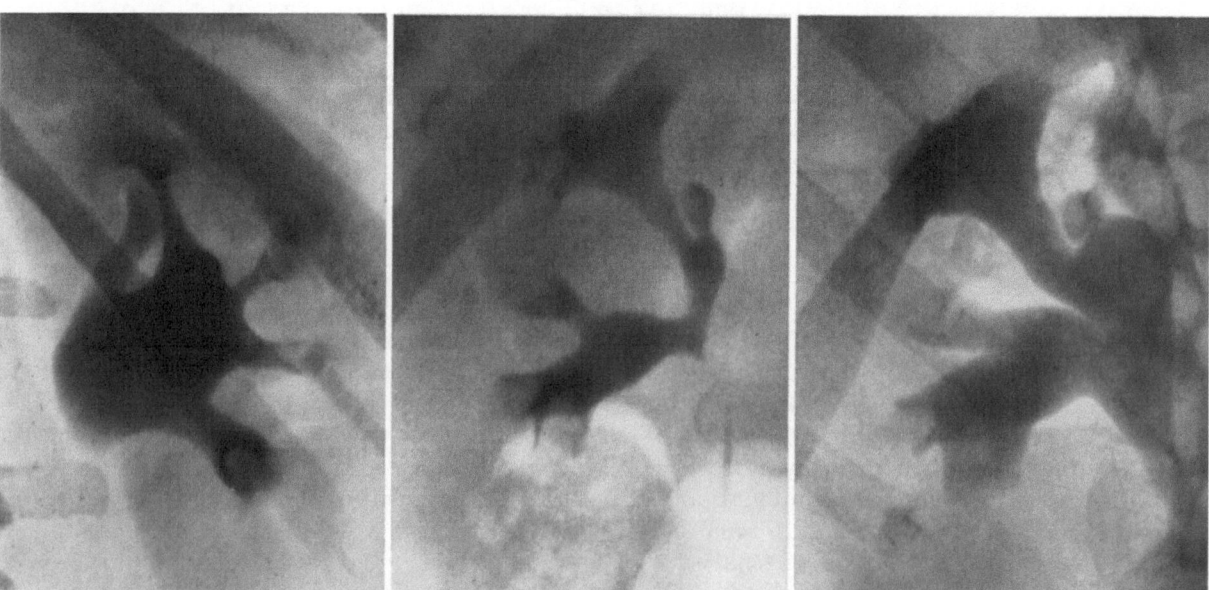

Fig. 47. Unusual anomalies of kidney pelvis with small extra branches from cranial part of confluence of kidney pelvis

1. Double renal pelvis

The embryonal renal pelvis has two parts separated by a sulcus, the so-called primary bifurcation angle (LÖFGREN, 1949). If these two parts persist more or less independently in the confluence, the result will be the formation of a deeply cloven renal pelvis which is usually regarded as a normal anatomic variant. If they do not fuse at all, the result will be an anomaly, the so-called ureter fissus or forked ureter. The kidney then has two separate pelves, each drained by its own ureter. The ureters unite, however, and from their point of union, which may occur at variable levels, there extends a common ureter to the bladder. Ureter fissus is regarded by many (cited NORDMARK, 1948) as being due to premature division of the ureteric bud or coming from an originally double ureteric bud. If this double bud persists, it will result in a double ureter. If the buds fuse partially, they will result in the formation of a forked ureter. Other authors claim that a divided renal

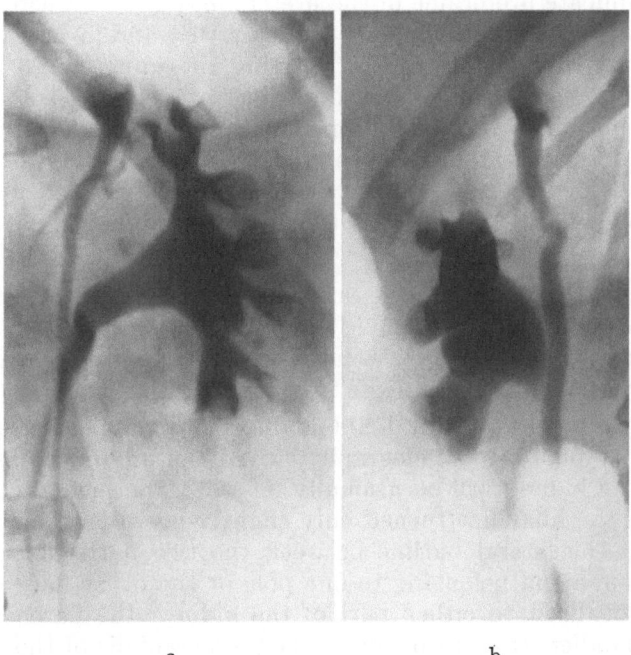

a   b

Fig. 48. Double kidney pelvis with small upper part. a) Caudal pelvis of ordinary anatomic form not modelled by cranial part of kidney, which is too small to influence large caudal part. Note pyelolymphatic backflow from uppermost calyx of caudal pelvis. b) Small pyelogenic cyst at edge of uppermost calyx of caudal pelvis

pelvis, forked ureter, and double ureter are different grades of one and the same anomaly, i.e. the ureteric bud divides a varying distance from its attachment to the Wolffian duct.

In double ureter the upper renal pelvis is usually the smaller (Fig. 48). As a rule, it consists of two small groups of calyces corresponding to the upper branch of the ordinary renal pelvis. It may also, however, be much smaller and have only one calyx which drains only a small amount of renal parenchyma. It then forms a transition to a blind ureter (see below). In bilateral double kidney the renal pelves on one side may be very different from those on the other. Thus, the upper renal pelvis on one side may have the common shape described above, while that on the other may have only one calyx.

The lower part of the renal pelvis may resemble a small normal single pelvis. It may sometimes be difficult particularly in children to distinguish the lower part of a double kidney from the renal pelvis in a normal kidney. This should be remembered in cases where no excretion of contrast urine occurs in the upper renal pelvis during urography. The distance from the calyces to the cranial renal pole is then usually but not always longer. This should lead the examiner's thoughts to the possibility of a second renal pelvis. In addition, the distance from the uppermost calyx to the medial surface of the kidney is usually increased. Therefore, in the absence of demonstrable excretion in the upper renal pelvis, the presence of a tumor in the upper part may be suspected. The upper calyces of the lower renal pelvis often appear to be flattened. This anatomic shape of the upper calyces can be thought to be due to pressure by a tumor. Thorough knowledge of the shape of the lower renal pelvis, especially the topography of its upper calyces, is therefore imperative if mistakes are to be avoided. The shape of the lower renal pelvis in a double kidney may vary considerably and sometimes represent the smaller part of the total volume of the renal pelvis. The lower part of the kidney is then often small and the changes as a whole may be caused by atrophy due to pyelonephritis (see chapter on generalized diseases).

In complete duplicate ureter one of the ureters may have an ectopic orifice. In males it is prone to empty into the prostatic part of the urethra and in females into the urethra, vagina or vulva. It is usually the ureter draining the upper renal pelvis that has the ectopic orifice. This is readily understood on an embryologic basis. In the course of embryologic development the orifice of the upper ureter is regularly situated farther down and closer to the middle of the bladder than the orifice of the lower ureter in complete duplication (Weigert-Meyers rule). Thus, since the ureter of the upper renal pelvis is located farther down, it will be closely related to the Wolffian duct and organs derived from it.

The detection of an ectopic ureteric orifice may be difficult. It has been stressed by SEITZMAN and PATTON (1960), for example, that the finding of unexplained pyuria in the male as well as urinary incontinence associated with an otherwise normal voiding pattern in the female, warrants complete urologic investigation.

Changes may also be observed in double kidney in the appearance of the actual renal parenchyma. Thus at plain roentgenography two hila or an unusually long hilum in the medial contour of the kidney will occasionally be seen. The medial contour is also strikingly straight, with the hilar lips turned only slightly inwards. A marked indentation is occasionally seen in the lateral outline between the two parts of the kidney (Fig. 49). The amount of parenchyma belonging to one pole or the other may vary widely. In the absence of lesions localized to either part of the kidney, the parenchyma of the upper half is usually the smaller. It corresponds to the pars cranialis of the normal kidney and, as a rule, comprises three pairs of pyramids, while the lower part corresponds to the pars intermedia and caudalis of the normal kidney and contains four pairs of pyramids (LÖF-GREN, 1949). The line of demarcation between the regions of the parenchyma is not sharp. This may be demonstrated clearly by the nephrographic effect on urography in acute urinary stasis due to stone in one of the ureters (HELLMER, 1942). If one part of a double kidney harbors a lesion, e.g. pyelonephritis, it may shrink and the upper part may show hyperplasia with a marked difference between the two parts.

The parts of the kidney on one side may also be entirely independent, with supernumerary kidneys as a result.

Multiple arteries to kidneys with a double pelvis are often, but not regularly, found at renal angiography.

NORDMARK (1948) studied the frequency of double renal pelvis. Of 4,744 urograms he found duplication of the renal pelvis in 201 (4.2 per cent) and duplication of the ureter in 138 (2.8 per cent). Bilateral double pelvis was seen in 1 per cent of the cases and double ureter in 0.4 per cent. Unilateral incomplete division of the ureter, forked ureter, was seen in 60 cases, unilateral complete division of the ureter in 59 cases, bilateral complete division of the ureter in 11, bilateral incomplete division of the ureter in 5, and complete division of one side and incomplete division of the other in 3 cases.

As mentioned, supernumerary kidneys also occur. Thus ureters may not only be duplicated but also triplicated. In all cases of triplication of the ureter on record the anomaly was unilateral. The three ureters may empty separately into the bladder or together, with a varying length of the different free ureteric segments. One or more of the ureters may be dilatated and empty ectopically. As a rule, they belong to a composite kidney, which may be caudally ectopic (PERRIN, 1927). One ureter may belong to a free supernumerary kidney (LAU and HENLINE, 1931) or it may be a blind ureter (CHWALIA, 1935). A good survey of these rare anomalies has been given by GILL (1925), SPANGLER (1936). A case of sextuplicitas renum, six functioning kidneys and ureters, was described by BEGG (1953). The latter author gives a critical survey on prevailing theories offered to explain how such an anomaly can arise.

To complete the list, mention should be made of ureter duplicatus caudalis, i.e. one renal pelvis but with branching of the ureter. This anomaly is difficult to understand.

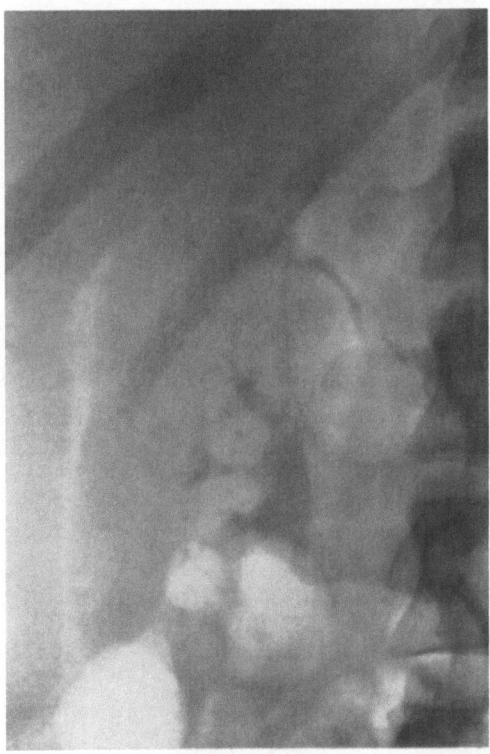

Fig. 49. Kidney with double renal pelvis with marked fat capsule laterally. At division of the two parts of the double kidney, a fat pad marks an indentation in the lateral contour of the kidney

2. Blind ureter

In double formation of the ureter, one of these may cease to continue the course of its development and never unite with the renal parenchyma. It persists as a blind ureter. It may be as short as 1—2 cm but it may also be even longer than a normal ureter (ENGEL, 1939). The long blind ureter is, in reality, the ureter to the upper part of a double kidney that fails to form and, as mentioned, this malformation approaches that of a double kidney with a very small upper part. The blind part may unite with the lower ureter to form a forked ureter. It may also be free, however, and can then empty ectopically. Though such a ureter does not drain any parenchyma and thus has no real function, contractions may occur in its wall. Such contractions may be so severe as to cause pain. Stagnation of urine in the blind ureter favors infection with fever, pain and stone formation, which can cause pyuria and haematuria.

A blind ureter is best detected by pyelography (Fig. 50). It can be diagnosed by urography, however, if it opens into the other ureter. It must not be confused with a ureteric diverticulum (Fig. 51), which is only a pouch which may be adjacent to a stricture in a ureter, for example.

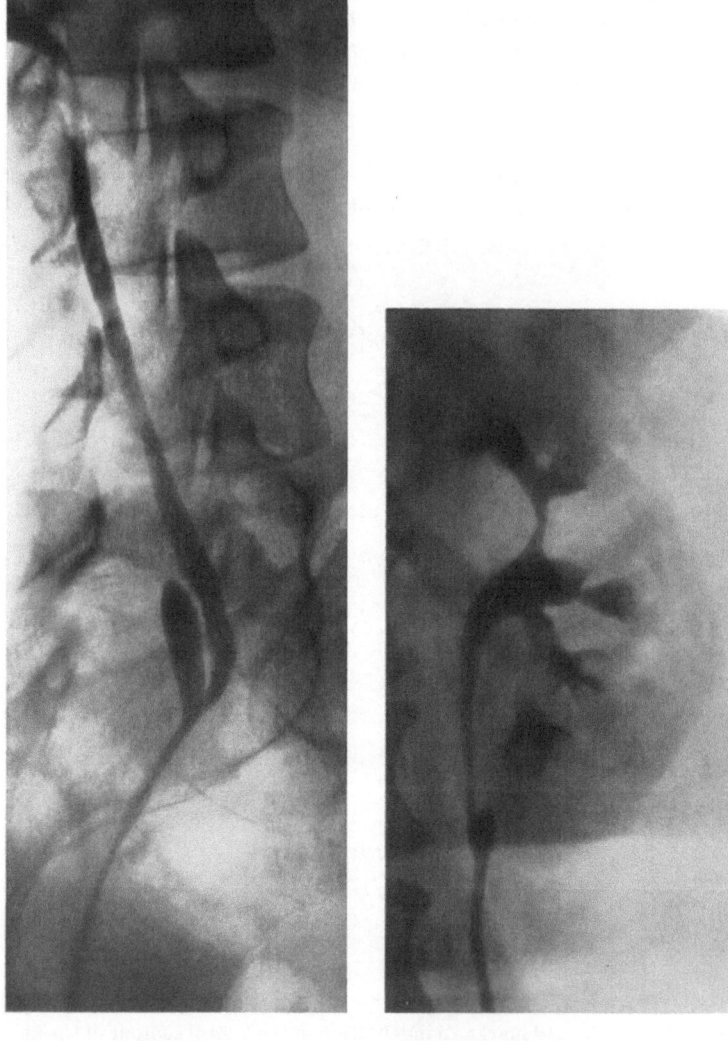

Fig. 50   Fig. 51

Fig. 50. Blind ureter in ureter fissus

Fig. 51. Small ureteric diverticulum

3. Anomalies of the calyces

An important group of anomalies which have received but scanty attention but which are of great importance are malformations of the calyces. These are important not only from a puraly diagnostic point of view, since they are likely to be mistaken for pathologic processes, but also because they may favor stone formation, for example. It is difficult to draw any definite line of distinction between normal variation and anomaly because, as mentioned, the range of normal variation is so wide and has not been the subject of sufficient systematic investigation. *Microcalyces* (Fig. 52) may be regarded as anomalous. They are very small. 5—10 mm long, calyx-shaped, tiny projections from the border of a calyx or consist of thin branches of a renal pelvis like an ordinary calyx. In these microcalyces stones may sometimes be observed and they may dilate. They may simulate a well defined sinus reflux.

Another anomaly consists of more or less distinct local evaginations from the border of the calyx (Fig. 53) usually from several calyces in the same kidney. Such small evaginations sometimes contain minute calculi (see Fig. 89). It is suggested that the term *calyceal evaginations* be reserved for this anomaly. Some of these changes represent border-line cases of a spongy kidney, for instance (see chapter on medullary sponge kidney).

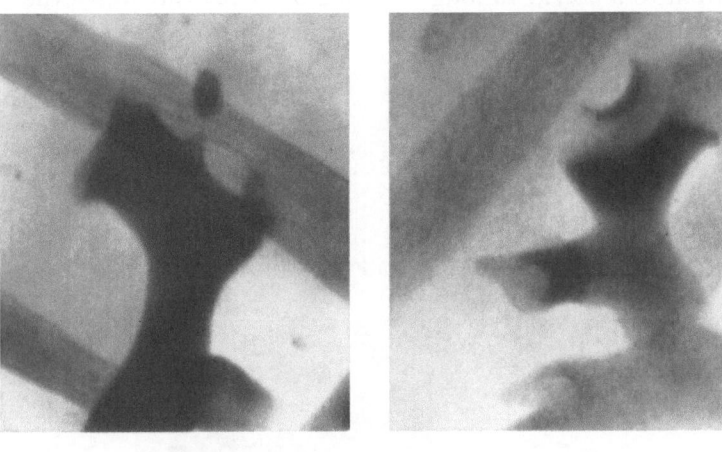

Fig. 52   Fig. 53

Fig. 52. Dilated micro-calyx

Fig. 53. Calyceal border evagination

4. Anomalies in the border between calyces and renal parenchyma

Anomalies are common along the border between the two components of the ureteric bud and of the metanephrogenic blastoma, thus the junction between the calyces and parenchyma. This region is also a common seat of pathologic changes. Diagnosis and differential diagnosis are therefore difficult in the presence of changes in this region. The most important form of anomaly is a cyst. A large number of bewildering names have been given to these formations, such as cystes urinaires (RAYER, 1841), pyelogenic cyst (DAMM, 1932; LJUNGGREN, 1942), calyceal diverticulum, Kelchdivertikel (ITIKAWA and TANIO, 1939; PRATHER, 1941), cyst of the kidney due to hydrocalicosis (WATKINS, 1939), calectasia (ENGEL, 1947), solitary renal cyst with communication to the renal pelvis (NATVIG, 1941), Kelchzyste (ESCH and HALBEIS, 1953), diverticules kystique des calices (FEY et al., 1951), ectopic calyx (KENT, 1954), etc. This long list is by no means exhaustive. It is sufficient, however, to show that the nomenclature is confusing. These terms have undoubtedly been used to cover many different pathologic conditions. It is obvious that many authors have used the same name for different processes and that other authors have used different names for one and the same condition. This may be explained by the fact that some different pathologic conditions may simulate one another macroscopically, i.e. at roentgen examination and at operation and, secondly, that various names have apparently been suggested without due consideration.

On roentgen examination the process appears as a cavity connected to a calyx. It is well outlined, more or less oval or round, of varying size from a few millimetres to a few centimetres in diameter, situated at any height in the kidney and usually connected with the renal pelvis by a narrow or wide, short or long channel. It may communicate with the fornix of a more or less well preserved calyx or with the middle of a calyx, or it may originate between two calyces.

The pathologic conditions capable of producing such a roentgen finding may be divided roughly into two groups: 1. changes in the renal parenchyma with formation of a cyst communicating with the renal pelvis and 2. changes in the renal pelvis, particularly a calyx which may intrude upon the renal parenchyma.

Group 1. Various types of papillary ulceration such as renal tuberculosis, pyelonephritis and papillary necrosis may lead to destruction of the papilla and a wide communication or fistulation to a calyx. In long-standing or healed processes the remaining cavity may be smooth and well-defined.

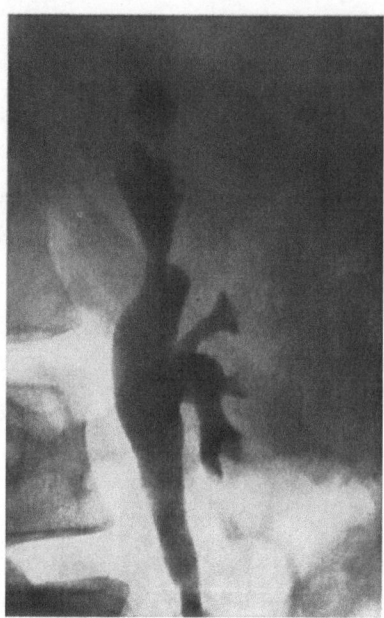

Fig. 54. Pyelogenic cyst in cranial kidney pole

If it is situated near the renal pelvis, a so-called meta-nephrogenic renal cyst which is laid down in the usual way may rupture into the renal pelvis, with which it then communicates. In such cases cysts are usually multiple and dislocate the branches of the renal pelvis. Meta-nephrogenic cysts communicating with the renal pelvis have cubical epithelium. The so-called pyelogenic cyst (see Fig. 54) may be of similar appearance, but it is usually single and, unlike multicystic changes, it does not deform the renal pelvis. The pyelogenic cyst is as a rule small, 1—2 cm in diameter, but may on occasion be much larger. It is round or oval and well defined. The cyst often contains calculi, sometimes numerous microliths. Such a case has been described by RUDSTRÖM (1941) with about 2,000 microliths. The communication of a pyelogenic cyst with the renal pelvis may be very narrow. Not until after prolonged compression during urography can a filling be obtained, and sometimes the cyst is situated deep in the parenchyma without any demonstrable connection with the renal pelvis. This is because the duct is so thin that it cannot be seen. The collecting tubules empty into the wall of the cyst, and it is possible that a filling may be obtained from the parenchymal side, which explains why cysts of this type are sometimes not demonstrable by retrograde pyelography. As a rule, however, it must be supposed that even in urography the cysts are filled in retrograde direction by constrast medium which is first excreted into the renal pelvis. Only in one instance have I seen a fairly large cyst communicating with the renal pelvis, which after prolonged compression became filled and then suddenly expanded and dislocated adjacent calyces. Microscopically the pyelogenic cyst has transitional epithelium. Without shedding much light upon this anomaly, DALLA et al. (1958) ascribed it to "calico-pyramidal dysplasia". Roentgenologically the term pyelogenic cyst undoubtedly covers changes of different origins.

Group 2. The actual border of the calyx is capable of wide variation and, as mentioned, can show bulges which will be referred to here as calyceal evaginations. Most of the changes in this group, however, consist of hydrocalyces. Papillary ulceration often involves both the renal parenchyma and the renal pelvis. This is the case in tuberculosis and pyelonephritis. In these diseases edema occurs in the stem of a calyx which may be accompanied by shrinkage resulting in stasis in the calyx, with distention, flattening of the papilla and ulceration, if infection is present. A common cause of hydrocalicosis is stone lodged in the stem of the calyx.

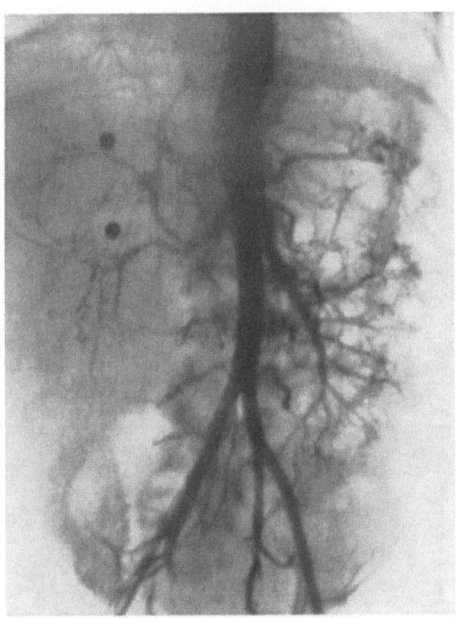

Fig. 55. Complete aplasia. Angiography: no renal arteries

It has been claimed (WATKINS, 1939 and others) that hydrocalicosis may result from achalasia of the muscle in the calyceal wall. The idea is interesting but as yet no supportive evidence is available.

The changes in juvenile hypertension described by ASK-UPMARK (1929) show anomalies of the calyx as well as of the corresponding part of the renal parenchyma. In these cases the calyx may be club-shaped and extend out to the periphery of the kidney. The appearance of the change simulates that of so-called local hypoplasia. A similar picture is seen in healed papillary necrosis.

Many of the lesions referred to above are difficult to distinguish from one another and undoubtedly a change of a certain type may be the end result of many completely disparate lesions.

II. Anomalies of the renal parenchyma

1. Aplasia and agenesia

Defective development of the kidney may vary from slight hypoplasia to severe aplasia and agenesia. (Fig. 55). Hypoplasia has been defined as a local or general maldevelopment of a kidney with apparently normal excretory capacity, as judged by urography (see below). The definition is arbitrary. Aplastic kidney is accordingly to be understood as a small malformed kidney showing only slight or no excretion during urography. Such a kidney is sometimes seen in plain roentgenography as a small formation resembling a kidney only in outline. Sometimes it does not show up in plain roentgenograms but can be demonstrated by the use of tomography or retroperitoneal pneumography. It may be demonstrable by renal angiography and will then be seen as a miniature of an ordinary kidney (Fig. 57). This type of defective formation of the kidney must be remembered in obscure cases of pyuria.

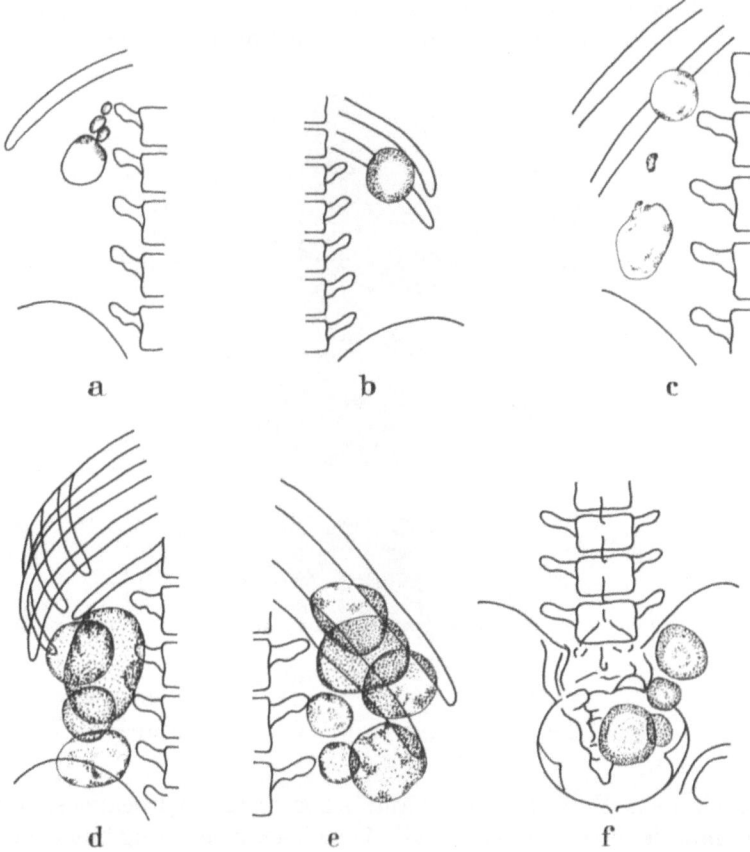

Fig. 56. Aplasia. Congenital unilateral multicystic kidney. Schematic drawing of some different types of this rare form of aplasia. (After STAEHLER)

In the gravest form of aplasia, one or more irregular cyst-like formations, usually calcified and of different size, are seen in the area normally occupied by a kidney. This is the result of a malformed primordium of the kidney. Such aplasia, known as Knollenniere in the German literature and as congenital unilateral multicystic kidney in the English (SCHWARTZ, 1936; SPENCE, 1955), is very rare (Fig. 56). Only about 20 cases are represented in the literature (BARTLEY et al., 1967). The entity differs from polycystic renal disease by its not being familiar and not being bilateral. On occasion such a kidney may have a normal ureter, but it is usually atretic, rudimentary, or missing. The vascularity is also rudimentary or missing. The deformed kidney may be ectopic; it may even show crossed ectopy (DEAK, 1956). One of the cases of calcified hydronephrosis published by LEWIS and DOSS (1958) resembles such an anomaly.

Severe malformation in the urinary tract may cause complete absence of renal function at birth.

It has been pointed out by ABRAMS and KAPLAN (1956), for example, that urography as a final procedure in connection with angiocardiography may help in detecting unsuspected absence of a kidney, ureteropelvic obstruction with marked hydronephrosis, congenital bladder-neck obstruction, double kidneys, and other anomalies (see C III 2h, Urography at health-check examinations).

2. Hypoplasia

The finding of a small kidney on one side and a normal-sized or compensatorily enlarged kidney on the other is not uncommon. The smallness of the kidney may be explained in different ways: it may originally be hypoplastic or it may have shrunk. Shrinkage may be due to different conditions such as tuberculous or non-tuberculous inflammation, stasis due to stone or to emboli, for example. The most common cause is pyelonephritis, sometimes in combination with anomaly or urinary stasis. Occasionally neither roentgen examination nor pathologic examination can explain the cause of the small kidney. Only if the shrinkage of a kidney has been followed roentgenographically is it possible to diagnose the small kidney as a shrunken kidney. Repeated roentgen examination will reveal the course of reduction of a normal-sized kidney and thereby yield definite evidence that the kidney is contracted. The more widely the value of roentgenologic follow-up during conservative treatment of a renal disease is realized, the more often it will be possible to ascertain, for instance, whether or not a small kidney is the end result of pyelonephritis.

Many pathologists have tried to find acceptable criteria regarding the origin of small kidneys, but those suggested are to a large extent contradictory. After a careful study of 183 unilateral small kidneys, of which half were available for pathologic examination, EMMETT et al. (1952) conclude: "There is no doubt in our minds that the unilateral 'hypoplastic' or 'atrophic' kidney represents several different and distinct pathological entities. We are sure that in some cases the lesion is congenital while in others it is the result of acquired, or a combination of congenital and acquired conditions. One of the commonest acquired conditions is infection ('chronic atrophic pyelonephritis'). We feel that in some cases of apparent chronic atrophic pyelonephritis the kidney may have been congenitally small to start with, but we know of no way to decide this problem accurately. For this reason it would seem that it might be more sensible to forego any attempts at classification according to origin and clinical findings and instead to employ some common 'blanket' term, such as 'atrophic kidney' or 'renal atrophy', to describe the unilateral small kidney, the cause of which is not apparent."

In a monograph on hypoplasia EKSTRÖM (1955) presented a material in which kidneys were said to be hypoplastic if one of the two kidneys was small (two thirds or less than that on the other side) with adequate excretion at urography. Kidneys of this type often show characteristic renal pelvic changes, which can also sometimes be found to a varying extent in somewhat small or normal-sized kidneys. Such cases were also included as local or partial hypoplasia. The material consisted of 156 cases of hypoplasia. Females were more common than males, namely 128 of the 156. In addition, in the females the condition was much more frequently seen on the right side. I feel that the sex distribution and the preponderance of the condition on the right side strongly suggest that the material was biased by non-congenital factors.

It is obvious that neither the size of the kidney nor its capacity for excreting contrast urine is a reliable criterion in the diagnosis of renal hypoplasia. This term therefore simply means unilateral small kidney with good function. Some cases may be congenital, while others are undoubtedly acquired. Changes seen in the so-called hypoplastic kidney are described with due reservation below.

EKSTRÖM (1955) distinguishes three grades of renal hypoplasia, namely general, partial, and local. Partial hypoplasia is to be understood as hypoplasia in one half of a kidney with a double renal pelvis. In the series of 156 cases of renal hypoplasia, the disease was general in 98, partial in 18, and local in 40. In 35 of the 40 cases of local hypoplasia, the entire contralateral kidney was hypoplastic; in 3 cases only part of the kidney was hypoplastic.

In two thirds of the cases with local hypoplasia the condition was localized to the upper pole.

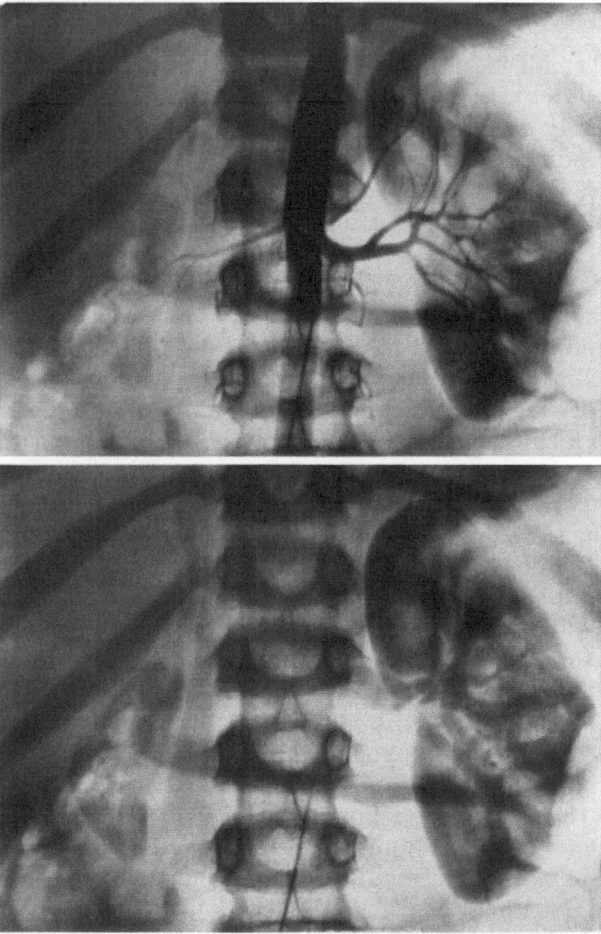

Fig. 57. Marked hypoplasia. Right kidney very small; left kidney fairly large. Urography: no excretion on right side; normal function and morphology on left side. Aortic renal angiography: normal conditions on left side (note separate upper polar branch to dorsal pyramids). Extremely small but otherwise normal kidney on right side. In final stage of renal angiography contrast urine was excreted also from right kidney showing small but otherwise normal kidney pelvis

a) General hypoplasia

(Fig. 57)

In the plain roentgenogram a small kidney is seen. It may be so small as to simulate agenesia. It may also occur as a small oblong formation, which closer examination by tomography or retroperitoneal pneumography, for example, will reveal to be a small kidney. As a rule, however, the kidney is somewhat larger, of ordinary shape and of smooth outline.

At urography and pyelography the renal pelvis will be found to be small for the size of the kidney. It may be of ordinary shape or it may be short, upright and with few calyces. These calyces are, on occasion, elongated and almost reach the surface of the kidney and they may be club-shaped, so-called dysplastic calyces. This implies that the corresponding papilla is missing. In fact, it is this form of calyx that is the most common characteristic feature of so-called hypoplasia. Sometimes the changes closely resemble the anomalies described by ASK-UPMARK in which the recesses of the renal pelvis extended towards an indentation in the outline of the kidney, where they terminated blindly. This last-mentioned change, however, is, said always to be located in the central portion of the kidney or in the lower pole.

The contralateral kidney is usually hyperplastic. The kidney is then somewhat larger than usual and often rounded and plump, but otherwise of normal shape.

In partial hypoplasia changes of the type described above are localized to one half of a double kidney. Then the upper part is as rule involved, and, on occasion, it is converted into a small or large hydronephrotic sac with extremely little parenchyma. Malformations such as ectopic ureteric orifice are sometimes seen in association with this condition. The disease may be localized to the lower part of the kidney however, with hyperplasia of the upper part.

b) Local hypoplasia

Local hypoplasia involves only a part of a kidney. If the change is small, the kidney many be of ordinary size but usually its outline will show an indentation or a reduction in the size of the pole at the seat of the hypoplasia. The calyces in the region involved resemble those described above and thus differ from those in the rest of the kidney. The calyces are short and broad or long and clubbed. Local bulges can sometimes be seen along the border of a calyx resembling calyceal border evaginations or pyelogenic cysts.

All types of hypoplasia can be bilateral with different distribution of the changes on the two sides.

It must be noted that roentgendiagnostic features described as characteristic for so-called hypoplasia may be caused by pyelonephritis and represent end stages with shrinkage.

Renal angiography. In the few cases in which at urography a small but normally functioning kidney was found, the appearance of the vasculature was a miniature of that of a normal kidney. Severe changes in the size, shape and outline of the kidney may also be seen, however. Experience is too limited to allow of a description of changes seen at renal angiography in cases of hypoplasia.

III. Malrotation

On their ascent up to their definitive position during embryonal life, the kidneys rotate on their longitudinal axis. This may be a true rotation, or only apparent and due to different regional growth of the renal parenchyma. From an originally ventral position the kidney pelvis then assumes a medial position. Sometimes this rotation is arrested at an intermediate stage, resulting in malposition of the kidney, which is termed malrotation in accordance with similar inhibitory malformations in the digestive tract. Arrested rotation may be a better term but the term malrotation is widely used. The confluence of the malrotated kidney faces more or less ventrally and, accordingly, one or more calyces are directed medially.

The malformation may be more or less marked. In fact, some cases of so-called intrarenaly positioned kidney pelvis diagnosed roentgenologically are in reality slightly

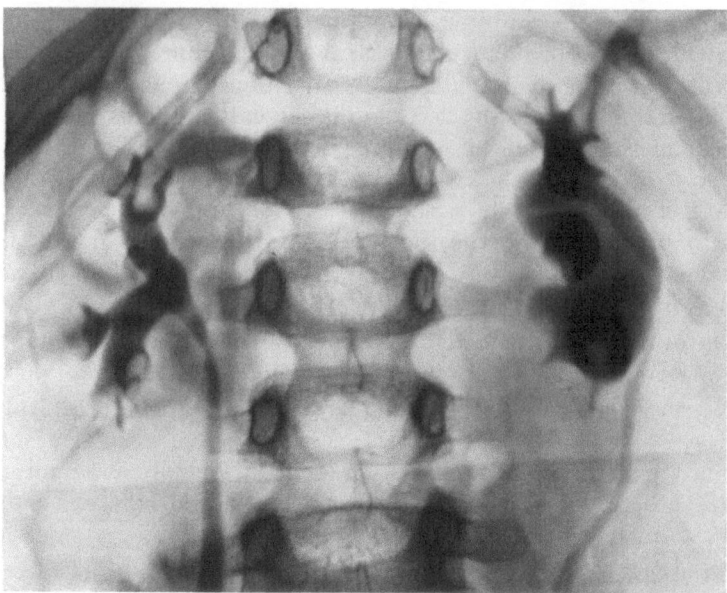

Fig. 58

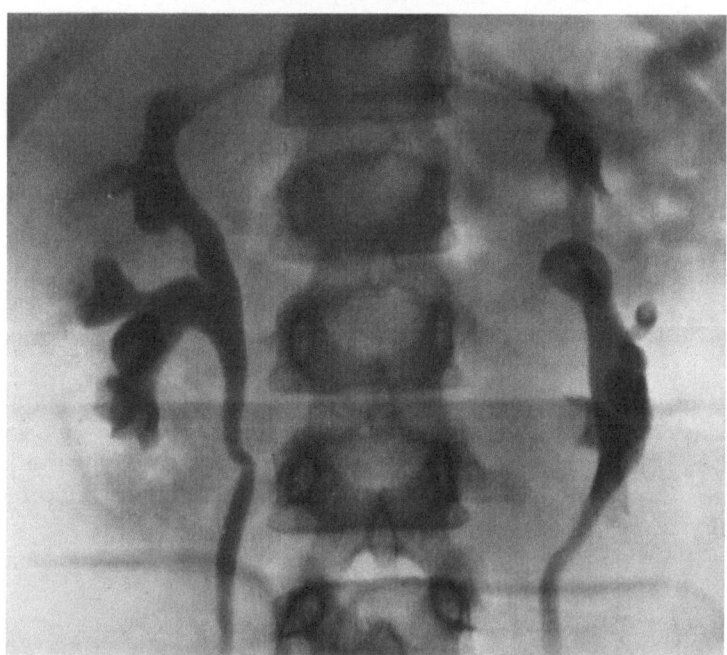

Fig. 59

Fig. 58 and Fig. 59. Malrotation. Urography: different types of unilateral malrotation

malrotated kidneys in which the kidney pelvis has been projected completely within the contour of the kidney. The malrotation may be unilateral or bilateral (Figs. 58, 59, 60).

Vascular anomalies are common in malrotated kidneys. Most malrotated kidneys have a short and straight supplementary artery running from a low abdominal segment to the posterior part of its lower pole. The course and straightness of this artery give the impression that it has arrested further rotation of the kidney (BOIJSEN, 1959).

Malrotation is often seen in association with other malformations, such as caudal ectopia and fusion.

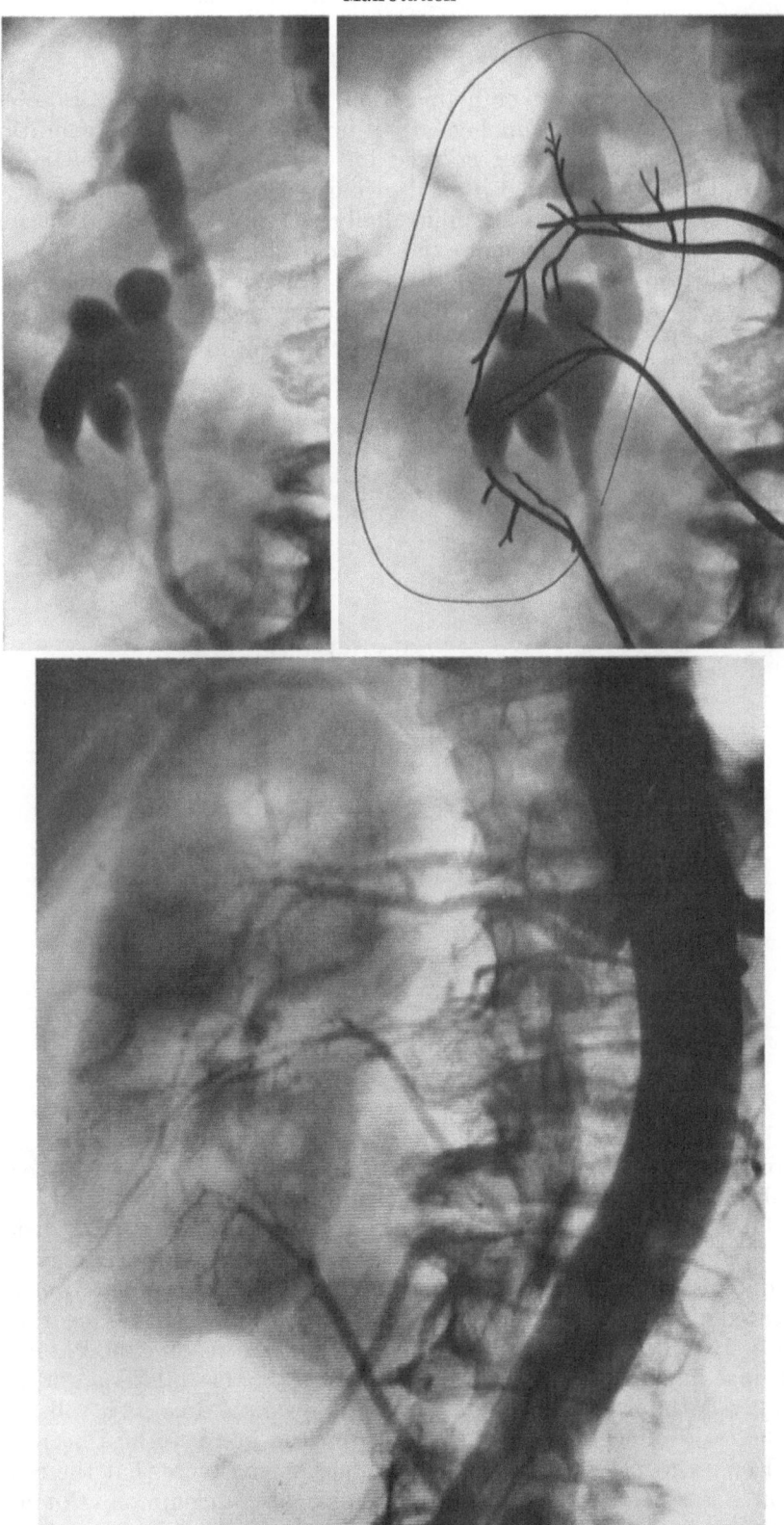

Fig. 60. Slight malrotation. Urography: so-called intrarenal kidney pelvis. Calyces in lower pole directed medially. Urogram and diagramatic superimposition of arteriogram showing the relation between kidney pelvis and arteries

IV. Ectopia

Ectopia means displacement or malposition. The term dystopia is sometimes used
to designate the condition, but etymologically it implies a more serious condition, for which
it should be reserved. It should not be used for the whole group. Renal ectopia means
that one or both kidneys are malpositioned owing to defective development. The kidney
may be displaced caudally, cranially or medially. Caudal and cranial ectopia are often
referred to under the common name of axial or longitudinal ectopia. Caudal displacement
of the kidney is the most common type (Figs. 61, 62). Various types may be recognized,
such as the pelvic type, which means that the kidney is located in the true pelvis; the
iliac type where the kidney is found in the iliac fossa or opposite the crest of the ileum;

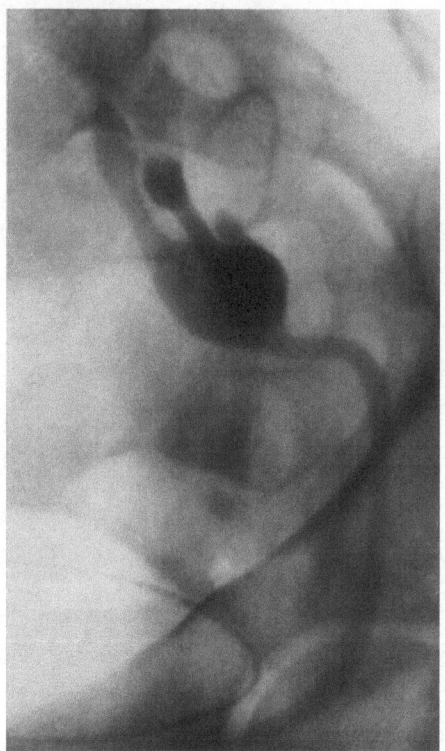

Fig. 61. Caudal ectopia. Pyelography. Malrotation, confluence of kidney pelvis situated anteriorly

and the abdominal type, where the kidney is fixed below the level of the second or third
lumbar vertebra and above the crest of the ileum (THOMPSON and PACE, 1937). An abdominal caudal ectopia may be difficult to distinguish from a caudal dislocation of a
kidney in an originally normal position, so-called mobile or ptosed kidney. In principle,
an ectopic kidney is understood as a kidney that has never occupied a normal position,
while a dislocated kidney has attained but not maintained its normal position (HARRISON
and BOTSFORD, 1946). Of 97 cases of caudal ectopia THOMPSON and PACE found pelvic
ectopia in 61, iliac in 8, and abdominal in 28. Of these, 4 were bilateral and in 8 cases the
ectopic kidney was the only one. The ectopic kidney may thus be a solitary kidney. A
collection of 66 cases of single ectopic kidney from the literature has been published by
BORELL and FERNSTRÖM (1954). Pelvic ectopia may be so severe that the renal pole may
be situated in a scrotal hernia. Bilateral ectopias are uncommon. COPPRIDGE (1934)
collected 21 cases of bilateral pelvic ectopia from the literature, to which he added one
of his own.

According to THOMAS and BARTON (1936) and CAMPBELL (1954) renal ectopia has been
found more frequently on roentgen examination (one out of 500 according to THOMAS

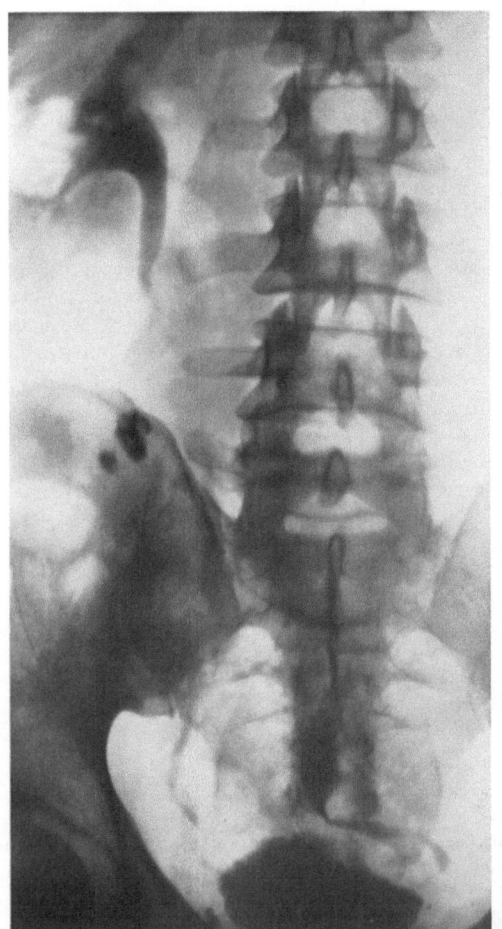

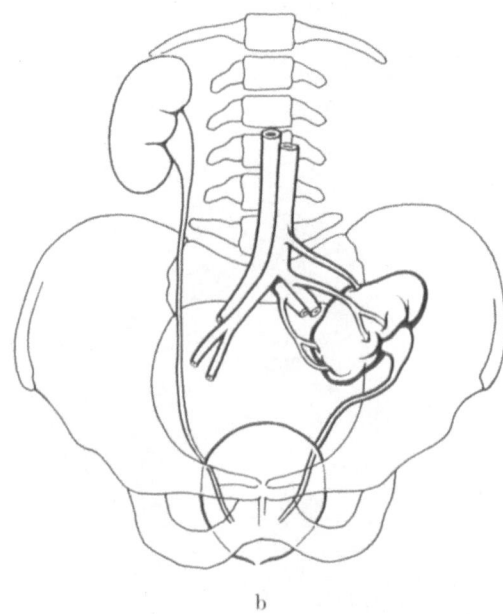

b

Fig. 62. Pelvic ectopia. a) Urography: good excretion of contrast urine from ectopic kidney to the left in pelvis. b) Schematic representation of similar case. (After STAEHLER)

a

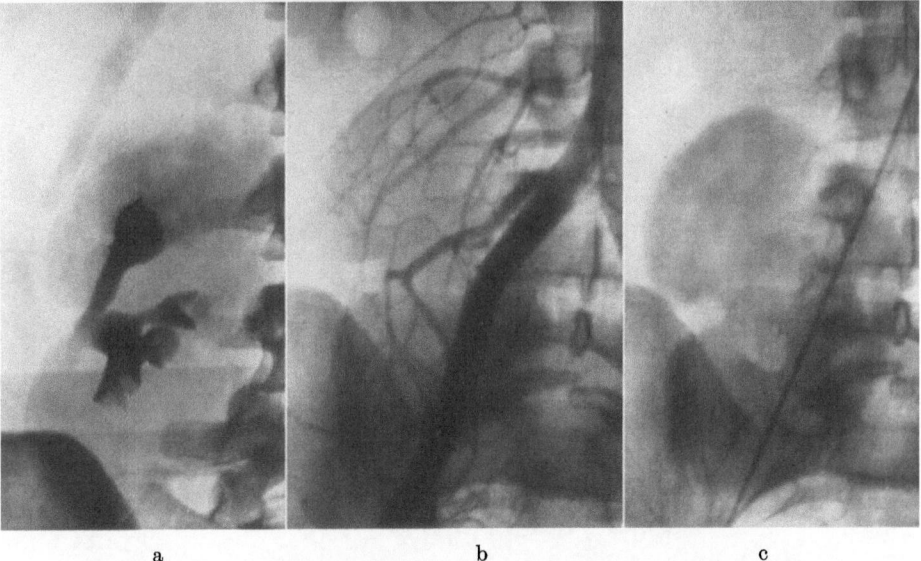

a   b   c

Fig. 63. Iliac caudal ectopia with marked malrotation. Examination because of recurrent severe pains on right side. a) Urography: kidney pelvis occupies a ventral, lateral position. Hilum of kidney points laterally. b) Aortic renal angiography: multiple arteries to right kidney, the most caudal artery taking its origin from the iliac artery. c) Nephrogram clearly demonstrates position of hilum. At operation, upper $1/3$ of kidney found to be pressed between an anterior and a posterior artery and vein, forming deep impressions in the parenchyma. Resection of this part of kidney. Patient completely free of pain

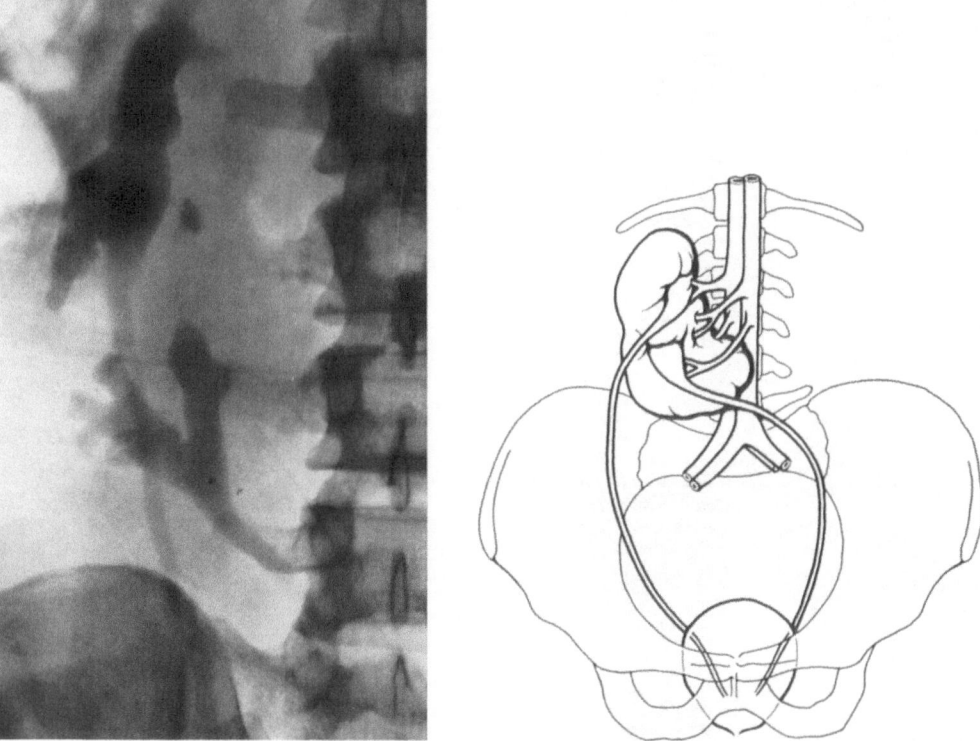

Fig. 64. Medial dystopia (crossed dystopia) and fusion. Both ureters open in bladder at normal site. Schematic representation of similar case. (After Staehler)

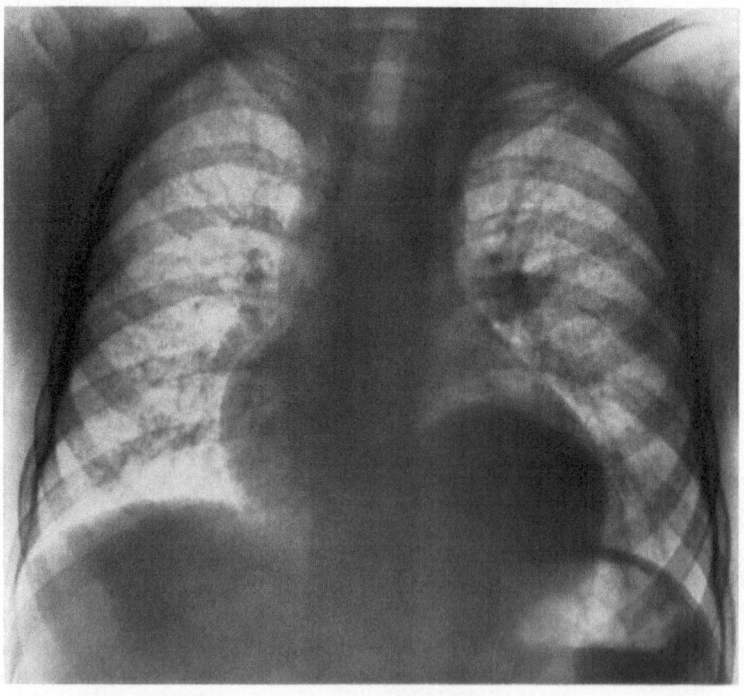

a

Fig. 65. Cranial dystopy. a) and b) chest examination: large expansive mass medially-posteriorly in left part of chest. c) Urography: expansivity represents the upper half of a cranially ectopic left kidney

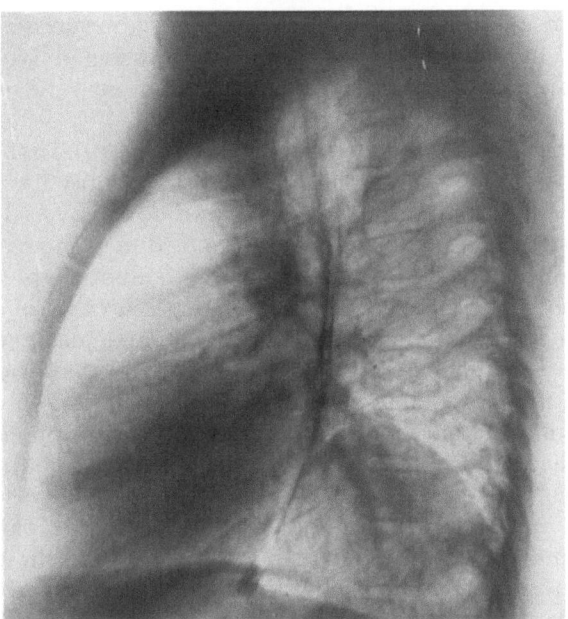

Fig. 65 b

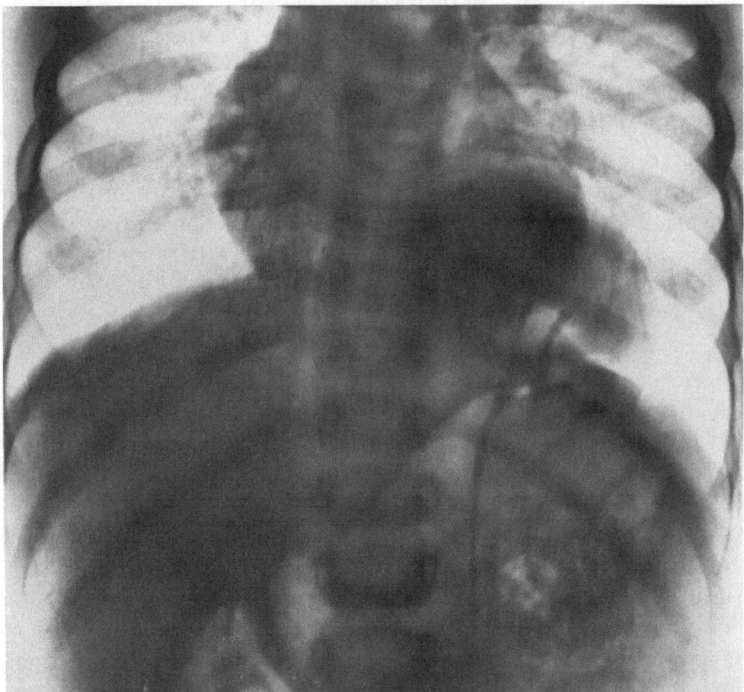

Fig. 65 c

and BARTON, 1936) than in autopsy series (one out of 700—1,000). The frequency with which the condition is seen at autopsy will, of course, vary with the thoroughness of the examination, the criteria used and the composition of the material, *i.e.* whether it consists mainly of urologic cases. An over-representation may be assumed in urologic cases because pathologic conditions such as stone and hydronephrosis are more common in renal ectopia.

Caudal ectopia is often combined with malrotation (Fig. 63).

Pelvic ectopy is of obstetric importance because it may complicate delivery. As a rule, a pelvic ectopic kidney is pushed out of the pelvis during delivery, but if the existence of the anomaly is known, delivery by caesarean section may be considered (ANDERSON et al., 1951).

Ectopia may also be cranial (SPILLANE and PRATHER, 1949). In this rare type of anomaly the kidney is localized more cranially than normally and may have reached the level of, or passed through, the diaphragm into the thorax and be discovered on roentgen examination of the chest. Its passage through the diaphragm is due to migration through the foetal hiatus pleuroperitonealis, which does not close but persists as a diaphragmatic defect, the so-called foramen of Bochdalek. In fact, in recent years such cases of ectopia have been discovered in association with mass chest radiography, particularly when the examination included lateral views, in which the kidney is seen as a mass in the posterior part of one of the sinuses. Unless this possibility is borne in mind, cranial ectopia may be mistaken for diaphragmatic tumor (Fig. 65). Cranial ectopia occurs on occasion in association with eventration of the diaphragm (BULGRIN and HOLMES, 1955).

Medial dystopia is usually called crossed dystopia. Both kidneys then lie on the same side (Fig. 64). The ureteric orifice is usually not ectopic, the ureter passing across the spine. The displaced kidney may be fused with or separated from the fellow kidney or the ectopic kidney may be the only kidney, the fellow kidney being hypo- or aplastic. The ectopic kidney, however, is often small and usually situated adjacent to the lower pole of the normally situated kidney. In only 7% of the cases is it adjacent to the upper pole (DAVIDSON, 1938). The kidney is also usually malrotated. According to ØDEGAARD (1946) it is more common in males than in females and the left kidney is more frequently ectopic than the right.

True crossed dystopia, i.e. the right kidney on the left side and the left kidney on the right, has been described by HARRIS (1939) under the name of double crossed ureters. He also reported that one of the ureters of a double kidney can cross the midline. The lower portion of a double kidney may thus be crossed. A kidney is then present also on the other side.

In this connection it might also be mentioned that the kidney may be located in a true lumbar hernia. This is a very rare type of hernia, and such a hernia containing a kidney is, of course, a great rarity (KRETSCHMER, 1951).

V. Fusion

Fusion here means that both kidneys are united. The commonest type is the horse-shoe kidney, in which the two lower poles are united, while the upper poles are separate. On occasion, though rarely, the upper poles of the kidneys may be united and the lower poles separate.

In plain roentgenograms of a horse-shoe kidney, kidneys with the caudal poles are seen to be directed towards the spine.

The longitudinal axes of the kidneys run parallel to that of the body, or converge caudally. The kidneys are often situated lower than usual and always rotate with their medial parts anteriorly. One can often see the outline of one kidney merge with that of the other. In such cases the kidneys are united by a bridge of parenchyma. On occasion, however, one or both renal poles are well outlined on either side of the spine, while their position and shape is otherwise characteristic of horse-shoe kidney. In such cases it may be assumed that the two kidneys are united only by a band of connective tissue. The anatomy of the renal parenchyma of a horse-shoe kidney can be studied best in the renal nephrogram. If the kidneys are united by a parenchymal bridge, it will show up distinctly in the nephrogram, while if the kidneys are joined only by a connective tissue-bridge, they will appear as separate formations in the nephrogram. At urography calyces on either side will be found to be directed medially and the renal pelvis to bend towards the midline (Figs. 66, 67). The course of the ureters varies with the sever

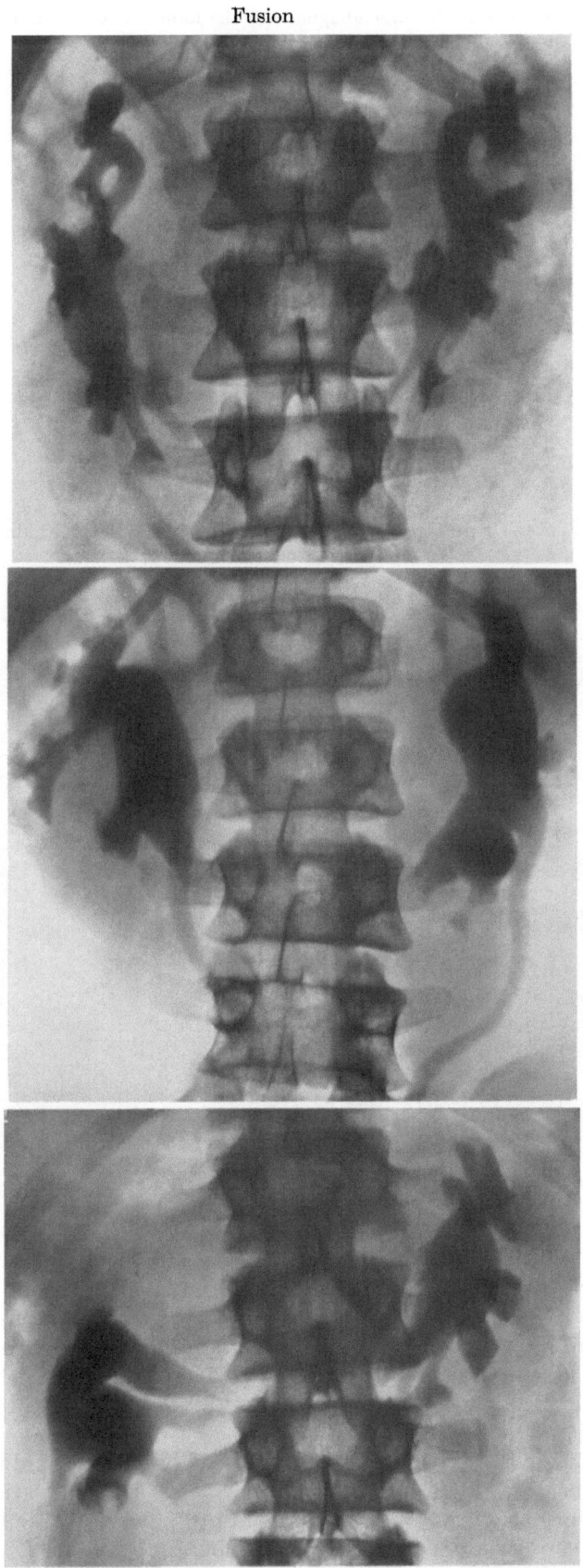

Fig. 66. Fusion. Urography: horse-shoe kidneys of different types

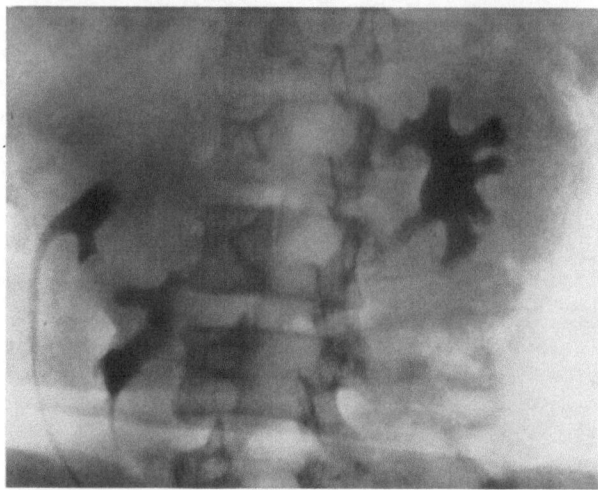

Fig. 67. Fusion. Urography: complex horse-shoe kidney with three kidney pelves

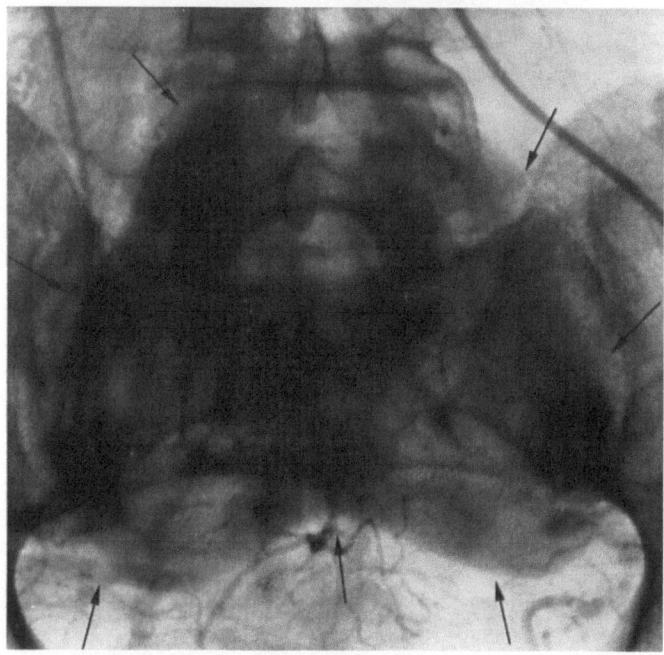

Fig. 68. Complete fusion of both kidneys to a conglomerate kidney with a common cranial pole. The conglomerate kidney is situated in the lumbo sacral region

ity of malrotation and deformation. The ureters extend from a lateral origin as a rule, and swing in a fairly sharp bend towards one another.

The degree of anomaly of a horse-shoe kidney varies widely from case to case. It may be slight, when two kidneys of almost ordinary shape but malrotated may be seen; or it may be severe: one kidney may be small, for example, and the other may be situated on the contralateral side with the course of the ureter resembling that in crossed ectopia (PETROVCIC and MILIC, 1956).

These last-mentioned, less charateristic types of horse-shoe kidney are transitional forms to severe types in which deformed kidneys are fused in various different ways. These types of malformations are referred to as lump kidney or cake kidney. Such fusion occurs in caudally ectopic kidneys particularly; therefore pelvic, fused kidneys are not very rare (Fig. 68). Such kidneys are markedly lobulated. It has been claimed (GLENN, 1958) that the calyceal configuration is abnormal (which is probably to be understood as hypoplasia) and that histologic examinations will reveal immature glomeruli, inter alia. Taken together these anomalies are purported to show that the development of the kidney has been arrested at approximately the ten-millimeter stage of embryonic development.

The pathologic conditions seen in horse-shoe kidney vary with the severity of the anomaly. Dilatation of the renal pelvis, often seen in horse-shoe kidneys, may thus vary widely from case to case. The obstructed drainage may result in stone formation and infection. Pelvic-fused, kidney, like pelvic-ectopic kidney, may be of obstetric importance. The reader is referred to a compilation of 94 cases of pregnant women with pelvic kidney by ANDERSON et al. (1951).

According to BOATMAN et al. (1972) about $1/3$ of patients with horseshoe kidney have associated congenital malformations, for example serious cardio-vascular and central nervous system anomalies.

In identical twins marked anomalies of the kidneys are usually identical. However, the literature contains sporadic reports of discordant abnormalities. LEITER (1972) gives a survey of the literature with presentation of one case where in a pair of identical twins one had normally paired kidneys, the other a horseshoe kidney.

VI. Vascular changes in renal anomalies

As mentioned in the introduction, vascular anomalies are common and important in association with other anomalies of the urinary tract. The more widely renal angiography is used, the greater will our knowledge become of associated vascular anomalies (OLLE OLSSON and WHOLEY, 1964), The frequency of vascular anomalies in connection with some of the severe anomalies described above is so high that they appear to be a regular accompaniment of all types of maldevelopment of the kidneys. Vascular anomalies appear to be the rule in malrotated kidneys. They usually consist of multiple renal arteries or of branches of a single renal artery with an anomalous course. The artery need not enter the kidney via the hilum; wide branches may instead pass directly into the renal parenchyma through the capsule from the side opposite the hilum. Both arterial and venous branches may embrace large or small parts of the kidney like tongs.

The branches then run along the dorsal and ventral surface toward the hilum. They may enter the hilum or they may pierce the renal capsule and pass directly into the parenchyma. The vessels may then lie so close to the renal parenchyma as to form ridges in it. We have seen a case in our department in which such a vascular tong pressed the kidney so as to cause stasis in the upper part of that organ, causing pain (OLLE OLSSON and JÖNSSON, 1962).

Horse-shoe kidneys almost always have multiple arteries, often a large number of these arising from the aorta and/or iliac arteries. This may cause hydronephrosis. Ectopic kidneys often have anomalous arteries, usually branching from an abnormally low segment. According to the anatomic literature, in cranial ectopia the artery extends from a high aortic segment.

In less severe anomalies such as calyceal anomalies and hypoplasia, vascular anomalies are less common.

Multiple renal arteries

Multiple renal arteries represent the most common vascular abnormality. The pattern of the renal vasculature in the kidney supplied by a single renal artery may vary widely, as mentioned above. The range of variation in the renal blood supply is widened still more by the numerous anomalies. In this respect multiple arteries are of significance.

Vessels deviating from the natural number are referred to in the literature by etymologically different names such as aberrant, accessory, abnormal, or supernumerary.

The nomenclature is all the more bewildering because some authors use one and the same name for different anomalies, while others use different names for the same thing. The nomenclature is misleading also in that it suggests the existence of an extra arterial supply to the kidney. There is no such extra supply, however. Like other arteries, multiple arteries are end-arteries. They often supply a large portion of the renal parenchyma, as a rule between 20 % and 50 % (McDonald and Kennelly, 1959). The vessels should therefore be referred to preferably as multiple or supplementary vessels.

Supernumerary renal arteries may have varying origins. In pelvic dystopy the renal artery may arise from the inferior mesenteric artery or the hypergastric artery or the middle sacral artery. Cases have been described in which a right accessory upper polar artery originated from the celiac artery and where supernumerary polar arteries to both kidneys had a common origin at the lower part of the lumbar aorta. The different types of unusual origin of renal arteries are reviewed with well motivated critical acumen by Jeffery (1972).

a) Anatomic investigations

The frequency of multiple arteries is given as 20%—25% in the anatomic literature. In a series of 2,562 kidneys Hou-Jensen (1930) found multiple arteries in 22.4%. As a rule supplementary arteries arise near the origin of the main renal artery but sometimes a fair distance from it, if it stems from the iliac artery, for example. Hellström (1928) found the longest distance to be 70 mm, while Seldowitsch (1909) found a vessel to originate 105 mm distal to the other arteries. Multiple arteries may course separately or together with a main artery into the renal hilum or directly into the parenchyma, depending on the distance of their origin from the renal artery (Graves, 1956).

In the anatomic literature opinions differ widely on the regions supplied by multiple arteries. A thorough investigation by Graves (1954, 1956) showed that the vessels are normal segmental arteries but arise extrarenally instead of intrarenally. He found multiple arteries coursing to the lower pole to be more common than others and related this to the fact that in 63% of these cases the lower polar artery was given off as the first branch of the renal artery when the latter was single (see below).

b) Angiographic studies

Edsman (1957) found multiple arteries in 21% of 1,240 kidneys. After exclusion of hydronephrotic kidneys the frequency was 20%. Our material (Boijsen, 1959) consisted of 638 kidneys, of which 152 (23.8%) had multiple arteries. After exclusion of hydronephrotic kidneys (64), multiple arteries were found in 20.6%.

Multiple arteries are not seen quite so frequently in angiographic studies as in autopsy series. According to Boijsen this can be explained by the fact that fine arteries coursing to the two cranial pyramids and supplying at most one renculus do not always show up in the film because they are too thin. The possibility of the existence of fine vessels not demonstrable in the angiogram should be borne in mind in contemplated partial nephrectomy.

Multiple arteries are of smaller caliber than the main renal artery as a rule, but not always (Fig. 69).

c) Level of origin

Of 101 kidneys in our material in which the level of origin of the supplementary arteries could be judged, 50 originated at a distance of up to 19 mm from the renal artery, of which 7 arose cranially thereto. Nineteen arose 20—39 mm, ten 40 to 50 mm and four 60—70 mm from the renal artery. Thus the frequency of multiple arteries decreased with increasing distance from the main artery. After a distance of 80 mm, however, the frequency again began to increase and as many as 18 kidneys were in that group (Boijsen).

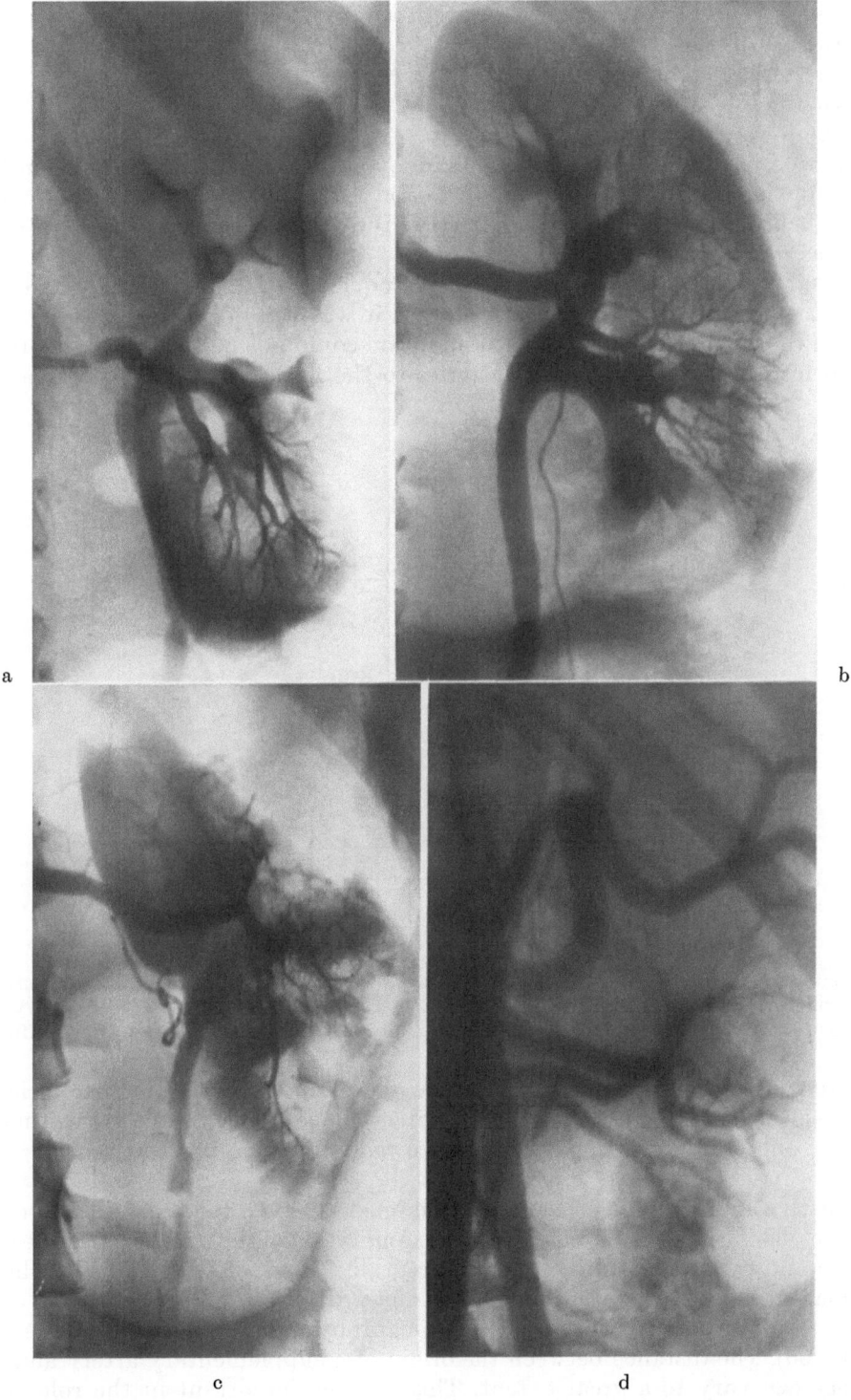

Fig. 69. Angiography in multiple renal arteries: three arteries to left kidney, a, b, and c. Each of the three arteries is catheterized selectively. d) Arteriographic phase: aortic injection demonstrating the three arteries to the kidney

The distribution of supplementary arteries in our material is:

    to the upper pole 14 %;

    to the middle ventral segment 5.5 %;

    to the middle dorsal segment 14 %;

    to the lower pole segment 72.5 %.

It is clear from the figures that some kidneys were supplied by more than two renal arteries. Supplementary arteries coursing to the lower pole were most common. Of 134 kidneys with only one supplementary artery, the latter supplied pyramids in the pars inferior in as many as 95 (71%).

Graves, as mentioned, ascribed the high frequency of supplementary arteries to the lower pole to the fact that in 63% of his cases it was the first artery to leave the renal artery when the latter was single. This assumption could not be confirmed in our material. The reason for the high frequency of arteries to the lower pole may be instead, that all

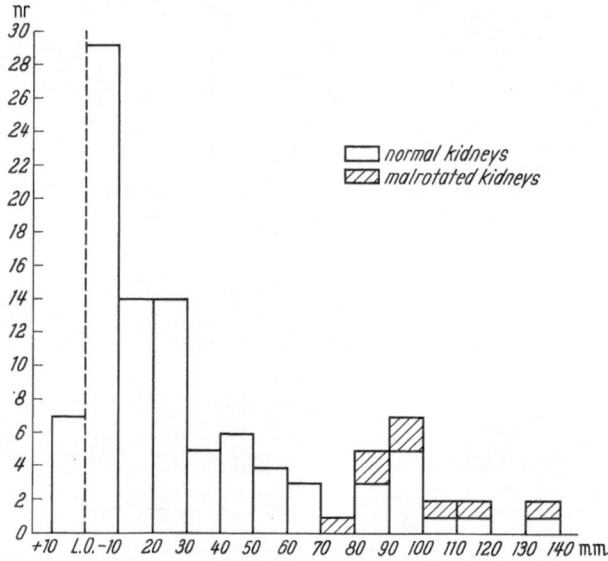

Fig. 70. Variations in distance between origin of supplementary artery to caudal pole and main artery in well rotated and malrotated kidneys with multiple arteries. L. O. Level of origin of the main artery. + and — denote origin of the supplementary artery cranially and caudally respectively to the main artery. (After Boijsen)

supplementary arteries near the main artery represent persisting mesonephric arteries. These vessels degenerate in craniocaudal direction so that the vessels situated most caudally are obliterated last and are therefore most likely to persist in adults (Boijsen, 1959).

At selective angiography special attention must be given to the possibility of multiple renal arteries. This can always be checked by examination of the pattern of the vessels in the arteriogram and by examination of the nephrogram for any defects. This is achieved best by examination of the kidney in more than one projection. Should multiple arteries be demonstrated or suspected, aortic renal angiography should be performed (see, for example, Fig. 60). The distance between the origin of a supplementary artery and the main renal artery can vary to a great extent. This may be important in the role of such an artery as the cause of hydronephrosis. The variations have been studied by Boijsen (1959) (see Fig. 70).

If the catheter for selective angiography is passed into a small supplementary artery and the entire dose of contrast medium deposited there, it will result in high concentration of the medium in a small portion of the kidney (Ljunggren and Edsman, 1955) with a pathologic nephrogram as a consequence.

If the tip of the catheter lies in the main renal artery but a supplementary artery is present, branches to a portion of the kidney will be missing in the arteriogram. The absence of such a filling is more obvious in the nephrogram, however. The region supplied by the supplementary artery not filled with contrast medium will then appear as a defect in the nephogram and will be diffusely outlined against the remainder of the renal parenchyma. Unless the possibility of a supplementary artery is borne in mind, this may result in an erroneous diagnosis. If the artery is very narrow, the region it supplies may be so small as not to show up in the nephrogram. Such fine supplementary arteries occasionally course to the upper pole and escape detection in the arteriogram and nephrogram, as previously mentioned. The clinical importance of supplementary arteries is discussed in Chapter K., I. 3.

VII. Renal angiography in anomalies

Renal angiography is often helpful in the investigation of renal and urinary tract anomalies. Fusion, double kidneys and malrotations of different types may occasionally offer differential diagnostic difficulties and in plain roentgenography, urography or pyelography may be suspected of representing tumor, for example. Renal angiography helps to solve the differential diagnostic problem. In hypoplasia, particularly if local, as well as in other types of parenchymal malformations, renal angiography may be useful in determining more exactly the amount of functioning renal parenchyma and its distribution. Angiography may be valuable for differentiation between aplasia and ectopia.

In cases of contemplated operation for malformation, knowledge of the frequently bizarre vasculature is important. As already pointed out, multiple arteries arising at different levels from the aorta and/or iliac arteries are common in renal malformations and increase in frequency with the complexity of the malformation. Horse-shoe kidney may consist of two separate kidneys united only by a narrow neck of connective tissue or may be a true conglomerate kidney. Any doubt in this respect can be cleared up by renal angiography, particularly the nephrogram, and at the same time the amount of renal parenchyma in different parts of a conglomerate kidney can be demonstrated. This is important in cases of contemplated operation for stone or hydronephrosis in part of such a kidney.

A case with an aberrant branch from the left renal artery supplying part of the right kidney in a patient with no connecting parenchyma between the two kidneys is described by LIBSHILTZ et al. (1972).

As mentioned in the chapter on vascular anomalies, malformations are sometimes dominated by the bizarre appearance of vessels, which makes angiography a rational method in the investigation of many anomalies. Clinically important changes, often combined with multiple vessels, as in hydronephrosis, require angiography.

To summarize, it may be concluded that anomalies are common in the calyces, renal pelvis, and ureter, and that grave anomalies such as ectopia, fusion, malrotation, hypoplasia are not uncommon. These anomalies are due to disturbances in embryo-dynamics and therefore often appear in combination. The earlier such disturbances occur in foetal life the more complex the anomalies will be. Anomalies of this type are often closely connected to the development of the vasculature. Renal angiography is therefore an important method in the investigation of anomalies.

It cannot be stressed enough that anomalies of the urinary tract are often multiple. It has even been questioned by FELTON (1959) whether it might not be wise to consider urography indicated in all cases of such readily demonstrable anomalies as cryptorchism and hypospadia. Of 61 patients with undescended testes urography showed unsuspected significant anomalies of the upper urinary tract in 13.5%, and in 9% of 45 patients with hypospadia.

It may finally be stressed that grave anomalies of the urinary tract are often seen in association with anomalies in other parts of the organism.

VIII. Ureteric anomalies

Ureteric anomalies have been described under the heading of blind ureter, and a deviating course of the ureter in association with renal anomalies has also been described in connection with fusion, ectopia and malrotation of the kidneys.

1. Retro-caval ureter

Another unusual but often characteristic and important deviation from the ordinary course is that shown by the ante-ureteric inferior caval vein, usually known as retro-caval, post-caval or circum-caval ureter. As indicated by the name, the right ureter passes behind or round the inferior caval vein from a position lateral and ventral to the vein to a point medial to it. Several variants of the course of the ureter in relation to anomalous veins can be seen. It should be observed that this abnormal course of the ureter is secondary to a venous anomaly, which is indicated by the correct name given above. Left-sided retrocaval ureter has been seen in connection with situs inversus (Brooks, 1962).

On occasion the distal portion of the right ureter contacts the inferior caval vein but is not displaced by it. In the anomaly under discussion the ureter is situated roughly at the level between its upper and middle third behind the vein, and is compressed between the latter and the posterior abdominal wall and aorta, respectively. In such cases the ureter will be bent medially and displaced backwards and its cranial segment and the renal pelvis will be dilated. The impression caused by the vein may be considerable. The medially bent portion of the ureter may cross the midline and the distal two-thirds may run relatively close to the midline.

The embryonic development of the caval vein is briefly as follows: The vein arises from a venous system originally consisting of three different venous trunks on either side of the midline and anastomosing richly with one another. Their arrangement in medio-lateral and dorso-ventral direction and their transverse anastomoses give them the shape of a tunnel through which the kidney passes during its ascent. The post-cardinal vein runs anteriorly and laterally to the ureter. During embryonic life that segment of the vein caudal to the kidney atrophies and the inferior caval vein develops from the right and left supra-cardinal veins. The ureter thus lies lateral to the vein. However, in some cases the caval vein is formed from the post-cardinal vein instead, in which case the ureter lies behind the caval vein and it will follow medially the anterior aspect of the vein. Thus the anomalous course of the ureter is caused by a persisting post-cardinal vein forming the inferior caval vein. The anomaly can vary widely with double caval vein in which, for example, the post-cardinal and supra-cardinal veins both persist and each forms its own caval vein. In one case retro-caval position of the ureter has been found to be bilateral in association with grave renal malformation. All cases on record are otherwise right-sided. A detailed description has been given by Sesboue (1952). One case of retro-caval ureter and solitary kidney has been described by Laughlin (1954). It is pointed out by Arne Nilsson (1960) that the changes in the size and shape of the kidney pelvis and ureter caused by this anomaly can be uncharacteristic. Cavography is a rational diagnostic method.

Other common anomalies may cause changes of the same type as retrocaval ureter (Dreyfuss, 1959).

The ovarian vein, if dilated, may cause indentation in one or both ureters (Melnick and Bramwit, 1971). Occasionally the indentation, displacement and dilatation of the right ureter may resemble changes caused by the retro-caval ureter.

Mehl (1969) reports a case of a young girl with multiple congenital anomalies including a ureteral stenosis secondary to iliac artery—iliac vein compression.

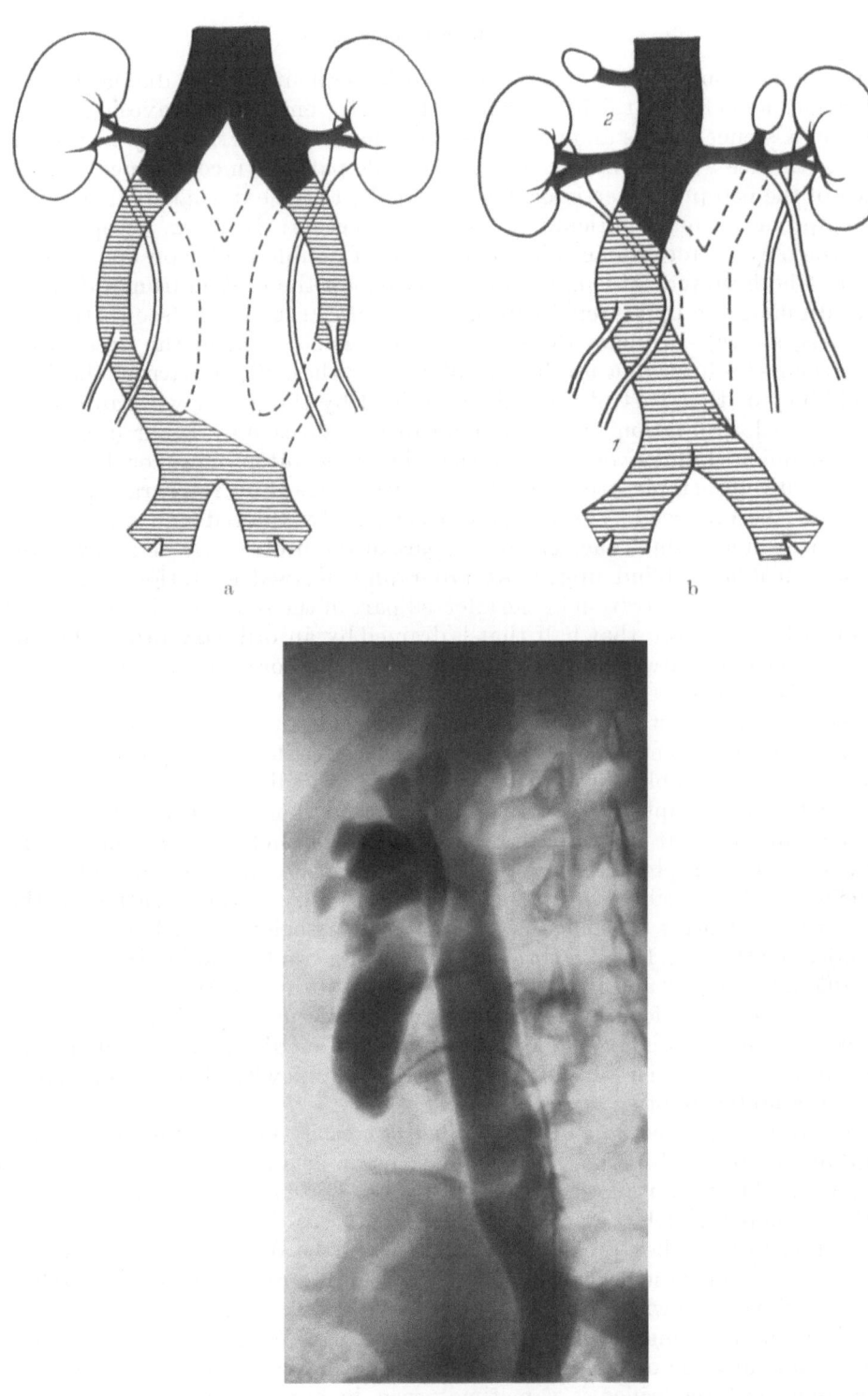

Fig. 71. a and b Schematic drawings of development of retrocaval ureter in two stages demonstrating venous segments partaking in formation of inferior caval vein anteriorly to ureter. 1. from posterior cardinal veins; 2. from subcardinal veins (after SESBOÜE). c) Retrocaval ureter. Simultaneous pyelography and cavography: kidney pelvis and proximal part of ureter markedly dilated; ureter (catheter) swings behind inferior caval vein

2. Ureters with ectopic orifice

An uncommon but important anomaly which frequently offers diagnostic difficulties is a ureter with an ectopic orifice, i. e. where the ureter empties extravesically. The possibility of the existence of this anomaly must be considered, particularly in the investigation of incontinence and in obscure pyuria. (In male patients incontinence is rare because the orifice of the ectopic ureter is located proximally to the external sphincter. The dominating symptom in male patients is urinary infection). Such an ectopic orifice may belong to the only ureter on one side, or, in cases of double ureter on one side, to one of the two or to both ureters. It is most commonly one of the ureters from a double kidney, the ureter draining the upper renal pelvis, that empties ectopically (see section on double kidney pelvis, above). In males the ectopic orifice is situated in the urethra or genital organs, in females in the vagina, urethra or vulva. Since the orifice is narrow, the flow of urine from the kidney or that part of the kidney drained by the ureter with an ectopic orifice often is impaired. Dilatation and functional disturbances may occur (see Chapter K). The corresponding kidney or part of the kidney is often more or less hypoplastic.

Ureters with an ectopic orifice can be readily diagnosed by retrograde pyelography if the orifice can be observed. The ureter is then usually dilated and the corresponding renal pelvis is seen as a small sac. The distal part of the ureter may be severely distended and resemble a dilated blind ureter. At urography delayed excretion will occasionally be found, with poor concentration in the affected part of the renal pelvis. In double kidney, excretion can be seen from that half that is drained by an ordinary ureter, in which case existence of a second dilated renal pelvis can be concluded or suspected. (A source of error in the diagnosis of suspected ectopic orifice of a ureter by urography is the so-called ureter jet. The stream of contrast medium from the jet should not be mistaken for an extension of a ureter). In male patients the ectopic ureter may have its orifice in the seminal vesicle, in which case it is possible through vesiculography to fill the ureter. (GOLDSTEIN and HELLER, 1956, for example). When the ectopic ureter has its orifice in the urethra, a filling can be obtained at urethrocystography. The parenchyma can be studied more closely by renal angiography (see Chapter K). A retrograde filling can be obtained via the ductus deferens and possibly via the seminal vesicles by catheterization of the orifice of a ductus ejaculatorius in colliculus seminalis in association with urethroscopy and contrast injection (ENGEL, 1948). A corresponding filling can be obtained by vesiculography (MEISEL, 1952). HAMILTON and PEYTON (1950) and PASQUIER and WOMACK (1953) described a case in which a cystic formation protruding into the urinary bladder was punctured in association with cystoscopy and in which contrast medium was injected. The cystic formation proved to consist of a dilated ureter and likewise dilated seminal vesicles, into which the ureter emptied.

The occurrence of an ectopic ureteric orifice can easily be explained from an embryologic point of view on the basis of the close relationship between the Wolffian duct and the urogenital sinus. The ureter arises as a bud from the Wolffian duct, from which the posterior urethra, seminal vesicles, ejaculatory ducts and vas deferens develop in males. In females Gartner's duct, when present, is a rudiment of the Wolffian duct, which also gives rise to the urethra and vestibulum vaginae. The Wolffian duct is intimately related with the urogenital sinus from which the major part of the proximal urethra is formed in males, and the vestibulum vaginae in females. More difficult to explain are those rare cases in which an ectopic ureteric orifice is seen within the uterus and in the rectum.

An ectopic ureteric orifice is sometimes seen in association with complex malformations.

3. Ureteric valve

A few cases of valve in the ureter have been described. The valve may have the form of an iris, with a central opening, and be unilateral or bilateral (WALL and WACHTER,

1952). It can be situated at any level of the ureter, also at the ureterovesical junction (FOROGHI and TURNER, 1959).

E. Nephro- and Ureterolithiasis

Stone in the upper urinary tract is a common disease. Often, however, it is not a disease sui generis but, rather, a sign of some other disease or a result of some other pathologic process. It can be not only an independent clinical entity but also a complication in other diseases. The occurrence of urinary calculi in association with infection, malformations, long bed rest, metabolic disorders, certain genetic characteristics, etc., makes the diagnosis of nephro- and ureterolithiasis richly faceted. Acute attacks of renal colic add to the diagnosis a dramatic touch; they spotlight fundamental aspects of the pathophysiology of the urinary tract and, in addition, present important differential-diagnostic problems.

Lithiasis is of great practical importance from a urologic point of view as it is a common cause of renal damage. This is clearly stressed by the fact that about one third of all nephrectomies are necessary because of stone (DODSON, 1956). The importance of a refined method of roentgen examination including evaluation of renal function is obvious if the disease is to be diagnosed with reliable detailed information on various relevant aspects in order to permit timely institution of adequate conservative therapy and avoid nephrectomy.

I. Chemical composition of stones

Demonstration of stones in the upper urinary tract in plain radiography depends on their chemical composition, *i. e.* on their content of radiopaque material. Most stones contain calcium and can therefore be demonstrated in plain roentgenograms.

Table 3. *Components identified in urinary calculi by x-ray diffraction and their frequency of occurrence.* (After LAGERGREN)

| Chemical name | Chemical formula | Mineralogical name | Percentage frequency of occurrence | | |
			Kidneyureter (460 cases)	Bladder (140 cases)	Total (600 cases)
1. Calcium oxalate monohydrate	$CaC_2O_4 \cdot H_2O$	Whewellite	52.4	26.4	46.3
2. Calcium oxalate dihydrate	$CaC_2O_4 \cdot 2 H_2O$	Weddellite	52.0	24.3	45.5
3. Calcium hydrogen phosphate dihydrate (CHPD)	$CaHPO_4 \cdot 2 H_2O$	Brushite	2.6	6.4	3.5
4. Tricalcium phosphate (TCP)	$Ca_3(PO_4)_2$	Whitlockite	1.3	1.5	1.3
5. Basic calcium phosphate, "apatite"	$Ca_{10}(PO_4)_6(OH)_2$	Hydroxyapatite	75.8	68.0	74.0
6. Magnesium ammonium phosphate hexahydrate (MAPH), "triple phosphate"	$MgNH_4PO_4 \cdot 6 H_2O$	Struvite	30.2	45.0	33.7
7. Calcium sulfate dihydrate	$CaSO_4 \cdot 2 H_2O$	Gypsum	—	0.7	0.2
8. Uric acid	$C_5H_4N_4O_3$		3.9	24.3	8.7
9. Ammonium hydrogen urate	$NH_4C_5H_3N_4O_3$		0.2	10.0	2.5
10. Sodium hydrogen urate monohydrate	$NaC_5H_3N_4O_3 \cdot H_2O$		—	0.7	0.2
11. Cystine	$[SCH_2CH(NH_2)\text{-}COOH]_2$		1.1	1.4	1.2

8*

The composition of the stones has been described by many authors. Most data available are based on chemical examination, however. Since practically all urinary calculi are crystalline, they should preferably be analysed by means of physical methods used in the study of minerals, particularly X-ray diffraction. TOVBORG JENSEN & THYGESEN (1938) used this method in their analysis of stones from 111 patients. The largest material studied by the method is that described by PRIEN & FRONDEL (1947). Their series consisted of 1,000 cases, afterwards increased to 6,000. In a report by PRIEN in 1963 the material is 25,000. The crystalline components of urinary calculi are: calcium oxalate monohydrate, calcium oxalate dihydrate, magnesium ammonium phosphate hexahydrate, carbonate-apatite and hydroxyl-apatite, calcium hydrogen phosphate dihydrate, uric acid, cystine and sodium acid urate.

Pure calcium oxalate calculi represented 36.1 per cent of the total; mixed calcium oxalate-apatite calculi comprised 31.0 per cent; together they composed 67.1 per cent of the total. These calculi usually occurred in acid, sterile urine.

Pure magnesium ammonium phosphate hexahydrate, pure apatite and mixed magnesium ammonium phosphate hexahydrate-apatite calculi represented 19.5 per cent of the total. These calculi usually occurred in alcaline, infected urine.

Calcium hydrogen phosphate dihydrate occurred in 1.6 per cent of calculi. Uric acid and cystine existed more frequently in pure than mixed form and occurred in 6.1 per cent and 3.8 per cent of the series, respectively.

Sodium acid urate occurred but once in the series and then only in microscopic amount. It was the only urate found.

PRIEN (1955) summarized: There are apparently only three important crystalline substances in calcium-containing calculi. They are calcium oxalate monohydrate, calcium phosphate (or apatite as it has been called) and magnesium ammonium phosphate. In addition, uric acid and cystine are of clinical importance.

LAGERGREN (1956) published 600 cases examined by x-ray crystallography, microradiography and x-ray micro-diffraction. His figures agree well with those given above (see Table 3). The survey shows the existence of 11 distinct crystalline substances occurring either in pure or in mixed form. It is clear from the table that 460 of the stones were renal or ureteric calculi and 140 were calculi of the urinary bladder. The percentage distribution of the components present in calculi of the kidney and ureter differed significantly from that of the calculi recovered from the urinary bladder. Uric acid stones, for example, were much more common in the urinary bladder than in the kidney or ureter.

The most common component of the calculi was apatite, but only 3.9% of the samples were made of pure apatite. In all cases but one, multiple concrements from the same individual were of identical composititition.

In order to obtain accurate information on stone composition in a short time and by use of a simple method, GIAN-CHINSEI (1961) has used infrared spectroscopy for analysis. He considers this to be the ideal method for studying the composition, which is fundamental to an understanding of the etiology of stone formation and essential to the treatment and prevention of stone. Stones usually contain the same components in the nucleus and outer layers, but occasionally the components vary. BOYCE et al. (1958) in a microradiographic comparison of crystalline structure by microscopic and histo-chemical studies, found that the organic matrix is a prerequisite to concrement formation and that crystal deposition is a secondary phenomenon. Size, shape, lamination, and radial striations are determined primarily by the mucoprotein matrix.

Analysis of urinary calculi may be of importance from a therapeutic point of view. It may give information as to specific causes of formation of certain types of stone and be a guide in preventing further formation (WINER, 1959). When the etiology of stone is unknown, "the chemical composition indicates the type of isohydruria which permits each particular crystalloid to be precipitated with its associated matrix. Isohydruria may be changed by proper utilization of drug and dietary means".

II. Age, sex, and side involved

On perusal of the records at our department, renal and ureteric calculi were found to be twice as common in males as in females. In males the disease was found to be most common between the ages of 40 and 50, in females between the ages of 20 and 30. However, the disease was roughly equally prevalent in all age groups except in the 0—10 year group, in which it had by far the lowest occurrence. Stone in the upper urinary tract is fairly uncommon in childhood, except in association with bed rest because of fracture. However, the possibility of calculi should always be considered in children with diffuse abdominal pain.

The frequencies given for urinary calculi in children are usually high but vary widely. The explanation may be that bladder stones are extremely common in tropical regions, particularly in boys.

Of 900 patients in our material, approximately 800 had stone on one side only and 100 on both. The unilateral cases occurred equally often on either side. The concrements were much more frequently situated in the caudal calyces and the confluence of the renal pelvis than in the middle and cranial calyces. The combination of stone in the kidney pelvis and stone in the ureter should always be kept in mind.

III. Size and shape of stones

Calculi vary widely in both size and shape; they range from minute stones hardly possible to detect, to large stones with branches filling the entire renal pelvis and additional cavities caused by parenchymal destruction in communication with the renal pelvis.

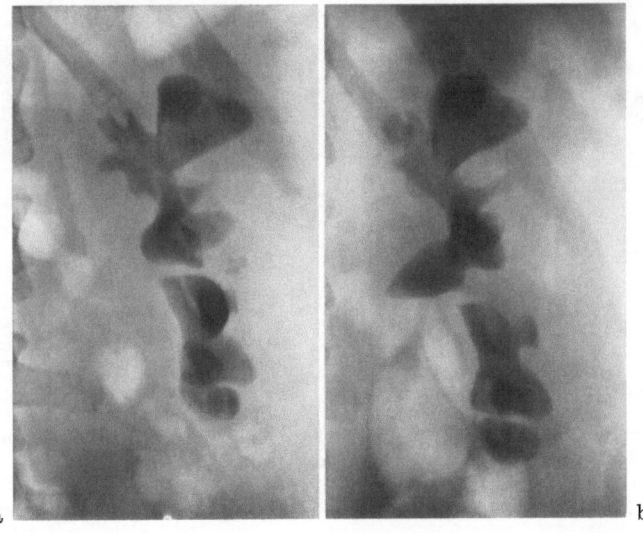

a   b

Fig. 72. Staghorn calculus with multiple fragments. In b) one fragment has changed position and plugs pelviureteric junction. (Patient examined because of pain)

Solitary stones are about 3 times as common as multiple stones. It is, however, sometimes difficult to decide whether a stone is solitary or not. Determination of the number of stones or their shape, requires films taken in different projections.

The kidneys may contain very small calculi in a papilla or one stone moulded to a calyx or a calyx with its stem. The cast may fill the entire renal pelvis or one of its branches. In such cases the shape of the stones will usually show that the calyces are more or less severely dilated. These calyx-shaped stones occasionally have amorphous calcareous extensions reaching the surface of the kidney and thereby demonstrating severe dilatation of calyces or primary tissue destruction with calcareous deposits. These milk of calcium renal stones consist of an amorphous mass of calcareous sand and are usually situated in a hydrocalyx or a pyelogenic cyst. The shape of the deposit usually changes with the posture of the patient. The phenomenon is analogous to limy bile in the gallbladder. Small calculi may be seen lateral to a large stone, which calculi shift position

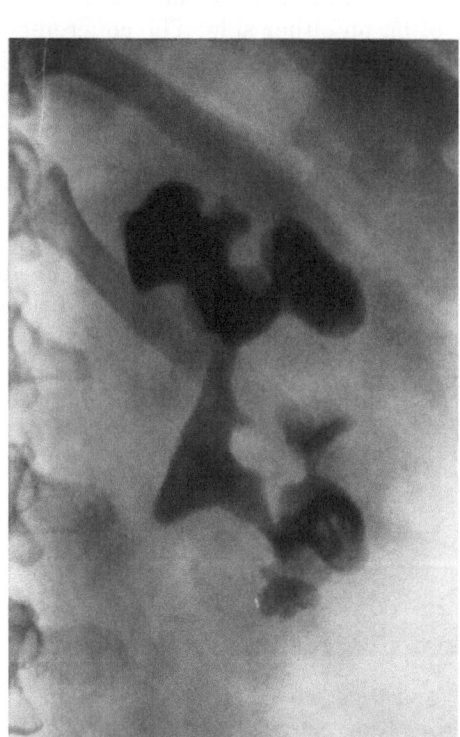

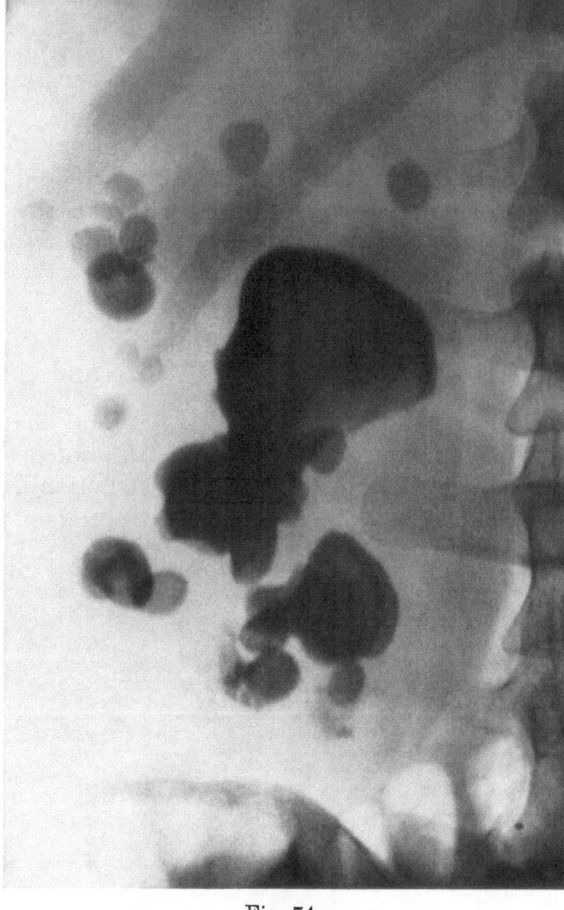

Fig. 73   Fig. 74

Fig. 73. Staghorn calculus, Shape of stone shows that calyces are dilated, whereas branches and confluence are narrow

Fig. 74. Multiple stones in pyonephrosis with peripheral stones in dilated calyces

within the kidney upon change of posture of the patient. Such stones are situated in a hydrocalyx or in some other space formed upon the obstruction of drainage by the jackstone. One or more stones, often fragmented stag-horn stones, are sometimes seen to shift within a dilated renal pelvis.

Concrement often completely fills the confluence and assumes the original anatomic shape of the latter (Figs. 72—74). Occasionally a well defined break can be seen in the middle of a stag-horn calculus or the shape of the stone is modelled not only to the basic anatomy of the kidney pelvis but can also be influenced by arterial branches, for example. Staghorn stones vary widely in shape and site of formation and extent, and any dilatation of the pelvis and calyces. That part of the concrement corresponding to the confluence is often slender, while the peripheral parts formed in the dilated calyces and in regions of parenchymal destruction are plump. The slender part is a cast of the contracted confluence and corresponds to what is said below about the shape of the confluence when it harbors a calculus.

In renal anomalies the site and shape of calculi may indicate the type of anomaly, e. g. double kidney (Figs. 75—78), horse-shoe kidney, malrotation. In papillary necrosis, shed tissue gathers calcium to form concrements. These stones are often of a characteristic papillary shape and thereby betray the nature of the fundamental disease.

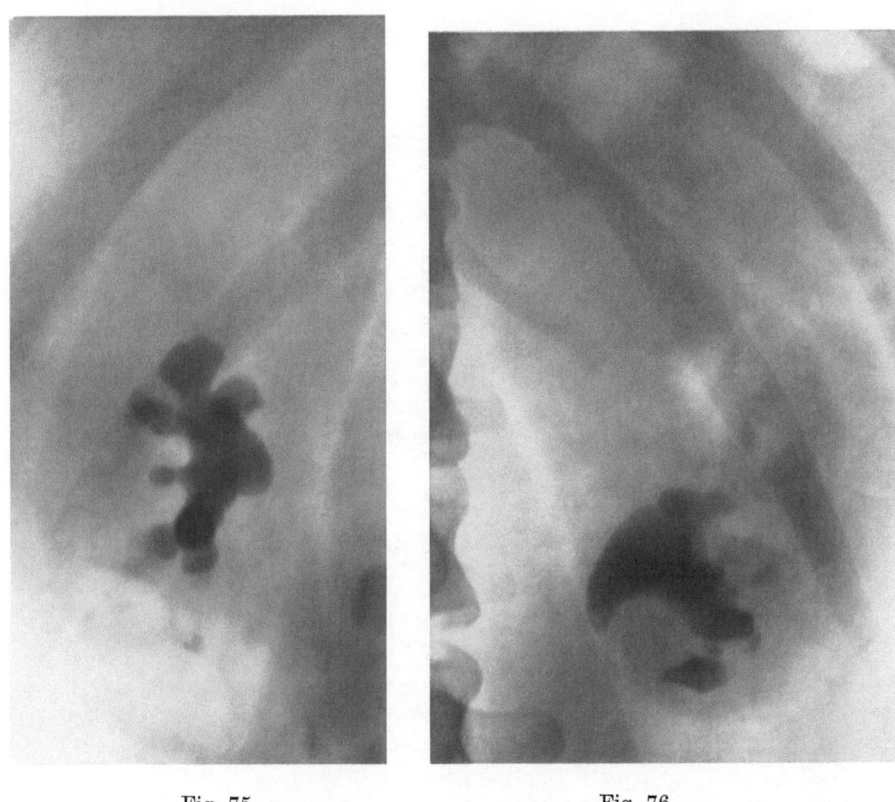

Fig. 75   Fig. 76

Fig. 75. Staghorn calculus filling caudal kidney pelvis in double kidney

Fig. 76. Stone in caudal kidney pelvis of double kidney. Stone in caudal calyx widened towards surface of caudal pole

Concrements vary in density, but owing to their calcium content they are often slightly opaque. The calculi are usually homogeneous, but not always. Occasionally they are irregularly vacuolized or they may contain radiating structures. Distinctly laminated calculi (Fig. 79) occur not only in the urinary bladder but also in the renal pelvis. In hydronephrosis they may even be very large (SAUPE, 1931; KJELLBERG, 1935).

A group of calculi of waxlike consistency and with a low calcium content should also be mentioned here. These concrements are made up of organic material which has begun to gather calcium deposits. The organic material may consist of a clot or a detached renal papilla. It is occasionally difficult to decide whether or not such formation should be classified as calculi (MEADS, 1939).

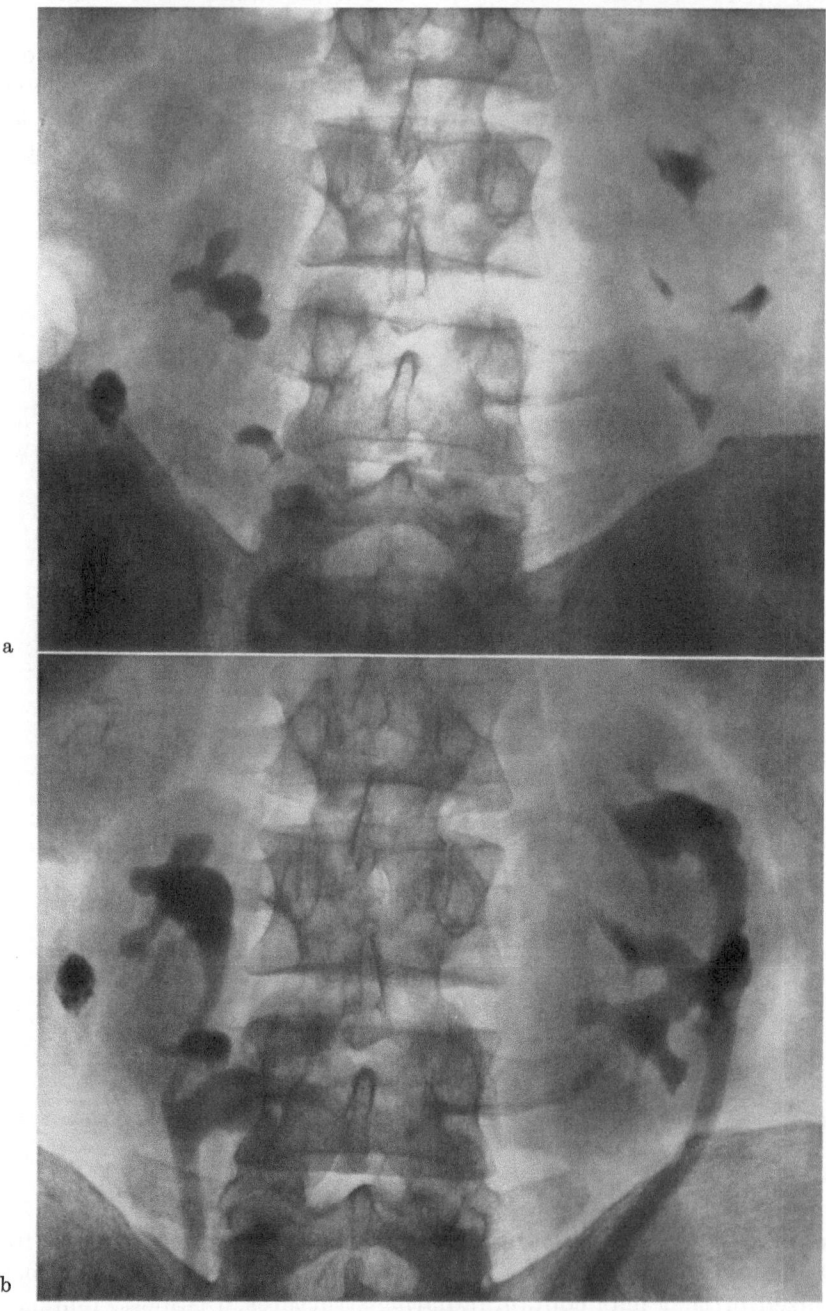

a

b

Fig. 77. Caudally fused kidney, so-called horseshoe kidney, with stones.
(a) Plain roentgenography, b) urography

Calculi are capable of changing in size and usually become larger (Figs. 80, 81). The increase in size is slow, as a rule, but occasionally a small stone may develop into a large stag-horn stone within a month or two. After surgical removal of a large stone, any small stones or fragments remaining may sometimes be seen to grow rapidly.

Stones occasionally decrease in size, however, because small parts separate and pass with the urine. Stones may also diminish in size in association with antibiotic therapy for infection or because of the use of urinary calculi solvents, for example Renacidin, a compound of multivalent organic acids (MULVANI, 1959; WEIS and MALLAMENT, 1962).

Stones also change in density, which usually increases. This may occur very rapidly by the deposition of calcium on organic substance, e. g. a coagulum or a shed papilla.

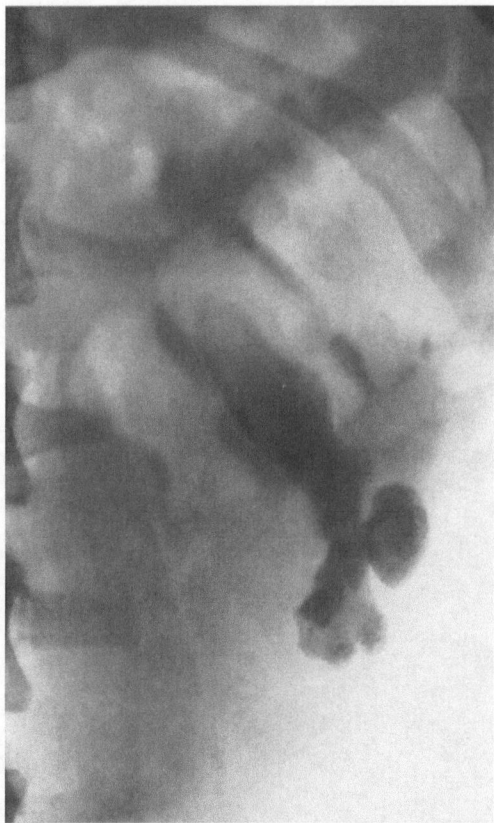

Fig. 78. Malrotated kidney. Shape of stone indicates the anomaly

The concrements may decrease in opacity in association with therapy, particularly antibiotic therapy. This, too, may occur rapidly.

Any change in the size, shape or opacity of a concrement may be only apparent and due to rotation or shifting of the stone. Rotation of a stone, particularly if it is elongated or flat, can give an erroneous impression of all types of such changes. A supplementary film taken at a different angle will reveal if any such change is true or only apparent.

Ureteric calculi are, as a rule, renal calculi that have been passed down into the ureter. They are usually small or relatively small. Roentgenograms taken with the beam parallel to the longitudinal axis of the small pelvis and with relatively soft roentgen rays will often demonstrate even very small stones in the distal part of the ureter. Bladder stones are often faceted or spiculated. It should be observed, however, that stones that appear to be spiculated may be smooth; the core may be spiculated but embedded in a less opaque, smooth-surfaced mass. Stones more than a few millimeters in diameter

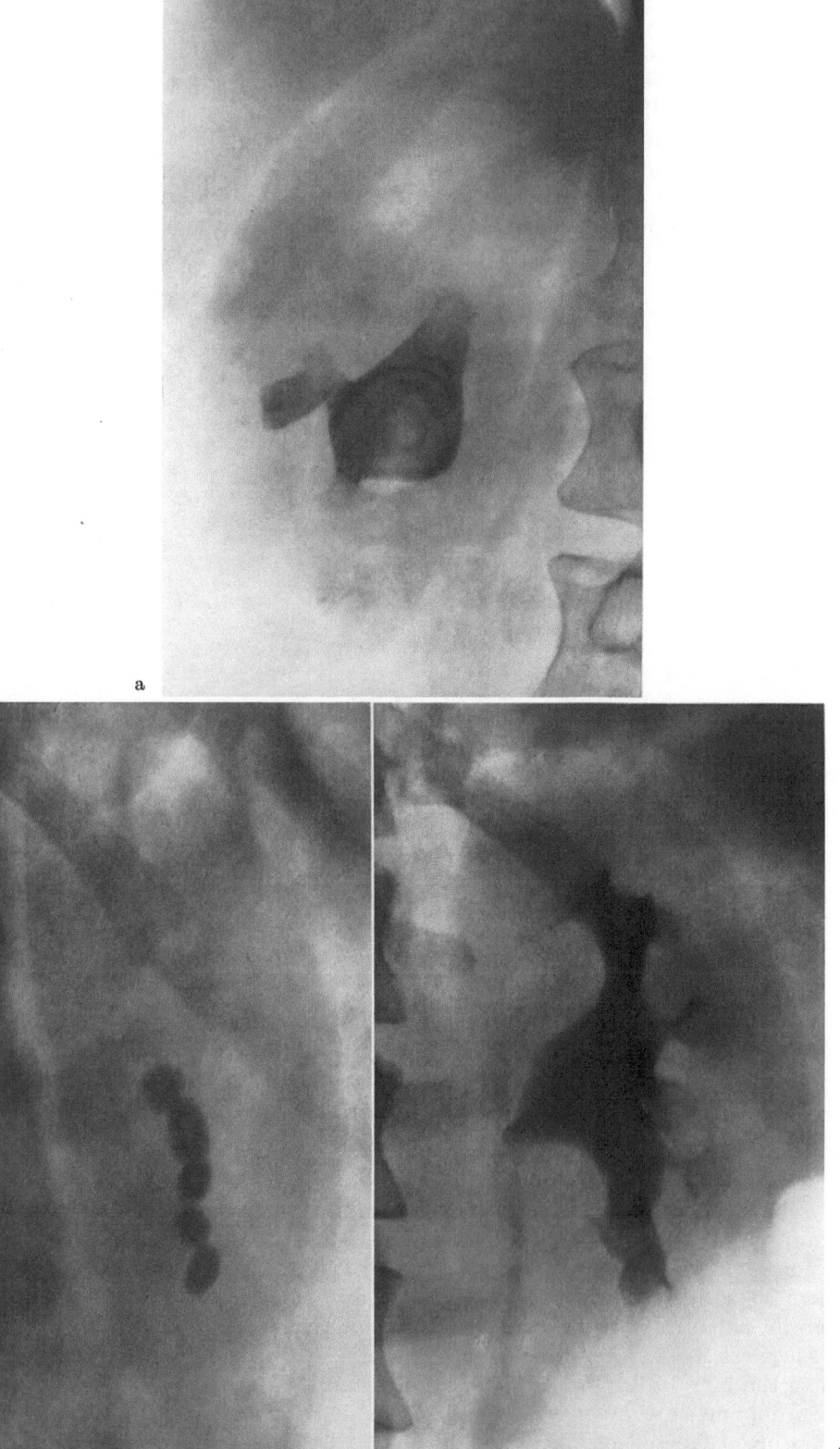

Fig. 79. a) Large laminated stone, b) (another patient) plain roentgenography: five laminated stones in left kidney, c) urography: stones are localized in caudal branch and calyces

occasionally are less dense centrally, indicating the presence of a lumen or groove permitting the passage of urine. At the distal part of the ureter phleboliths are often seen in thrombi in pelvic veins. Variations in size and number are great, as are differences between the two sides. Phleboliths are usually denser than ureteric stones and they often exhibit a characteristic layer formation in their structure. It is occasionally impossible to deter-

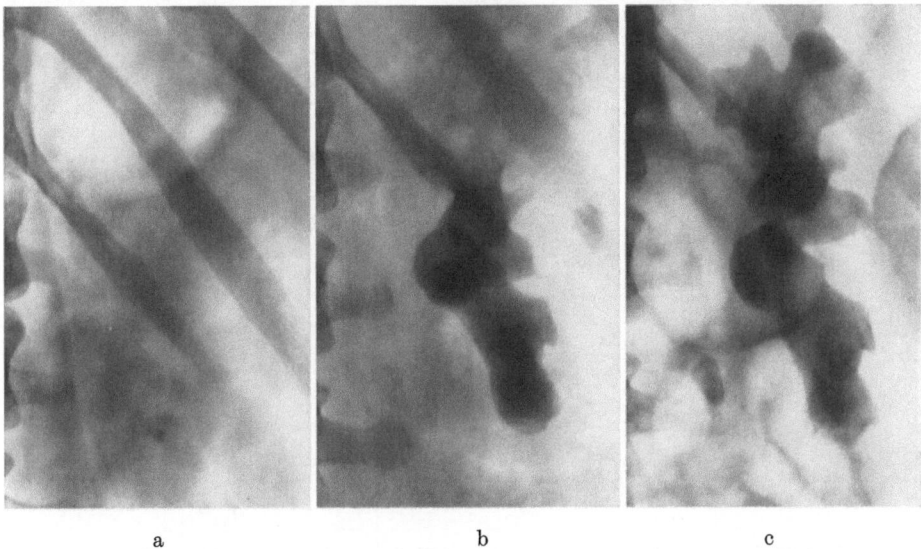

a   b   c

Fig. 80. Development of stone: from a) to b), seven years; from b) to c), one-half year

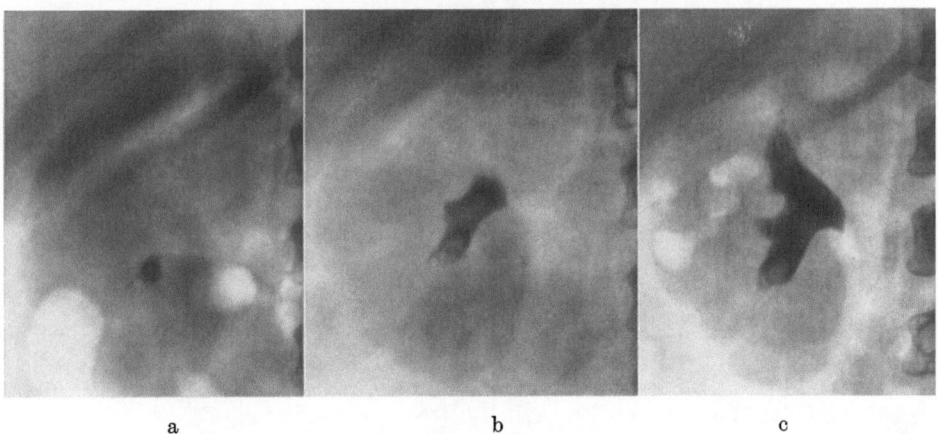

a   b   c

Fig. 81. Development of stone in girl patient 5 years of age, confined to bed because of chronic rheumatoid disease: from a) to b), two months; from b) to c) seven months

mine if a calcification is a stone or a phlebolith, or if among many calcifications one may be a stone. Urography (or pyelography) can solve this problem (Fig. 82).

Small stones lodged in the ureter often move freely up and down if the ureter is dilated. They may also rotate. This point should be recollected when judging the size of a ureteric stone. Oblong stones usually lie longitudinally in the ureter, which is sometimes obvious in the lower part of the ureter, which bends medially, sometimes cranially.

Large stones may be seen to pass into the ureter. As a rule they are lodged high up in the ureter, but occasionally may pass fairly low. Ureteric stones are sometimes very long and can fracture (BURKLAND, 1953).

Stones sometimes form in the ureter, *e. g.* in a diverticulum or more commonly in or above a ureterocele. Such stones may be solitary or multiple. The shape and position of the calculi in plain roentgenograms are often sufficient to show that they are situated in a ureterocele (Figs. 83, 84).

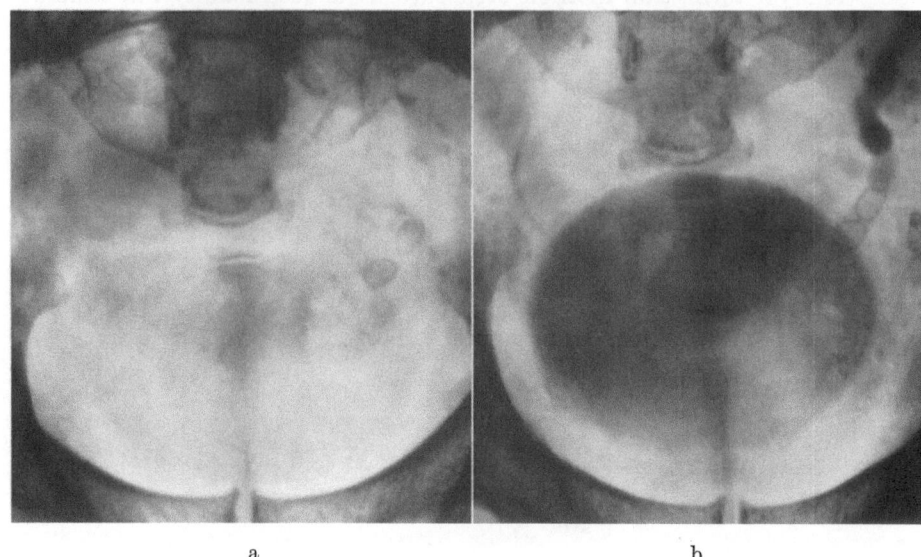

a   b

Fig. 82. Stones in distal part of ureter. a) Plain roentgenogram, b) urography

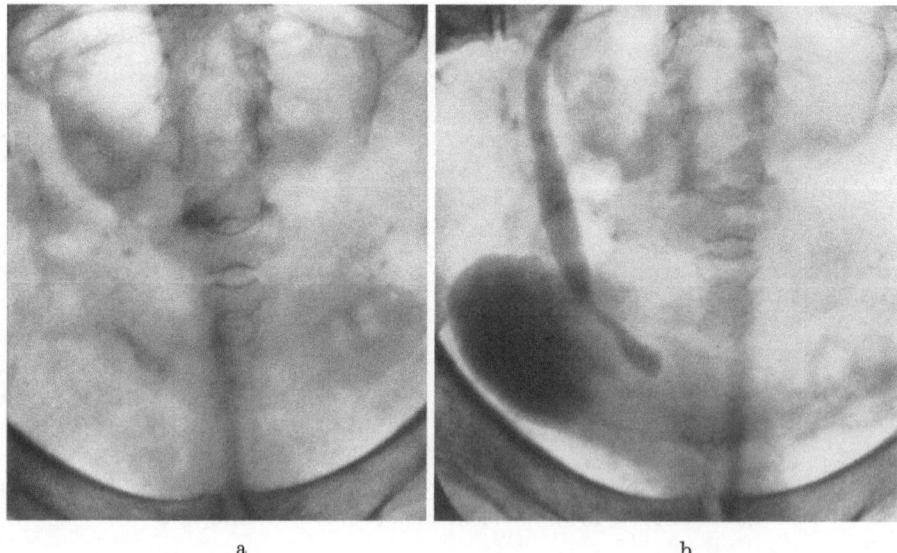

a   b

Fig. 83. Stone in ureterocele. a) Plain roentgenogram, b) urography

The roentgenologic appearance of urinary calculi has undoubtedly not received the attention it deserves. It is true that the density of a calculus, its shape and sometimes its size will permit certain conclusions regarding its chemistry. Thus cystine stones and urate stones can often be recognized as such because of their low opacity and smooth surface. Opaque, spiculated calculi are often oxalate stones. Large stag-horn calculi usually consist of phosphate or carbonate (WILDBOLZ, 1959). However, a more careful chemical analysis of the type of stone is probably often possible if clinically necessary.

Mention must be made here of stones with a density too low for detection at roentgen examination. Usually "non-opacity" of stones is due to incorrect technique at examination, regarding both the preparation of the patient and the performance of the actual examination. Occasionally, however, the calcium content of a stone makes it insufficiently absorptive of radiation, which makes demonstration impossible. Examination using contrast medium is then necessary.

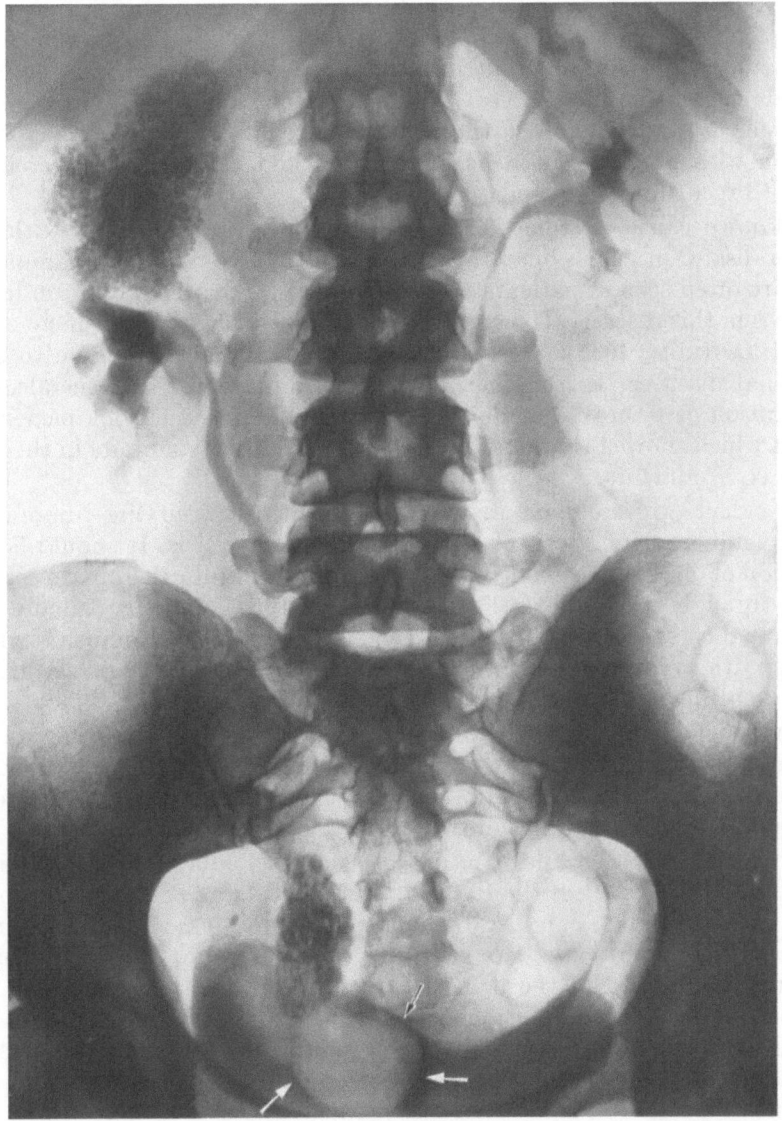

Fig. 84. Innumerable small stones in dilated cranial pelvis of double kidney and in distal part of dilated ureter. Dilatation due to large ureterocele protruding into bladder and demonstrable as filling defect (arrows) in contrast urine in bladder

Occasionally short-swing tomographic cuts can reveal small renal calcifications which it is not possible to detect in ordinary plain films (MADSEN, 1972).

A ureteric stone may have a density corresponding to that of the skeleton. If a stone is lodged in that part of the ureter where it passes over the pelvis, it may then not be demonstrable. Even here contrast examination is useful for diagnosis or for the exclusion of stone as the cause of blockage of flow in the ureter.

A ureter stone may be very small and flat and thus escape detection because of rotation, unless suitable projections are used.

All of these factors must be kept in mind continuously in diagnosis and in checking stones in the kidney and the ureter.

IV. Stone in association with certain diseases

Renal calculi are common accompaniments of certain diseases. In some countries the most important background for stone formation is pyelonephritis with papillary necrosis. Stones of this type often have a very characteristic shape and at urography and angiography changes in the papillae and the rest of the renal parenchyma may be seen. Stones in association with papillary necrosis have a marked tendency to increase in size and density and to recur after removal.

A well known cause of stone formation is parathyroid adenoma with ostitis fibrosa cystica generalisata, in which bilateral renal calculi are common. Intrarenal calcifications and calculi are often seen in patients with sarcoidosis. The serum calcium level is elevated in many cases in this disease. The coexistence of peptic ulcer and urinary calculi has been discussed (Hellström, 1935). The metabolism of oxalic acid is liable to disturbance in gastrointestinal diseases. In reference to the combination of peptic ulcer and urinary calculus, mention can here be made of experimental investigations performed for other purposes but which showed that oxalate is absorbed in large amounts in the small intestine in very acid environments.

Urinary calculi are common in association with decalcifying tumors such as myeloma and skeletal carcinomatosis and in chronic osteomyelitis. It should be noted that in the destruction of one gram of bone tissue, 100 milligrams of calcium are set free and must be excreted through the kidneys (Pierson, et al., 1954). Urinary calculi are also fairly common in renal osteodystrophy. This disease is difficult to distinguish roentgenologically from hyperparathyroidism. Hypercalciuria is common in Cushing's syndrome and 13 % of patients with this syndrome have kidney stone (Herks et al., 1959).

Vitamin A-deficiency regularly produces renal stones in experimental animals and it has been shown that patients with urinary stone may also have latent vitamin A-deficiency (Ezickson and Feldman, 1937). The relationship, if any, between vitamin-A-deficiency and concrement formation is still obscure, however.

In the metabolic disorder known as oxalosis or oxalaemia, occurring mainly in children, calcium oxalate is deposited in the renal tubulus, and large concrements sometimes form in the renal pelvis. Oxalate can also be deposited in the bones and in the intestinal wall (Ostry, 1951; Zollinger and Rosenmund, 1952; Dunn, 1955). In this disease the oxalate normally excreted in the urine is precipitated and forms calculi. In animal experiments chronic oxalic acid-poisoning has been shown to result in a filling of the tubules with calcium oxalate crystals (Ebstein and Nicolaier, 1897). As mentioned, certain metabolic disorders are sometimes seen in association with cystine and uric acid concrements.

Uric acid calculi, although rare, are produced continually because of the metabolic disorder responsible for their formation. In urine of average pH (6 or higher) uric acid is present largely as the soluble sodium and potassium urates, whereas in highly acid urine the relatively insoluble free acid may predominate and may precipitate from solution. Allyn (1957) described a patient who had passed 2,000 renal calculi, as many as 15 a month, for about 25 years. As a rule, calculi of this type cannot be seen in plain roentgenograms even of good quality. In leukemia and osteomyelosclerosis such stones are formed by rapid destruction of protein-rich tissue. Excretion of uric acid in the urine is increased in leukemia and in treatment of the disease with nitrogene mustard-like components, the increase in uric acid excretion is marked (MacCree, 1955).

In cystinuria, a familial intermediary metabolic disorder due to inborn faulty metabolism, which appears to be more common in males than in females, cystine stones are prone to form in the urinary tract. When a cystine stone is found, there is every reason to examine close relatives of the patient, because of the familial occurrence of cystine calculi. Such stones are capable of growing rapidly but also of responding promptly to adequate therapy. If the urinary tract is infected, they may become encrusted with calcium.

In tuberculosis, sand or seed-like concrements form in the renal pelvis. Such microliths may also form in the presence of a tumor, e. g. papilloma, in the renal pelvis.

In medullary sponge kidney calculi are common and they are often of characteristic appearance and location. The more one is familiar with the appearance of concrements in papillary necrosis and medullary sponge kidney, for example, the more often these diseases can be diagnosed on the basis of the appearance of the calculi.

Long bed rest is known to favor stone formation, as is apparent from the term "recumbency stones". In patients lying on their backs, stones will more often form in the cranial calyces, but in patients not confined to bed, stones are more common in the caudal calyces. Of 100 patients with fractures of the lumbar spine without neurologic symptoms, urinary calculi formed in 10 (CONWELL). Among 800 patients who had been invalids for a long time KIMBROUGH and DENSLOW (1949) found 15 with urinary calculi that had formed within 74 to 1.200 days and among 1507 patients with injury to the spinal cord, COMMAR et al. (1962) found renal stones in 124 (8.2%). On examinations of 1,104 paraplegic patients, COMARR (1955) found renal calculosis to be more frequent in patients with lower motor neuron lesions and that the incidence of renal calculosis was higher among patients with complete neurologic lesions than with incomplete lesions. Urinary calculi are common in patients with orthopedic diseases. Of some 300 patients with different types of spondylitis, about 3% were found to have lithiasis. The incidence of stones in spondylitis is higher in patients with an active inflammatory process such as an abscess, and the incidence of stone formation can be reduced in such patients by regular postural changes (STÅHL, 1942). Finally, mention should be made of stone formation in generalized malformations such as Klinefelter's syndrome.

V. Stones induced by side-effects of therapy

Vitamin D intoxication can cause nephrolithiasis in childhood because this vitamin facilitates absorption of calcium from the intestine. Formation of calculi in association with treatment of infections with sulphonamides has been seen as deposits of sand in the mucosa of the renal pelvis demonstrable in the roentgenograms as a faint calcification. This type of calculi was common when only less soluble sulphonamides were available. Now that readily soluble preparations are obtainable, such concrements are only of historical interest.

Acetasolamide (Diamox) has been used in ophthalmiatrics, because it reduces the secretion of the aqueous humor in the eye. It also, however, produces diuresis by a complex process, inhibiting the enzyme carbonic anhydrase in the kidney tubuli. The treatment of glaucoma with this substance is sometimes accompanied by attacks of renal colic due to concrements of low opacity. It is believed that the formation of these concrements is due to a decrease in urinary excretion of citrate, which substance aids in maintaining calcium in the urine in a soluble complex (PERSKY et al., 1956; MacKENZIE, 1960).

According to HAMMARSTEN (1958), concrements induced by therapy are seen also in conditions with increased precipitation of calcium in the urine, not only vitamin-D intoxication, in patients receiving large doses of parathormone or AT 10, and formation of uric acid ammonium urate stones can be seen on medication with substances producing a strongly acid urine. Mandelic acid is likely to give rise to calcium oxalate concrements by being split to glycolic acid, which can be oxidized to oxalic acid. Finally, antacids containing silicates can cause silicate calculi (HAMMARSTEN, 1953; HESSEN, 1963).

Renal insufficiency together with hypercalcaemia causes the milk-alkali syndrome due to excessive ingestion of milk and absorbable alkali usually taken as treatment for peptic ulcer (BURNETT *et al.*, 1949, KEATING jr., 1958).

VI. Formation of stones from a roentgenologic point of view

Calcifications in the renal pelvis or lower urinary tract are usually called concrements to distinguish them from the many varying types of parenchymal calcifications. In the discussion of the etiology of calculi, however, calcifications in the renal parenchyma lining the renal pelvis are important. In 1937 RANDALL suggested that the source of renal calculi should be sought in the fornix calyces or in the papillae. In a careful study of autopsy specimens he sometimes observed calcium deposits on the tips of the renal papillae under the epithelium and in one case he found such a calcium deposit to have become detached and forming a concrement. On examination under a magnifying glass of small stones that had been passed by patients with concrements, he found them to have a grooved surface corresponding to the attachment to a papilla. ROSENOW (1940) and VERMOOTEN (1941) confirmed RANDALL's findings.

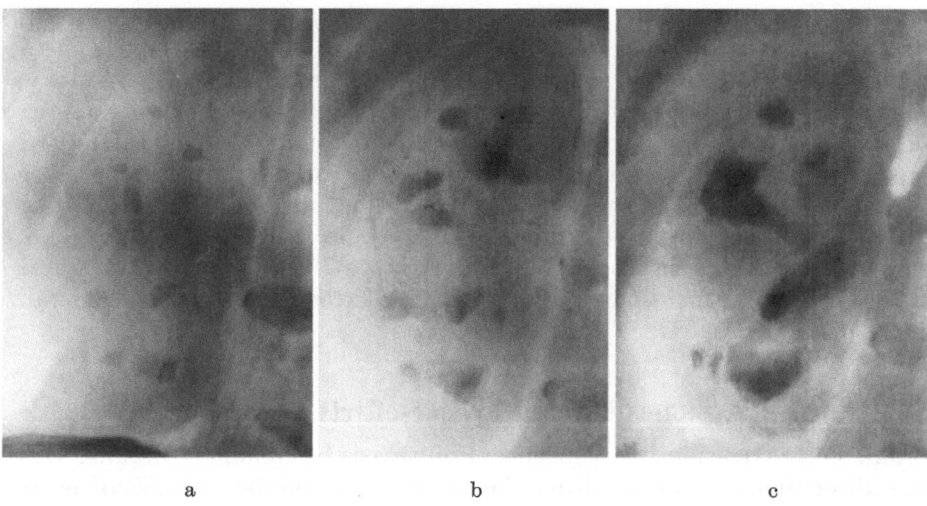

a   b   c

Fig. 85. Stone in papillary necrosis: a) multiple papilla-shaped stones; development of stones from a) to b), six months; from b) to c) 11 months

CARR (1954) made a further contribution to the theory of the formation of renal calculi. He claims his observations argue for the assumption that renal calculi form at the edge of the calyx when the lymphatic drainage mechanism breaks down because of overloading of the mechanism by an excessive number of microliths, such as occurs in hyperparathyreoidism and other disorders of calcium excretion, and, possibly absence or deficiency of protective colloids etc., and because of impairment of the mechanism of lymphatic drainage due to previous inflammatory changes with subsequent fibrosis. Small calcifications collected outside the fornix calyces have been identified by x-ray diffraction as ordinary types of concrements. CARR's theory includes some of RANDALL's observations.

Roentgen examination provides some support for these views by the demonstration of very small, often multiple papillary incrustations. Occasionally such incrustations are seen by themselves but they can also be seen in association with concrements moving freely in the renal pelvis. In this connection, the entity medullary sponge kidney should be borne in mind, as well as any type of tubular ectasias and tubular acidosis.

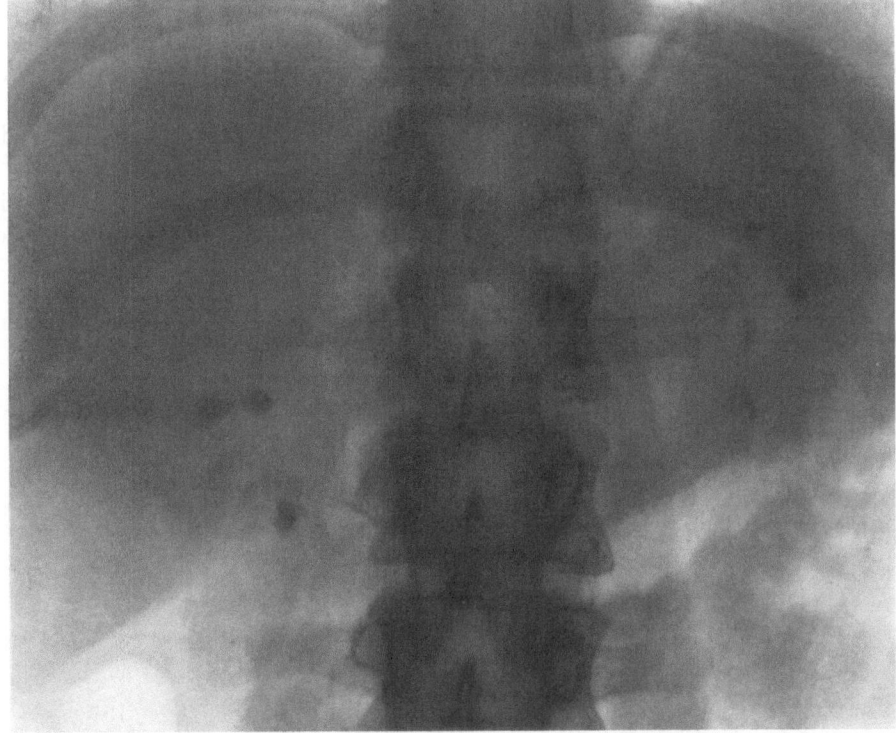

a

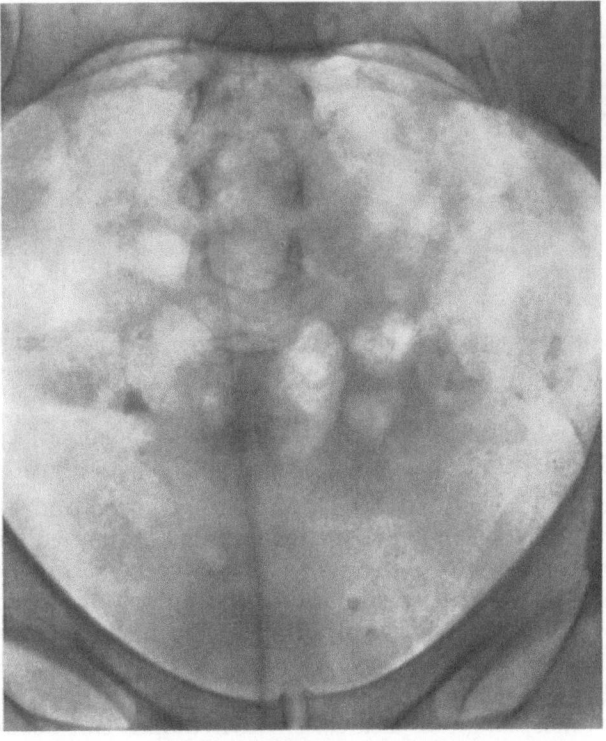

b

Fig. 86. Calcified shed papillae in both kidneys in papillary necrosis. One calcified papilla is stuck in the right ureteric orifice (b)

Kidney stones can contain three similar types of nephrocalcinosis: intratubular calcified conglomerates of cell debris, structured microcalculi, and interstitial calcifications (RANDALL's plaque). These calcifications represent nuclei on which ions of urine may crystallize if urine is supersaturated or otherwise in a state where crystallization is possible. Such crystallization is rare in normal humans, however (DRACH and BOYCE, 1972).

HAGGITT and PITCOCK (1971) found in an electron microscopic study bodies dense with electrons occupying the basement membranes of collecting ducts and the interstitium

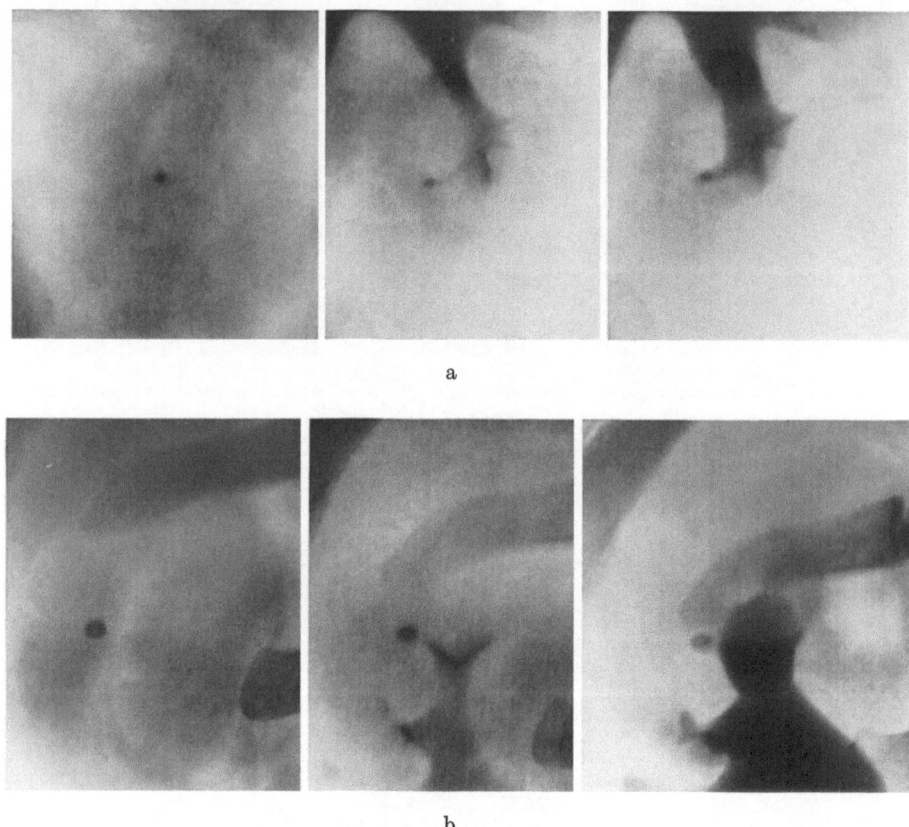

a

b

Fig. 87. Formation of stone according to Randall-Carr theory: small stone in fornical angle of calyx

in every patient. The authors believe that this high frequency of calcifications can help explain the formation of stone in persons with morphologically normal urinary tract.

Since urinary calculi are usually unilateral, stone formation can scarcely be simply a matter of general metabolism and the urinary crystalloid-colloid balance (TWINEM, 1940). Importance must therefore be attached to localizing factors. Such factors have long been known, but those which can be demonstrated explain only a small percentage of the stones. The anatomy of the calyx is one of these localizing factors. Small calyces with small stems may contain stones (Fig. 88), small diverticula-like bulges in the edge of the calyx, so-called calyx border evaginations, and pyelogenic cysts (Figs. 89—93) may also contain small stones, single or multiple. Such bulges can occur in many calyces, of which only a few harbor calculi. In addition, it is known that gross anomalies such as horse-shoe kidney, predispose to the formation of calculi, as do urinary obstruction and infections.

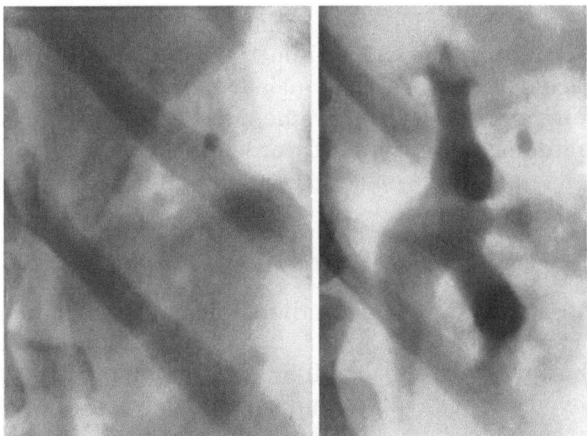

Fig. 88. Stone in narrow-stemmed microcalyx

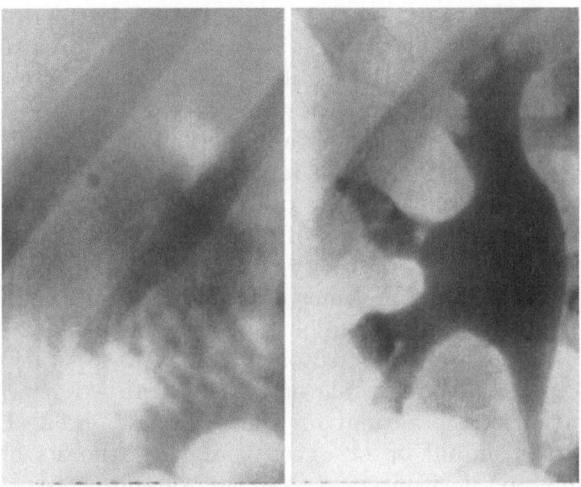

Fig 89. Stone in calyceal border evagination

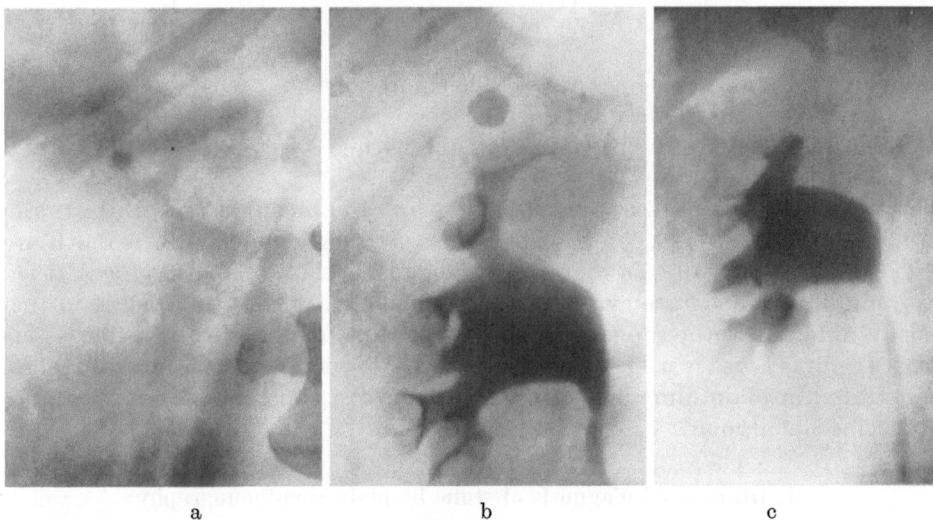

a   b   c

Fig. 90. Stone in pyelogenic cyst. Communication with kidney pelvis not seen. a) Plain roentgenography,
b) urography, c) following cranial polar nephrectomy

9*

Against the background of the above remarks, renal stones may be classified as primary or secondary, the primary being due to some factor outside the urinary tract, the secondary to a localizing factor in the urinary tract.

Recurrence of stone after passage or removal is common. It is favored by the fact that the localizing factor or the original disorder may be unknown or inaccessible to treatment, or that it has not been observed.

VII. Plain roentgenography

As mentioned, most calculi contain radiopaque material and are therefore demonstrable in plain roentgenograms.

Opinions differ, however, on the possibility of demonstrating cystine stones in this way. It is widely believed that calculi are not opaque enough to be demonstrated in plain roentgenograms. Renander's investigation (1941) of 15 cases, however, shows that these stones can always be seen in good-quality plain films. Photometric examination of urinary calculi showed the following roentgen densities in air: for cystine 3.8, uric acid 1.1, calcium oxalate 4.9, ammonium magnesium phosphate 5.1, calcium diphosphate 7.6, all in relation to water. Without going into the accuracy of the measuring technique, these figures show the relative density of these substances. The value in water, i. e. the value corresponding to roentgen examination in practice, was 2.7 or 30% lower than for cystine in air. For ammonium magnesium phosphate it was 3.2 and for calcium diphosphate 5.7.

The possibility of demonstrating calculi depends not only on their chemical composition but also on their size. It is obviously more difficult to demonstrate a small stone than a large one. But with an effective technique often even small calculi will be demonstrated. However, if the patient is obese and stocky, some small stones, and even large ones of certain chemical composition, are sometimes not demonstrable by the very best technique because of low primary absorption and high secondary radiation. In some of these cases roentgen examination of the surgically exposed kidney at operation may be important.

Whether a stone will be demonstrable or not naturally depends on the examination technique and preparation of the patient for the examination. As far as the examination technique is concerned, it should be observed that the calculus may be projected onto bone, e. g. if a ureteric stone is situated in that part of the ureter passing over the pelvis (see Fig. 116). If the floor of the pelvis is low, as it often is in multiparae, a stone in the lower section of the ureter may be projected onto the the anterior portion of the pelvic bone. The different parts of the pelvic ureter can, however, be projected free by changing the angulation of the beam.

Non-opaque stones sometimes rapidly become encrusted with such a thick layer of calcium as to be demonstrable in plain roentgenograms. I have seen radiolucent stones demonstrated by pyelography become so opaque within 3 weeks as to be readily demonstrable in plain roentgenograms.

Several authors have assessed the percentage of radiolucent stones. Boeminghaus and Zeiss (1935) thus gave 2—5% of so-called roentgen negative calculi, while Kneise and Schober (1941), gave 5—10% as more probable, and Wildbolz (1959) 10 %. It is obvious that anything like an accurate evaluation is difficult because of differences in the technique used by different authors and particularly because it is hardly possible to check the reliability of figures given. Suffice it here to say that a certain percentage of stones cannot be demonstrated in plain films but that this percentage can be markedly reduced by the use of first-class technique.

1. Differential diagnosis of stone by plain roentgenography

In view of the wide variety of types of calcification in the renal pelvis, and renal parenchyma in the neighbourhood of the kidney, and in regions which may be projected

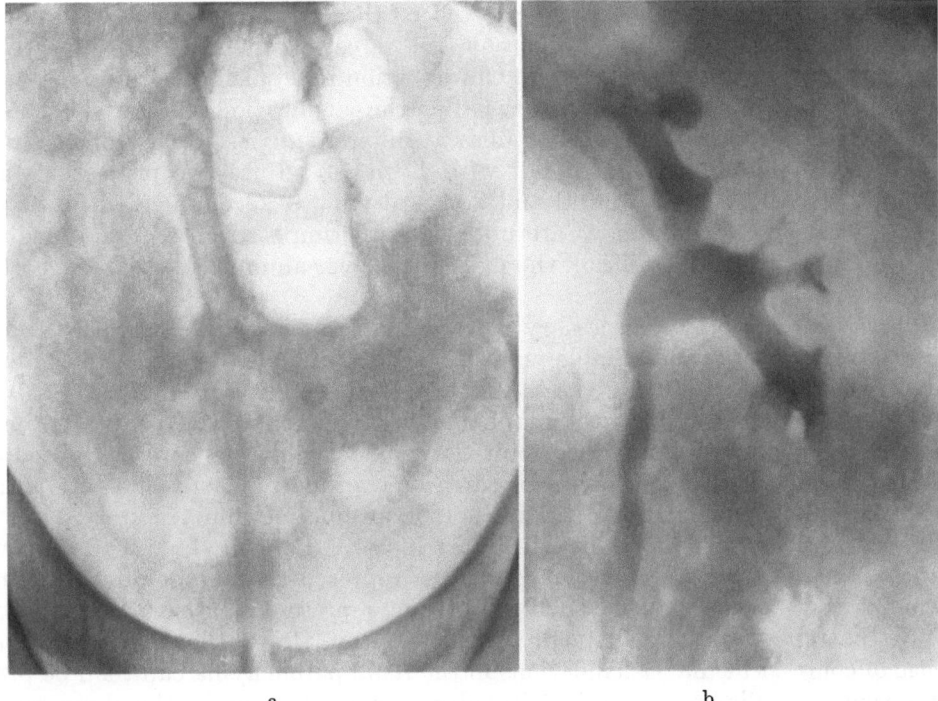

a   b

Fig. 91. a) Plain roentgenography: stone in distal part of left ureter; b) urography: pyelogenic cyst in cranial part of left kidney with size and width of neck corresponding to size and shape of ureteric stone

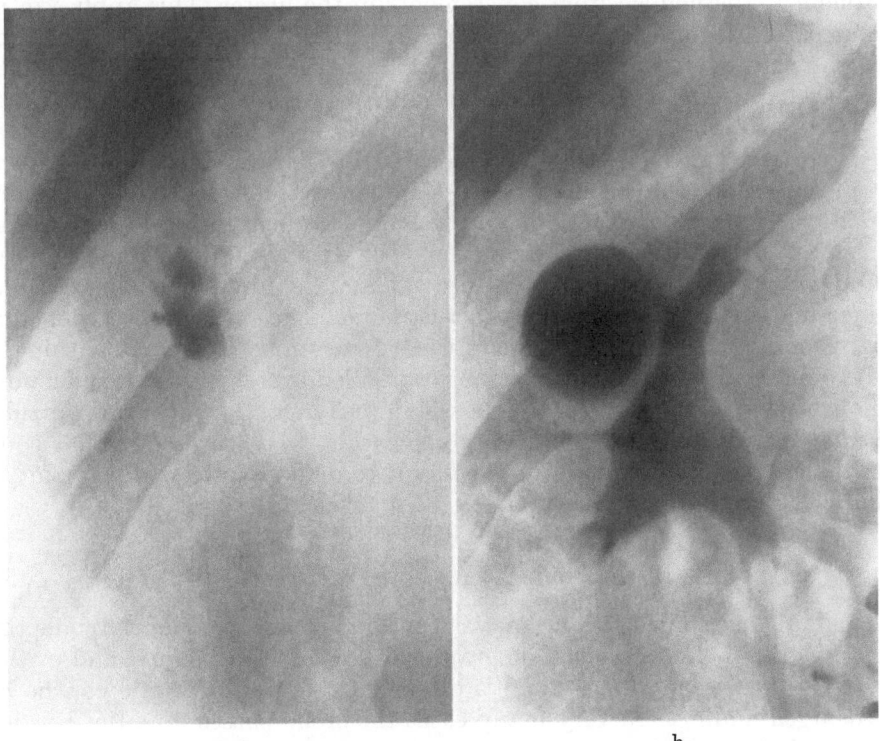

a   b

Fig. 92. a) Plain roentgenography; b) urography: large irregular stones in large cyst communicating with kidney pelvis

onto the kidney, much space could be allotted to the differential diagnosis of stones in plain roentgenograms. All of these different factors can be reduced, however, to prime factors by a simple examination scheme. On detection of a calcification that is projected onto the kidney, the first step is to decide whether the calcification is situated in the kidney or outside it. This can be done by taking films at different angles, usually one frontal view and one or more oblique views. It is not wise, however, to use two projections at right angles to one another, e. g., a frontal and a lateral view as recommended by Sgalitzer (1936). In lateral views the kidneys are not only superimposed on one another but also projected onto the spine. In addition, the patient receives an unnecessarily large radiation dose.

It is, above all, not only unnecessary but also indefensible to use complicated methods instead of the very simple and reliable procedure, i. e. oblique views, to solve the problem. A handbook of urology of 1959 gives illustrations and description of a case in which in addition to plain radiography, pyelography, stereoroentgenography, pyelography with gas, and urography were performed to show that some calcifications were situated outside the kidney. The question could have been answered properly, easily, cheaply and safely by simply extending plain radiography to include an oblique film.

If the calcification is found to be within the kidney, the next step is to decide whether it is situated in the renal parenchyma and thus represents a parenchymal calcification or whether it is situated in the renal pelvis and thus represents a stone. This can often be decided by the appearance and shape of the calcification. If not, the decision can be made by the use of contrast media. Calcifications in the renal parenchyma can then be projected outside the contrast-filled renal pelvis. Difficulties are offered only by the above mentioned small calcifications situated at the border between the renal parenchyma and the renal pelvis.

Calcifications close to the ureter and resembling ureteric calculi in shape and size may be difficult to distinguish from concrements in the ureter. This applies in particular to the distal parts of the ureters where the differential diagnosis may be made difficult by phleboliths. However, as a rule differentiation offers no difficulties. The phleboliths are often of characteristic appearance. They are round, laminated, dense, multiple and bilateral. Their size, form, density and number can vary, however, Occasionally their position is such as to exclude their being located in the ureter. The ureteric stones are oval as a rule and homogeneous, less dense, singular and unilateral. They are oriented in the direction of the ureter. If the phleboliths are not numerous, a differential diagnosis is easy in most cases. But if they are numerous, the diagnosis of a possible ureteric stone among innumerable phleboliths may be difficult and require further investigation with contrast medium or insertion of a contrast catheter. The decision then depends on the possibility of showing whether or not one of the calcifications is situated within the ureter. This can be done by taking films of the contrast filled ureter in different planes. In urography the urinary stasis may be of diagnostic importance. Calcifications outside the urinary pathways may be situated immediately adjacent to the ureter so that considerable changes in the angles of projection are necessary to demonstrate with certainty that the calcification is situated outside the ureter.

2. Disappearance of renal and ureteric stones

Renal and ureteric stones are often passed spontaneously, frequently while the patient is under observation including roentgenographic follow-up. If the nurse and/or the patient are observant, the passage of the stone is often noticed and the stone can be compared with the roentgen findings. In very many cases the stone passes unnoticed or is not presented for examination. When a stone has been demonstrated but is no longer detectable on check examination, it does not necessarily mean, however, that the stone has passed. Several factors may explain why the stone is not demonstrable in the film:

1. The stone may have shifted. A renal calculus may have been passed into the ureter or the bladder. On check radiography for renal stone it is, of course, not sufficient to examine the kidneys only, if the stone is no longer demonstrable. Examination must include the entire urinary tract. A ureteric concrement may also pass into the bladder or urethra. The possibility of the stone having passed into the urethra should be considered, since in males the urethra is usually not included in plain roentgenograms of the urinary tract.

A ureteric stone, on the other hand, may occasionally migrate up the ureter. If the ureter is dilated above a concrement, the stone may be dislodged and the stone may be displaced up into the renal pelvis, particularly if the patient is confined to bed or if the ureter has been catheterized.

2. A calculus may have shifted and may be projected onto bone, e.g. a ureteric concrement lodged in that part of the ureter passing over the pelvic bones. Careful study of these cases will often reveal the concrement, however. Special projections should preferably be used to project this part of the ureter free. This is possible by turning the patient slightly on the side and using views more or less strongly angulated, craniocaudally and caudocranially.

3. A small calculus may be flat and rotation of the otherwise easily observable calculus may make it less observable.

4. The calculus may have become less opaque. Just as the calcium content of a stone may increase rapidly, so may it rapidly diminish during treatment of a urinary tract infection, for example.

5. The calculus may disappear upon suitable medical treatment. This holds for urate concrements particularly (SMITH et al., 1959).

6. The examination technique may be less satisfactory for some reason, or intestinal contents may be abundant.

3. Perforation

Occasionally a stone may cause decubital lesions in the wall of the renal pelvis, with perforation as a result (RENANDER, 1940). A stone in an occluded calyx may also perforate the renal parenchyma (COUNCILL and COUNCILL, 1950). In such cases stones may be seen in uncommon positions or give rise to extravasation of contrast medium at urography or pyelography. Such perforations may also lead to perinephritis (see Chapter L). Perforations to the digestive tract or to the skin surface are less common. A broncholithiasis is reported by GORDANSON and SARGENT (1970) where a renal stone had passed over into the lung through a nephro-bronchial fistula.

VIII. Roentgen examination in association with operation

The importance of roentgen examination immediately before, during, and after operation is obvious from what has been said above about the size, density, passage, and recurrence of stones. It is known that calculi are likely to migrate in the urinary tract. Therefore, as a precaution, we always take films of the urinary tract immediately before operation. Such films often reveal that the stones which are to be removed have shifted within the kidney. We have also observed that a concrement in the ureter previously demonstrated on various occasions has found its way up into the renal pelvis or that a stone regularly seen high up in the ureter on previous examinations has been passed down to the distal part of the ureter, or even into the urinary bladder. Such check radiography immediately before operation has often facilitated a better planning of the operation or even made operation unnecessary. Occasionally it could be shown that the stone had passed unnoticed.

Roentgen examination during the actual operation is occasionally necessary in order to locate stones, to find stones of low density, and to check the result of extraction (see Chapter C II, 3 regarding technique).

IX. Urography and pyelography

The purpose of urography and pyelography is first to decide whether calcifications demonstrated within the kidney in plain roentgenograms are situated in the renal parenchyma or in the renal pelvis. If at examination the calcifications are shown to be concre-

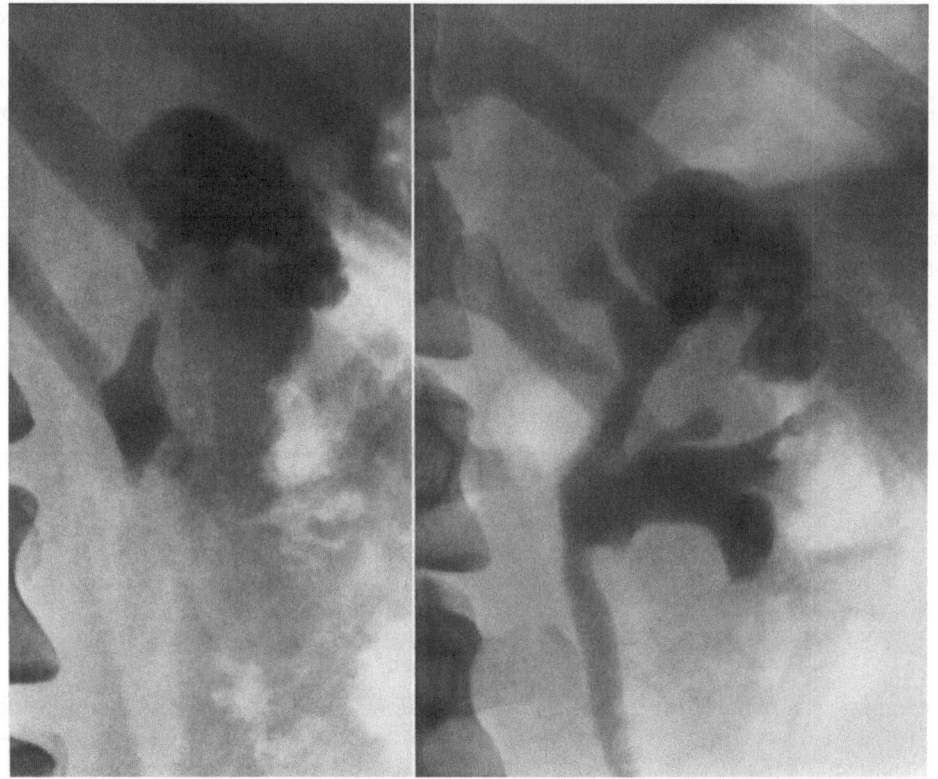

a   b

Fig. 93. Staghorn calculus in left kidney pelvis and enlarged, partly collapsed communicating cyst in cranial part of kidney. a) Plain roentgenography, b) urography

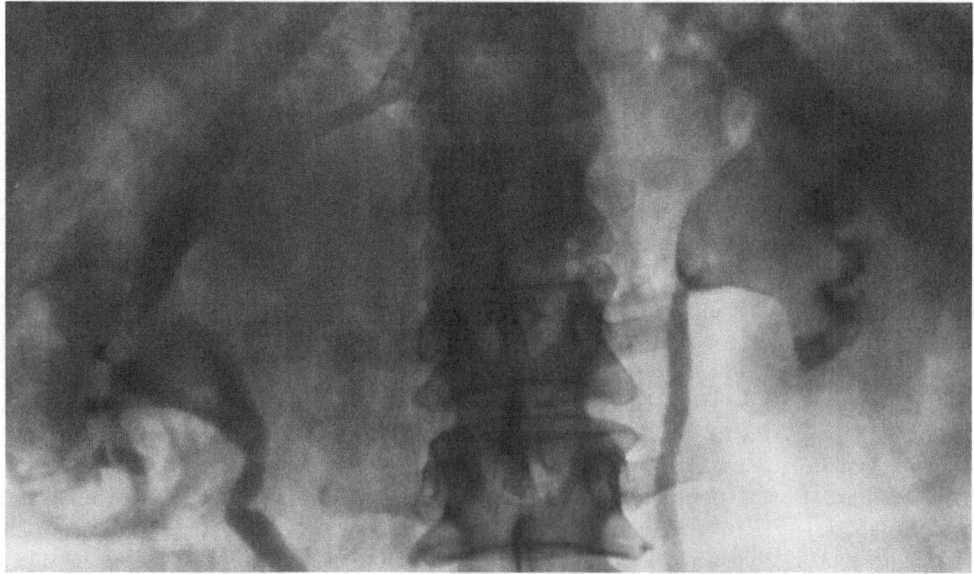

Fig. 94. Non-opaque stones. Urography: on left side only thin layer of contrast urine around stone; pelviureteric junction narrow (phenomenon often seen in presence of large stones in confluence)

ments, the next step in the examination is to study the shape of the renal pelvis, the functioning capacity of the kidney, the position of the stone in the renal pelvis, and any influence of the stone on the drainage of a single calyx or of the entire renal pelvis. Attention must be focused on details, inter alia the anatomy of the calyces. Reflux phenomena must be kept in mind (see Chapter I). Pyelonephritis may complicate the stone disease and be responsible for marked concomitant impairment of functional capacity and changes in the morphology of the kidney and kidney pelvis (see chapter on Pyelonephritis). All types of anomalies or renal diseases should be looked for (see discussion above in connection with pathogenesis of stone).

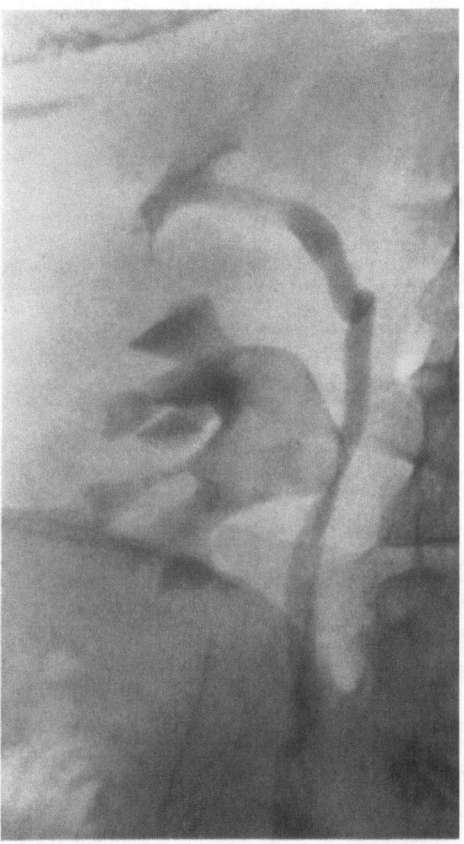

Fig. 95. Urography: double kidney, large non-opaque stone in caudal kidney pelvis distending confluence

To detect concrements appearing as filling defects in the contrast medium, the concentration of the medium in the renal pelvis must be suitable. In pyelography this can be secured by choosing a suitable concentration and amount of contrast medium to be injected. In urography it can be secured by exposing the films at an optimal moment in relation to excretion or to release of ureteric compression and by using a suitable kilovoltage.

It is often difficult, nevertheless, to detect stones in the contrast-filled renal pelvis, even when they have been seen clearly in plain roentgenograms. This stresses the necessity of taking plain roentgenograms before starting contrast radiography. It cannot be stressed often enough that plain roentgenograms produced and studied on the basis of general principles and the specific problems of the patient under examination, are a necessary part of the urographic examination. It must also again be stressed that urography should not be performed according to standardized rules but with a technique tailor-made for the actual problem confronting the patient and the roentgenologist.

In the differential diagnosis, thin stones (Figs. 94, 95) must be distinguished from polypoid tumors of the renal pelvis, gas in the renal pelvis after instrumental intervention or due to fistulation between the digestive tract and the urinary pathways, and gas

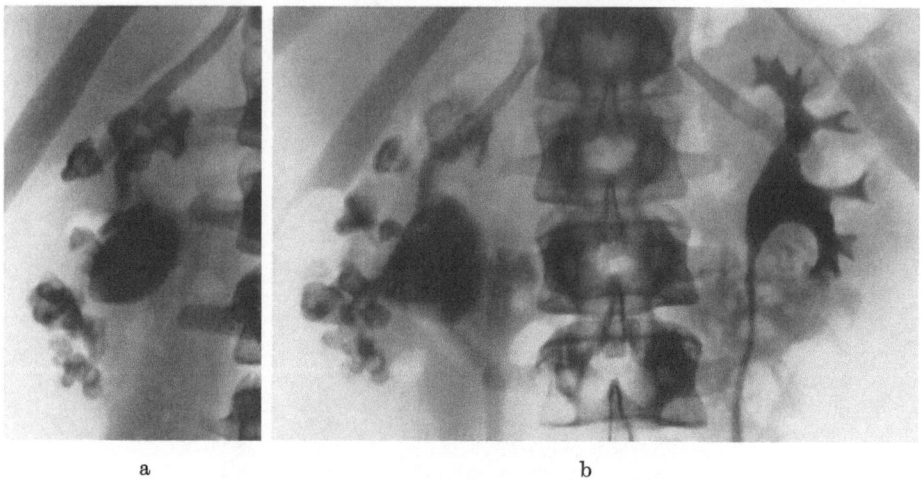

a   b

Fig. 96. Excretion of contrast urine. a) Plain radiography, b) urography: slight excretion

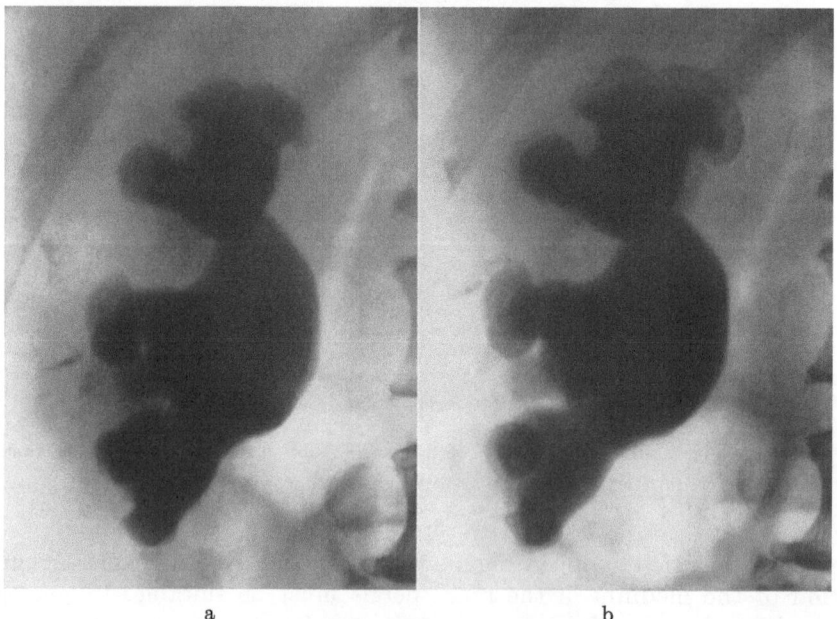

a   b

Fig. 97. Excretion of contrast urine. a) Plain radiography, b) Urography: only thin rim of contrast urine of low concentration around stone

formation due to fermentation in the renal pelvis. Such stones must occasionally also be distinguished from polyp-like parts of a renal carcinoma bulging into the renal pelvis.

The possibility of filling defects in the urinary pathways, renal pelvis, ureter or bladder in patients with haematuria which may be due to blood clots must always be borne in mind. Check examination will generally indicate if any such filling defect was due to stone or to a clot.

A gas bubble in the digestive tract can be projected onto the renal pelvis and simulate a filling defect caused by a stone. The examiner must make sure of the localization, of course, by using proper projections, and must check whether or not any filling defect is caused by an actual pathologic process in the renal pelvis.

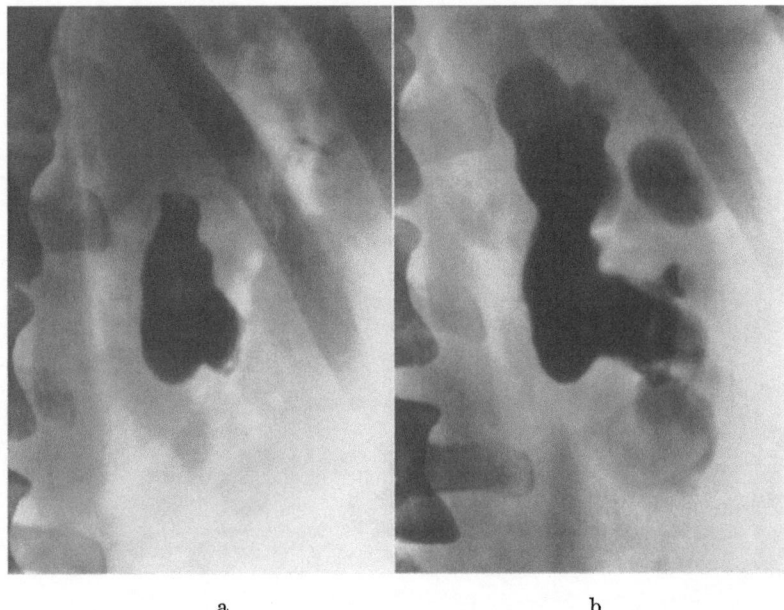

a   b

Fig. 98. Excretion of contrast urine. a) Plain radiography, b) urography: fairly good excretion in dilated calyces

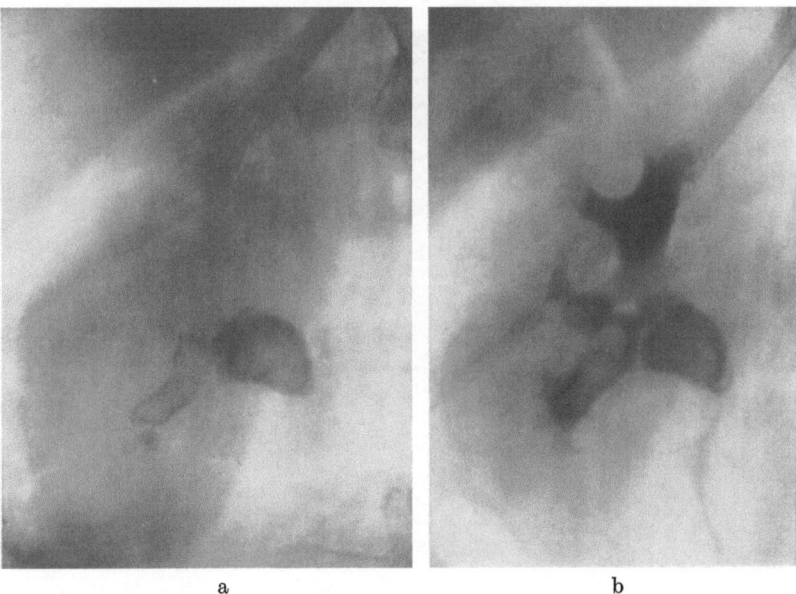

a   b

Fig. 99. Excretion of contrast urine a) Plain radiography, b) Urography: good excretion and no dilatation despite large stones

Even if the renal pelvis is full of large stones, contrast medium may nevertheless be excreted during urography. The excretion is usually delayed and of low concentration and often discernable only as a brim around the stone or part of its circumference (Figs. 96—98). Large stones do not necessarily always produce stasis, however (Fig. 99). With optimal filling, irregular indentations and contraction will occasionally be seen in the confluence of the renal pelvis, caused by mucosal lesions and shrinkage (Fig. 100—102). The possibility of cancer formation in the renal pelvis which may be a complication of stone should be borne in mind (see Chapter O).

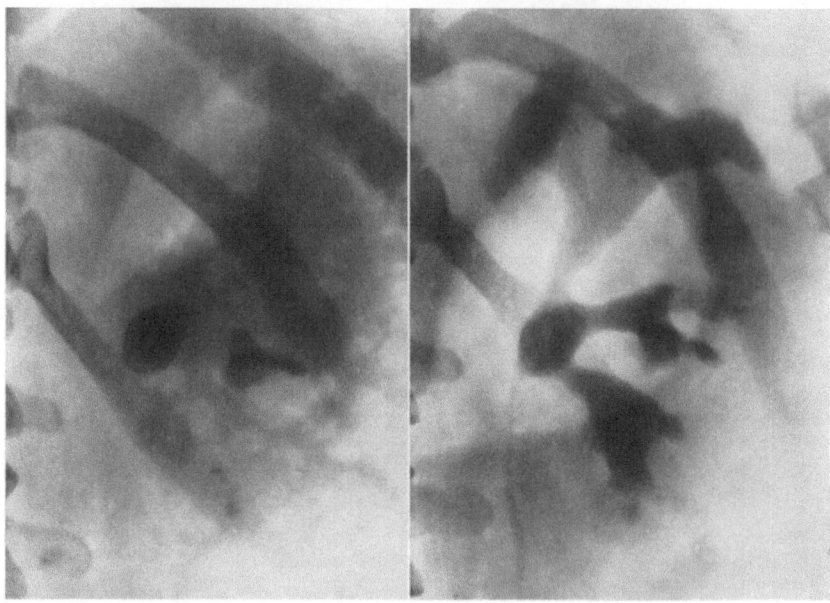

Fig. 100. Stone in confluence and in deformed calyces in caudal pole. Urography: marked narrowing of confluence around stone; dilatation of branches and calyces with papillary necroses

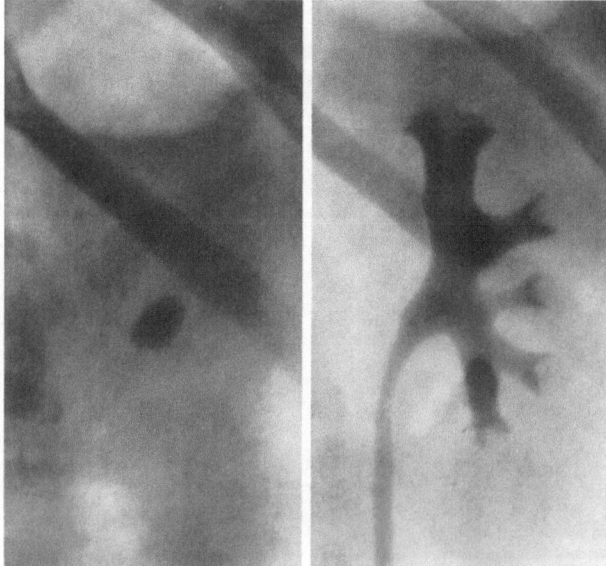

Fig. 101. Stone in confluence. Narrowing around stone and slight peripheral dilatation

The mucosa of the renal pelvis may be coarse when the pelvis houses stones. Occasionally the mucosa has a granulated appearance, so-called pyelitis granularis (Fig. 103). These mucosal changes may, at angiography, appear as a marked local hypervascularity (Fig. 107).

When stones are present in the confluence, the latter may be decreased in volume because of contraction and shrinkage. It is a striking fact that the confluence is often narrow and the calyces wide. This is particularly conspicuous in those cases in which the shape of the renal pelvis was known before the formation of stone (Fig. 104). The ureter is

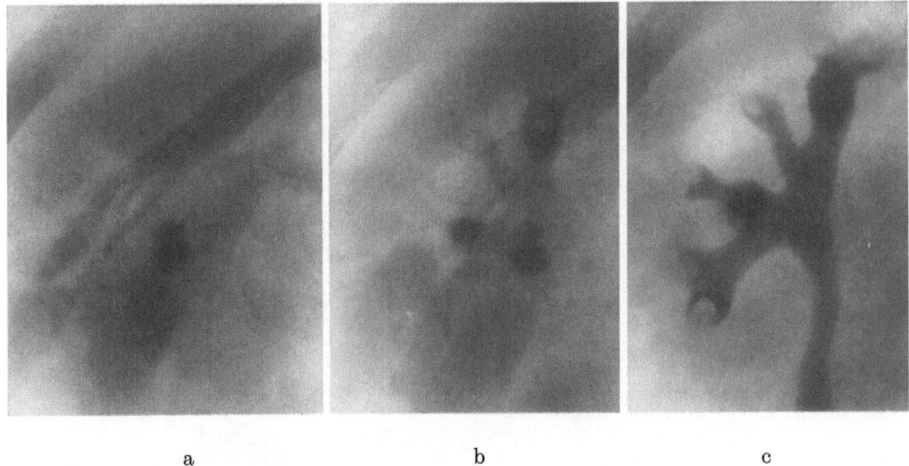

a   b   c

Fig. 102. Stone in confluence with narrowing of latter around stone. a) Plain radiography; b) urography at early stage: contrast urine in cranial (lowermost) calyces; c) ureteric compression: stone masked by contrast urine. Note coarse mucosa in confluence and cranial part of ureter

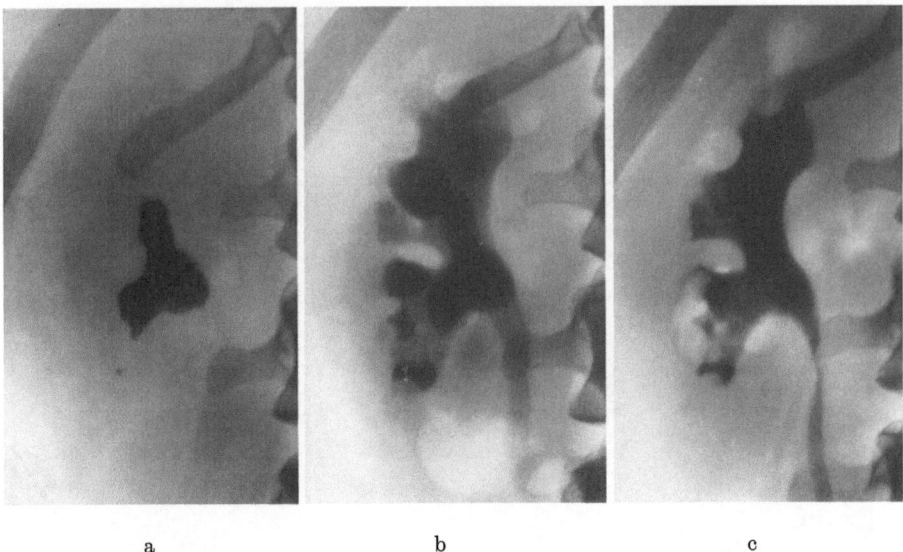

a   b   c

Fig. 103. Irregular surface of stone in a) corresponds to granular pyelitis seen in c) after release of ureteric compression

usually dilated distally to the renal pelvis thus altered, although no obstruction can be seen in the ureter.

Concrements are capable of obstructing the drainage of a single calyx, a major portion of the renal pelvis, or of the entire renal pelvis with the formation of a hydrocalyx or hydronephrosis as a consequence (Figs. 105—108). The delay of excretion of

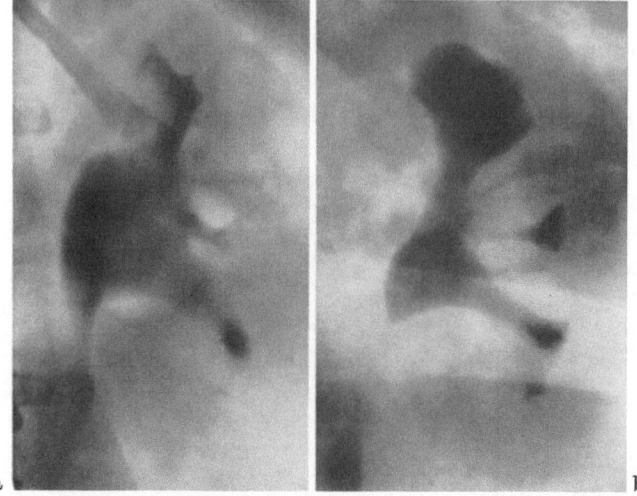

Fig. 104. Stone in confluence causes marked narrowing. Urography: a) before and b) after formation of stone

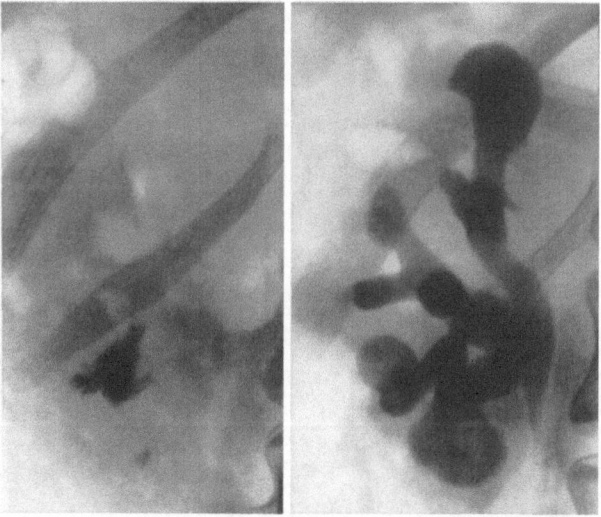

Fig. 105. Stone in caudal branch causing hydrocalicosis

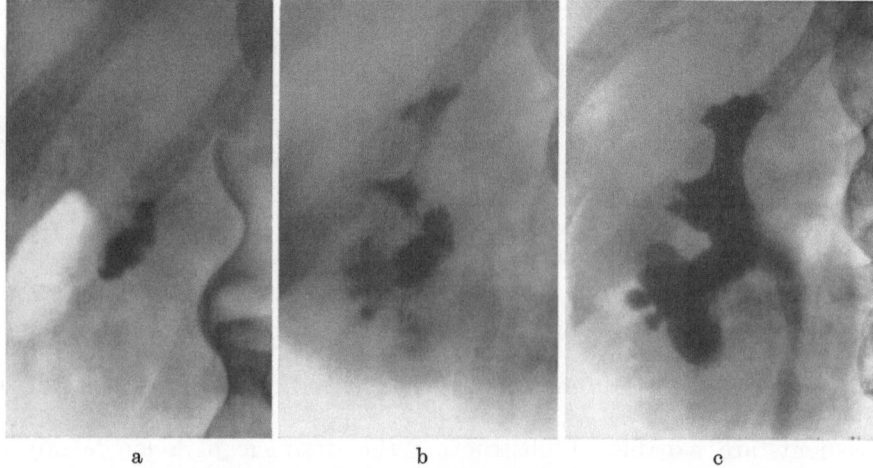

Fig. 106. Stones in caudal branch causing dilatation of caudal half of kidney pelvis. In c) during ureteric compression, stones are masked by contrast urine

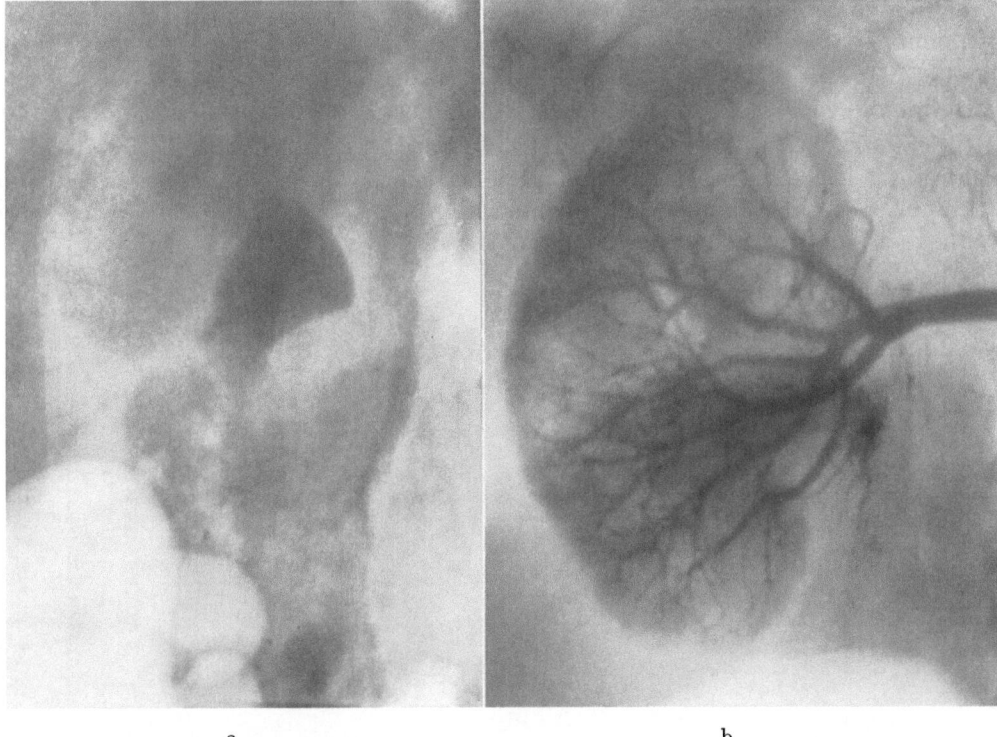

a   b

Fig. 107. a) Plain roentgenography: large stone in confluence; b) angiography, arterial phase: marked hypervascularity in region of confluence with hypertrophy and tortuosity of kidney pelvic arteries

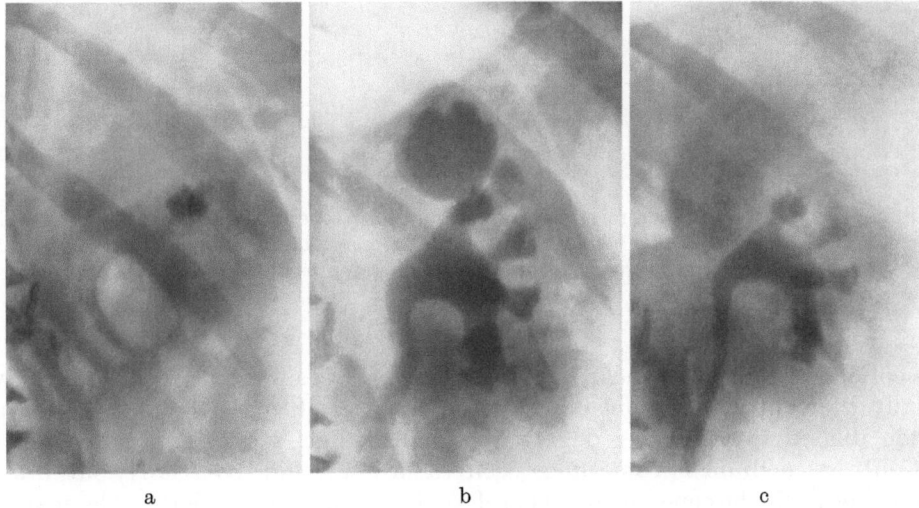

a   b   c

Fig. 108. Stone in upper branch causing dilatation of cranial calyces b) and finally complete block. (Two-year
interval between b) and c). Note displacement of filled cranial calyx by dilated, unfilled part of kidney pelvis
in c)

contrast medium in such blocked parts of a kidney may be temporary or permanent. Oddly enough, as mentioned above, even large stones do not always interfere with drainage.

The kidney is usually changed in size and shape in stone pyonephrosis and there is no excretion of contrast medium due to stasis and parenchymal destruction (Fig. 109).

Ureteric stones may be situated anywhere between the pelviureteric junction down to the ureteric orifice in the bladder. Small concrements are usually situated in the distal part. Larger concrements are often impacted high up. Large concrements may, however, sometimes pass down to the lower third of the ureter.

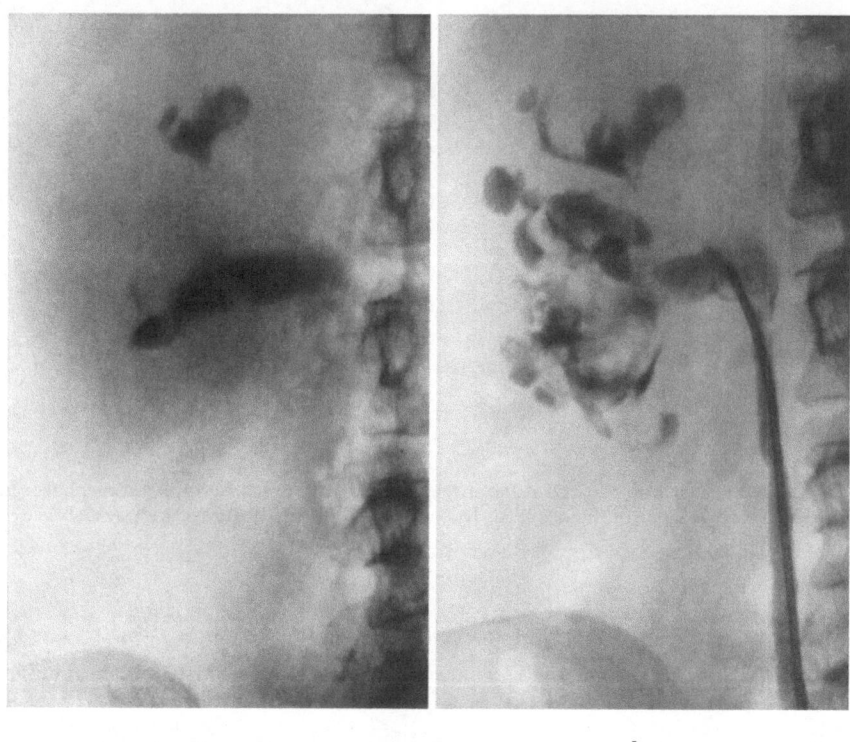

a   b

Fig. 109. Stone pyonephrosis. a) Plain roentgenography: multiple stones. Shape of cranial stones indicates papillary necrosis. Remaining cavities are filled with parts of the stone moulded to cranial calyces. b) Pyelography: papillary necrosis; detritus in kidney pelvis partly calcified

The column of contrast urine in the ureter is seen to cease at the level blocked by stone, but usually the contrast medium flows more or less easily past the stone. The ureter is then often dilated to a varying degree above the stone, while it is of ordinary width below. Contrast medium is sometimes seen to flow around even fairly large stones or through a groove in the concrement. Therefore, if it is not certain that a calcification really is a stone, ureteric compression may sometimes be applied for a time to secure an accumulation of contrast urine, which owing to its volume causes a slight stasis above a stone on release of compression. If a stone is found in the lower-most part of a ureter, full attention should be given to the possibility of a ureterocele which may be very small and the demonstration of which may be haphazard.

The distal part of the ureter may be widened by the stone itself or by swelling of the ureteric wall caused by a stone (which can have passed recently). This causes a broadening of the interureteric ridge at the orifice of the ureter (EDLING, 1941).

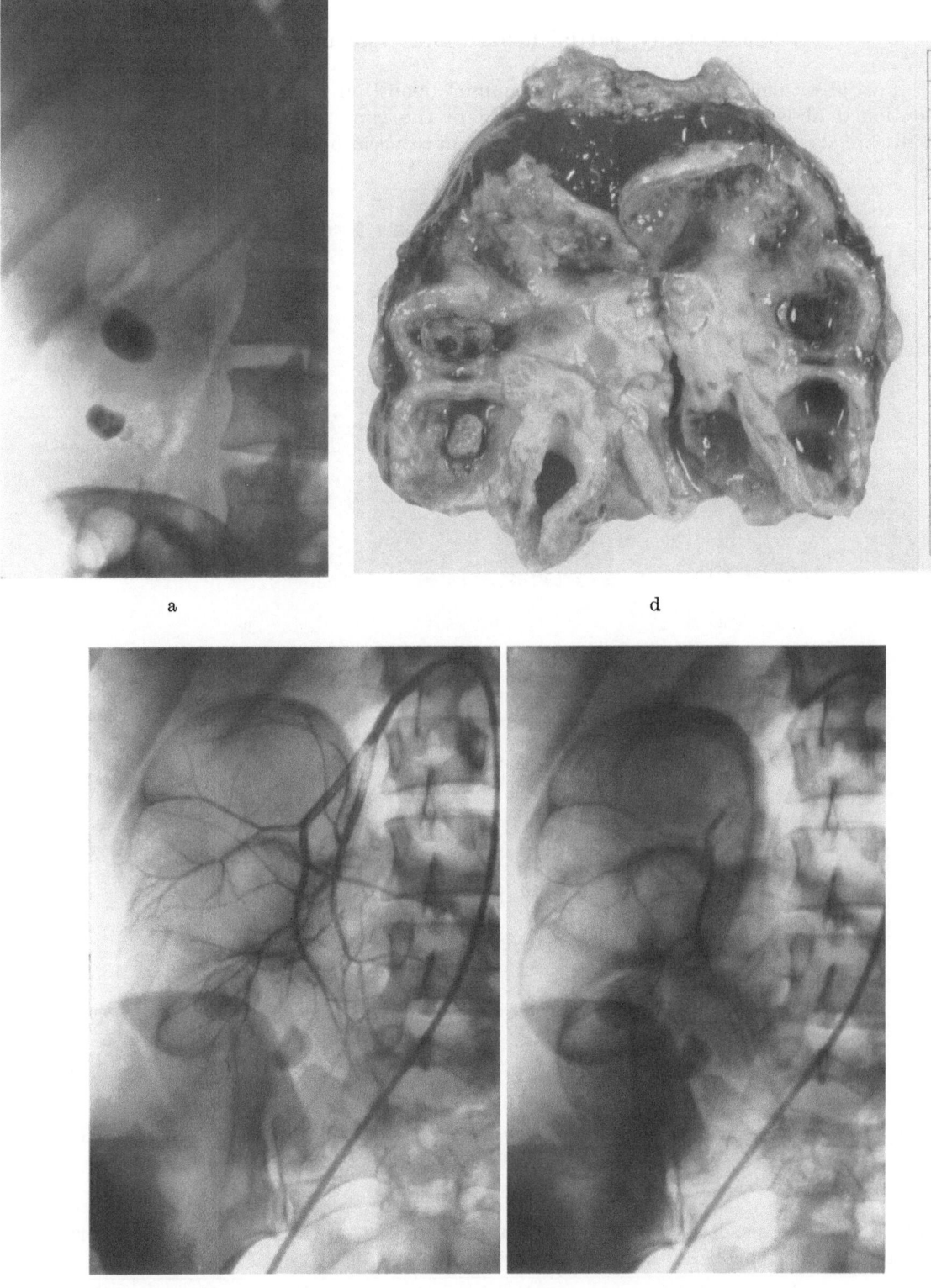

a

d

b

c

Fig. 110. Hydronephrosis with laminated stones. a) Urography: no excretion; b) renal angiography, arterial phase: arteries thin and stretched; capsular branches stretched along dilated kidney pelvis; c) nephrographic phase: atrophy of almost entire kidney parenchyma; d) operation specimen

X. Nephrectomy, partial nephrectomy and ureterolithotomy

Partial or polar nephrectomy is a common operation for renal stone (Fig. 111). As mentioned above, calculi are often situated in the caudal pole of the kidney. Concrements are also often seen in malformed calyces, in calyceal border evaginations, pyelogenic

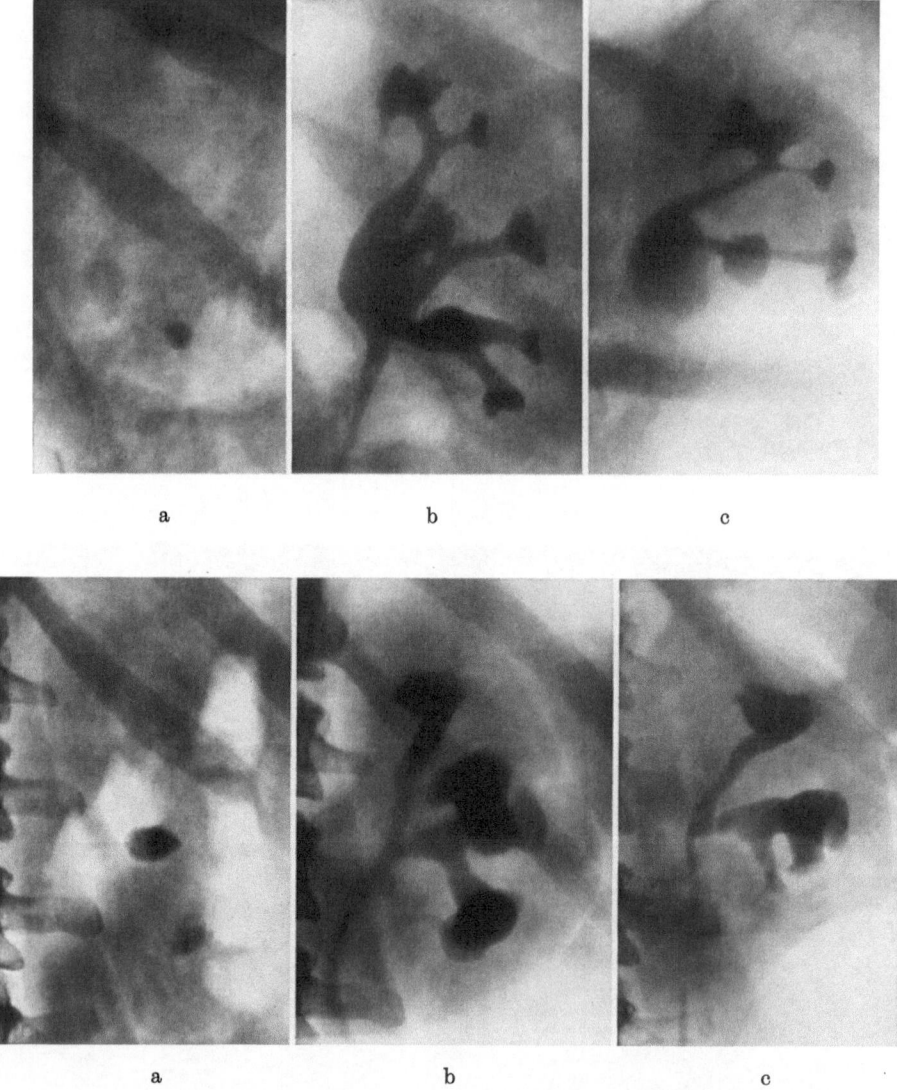

a   b   c

a   b   c

Fig. 111. Partial nephrectomy for stone (two patients). a) Plain radiography: Stone in confluence and caudal calyces. b) Urography. c) Urography after partial nephrectomy

cysts, hydrocalicosis, etc. The wide use of partial nephrectomy has increased the importance of detecting such localizing factors roentgenologically.

Angiography is useful for pre-operative investigation of the vasculature, particularly in the poles of the kidney. It may also be of importance for demonstrating impaired supply to the region in which the stone is lodged and for demonstrating, in the nephrogram, parenchymal atrophy around the stone due to stasis and/or infection.

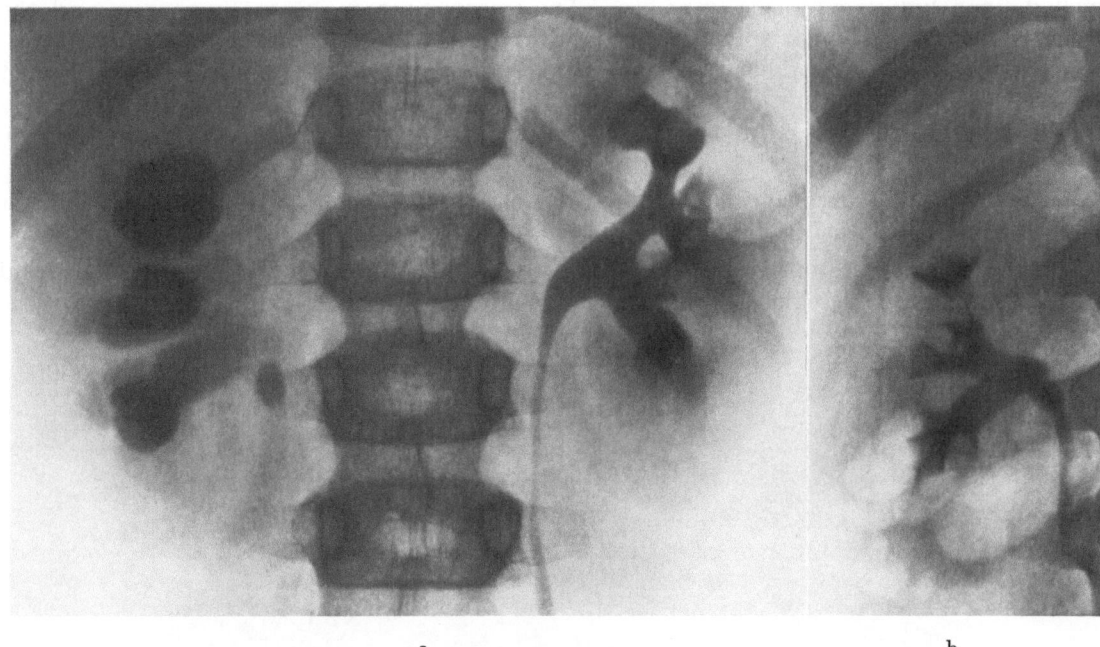

a   b

Fig. 112. Urography: a) stone on right side at pelviureteric junction, marked dilatation of right kidney pelvis; b) after operative removal of stone, only slight indentation at site of pyelotomy

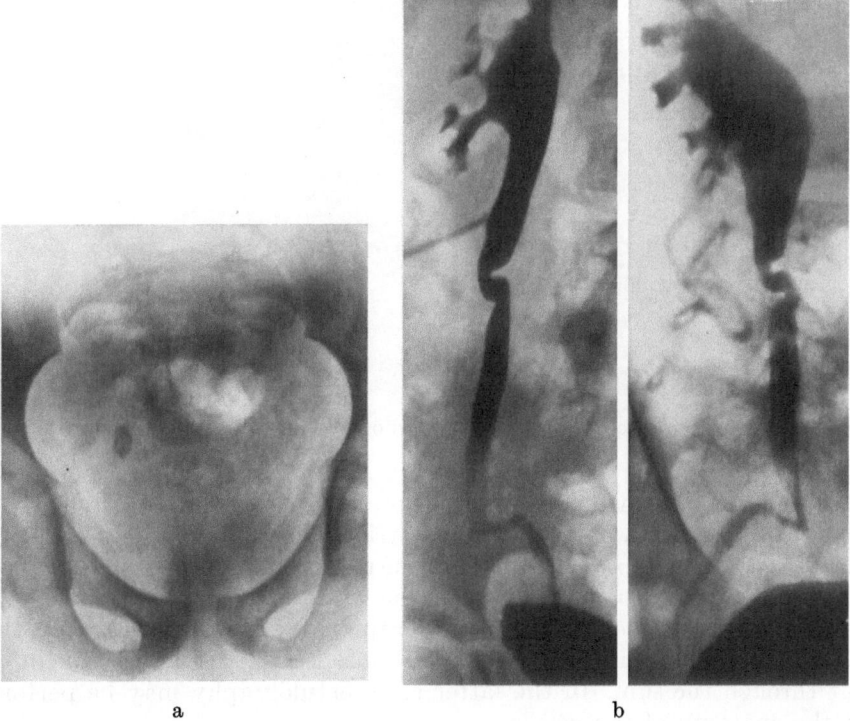

a   b

Fig. 113. Ureteric stricture after ureterolithotomy and ureteritis. a) Plain film: large ureteric stone; b) post-operative antegrade pyelography four months after operation: marked strictures and angulation due to adhesion

At post-operative check radiography following partial nephrectomy, a diminished but well defined kidney will usually be seen. The resected region is usually plump, and the kidney is often somewhat rotated, with the long axis in a straight craniocaudal direction. Its outline is sometimes blurred by post-operative fibrosis of the fatty capsule. At urography, ordinary excretion of contrast medium can be seen and the amputated region of the renal pelvis can be demonstrated, varying in size according to the extent of the operation.

In the event of fistulization, perirenal edema may be seen and the excreted contrast medium will fill the fistula or impaired excretion will be seen.

After ureterolithotomy, the ureter usually rapidly resumes its normal shape and width. Occasionally irregularities and slight luminar changes may be seen. Recovery is,

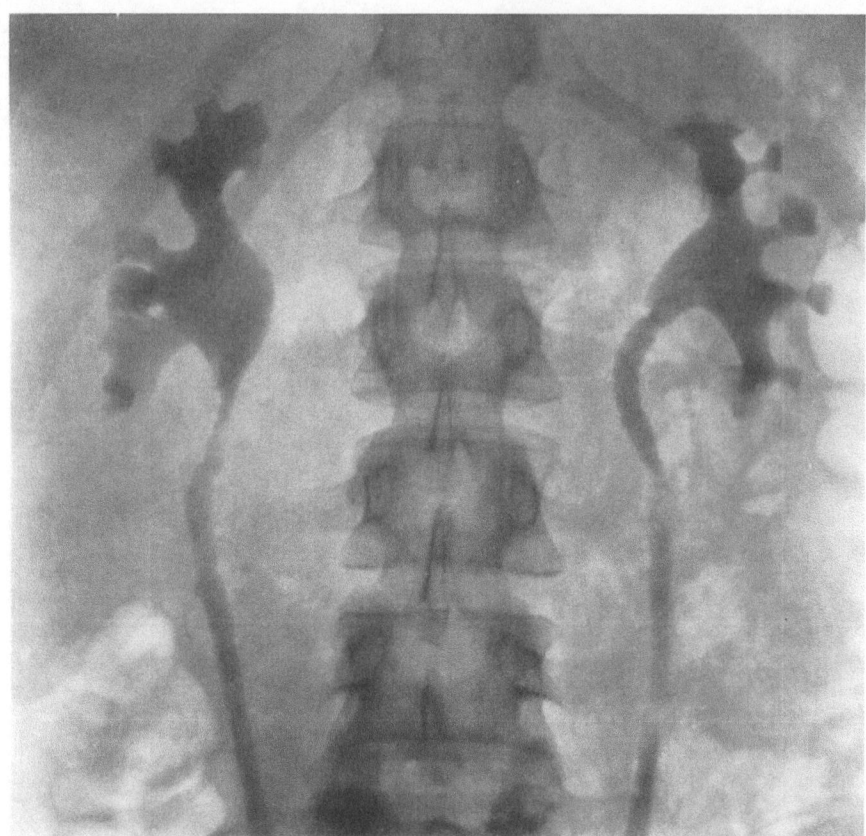

Fig. 114. Urography: irregularities in upper part of both ureters after bilateral pyelostomy

as a rule, so complete that after one month no change is demonstrable at the site of the operation. Occasionally, however, a marked stricture is seen at the site of intervention (Figs. 112—115). Proximal to such a stricture the ureter is dilated. In the event of complications such as large decubitus ulceration in the ureteric wall or infection, large or small fistulae may develop. At pyelography or urography, contrast medium may then be seen to escape into the periureteric tissue. If the fistula is large, it may break into the intestine or out through the skin. In the latter case, fistulography may be performed to demonstrate the anatomy of the fistula.

Stones may have been left or new stones may have formed and maintain an infection of the ureteric stump after nephrectomy for stone. It is sometimes possible to obtain a filling of such a stump by catheterization or by reflux from the urinary bladder.

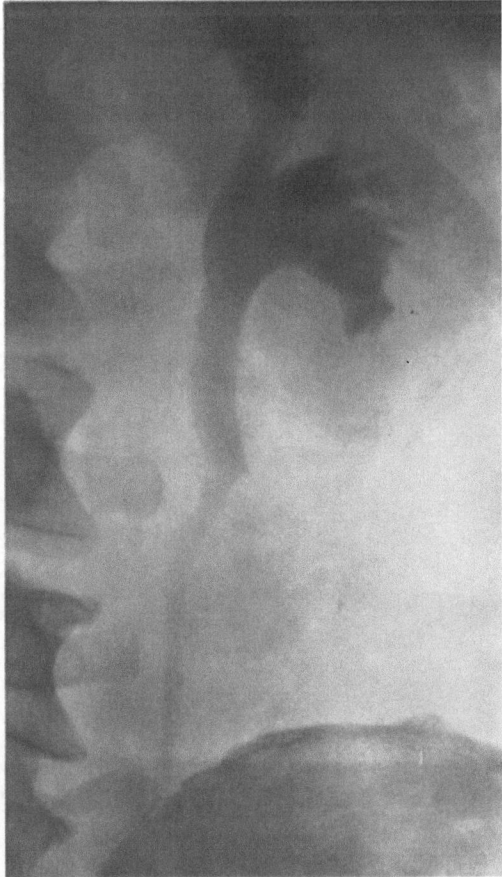

Fig. 115. Urography: adhesion of upper part of left ureter to kidney after pyelotomy

XI. Roentgen examination during renal colic

Acute renal colic is a dramatic experience for the patient and often gives rise to important differential diagnostic problems. The patho-physiology of the attack in its different phases can be well demonstrated urographically.

In acute renal colic, urography is therefore of great diagnostic and differential diagnostic value, particularly because of the reliability of the results of the examination during the acute attack.

For reasons given below, the examination should be carried out as soon as possible. The patient is taken, so to say, straight from the street to the examination table. There is no time and generally no need for an enema or purgatives. In addition, diseases of differential diagnostic importance such as appendicitis prohibit enema.

1. Plain radiography

In such emergency cases the large intestine often contains fecal material and meteorism may exist, which is sometimes considerable. If the attack is severe, it will often be accompanied by lumbar scoliosis with the concavity facing the side of the attack, and the contracted musculature in the flank will be seen to bulge onto the extraperitoneal fat.

The kidney on the side involved is usually somewhat large and plump due to renal stasis. (It has been claimed by FELTER, 1953 that the dilated renal pelvis is capable of compressing the veins in the sinus and that the increase in size of the kidney is therefore due in part to venous stasis). Because of meteorism it is often not possible to outline the kidneys and occasionally a slight perirenal edema adds to these difficulties.

The stone responsible for the attack is usually demonstrable. It may be situated at the pelviureteric junction but is most commonly in the ureter, most frequently in the distal part. Occasionally no concrement can be observed because it is too small and/or not opaque enough to be demonstrated, or it may be masked by intestinal contents. It may also be due to projection of the stone onto bone, if it happens to be situated in that part of the ureter crossing the pelvis (Fig. 116). It should also be borne in mind that in multiparae the floor of the pelvis is often low. Low ureteric stones may therefore be projected low down and be masked by the anterior portion of the pelvic bone. The stone may

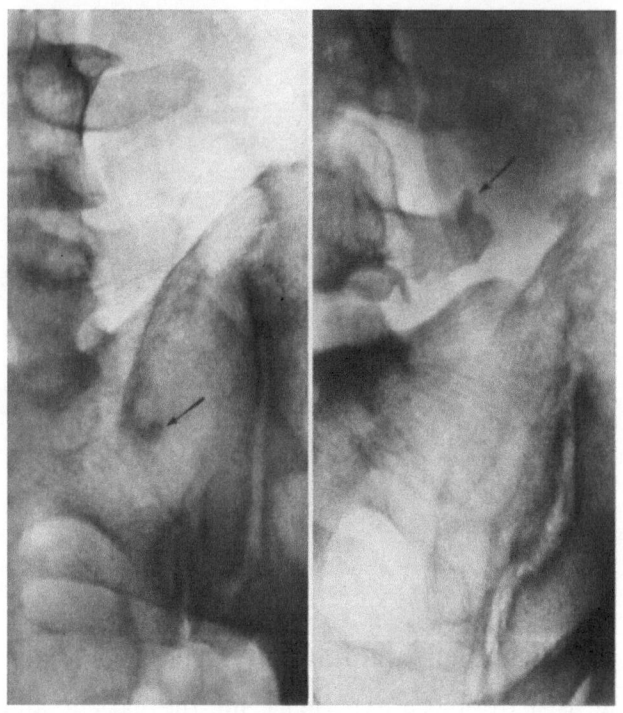

a   b

Fig. 116. Stone projected onto bone. Plain radiography in two different projections. In b) tube is tilted cranially and stone is projected free (arrow)

also have been passed, but pain persists. Finally, the absence of any demonstrable concrements may be due, for example, to the fact that the attack is not caused by a stone but by a clot (see below).

During the examination, a stone may occasionally be seen to shift (see Fig. 118), e.g. a concrement lodged at the pelviureteric junction may be displaced up into the renal pelvis and the attack may then cease, or a high stone may be seen to pass on distally, or a distal stone to pass into the urinary bladder.

Severe retroperitoneal edema is occasionally demonstrated, which may blur the entire outline of the kidney, or part of it. This is due to urinary reflux with retroperitoneal uroplania (see Chapter I).

2. Urography

After the plain films have been examined, contrast medium is injected for urography. The first film should be taken soon, 1—3 minutes after the injection, other films some minutes later. With these films as a guide, the examination may be continued. Ureteric

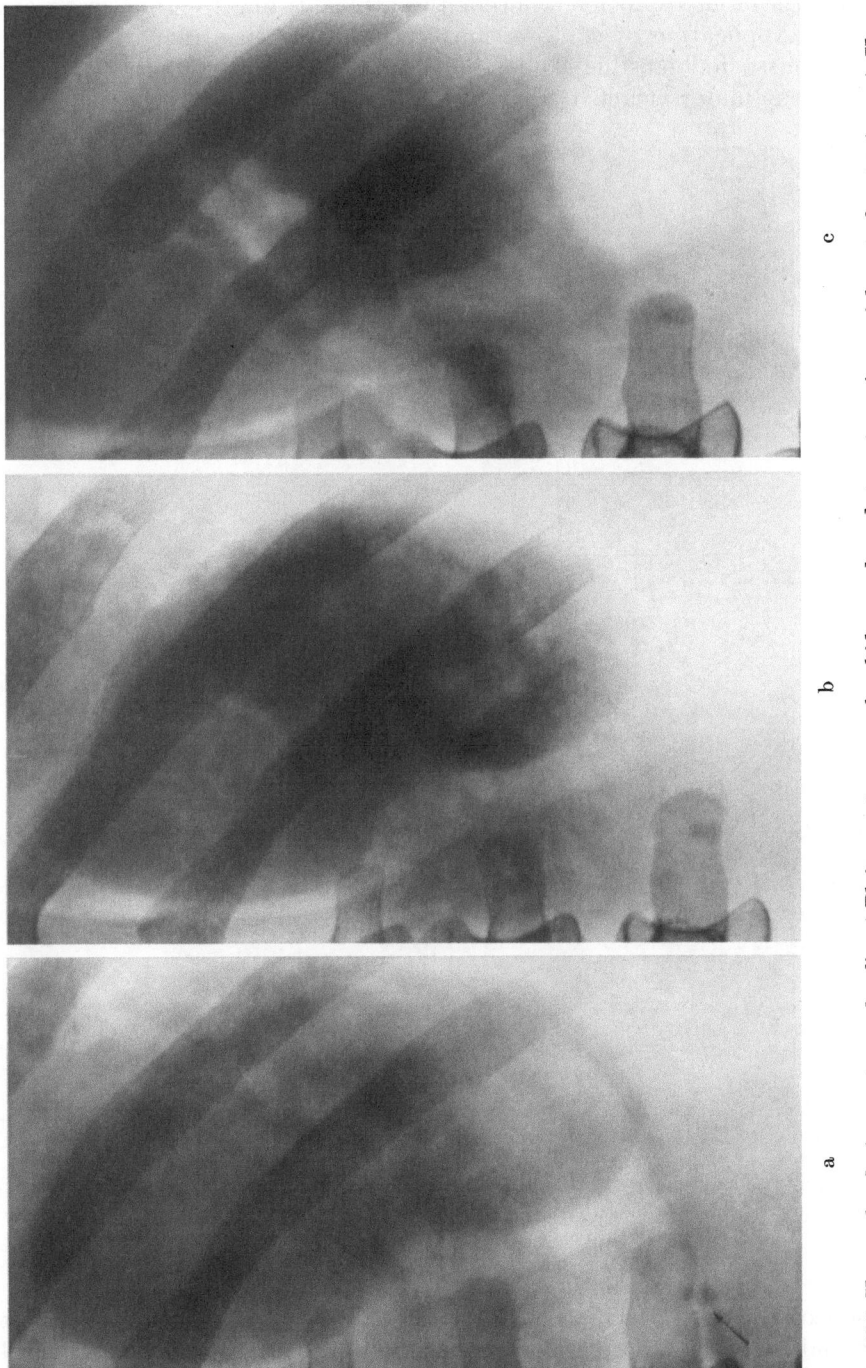

a   b   c

Fig. 117. Urography during acute renal colic. a) Plain roentgenography: kidney enlarged, two stones in cranial part of ureter (arrow). Urography during acute pain: ordinary excretion on right side, no excretion on left side. b) Two hours after injection of contrast medium: nephrogram caused by contrast urine in excretory system. c) Seventeen hours later: very slight excretion with filling of dilated kidney pelvis and of ureter down to stone; reabsorption of contrast medium

compression is not applied, of course. The main reason for this is that compression influences the examination findings. Compression causes stasis and should therefore not be used in the investigation of supposed urinary stasis. Another reason is that the examination is often performed in order to decide whether the attack is due to stone or to appendicitis, for example. Application of compression to the abdomen of a patient with acute appendicits is, of course, indefensible. Thus application of ureteric compression in the examination of a patient under attack is a grave fault.

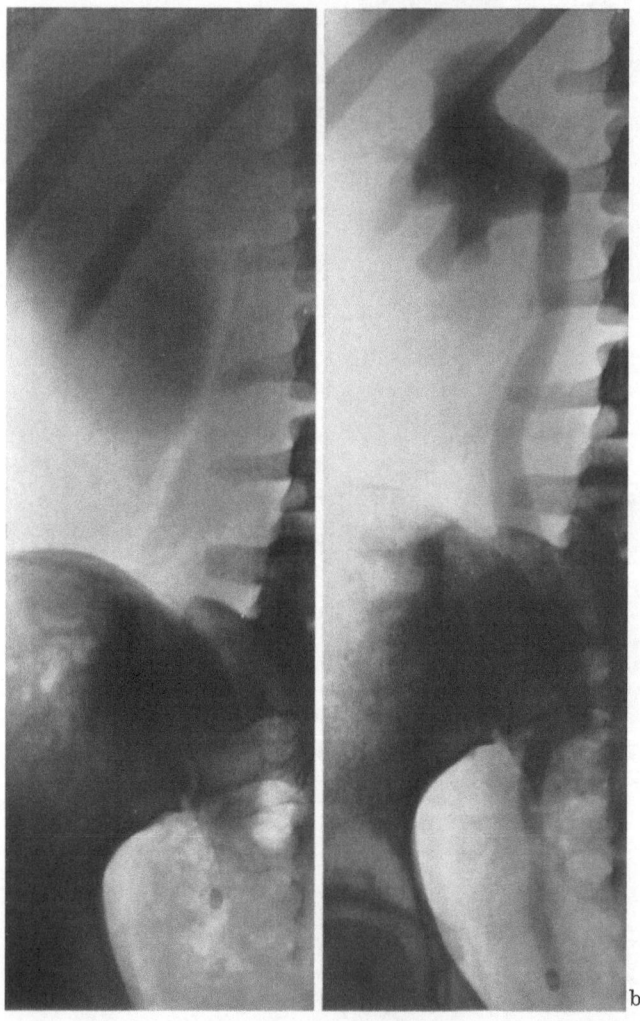

Fig. 118. Right-sided renal colic; stone in distal part of ureter. a) Plain roentgenography. Urography: excretion of contrast medium delayed; filling of dilated kidney pelvis and ureter down to stone, which has moved distally 2 cm. b) Four days after contrast injection

Examination of the first urogram during the actual attack is usually sufficient to make a differential diagnosis. Absence of excretion on the affected side, with ordinary excretion on the other side, indicates stasis and it may be concluded that the pain is due to renal colic. If excretion starts at the same time on both sides in a patient complaining of pain, the cause of the attack is not located in the urinary pathways but elsewhere. In other words, the attack in this case is not renal colic.

On examination during an attack of renal colic, urinary stasis will be demonstrated by delayed excretion of contrast medium (Figs. 117, 118). This delay may be several hours

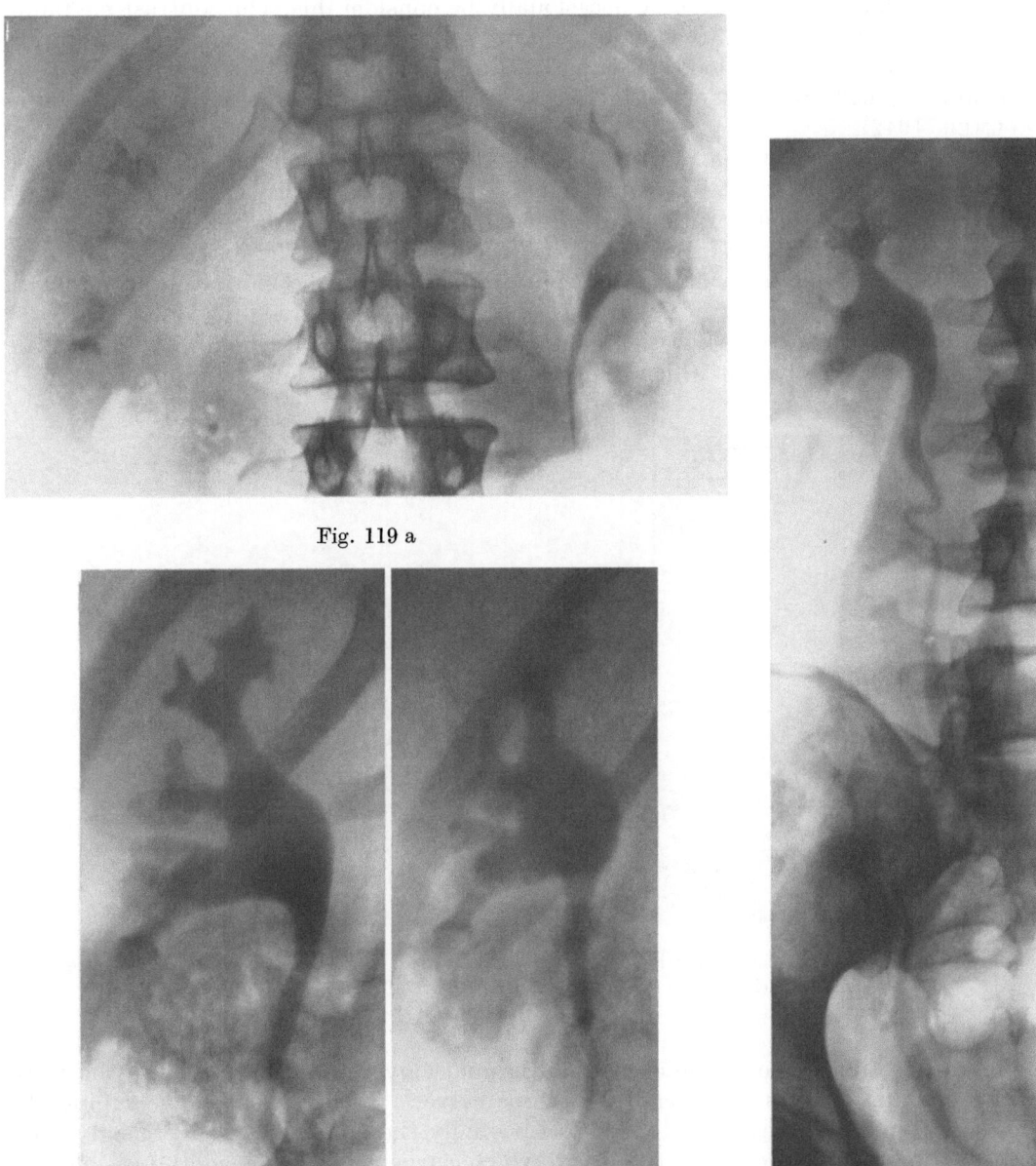

Fig. 119 a

Fig. 119 b   Fig. 120

Fig. 119. Examination during acute pain on right side. Urography during slight pain without preparation of patient. Plain roentgenogram: right kidney plump; small stone in cranial part of ureter. a) Urography six minutes after contrast injection: slightly dilated calyces filled (analgetics given); b) frontal, oblique view 20 minutes later: slightly dilated calyces filled; cranial part of ureter also slightly dilated down to concrement; contrast urine flows past stone in ureter of ordinary width

Fig. 120. Renal colic. Pain subsided during examination. Slight stasis with continuous filling of ureter down to very small stone at ureteric orifice (arrow)

or, exceptionally, a day or more. In these cases the renal parenchyma will usually show increased density. The increase may occasionally be considerable. The contrast medium is accumulated in the lumina of the nephrons. This is due to the increased pressure, but may be accentuated by a fall in blood pressure. In the enlarged kidney with increased density, the renal sinus will appear as a distinct, irregular filling defect in the renal parenchyma (Hellmer, 1942).

The accumulation of contrast medium in the renal parenchyma may persist for a short while or for one or several days if the stasis persists. The density of the kidney will gradually decrease with re-absorption of the contrast medium. More often, however, the density decreases rapidly. As soon as the attack subsides and the excretion of contrast medium into the renal pelvis starts, the contrast medium in the kidney empties into the urinary pathways.

As a rule, even in severe stasis, small amounts of contrast medium will gradually flow into the renal pelvis in which contrast medium of very low concentration can be

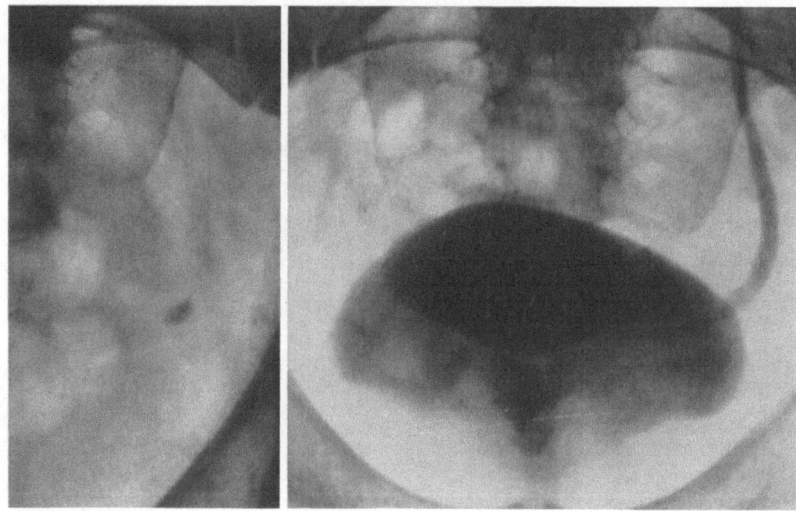

Fig. 121. Left-sided renal colic. Examination after pain had subsided. Slight stasis with filling of entire ureter. Contrast urine passes stone in extravesical part of distal end of ureter

demonstrated. First some of the dorsal and cranial calyces are filled because the heavy contrast medium collects most readily in these calyces when the patient is supine. The calyces are usually markedly dilated but occasionally the dilatation is surprisingly small.

As soon as the diagnosis is established, which, as mentioned, is usually possible after examination of the first urograms, and it has been shown that the attack is due to urinary tract disease, the patient may be given an analgetic and the examination continued at leisure. The analgetic should be given as soon as possible after it has been clearly demonstrated that stasis is present and it is thus decided that the pain is induced by renal colic. It is just as wrong to postpone giving the patient an analgetic to relieve severe pain at this stage as it is to give analgetic before the differential-diagnostic problem is solved.

It is believed (Herzan and O'Brien, 1952) that a glass of ice water will produce immediate relief and induce the excretion of contrast medium. We have tried this and found that it is occasionally effective, although only occasionally.

As soon as the pain has ceased, contrast medium will be excreted. The last step of the examination is to demonstrate the stone (Figs. 119—121). It may be useful to follow the excretion until it is well under way and the contrast urine has filled the ureter down to the site of the stone. The interval between the exposures is dictated to some extent by the findings but mainly by rule of thumb. The patient should preferably walk about to promote the flow of the heavy contrast urine down into the ureter towards the obstructing calculus. If the concrement is close to the bladder, the contrast urine in the bladder covers the region (Fig. 122). Then the patient should urinate in order to permit a completely free projection of the lower ureter and the concrement. If several calcifications are demonstrable and a differential diagnosis is to be made between concrements and phleboliths, oblique films must decide which calcification is the concrement.

During or immediately after a less severe attack, the excretion of contrast medium may be only moderately or very slightly delayed. In addition, the renal pelvis is usually slightly dilated and the ureter is filled down to the level of a stone, if any, and the emptying of the renal pelvis and the ureter is delayed.

When signs of stasis are present at urography in connection with acute renal colic, a contrast filling of the gall bladder is often seen. This occurs more often with the contrast

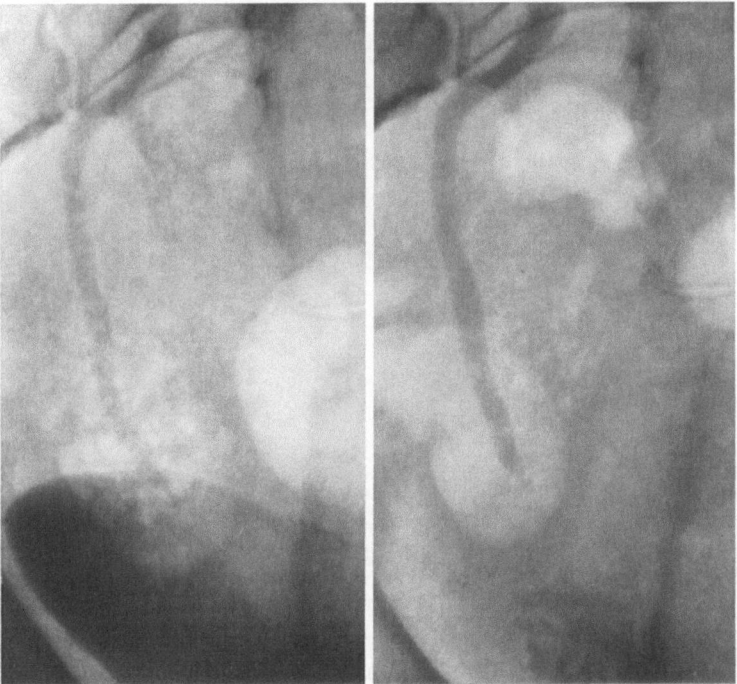

Fig. 122. Stone in distal part of right ureter. Urography: continuous filling of ureter down to stone. Distal end of ureter shown better after voiding of contrast urine from bladder

medium sodium metrizoate than with the diatrizoate media (OLLE OLSSON, 1971). We have encountered several cases in which during urography in connection with an attack of pain, marked or only slight stasis was present on one side and at the same time filling of the gall bladder was observable during the actual examination. When this happens, it may be used as an extra sign of diagnostic importance when the acute examination is performed for the purpose of clinical differential diagnosis between an attack of cholelithiasis and urolithiasis and if signs of stasis at urography are slight or absent when the examination is performed after cessation of pain. Filling of the gall bladder during the actual examination can be slight but may occasionally be marked. If minimal, increase in concentration will usually occur during the following hours and good filling may persist and be seen on the following day.

Symptoms of obstructed drainage in renal colic are the same on obstruction of one half of a double kidney. Thus, in the presence of obstruction of one part of a forked ureter or in one of the ureters in the presence of double ureter, stasis is limited to that part of the kidney drained by the ureter in question (Fig. 123). In severe stasis markedaccumulation of contrast medium may be seen in the corresponding part of the kidney (HELLMER, 1942). The possibility of a double kidney, which is not an uncommon anomaly, must therefore always be borne in mind on examination of a patient during an acute attack.

It cannot be stressed enough that in the performance of urography for such a differential diagnosis e.g. renal colic-appendicitis, ureteric compression should never beapplied.

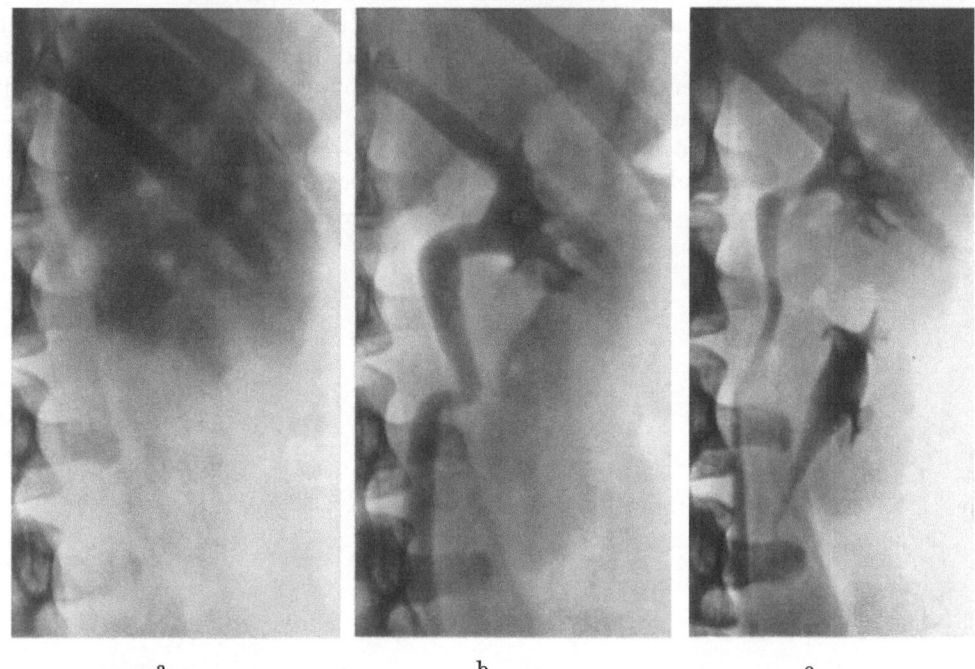

a   b   c

Fig. 123. Renal colic, left side. Stasis in upper part of double kidney. Urography during attack: low stone in left ureter; three minutes after contrast injection: normal excretion, right side, caudal pole left side. a) $1^1/_4$ hours later, nephrography of kidney parenchyma belonging to cranial part. Note irregular border to caudal part. b) $2^1/_4$ hours later: excretion into dilated cranial pelvis and corresponding ureter. c) Urography after pain had subsided: ordinary excretion

3. Discussion of signs of stasis

The signs of stasis as described by HELLMER (1935) and by WULFF (1936) are as follows: increase in size of the kidney, delay or absence of contrast excretion, increase in density of renal parenchyma, dilatation of renal pelvis and ureter, delay in emptying of renal pelvis and ureter. The frequency of positive roentgen findings decreases with increasing length of time after the attack. If the patient is examined during the attack, stasis will be demonstrable in almost all cases. Signs of stasis will be detectable in only 88% of cases if the examination is performed within three hours after the cessation of the attack, in 80% after six to twelve hours, and in only 50% after 24—48 hours. Since the examination yields most information if it is performed during the attack, it should when possible be started while the attack is still in progress. Since the roentgen examination under such circumstances gives clear-cut information, the diagnosis can be made in a very early stage of the examination. The first or second urogram is usually sufficient to decide whether or not stasis is present, and thus whether or not the pain is due to renal colic. Therefore, if stasis is seen in the first urogram, it may be concluded that the attack is due to urinary tract obstruction and that the differential diagnostic problem is solved. These remarks apply in particular to the differential-diagnostic problem caused by appendicitis.

It has been claimed (ARNESEN, 1939) that in acute appendicitis changes will be seen at urography that may be confused with the signs of urinary stasis seen during renal colic. ARNESEN'S opinion cannot be accepted: no signs of stasis of any type have ever been observed in the many hundreds of cases of appendicitis examined in our department. In appendical abscess, in which the ureter may be involved, the flow in the ureter may, of course, be impaired, but never in acute appendicitis.

The signs referred to above represent different degrees of stasis, the markedly delayed excretion of contrast medium, and the accumulation of contrast medium in the renal parenchyma representing signs of severe stasis. At repeated urography during one and the same attack, an increase in the severity of stasis is said never to be seen (ARNESEN, 1939).

An exception to this rule, however, are cases in which during examination in slight or no pain, a severe attack of pain starts, in connection with which reflux can be seen (OLLE OLSSON, 1971).

The longer the interval after the onset of attack, the more the appearance of the roentgenogram will be dominated by signs of mild stasis, such as slight dilatation of the ureter and a continuous filling of the ureter with contrast medium down to a small stone near the ureteric orifice.

HOLMLUND (1968) in model and experimental studies in rabbits in comparison with clinical findings has observed the mechanism of the passage and arrest of ureteral stones. He found that in the ureters of rabbits a bar was present when a concrement had been lodged in the same place for more than 24 hours. In human ureters a bar was verified in patients with a large stone lodged in the upper or middle part of the ureter for a substantial length of time. When a stone was lodged in the most declivous part of the obstructed ureter, small particles with high specific gravity could occasionally be packed just abov the stone, hindering the urinary flow. The bar and these small particles could be seena filling defects above the stone during urography (ARNALDSSON and HOLMLUND, 1971).

Urography performed during an attack of renal colic will not always make demonstration of a concrement possible. This may be due to the stone's being situated at a site where it is capable of remaining concealed, e.g. it may be projected onto bone. The stone may also be too small to be detected, or it may not be opaque enough, or it may have passed. Thus occasionally the stone may have passed despite persistent stasis, such stasis being of functional origin or due to edema of the ureteric orifice.

Another possibility which must always be borne in mind is that the absence of a demonstrable concrement may be explained by the fact that the renal colic may be caused by a clot, for example, and not by a stone. It should be emphasized that signs of stasis are signs of renal colic and not of urinary stone. The colic is most often caused by stone, but this does not mean that this is always the case. A diagnosis of urinary calculus can be made only if the concrement has been demonstrated on the roentgenogram (or if it has been passed). In the presence of stasis without a demonstrable concrement, the examination must be repeated after a few days, when the patient is free of pain and can be prepared for the examination. This re-examination has to be performed as a morphologic examination with ureteric compression. The reason for this is that certain diseases can cause renal colic without stone. This may occur, for example, in renal tuberculosis and in renal tumor. ROSENDAL (1948), on examination of a series of renal tuberculosis, found that as many as seven out of 59 cases had colic-like attacks in their history. A renal tumor may bleed and consequent clot formation may cause colic-like pain. Urinary stasis in such a case is demonstrable on examination during an acute attack, but since meteorism is often present and ureteric compression cannot be applied, the morphology of the renal pelvis cannot be properly investigated. Therefore, in such cases examination of the anatomy of the kidney pelvis must be postponed until repeat urography after the pain has ceased (OLLE OLSSON 1949).

Occasionally a combination of stone and blood-clot may be seen (Fig. 130).

4. Backflow in acute renal colic (see Chapter P)

5. Reflex anuria

Reflex anuria is to be understood as reflex cessation of urinary excretion on the side involved. More commonly, however, it is used to designate the non-excretion of urine on the contralateral side. As pointed out previously, the pathophysiology of the excretion of contrast medium during renal colic has been clarified experimentally and clinically. It is in general due mainly to the secretory pressure in the kidney, on the one hand, and to the intrapelvic pressure, on the other. Thus, no reflex cramps in hypothetic sphincters or elsewhere need be supposed to explain this condition.

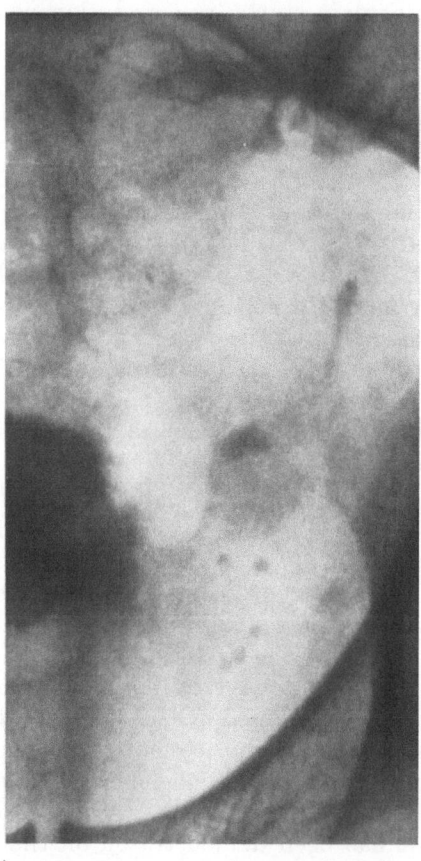

a

Fig. 124. Renal colic, left side. a) Plain roentgenography: large stone in ureter distally; b) acute urography: conglomerate kidney with crossed ectopy; contrast excretion only in caudal kidney pelvis corresponding to dystopic right kidney; c) after pain had subsided, excretion in left kidney also, with dilatation of kidney pelvis and ureter

Much has been written about this reflex cessation of the excretion on the contralateral side. The many thousands of cases of urographic examination during renal colic in our department alone is sufficient evidence to dismiss the term "reflex stone anuria" from the medical dictionary. We have in our department never seen any absence of secretion on the contralateral side in cases with unilateral stone. In stasis — also in cases of severe degree in one part of a double kidney or in one part of a fused kidney (Figs. 123, 124) — we have never seen reflex cessation of the contrast excretion, even in the half of the kidney the ureter of which had not been obstructed.

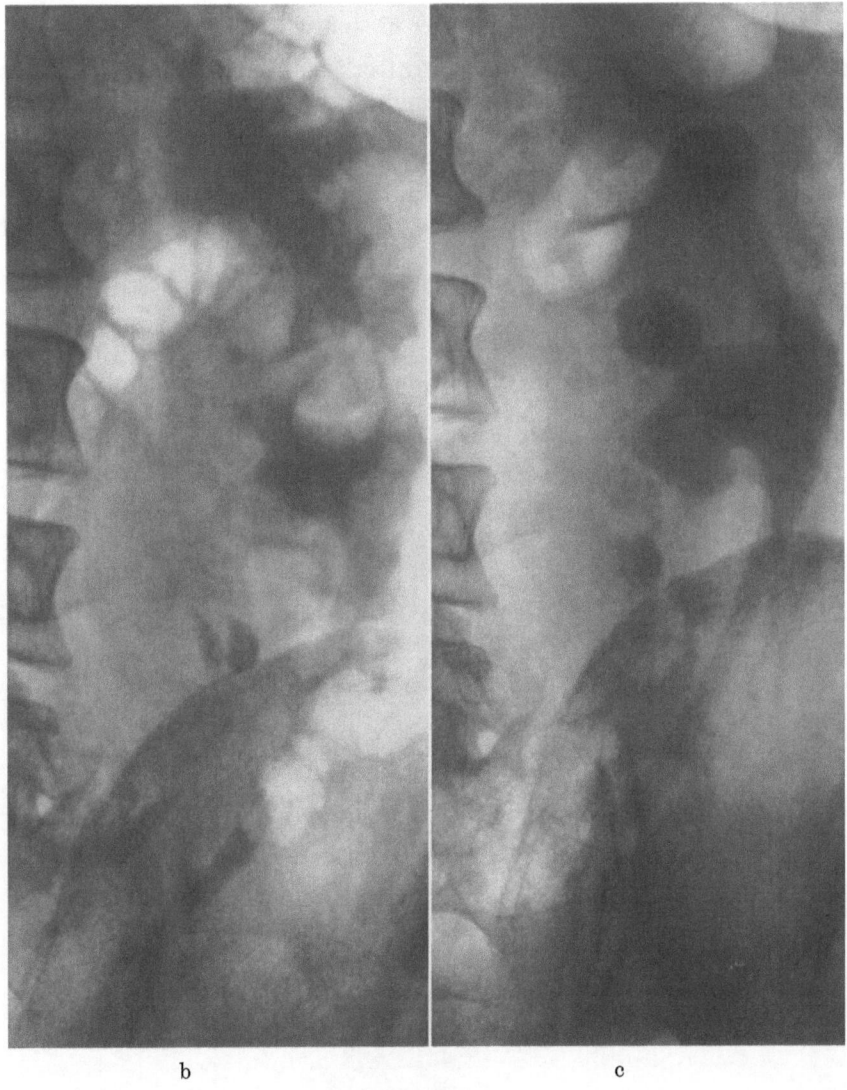

b   c

Fig. 124

WULFF (1941) has shown also in animal experiments that the possibility of reflex stone anuria may be ignored.

6. Cessation of pain

Cessation of pain usually indicates that passage is restored, which in turn can be due to passage of the stone. Nevertheless, stasis may persist. It is believed that lingering stasis is due to spastic contraction of the distal part of the ureter.

Here too it is not necessary to assume more or less hypothetical sphincter activity. The narrowing is due, as a rule, simply to edema of the mucosa at the site of the stone. As to the distal part of the ureter, the contrast filling is occasionally seen to terminate somewhat short of the concrement. This is often ascribed to spasm around the calculus, but is due instead to edema of the mucosa around the stone.

Detrusor spasm on the same side of the urinary bladder as the concrement has also been described in low concrements and is manifested by asymmetry of the bladder, which is better filled on the opposite side (ENDFEDJIEFF, 1958). The phenomenon corresponds to the so-called Constantinescus symptom, which is ascribed to reduced supply of urine from a kidney with impaired excretory capacity.

7. Passage of stone

Stones are often passed during or soon after renal colic. They occasionally remain impacted, however. The question then unsought presents itself: Is there any reasonable chance of the stone being passed spontaneously, or is surgical intervention necessary? In a material of 541 cases of ureteric stone in our department, Sandegård (1956) made the following observations: In the absence of indications for active intervention for reasons other than size, shape, or localization of the stone, the actual situation is influenced by the following facts:

a) Small stones (roentgenographic width < 4 mm) in the lower half of the ureter will usually (in 93 % of cases) be passed spontaneously.

b) Small stones in the upper half of the ureter will usually (81 %) be passed without serious complications. Occasionally (19 %) these stones persist in the upper half and can produce considerable obstruction.

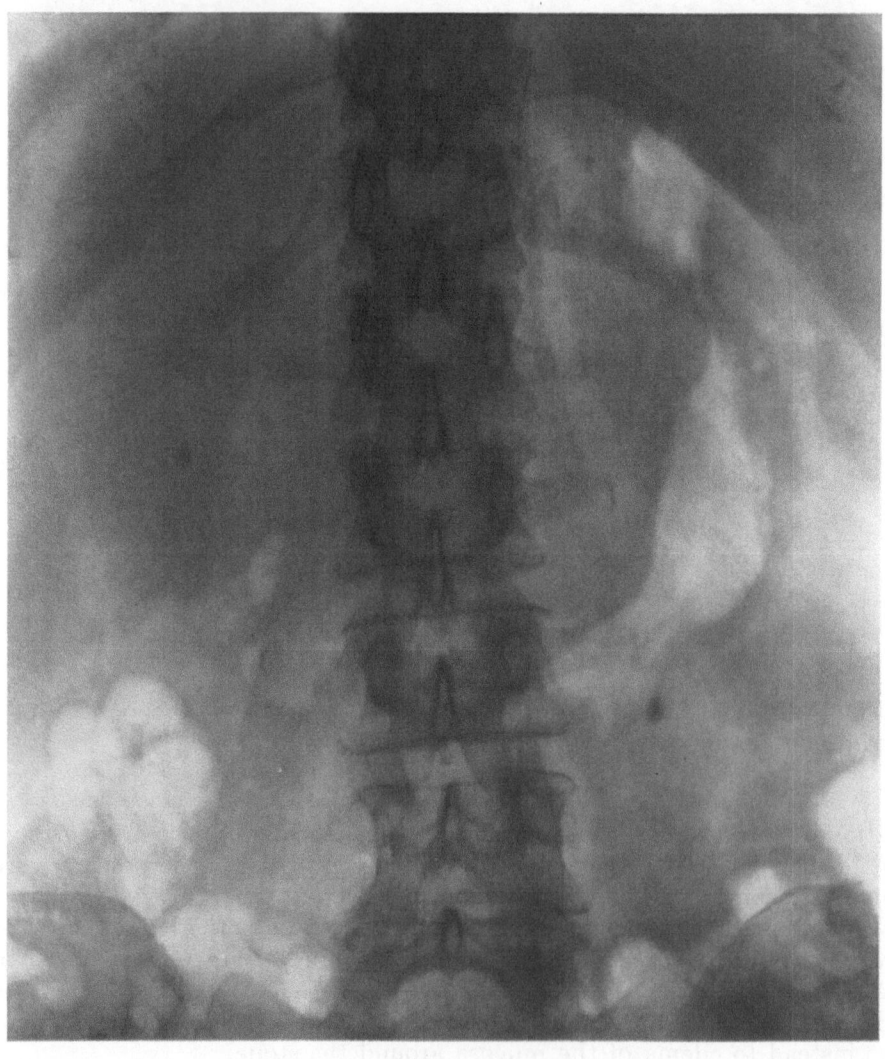

a

Fig. 125. Urography in connection with left-sided renal colic: a) plain roentgenography: stone in middle of left ureter; stone also in caudal pole of right kidney. b) Acute urography: delayed excretion of contrast medium; filling of dilated kidney pelvis and cranial part of ureter to stone. c) Pain subsided and stone passed a few days later. Check examination, plain roentgenography: stone which passed without pain was right-sided renal stone! d) Left-sided ureteric stone is localized in distal part of ureter. e) Very marked stasis despite cessation of pain

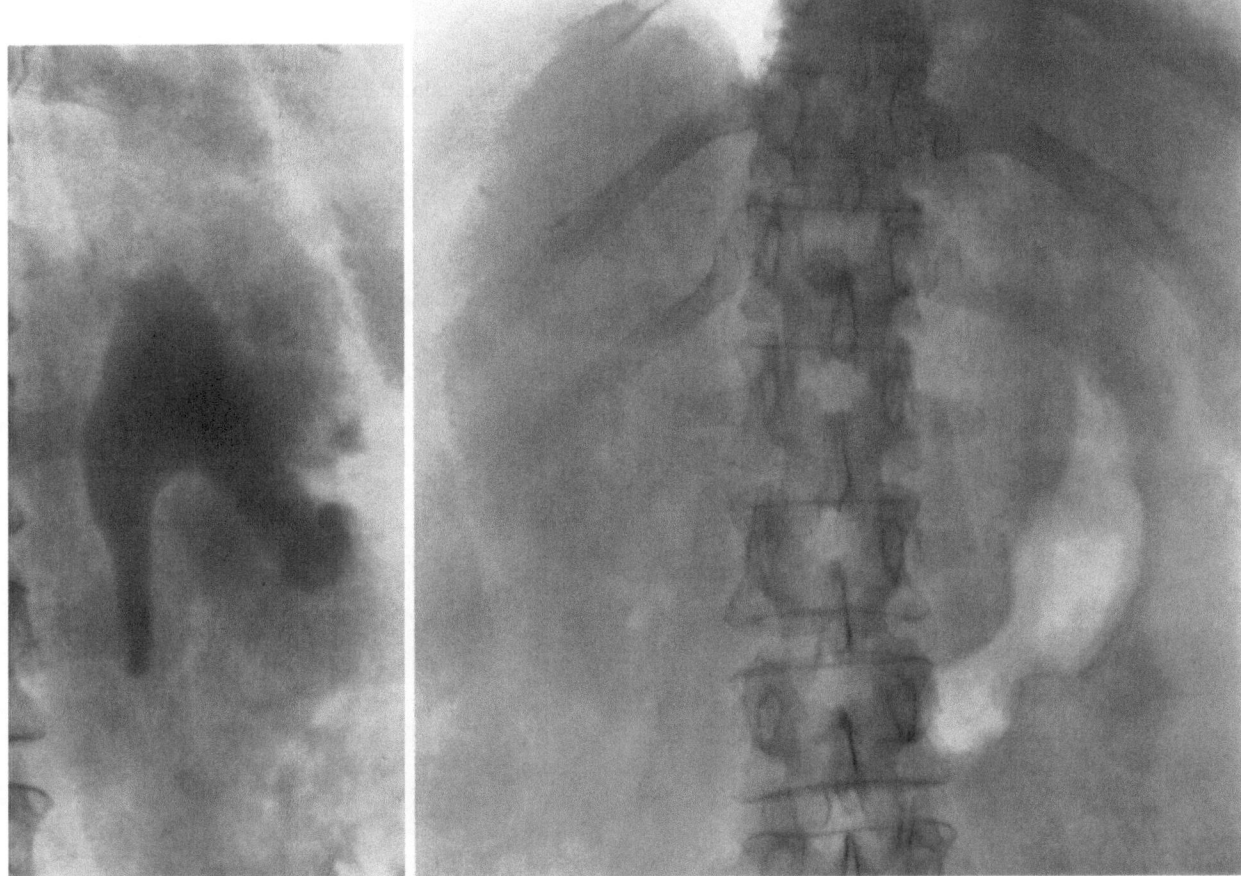

Fig. 125 b   Fig. 125 c

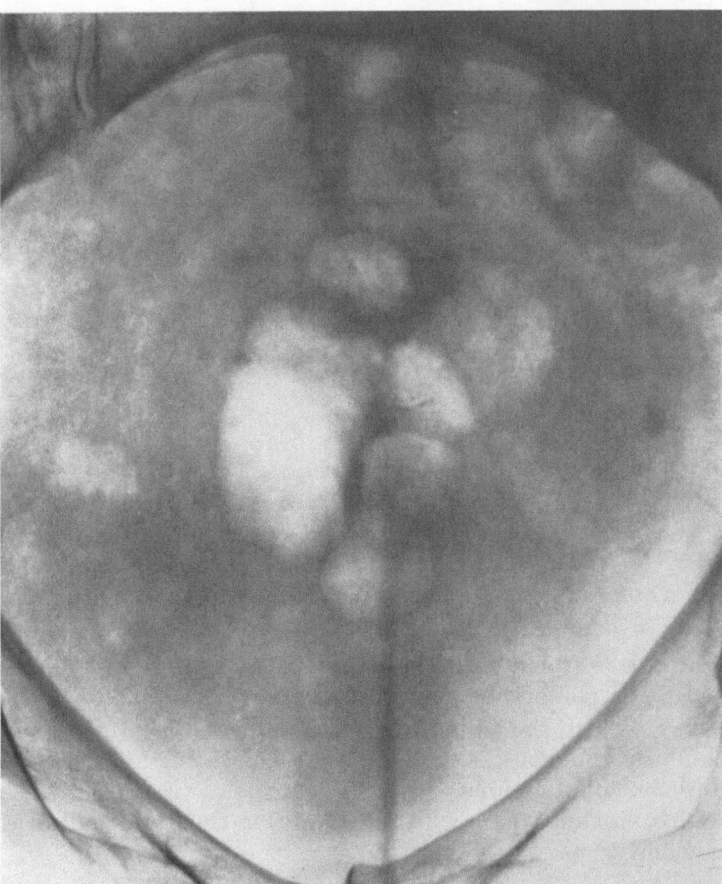

Fig. 125 d

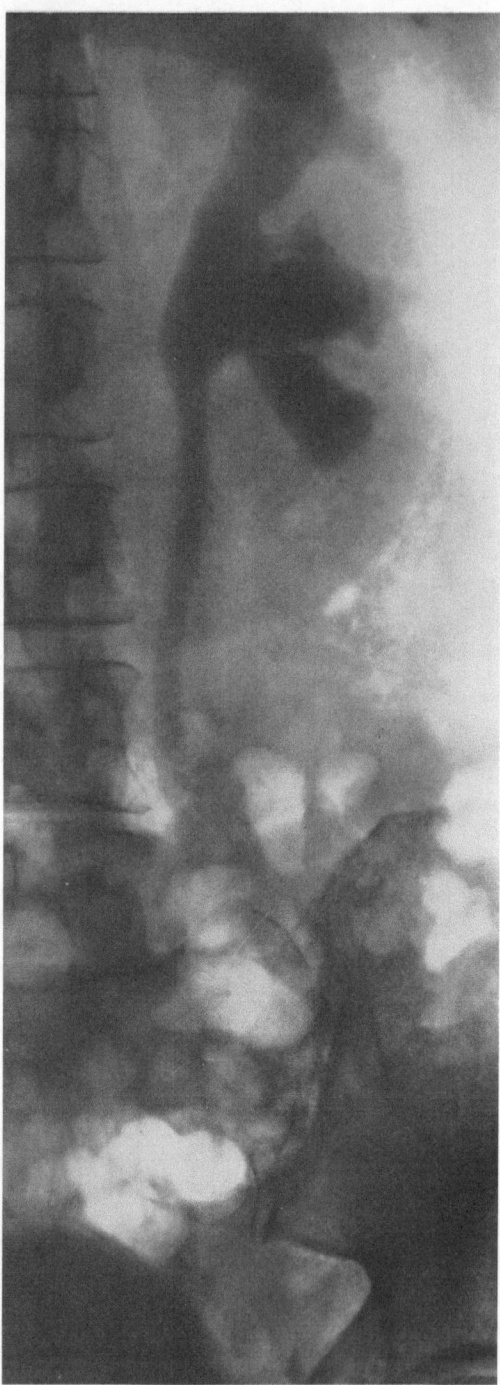

Fig. 125 e

c) Medium-sized stones (roentgenographic width 4—6 mm) in the lower half of the ureter will often (53 %) be passed spontaneously.

d) Medium-sized stones in the upper half of the ureter often (52 %) migrate down to the lower half within a few months. As long as the stone is in the upper half, it involves a definite risk of serious complications.

e) Large stones (roentgenographic width ≧ 6 mm) in the lower half of the ureter may (22 %) pass spontaneously.

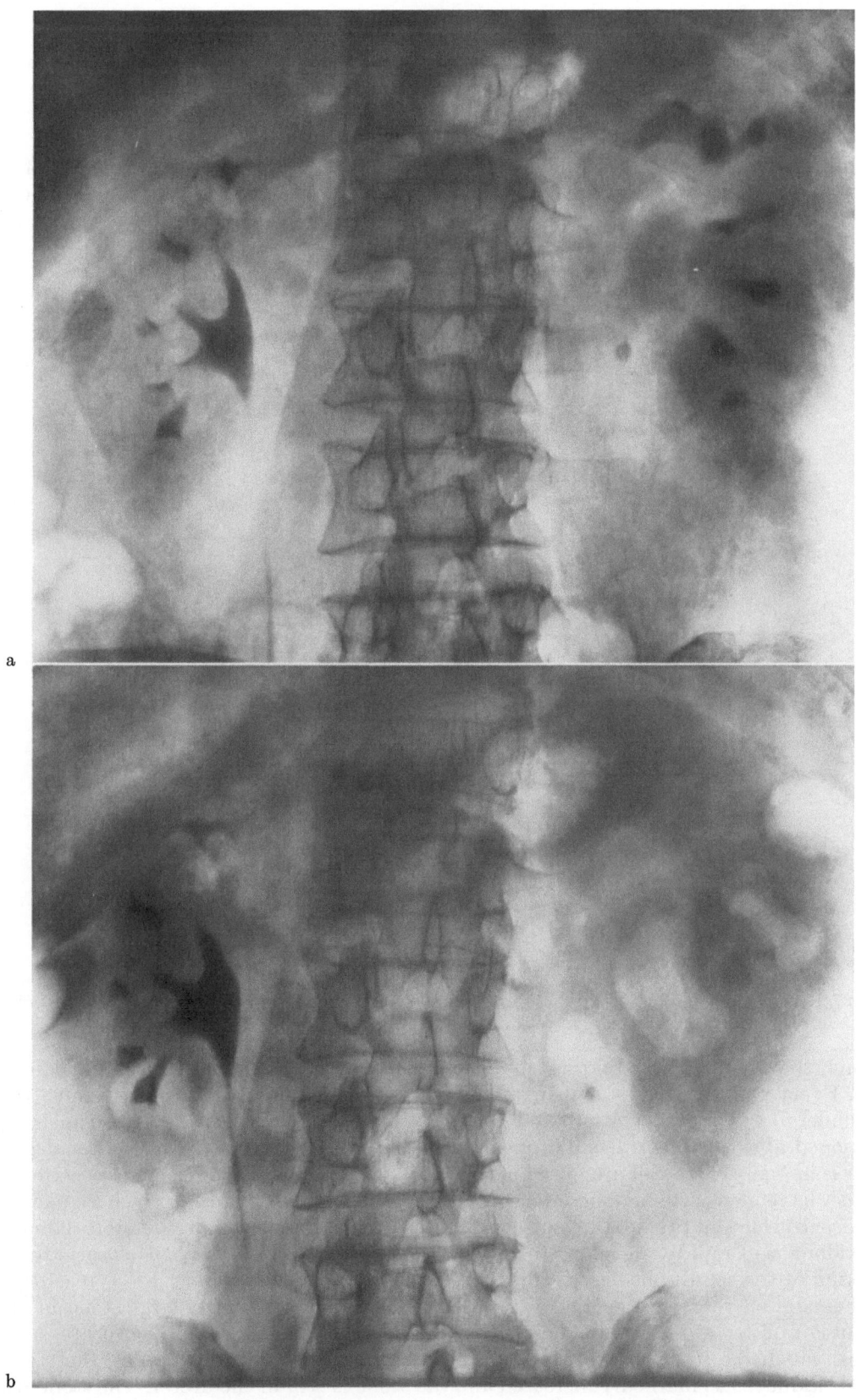

Fig. 126. a) Left-sided renal colic. Acute urography: stone in uppermost part of left ureter; marked stasis.
b) Check examination four weeks later (pain subsided soon after previous urography): changed position of stone;
stasis much more marked than at original examination

f) Large stones in the upper half of the ureter seldom (4 %) migrate down to the lower half. As long as the stone is in the upper half, it involves a considerable risk of serious complications.

8. Stasis in relation to pain

It cannot be stressed often enough that in ureteric stone the disappearance of pain does not necessarily mean the restoration of ureteric passage, even less the passage of the stone. Disappearance of pain usually means normalized conditions for passage of urine

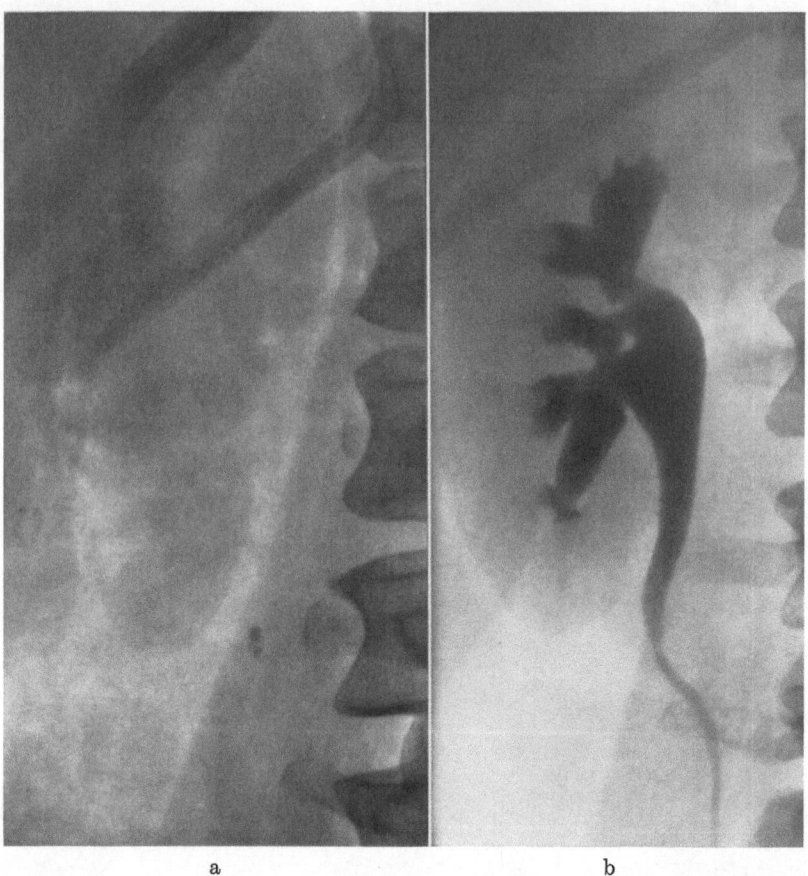

a   b

Fig. 127. Roentgen examination because of hematuria. a) Plain roentgenography: stone in cranial part of right ureter; b) urography: slight stasis down to stone; no pain at any time

through the ureter. Marked stasis is still present in many cases, however, after pain subsides. Every patient who, at acute examination, has been found to have stasis must therefore undergo a new examination after a few days in order to check the state of stasis or, as mentioned above, if stasis has disappeared, to check the morphology of the renal pelvis. Stasis is in many cases still present at such a check examination and in some cases the signs of stasis have increased, making intervention necessary. If in such cases no check examination is performed and the pathologic condition is thus not detected, irreversible damage to the kidney will rapidly develop. In order to spotlight the necessity of close individual checking of the conditions described above, I will relate a case history I saw recently:

Female, 58 years of age (Fig. 125). Left-sided renal colic. Fairly large stone in upper part of left ureter, stone also in lower part of right kidney pelvis. Pain disappears. A stone passes, which the patient presents. At check examination with urography, the stasis in the left kidneys has markedly increased and the stone is still in the ureter. The stone which passed was from the right kidney pelvis and had passed without pain.

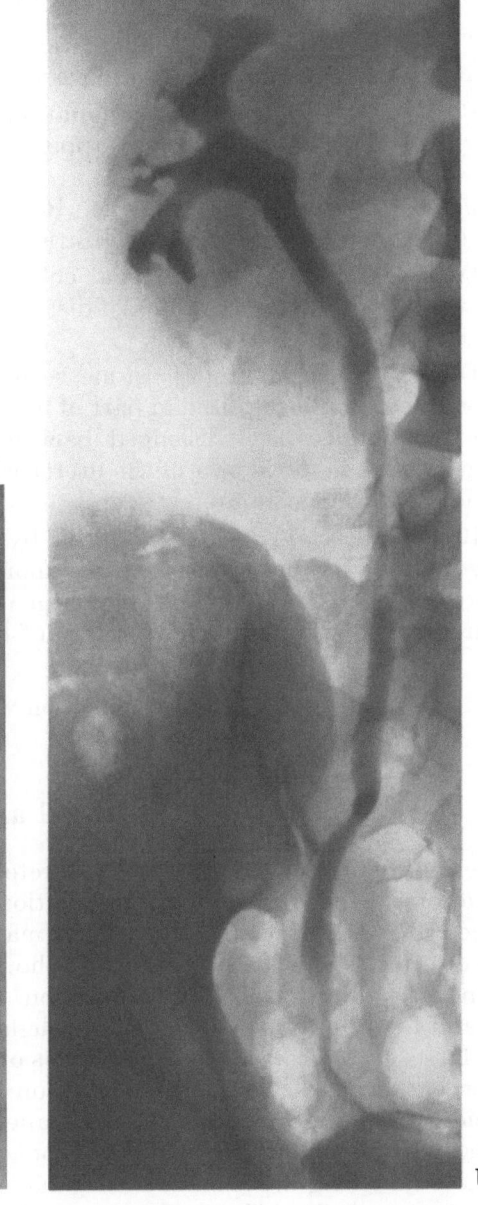

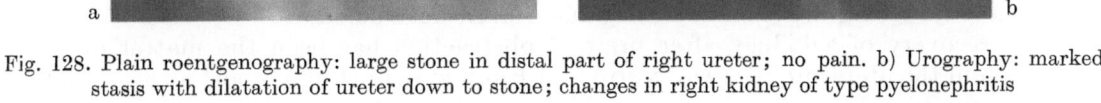

Fig. 128. Plain roentgenography: large stone in distal part of right ureter; no pain. b) Urography: marked stasis with dilatation of ureter down to stone; changes in right kidney of type pyelonephritis

It is not only in the post-pain period of renal colic that stasis can persist without pain. Hematuria was the indication for roentgen examination of a colleague 40 years of age. The patient and the referring nephrologist coupled the hematuria to a suspected glomerulonephritis. At plain roentgenography a fairly large stone was found in the upper part of the right ureter, causing moderate stasis (Fig. 127). This was the cause of the hematuria. The patient had at no time had pain.

In another patient examined because of prostatic hyperplasia, a large ureteric stone was found in the distal of part the left ureter, with marked stasis and dilatation of the left kidney pelvis and the ureter. Marked swelling of the ureteric orifice was also seen. The patient had had no attacks of pain whatsoever.

9. Master rules in acute renal colic

1. The patient is in pain. Roentgen examination: signs of stasis. Renal colic. Analgetics given as soon as possible to relieve pain.

2. Patient in pain. Roentgen examination: no signs of stasis. Pain not caused by renal colic but by other pathologic process, appendicitis, for example, or torquated ovarial cyst, etc.

3. Patient not in pain after colic. Roentgen examination: no signs of stasis. No definite conclusion possible as to localization of colic in the urinary tract or outside it.

4. Disappearance of pain in renal colic, with or without stone: Check stasis after a few days. Stasis can persist in spite of disappearance of pain and if not detected can cause irreversible kidney damage.

5. Disappearance of ureteric stone seen at previous examination. Stone may have passed or stone may be localized in part of ureter passing skeletal parts, for example pelvic bone, or it may have been dislodged back into the kidney pelvis. Therefore check examination of stone in distal part of the ureter when stone is not seen should always include the kidney and the entire ureter.

6. Renal colic caused not necessarily by stone, except if stone is demonstrated or presented. Instead: a coagulum from a tumor, for example, or a vascular malformation. Therefore, when stone not found at roentgen examination or seen after passage, always check urography with morphologic study of the kidney pelvis.

10. Backflow in connection with stone (see Chapter P)

XII. Renal angiography

The finding of a concrement in the ureter permits no direct conclusions concerning the duration of the obstruction. Obstruction may be partial or intermittent and, as mentioned above, even fairly large stones may be grooved or channeled and permit the passage of urine. In such cases urography should be performed at regular intervals during expectancy, in order to check renal function. As a rule the excretion of urine will appear normal and the urinary pathways will be slightly dilated at most, even if the concrement is fairly large. In some cases, however, signs of stasis appear, occasionally of severe stasis, and intervention is indicated. If renal function is markedly impaired or absent, the question is to decide whether the impairment is permanent or temporary. This question is important, particularly in cases in which the onset is not acute and in which it is therefore not possible to estimate how long a period flow may have been obstructed.

The recovery of a kidney after ureteral obstruction has been the matter of much discussion in the literature. Papaioannou and Brunschwig (1965) report a case of return of function after $1^1/_2$ years of complete blockage. This blockage, however, was verified only by urography, with fairly short examination times. Graham reports recovery of "useful renal function" after 46 days of obstruction. In a study from 1964 Brunschwig et al. stress the difficulty, in several cases of occlusion, of stating definitely the average occlusion time. Of 11 patients in whom it was possible to fix rather accurately the dates of complete renal occlusion, there was return of function in seven patients, with periods of occlusion varying from two to four weeks and in one patient $3^1/_2$ months. In two patients with occlusion lasting 165 days, impaired function returned. In one patient with 100 days of occlusion, function returned slowly and remained impaired.

From these and many other reports it is evident that urography is not a reliable method of studying capacity for recovery after ureteral obstruction. Renal angiography can help to decide on this point.

Renal angiography is of less value in the diagnosis of stone, but it may be very valuable in the evaluation of the condition of the renal parenchyma in stone with complicating infection, and in urinary stasis due to stone. In urinary stasis and in infection the entire parenchyma or only part of it may be affected. Thus in contemplated partial nephrectomy because of stone, renal angiography may be useful for judging the state of vascularization of the kidney, the extent of involvement of the parenchyma, and for planning of the operation. The method is of still greater value, however, in the estimation of the time drainage has been obstructed and of secondary impairment of kidney function.

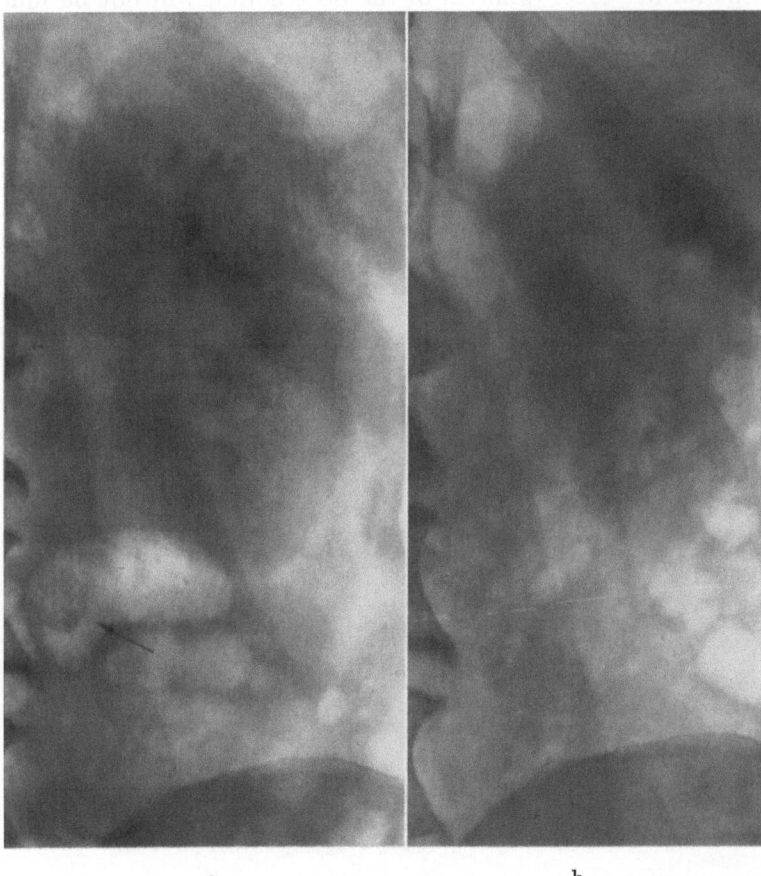

a   b

Fig. 129. a) Acute urography: stone in middle of left ureter (arrow); marked stasis. Cessation of pain. b) Check examination some days later: stone has disappeared from ureter and is found in caudal pole of left kidney

It is well known that prolonged urinary stasis is accompanied by atrophy of the renal parenchyma with gradual loss of renal function. Even if stasis is relieved in such cases, renal function may be definitely impaired. In experiments on rabbits IDBOHRN (1956) at our department showed that in complete unilateral ureteric stasis, pathologic-anatomic changes occurred with destruction of parenchyma proceeding parallel to the length of the stasis during the first 11—12 weeks. After this period of stasis the interstitial tissue had undergone fibrosis-hyalinosis and the tubules were markedly atrophied. After a period of stasis of more than 11—12 weeks the changes progressed only slightly. In further experiments in the same research program (WIDÉN, 1958) on dogs in which urinary stasis had been induced for periods of seven to 79 days and afterwards released, examination three to seven months after release showed that the kidneys were atrophic, the degree of atrophy varying with the period the ureter had been ligated. As a rule the tubules were more atrophic than the glomeruli. Atrophy of the parenchyma was accompanied by a narrowing of the renal artery and changes in the parenchyma as judged by urography (Fig. 131).

Examination of the renal blood flow by physiologic methods (IDBOHRN and MUREN, 1956) showed flow of blood through the kidney to be reduced.

If a ureteric concrement completely obstructs the ureter, and it is not known how long it has done so, absence of excretion in urography may depend either on such long-standing obstruction that the kidney is no longer able to function because of atrophy of functional elements, or on the pressure in the renal pelvis being so high as to prevent excretion. In the former case, removal of the obstruction will not be followed by return

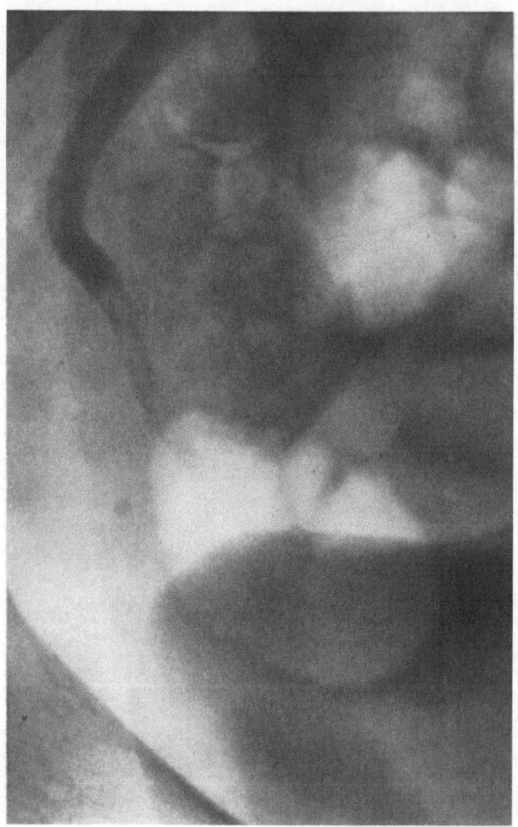

Fig. 130. Right-sided renal colic. Stone in distal part of right ureter. Stasis with filling of ureter down to stone. Coagulum 3 cm long immediately cranial to stone

of function, but in the latter, removal will give the kidney the possibility of recovering. In the former case at renal angiography decrease in the width of the renal artery, together with reduction of the capillary bed of the kidney, may be seen as a sign of atrophy. In the latter case, the renal artery will be of normal or nearly normal width and thereby indicate good potential renal function.

Many authors claim that there is a parallel between the degree of atrophy of a kidney and the decrease in the width of the renal artery. This conception is not correct, however. To clarify the question, as mentioned above, IDBOHRN studied the angiographic changes in animals at varying intervals after complete unilateral ureteric obstruction and WIDÉN studied the same question a considerable time after stasis had been relieved (Fig. 131). Both investigators showed that patho-anatomic changes with atrophy of the renal parenchyma increased rapidly; the caliber of the artery, however, decreased only slowly. When the caliber of the renal artery had diminished by 50 % all renal function had perma-

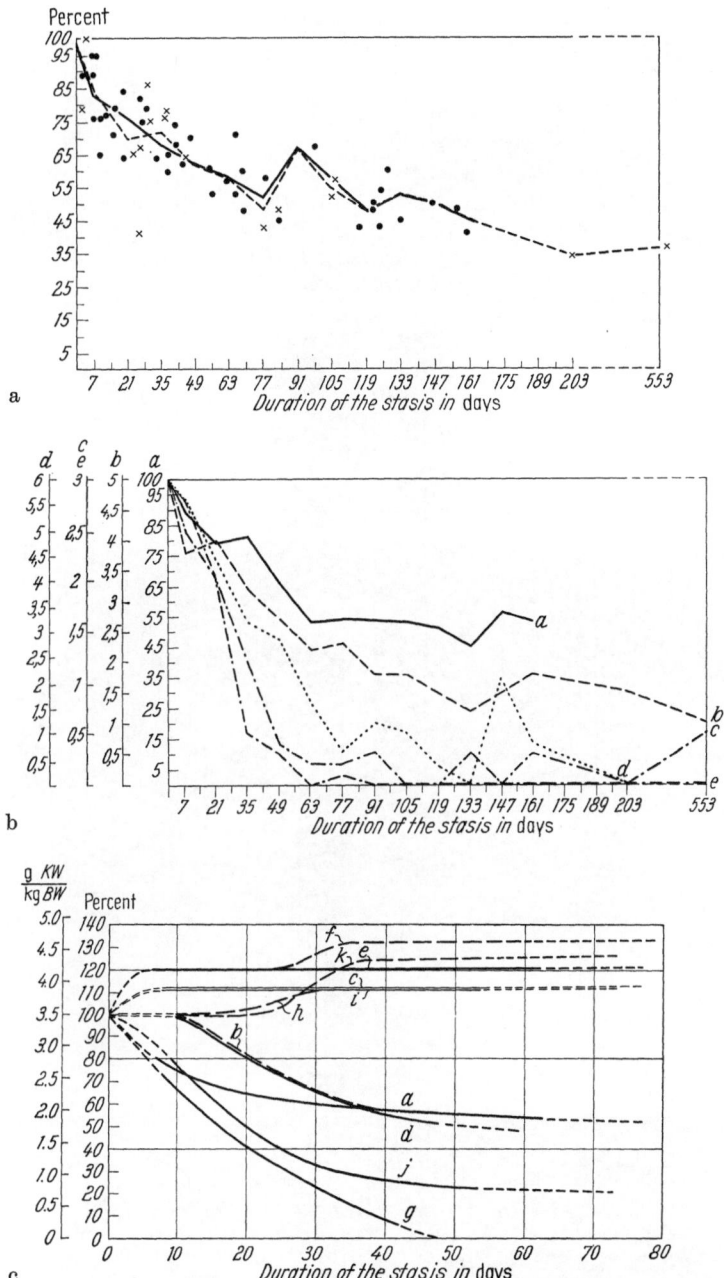

Fig. 131. a) Caliber of renal artery in rabbits after ligation of corresponding ureter. Fairly even decrease in caliber of artery until the 11—12th week, when the caliber is about 50% of original width. (After IDBOHRN); b) Comparison between caliber of renal artery (a), intrarenal arteries (b), nephrographic effect (c), function after ureterostomy (e) and histologic changes (d). (After IDBOHRN). c) Renal angiography in dogs after varying length of time after ligation of corresponding ureter and 3—7 months after release of ureteric occlusion and re-establishment of passage in ureter. The caliber of the renal artery on the ureter-ligated side recovered its original value when the ureter had been completely blocked less than 10 days. Angiographic, functional and morphologic changes in relation to duration of stasis. a Caliber of renal artery on ligated side during ligation period. b Caliber of renal artery on ligated side during post-release period. c Caliber of renal artery on contralateral side during ligation period and post-release period. d Size of kidney on ligated side during post-release period. e Size of kidney on contralateral side during ligation period and during post-release period after ligation of less than 30 days duration. f Size of kidney on the contralateral side during post-release period after ligation period of more than 30 days. g Inulin and PAH clearance on ligated side during post-release period, in per cent of half the total preoperative value. h Inulin clearance on contralateral side during post-release period, in per cent of half the total preoperative value. i PAH clearance on contralateral side during post-release period, in per cent of half the total preoperative value. j Weight of kidney (g/kg body-weight) on ligated side. k Weight of kidney (g/kg body-weight) on contralateral side. (After WIDÉN)

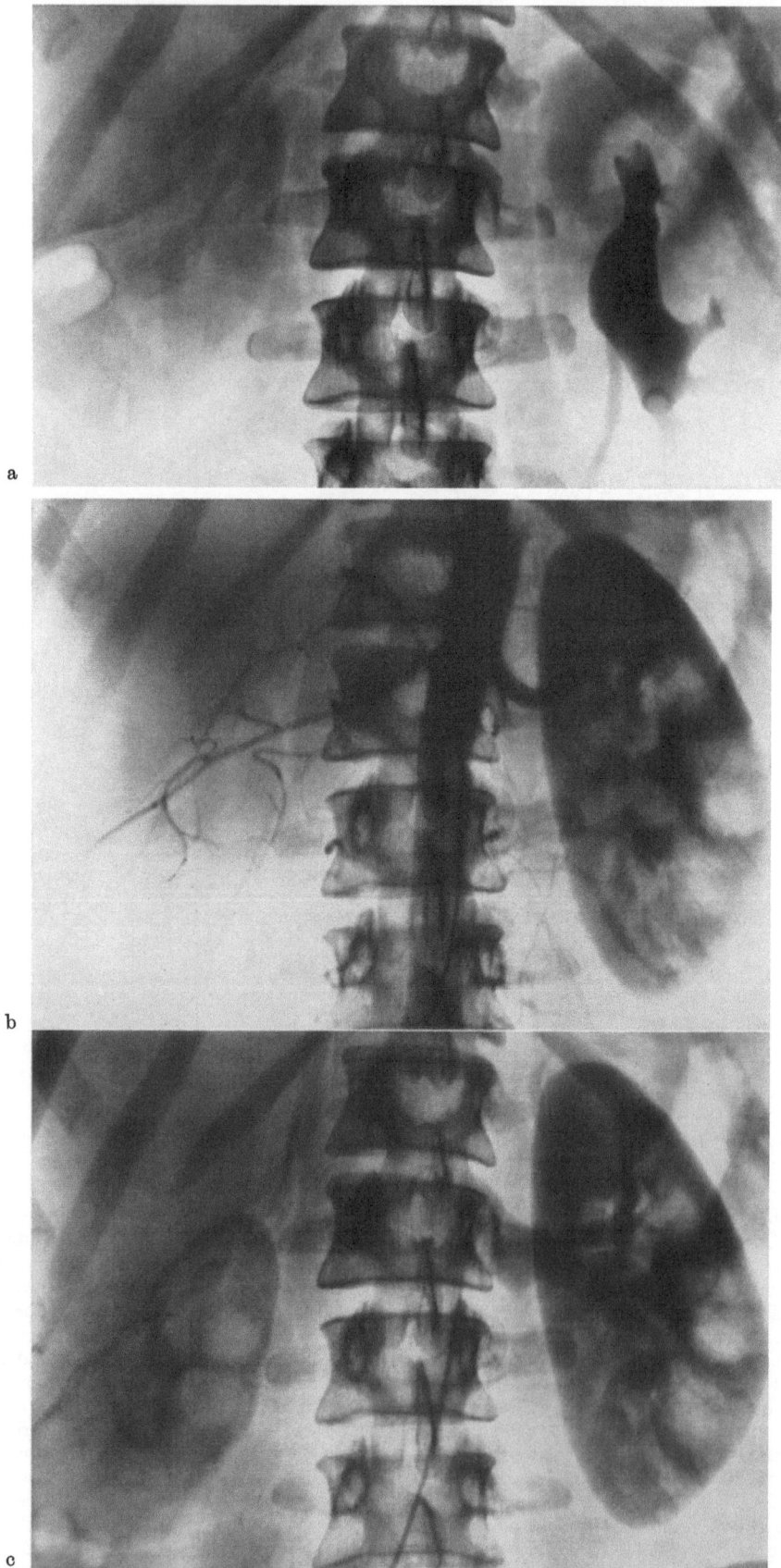

a

b

c

Fig. 132. Kidney atrophy due to ureteric obstruction. Gynaecologic operation some years previously. Afterwards "silent kidney". a) Urography: No excretion from small right kidney. b) and c) Angiography: Marked atrophy of arteries to right kidney, which is small, of irregular outline and has no parenchyma left. Nephrectomy

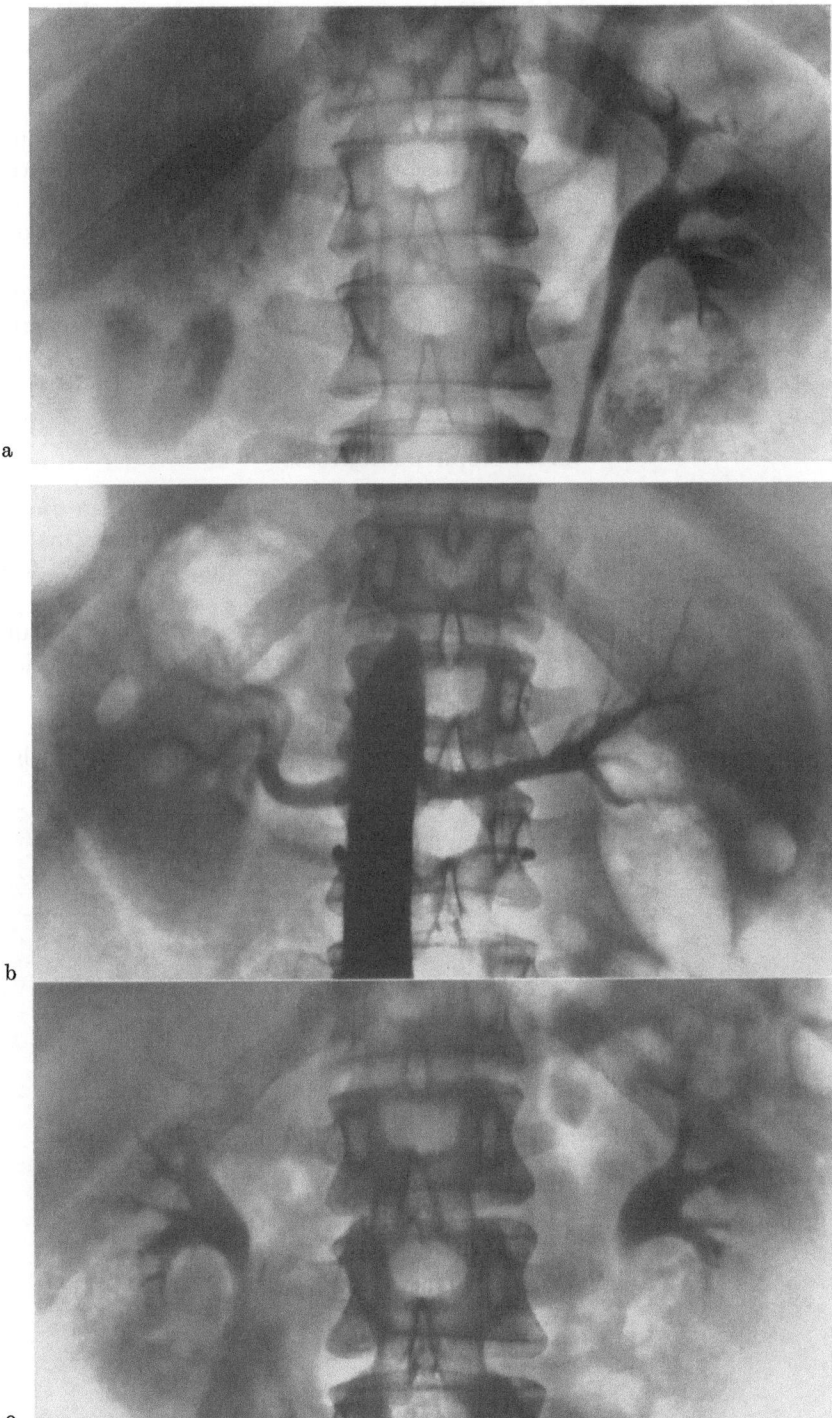

Fig. 133. Ureteric obstruction due to stone. Repeated attacks of pain for months. a) Urography: Ordinary excretion left side. No excretion right side. b) Renal angiography: Renal arteries have ordinary caliber. Nephrographic phase shows normal conditions. Potential kidney function good. Removal of ureteric stone. c) Urography: Normal conditions

nently ceased. Only after complete ureteric occlusion of less than 30 days duration was any recovery of renal function noted. After 30 days of complete occlusion the artery showed no tendency to recover. The investigations showed that renal angiography, with determination of the width of the renal artery and its branches and evaluation of the renal parenchyma by the nephrogram, provides a reliable method for judging potential renal function. If the caliber of the renal artery has diminished to half its normal width, in practice to half the width of the contralateral renal artery, removal of the obstruction will not result in recovery of renal function (Fig. 132). It is not only the width of the main branch of the renal artery that should be considered, but also the appearance of intrarenal branches and, as mentioned, of the nephrogram.

The reactive changes around a stone in the kidney pelvis may occasionally be sufficiently marked as to cause angiographically demonstrable changes. Thus a marked hypervascularity may be seen in the wall of the kidney pelvis and the ureter, with widened tortuous vessels (Fig. 107).

XIII. Nephrocalcinosis

In the discussion of renal stone it has been pointed out that certain diseases predispose to stone formation and in addition are often associated with calcifications in the parenchyma. In parenchymal calcifications smaller calcifications may become detached and appear as concrements.

Nephrocalcinosis is not a clear-cut clinical entity. It is used in the literature to designate calcifications in the kidneys as seen at autopsy or at roentgen examination. Here we are concerned only with the roentgenographic appearance. Since it appears so often in the literature it will be dwelt on here, but reference is made to the different diseases associated with concrement formation and parenchymal calcifications and described elsewhere. In

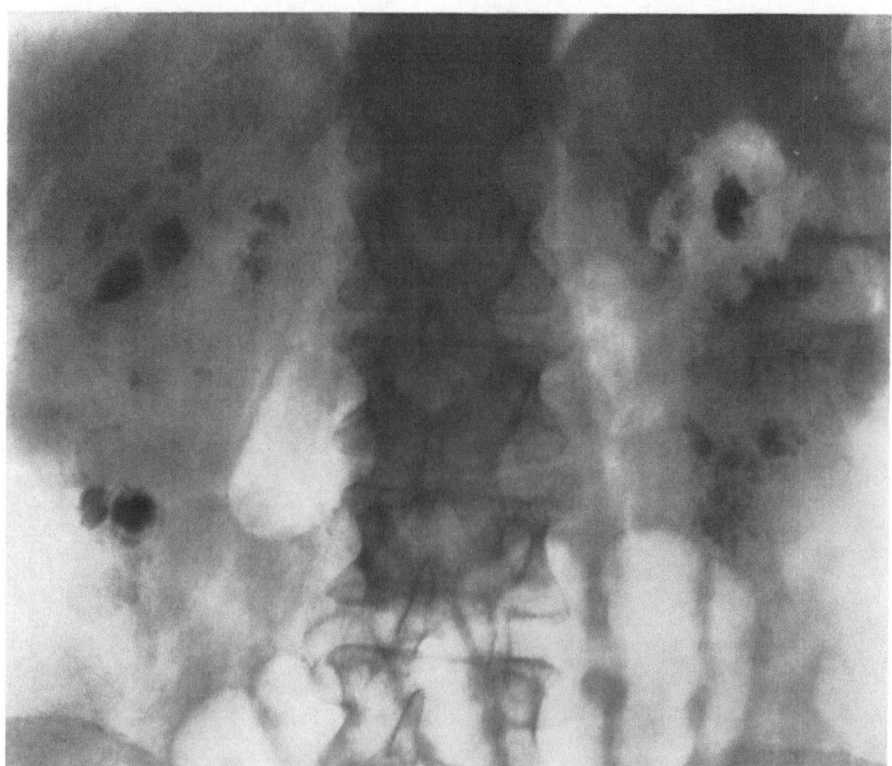

Fig. 134. Nephrocalcinosis in sarcoidosis

addition, it is stressed that nephrocalcinosis is not a disease *sui generis* and that every single case should be examined and evaluated individually in the light of the fundamental disease.

Renal calcifications are generally classified as metastatic calcifications when they are due to hypercalcemia in otherwise normal kidneys, and as nonmetastatic or dystrophic calcifications, when a primary renal lesion is present. The division may be useful for purposes of classification, but it is not always possible to make a distinction in a given case, because the renal parenchyma is often damaged, even in cases classified as metastatic.

Nephrocalcinosis is, generally speaking, a roentgen diagnosis. Diagnosis of the condition depends according to MORTENSEN *et al.* (1953) upon the following roentgenographic characteristics: 1. location of deposits of calcium in the renal parenchyma and 2. the diffuse distribution of such deposits. Obviously the description is diffuse and is worded so as to cover many widely different conditions.

Parenchymal calcifications occurring in association with renal tuberculosis and renal tumor, for example, are usually not included under the name of nephrocalcinosis. This term instead embraces such renal changes as those seen in osteitis fibrosa generalisata. This condition was the first in which the term nephrocalcinosis was used by ALBRIGHT *et al.* (1934). It also includes parenchymal changes in sarcoidosis and in some generalized diseases of the renal parenchyma, but only if the disease produces renal calcifications. The term also embraces certain conditions associated with changes in the blood chemistry, particularly hypercalcemia. Some cases described in the literature under the heading of nephrocalcinosis should have been assigned to other groups such as medullary sponge kidney.

1. Hyperparathyroidism

Hyperparathyroidism, usually due to adenoma of a parathyroid gland, is often accompanied by nephrocalcinosis and renal concrements. The renal changes are the most serious organic complication in this disease. Therefore, in all cases of hyperparathyroidism the kidneys must be examined, just as the possibility of hyperparathyroidism should always be considered in all cases of urinary calculi and nephrocalcinosis. HELLSTRÖM (1955) stated that in 56 of his 70 cases of hyperparathyroidism, renal concrements were found roentgenologically: in one third of the cases, stones only; in one third, parenchymal calcifications only; and in one third both in combination. According to ALBRIGHT and REIFENSTEIN (1958), on the other hand, hyperparathyroidism is the cause in 5 % of all cases of urinary stone. The concrements and calcifications vary widely from case to case and from side to side. One or both kidneys are often reduced in size.

Renal lesions can occur without bone lesions, the former being an index of the severity of the disease and the latter, an index of its duration (ALBRIGHT *et al.*, 1934).

It is assumed that the roentgen pathology of the bone lesions characteristic of hyperparathyroidism and the method for diagnosing parathyroid adenoma are known; they are therefore not described here.

2. Sarcoidosis

The term sarcoidosis is to be understood here as the obscure disease, also known as Besnier's, Boeck's, or Schaumann's disease, or lymphogranuloma benignum if the changes are localized to the glands, or ostitis multiplex cystica Jüngling when the lesions are seen in the bones.

It is common knowledge that autopsy has revealed calculi and parenchymal calcifications in a high percentage of patients with sarcoidosis. The calcareous formations may involve only a small part of the kidney or renal pelvis or the major part of the kidney. A few descriptions of the roentgen anatomy in this disease are on record. DAVIDSON *et al.*, (1954) described the largest series (7 cases) illustrating bilateral nephrocalcinosis; the lesions were irregular and they varied in extent from case to case and from side to side in one and the same patient. The kidneys are also sometimes reduced in size (SCHÜPBACH and WERNLY, 1943). Calcium deposits in the soft tissue resembling the changes seen in peritendinitis calcarea may also occur.

In a survey of 306 patients with sarcoidosis MURPHY and SHIRMER (1961) found, however, that the frequency of urolithiasis in sarcoidosis was no greater than that in the general population.

It is presumed that the reader is familiar with the changes of roentgendiagnostic importance in sarcoidosis outside the urinary tract.

3. Hypercalcemia

The findings described above in nephrocalcinosis resemble those in other conditions of hypercalcemia such as bone-destroying tumors.

The largest series of these conditions consists of 91 cases (MORTENSEN and EMMETT, 1954: 48 from the literature and 43 personal cases), of which almost half had hyperparathyroidism. Two thirds of the remaining cases consisted of hyperchloric acidosis and chronic pyelonephritis in equal proportions. The group hyperchloric acidosis included cases of the type described by BUTLER et al. (1936) and by ALBRIGHT et al. (1940), who called the disease nephrocalcinosis with rickets and dwarfism.

Nephrosclerosis occurring in association with sulphonamide therapy has been described by many authors (GREENSPAN, 1949; ENGEL, 1951).

4. Glomerulonephritis, pyelonephritis, and tubular nephritis

Glomerulonephritis, pyelonephritis, and tubular nephritis are sometimes associated with nephrocalcinosis. Widespread calcifications have been observed on occasion in chronic glomerulonephritis (ROSENBAUM et al., 1951). In pyelonephritis calcifications may be seen in the pyramids (ALBRIGHT et al., 1938) (papillary necrosis must here be kept in mind.). In tubular nephritis cortical calcifications have been observed by MOËLL in some of our cases. In this conjunction cortical calcifications in gross renal cortical necrosis should be remembered. In fact, nephrocalcinosis will prove to be fairly common in generalized diseases of the renal parenchyma if the examination aims at demonstrating diffusely spread, fairly thin calcifications.

The group of diseases under discussion is sometimes associated with bone lesions of somewhat varying type, so-called renal osteodystrophy, osteonephropathy etc. The fundamental diseases are of two different types. A smaller group consists of rare cases with selective tubular disturbances, and a second, larger group, of cases with chronic renal insufficiency due to glomerulonephritis, pyelonephritis or malformations of the kidneys and urinary tract. The roentgendiagnostic findings consist partly of skeletal changes, partly of changes of the type mestastatic calcifications and arterial calcifications. The type and severity of roentgenologic osseous changes vary with the patient's age and severity of renal insufficiency and the duration of such insufficiency. Bone lesions are partly changes of the type seen in rickets and partly changes resembling those occurring in osteitis fibrosa cystica. The former type is seen before the closure of the epiphyseal lines, the latter in adult age.

Renal rickets is caused by incomplete reabsorption of excreted calcium in the kidneys. The rachitic process is most marked in those joints which at the time are in the state of greatest development.

In some cases osteosclerosis is predominant and involves the major part of the skeleton, although it is occasionally limited to the spine, particularly the lumbar portion. These last-mentioned changes can often be detected at plain roentgenography of the urinary tract and indicate roentgen examination of the entire skeleton or places of predilection (Fig. 135) (CRONQVIST, 1961).

Young patients show changes, which in localization and type resemble those seen in rachitis. In adults the most characteristic changes are seen in the phalanges, in the medial part of the proximal third of tibia, in the corresponding part of the humerus and in the

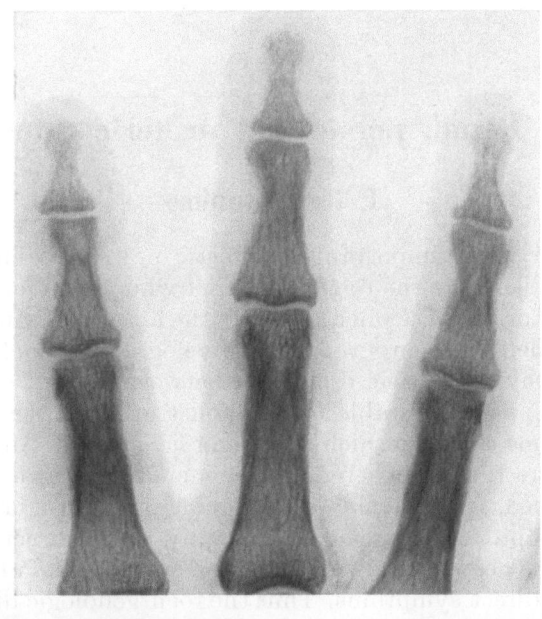

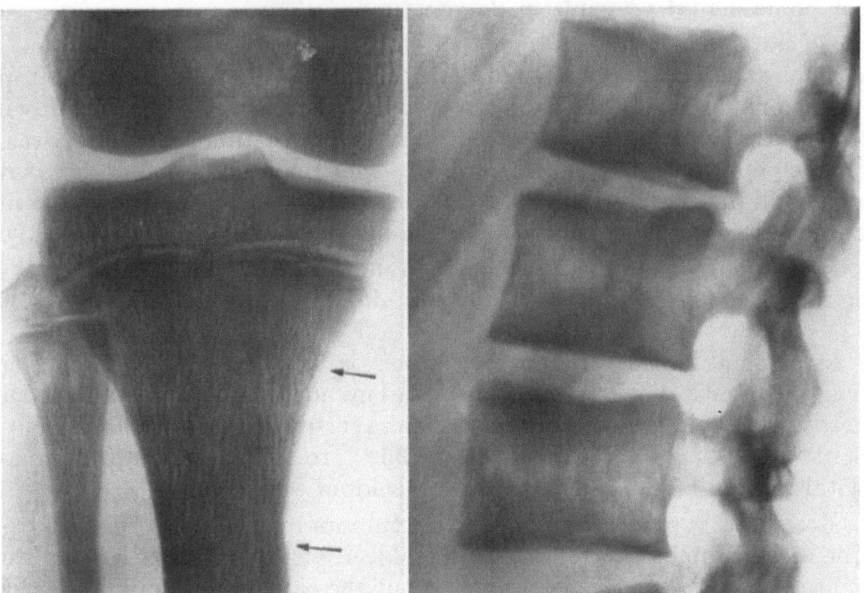

Fig. 135. Renal osteodystrophy. Characteristic type and localization of bony lesions. a) Cortical erosions in phalanges, especially middle phalanx and b) in proximal end of tibia medially (between arrows). c) Irregular sclerosis of vertebral bodies

clavicle, the acromion, and the ulna. In these bones diffusely outlined zones of cortical rarefaction are seen in the cortex.

In advanced cases the skeletal changes are the same as in hyperparathyroidism and can be differentiated from this disease only by blood studies. I doubt whether a differential diagnosis is always possible since hyperparathyroidism is often complicated by renal insufficiency.

It must be mentioned that renal osteodystrophy of different kinds is very common in connection with prolonged dialysis, the incidence increasing with increasing length of period of dialysis (COHEN et al., 1970).

F. Renal, pelvic and ureteric tumors

I. Renal tumors

Renal tumors offer many important diagnostic problems. The clinically raised suspicion of tumor is a challenge to the roentgenologist who must demonstrate unequivocally the presence of a tumor or, likewise unequivocally the absence of tumor. The main methods used to meet this challenge are urography (or pyelography), including plain roentgenography, and angiography. The basic difference between these two methods is that urography aims mainly at, and is suitable for, demonstration of the kidney pelvis, and not of the kidney parenchyma itself in which the tumor is localized. Angiography, on the other hand, helps demonstrate the renal parenchyma, including the tumor, the vasculature of which can also be studied. In principle, in tumor diagnosis urography-pyelography offers indirect diagnostic symptoms, whereas angiography offers direct diagnostic symptoms. Roentgen diagnosis at its best relies always on direct symptoms. Pathognomonic symptoms are practically always direct symptoms. Thus the roentgenologic diagnosis of renal tumor represents a fundamental principle in diagnostic radiology.

The most important type of renal tumor in adults is renal carcinoma, formerly called hypernephroma because of a belief that it had its origin in intrarenal ectopic adrenal remnants in the renal cortex. Grawitz advocated this view, hence the term "Grawitz tumor". Many other theories have been presented; therefore for a time the tumor was given the "neutral" name nephroma (JOHNSON, 1946). The most common name today is renal carcinoma. The general opinion now is that renal carcinoma has its origin in cells in the renal tubules or in adenomas. This theory was originally proposed by STUERCK (1908).

To produce tumors experimentally, dimethylnitrose amine can be used. We use this preparation for special angiographic studies in animal experiments (Ekelund and Jonsson, 1971).

Renal carcinoma in the pre-invasive stage is encapsulated in connective tissue. Upon growing, it breaks through the capsule and invades the kidney and the surrounding area. It metastasizes via the renal vein and paravertebral venous plexuses in 43—75 % of cases (SCHMIEDT, 1968), to the liver in 30—35 %, to the chest in approximately 50 %, to the skeletal system in 33—40 %, and more seldom to the brain.

The predominant type of malignant renal tumors in adults is different from that in children. The most common type of tumor in children is the embryoma or nephroblastoma, also known as WILMS' tumor. It represents 8 % of the cases in the series referred to above.

Renal tumors can be diagnosed by different roentgen-diagnostic methods, particularly plain roentgenography, urography or pyelography. The value of renal angiography, however, is becoming more and more obvious. The main purpose of roentgen examination is to demonstrate the presence of a tumor and, if a space-occupying lesion can be shown, to contribute to the differential diagnosis. Further, if plain roentgenograms and pyelograms show no signs of a pathologic condition in a patient in whom tumor is nevertheless suspected, roentgen examination can demonstrate or exclude the possibility of such a growth by other roentgen-diagnostic methods.

1. Renal carcinoma

The tumor can vary considerably in size and may be well defined or show signs of invasion. Occasionally it can infiltrate the entire kidney, including the renal pelvis and often encroaches upon neighboring tissues. Haemorrhage in a tumor is common, with different sized necrotic foci, and with cystic formations as a consequence. In some cases only small parts of the tumor show such cysts, while in others, although seldom, the entire tumor may be converted into a cyst or cysts with specific tumor tissue occurring only in the form of a protrusion in the wall of the cystic formation.

All roentgen-diagnostic methods must be thoroughly considered in the diagnosis and differential-diagnosis of renal carcinoma.

a) Plain roentgenography

A small tumor situated deep in the renal parenchyma need not cause any change in the size or shape of the kidney. If it is situated near the surface of the kidney, it may cause a small bulge in its outline, often seen only in tangential projections. Such a bulge may resemble a persistent fetal lobation, for example. A tumor situated in a hilar lip may make the latter appear somewhat thicker than usual, a change which cannot always be classified as clearly pathologic owing to the wide normal variation in the anatomy of the kidney, particularly of the lower hilar lip. Adaption of the kidney to adjacent organs, for example to the spleen, sometimes may give the kidney a shape which makes it impossible to exclude expansivity.

A relatively large tumor will produce a distinct local enlargement of one of the poles of the kidney, for example. The tumor may be round, oval, or lobulated but nevertheless well defined, or it may be well outlined in one part and diffuse in another. Large tumors occasionally infiltrate the entire kidney, when the kidney is seen as a nodose mass which may be very large.

A renal tumor may also cause a generalized increase in the volume of the kidney. The kidney becomes plump and large, but is of otherwise normal shape and well defined. The tumor may assume considerable proportions and compress adjacent organs. The liver, for example, may appear as a cap over the tumor and the diaphragm may be displaced upwardly and its mobility may be reduced.

In a material of 164 cases of renal carcinoma from our department (FOLIN, 1961) the kidney with tumor was well outlined in 150 cases, had normal size in 10 patients, was generally enlarged in 21, and was irregular in 119.

The kidney may be displaced in cranio-caudal and medio-lateral direction by the tumor, or rotated around different axes. A large tumor in the upper pole of the kidney will often tilt the kidney. A tumor situated dorso-medially to the kidney will rotate the latter in such a way that the hilum will face anteriorly.

Renal carcinoma, regardless of its size, occasionally contains calcifications (Fig. 136). These may vary widely in number, appearance and size, from punctate calcifications to calcium skeletons in the entire tumor. They may also be shell-like and localized in the periphery of a more or less spheric tumor. Calcifications in the entire circumference of the tumor or in small parts of it are more often seen in large tumors, but also, in exceptional cases, in very small ones. The calcifications have a certain relation to the age of the tumor (as has the size of the tumor). The frequency of calcifications is higher in older material of renal carcinomas than in recent material because formerly patients came for examination at a later stage of the disease. Thus in renal carcinomas seen in our department during the years 1933—1945 calcifications were demonstrable in more than 25 % of the cases, whereas in a corresponding material from 1951—1960 they were found in only 5 %, since the diagnosis of renal carcinoma was made at an earlier stage.

In 50 out of 67 cases of renal mass lesion seen in roentgenograms of varying quality ETTINGER and ELKIN (1954) recognized the mass in 48 cases because of the changed

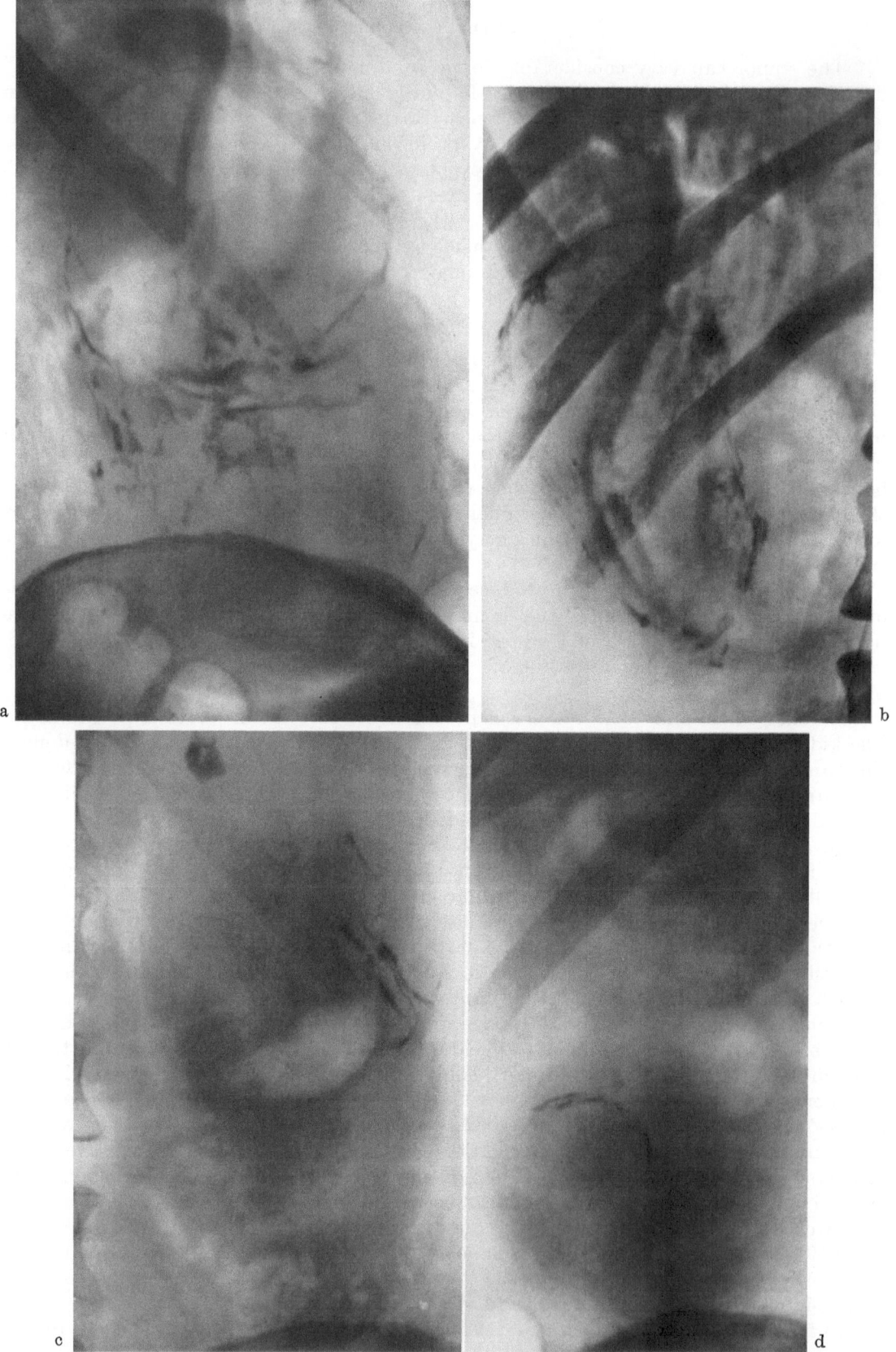

Fig. 136. a) and b) and c): Different types of combined peripheral and central calcifications indicative of solid tumors, practically pathognomonic of renal carcinoma. d) Calcification in tumor periphery not indicative of solid tumor. Calcifications of this type are also seen in simple cysts.

outline of the kidney, and in two because of calcifications. The calcifications in the renal tumor are sometimes characteristic but they may also be non-characteristic and not distinguishable from other calcifications in the renal parenchyma and the renal pelvis.

The finding of a renal mass is often accidental in association with other examinations, such as of the gallbladder, particularly if the examiner has made it a rule to pay attention to the appearance of the right kidney, which is included in survey films of the gallbladder.

If the kidney outline is difficult to demonstrate, tomography or zonography may sometimes be useful. Retroperitoneal pneumography has been used (COCCHI, 1957) but in my experience this method is unnecessary in this situation.

The changes seen already in plain roentgenograms are sometimes sufficient to permit a diagnosis of renal carcinoma, particularly if the tumor is large and irregular and/or if it contains characteristic calcifications.

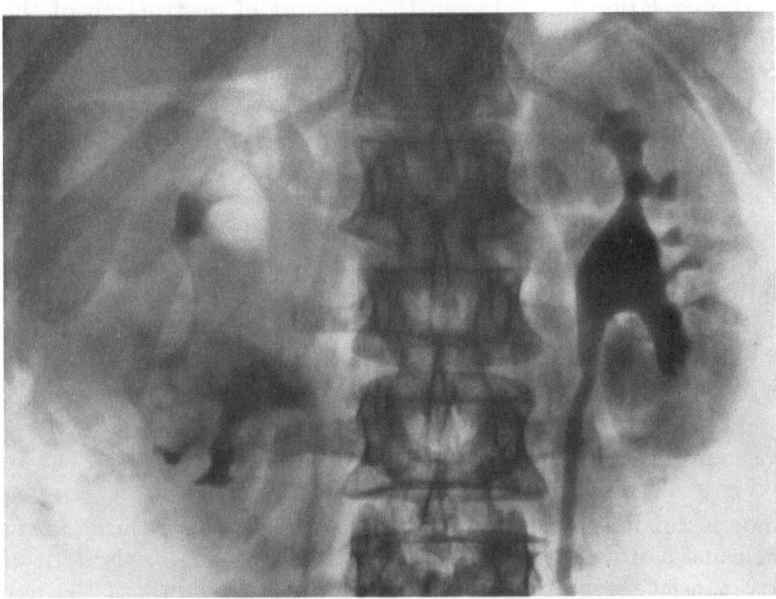

Fig. 137. Renal carcinoma, definite diagnosis possible at urography. Right kidney pelvis irregularly enlarged, contrast excretion diminished, kidney pelvis wall infiltrated

On occasion a large renal carcinoma may encroach directly upon and destroy parts of the skeleton. One or more metastatic foci are not infrequently seen in skeletal parts included in plain roentgenograms of the urinary tract. Such changes in combination with the finding of a space-occupying growth in the kidney permit a diagnosis of tumor. If a space-occupying lesion has been demonstrated in a kidney it may be useful to examine the chest because the demonstration of metastases in the lungs will make the diagnosis of tumor a firm one.

Large tumors can encroach upon the diaphragm and give rise to metastases in the pleura, demonstrable by the presence of fluid in the corresponding pleural cavity.

It is a well-known fact that on occasion lung changes of the type multiple metastases disappear entirely after nephrectomy. Such cases have been described by BUMPUS (1928), BEER (1937), MANN (1948), ARCOMANO et al. (1958), KESSEL (1959). The metastases had not been verified pathoanatomically. In this connection it may be convenient to call attention to a case published by ANDRESEN (1936): Roentgen examination of the chest of a male aged 43 years revealed changes suggestive of metastases. On examination of the kidneys a space-occupying, well defined lesion was found in one kidney. Renal carcinoma with lung metastases was assumed. The lung changes, however, diminished and operation on the kidney mass was decided upon. It disclosed a benign cyst!

A case has been described by LJUNGGREN et al. (1959) in which histologically verified, widespread bilateral pulmonary metastases disappeared completely *before* nephrectomy, which was performed later and disclosed a renal carcinoma. ADOLFSSON (1967), on the other hand, reports a patient with pulmonary metastases from a renal carcinoma in which the primary tumor underwent complete regression.

b) Urography/pyelography

Of the patients in our material of renal carcinoma 50% had at urography ordinary excretion conditions, permitting detailed study of the morphology of the renal pelvis after ureteric compression. In 18 out of 157 cases no excretion of contrast medium could be seen, and in 60 patients the excretion and its density were reduced in varying degrees. There was a certain relationship between the amount of destruction of the renal parenchyma through tumor and the density of the excreted contrast urine. Thus the kidneys without excretion were markedly destroyed by tumor. In exceptional cases, however, a small tumor may cause cessation of excretion because it blocks the flow in the kidney pelvis or in the ureter. Such blockage of passage may also cause dilatation of the kidney pelvis; otherwise such dilatation may be present for other reasons. A dilatation may counteract impression by a tumor in the kidney pelvis and thus cause non-detection of an expansivity (OLLE OLSSON, 1962).

Parts of the renal parenchyma not involved by the tumor will often show a somewhat increased nephrographic density at ordinary urography, while those parts harboring a tumor will retain their original density. This difference in density between normal and pathologic parts of the kidney can be enhanced by the modification of the method with a much larger dose of contrast medium (nephro-urography see chapter: Examination Methods.)

Both at pyelography and morphologic urography deformation of the renal pelvis by a space-occupying growth will be shown (see Figs. 137, 138).

If the tumor is small and near the surface of the kidney, the deformation may be only slight and consist of a flattening or dislocation of a single calyx. In central tumors the change may consist essentially of a separation of the stems of the calyces, while if the tumor is larger, the calyces may be markedly compressed. If the tumor is very large the renal pelvis may assume a grotesque shape with extension or shortening by considerable compression of its branches. A single expanding process is capable of producing all types of deformations in different combinations, depending on the direction of the pressure the expanding growth exerts in relation to the direction of the branches. The tumor may shorten a calyx stem and cause a flattening of the calyx itself if the tumor exerts its pressure in the longitudinal direction of the calyx. A calyx in the immediate neighborhood which is perpendicular to the direction of pressure of the same tumor may be elongated and compressed, for example. Rotation of the kidney also produces typical changes in the shape of the renal pelvis. A tumor situated in the lower pole of the kidney, particularly in its medial part, will press against the ureter and displace it. Such compression of the ureter may cause a dilatation of the renal pelvis.

The deformation of the renal pelvis as seen in the pyelogram is due in part to the fixation of the kidney, which permits only a limited amount of movement. An expanding process in or beneath the kidney is likely to cause deformation of the kidney and the renal pelvis in an early stage because the kidney can only give way to a certain extent. In addition the intrapelvic pressure is ordinarily low and is easily overcome by a growth pressing upon the pelvis. This is conspicuous on comparison between clinical pyelograms and pyelograms of autopsy specimens, the deformation due to rotation and stretching being much less in the latter.

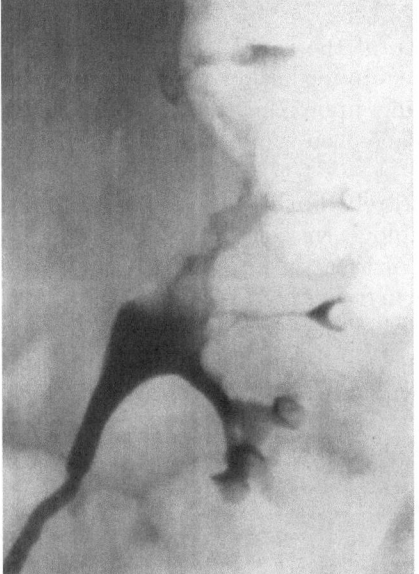

a

b

Fig. 138. Renal carcinoma infiltrating kidney pelvis. a) Pyelography, b) Operative specimen

Encroachment of the lesion onto the wall or into the lumen of the renal pelvis is seen in our material in approximately 35 % of the cases. In the former situation, single calyces or large parts of the renal pelvis may be irregularly narrow and their wall rigid as a sign of invasion by a malignant tumor (Fig. 138). In the latter situation a more or less irregular filling defect is seen in the renal pelvis (Fig. 139). This defect resembles those produced by papilloma of the renal pelvis or by radiolucent stones. Such a defect in a patient with a space-occupying lesion therefore does not necessarily mean that the lesion is a tumor encroaching upon the renal pelvis. Stones, for example, may be co-existent with any type of space-occupying parenchymal lesion. The filling defect may also be due to a blood clot.

Occasionally, although rarely, both at pyelography and urography, reflux will be seen of contrast medium in pathologic vessels belonging to a tumor or in the outer layer of a tumor, owing to distention of a calyx into the tumor capsule (OLLE OLSSON, 1948).

Incidence of renal pelvic deformity: Most tumors produce a more or less characteristic deformity of the renal pelvis. The deformity is occasionally very slight. Demonstration of the changes in the renal pelvis depends to a certain extent on the original shape of the renal pelvis. If it has well formed branches, even a slight deformation will be more conspi-

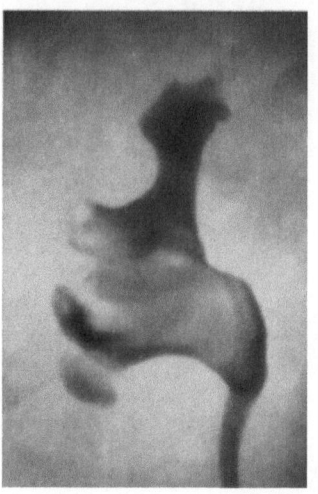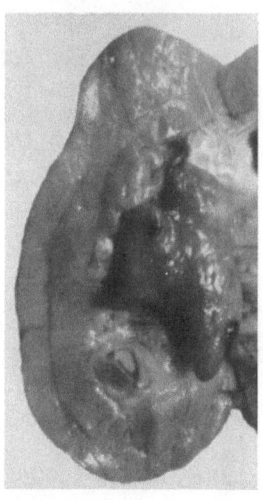

a   b

Fig. 139. a) Small renal carcinoma infiltrating and with a large protuberance projecting into the kidney pelvis. b) Operative specimen

cuous than in cases where the renal pelvis has a large confluence and short calyces.

Sometimes deformity of the renal pelvis may not be demonstrable despite the fact that changes in the outline of the kidney are seen in the plain roentgenogram (see Fig. 159).

Cases have also been described in the literature as "hypernephroma too early to diagnose". Accompanying illustrations, however, show that the examinations were not properly performed and were therefore inconclusive. It is obvious that the demonstration of changes in the shape of the renal pelvis depends largely on the examination technique. If the technique is slipshod, or standardized without necessary variation, at urography and pyelography many changes will be missed. Only an adaptable technique with suitable projections will demonstrate the deformation to its full extent.

Cases are on record, however, in which no signs of tumor were found at careful and complete examination and check examination with plain roentgenograms or urography or pyelography, but in which further examination by renal angiography (see below) gave the diagnosis (LÖFGREN, OLHAGEN, 1954) (Fig. 152, 161). Cases of this type are demonstrated more often with the increasing use of renal angiography.

c) Renal angiography

The crucial points on the importance of angiography in the diagnosis of renal tumors are:

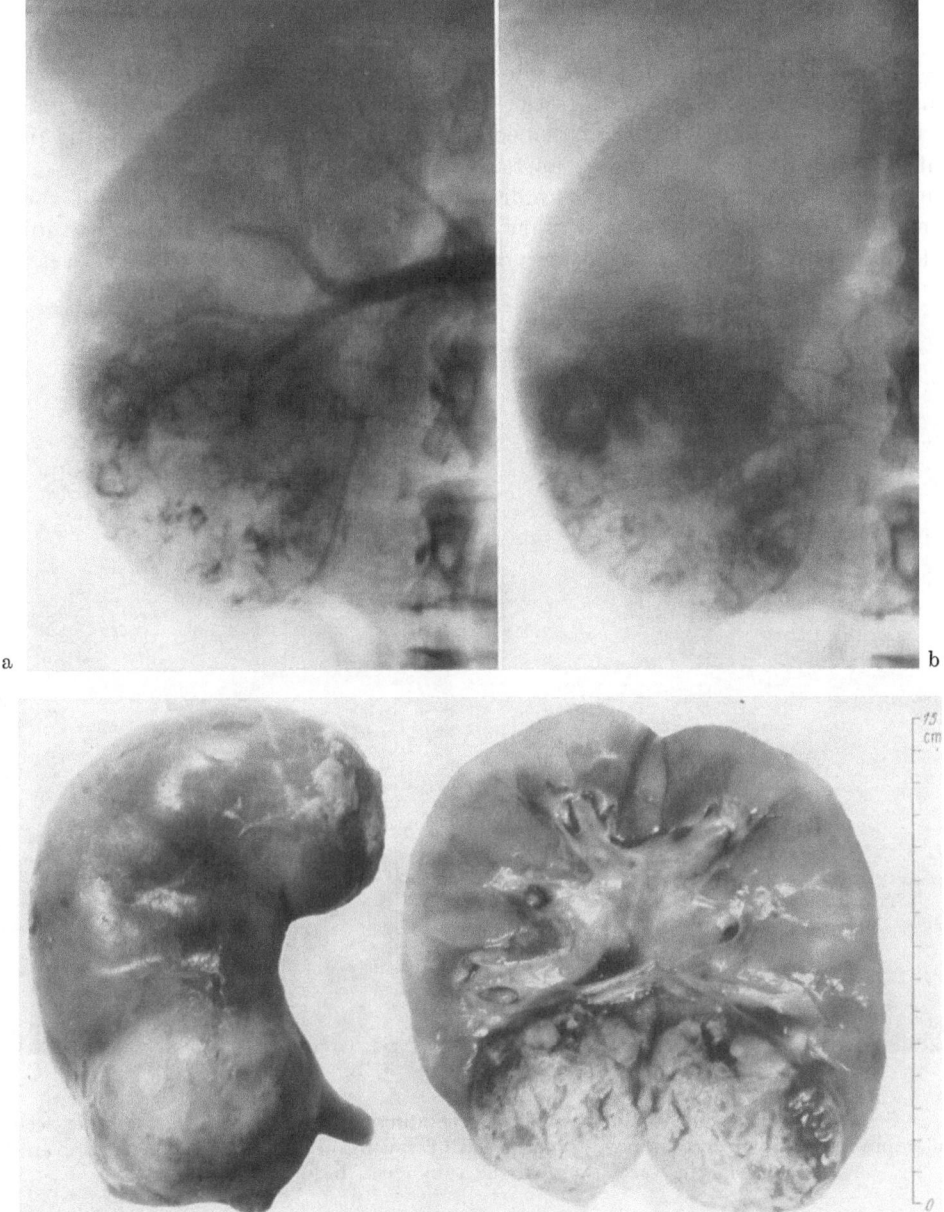

Fig. 140. Urography. Displacement and deformity of kidney pelvis indicative of space-occupying lesion. Impossible to decide if the latter was a cyst or a carcinoma. a) and b) Renal angiography, arteriographic and nephrographic phases: well defined tumor with much pathologic vasculature — renal carcinoma. c) Operative specimen

1. urography/pyelography gives negative results
2. urography/pyelography is indecisive as to the existence of a pathologic process
3. urography/pyelography is indecisive as to the nature of an existing pathologic process.

The problem can be solved by the use of angiography.

The renal artery to the kidney harboring a tumor is usually somewhat wider than its fellow artery. Highly significant statistical evidence is reported by FOLIN (1967) in a large material of renal carcinoma where the diameter of the renal artery on the tumor side was

7.6 ± 0.4 mm and on the other side 6.2 ± 0.5 mm. In 53 cases in which the two arteries could be directly compared, 37 had a wider artery on the affected side, in 14 the arteries were equally wide and in two the artery was narrower on the tumor side because the kidney harboring a small tumor was destroyed by pyelonephritis. The main artery and its branches are likely to be displaced in various ways by the expanding process. If the tumor is very large, the lumbar aorta may be displaced.

The region occupied by the tumor shows a pathologic pattern of the vessels, which run an irregular course and vary abruptly in width. (See, for example, Figs. 140—145, 151—153). Numerous fine or markedly irregular tortuous vessels with

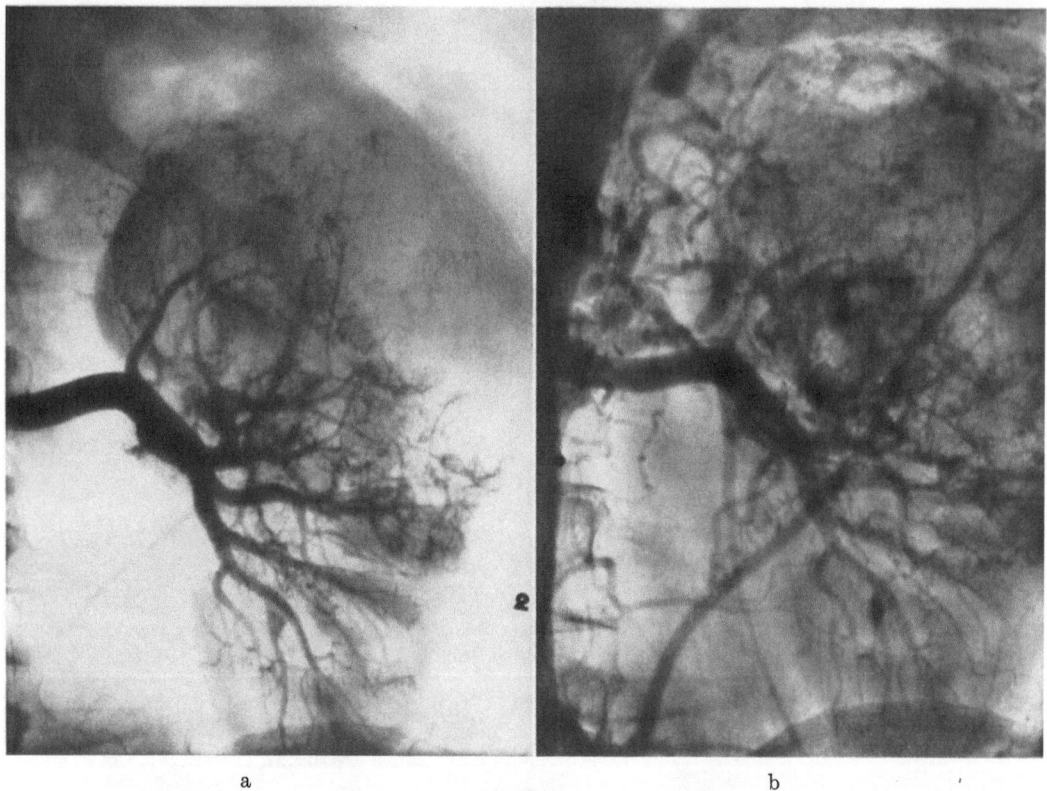

a   b

Fig. 141. a) Selective angiography: tumor vessels corresponding to medial part of large tumor seen at plain roentgenography. b) Lumbar aortography: tumor is fed by several other arteries. When latter are filled, all pathologic vasculature in the tumor can be demonstrated

aneurysm-like dilatations or irregularly outlined accumulations of contrast medium (so-called pooling or laking) are common findings. The contrast medium frequently passes rapidly into the veins via arteriovenous fistulae within the tumor. Such fistulae, which were known long before angiography, are capable of producing the same clinical symptoms as large arteriovenous aneurysms. The polycythaemia frequently seen in renal carcinoma has been ascribed to this direct shunting from the artery to the vein. It may also be caused by other factors, however.

Large tumors are often fed not only by the main renal artery but by other arteries as well, such as lumbar arteries, the phrenic artery, the intercostal arteries, the suprarenal artery, etc. (Fig. 141). In such cases only part of the tumor is demonstrated at selective angiography, whereas at aortic injection with filling of all pararenal arteries, all tumor vascularity will be demonstrated.

A tumor may be localized within the nutritional area of one of multiple renal arteries. (See below). As pointed out in the chapter Examination Methods, it is necessary to be

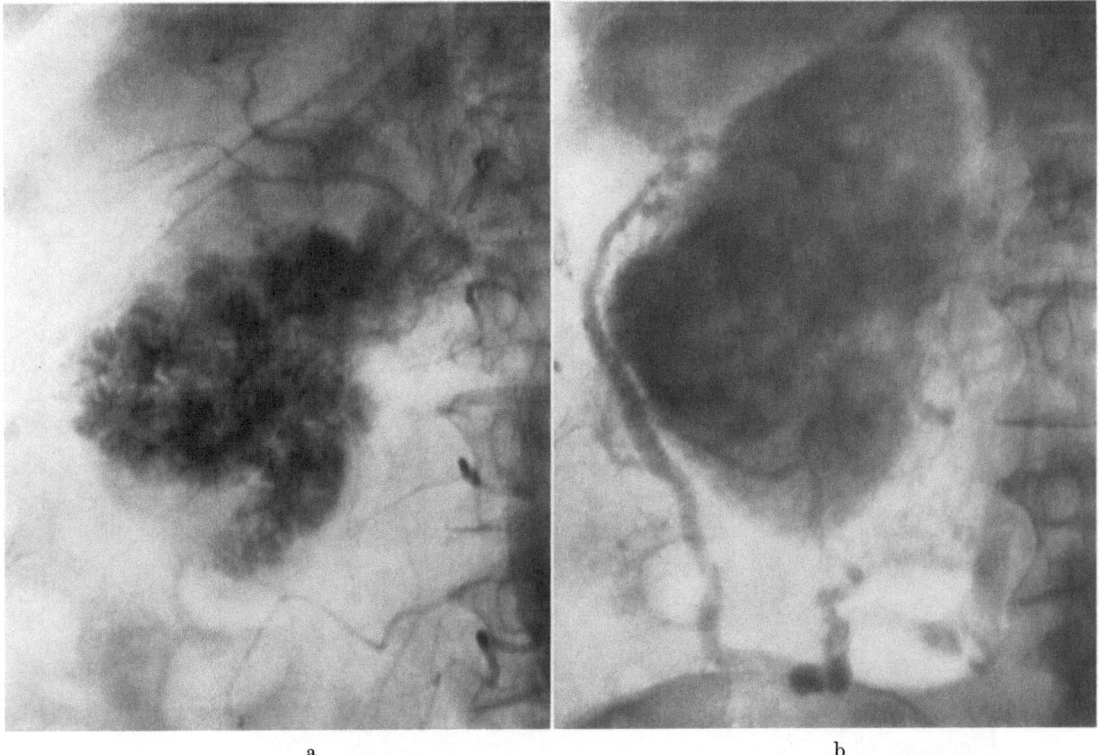

a   b

Fig. 142. Angiography: a) late capillary phase: large renal carcinoma with extension medially-cranially, corresponding to renal vein — tumor thrombus in renal vein. b) Venous phase: non-filling of renal vein, filling of many collateral veins around the kidney

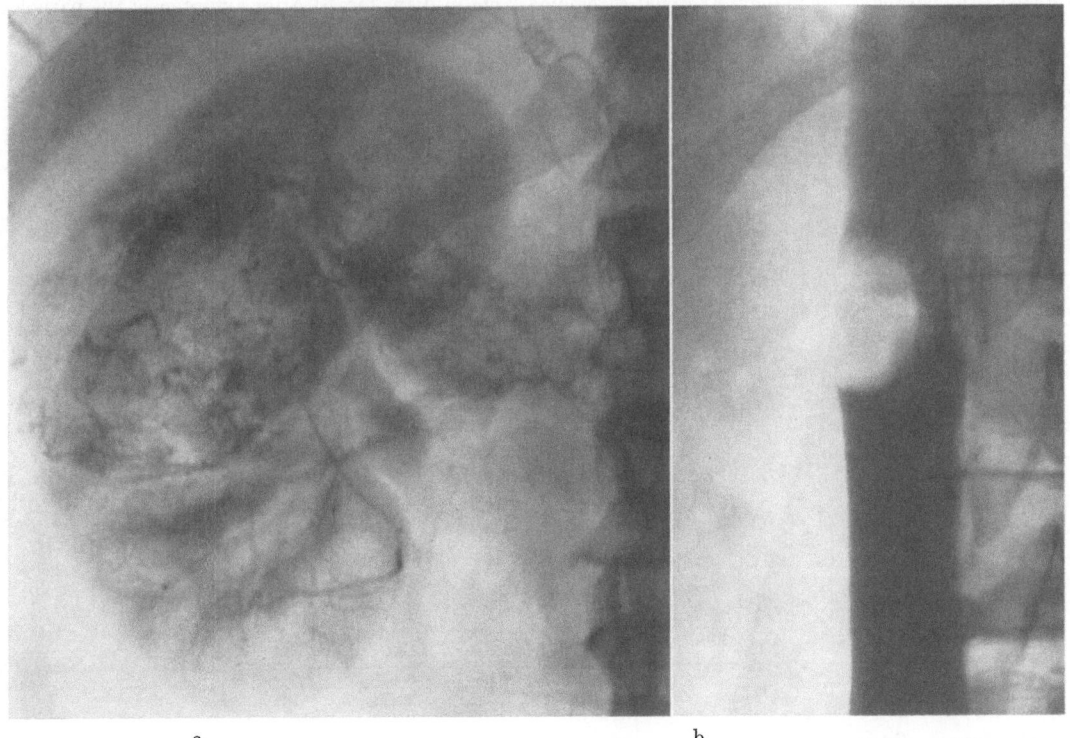

a   b

Fig. 143. a) Well defined renal carcinoma in middle of right kidney. Extension of tumor tissue medially, corresponding to renal vein. b) Cavography: large tumor thrombus from renal vein extending to inferior caval vein

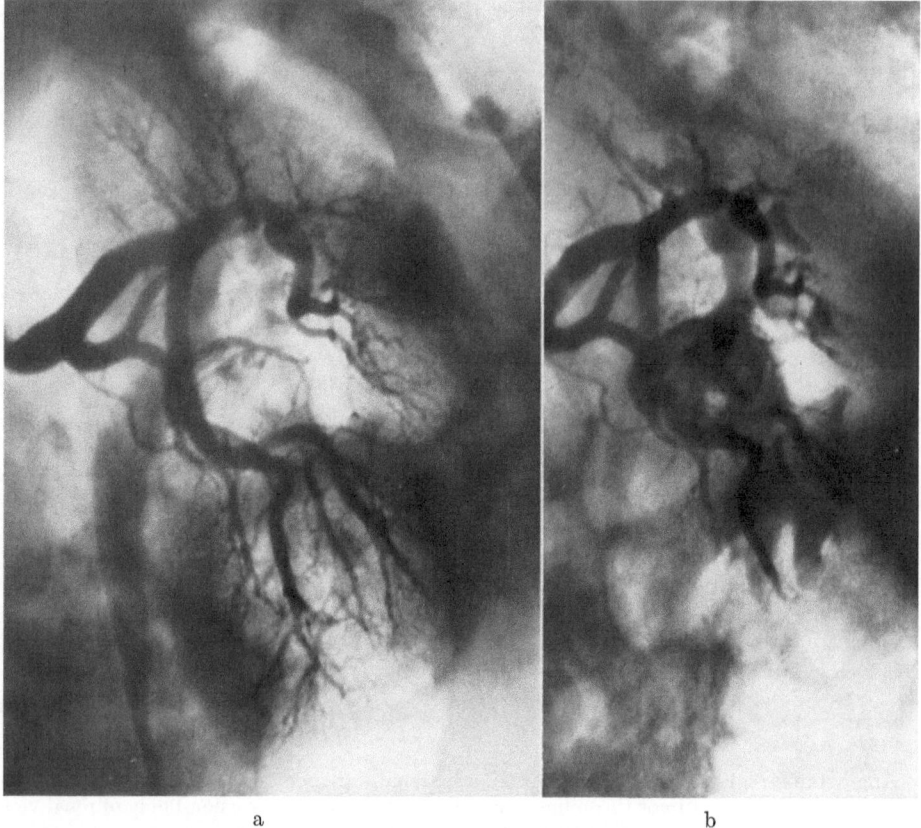

a b

Fig. 144. Angiography, left kidney: a) Renal carcinoma 2 cm in diameter. b) After angiotensin the pathologic vasculature in the tumor is better demonstrated

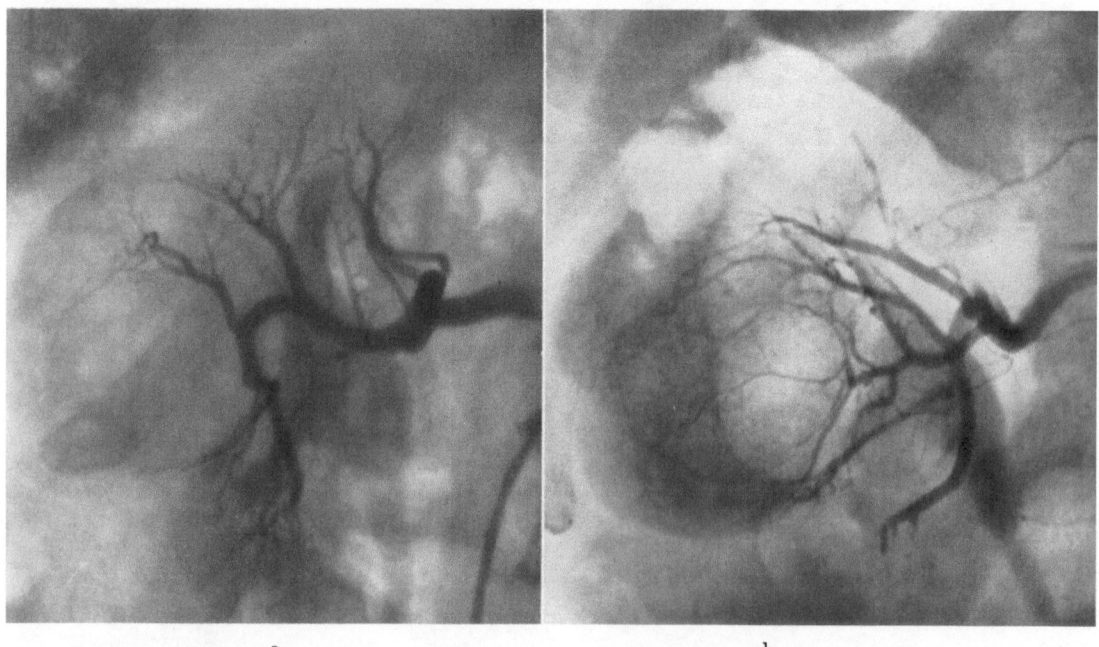

a b

Fig. 145. a) Large expansivity with very few pathologic vessels in right kidney. b) After angiotensin the pathologic vasculature is much better demonstrated

familiar with the vascular anatomy of the kidney in its roentgenologic aspects to understand the picture fully. On the other hand, a non-filling of an area of the renal parenchyma fed by a small supernumerary artery must not be mistaken for a pathologic process.

The larger the tumor, usually the more marked are the pathologic vasculature changes. Even small tumors may have marked changes. Large tumors, on the other hand, may necrotize to a great extent and the pathologic vasculature diminishes correspondingly.

Renal carcinoma has a tendency to become necrotic partly because of arterial thrombosis. This has been studied from a patho-anatomic point of view by BARTLEY and HULT-QUIST (1950), who found fibrosis and other regressive changes. Vessels are never seen within the necrotic parts. This implies that some carcinomas are very poor in vessels or have no pathologic vessels whatsoever. In autopsy material LASSER and STAUBITZ (1957) found arterial thrombosis to be capable of preventing the passage of contrast medium to a tumor (Figs. 146, 147).

There is occasionally a scarcity of pathologic vasculature in both small and large tumors. In order to demonstrate the vasculature in such cases the technical performance of the examination in all its many details must be as expert as possible.

WOODRUFF et al. (1956) claim that less than one third of all renal tumors will show no pathologic vessels and LÖHR et al. (1968) found in one third of the tumors examined either that there were no pathologic vessels or that such vessels could be observed only with difficulty. EDSMAN (1957) found pathologic vessels in 75 out of 80 cases of malignant renal tumors. Of the five without pathologic vessels, in nephrograms it could be demonstrated that in three cases the growth was a solid tumor of irregular outline against the renal parenchyma and that in one case there were no pathologic vessels and no accumulation of contrast medium. The latter case was therefore diagnosed as cyst. The fifth case was a very small tumor described as being of the size of a coffee bean, situated cortically and found accidentally at operation on the kidney.

In our material presented by FOLIN (1967), in 135 patients of whom 58 were examined with aortic injection and 92 with selective technique, a moderate or large number of tumor vessels were found in 81 % at aortic and in 93 % at selective examination. In five patients no tumor vessels were seen at aortic injection. Two of these cases were also examined with selective technique, whereby tumor vessels were demonstrable.

Occasionally in addition to a selective angiography of a kidney with tumor, it may be advisable also to perform aortic angiography in the same session, in order to fill all arteries contributing to the feeding of the tumor, thus giving complete information concerning the size and spread of the tumor.

Pharmaco-angiography: In connection with angiography, enhancement of findings of pathologic vasculature may be achieved and subliminal symptomatology may be transcribed into well detectable signs by use of certain drugs (as described previously).

BILLING and LINDGREN (1944) described the appearance of the arteriogram on the basis of post mortem angiography and patho-anatomic examination of 14 kidneys with renal carcinoma. The appearance of the arteries differed markedly from the normal pattern, and the branches anastomosed richly. Otherwise normal branches of the renal artery terminated in aneurysm-like dilatations giving off several pathologic twigs. The widest pathologic vessels were barely 4 mm in diameter. The irregular caliber and course of the vessels is due to the fact that pathologic vessels have no elastic lamellae, which are always present in dislocated but otherwise normal vessels.

In the nephrographic phase the tumor may be well outlined against non-affected renal parenchyma, especially if the tumor is small and encapsulated. The border towards normal parenchyma is more often irregular, however. The renal parenchyma is occasionally totally replaced by tumor tissue. Only four out of 125 tumors reported by Folin were well outlined against the renal parenchyma in the nephrographic phase.

A filling of the renal vein is obtained in the venous phase of angiography. The renal vein may fill earlier than normally in the presence of much pathologic vasculature and a

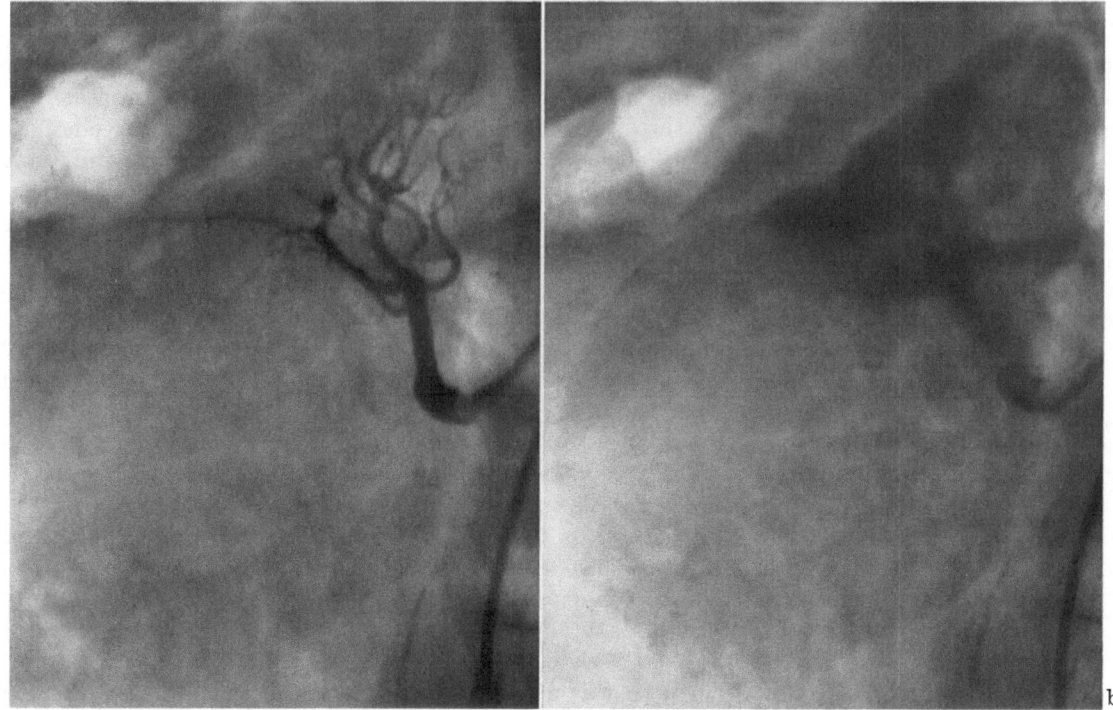

Fig. 146. a) Large renal carcinoma with very low vascularity. Only a few pathologic vessels in cranial part of tumor. b) Nephrographic phase: tumor is irregularly outlined against normal renal parenchyma

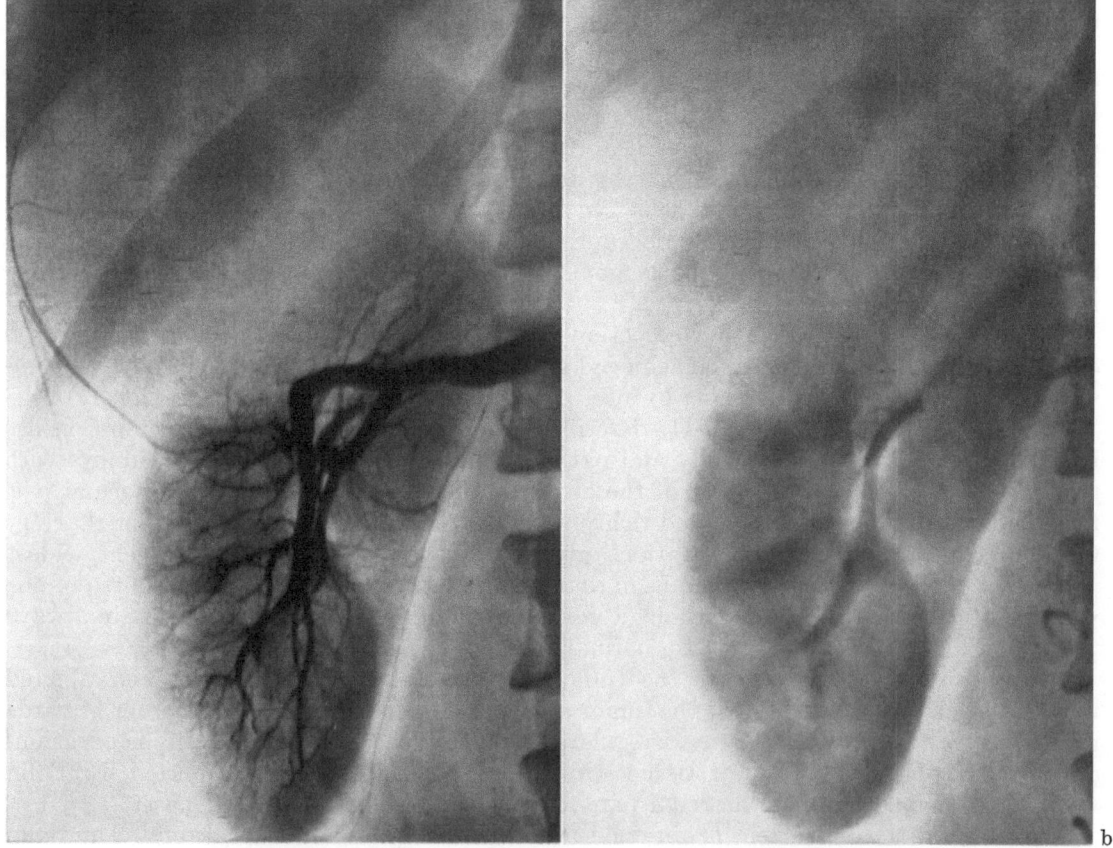

Fig. 147. Large renal carcinoma with low vascularity. Tumor is poorly outlined against renal parenchyma as compared with a cyst. a) Arterial phase. b) Nephrographic phase

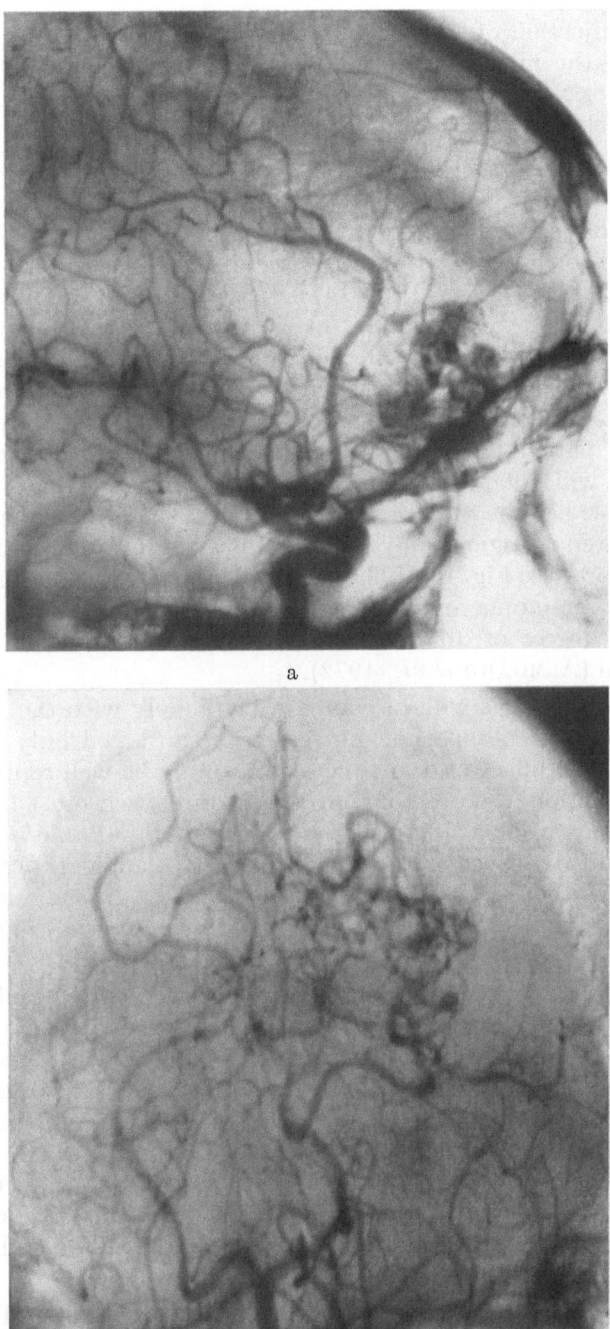

Fig. 148. Richly vascularized metastases. Cerebral metastases from renal carcinoma diagnosed by angiography: a) Carotid angiography: one tumor in frontal lobe. b) Vertebral angiography: one tumor in occipital
lobe

correspondingly great number of arteriovenous fistulae. Full filling of the vein excludes tumor thrombus, whereas non-filling may be due to thrombus or to insufficient amount of contrast medium injected. A thrombus may be seen directly as a filling defect in the vein. It may also be diagnosed indirectly as non-filling of the vein but filling of collateral veins (Figs. 142—143). Since nonfilling of the vein may be due to an insufficient amount of contrast medium, injection of a large amount of contrast medium (for example 25 cc) into the renal artery as the final part of the angiographic procedure is made in patients in whom a firm diagnosis of renal carcinoma is established during angiography. If the vein is patent, it fills well and can be studied in detail.

Other types of malignant tumors show essentially the same characteristics as renal carcinoma (see Fig. 158).

Avascular tumors can offer differential diagnostic difficulties because the most characteristic feature, i. e. pathologic vessels, is missing (ABOULKER, 1955; OLLE OLSSON, 1956; MACQUET et al., 1957 (Figs. 144—147). LINDBLOM and SELDINGER (1955) described huge avascular malignant renal tumors in three of 16 cases. Some authors claim that renal angiography is a less reliable method for demonstrating renal tumor because of the frequently poor vascularization of such tumors. This view is incompatible with our experience. We have found that pathologic vessels are common, that even in the presence of massive necrosis part of the tumor shows pathologic vessels, and that even a poorly vascularized tumor will not produce angiographic changes of the type that is most characteristic of cyst (see below). Small tumors of clinical significance have pathologic vessels and in these cases renal angiography is sometimes the only diagnostic method capable of yielding information (see Fig. 161). There is statistical significance in the relation between vascularity of renal carcinoma and the degree of malignancy. Highly vascularized tumors usually have a low degree of differentiation, whereas tumors with poor vascularity are highly differentiated (ALMGÅRD et al., 1972).

The angiographic findings will, of course, vary largely with the technique used. EDSMAN points out that, as a rule, pathologic vessels are observed only in the arterial and in the early nephrographic phase and this phase thus must be well represented in the angiographic series. In addition, the dose of contrast medium used must be of suitable size and concentration to secure a good filling of the arteries and suitable density of the nephrogram. Most important, however, is the use of a selective angiographic technique avoiding superimposition of irrelevant vessels. *A good technique, i. e. good selectivity and timing, is necessary for full utilization of the possibilities of angiography to diagnose malignant renal tumors.*

Perusal of the literature and the descriptions of accompanying illustrations will show that the technique employed often leaves much to be desired. One might even go so far as to say that many of the examinations referred to in the literature are not worthy of the name renal angiography. Often they do not represent a roentgen examination but simply a roentgenogram and often a very inconclusive one. In my opinion, this is the most important reason why many authors underestimate the value of renal angiography in the diagnosis of tumors. It should therefore be stressed once more that the value of renal angiography depends on the technique employed. In other words, full utilization of the possibilities of angiography requires that the examiner be thoroughly familiar with all types of angiography.

It must be pointed out on the other hand that in a small number of cases it is impossible at renal angiography to demonstrate pathologic vasculature. In some cases, also, the tumor in the nephrographic phase is very well outlined and has an even contour. In such cases the differential diagnosis between tumor and cyst is angiographically impossible. Puncture of the expansivity in such cases must be performed (see below discussion on differential diagnosis between tumor and cyst).

In order to try to find means of increasing diagnostic stringency in renal tumors we have started angiographic experiments in animals with tumors induced by dimethylnitrosamine (EKELUND and JONSSON, 1971). This will make possible closer studies of pathologic vasculature and influences on this vasculature. The drug-induced tumors represent different histo-pathologic types from well differentiated tumors to anaplastic tumors. In this respect they resemble tumors encountered at clinical angiography.

d) Phlebography

Renal carcinoma has a tendency to invade the renal vein. Occasionally tumor growth and thrombosis are so massive as to cause stasis in the region drained by the inferior caval vein. This may occasionally dominate the clinical picture to such an extent as to be the indication for roentgen examination with the discovery of the renal tumor as a consequence.

In complete obstruction of the inferior caval vein at phlebography the normal filling of the vein is missing and a filling is obtained of the usually numerous collateral veins instead. If obstruction by thrombosis is not complete, the vein may be dilated distally, but it may also be distended by the tumor masses. These appear as massive, well circumscribed filling defects which may assume considerable dimensions. The tumor may have grown along one of the walls of the vein and obstructed a fair length of the lumen. Small changes will produce well defined filling defects caused by protuberances encroaching upon the lumen of the renal vein or from the renal vein into the caval vein (Fig. 143).

The actual tumor or metastases to the lymph nodes may displace or compress the renal veins and/or the caval vein.

e) Nephrotomography

EVANS et al. (1954) have described the following technique "providing precise delineation of functioning renal parenchyma":

"1. The patient is positioned supine on a roentgenographic table equipped for tomograms.

2. Preliminary plain films and tomograms are obtained, to be used as control films and to check the roentgenographic technique.

3. A 12-gauge Robb-Steinberg angiocardiographic needle is inserted into an antecubital vein.

4. Arm-to-tongue decholin circulation time is determined by employing the same injection technique as for the contrast substance.

5. Prior to the injection of the urokon, it is advisable to rehearse the injection with the patient and warn of the sensations to be expected, so that there will be no movement or breathing during the exposures. We feel that sensitivity testing is of little value. This opinion is based on a very extensive angiocardiographic experience in our department and the survey on angio-cardiographic mortality conducted by DOTTER and JACKSON.

6. With the roentgen tube in mid-position, 50 cc of urokon sodium 70% is rapidly injected (in 1.5 to 2 seconds) into the abducted arm. A film is then exposed at the predetermined circulation time. The first roentgenogram will demonstrate the renal arteries. This is followed as rapidly as possible by a second film which secures the nephrogram. Immediately after the second exposure a tomogram is obtained. The elapsed time between the first exposure and the completion of the tomogram should not exceed 25 seconds.

7. After inspection of the films, a second injection may be considered necessary. A repeat circulation time is advisable before the second injection because we have found that the circulation time is delayed after the first injection, presumably due to an increase in the peripheral resistance. If this is not done, opacification of the abdominal aorta and renal vessels will not be secured."

The method is called nephrotomography. The same authors in 1955 published the results of 100 examinations with this method. The material included 32 solitary cysts of the kidneys, of which 30 were proven surgically, and 11 renal carcinomas, all but one confirmed. The surprisingly great number of operated cysts can be explained by a slight unreliability of the method expressed in the summary: "Cysts can be diagnosed with relative certainty ....". Further results with nephrotomography are discussed in the section on roentgendiagnostic differential diagnosis in expansive lesion.

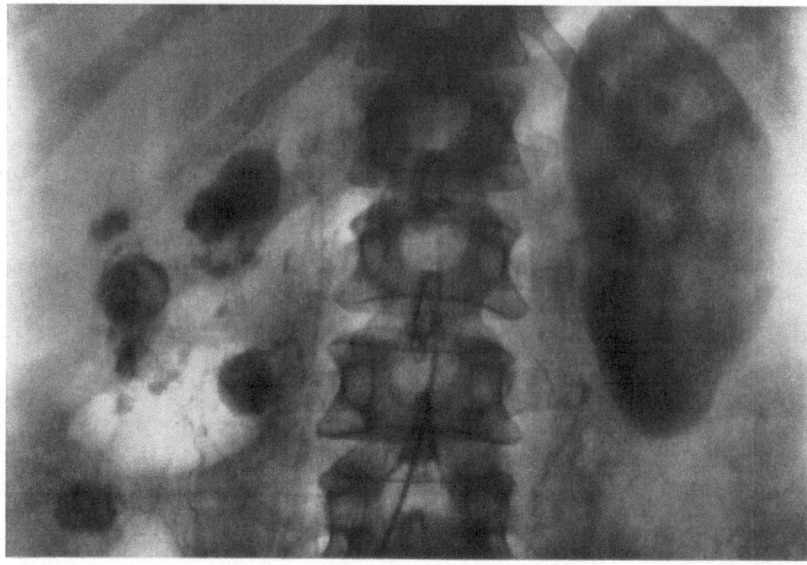

Fig. 149. Local recurrence of operated renal carcinoma. Tumor tissue richly vascularized, like original tumor

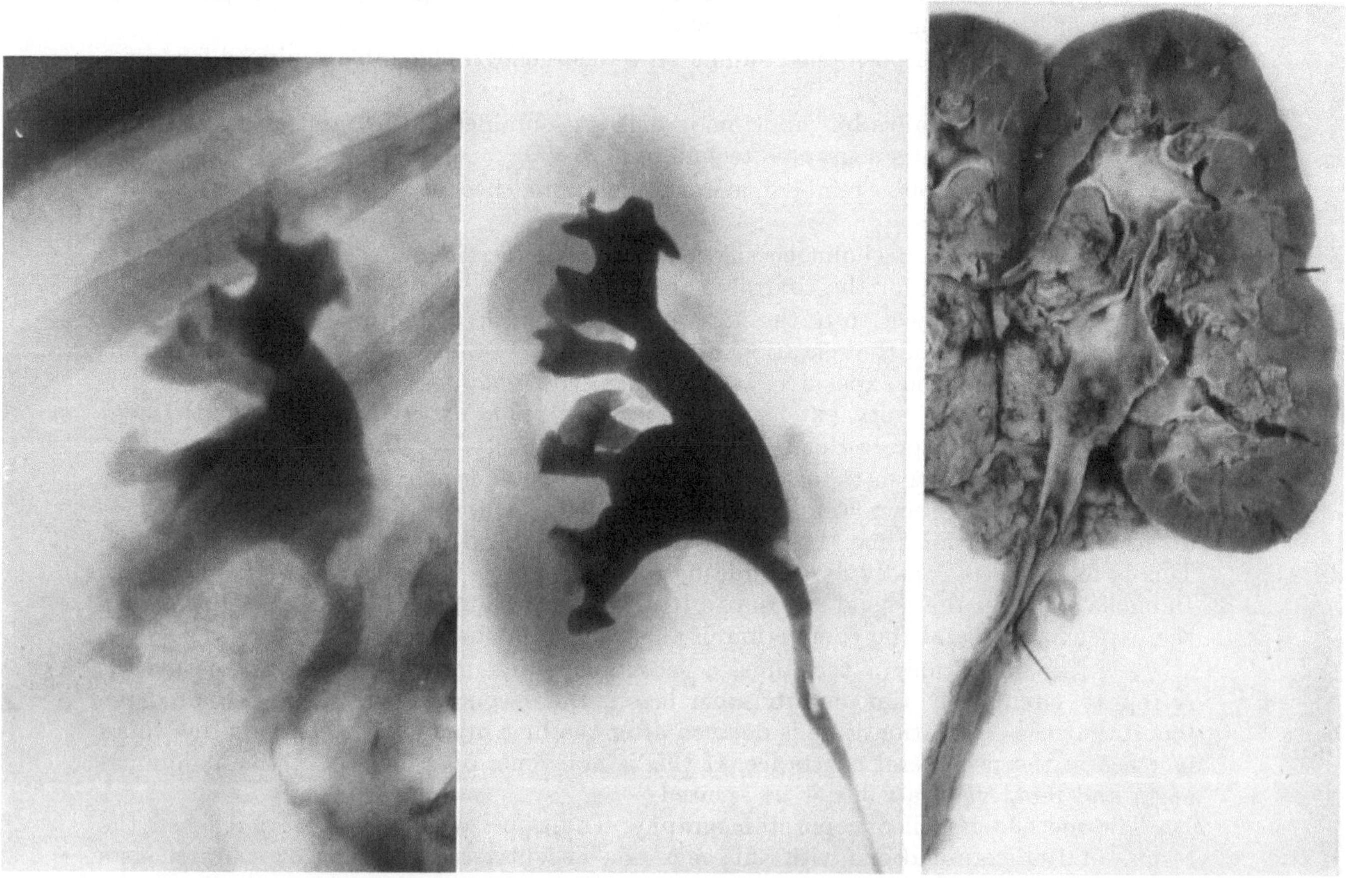

a   b   c

Fig. 150. Renal carcinoma with implantation metastases in ureter. a) Urography: Besides deformation of kidney pelvis with flattening (seen better in other projection) there are two sessile papilloma-like tumors in upper part of ureter. b) Pyelogram of specimen. c) Specimen: Tumor in parenchyma. Implantation metastases in ureter. Histology: Papillary metastases of renal carcinoma

f) The growth of renal carcinoma

The growth of a renal tumor is demonstrable in cases that have for some reason or other not been operated upon. The growth process varies widely from case to case. JOHNSSON (1946) described four cases examined during expectancy. In one case the tumor grew only 3 cm in diameter in the course of five years but retained its round shape and was well defined. After an additional five years the patient was examined again but not operated upon. The tumor had now broken through the capsule, invaded contiguous tissue and metastasized to the lungs. In another case where examination was repeated after an interval of one year, an increase in diameter of only 0.5 cm was demonstrable and the tumor was well defined. Two other patients were re-examined after eight and five months, respectively, but no further roentgenologic changes could be demonstrated. Many cases show rapid progress, however, We have seen a case from another hospital where a renal carcinoma had been examined repeatedly without its nature having been detected. At the first examination the tumor was small and contrast excretion was adequate. Two months later the growth had increased in size and the excretion of contrast medium was delayed. Another six months later the patient came to our hospital. At that point the tumor was very large and the kidney no longer functioning. These cases stress the fact that expectancy is not justified in the differential diagnosis between malignant renal tumors and benign lesions. A renal tumor may show only very slow progression and be encapsulated for a long time. However, when the tumor breaks through the capsule and appears in the roentgenogram as a definite tumor, an invasion has started. The change that makes the differential diagnosis possible by expectancy thus means a worse situation for the patient.

Although regressive changes are common in tumors, I have observed in only one single instance a renal carcinoma decrease in size.

g) Multiple tumors

(Figs. 151—153)

Renal carcinoma is occasionally bilateral. BAILEY and YOUNGBLOOD (1950) described such a case and referred to 11 others from the literature. They stated that it is not possible to decide whether each tumor is primary or whether one tumor is a solitary secondary growth.

Multiple dissimilar tumors occasionally occur in one and the same kidney. Most of the cases on record, however, were probably not dissimilar but represented different patho-anatomic evaluation of different parts of one and the same tumor arising from the same mesenchymal tissue but differentiated to a varying extent in different parts of the tumor. Co-existence of malignant and benign tumors and of tumors of the renal parenchyma in association with tumor of the renal pelvis has also been described. A survey of cases of this type has been given by PENNISI et al. (1957).

Co-existence of tumor and cyst is not uncommon (Fig. 152).

Multiple expansivities, unilateral or bilateral, are found occasionally at roentgen examination. This is characteristic of polycystic disease bilaterally and of multicystic disease unilaterally. It is well known that embryoblastoma may be bilateral.

We have also encountered other types of multiplicity: simple, single cyst may be multiple. I have seen a patient with hematuria in which at urography an irregular expansive lesion was found in the upper part of the right kidney. Because of the irregularity, the lesion was assumed to be a renal carcinoma. At angiography, however, it was shown that the expansivity consisted of two adjacent simple cysts. The hemorrhage was caused by an arterial aneurysm with a small rupture in its wall. Another combination encountered is hemangioma and carcinoma in the same kidney.

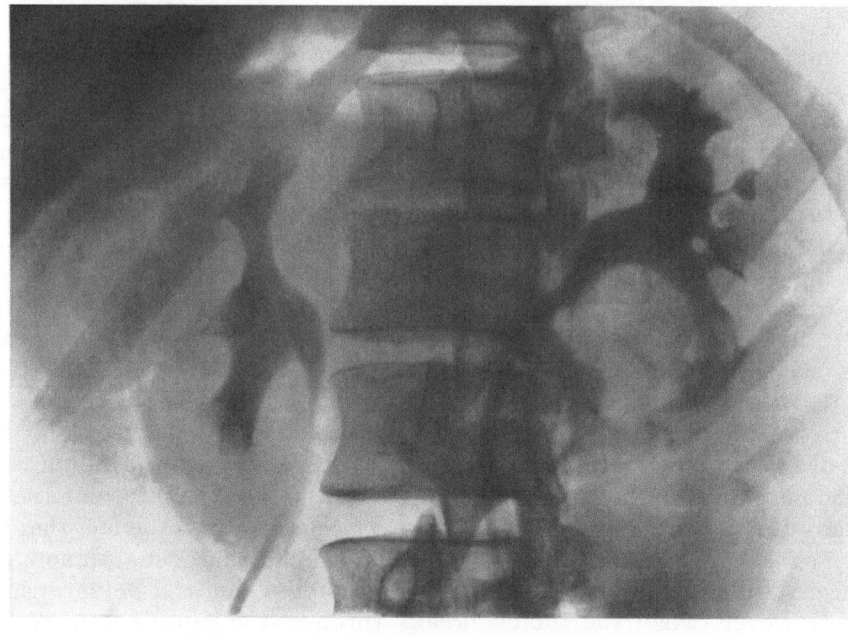

a

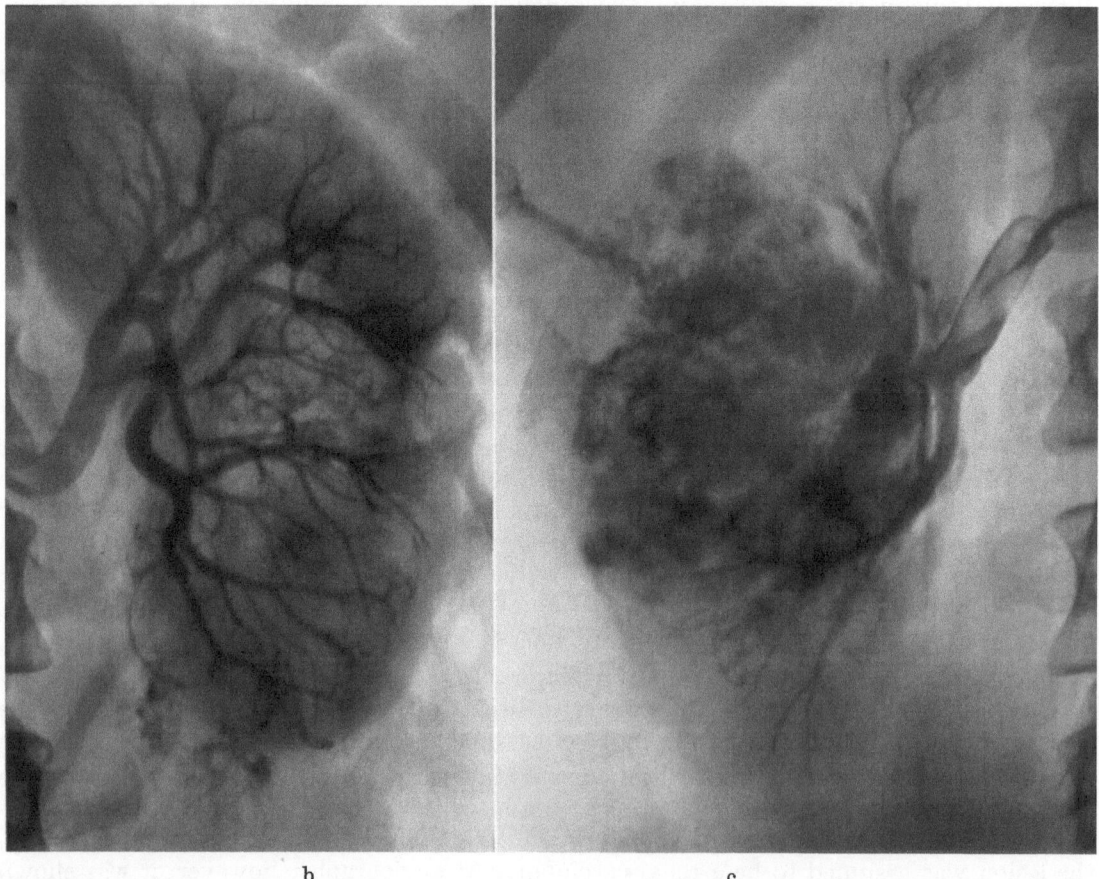

b   c

Fig. 151. Bilateral renal carcinoma. a) Urography: expansivity in lower medial part of left kidney and in middle
of right kidney. Selective angiography: b) left: renal carcinoma in lower kidney pole; c) right: large renal
carcinoma

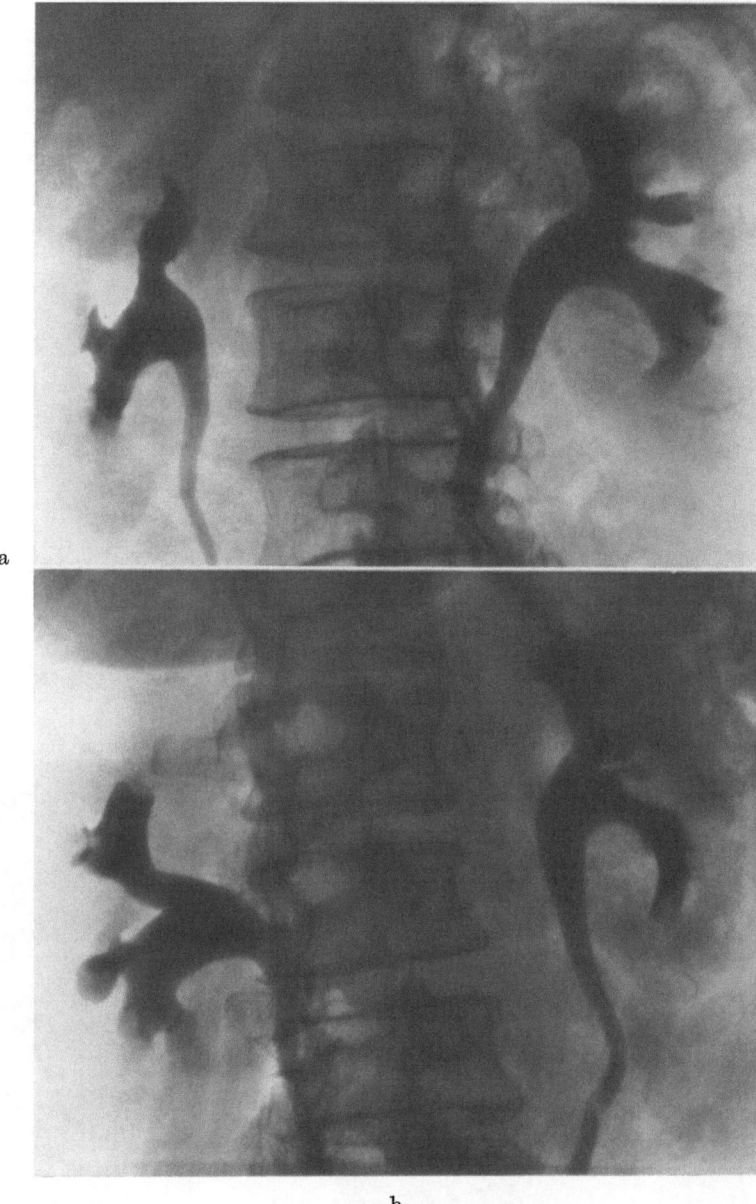

a

b

Fig. 152. Multiple expansivities, renal carcinoma on right side, renal cyst on left. a) and b) Urography in different projections: a slight expansivity can be noted on left side with distention of lower branch. No expansivity is seen on right side. c) Angiography, left side: corresponding to expansivity, well defined cyst in lower hilar lip. d) right side: small renal carcinoma laterally below middle of kidney. No influence on renal contour or on renal pelvis

Multiple carcinomatous tumors are rare. In our material we have had one case with two tumors in one kidney, one case with bilateral renal carcinoma, and one case with a renal pelvic carcinoma in one kidney and a renal carcinoma in the other. Carcinoma in one kidney and cyst in the other can be encountered. We have also had several cases with carcinoma and one or more simple cysts in the same kidney. Changes were well demonstrable at angiography in one patient who was found to have in the same kidney a renal carcinoma, a simple cyst, and a multilocular cyst.

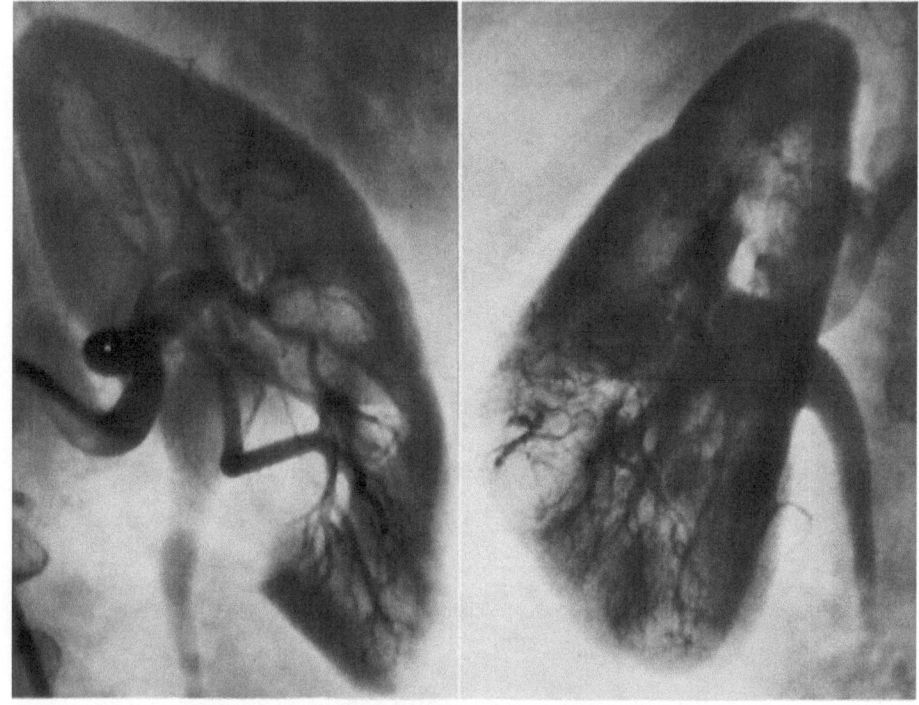

Fig. 152 c   Fig. 152 d

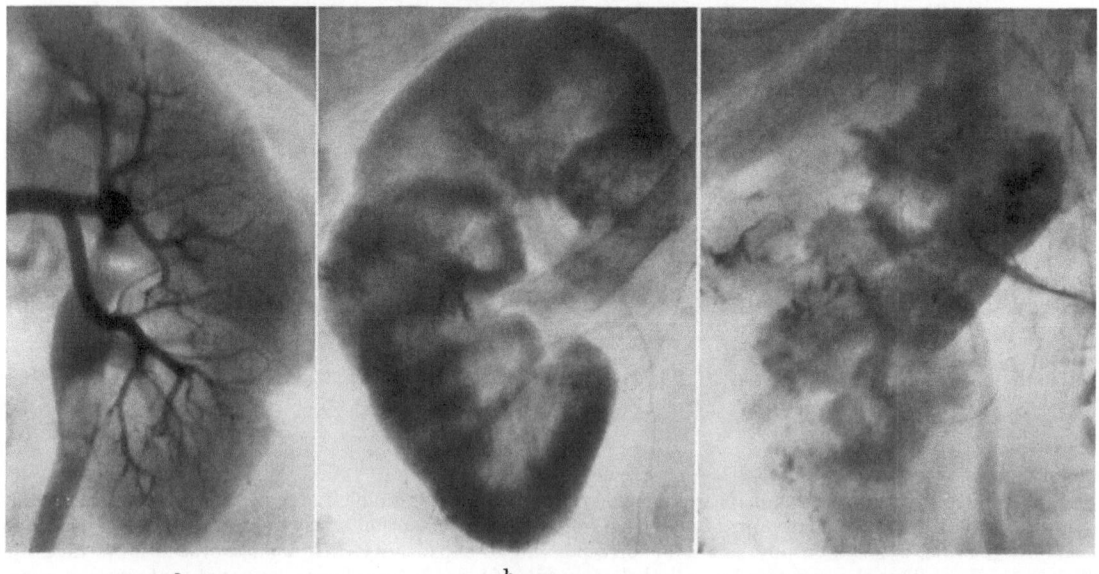

a   b   c

Fig. 153. a) Multiplicity of renal tumor. Left side, renal pelvic carcinoma. Note normal vasculature at angiography, filling defect in lower part of kidney pelvis. b) and c) Right kidney, angiography in nephrographic phase in each of two renal arteries: In upper hilar lip: renal carcinoma 2 cm in diameter. Lateral part of tumor is filled from one of two renal arteries, the medial part from the other renal artery

Multiple pathology of other types may also be mentioned here. Naturally a kidney harboring a carcinoma or a cyst may be pyelonephritic and show changes characteristic of both at urography or angiography. Renal carcinoma and cyst with renal arterial aneurysms or with hemangioma in the same kidney are also included in our experience.

2. Malignant renal tumors in children

Renal carcinoma is not strictly limited to adults. In the material of Riches *et al.* referred to above, the youngest patient was 11 years old. Cases of renal carcinoma in childhood have also been described by HEMPSTEAD *et al.* (1953), BEATTIE (1954) and POOLE and VIAMONTE (1970), for example.

The most common malignant renal tumor in childhood is that usually known as Wilms tumor after Wilms, who was the first to give a detailed description of this previously unknown tumor in 1899. The tumor is known under various other names such as adenosarcoma, adenomyosarcoma, dysembryoma, but it is usually called embryoma or nephroblastoma. Half of the cases occur in children between the ages of two and four years. Occasionally the tumor is present at birth. SALLER described such a case in which the new-born had not only such a tumor but also metastases and LATTIMER *et al.* (1958) reported nephrectomy in a four-day-old infant. The tumor can be of roentgen-diagnostic interest during the prenatal period; tumors of this type have often been observed at autopsy of fetuses. They are known to be a cause of dystocia.

The kidneys are the most common seat of tumors in children, apart from the eyes.

Tumors of the embryonal type, as pointed out by DEUTICKE (1931), for example, have been known to occur in several members of the same family.

The embryoma usually metastasizes to the liver and lungs but not to the skeleton. It may also spread to the other kidney. Large space-occupying processes are then seen in both kidneys. A case of this type has been described by AGERHOLM-CHRISTENSEN (1939) in an 8 month old child. True double-sidedness may also occur (CAMPBELL, 1948) (Fig. 152). In such cases it may not be possible to distinguish it roentgenologically from polycystic kidney at urography.

Since the tumor appears at such an early age, the diagnosis is usually based on objective findings. Haematuria is rare, and the patients are usually referred for roentgen examination because of a palpable tumor.

a) Plain roentgenography

By the time the patient is referred for roentgen examination the tumor is, as a rule, large, irregular, and often not well outlined. Smaller, well defined tumors are also seen, however. The tumor often contains irregular calcifications which may be limited to a small part of the tumor or may be scattered throughout the entire growth.

b) Urography, pyelography and angiography

At urography/pyelography deformation is seen of essentially the same type as that in renal carcinoma in adults (Fig. 154).

In the differential-diagnosis hydronephrosis and polycystic kidney (which may also occur in children) are particularly important, also extrarenal expanding processes such as an enlarged spleen. The most important lesion from a differential diagnostic point of view, however, is another growth, namely sympathico-blastoma. If the growth contains calcifications, the differentiation between these two types of tumor is particularly difficult. Sympathico-blastoma, in contrast to embryoma, often metastasizes in a typical way to the skeleton. The tumor vascularity, the type of pathologic vasculature, and the irregular and indistinct definition of the tumor in relation to the surrounding renal parenchyma are essentially the same as in renal carcinoma. The vasculature, however, may appear to be somewhat different from that found in malign tumor in adults, as has been stressed by MENG and ELKIN (1969). The important aspect, however, is that in nephroblastoma examined angiographically tumor vessels of different degrees have been found.

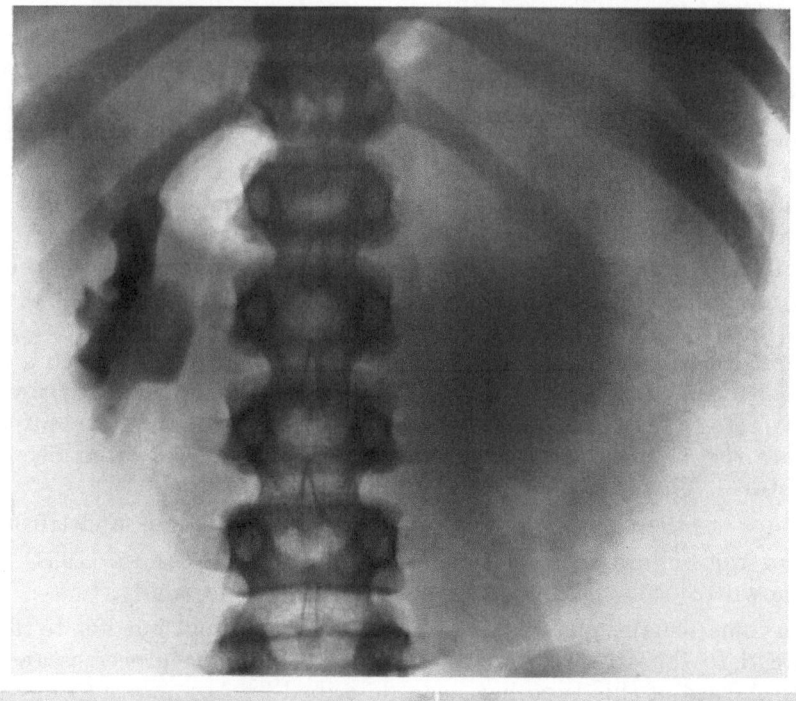

a

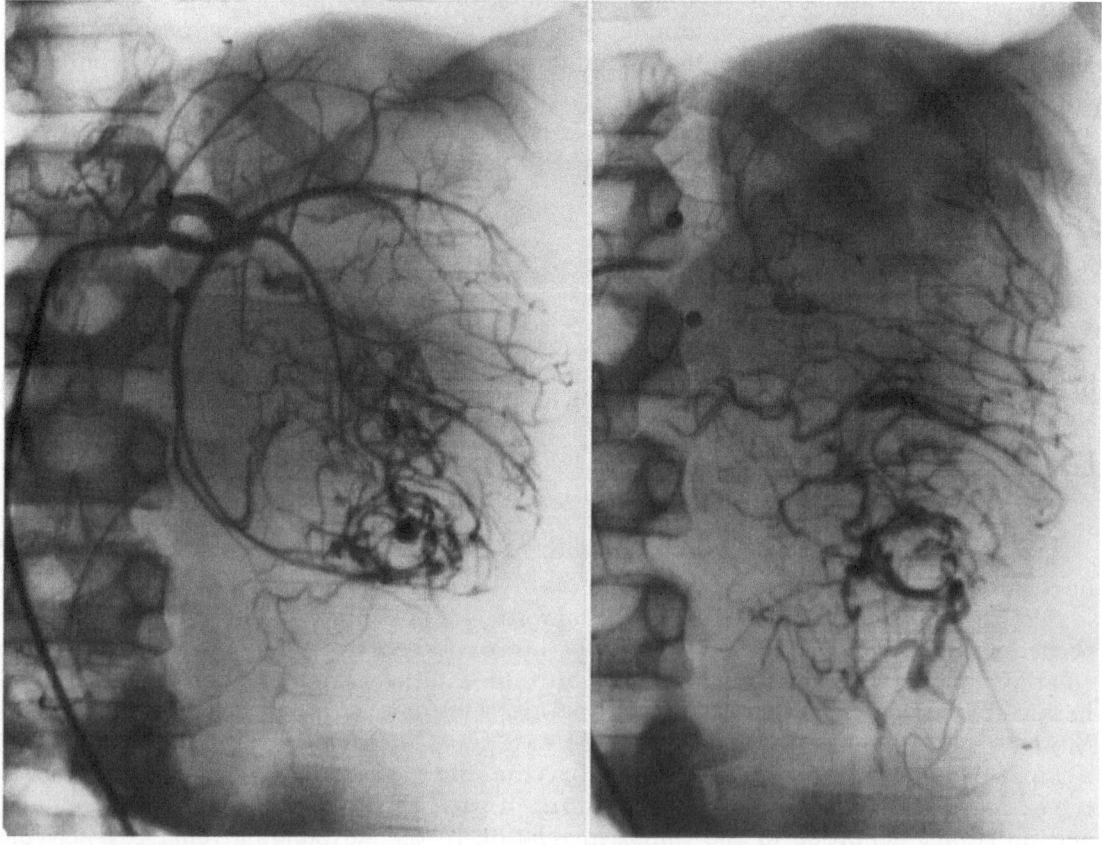

b   c

Fig. 154. Embryoblastoma in 14-year-old boy. a) Urography: right side normal. No contrast excretion on left side, where a large mass can be seen. b) and c) Renal angiography: b) Arterial diastole; c) Arterial phase, next systole: Marked displacement of intrarenal vessels around a huge tumor. Numerous pathologic vessels. Vascular changes of same appearance seen in renal carcinoma.

3. Other types of malignant tumor

Other types of malignant tumor in the kidney are rare. Sarcoma is occasionally seen. The specific type of Kaposis sarcoma may affect the kidney as a part of a systemic disease. Usually this tumor is localized to the skin.

Lymphoma may affect the urinary tract. LALLI (1969) reviewed nearly 3,000 necropsy reports and found 96 lymphoma cases, of which 50 showed evidence of urinary tract involvement. Such involvement occurs during the terminal stages of the disease, with lesions which are usually too small to be found roentgenologically. If the infiltration is marked, a general enlargement of the kidney is more usually seen than a localized mass.

The angiographic findings in lymphoma consist sometimes of pathologic vasculature and rapid arteriovenous shunting (SELTZER and WENLUND, 1967; CHIO and KOHLER, 1969), but often only displacement and stretching of arteries may be seen. The renal involvement can also be studied by lymphangiography.

Renal involvement by reticulum cell sarcoma (Fig. 158) and lymphosarcoma and by leukemia is more common. The renal infiltration causes increase in the size of the kidneys. At urography the calyceal system usually has normal shape. In children the infiltration may be irregular, causing displacement of calyces of a type seen in polycystic disease (TRUCKEN-BRODT, 1971).

In thalassemia major without urinary tract symptoms, the kidneys are evenly enlarged bilaterally, which is caused by tubular dilatation (GROSSMAN et al., 1971).

The kidney may occasionally be the target organ for metastases of malignant tumors from outside the urinary tract (AGNEW, 1958). Metastases are said to be extremely uncommon (ROY and WALTON, 1970) but BOSNIAK et al. (1969) found them to be common. The latter authors report on four cases of metastatic neoplasm which presented as a single large renal mass. The primary lesions were epidermoid carcinoma of the lung in two cases, myxolipous sarcoma of the leg in one case, and corium carcinoma in one case. All of the cases presented angiographically with low vascularity without definite tumor vessels but with infiltration of some arterial branches. The tumors were not well outlined against the surrounding renal parenchyma.

4. Metastases from renal carcinoma

Renal carcinoma may metastasize anywhere in the body. Occasionally the metastasis is the lesion which is first diagnosed when, for example, a pathologic fracture brings the patient under medical observation. The primary tumor may be too small to be diagnosed urographically but can be seen angiographically.

Local metastases around the kidney in the perirenal tissue and in glands can also be studied angiographically, specifically tumor recurrence after nephrectomy.

In findings of suspected metastases in the chest the kidney should be suspected as an origin of primary tumor and the hilar lesions as metastases, particularly if a glandular mass is found in a lung hilum. Skeletal and cerebral metastases should also direct the examiner's attention to the kidneys as a possible source of primary tumor. This also holds in cases of unexplained fever, particularly periodic fever, and polycythaemia. Metastatic growths from renal carcinoma are often characteristic, with large arterio-venous fistulae like those in many of the primary tumors. They are therefore well demonstrable by angiography (Fig. 148, 149). This applies to local metastases in lymph nodes and retroperitoneal tissue, lung metastases and cerebral metastases and also to the rare metastases from a renal carcinoma to the homolateral and heterolateral adrenal.

A renal carcinoma may, although rarely, metastasize to the ureter (Fig. 150) or the urinary bladder and produce symptoms simulating a bladder tumor.

5. Benign renal tumors

(Figs. 155—158)

Benign renal tumors of clinical interest are rare. As a rule, these tumors are small and are nearly always found accidentally on patho-anatomic examination of a kidney removed for some other reason or on routine pathologic examination of the kidneys at autopsy. The above mentioned material by RICHES *et al.* consisting of 2,314 cases of renal

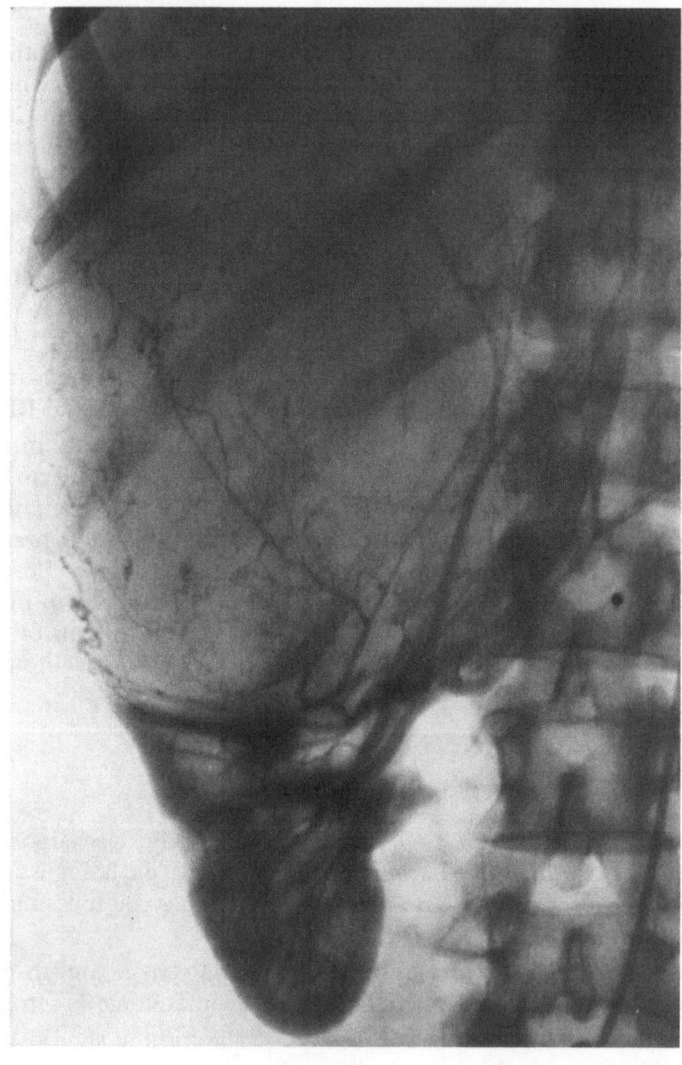

a

Fig. 155. a) Large hamartoma of right kidney. b) Large lipoma, left kidney. c) Urography. d) Angiography

and ureteric tumors included only 12 benign tumors of the renal parenchyma, namely 5 adenomas and 3 haemangiomas. In 1956 FOSTER reported that a perusal of the literature on all benign kidney tumors large enough to be of clinical significance revealed a total of 135, namely 57 adenomas, 24 lipomas, 22 myomas, 17 fibromas, seven angiomas and eight mixed tumors. Occasionally, however, an adenoma may have the same type of patho-logic vasculature as that in some renal carcinomas. Actually, patho-anatomic differen-tiation between a small renal carcinoma and an adenoma is a semantic problem!

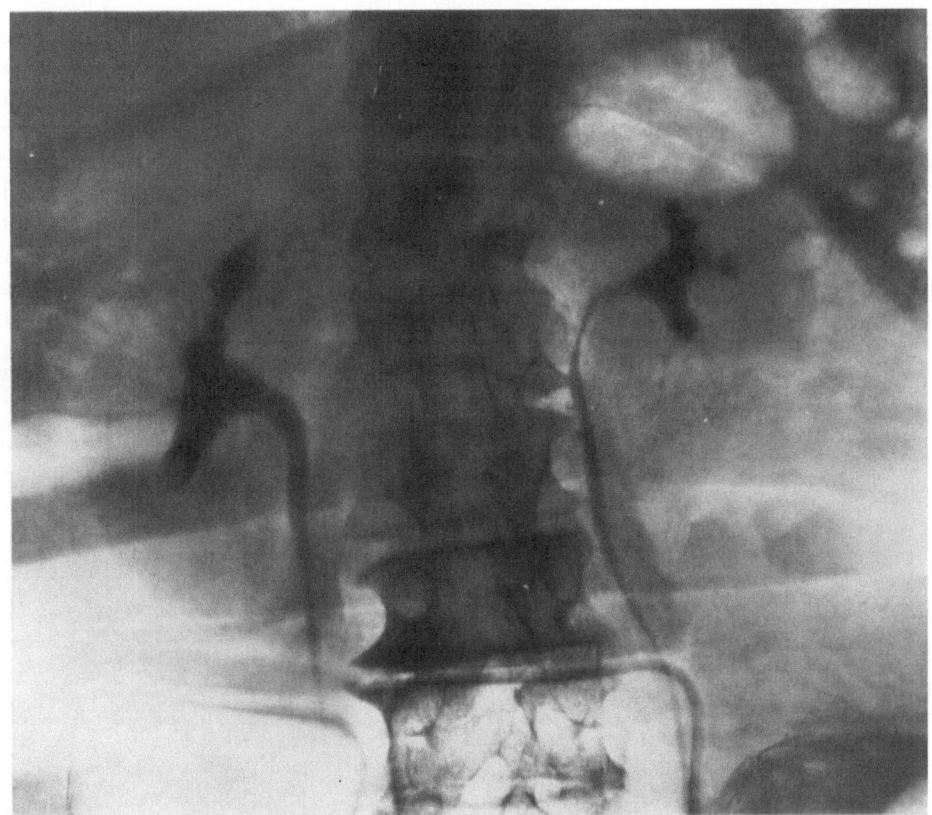

Fig. 155 b

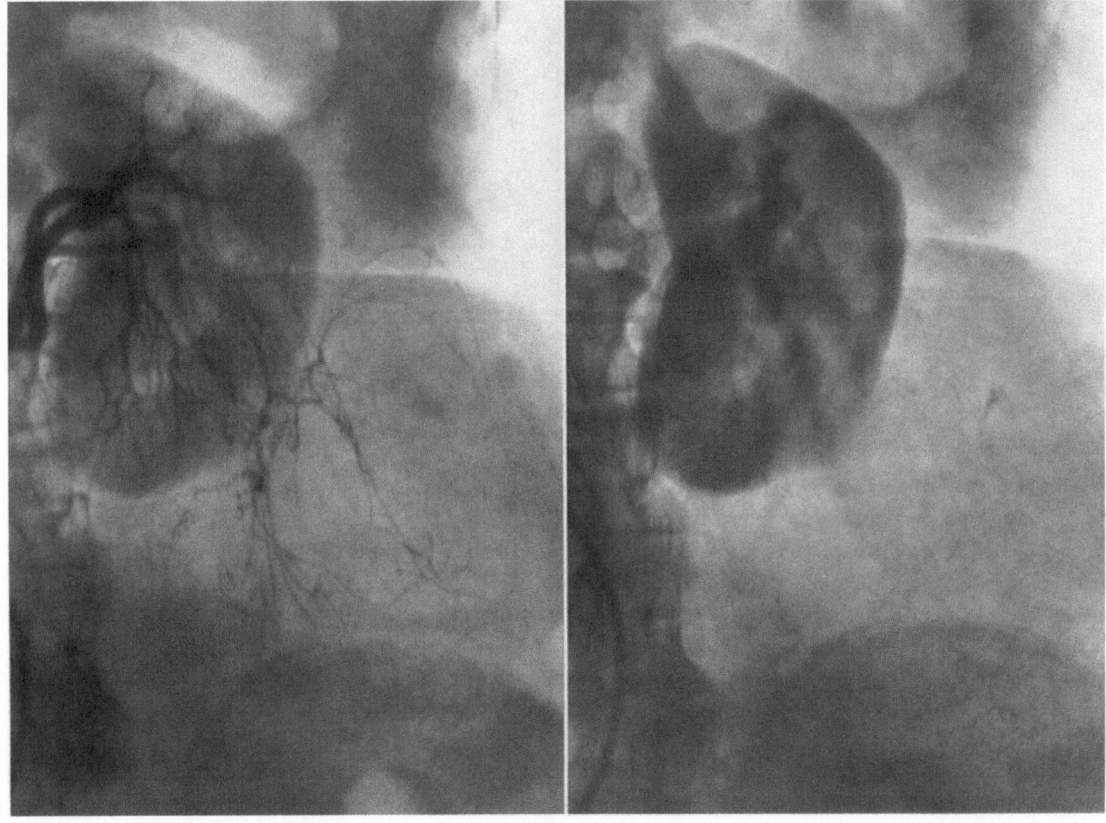

c   d

The majority of benign tumors of the renal parenchyma are adenomas, as seen above. Small solitary cortical adenomas are common in arteriosclerotic kidneys (TWISS, 1949), but they are of no roentgen-diagnostic interest. Like some fibromas, lipomas and mixed tumors, adenomas can be demonstrated by plain roentgenography and urography or pyelography. The findings are the same as in a well outlined renal carcinoma (BAUER *et al.*, 1958). The adenoma usually appears in the angiogram as an avascular tumor which cannot be distinguished from a well demarcated avascular renal carcinoma. Adenomas increase in size very slowly. MISHALANY and GILBERT (1957) described a case of probable ossified cortical adenoma which simulated hydatid cyst in the plain roentgenogram and in the pyelogram and which was therefore diagnosed as such. MEISEL (1954) described a case in

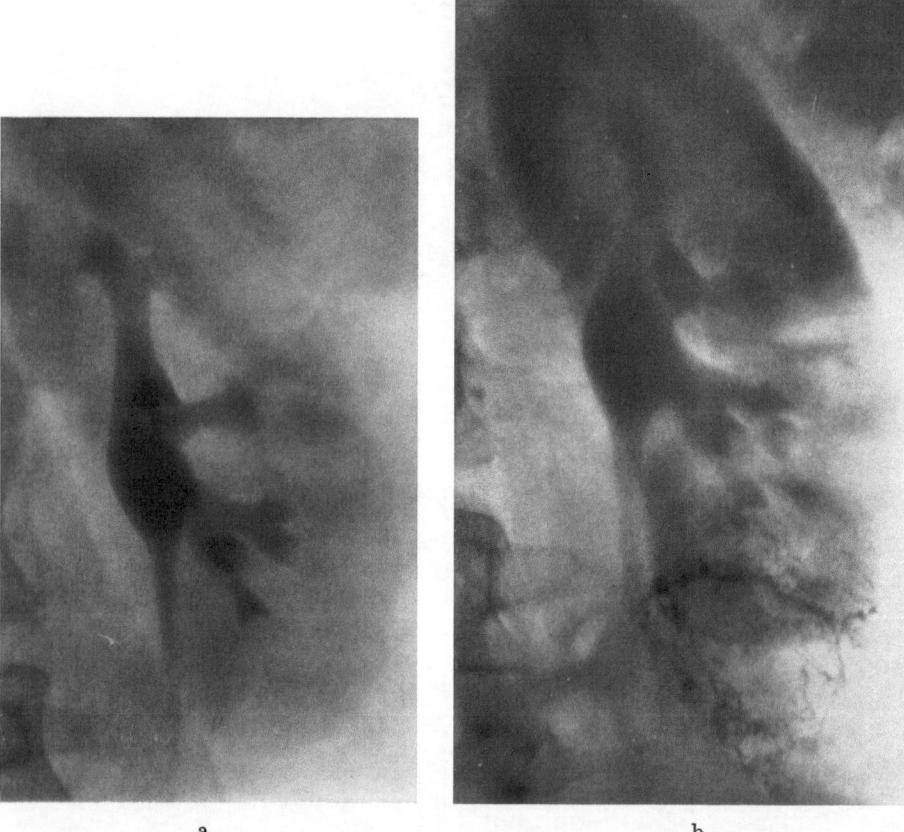

a   b

Fig. 156. Angiolipoma of left kidney. a) Urography: slight irregularity in lower kidney pole, left. b) Angiography: irregular vascularity in lower kidney pole—tumor. Impossible to exclude malignancy. Patho-anatomic diagnosis = angiomyolipoma

which both kidneys were studded with small adenomas so that the pyelogram simulated that of a polycystic kidney.

In the Pringle syndrome of adenoma sebaceum, teleangiectases in the face, and subungual fibroma and pigment nevi, a combination with tuberous sclerosis is common. Therefore adenomas in the kidney may be found also in Pringle's syndrome (DEININGER and TRAPP, 1971).

Fibromas are usually very small but may sometimes be very large. Thus FOSTER (1956) described a case of a tumor in an 8 year old child in whom the tumor weighed 43 pounds while the patient together with the tumor weighed 94 pounds.

The fairly uncommon lipoma must be distinguished from such conditions as replacement lipomatosis (see chapter L). Lipomas are true tumors and often appear as mixed tumors, angiomyolipomas, so-called hamartomas, fibromyxolipomas, etc. Angio-myolipoma is the most important benign tumor from the point of view of roentgen-diagnostics and differential diagnostics. This tumor can be of two different types: one is hamartoma in connection with tuberous sclerosis, usually small, multiple tumors situated anywhere in the body, for example in the brain, the heart, or in the kidneys. At angiography a pathologic vasculature is seen which is not definitely distinct from that seen in some cases of renal carcinoma. The vessels in the tumor also respond to epinephrine in the same way as tumor vessels in renal carcinoma (PALMISANO, 1967). Eighty percent of pa-

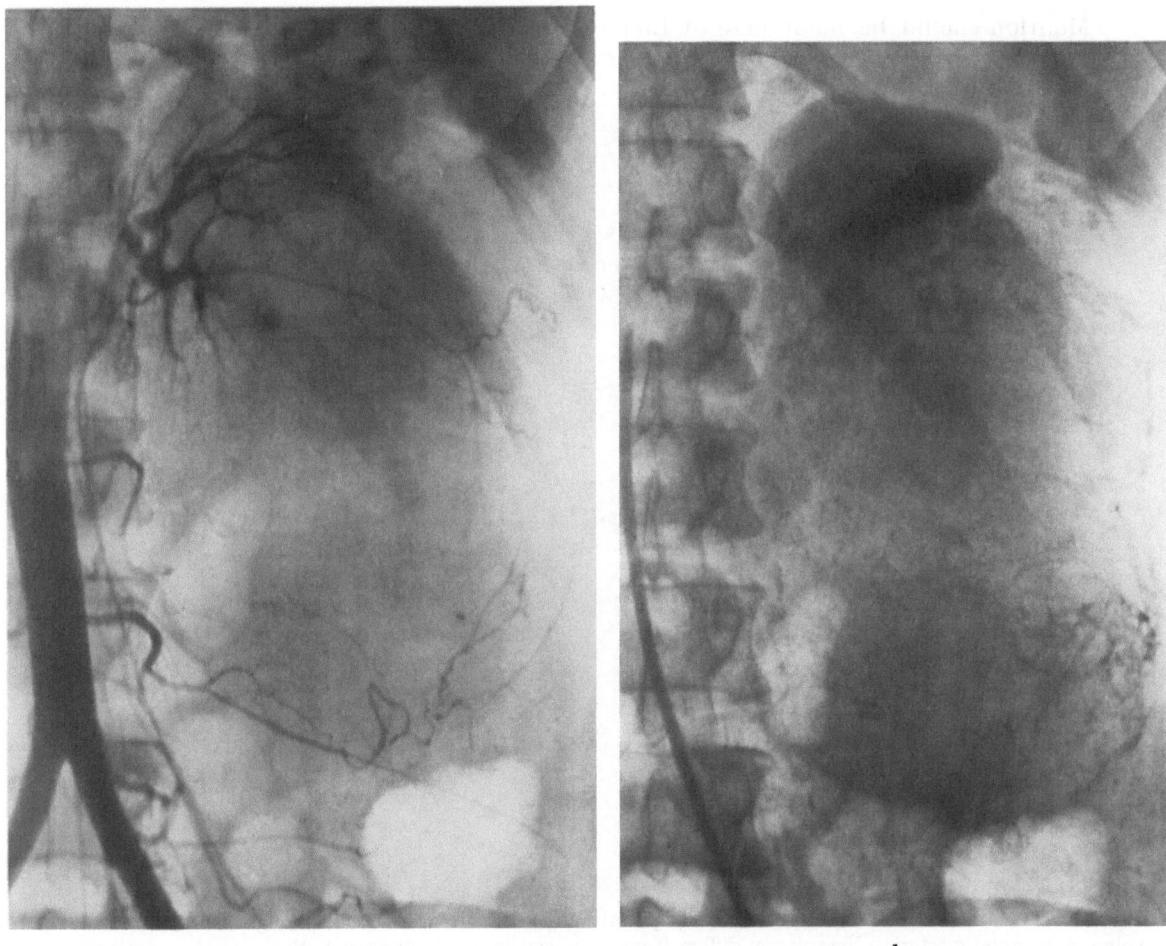

a   b

Fig. 157. Angiomyolipoma. Very large irregular tumor in left kidney. Angiography: normal kidney parenchyma is seen only as a cap on left kidney. In remainder of kidney: pathologic vasculature in a huge tumor. Vasculature differs from what is usually seen in renal carcinoma. Patho-anatomic diagnosis: angiomyolipoma. a) Arterial phase. b) Nephrographic phase

tients with tuberous sclerosis are said to have renal tumor of this type. The term "disseminated hamartosis" has been used to describe this type of tumor. The other type is the isolated angiomyolipoma which has a tendency to arise multifocally, however, and is occasionally bilateral (BECK and HAMMOND, 1957; TAYLOR and GENTERS, 1958; ALLEN and RISK, 1965) and often calcifies. WEAVER and CARLQUIST (1957) described such a growth in a 12-year-old girl. The tumor was twice as large as the actual kidney and had a circumscribed protuberance growing into the renal pelvis. The tumors sometimes become malignant and then resemble renal carcinoma roentgenologically. In plain roentgenography these lipomatous tumors do not differ from any other expanding process, such as a circumscribed renal carcinoma. Only if the growth is very large and contains calcifications, as in tuberous sclerosis, or if it has a high fat content diminishing the density, can it be diagnosed as a lipoma. Fat is actually in some instance the general and predominant content of the tumor. This may give the tumor a particular appearance in plain films, with low density of the entire tumor because of the distribution of fat throughout the mass (ADELMAN, 1965, KEATS and SECHNIANA, 1968). A case with tuberous sclerosis and multiple hamartomas in the kidneys and in the liver is reported by KAUDE and CHANG (1971).

Mention should be made here of Lindau-von Hippel disease in which, in addition to angiomatous lesions of the cerebellum, cysts may be found in the pancreas, liver, and kid-

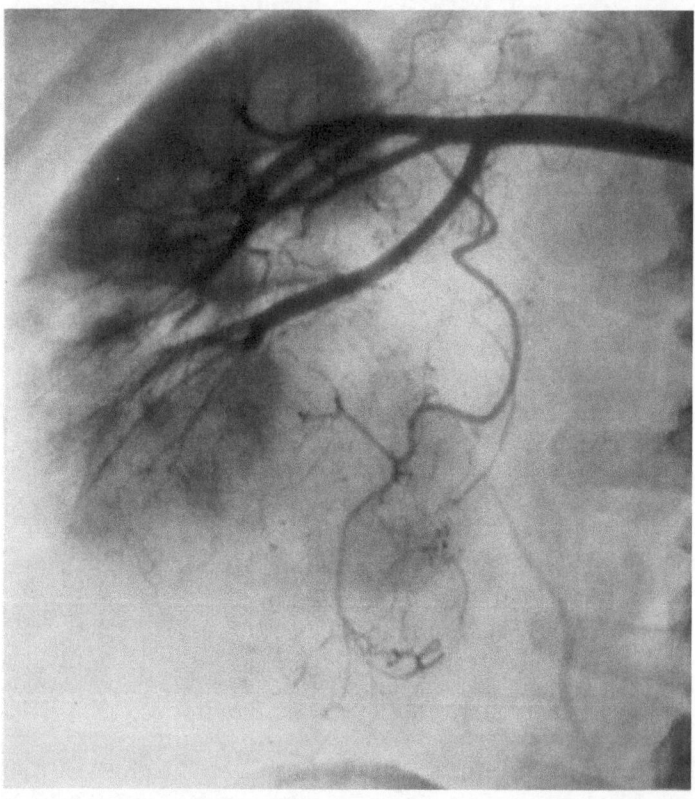

Fig. 158. Huge tumor in right kidney. Angiography: pathologic vasculature is seen, coming mainly from widened pelvic and ureteric arteries. Vascularity differs from that seen in renal carcinoma. Patho-anatomic diagnosis: reticulum cell sarcoma

neys and in which solid tumors, benign or malignant, in the kidneys may occasionally be part of the syndrome (MALEK and GREENE, 1971).

A very rare renal tumor which may assume a considerable size is neurinoma, also known as schwannoma, neurilemmoma or neurofibroma (PHILLIPS and BAUMRUCKER, 1935). Another very rare tumor is osteoma consisting of spongy bone. It resembles a calculus or any type of parenchymal calcification (CALDERÓN et al., 1965).

Hemangiomas are very rare. BELL (1938) reported that he found only one case of hemangioma in a total of 30,000 autopsies. Hemangiomas vary in dimension: they may be very minute or up to more than one dm in diameter. Hemangiomas are usually cavernous but may also be capillary. They are sometimes bilateral and can become malignant. A survey of the cases on record in the literature has been made by WALLACH et al. (1959).

The diagnosis is not specific. A haemangioma may cause a slight displacement of parts of the kidney pelvis, as occurs in any other type of expansive lesion. At angiography the irregular vasculature and early filling of wide, irregular veins are findings characteristic of haemangioma. (See chapter on renal vascular lesions).

Mention can be made here of the extremely rare cholesteatoma in the kidney, usually in a pyonephrotic renal pelvis. The renal parenchyma may also be invaded, however. Cholesteatoma is associated with extensive leukoplakia. It is not a true tumor but part of a chronic pyelonephritis (KARKSKY et al., 1962).

A case of multiple eosinophilic granuloma with a well circumscribed expanding process in one kidney was described by AHLSTRÖM and Welin (1943). The tumor was believed to be a granuloma in the kidney. Verification was not available at the time of publication. Later pathologic examination of the growth in the kidney, however, has shown it to be a simple cyst. There are also pseudotumors of the kidney, for instance bleeding which is occasionally seen secondary to anti-coagulant therapy (SURTOKMIYA and LEDDING, 1967). This is mentioned here because of aspects relating to differential diagnostics.

6. Roentgenologic differential diagnosis in expansive lesions

The correct roentgenological diagnosis of a renal carcinoma is extremely important for a specific reason: good late results of nephrectomy for carcinoma are directly related to the possibility of nephrectomy en bloc. ROBSON (1963) relates the operative prognosis for renal carcinoma to five factors and/or a combination of these: 1) involvement of adjacent structures by direct extension, 2) presence or absence of distant metastases, 3) involvement of regional lymph nodes, 4) gross invasion of the renal vein or its main branches, 5) pathologic grade of the tumor. Rational surgical approach offers a significant improvement in survival rates. This involves removal of the renal tumor en bloc with the lymphatics. WAHLQVIST (1969) stresses this further. He advocates that, in view of the risk of manifest tumor spread, primary operation for renal carcinoma should comprise the kidney with the primary tumor, homolateral suprarenal gland, perirenal fat, retroperitoneal lymph nodes along the aorta and inferior vena cava, as well as along the homolateral common iliac vein and artery.

Operation with removal of the tumor and adjacent tissue en bloc means that the preoperative diagnosis must be clear-cut. Exploration of any kind with dissection for inspection and palpation will diminish the patient's chances of long-time survival.

This need for a correct preoperative diagnosis places a great responsibility upon the roentgenologist. Three main types of examination methods are at his disposal for diagnosis and differential diagnosis: the basic type consisting of plain films of the urinary tract together with urography or pyelography, nephrotomography and renal angiography.

The answer to the question as to how the first method (plain films and urography/pyelography) fills the requirements is as follows: JOHNSON in 1946 reported on our material of roentgen examination in 84 cases of verified renal carcinoma. There were roentgenologically demonstrable remote metastases in 26 cases, definite signs of tumor, for example infiltration by the tumor of the wall of the kidney pelvis, in 28 cases. This means that out of the 84 cases, 54 could be diagnosed definitely as tumor at roentgen examination with urography. Thirty cases could be diagnosed only as expansive lesions and the definite diagnosis of carcinoma was not made until exploratory operation. In an additional 48 cases an expansive lesion was diagnosed which clinically was believed to be a cyst and the patient was not operated upon. A check of 38 of these cases within 10 years after operation revealed that 17 had died, of which six had a definite autopsy diagnosis of renal carcinoma. This demonstrates that urography is by far not sufficient for roentgenologic diagnosis and differential diagnosis of expansive lesions of the kidney.

Expectancy at check examination is an unacceptable method because the signs definitely expected to support the diagnosis of malignancy are at the same time signs of increased tumor spread.

Exploration is not an acceptable method because, as mentioned above, late operative results in renal carcinoma are directly related to the operation method. Nor is exploration acceptable in cases of cyst: KROPP et al. (1967) report on a review of 126 consecutive adult patients subjected to exploration within a ten-year period for presumed renal mass which proved to be cystic. There were two post-operative deaths giving a mortality rate of 1.6 %. Operational complications were present in 38 cases and it was necessary to perform nephrectomy in two cases!

It must be pointed out that in several cases of renal carcinoma the tumor is not large enough to cause changes observable at urography and that anatomic variations in the shape of the pelvis may in some instances lead to a wrong diagnosis or suspicion of expansivity.

Nephrotomography has been used in order to increase the possibilities of roentgen diagnosis and differential diagnosis. Through this procedure malignancy can be demonstrated in many instances. No differential diagnosis will be arrived at in a great many cases, however. WITTEN et al. in 1963 reported the use of nephrotomography in its most important application, which is to distinguish renal cyst from renal neoplasm. The authors make it emphatically clear in their conclusions that surgical exploration is not to be abandoned in questionable cases (" ... indeed, we employed this device in 82 of our 330 cases, including seven in which both nephrotomography and renal exploration revealed normal kidneys.") This is a good illustration of the unreliability of nephrotomography.

The better method is *renal angiography*. This method is available in two variations: aortic renal angiography and selective renal angiography. The results of renal angiography in the diagnosis of renal carcinoma have been reported above. The crucial point in the angiographic diagnosis is the demonstration of tumor vessels. As mentioned above, the renal carcinoma, small or large, usually has an abundance of tumor vessels. In a certain percentage of cases, however, tumor vessels are few or entirely absent. Such a tumor may cause diagnostic difficulties because it may be diagnosed as a cyst, which is, of course, a very serious mis-diagnosis.

In the chapter on angiography in tumor, some statistical hints have been given as to the frequency of low vascularity in the tumor, or the absence of vascularity. The finding for the individual patient, however, is the important thing. In our material of renal carcinoma (FOLIN, 1967) only one patient had no demonstrable tumor vessels at selective renal angiography. Later we have experienced another 3 cases. MEANEY (1969) reports that out of 497 non-selective examinations because of renal masses, 10 cases of malignant tumor were incorrectly diagnosed, eight cases as renal cysts. Our material is represented in the following table (FOLIN, 1967):

Table. 4. *Angiography in renal carcinomas*

	renal carcinoma	129
135	adrenal carcinoma	2
	probable cyst	2*
	no tumor	2**

 * Unsuccessful examination. Therefore immediate puncture: Tumor.
** Tumor 1 cm in diam. in kidneys destroyed by pyelonephritis.

In no case delay in operation because of angiography.

Although through the use of selective renal angiography, in the great majority of cases, diagnosis of an expansive lesion definitely can be made as tumor, it is important that in any case where the slightest doubt is present, puncture should be performed.

In the differential diagnosis between malignant and benign tumor with high vascularity, HÄRTEL et al. (1973) find the positive diagnosis of benignity of a tumor possible: in benign tumors there are no intratumoral shunts and never an invasion of the venous system. In some cases it may be possible to diagnose the tumor as benign and thus indicate resection instead of nephrectomy. OWMAN (1973) refers to previous papers on the possibility of a differential diagnosis between renal carcinoma and angiomyolipoma. On the basis of five own cases with very marked variation in tissue types within the tumor, a real differential diagnosis was not possible on the basis of the angiographic characteristics.

Other expanding processes involving the kidney may be of varying origin. They may be due to changes in the actual kidney or to pararenal or extrarenal processes. Splenomegaly, a conglomerate of lymph nodes, and various types of retroperitoneal tumors and abscess from spondylitis are examples of extrarenal processes capable of simulating a space-occupying process in the kidney. The kidney may be markedly displaced or deformed by such a process. Urography, pyelography and angiography, in a combination chosen according to conditions in a given case, can always solve the problem and decide whether or not such an expanding process is extrarenal.

Processes with a pararenal position may be difficult to distinguish from expanding renal processes. In plain roentgenography and urography, inflammatory pararenal processes may resemble renal tumors. Paranephritis often originates from a renal carbuncle, which is itself a space-occupying intrarenal lesion. Even without such expansiveness paranephritis may be so local as to simulate a space-occupying lesion in the kidney. Pararenal lipomas, solitary or multiple, can as a rule be readily identified. Pararenal sarcoma is often not well outlined against the kidney, but the border of the kidney can be recognized in angiograms since the vessels are of normal appearance within the kidney, which is well defined in the nephrogram, while pathologic vessels are located outside the kidney. Adrenal tumors often stand out distinctly against the kidney, which is often deformed in a characteristic way by such tumors, i.e. with a flattened upper pole in which an impression is occasionally also made by the tumor, which, in addition, displaces the kidney caudally. The outline is occasionally less clear, however. Angiography decides the diagnosis except in a few cases in which the patho-anatomic diagnosis is sometimes also doubtful.

Intrarenal expanding processes may consist of tumors of different types, cysts, partial or total hydronephrosis, or inflammatory changes. All of these possibilities should be borne in mind in the evaluation of the roentgen findings. Experience has shown that this applies, above all, to the differentiation between a tumor and a large hydronephrotic kidney. It also holds if the upper pole of the kidney is enlarged. It may be due to hydronephrosis of one of the renal pelves in a double kidney or to hydrocalicosis. If no excretion is seen during urography, renal angiography will clarify the situation. If one branch of the renal pelvis is occluded and the rest of the pelvis dislocated, the possibility of an inflammatory process, particularly tuberculosis, must be considered. Irregular calcifications in the occluded part seen in plain roentgenograms often suggest the diagnosis.

Thorough differential diagnostic efforts are also called for in certain other lesions. VOEGELI (1971) in a study of our material of renal abscesses points out the difficulty in some cases of excluding the possibility of tumor in the vascular changes in a chronic abscess. This also holds for other chronic inflammatory lesions such as renal tuberculosis.

7. General views on diagnostic difficulties in renal tumor

It is evident from the above that the difficulties in diagnosing renal carcinoma are related to different conditions and are encountered at different levels of the diagnostic procedure.

One difficulty has relation mainly to tumor size. In an autopsy material reported by WEHLIN it was found that renal carcinoma was diagnosed in 350 cases. Cases unknown

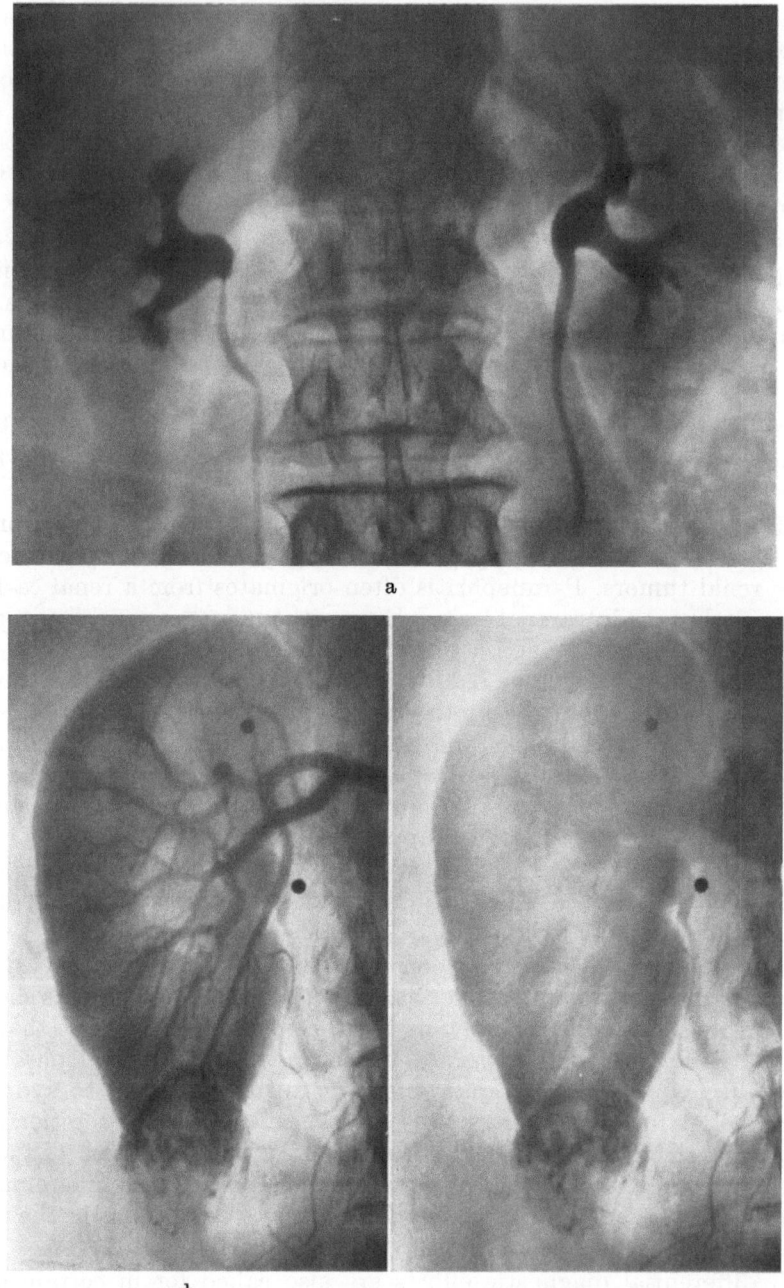

Fig. 159. Renal carcinoma affecting shape of kidney but not shape of kidney pelvis. a) Urography: expansivity in lower pole of right kidney. No displacement whatsoever of corresponding renal pelvis. b) and c) Angiography: well defined, richly vascularized carcinoma in caudal kidney pole

before autopsy were 237. Urography had been performed in 42 of these, with negative results. It would appear that one explanation for this is that not enough attention had been paid to plain films and a study of the renal outline, small bulges having escaped detection (Fig. 159). The more important explanation may be the variations in anatomical shape of the renal pelvis. A small tumor may cause an impression in the renal pelvis that cannot be distinguished from a normal variation of the configuration. Another difficulty is that a normal variation of the anatomy of the kidney pelvis can have the same appearance as a local deformation due to expansive lesion. Renal angiography in such a case is necessary and decisive (Fig. 160).

Through wider use of renal angiography we encounter more and more cases of small renal tumors showing completely normal conditions at plain roentgenography and urography.

Another difficulty faces us on a higher level: an expansive lesion is found but the nature of this lesion is misdiagnosed. The main problem in this connection is centered on angiographic symptomatology and differential diagnosis between tumor and cyst. The literature

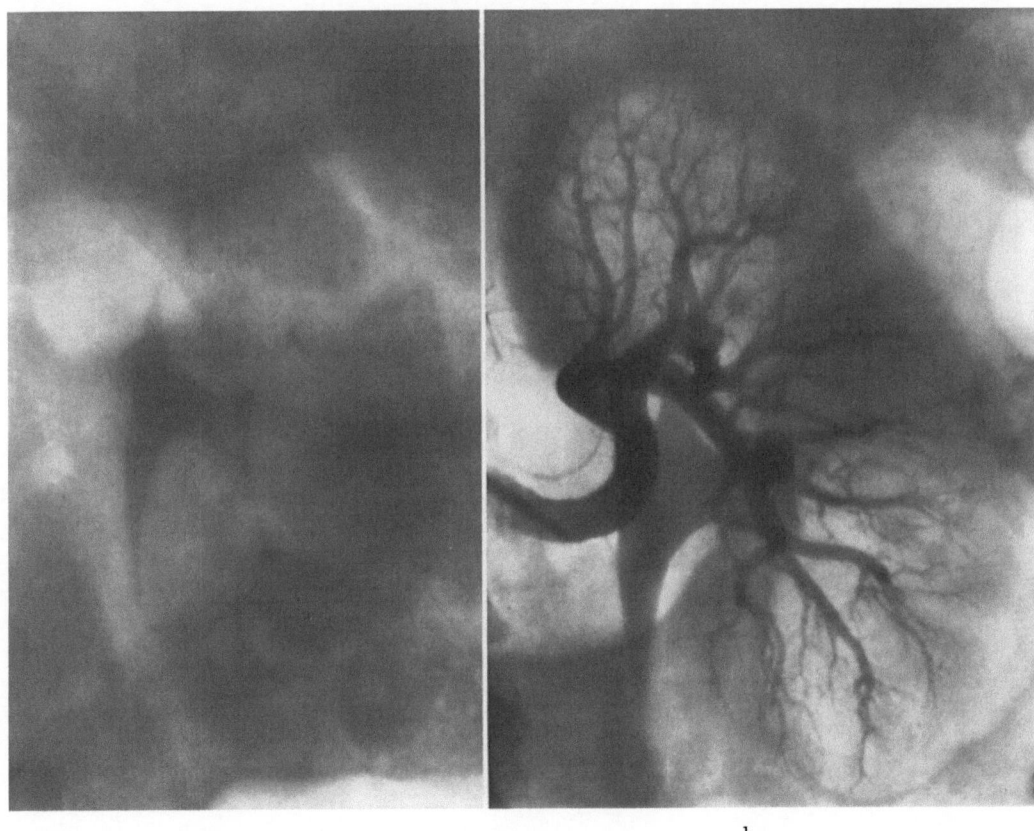

a   b

Fig. 160. Anatomic shape of kidney pelvis mimicking expansivity. a) Urography: middle and caudal calyces look impressed and extended. b) Selective angiography: nothing pathologic

on this problem is abundant and partly — whether opinion is positive or negative—demonstrates incompetence in examination technique and principles.

This is an important problem for competent and critical roentgenologists, however. MEANY (1969), for instance as mentioned above, thus reports four cases of renal carcinoma in which the tumor appeared angiographically to be identical with renal cyst. We have in our department continuously emphasised the necessity of using the best possible technique for the examination, including selective examination, meticulous collimation, the necessary number of films of highest quality in correct angiographic phases, suitable variations in examination technique based on continuous study of the films during the actual examination, and experienced study of the films with attention to every diagnostic detail. Nevertheless, we will occasionally encounter a case where it is impossible definitely to make a differential diagnosis between tumor and cyst. We also advocate the rule of performing percutaneous puncture of every lesion which we diagnose as cyst.

8. Short summary of tumor diagnosis and differential diagnosis

a) *Plain roentgenography*

Tumors and cysts may closely resemble one another in both size and shape. Thus a round, well circumscribed space-occupying process may be due either to a cyst or a pseudo-encapsulated renal carcinoma. If the expanding process is irregular in outline, it argues for carcinoma. However, it should not be forgotten that on occasion cysts can be multiple and lie adjacent to one another and produce a polycystic border.

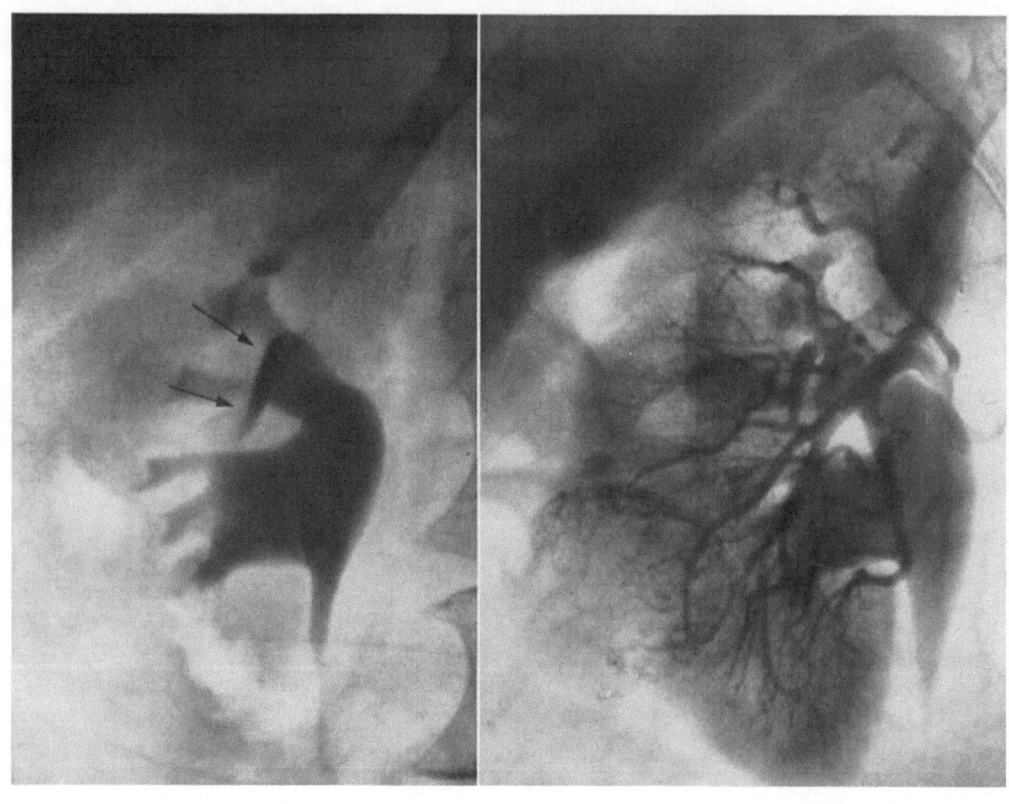

a   b

Fig. 161. Anatomic shape of kidney pelvis suggesting expansivity. a) Urography: one calyx in upper part of kidney (see arrows) looks flattened. b) Angiography: nothing pathologic in region corresponding to the calyx mentioned above but well defined renal carcinoma below middle of kidney. No deformity of kidney pelvis in this region

During expectancy both tumors and cysts may increase in size. If the outline becomes irregular during such expectancy, a tumor may be assumed. Unlike a tumor, a cyst may decrease in size or disappear entirely.

Peripheral calcifications may be seen in cysts and in tumors. Central calcifications which, of course, cannot occur in a cyst, are not uncommon in tumors. Occasionally the tumor may show characteristic calcifications in the form of a calcium skeleton pathognomonic of tumor.

On examination of plain roentgenograms of the kidneys, attention must also be paid to the skeletal parts included in the films. If bone destruction is demonstrable, the space-occupying lesion in the kidney is a tumor. This also holds for other extra-renal metastases.

b) Pyelography and urography

Most pyelographic changes are common to both tumor and cyst. A tumor can, however, be diagnosed with certainty if it has infiltrated part of the wall of the renal pelvis or if a tumor protuberance has grown into the renal pelvis. A calculus or a blood clot should not, however, be taken for such a protuberance.

A tumor may interfere with the excretion of contrast urine during the examination. If the excretion is normal, it permits no decision as to whether the enlargement of the kidney is due to a tumor or cyst. If excretion is delayed or absent, it suggests a tumor.

c) Puncture

An expanding process can be punctured percutaneously. A cyst contains clear fluid. After aspiration of the fluid contents of the cyst or part of it, contrast medium can be injected and it can then be checked whether the contrast-filled cyst occupies the entire region of the space-occupying process. If the cyst fluid is blood-stained, or if the wall of the cyst is uneven, or if the cyst does not correspond to the entire space-occupying lesion, a tumor must be suspected. On injection of contrast medium into a tumor a filling will be obtained of the interstitial spaces. Such a filling can be so irregular as to permit a diagnosis of tumor, but it may cause diagnostic difficulties if the contrast medium is injected into the normal renal parenchyma outside the wall of a cyst. Puncture is therefore decisive only if it produces positive signs of a cyst. (Cyst fluid should always be sent for patho-anatomic examination for tumor cells as an extra precaution.)

d) Renal angiography

Most tumors show pathologic vessels. The outline of the expanding process is also often irregular. A cyst will produce a region free of contrast medium with a sharp border against normal parenchyma. In the free periphery of the cyst no vessels are seen. If the cyst is surrounded by renal parenchyma, the diagnosis may be difficult and the cyst therefore not easy to distinguish from an avascular tumor. In such cases puncture should be resorted to. The frequency of cases requiring puncture will decrease, however, with improvement of the technique and experience. With reference to the chapter on the technique of renal angiography and to the description of the findings in renal angiography in tumor and in cysts, it must be stressed that the value of angiography depends largely on the technical performance of the examination.

c) Metastases

Sometimes the tumor has metastasized by the time the patient is referred for roentgen examination. As mentioned, those parts of the skeleton included in plain roentgenograms of the urinary tract must receive attention. For the same reason we always examine the chest in patients with a space-occupying lesion in a kidney. Lung metastases confirm the diagnosis of tumor. Because of absence or neglect of symptoms, renal carcinoma has often metastasized by the time the patient is examined.

To summarize, it may thus be stated that the following factors are of the greatest importance in differentiation between malignant tumor and benign cyst:

Irregular outline of the growth argues decidedly for tumor.

Characteristic tumor calcifications may occur.

Infiltration of or growth into the renal pelvis is a sign of tumor.

Encroachment upon the skeleton or metastases is a sign of tumor.

Severly impaired excretion of contrast medium as seen during urography argues for tumor.

14*

Pathologic vessels in renal angiography are pathognomonic of tumor.

Failure of puncture to aspirate fluid suggests tumor.

If these factors — with the reservations given above — are considered in the order given in the various examinations, differentiation between tumor and cyst will nearly always be possible. Establishment of a differential diagnosis should very seldom require surgical exploration.

II. Tumors of the renal pelvis and the ureter
(Figs. 162—175)

In the collection of RICHES et al. of 2,314 tumors of the kidney and ureter, 336 were tumors of the renal pelvis and ureter. Twenty-one were primary tumors of the ureter.

1. Tumors of the renal pelvis

Of the 315 tumors of the renal pelvis, 241 were malignant, the majority transitional cell papillary carcinoma, and less than half as many were squamous cell carcinoma. The youngest patient was 9 years old. Simple papillomas of the renal pelvis were found in 24 cases. Almost one third of the cases of squamous cell carcinoma had renal calculi. This type of tumor is often seen in patients with chronic inflammatory changes and sometimes with co-existent leukoplakia in some parts of the mucosa of the renal pelvis. An important observation of roentgendiagnostic interest is also that the operable cases of transitional cell papillary carcinoma involve the ureter and/or bladder or both in some 50 per cent of all cases. STRICKER (1926 cit. MacLean and Fowler) found that in 47 % of 175 cases of papillomatous neoplasms of the renal pelvis, neoplasms were also present in the ureter and urinary bladder. Simultaneous involvement of the renal pelvis, ureter and urinary bladder is likely to occur and is characteristic of all the papillary tumors. If this type of tumor is suspected, it is necessary to investigate the entire urinary tract. Of 26 cases of primary carcinoma of the ureter, WHITLOCK et al. (1955) found one third of the tumors of the ureter to be situated in the lower third. In half of these cases where the tumor occupied the distal part of the ureter, a portion of the tumor could be seen protruding from the ureteric orifice at the time of cystoscopic examination. Tumors of the bladder were seen in 14 out of 33 cases prior to and after operation for a primary carcinoma of the ureter, and multiple ureteric tumors were seen in 17 cases.

Papillary tumors are often multiple, with several tumors in the renal pelvis, and tumors may also occur in the ureter and/or in the urinary bladder, as mentioned above. Carcinogenic substances excreted by the kidneys can cause tumor growth at various sites, but tumors distally in the urinary tract may also have been implanted there by material shed from growths more proximally located.

In a material of patients with uroepithelial tumors of the kidney pelvis, NILSSON et al. (1971) found tumor in the urinary pathways outside the kidney pelvis in 25 % of the cases, in the ureter on the homolateral side in 10 %, and in the bladder in 23 %. In these cases the bladder tumor was usually localized on the same side as the renal pelvic tumor. In 23 % of the cases a bladder tumor was found after the operation of the kidney pelvic tumor. In two cases the renal pelvic tumor was bilateral.

An increased incidence of epithelial renal pelvic tumors has been found in patients with renal papillary necrosis in connection with abuse of drugs containing phenacitin (HULTENGREN et al., 1965; BENGTSON et al., 1968). In an area of Sweden where workers from a certain factory were known for heavy "analgesic" consumption, ANGERVALL et al. (1969) reported on a series of renal pelvic tumors in 15 patients, 10—12 of whom had been abusers of drugs containing phenacitin and 9 of whom were employed at the above-mentioned factory. Two patients had, in addition, urinary bladder carcinoma. All but two of the patients were males, which fits with the epidemiology of "analgesic" abuse in that particular area (Figs. 167, 168).

TAYLOR (1972) found in a survey that over half of patients with carcinoma in the renal pelvis showed analgesic abuse. Out of 110 patients with analgesic nephropathy 11 had carcinoma of the urinary tract, 7 of the tumors occurring in the renal pelvis, whereas in most series carcinoma of the renal pelvis accounts for 7—8 % of all renal carcinomas. In this series renal pelvic tumors account for 30 % of all primary tumors of the kidney in adults. The analgesic in this material was in most cases mainly phenacitin.

A case of polypoid tumor of the renal pelvis which was found patho-anatomically to represent a leiomyoma is reported by LITZKI et al. (1971). A polypoid tumor can also be a fibroma, in exceptional cases (IMMERGUT and COTTLER, 1951). A peripelvic fibroma is reported by GROSSMAN and KOPILNICK (1971).

Another type of tumor of the renal pelvis should also be mentioned. PLAUT (1929) described a case of stone-producing tumor of the renal pelvis. Since then other cases of this type have been described, f. i. by ARCADI (1956) and BRØNDUM-NIELSEN (1957). These tumors may be benign or malignant. They may be associated with calculi and be difficult to distinguish from stone pyonephrosis.

MACLEAN and FOWLER (1956) described a case of primary liver cancer that had metastasized to the renal pelvis.

Urography and pyelography

With reference to what has been said above, these two types of examination should include the entire ureter and urinary bladder.

Cancer of the renal pelvis may appear roentgenologically as an infiltration of the renal pelvis wall and as a polypoid tumor bulging into the renal pelvis (Fig.162, 163, 164). It may invade the renal parenchyma and will then be difficult or impossible to distinguish roentgenologically from a primary renal carcinoma encroaching upon the renal pelvis. The infiltration into the wall of the renal pelvis results in deformation, with irregular decrease in the lumen and rigid walls. Strictures produced by such infiltration can lead to dilatation of single calyces, groups of calyces, or of the entire renal pelvis, depending on the level of the stricture. One or several calyces may be destroyed. Stenosis of the stem of a calyx or of a branch may resemble that seen in tuberculosis (HEIDENBLUT, 1955).

Certain types of carcinoma of the kidney pelvis may initially or later resemble pyelonephritic changes with or without stone (Fig. 166). Pyelonephritis may also be coexistent with tumor and complicate the roentgen-symptomatology.

Papillomas appear as filling defects in the contrast medium. On observation of such a filling defect, it must first be decided whether the defect is localized to the kidney pelvis and not outside it, simply representing an intestinal gas bubble superimposed upon the renal-pelvis. This can be readily checked by using oblique projections.

Filling defects in the renal pelvis may be due to a wide variety of factors. As mentioned in the section on normal anatomy, vessels and the border of the kidney parenchyma may cause impressions in the outline of the renal pelvis with a filling defect as a result. Such defects are, however, fairly characteristic and are seldom difficult to distinguish from tumors of the renal pelvis. Calculi, blood clots, gas bubbles etc. are all capable of causing filling defects resembling tumors in the renal pelvis. Even if they are of fairly low density calculi can, as a rule, be diagnosed already in plain roentgenograms of good quality, but, as stressed in the section on renal calculi, some stones may be of such a low density as not to show up in plain roentgenograms. Tumors cannot be seen in plain roentgenograms except in very rare cases when a papillomatous tumor of the renal pelvis

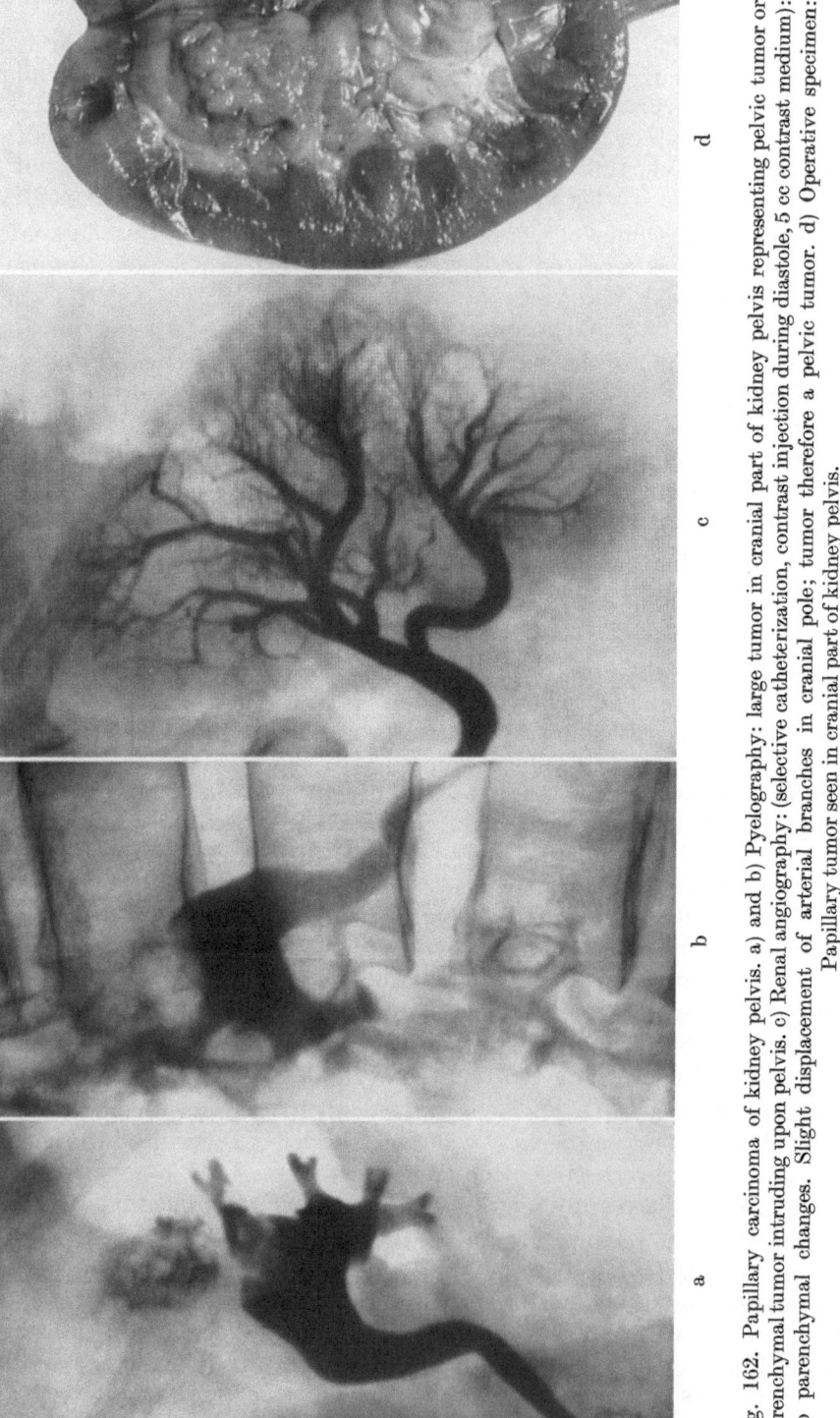

Fig. 162. Papillary carcinoma of kidney pelvis. a) and b) Pyelography: large tumor in cranial part of kidney pelvis representing pelvic tumor or parenchymal tumor intruding upon pelvis. c) Renal angiography: (selective catheterization, contrast injection during diastole, 5 cc contrast medium): No parenchymal changes. Slight displacement of arterial branches in cranial pole; tumor therefore a pelvic tumor. d) Operative specimen: Papillary tumor seen in cranial part of kidney pelvis.

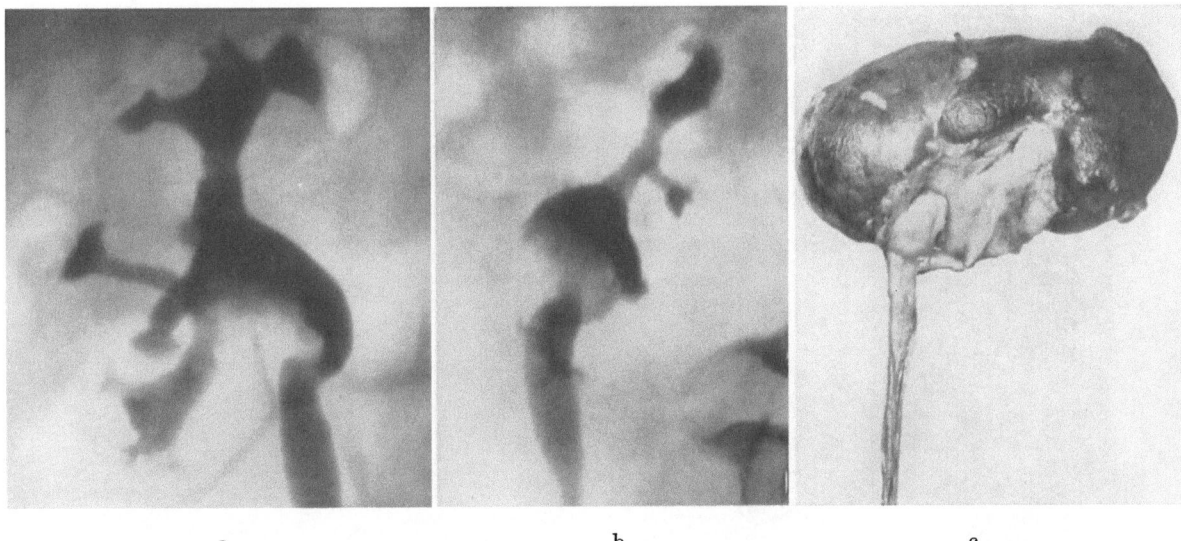

a   b   c

Fig. 163. Malignant papilloma of kidney pelvis. a) and b) Pyelography: Irregular broad-based malignant tumor of kidney pelvis. c) Operative specimen

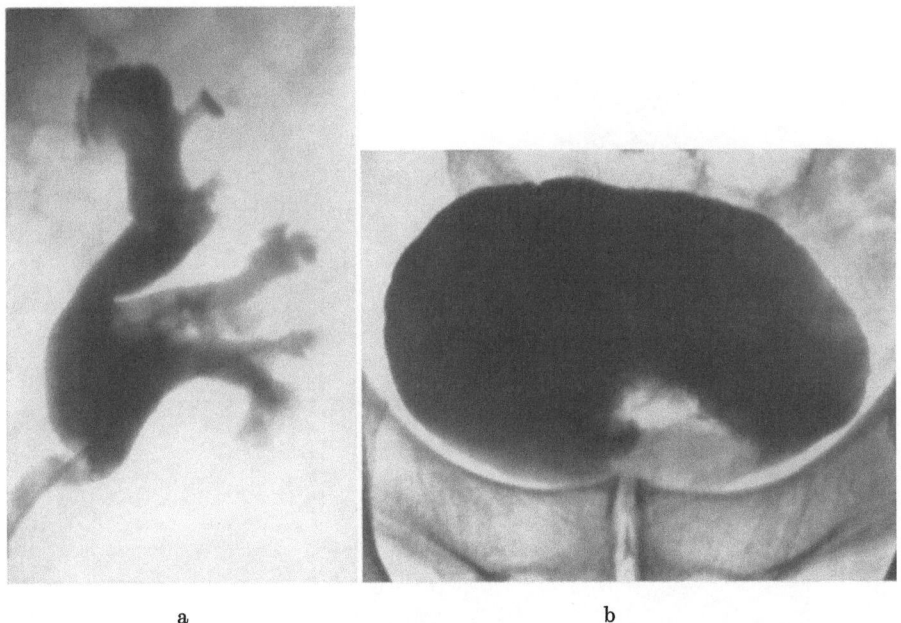

a   b

Fig. 164. Papillary carcinoma of renal pelvis and of bladder. Pyelonephritis. a) Pyelography: irregular tumor with clefts on surface in kidney pelvis laterally at base of middle branch and middle cranial branch. Changes in most papillae characteristic of pyelonephritis with papillary necrosis. b) Cystography: irregular papillary tumor in base of bladder

has collected a layer of calcium on its surface. Calculi tend to assume the shape of the renal pelvis and are surrounded by a thin layer of contrast medium. Since patients with suspected tumors are often referred for roentgen examination because of haematuria, blood clots are of great importance in the differential diagnosis of changes in the renal pelvis, ureter

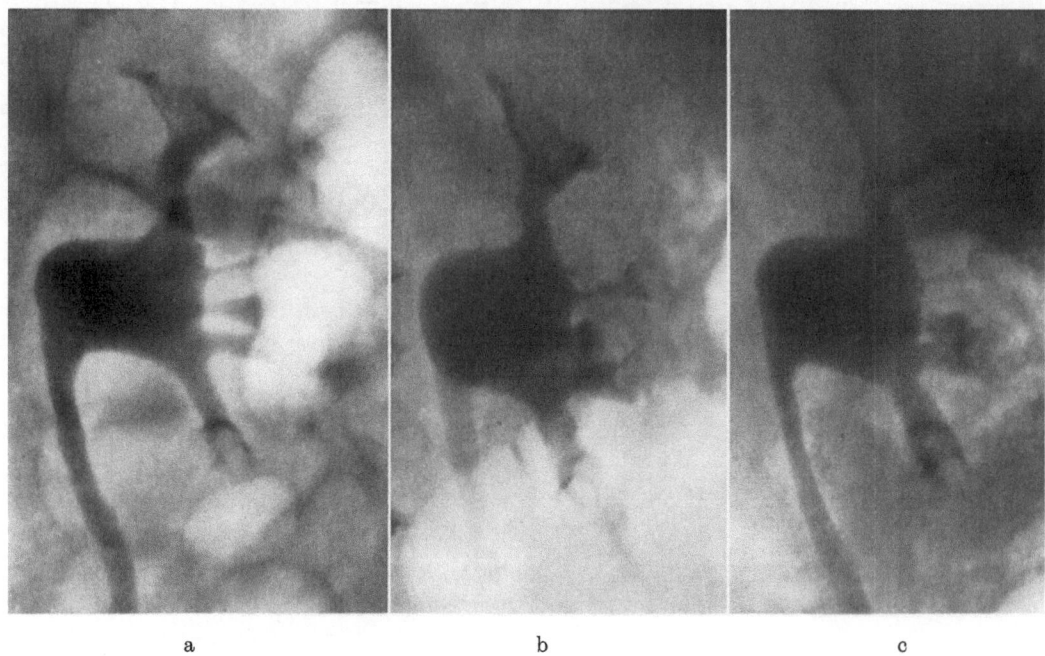

a   b   c

Fig. 165. Small renal pelvic carcinoma in uppermost calyx. Tumor increases in size slowly. One-year interval between examinations a)—b) and b)—c)

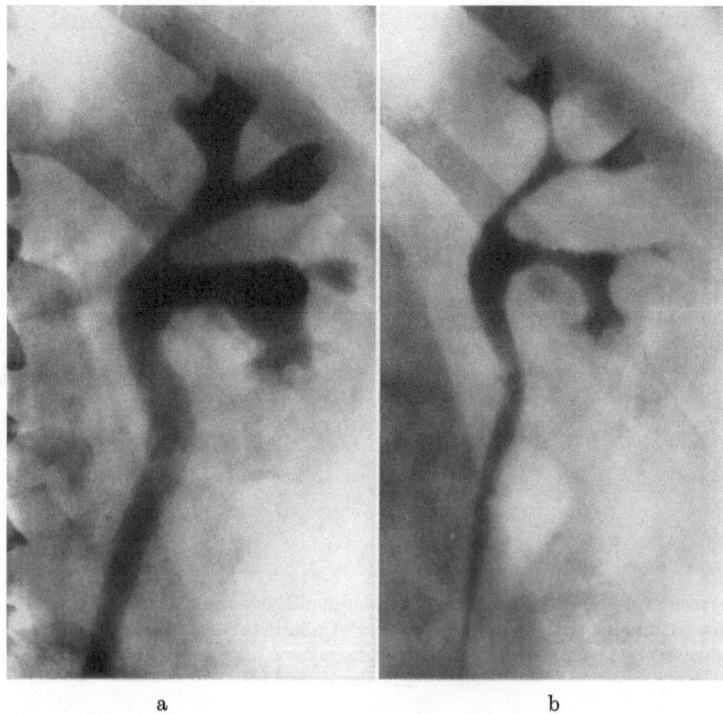

a   b

Fig. 166. Pyelonephritic changes with malignant degeneration. Pyelonephritis for 5 years. Urography: granular to papillary changes in mucosa of kidney pelvis and ureter. Plasticity of wall normal. (Note distention during ureteric compression (a) compared with (b) after removal of compression.) Two years later: pain and hematuria, left side. Nephro-ureterectomy. Histology: chronic pyelonephritis and secondary malignant degeneration in kidney pelvis and ureter. Another two years later: bladder carcinoma

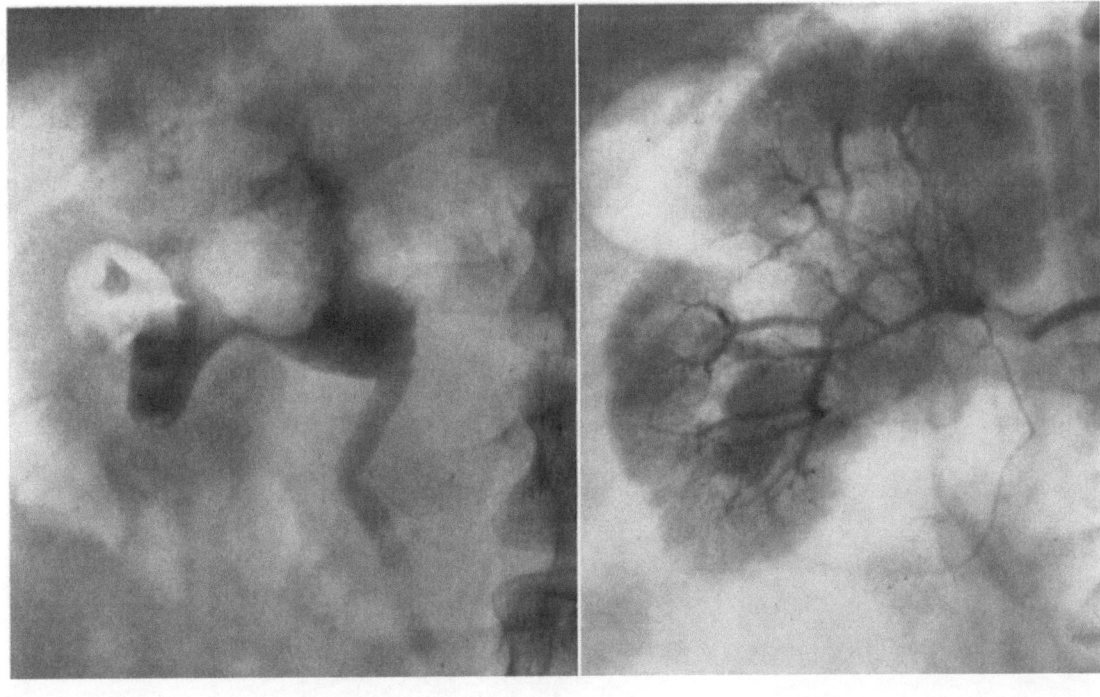

a   b

Fig. 167. Renal pelvic carcinoma. For 20 years, abuse of phenacitin. a) Urography: large tumor filling central part of confluence of kidney pelvis. Infiltration into kidney pelvic wall cranially-medially. b) Angiography: slight pathologic vasculature corresponding to pelvic tumor. Marked pyelonephritic changes in kidney parenchyma.

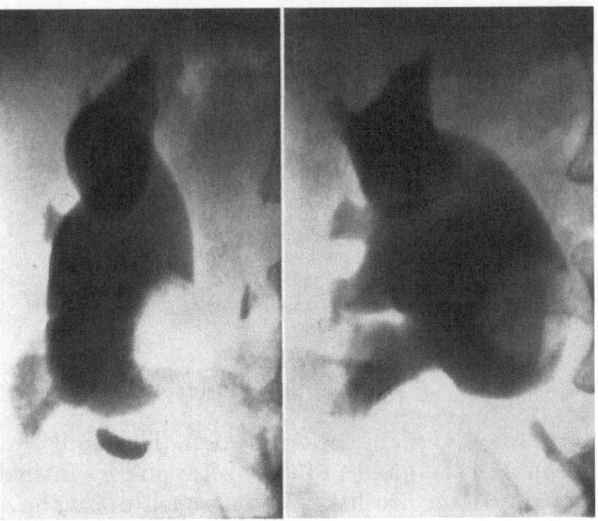

Fig. 168. Tumor of same type as in Fig. 32, anaplastic carcinoma in kidney pelvis in patient with several years abuse of phenacitin

and urinary bladder. Check examinations for any change in the shape or size of the defect may sometimes be necessary before a differential diagnosis is possible.

Renal angiography is not widely used for the diagnosis of tumors of the renal pelvis. According to the literature, these tumors produce no angiographic changes. Truly selective angiography, however, will be useful (although not in all cases) in demonstrating pathologic changes in tumors of the renal pelvis because in selective angiography the arteries to the renal pelvis and to the ureter can be studied (Boijsen, 1959). Renal angiography can thus contribute to the diagnosis and differential diagnosis of tumors of the renal pelvis. Angiography has specific importance in cases with extensive hydronephrosis, in deciding whether or not the hydronephrosis is due to tumor (Fig. 170). If a renal pelvic carcinoma is the cause of the tumor, the hydronephrotic kidney pelvis is filled with tumor mass. These tumors can be diagnosed angiographically by their content of tumor vessels. The characteristic findings are thus a combination of distension and atrophy of arteries typical of hydronephrosis and small conglomerates of tumor vessels related to those atrophic and distended arteries.

In some cases where by ordinary roentgen methods a tumor in the renal pelvis can be demonstrated, it is impossible to decide whether the tumor is primary in the kidney pelvis or whether it represents an invasion into the pelvis of a small renal carcinoma (see Fig. 139). Renal angiography in such cases solves the problem.

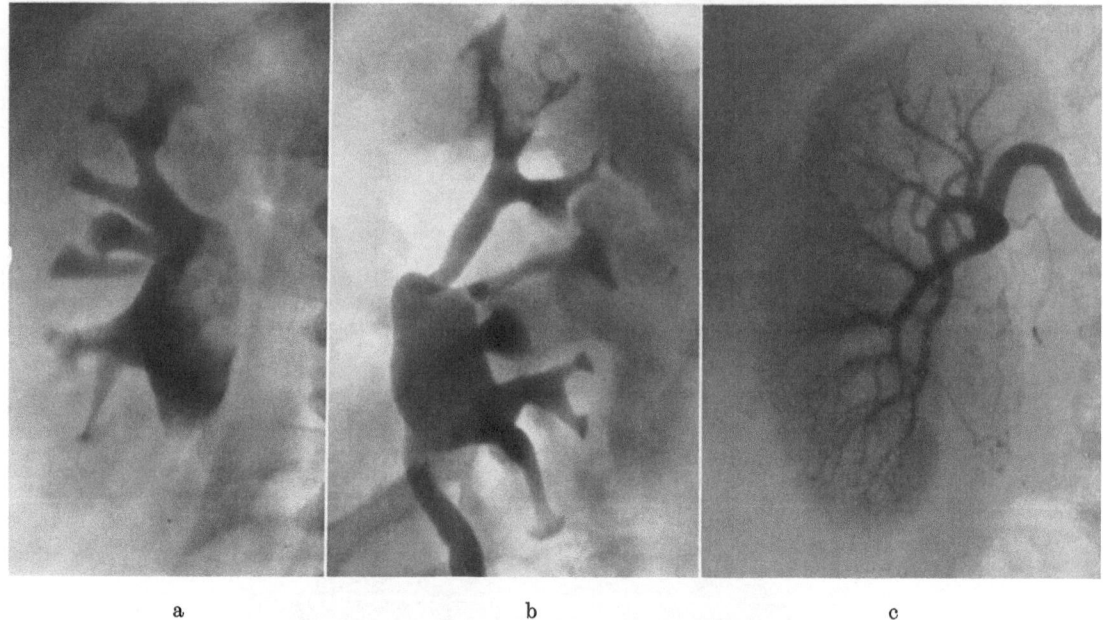

a   b   c

Fig. 169. Bilateral renal pelvic carcinoma. a) Urography, right kidney. b) Urography, left kidney. c) Angiography, right kidney

2. Tumors of the ureter

Tumors of the ureter may be malignant or benign. The malignant tumors may be primary or secondary. Because of the length of the ureter and its intimate relation to several other organs, tumors of the latter are likely to encroach upon the ureter, e.g. tumors of the colon and rectum, uterine and ovarian carcinoma. Metastasizing tumors in the retroperitoneal space also often involve the ureters. This is the case, for example, in metastases from seminoma testis to the retroperitoneal lymph nodes or in lymphogranulomatosis. The enlarged lymph nodes often only displace the ureters and sometimes cause indentations in them and compress them along a varying length. Changes of the same type occur in the same diseases in another long transport channel, namely the inferior caval vein, and can be seen at cavography.

Primary malignant tumors of the ureter are rare. Abeshouse (1956) has collected 454 cases from the literature. The malignant tumors produce an ill-defined narrowing along a

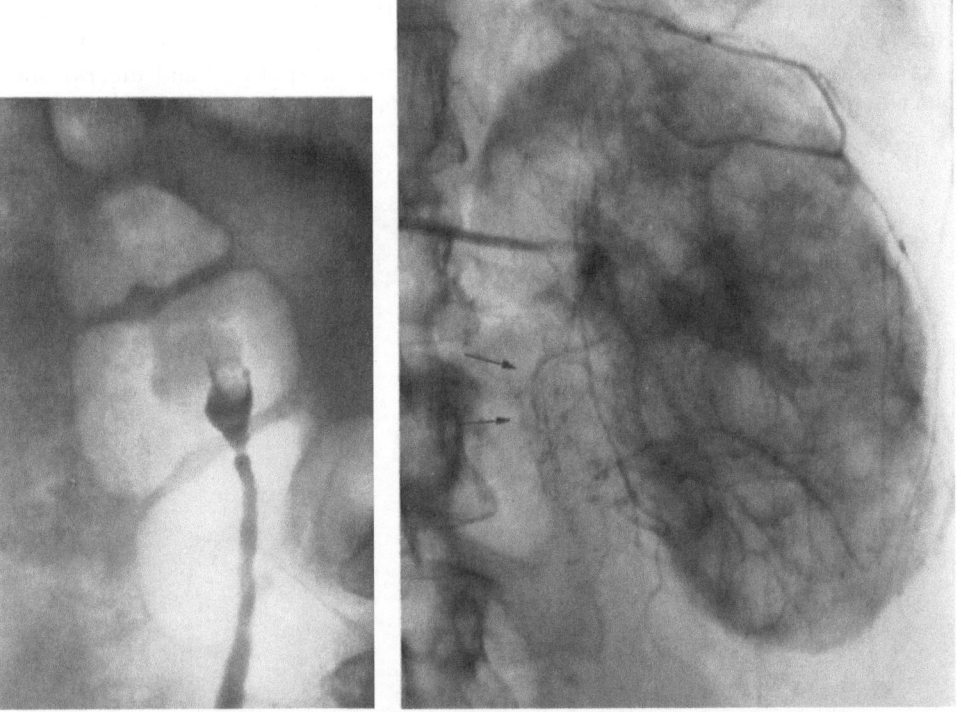

a   b

Fig. 170. Renal pelvic carcinoma with hydronephrosis. a) Pyelography: tumor at pelviureteric junction
b) Angiography: marked thinning and stretching of arteries and veins. Islands of pathologic vasculature. Marked
pathologic vascularity in branches from widened pelvic and ureteric artery (see arrows)

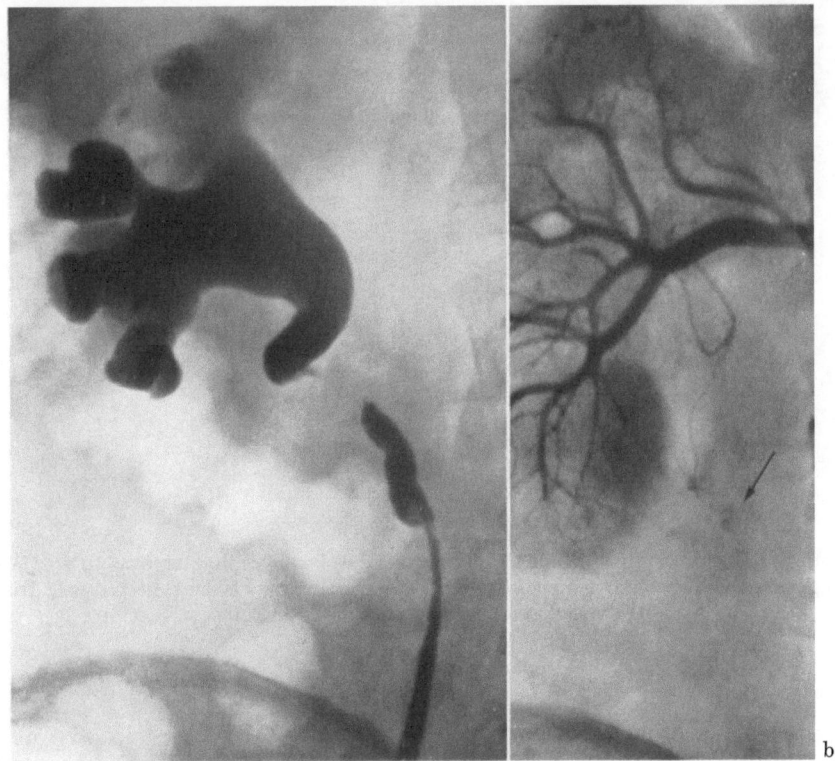

a   b

Fig. 171. Metastasis in wall of cranial part of right ureter by pancreatic carcinoma. a) Pyelography: 2 cm-long,
markedly irregular narrowing. b) Angiography, arterial phase: pathologic vasculature from ureteric artery
in tumor (arrow)

varying length of the ureter, or complete obliteration. The obstruction may be abrupt or gradually increasing along a length of a few centimeters. In the region of the infiltration by the tumor the lumen of the ureter is very irregular and superficial ulcerations can be seen, but the infiltration may also be seen as an increasing stricture. The roentgen-anatomic

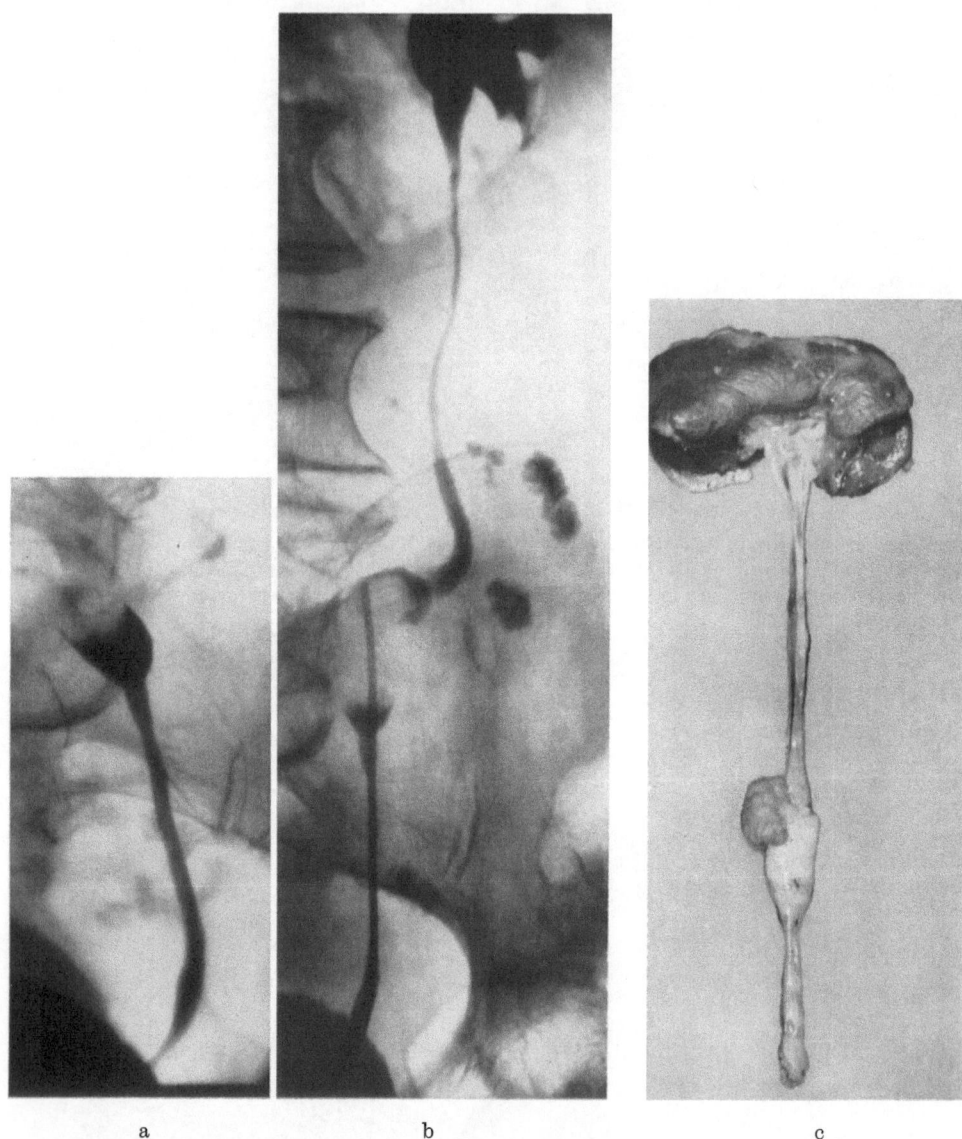

a   b   c

Fig. 172. Ureteric papillomas with incipient malignancy. a) and b) Pyelography: large polyp $3 \times 1^1/_2$ cm distending but not dilating ureter. c) Specimen: Tumor has broad attachment to thickened ureter wall. Histology: cancer ureteris. Papilloma with slightly infiltrative character.

findings in cancer of the ureter are of the same type as those well known in other types of malignant infiltration of other ductal organs (Fig. 174). In malignant papillomas the tumor may have the same appearance as a benign papilloma. A broad base and signs of infiltration must make the examiner suspect malignancy (Fig. 172).

The severity of the dilatation above an obstruction varies from case to case and with the duration and severity of stasis. There may be no dilatation at all, or it may be very slight.

The development of carcinoma of the ureter may be slow. One case described by GLENN (1959) was still of identical roentgen appearance on examination after an interval of eight years.

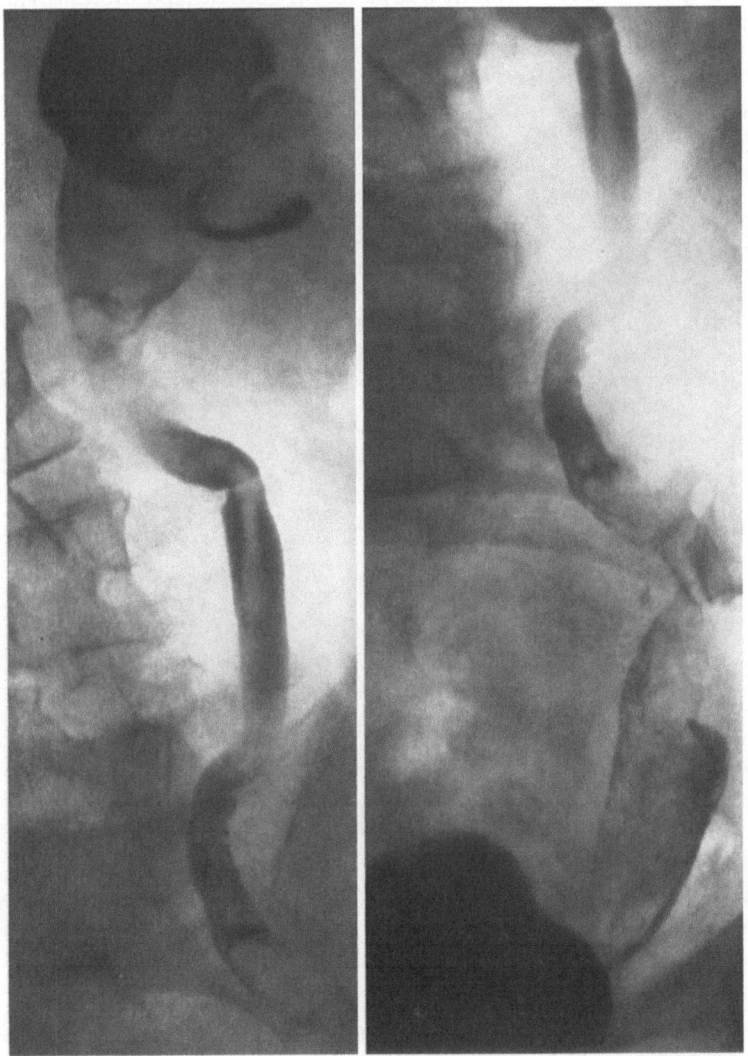

Fig. 173. Tumor at pelviureteric junction. Pyelography: marked distention of kidney pelvis and ureter by coagula from bleeding tumor

In strictures of the ureter the possibility of malignant tumor must be borne in mind.

As a rule, primary malignant tumors of the ureter affect only one of the ureters. Cases of bilateral primary carcinoma of the ureter are on record (RATLIFF et al., 1949, FELBER, 1953, GRACIA and BRADFIELD, 1958, GILLENWATER et al., 1966). Multiple carcinomas of the ureter may also be multiple in one and the same ureter. The multiplicity may also be asynchronous. In suspected retroperitoneal fibrosis with unilateral or bilateral changes, ureteric carcinoma must be one of several differential diagnostic possibilities to consider.

Secondary malignant tumors of the ureter are, as a rule, growths from malignant processes in surrounding organs. As mentioned, this is common in rectal cancer or gynecologic cancer, for example. While, as mentioned, the primary malignant tumor in the ureter is, as a rule, unilateral, secondary growths usually involve both ureters and often at the same level. The other type of secondary malignant tumors of the ureter is malignant metastasis to the ureter, which is rare. One case has been described (Robbins and Lich, 1958) in which carcinoma from the uterine cervix metastasized to the proximal part of the ureter. A renal carcinoma may metastasize to the ureter (see Fig. 150). In all reported cases of this type, ureteral involvement was part of a generalized metastatic process (Gross and Minkowitz, 1971).

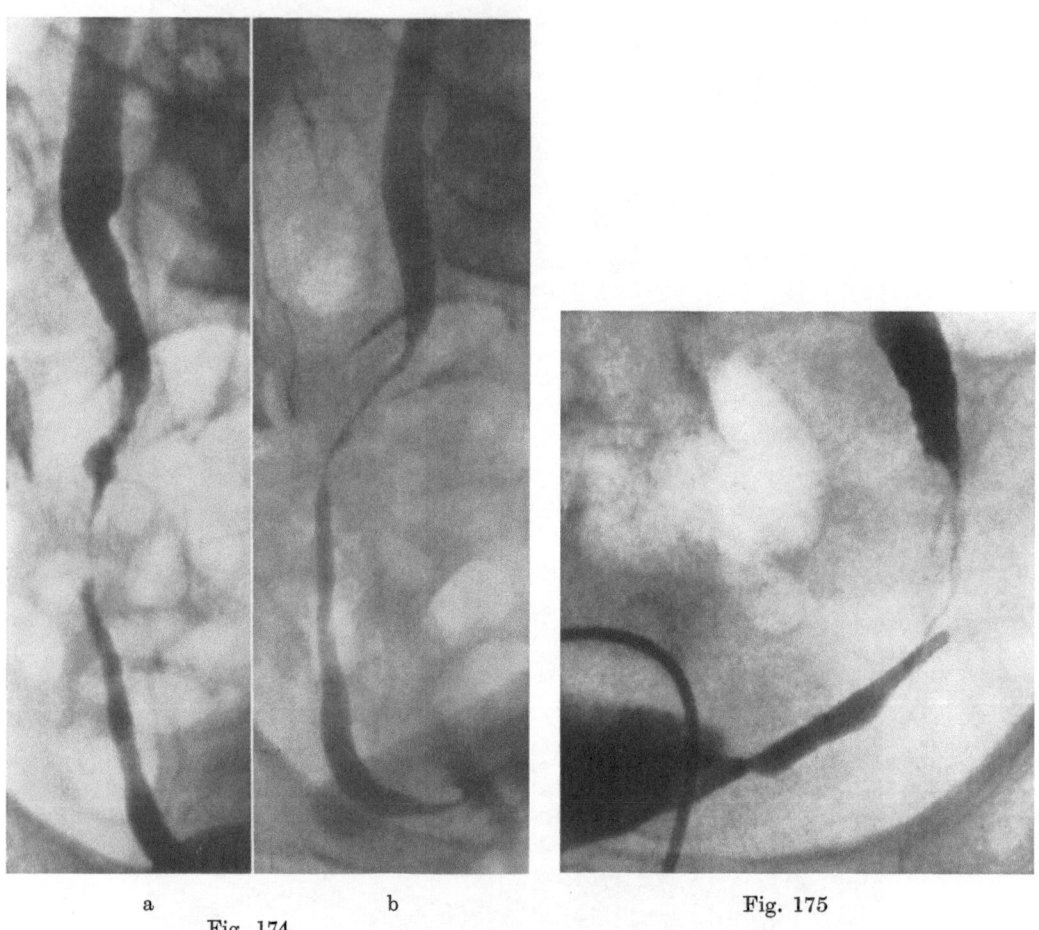

a   b   Fig. 175
          Fig. 174

Fig. 174. Ureteric carcinoma. a) 5 cm-long, irregular infiltration in part of ureter just below ileosacral joint. b) Decrease in changes after radio-therapy

Fig. 175. Ureteric carcinoma. Irregular infiltration in 3 cm-long part of left ureter in small pelvis. Slight dilatation above infiltration

Primary benign tumors of the ureter are still rarer than malignant ones. Abeshouse's above-mentioned collection included 138 primary benign tumors of the ureter. They are of the same type as tumors of the renal pelvis and tumors occuring elsewhere in the urinary tract. Papillomas and polyps are thus the most common. They are round or oval, usually pedunculated, assume the form of the ureter, and are sometimes very long. They may be very small to very large. Howard (1958) thus described a case of a pedunculated ureteric polyp, which measured 10×3 cm and which distended and filled a large part of the ureter but nevertheless permitted good passage of urine and thereby spared renal function which proved to be good, as judged by excretion urography. The renal pelvis was moderately dilated.

It is well known and has been stressed previously that papillomatous tumors have a marked tendency to form multiple and recurrent growths in the entire urinary tract. Papillomas may thus be multiple or solitary. If multiple, they may be seen crowded together at the same level or they may arise at different levels of the ureter.

Roentgenologically, these tumors appear as an obstruction in the ureter. The obstruction is often manifested by a concave outline of the end of the column of contrast medium in contradistinction to the abrupt termination or the tapering of the contrast column in ureteric stricture. The tip of the papilloma may simulate a concrement in the ureterogram. Sometimes the contrast fluid flows around the tumor, whose size and shape can then be assessed (Fig. 172). The ureter may be markedly widened by the tumor *per se;* in other words, the actual tumor mass distends the ureter. A tumor blocking the ureter causes dilatation of the ureter proximal to the tumor, and of the kidney pelvis. On the other hand, large ureteric tumors may sometimes cause only slight or no dilatation of the renal pelvis.

A ureteric tumor can also prolapse out into the bladder if it is pedunculated. A hemangioma of this type measuring 6.5 cm in length was described by BRODNY and HERSHMAN (1954) in a patient in whom at urography ordinary excretion and a filling defect in the distal part of the ureter were found. The hemangioma may cause intussusception of the ureter occasionally (HUNNER, 1938; MORLEY et al., 1952).

Angiography may be useful in exceptional cases in diagnosing a tumor by demonstrating the pathologic vasculature. It should be pointed out here that the arterial supply of the ureter comes from all arteries in the vicinity of the ureter. Thus branches can come from the renal artery, the internal spermatic artery or the ovaric artery, the iliac artery and, in women for instance, from the uterine artery.

G. Renal cysts and polycystic disease

Renal cysts are common and of many patho-anatomic types. They have been classified according to various criteria such as macroscopic characteristics, histologic appearance, clinical significance, site, appearance of fluid content, multiplicity etc. Of the various types of cysts, the pyelogenic and aplastic have been described in the chapter on Anomalies and cystic degeneration of renal carcinoma in the chapter on Tumors. The common small retention cysts situated in the outer part of the cortex are, broadly speaking, of no roentgenologic interest. They may sometimes be demonstrated in the nephrographic phase of renal angiography. In the cerebrohepatorenal syndrome (Zellweger's syndrome) in infants, for example, cortical cysts of the kidneys are always present. This leaves three groups of roentgen-diagnostic importance, namely serous cysts, hydatid cysts, and polycystic disease.

I. Serous cysts

Serous cysts fall essentially into three groups: simple cysts, peripelvic lymphatic cysts, and multilocular cysts.

1. Simple cysts

Simple cysts are usually solitary and unilateral. Multiple cysts of this type can occur in one or both kidneys, however, The name solitary cyst, which is commonly used in the literature, is therefore sometimes misleading. Simple cysts occur at all ages, but they are uncommon in childhood. They are often found incidental to examination of the urinary tract or abdomen for some other reason. In our material a great many cysts have been detected accidentally on routine urography of patients with prostatic hyperplasia. In children, positive palpatory findings often lead to the discovery of such cysts.

A simple cyst may be a so-called capsular cyst and be situated almost entirely extra-renally. It may also be partly or completely embedded in renal parenchyma. It can vary widely in size.

a) Plain radiography

The findings made on plain radiography vary from case to case depending on the size and site of the cyst. If the cyst is situated mainly outside the kidney, it will be seen as a round or oval, usually very well defined smooth formation adjacent to the kidney. If the cyst is partly embedded in renal parenchyma, a bulge will be seen in the outline of the kidney. Sometimes the cyst is embedded in parenchyma near the surface of the kidney, when the bulge may be almost circular. Sometimes the cyst is seated deeper in the paren-chyma and causes only a slight bulge in the outline of the kidney. Exposures should, of course, be taken at different angles in order to secure a projection of the cyst in profile to judge its attachment and size. If the cyst is situated entirely within the kidney, it may cause a generalized enlargement of the latter. A small intrarenal cyst may produce no pathologic changes demonstrable by plain roentgenography.

In the event of multiple cysts, similar changes may be seen in two parts of the kidney. If the cysts are close together, they will cause a coarse lobulation of the outline of the kidney. Sometimes the whole kidney undergoes cystic degeneration and a well defined lobulated mass, often of considerable size, will be seen instead.

It has been claimed that cysts may be detected in plain roentgenograms as an area of less density than the kidney and that this is sufficient to make a diagnosis of cyst. For this to be possible the density of the normal tissue would have to be increased or the con-tents of the cyst would have to consist of fat. But, as a rule, neither of these conditions is satisfied by a simple cyst. Such claims are based mainly on non-roentgenologic reasoning.

Sometimes, though very seldom, a cyst can be diagnosed because its content is fatty. We have seen this type of cyst only once in our large material of simple cysts. It has also been stated that even large cysts sometimes escape detection in plain roentgenograms. This may be true, but is not due to any specific roentgen-diagnostic character of cysts. It can only happen if the patient is not properly prepared or if the examination is not pro-perly performed. Plain radiography has to be performed efficiently, and such an exa-mination must always be carried out preliminary to urography or pyelography.

Sometimes a cyst may be seen to grow during long expectancy. Of 16 patients with cyst re-examined in our material (JOHNSSON, 1946), the cyst was found to increase in size in 6. In one, the cyst attained fairly considerable proportions. In one case the cyst had become smaller. A cyst can also disappear completely by rupturing and emptying into the renal pelvis or the retroperitoneal tissue.

The wall of the cyst may calcify. In such cases more or less opaque calcifications are seen in the periphery of the cyst, occasionally as a ring encircling the entire cyst, though more commonly as small bow-shaped calcifications corresponding to parts of the peri-phery of the cyst. FRIMANN-DAHL (1964) has found that in patients with a complete calcification of the cyst wall, the cyst is often combined with carcinoma. In simple cysts as well as in other types, heterotopic ossification occurs, although rarely.

b) Urography and pyelography

The shape of the renal pelvis varies with the position and size of the cyst. In principle the changes are of the same type as those seen in well defined solitary tumor and described above (Figs. 176, 177, 180).

As mentioned, the deformation will vary to a large extent with the primary anatomic shape of the renal pelvis. It has been stated by BRAASCH and EMMETT that "in most

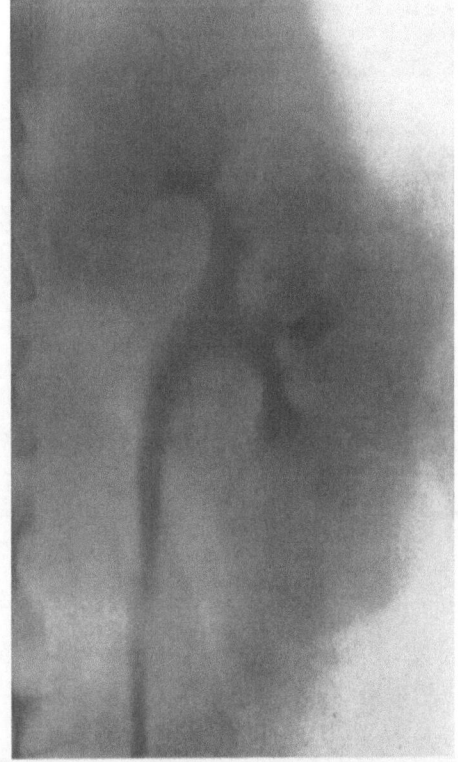

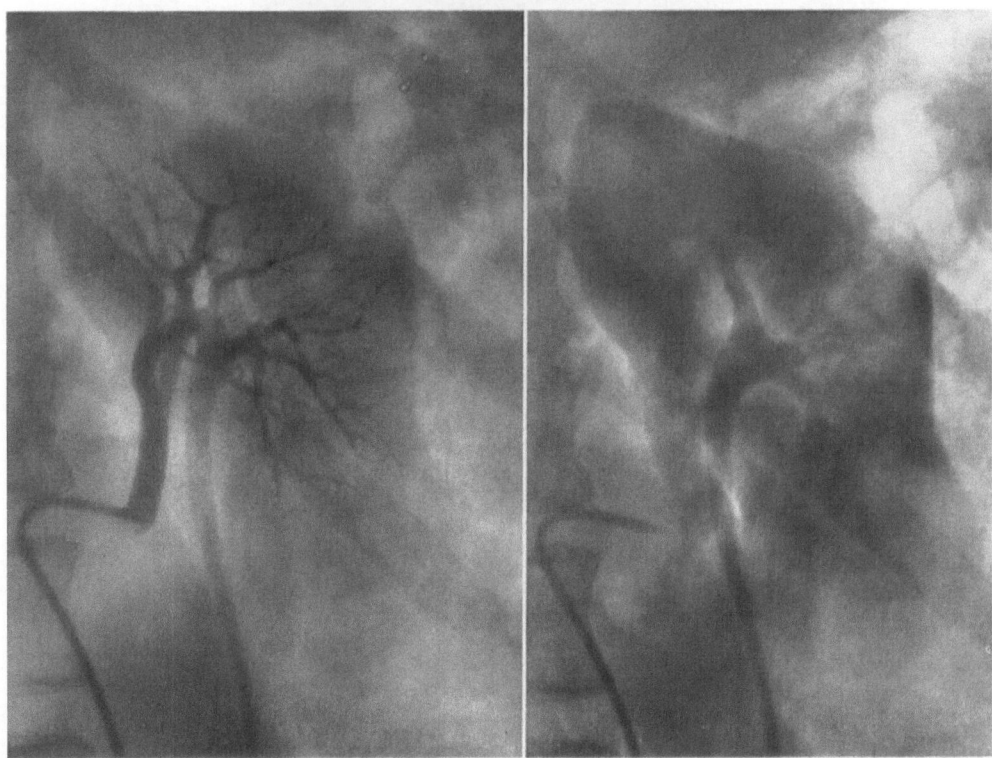

Fig. 176. Cyst. Series demonstrating roentgen-diagnostic procedure in definite diagnosis and treatment of cyst. a) Urography with tomography: well defined, rounded expansivity in caudal kidney pole. b) Angiography: characteristic defect in kidney parenchyma caused by cyst with lipping of border of parenchyma along base of cyst. No pathologic vasculature whatsoever in cyst. Series of films made after injection of angiotensin to definitely exclude presence of pathologic vasculature. c) Puncture of cyst and filling with contrast medium. Different projections to exclude protrusions of tumor tissue into cyst. Cyst size corresponding to size of process seen at angiography. d) Injection of Lipiodol into cyst cavity. e) Check examination one year later: Lipiodol in cavity helps demonstrate cyst, which has diminished considerably in size

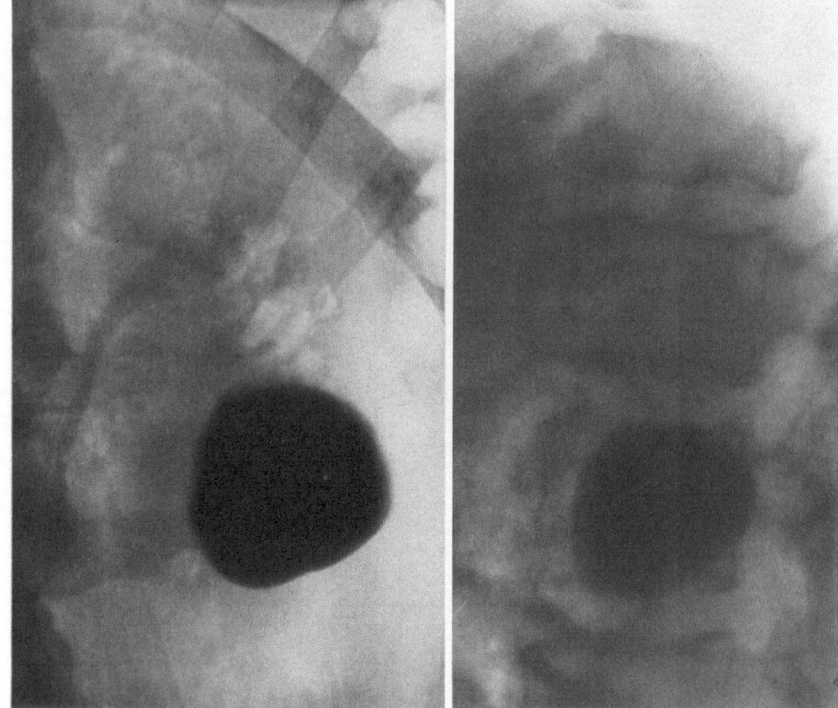

Fig. 176 c

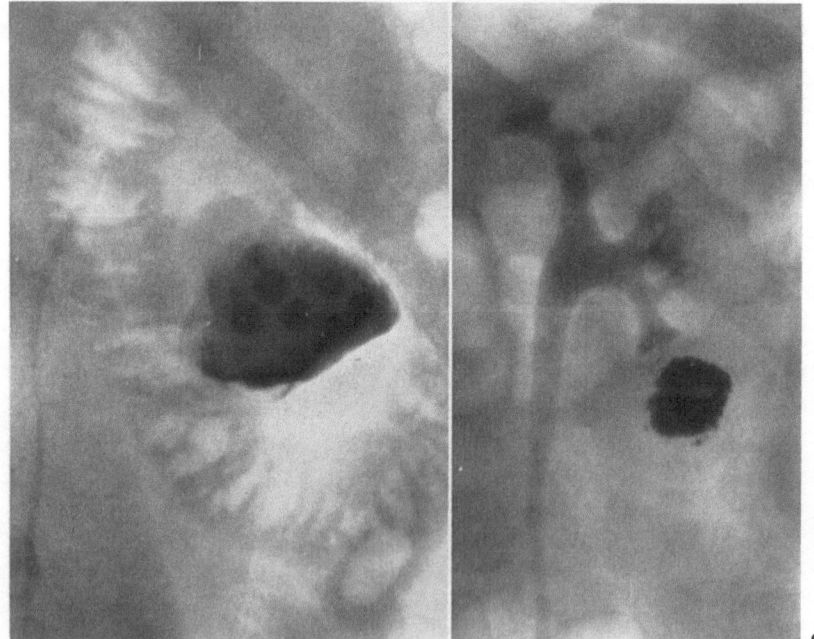

d   e

Fig. 176

cases of cysts the normal terminal irregularities of minor calyces involved will be well
retained". Although I am not quite sure what is to be understood by "normal irregularities" I feel that a cyst and a well defined carcinoma of the same size and position
will produce the same deformation. Under such conditions it is not possible to make a
differential diagnosis on the basis of the findings in the plain roentgenogram, pyelogram
or urogram. A guess is never a diagnosis.

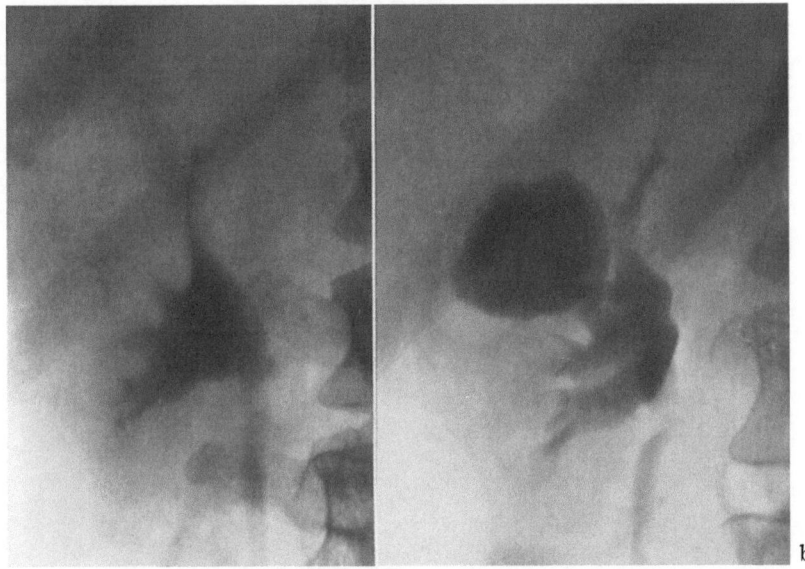

a   b

Fig. 177. Cyst rupturing into kidney pelvis. a) Urography in connection with acute renal colic after pain subsided: slight displacement of cranial part of kidney pelvis. b) Urography a few days later: filling of cyst communicating with kidney pelvis. Cyst walls slightly folded

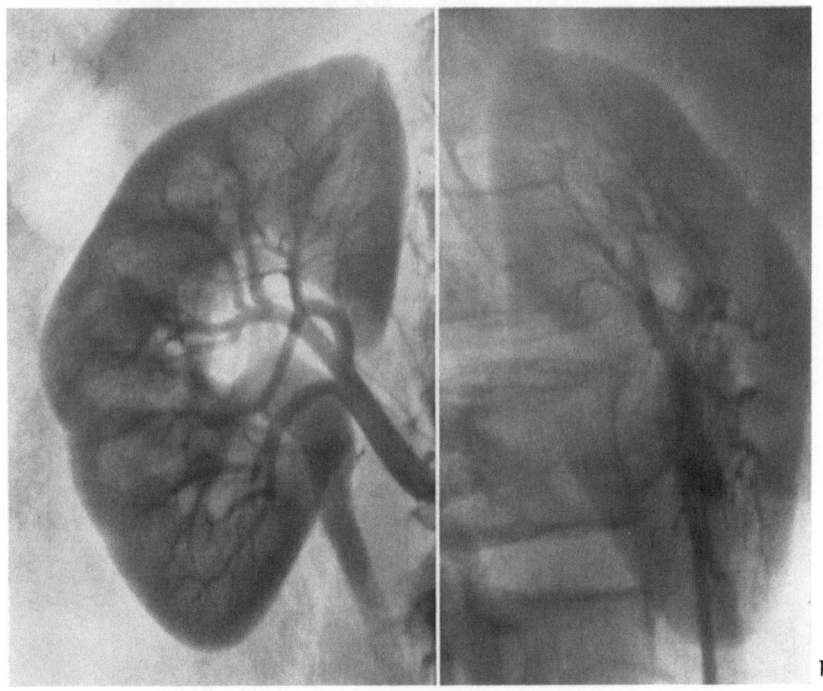

a   b

Fig. 178. Cyst 3 cm in diameter in posterior part of kidney parenchyma. Demonstrable best in b) true lateral projection of kidney

It is often to be read in the literature that cysts do not cause any changes in the shape of the renal pelvis. This is not true. On the contrary, cysts nearly always produce demonstrable changes in the shape of the renal pelvis. The more the cyst is developed in the periphery of the kidney the less it will deform the pelvis, however. Sometimes it will only cause a slight flattening or displacement of a single calyx. This holds especially for the

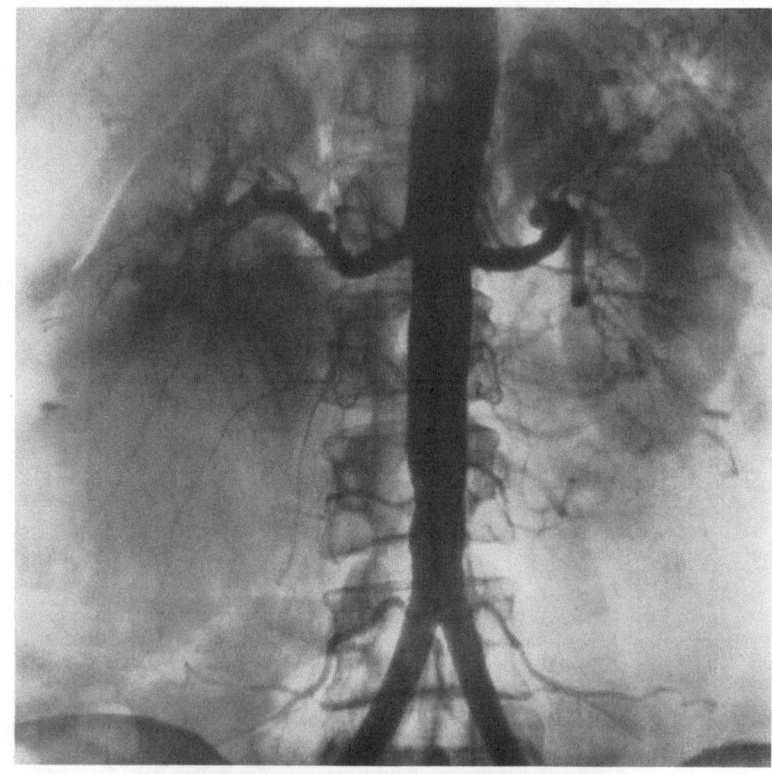

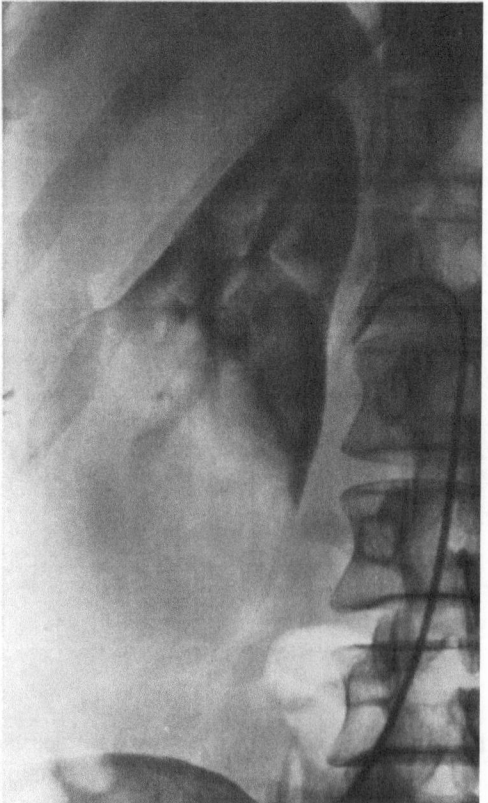

Fig. 179. Large cyst in caudal half of right kidney. a) Aortography: displacement of intrarenal arteries. Note hyperplasia and distention of lumbar arteries. b) Nephrographic phase at selective angiography of right kidney: sharp border of cyst toward kidney parenchyma, marked lipping of border of kidney parenchyma around cyst

above-mentioned encapsulated cysts. A necessary condition for demonstrating changes in the renal pelvis, particularly small changes, is the use of projections capable of demonstrating the changes. Examinations consisting only of standard frontal projections cannot be regarded as satisfactory. The urographic and pyelographic technique should always be adjusted according to the findings at plain roentgenography.

At urography and pyelography it may sometimes be necessary to vary the density of the contrast medium to demonstrate small space-occupying lesions. It should also be observed that dilatation of the renal pelvis by a pathologic process or by the examination procedure may mask a small impression in the renal pelvis.

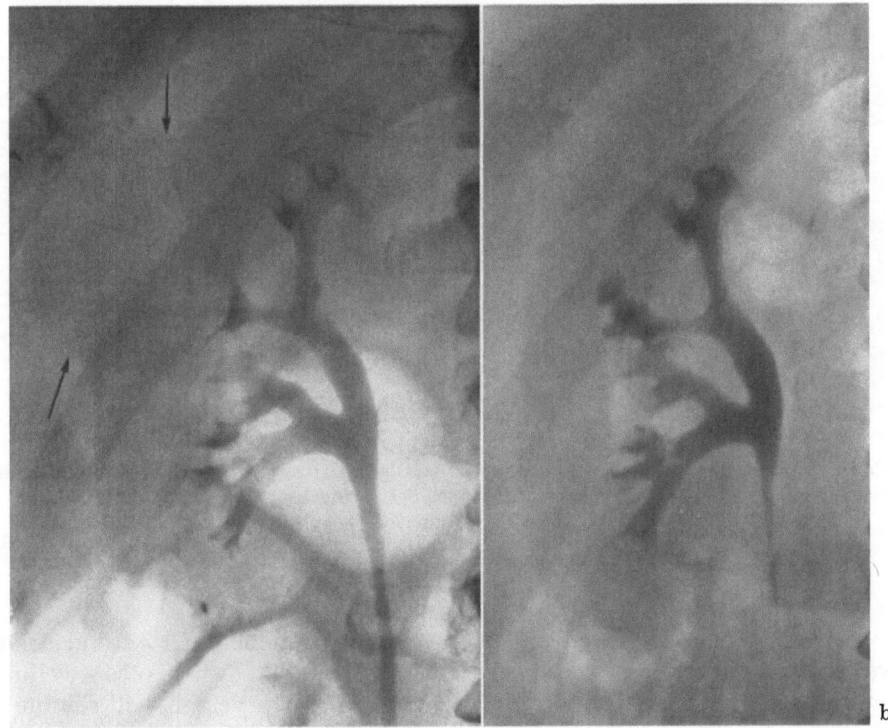

a   b

Fig. 180. Cyst roentgenologically disappearing after puncture and emptying of fluid content. a) Urography, right kidney: Large spheric expansivity at middle of kidney (arrows) without calcification. Flattening of one calyx. Puncture of cyst and emptying of clear fluid. b) Urography one year later: kidney surface and urogram completely normal

Typical of urography is excretion of contrast urine. Only if a major portion of the renal parenchyma has been replaced by cysts will impairment of renal function be demonstrable urographically. Function may then be completely lost. Small cysts and even many large cysts without complicating urinary stasis will, however, produce no demonstrable impairment of excretion. Sometimes the density of the renal parenchyma in the nephrogram will be increased, while the region involved by a cyst will show no such increase in density. This nephrographic effect can be increased by injection of a large amount of contrast medium or by protracted ureteric compression.

At check examination of a patient at intervals of several years, the cyst may be observed to change in size. This may cause a marked change in the pyelogram, particularly if a cyst has collapsed (see Fig. 181).

Such a collapse may be due to a break-through of the cyst wall to the kidney pelvis and attendant drainage. This may lead to a complete disappearance of the cyst or to a more or less marked decrease in the size of the cyst.

At urography and pyelography, filling defects will occasionally be seen in the renal pelvis, caused by stone or blood clots in association with haematuria. It is important not to mistake such filling defects for tumor growing into the renal pelvis, with the erroneous diagnosis of renal carcinoma as a consequence.

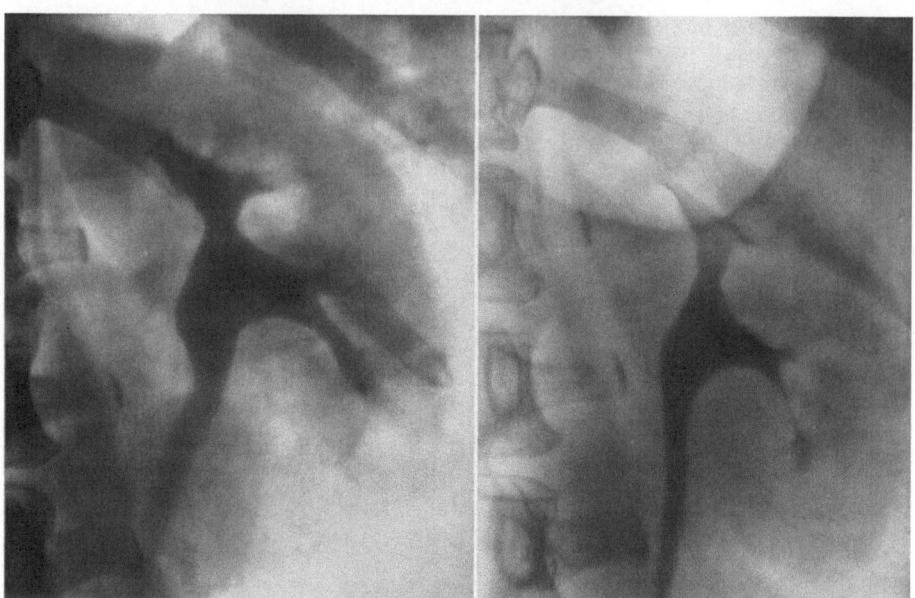

Fig. 181. Probable peripelvic cyst disappearing spontaneously. a) Urography: expanding lesion medially in caudal pole displacing kidney. At renal angiography the space-occupying lesion was thought to be a cyst. b) Check urography two years later: cyst has disappeared

c) Renal angiography

The arteries will be displaced and thin arterial branches will extend around a cyst if the cyst is situated intrarenally. In the venous phase the cyst is often well outlined by fine, stretched veins. If the cyst is mainly extrarenal, such vessels will seldom be seen in the free periphery of the cyst. The most important phase is the nephrographic, which should include a sufficiently large number of films. A cyst appears in the nephrogram as a filling defect. Since part of the cyst bulges outside the kidney, the filling defect will be seen as a pit in the renal parenchyma. This is best demonstrated in profile projections of the filling defect. Characteristic of cysts is that this filling defect is bordered by parenchyma which will be beak-shaped in the different projections. This is because the cyst pushes aside and lifts the edge of the parenchyma. The edge of the defect may be somewhat irregular, but it is always sharp in suitable projections (Figs. 176, 177).

If a cyst is small and surrounded by renal parenchyma it may be difficult to detect. Tomography is helpful in such cases.

It must be noted that a cyst can also receive nutrition through extrarenal arteries, for example lumbar arteries.

In a large cyst branches of lumbar arteries at the level of the cyst may also be displaced and extended.

We have occasionally noticed that widened veins and varices appear in the wall of a cyst in connection with angiography in patients with expansive lesions. This may explain bleeding in connection with cyst causing haematuria.

It is important to perform the examination with the selective technique. Superimposition of vascular branches not belonging to the renal arteries may give the appearance of vascularization. It may also be necessary to use several projections to demonstrate the above-mentioned pitting in the renal parenchyma due to the cyst and to avoid super-imposition of gas bubbles in the gastro-intestinal tract. Tomography is often valuable as a part of the procedure, particularly to demonstrate changes in the nephrographic phase.

d) Puncture of cyst

For diagnostic and therapeutic purposes the cyst may be punctured and its contents aspirated. Contrast medium such as gas (FISH, 1939) or water-soluble contrast medium (JOHNSSON and LINDBLOM, 1946; AINSWORTH and VEST, 1951) may be injected (see Fig. 176). This method has been elaborated in detail by LINDBLOM (1946, 1952) and has been used in a large number of cases.

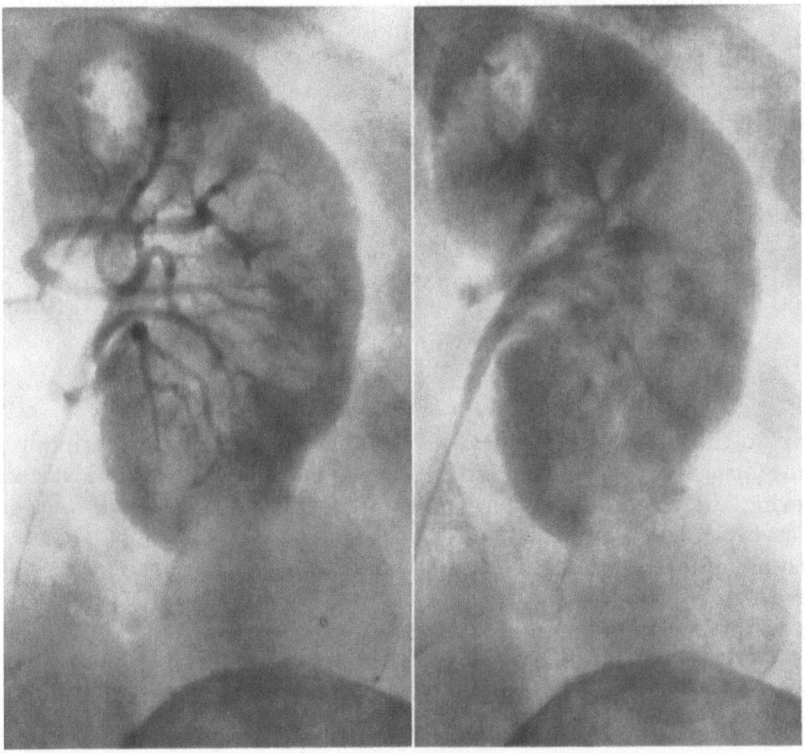

Fig. 182. Cyst with regressive carcinoma. Spheric formation at caudal kidney pole with thin calcification around entire wall. Angiography: a) irregular arteries are seen in caudal pole in arteriographic phase. b) Shallow indentation at site of cystic formation is slightly irregular. No lipping of border of normal kidney parenchyma

With the guidance of urography, which may be performed in association with puncture, the expanding process is punctured percutaneously from behind. A puncture can also be made in direct connection with angiography upon the finding of a cyst or a suspected cyst. The correlation between the cyst and the defect in the nephrogram caused by the cyst is in this situation direct. If fluid is produced, it is aspirated and a small amount of contrast medium is injected. If the cyst is large, contrast medium should be injected before all the cyst content has been aspirated. If too much fluid is aspirated, the cyst will collapse and the needle may slip out and thereby make it impossible to inject contrast medium. The next step is to take films in different projections to ascertain the size of the cavity, its shape and any mural growths. It should be carefully checked that the image of a contrast-filled cavity coincides with the filling defect seen in the nephrogram, since part of a tumor can undergo cystic degeneration, and a kidney may harbor both a tumor and a cyst.

It may be difficult to puncture a very small cyst or a ventrally located cyst percutaneously. Puncture is thus useful as a differential diagnostic measure against tumor only if it proves the existence of a cyst. If puncture yields no cyst fluid, it may mean that the expanding process is a solid tumor, but it can also mean that the cyst is not properly punctured, the puncture having been made into normal renal parenchyma.

Puncture and injection of contrast medium will often show that the cyst has a somewhat irregular outline. It may be more or less distinctly lobated or dumbbell shaped. The wall is quite smooth, however, and the filling complete. Should any mural growth be observed, the lesion cannot be diagnosed as a simple cyst. According to GORDON (1958) all cysts containing blood or heavily blood-stained fluid must be regarded as potentially malignant and accordingly should be surgically explored. As an extra precaution we have the fluid examined histologically for neoplastic cells. FRIMANN-DAHL has proposed the injection of lipiodol into the cyst as an indicator for check examination and to bring about sclerosing of the cyst wall and shrinkage.

A puncture may occasionally cause mild local pain or a sensation of pressure. A slight rise in temperature may also occur. After puncture and emptying of the cyst content the cyst may completely disappear roentgenologically (Fig. 180).

The most important differential diagnosis is renal carcinoma versus simple cyst. This is discussed in a special section of the chapter on renal tumors. Renal abscess, although rare, may also be taken into account. The appearance of such an abscess may simulate that of a simple cyst at plain radiography, urography and pyelography, as well as at renal angiography. Occasionally, however, the vasculature in an old abscess may make it impossible to differentiate it from a tumor (VOEGELI, 1971).

e) Flow studies

According to the literature, surgical procedures on kidneys harboring a cyst are very common. These procedures are often exploratory and as such are in most cases not necessary, considering the availability of refined angiographic technique. Occasionally, when operation is assumed to be clinically indicated, studies on renal flow (GÖTHLIN and OLIN, 1971) seem to have definite value in leading to a decision. In those cases where increased vascular resistance in a kidney harboring a cyst is demonstrable, this resistance can be decreased by emptying or removing the cyst.

2. Peripelvic lymphatic cysts

A special variant of renal cyst is the so-called peripelvic lymphatic cyst. This type of cyst, as indicated by its name, is localized to the sinus and hilum of the kidney and can protrude through the hilum. It varies widely in size from a small cystic process to a large formation prolapsing through the hilum. It consists of one or more thin-walled cystic formations related to the lymphatics and is conceived as a lymphatic retention cyst. DUBLIER and EVANS (1958) described the roentgen findings in this disease as characteristic. In plain roentgenograms, and in urograms or pyelograms, however, the findings cannot always be distinguished from those produced by simple cysts or tumor (Fig. 181). Renal angiography can distinguish them from tumor. In contrast to the simple cyst, the peripelvic cyst does not produce demonstrable changes in the renal parenchyma. Thus, an extrarenal process situated near and deforming the hilum, but producing no angiographic signs of involvement of the renal parenchyma, can be diagnosed as a peripelvic renal cyst.

3. Multilocular cysts

Another variant is the multilocular cyst. It consists of a well defined cyst in a firm capsule occupying a major portion of the kidney. The capsule encloses numerous cystic cavities with a mucin-like fluid. This type of cyst is extremely rare but has been described under the same headings as other unilateral cystic processes. It is important because it occurs in childhood and because it has been confused, clinically and roentgenologically, with Wilms' tumor (FRAZIER, 1951).

II. Hydatid cysts

Hydatid cyst or echinococcus cyst is a parasite cyst of interest mainly in those countries where the parasite is common. With increasing international traffic, however, the disease must be borne in mind in other countries. It has also been called *une maladie cosmopolite*. On the whole, it follows the industry of sheep and cattle-raising. The dog is the host of the tenia echinococcus granulosus, while man and various ruminants are intermediary hosts for the cystic stage of the worm. The infestation is caused by ingestion of the ova. Hydatid cyst is most common in the liver, next in the lungs, but it may also occur elsewhere in the body (slightly more than 2 % are supposed to be found in the kidneys). It is usually solitary, The hydatid cyst consists of a cystic sac surrounded by a fibrous capsule formed as a reaction of the host. The cyst is usually round but may be irregular in shape. It can grow but can also shrink or rupture and empty itself. Infection of the cyst is not uncommon. The connection between the actual parasite and the surrounding fibrous capsule may be more or less firm. The capsule often calcifies.

At plain radiography the findings are the same as in simple cysts. Capsular calcifications are common; they are seen in approximately 60% of the cases and are irregular and fragmentary but arranged in the form of a spheric shell.

The urographic and pyelographic findings are the same as those produced by simple cyst or by a well defined solid tumor. If the fibrous capsule is not intact, contrast medium can escape between it and the parasite cyst. Reproductions presented to illustrate this, however, usually show only a strongly distended calyx whose fading edge has been erroneously regarded as representing contrast medium inside the fibrous capsule. If the cyst perforates into the renal pelvis, contrast medium may enter the actual cyst.

If the calcifications are characteristic, the diagnosis is easy. Otherwise differentiation must be made from the same conditions as occur with simple cysts. Clinical serologic findings typical of hydatid cysts can decide the differential diagnosis, of course. In cases where hydatid cyst is suspected, cyst puncture should not be performed because of the risk of spreading.

III. Polycystic disease

Polycystic disease is a bilateral congenital hereditary disease in which both kidneys may be full of cysts of varying size.

The cystic formation on one side may differ considerably from that on the other. Polycystic disease many undoubtedly also occur on one side only. This is, however, uncommon and naturally seen less frequently post mortem than at roentgen examination, because small changes on one side may escape detection or produce non-characteristic and inconclusive changes.

Double-sidedness is thus not a *conditio sine qua non* of this disease. Congenital or hereditary occurrence is often a significant characteristic. However, IVEMARK and LINDBLOM (1958) distinguish a special type, adult polycystic kidney, which as a rule, occurs later in life, generally in the fourth decade and with renal colic as its first symptom. On the basis of various observations they suggest that the cysts may be intrarenal haematomas due to rupture of aneurysm-like formations, which they claim to have shown both histologically and by micro-angiography. Definite proof of the existence of such a group is, however, not yet available. One might also well imagine that the vascular changes

and hemorrhage are not primary but secondary, that the vascular changes due to polycystic disease in association with hypertension, for example, might cause the bleedings
with consequent changes. Personally, however, I believe that bleeding plays a role in the
symptomatology and that the progress of the disease with increasing size of the cysts is
due to a mechanism resembling that underlying the increase in the size of a subdural
haematoma, namely the breaking down of haemoglobin molecules into several smaller
ones with an increased osmotic effect in the cyst.

The frequency of polycystic disease in autopsy studies is, according to Bell, one in
350 and one in 620, varying in different materials. Campbell reports that approximately
one in 250 individuals is born with polycystic disease. Many cases are not detected until
autopsy. In a series published by Dalgaard, out of 350 patients 134 were not discovered
until autopsy.

There seems to be a certain correlation between polycystic disease and aneurysms
of the cerebral arteries causing subarachnoid bleeding. Thus Ask-Upmark (1948) among
50 patients with subarachnoid bleeding found 5 with polycystic renal disease.

a) *Plain radiography*

Both kidneys are enlarged and their surface is bulgent. Sometimes the enlargement is
enormous and equally severe on both sides. Sometimes it is less marked, and sometimes
the kidney on one side may be much larger than that on the other. The kidneys, or one
kidney, may have a size or shape not different from ordinary conditions.

Calcifications are often seen partly as a thin shell around single cysts and partly as
small irregular calcifications (Fig. 183).

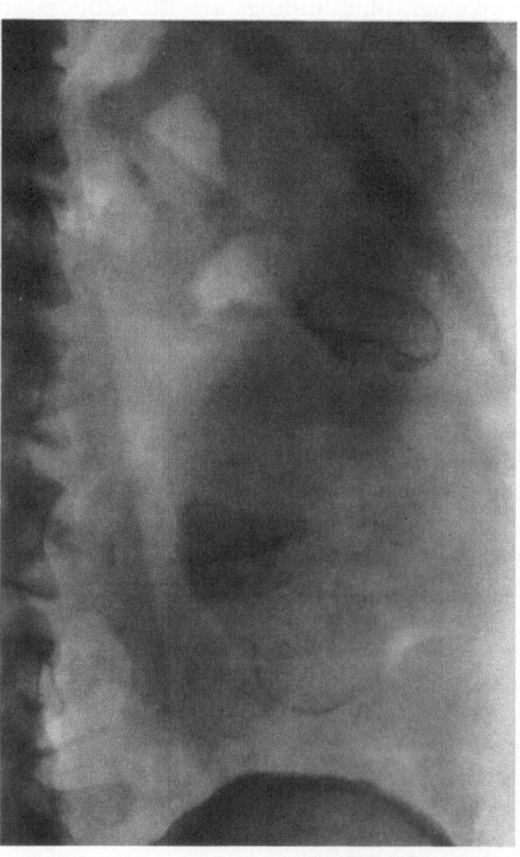

Fig. 183. Polycystic kidney. Very large bulging kidneys. Multiple calcifications in cyst walls, left kidney.
Calcified cysts partly deformed by impression from adjacent non-calcified cysts

b) *Urography and pyelography*

The characteristic changes in the renal pelvis are multifocal bulges (Figs. 184, 185, 186). In severe cases the findings may be completely characteristic with grotesque deformation of the renal pelvis by different sized multiple, space-occupying processes. The stems of the calyces may be markedly elongated or one or more calyces may be flattened. The confluence may be compressed or show small impressions. The changes may, however,

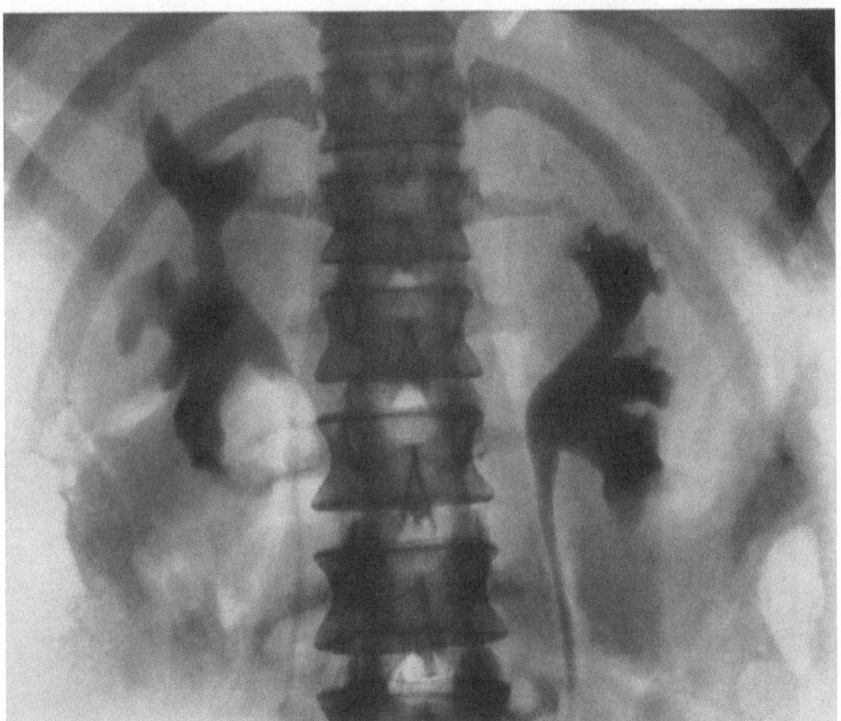

Fig. 184

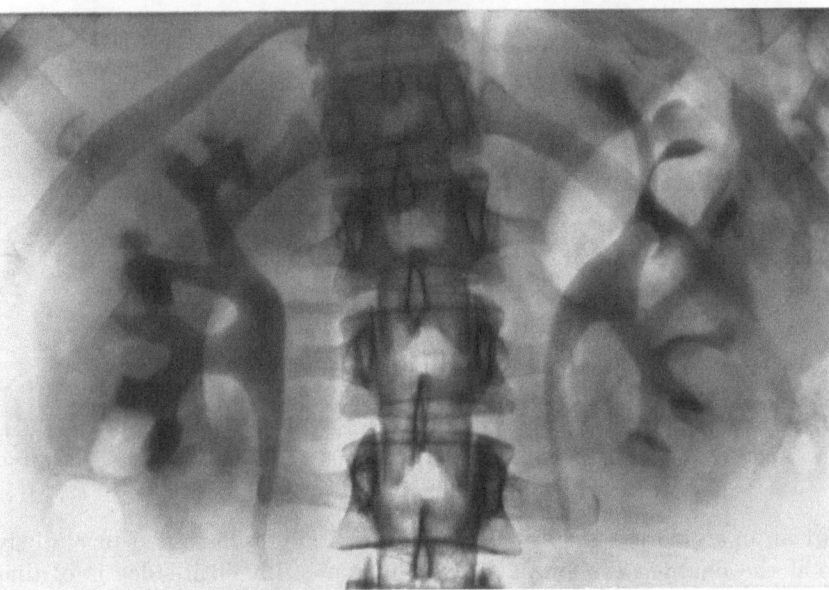

Fig. 185

Fig. 184, 185. Polycystic kidneys. Enlarged kidneys with bulging outline. Urography: good excretion of contrast medium. Marked deformity of both kidney pelves. Increased distance, kidney pelvis to kidney surface

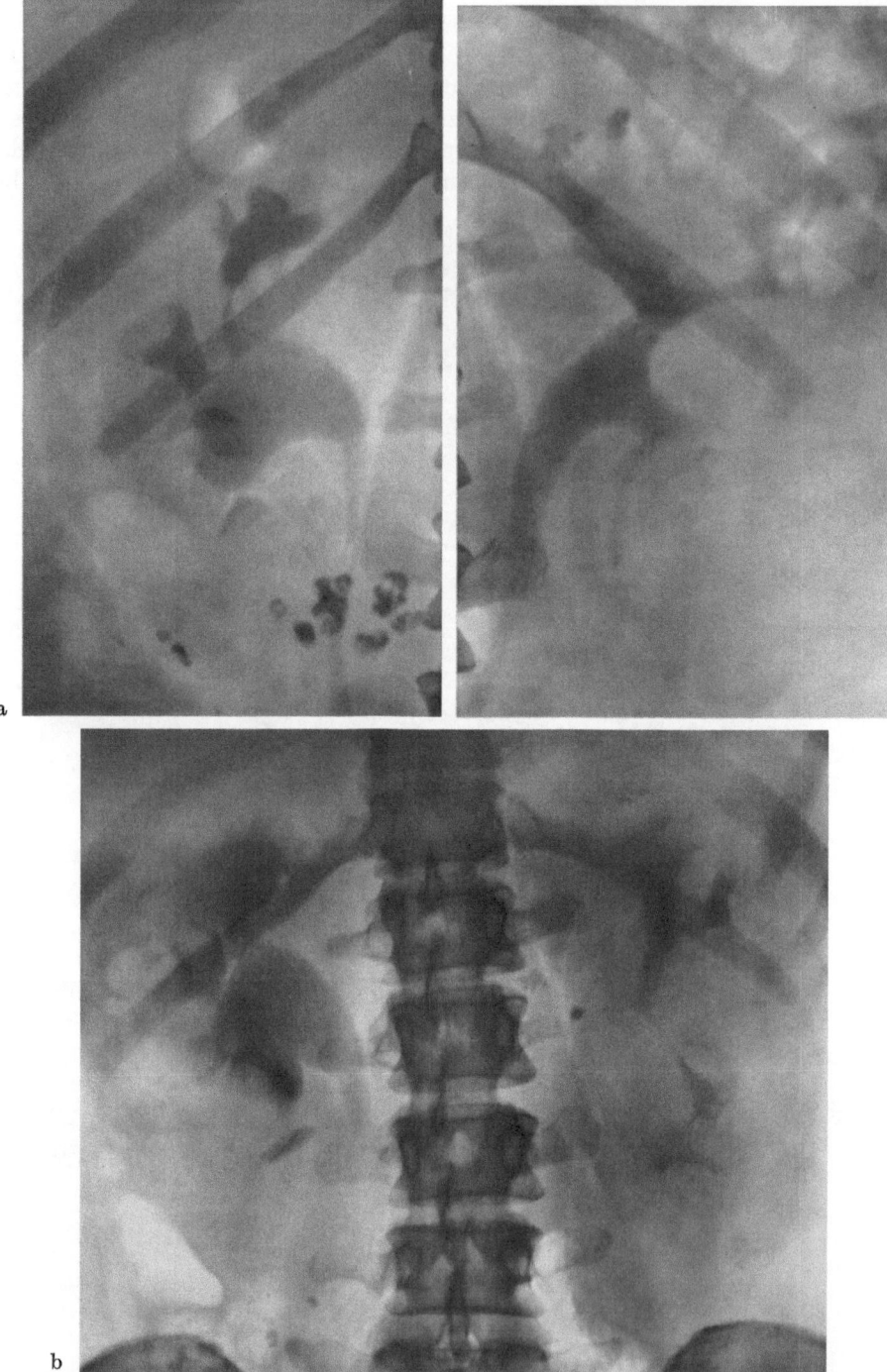

Fig. 186. Polycystic kidneys—progression. Urography: a) moderate bilateral changes. b) Nine years later: advanced changes. Another four years later plain roentgenography because of uremia demonstrated enormous kidney enlargement

be slight and on one side the only change may be a single flattened or slightly elongated calyx. Even if the changes are small, their occurrence on both sides is of diagnostic importance. On cyst formation the distance between the periphery of the kidney and the nearest calyx increases. While the distance seldom exceeds 2—2,7 cm in a normal kidney except in the renal poles, in cystic kidneys it may be more than 3 cm (Billing 1954).

Single cysts may be in open communication with the renal pelvis and be filled in association with urography or pyelography, or they may be perforated by the catheter or they may rupture.

On repeated examination at long intervals cystic kidneys will be seen to increase in size and to change in shape (Fig. 186). The deformation of the renal pelvis also changes on development of new cysts and collapse of others. The change may be considerable, from slight or relatively slight to grotesque deformations.

In urography the contrast density is often reduced because of poor concentrating power of the kidneys. As a rule the density is sufficient for diagnosis, however.

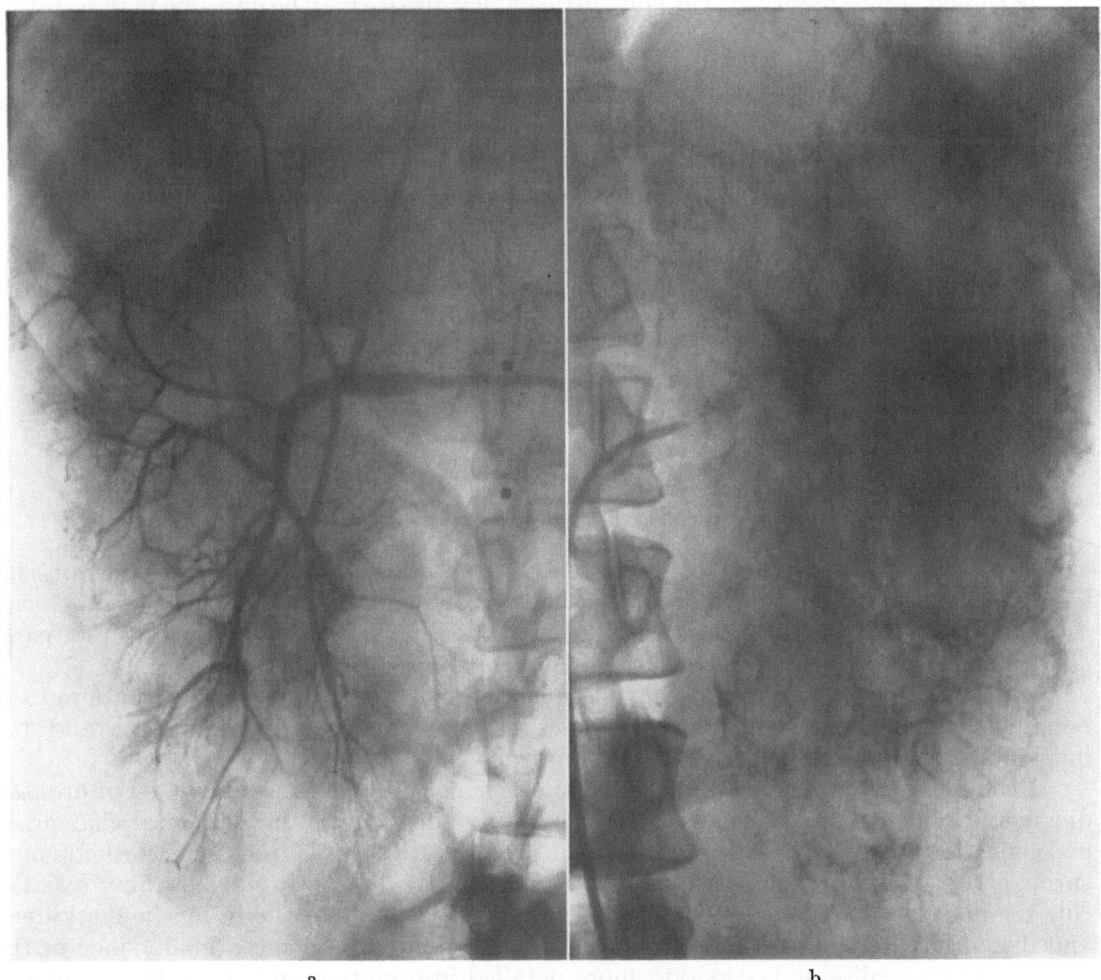

a   b

Fig. 187. Polycystic disease. Angiography: both kidneys very enlarged and irregular. Same findings on both sides. a) Arteriographic phase, right kidney: distention and displacement of intrarenal branches. b) Nephrographic phase in opposite kidney: many large cysts and innumerable small cystic formations

c) *Renal angiography*

In advanced cases the intrarenal arterial branches are distended; sometimes they are markedly stretched and narrow. In the nephrogram filling defects are seen resembling those seen in simple cysts. It is characteristic of the disease, however, that the cysts are multiple and of different sizes. A particularly characteristic, pathognomonic angiogram is seen in patients with numerous small cysts. Then the entire cortex of the kidney shows small filling defects, giving the kidney an irregular, notchy outline in the nephrogram (BILLING, 1954) (Fig. 187).

As a rule, however, the diagnosis can be made without renal angiography. The examination may be of prognostic value in so far as it gives a much better impression of the extent of the cystic process and of the amount of funtioning renal parenchyma than pyelography or urography. Since renal function is often impaired in polycystic disease, the range of indications for renal angiography in this disease should be kept narrow, and when the examination is indicated, it should be performed using the selective technique, and the method used should be such as to require only a small amount of contrast medium.

Sometimes a kidney with polycystic disease may be the seat of a tumor. Cases have been described with bilateral cancer (BORSKI and KLIMBROUGH, 1954; PUIGVERT, 1958).

It should also be observed that polycystic kidney disease may be only one manifestation of several in Lindau's disease. ISAAC et al. (1956) have described such a case with cystic disease of the kidneys and pancreas with renal and cerebellar tumours. RALL and ODEL (1949) pointed out co-existent cystic degeneration of other organs. The liver, the ovaries, the pancreas and the spleen may be the sites of concomitant polycystic disease (WARD et al., 1967). ROLLOF et al. (1971) report the combination of pulmonary cystic adenomatoid malformations and macrobullous polycystic kidneys, which combination they believe to be fortuitous, however.

It should be pointed out that polycythemia or erythrocytosis may be seen in patients with polycystic disease, as in patients with renal carcinoma and simple renal cyst due to increased erythro-poietic activity (MURPHY et al., 1964). Finally, ASK-UPMARK and INGVAR (1950) and others have pointed out that intracranial aneurysms seem to be common in patients with polycystic renal disease.

H. Renal tuberculosis

Renal tuberculosis is part of the primary stage in the cycle of the tuberculous infection. Because of anti-tuberculosis vaccination of children and the increase in socio-hygienic standards, the disease has diminished markedly in many countries. In other parts of the world, however, the disease is still common.

In countries with a low frequency of tuberculosis it is necessary to keep in mind the possibility of this disease in certain types of lesions in the urinary tract and the importance of not letting the disease go undiagnosed as such.

Roentgen examination for renal tuberculosis is not only an important field of urologic diagnostic radiology but also of particular interest in so far as fundamental changes in our concept of this disease and its treatment are reflected by the roentgen methods used through the years in the investigation of the condition. Formerly nephrectomy was the rule for unilateral renal tuberculosis regardless of the extent of the lesion in the kidney and demonstration of the lesion was all that was required. Advances made since in the treatment of the disease necessitate more detailed information and place high demands on diagnostic radiology.

Patho-anatomically the tuberculous infection of the kidney may assume various forms, of which the so-called ulcero-cavernous type is most important from a clinical point of view. One of the purposes of roentgen examination is to detect this ulcero-cavernous tuberculosis and to distinguish it from other types of tuberculous infection of the kidney. Roentgen examination is also important in the assessment of the extent of the process within the kidney and urinary tract and of the effect of conservative treatment.

Ulcero-cavernous renal tuberculosis is also often called surgical renal tuberculosis because in this particular type, nephrectomy was the rational therapy before specific anti-tuberculous chemotherapeutics or tuberculostatis came into use. This disease is characterized by the fact that in the course of their development the lesions are transiently or permanently in open communication with the renal pelvis, where they can deposit infectious material. This explains the clinical picture with so-called aseptic pyuria and bacilluria. This type of tuberculosis is associated with the risk of canalicular infection of the entire urinary tract and — in males — of the genital organs.

I. Remarks on pathology

Ulcero-cavernous renal tuberculosis usually begins as a focus in a papilla. Communication is established between this focus and the renal pelvis either by fistulation of the lesion into the renal pelvis, if the lesion is located deep in the papilla, or by a broad ulceration of the papilla toward the renal pelvis, if the caseation is superficial. The process may in this way involve one or more papillae, often all of the papillae in the kidney. The ulceration can be localized to the tip or side of a papilla or up in the fornix, or it may result in caseation of the major part of a papilla or papillae. The earliest patho-anatomic form of ulcero-cavernous tuberculosis to be met with in roentgen examination is ulceration of a single papilla. In more widespread changes ulceration of several papillae can occur and cavities may be formed in the renal parenchyma. They may be small and solitary or represent complete destruction of the kidney in tuberculous pyonephrosis. Edema and ulceration occur in the mucosa of the renal pelvis, in the ureters and in the mucosa of the urinary bladder.

Regressive changes may occur in the renal parenchyma as well as in the urinary tract. They are manifested by demarcation of necrotic tissue, part of which is often calcified. Fibrous tissue is formed which, as in all forms of tuberculosis, is characterized by a marked tendency to shrink. This gives rise to local scars in the renal parenchyma with local scar formation in the surface of the kidney or contraction of the entire kidney. Regressive changes located in the renal pelvis may lead to occlusion of small or large parts of the kidney pelvis, usually at the level of the originally narrow parts such as the stems of the calyces, the pelvi-ureteric junction, or the ureteric orifice in the urinary bladder, and to local or general shrinkage of the bladder. This shrinkage due to scar formation may thus result in various types of obstruction and in considerable distortion of various parts of the renal pelvis, including dilatation, and of the entire urinary system. The pathologic process may be unilateral or bilateral and the localization and extent may in bilateral cases vary markedly between the two sides.

II. Roentgen examination

The roentgen findings can be readily understood in the light of the gross pathology of ulcero-cavernous renal tuberculosis outlined above. The pathologic changes can be demonstrated by various methods, namely plain roentgenography, pyelography, urography, and angiography. Urethrocystography and occasionally vesiculography may also be important.

1. Plain roentgenography

The size and shape of a kidney can be changed by a tuberculous process. Calcifications can occasionally also be seen in plain roentgenograms. If the kidney is considerably shrunken it may be very small, yet its outline may be more or less regular and fairly sharp. The final stage of such a process is the so-called tuberculous contracted kidney (Fig. 188, 191. See also fig. 196). The shrinkage may also be local and limited to one of the poles, for example, or it may only produce local indentations in the surface of the kidney. On the other hand, the kidney may also be of ordinary size or enlarged, with an irregular bulgent surface due to cavities or calyces dilated as a result of strictures. The change may be local, with formation of one or more adjacent caverns causing a single bulge in the surface of the kidney.

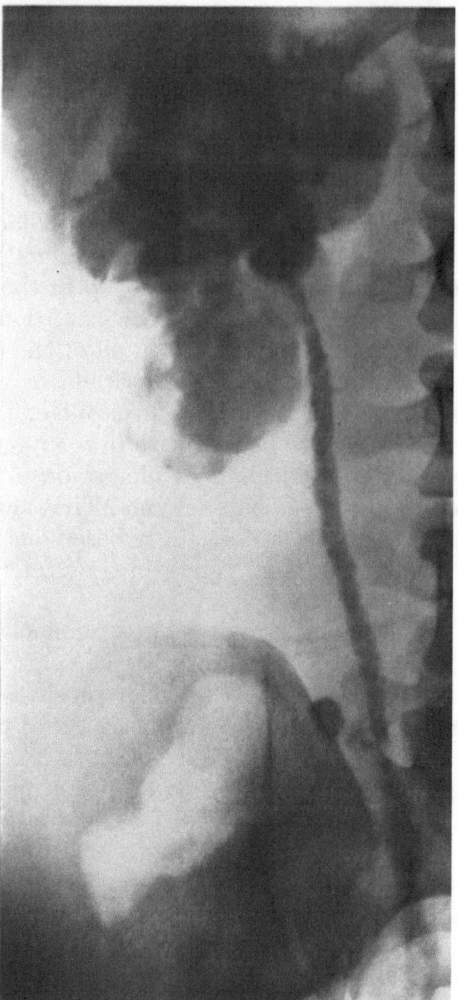

Fig. 188. Complete calcification of tuberculous kidney and ureter

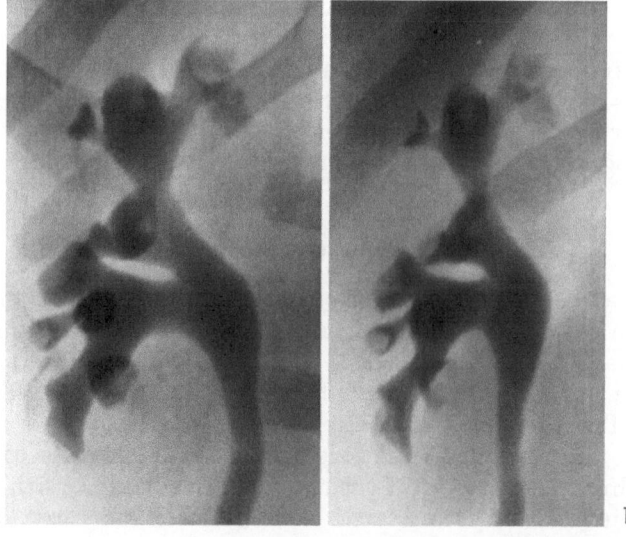

a   b

Fig. 189. Solitary papillary ulceration. Urography: a) small cavity in uppermost medial part of right kidney
and in adjacent papilla. b) Oblique view: lesion located in dorsal part of upper pole

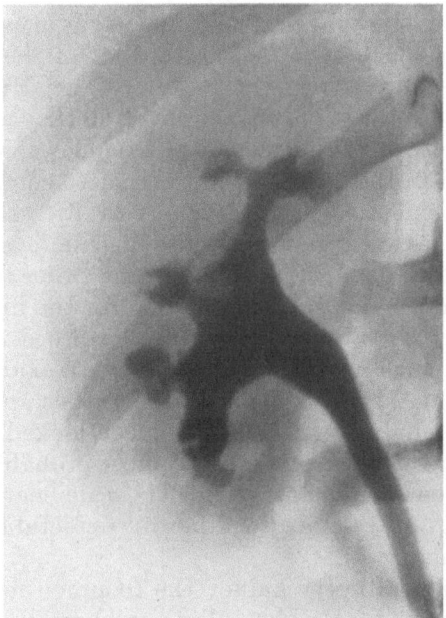

Fig. 190. Solitary papillary ulceration. Urography: small cavity next to lowermost papilla communicating with calyx

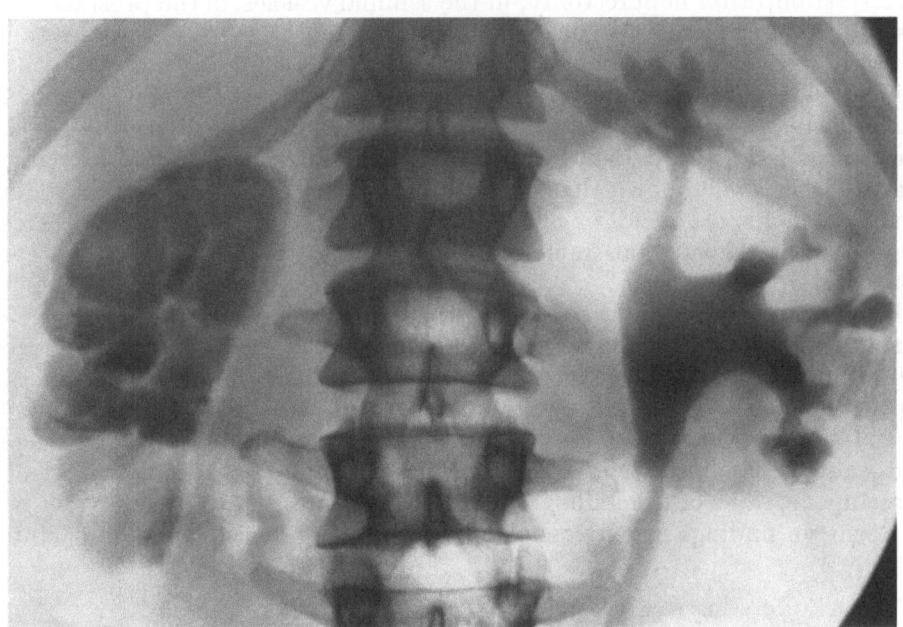

Fig. 191. Bilateral tuberculosis. Urography: calcified tuberculous pyelonephritis on right side. Putty kidney. Small, mainly irregular, cavities in most pyramids of left kidney. Slight irregularity of outline of kidney pelvis due to tuberculous pyelitis

Calcifications are often seen in the parenchyma (see Figs. 188, 191, 194, 210). They may involve the entire kidney and even the ureter and produce the characteristic putty kidney. Sometimes only part of the kidney will assume the appearance of a putty kidney. On auto-amputation of the upper branch of the renal pelvis, for example, the corresponding portion of the kidney may calcify in the same manner as a putty kidney. Irregular calcifications may be widespread. The tuberculous calcifications are usually seen only in small regions however. They may appear as amorphous masses in a well defined area corresponding to a bulge or indentation in the contour of the kidney and then represent calcium deposits in the caseous contents of a cavity. They may also be localized to the wall of a cavity and then give an outline of it. More often they are seen as calcified necrotic areas. The calcifications are usually dense and of irregular shape. They may be small or large and local or scattered in the kidney. They are most commonly unilateral or at any rate much more marked on one side. Tuberculous cavities sometimes contain multiple concrements resembling those seen in so-called pyelogenic cysts.

The frequency given for parenchymal calcifications varies from one author to another. In half of our cases patients coming for examination for the first time had an already old process in spite of the fact that in several cases the process was detected in patients without symptoms of renal tuberculosis in connection with examination for other purposes (Olle Olsson, 1944). In patients with genital tuberculosis and tuberculosis of the bone and joints, a concomitant renal tuberculosis should be looked for. The high incidence of calcifications in comparison with older material is most probably due to advances in technologic background for roentgen examination. The calcifications vary widely in type, form, and density from minute calcifications hardly detectable to massive formations of the type seen in putty kidney.

In putty kidney and partial putty kidney the roentgen findings are pathognomonic. Other types of calcification in renal tuberculosis are usually not diagnostically characteristic and may not differ from parenchymal calcifications of other origin.

Calcifications in tuberculous material are sometimes seen in the ureter, particularly in the ureteric stump after nephrectomy, in the seminal vesicles, in the prostatic gland, and on occasion in the wall of the urinary bladder. They are very rare in tuberculous epididymitis.

Calcification is a late pathologic sign, of course, yet it may be seen in patients with only a short history or no history at all. We have not infrequently seen calcifications as part of advanced lesions in patients who cannot remember ever having had any urinary symptoms. It is also well known that a putty kidney is often an incidental finding in patients who have no history at all or only slight non-characteristic symptoms. This implies that even advanced tuberculous infection of the kidney may sometimes be completely asymptomatic.

In all roentgen examinations for renal tuberculosis due attention should be given to those parts of the skeleton included in plain roentgenograms of the urinary tract. Since renal tuberculosis and skeletal tuberculosis belong to the same phase of infection, they often appear together. Sometimes spondylitis in the lumbar spine with or without abscess can be seen (see Fig. 209). The abscess may displace one or both kidneys. Ileosacral tuberculosis may also be demonstrated. Pleural changes in the base of the thorax are often seen in plain roentgenograms of the kidneys. It is taken for granted that the reader is familiar with the roentgen findings in extrarenal tuberculosis e. g. chest, bone and joints.

2. Urography and pyelography

Ulcero-cavernous renal tuberculosis can be diagnosed by urography or pyelography because of the fact that the foci are in open communication with, or cause changes in, the renal pelvis. This also holds for the earliest form of renal tuberculosis, i. e. ulceration of a single papilla. Contrast urine in the renal pelvis will fill the ulceration. This often has the appearance of a small round or oval cavity with a somewhat irregular outline and in more or less wide communication with the calyx (Figs. 189, 190; see also Fig. 193). The connection may on occasion consist only of a fine duct. A more superficial ulceration of the papilla will be seen only as an irregularity in the outline of one calyx. In more extensive lesions a filling will be obtained of sometimes large cavities of more or less irregular

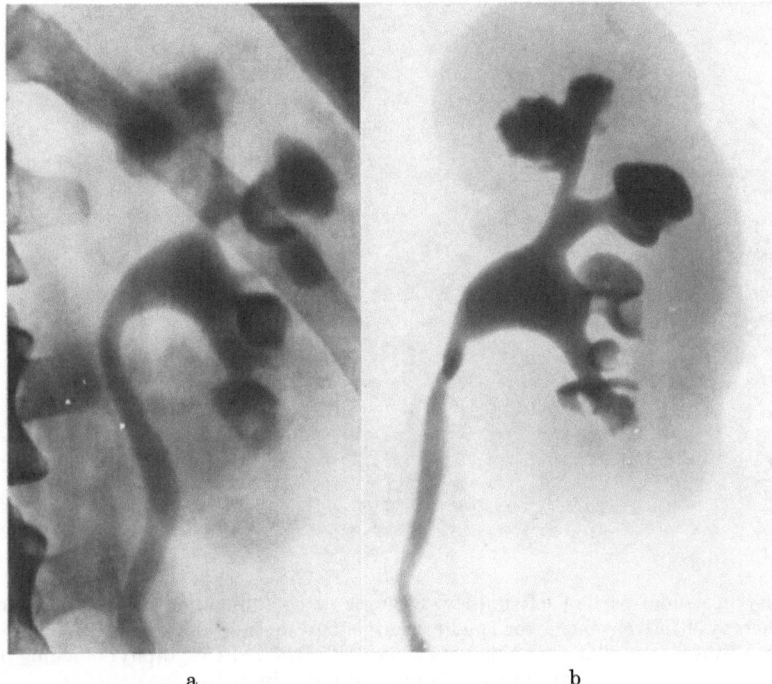

a   b

Fig. 192. Widespread unilateral chronic renal tuberculosis with irregular cavities in communication with most calyces. a) Urography: density of contrast urine somewhat decreased. b) Pyelogram of operation specimen for comparison with urogram

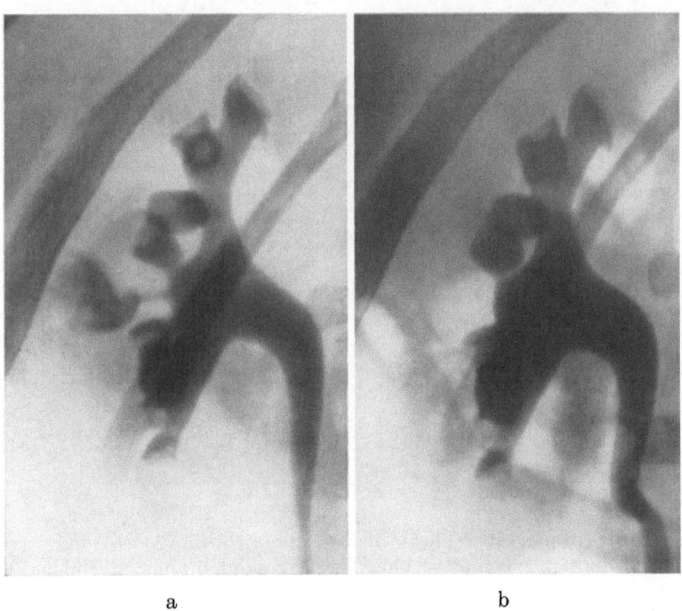

a   b

Fig. 193. a) Irregular cavity in communication with micro-calyx in middle of kidney. b) One year later, chemotherapy: complete blocking of calyx

outline in the renal parenchyma (Figs. 191, 192; see also Figs. 194, 195, 209). In some cases a filling may be obtained of only a small cavity, while at pyelography will be seen displacement of the adjacent calyces, indicating more extensive involvement. This discrepancy may be due to the cavity being very thick-walled or being filled with necrotic material permitting the flow of only a small amount of contrast medium into it. Some-

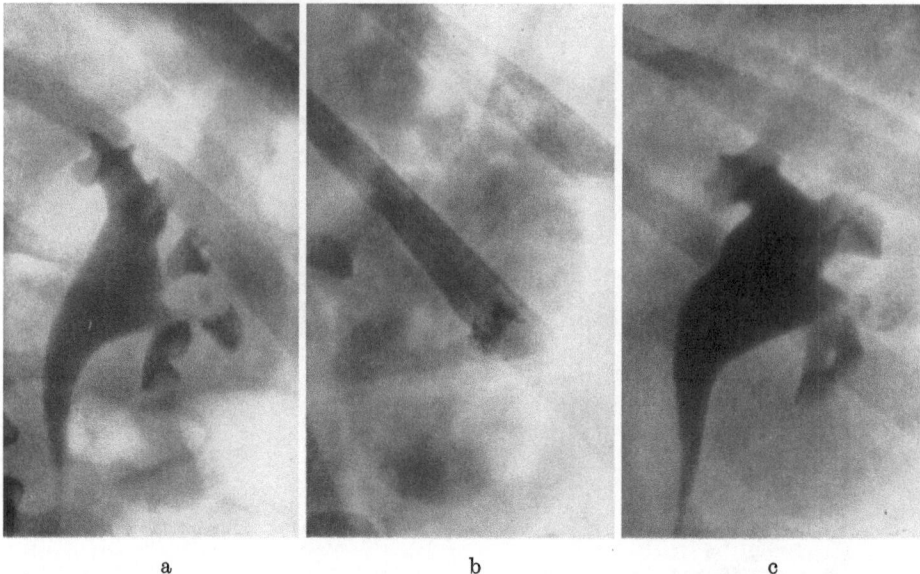

a　　　　　　　　b　　　　　　　　c

Fig. 194. a) Cavity in caudal part of left kidney. Stenosis of corresponding calyx and shrinkage of caudal branch. Chemo-therapy. b) Five years later, plain roentgenogram: irregular calcification at site of cavity. Indentation in lateral contour of kidney corresponding to calcification. c) Urography: blocking of calyx at site of calcification. Pursing of lower branch

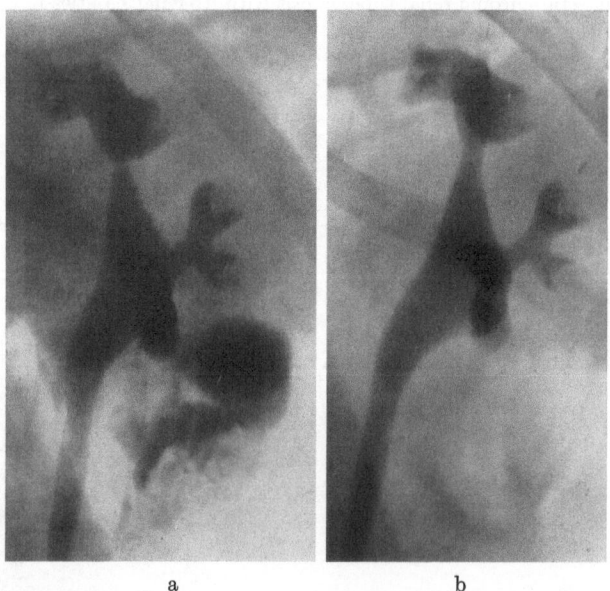

a　　　　　　　　b

Fig. 195. Rapid blocking. a) Chronic tuberculosis in lower pole with large irregular cavities. b) Three months after institution of chemo-therapy: complete blocking of caudal branch. Shrinkage of caudal kidney pole

times no filling at all is obtained of the cavity, which then appears only as an expanding process by the displacement of the calyces (see Fig. 209), or it may even remain concealed. Cases are on record (Olle Olsson, 1943) in which fairly large intrarenal tuberculous foci were shut off from the renal pelvis by stenosis in a branch in such a way that the roentgen anatomy of the renal pelvis appeared normal.

A special type of ulceration is that in which several, sometimes all, papillae are the seat of small relatively superficial ulcerations. This type of ulceration must not be mistaken for so-called medullary sponge kidney (see Chapter O). In long-standing processes the

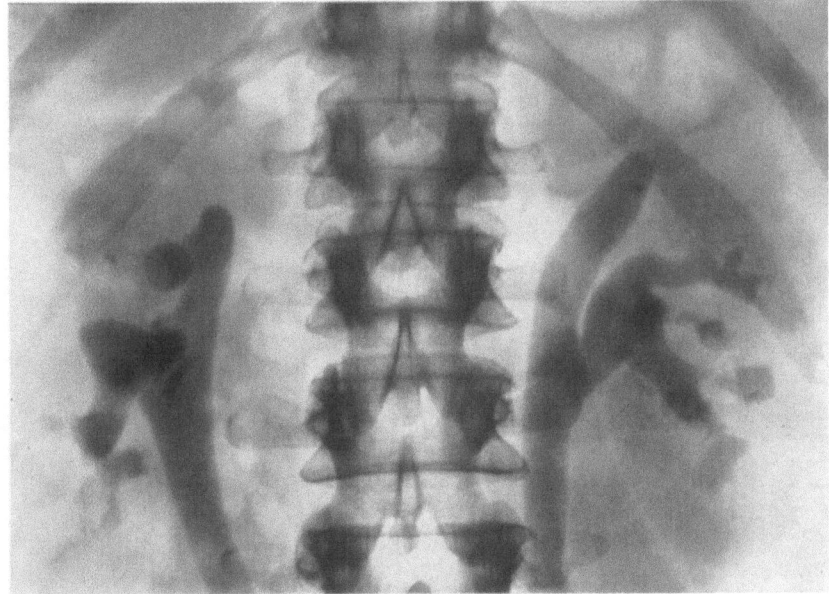

a

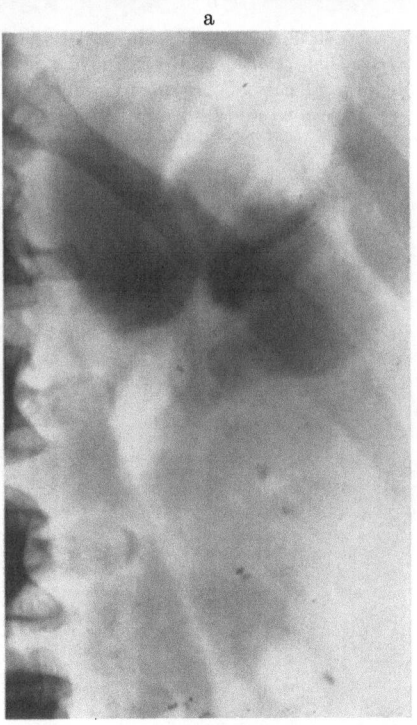

b

Fig. 196. Widespread, long-standing, bilateral renal tuberculosis. a) Urography: complete auto-amputation of cranial branch bilaterally and of middle calyx group on right side. Multiple small and larger cavities in communication with most calyces on both sides. b) Plain roentgenogram 8 years later: partial putty kidney. Left cranial pole completely calcified

wall of the cavern may be quite smooth, and such a cavity may contain one or more concrements.

Even such an early change as ulceration of a single papilla may be associated with a narrowing of the calyx draining the papilla. This stenosis is initially due to edema but in more advanced cases to granulation tissue and finally to shrinkage. Then the calyx often becomes dilated and the obstruction of the flow results in increased destruction of

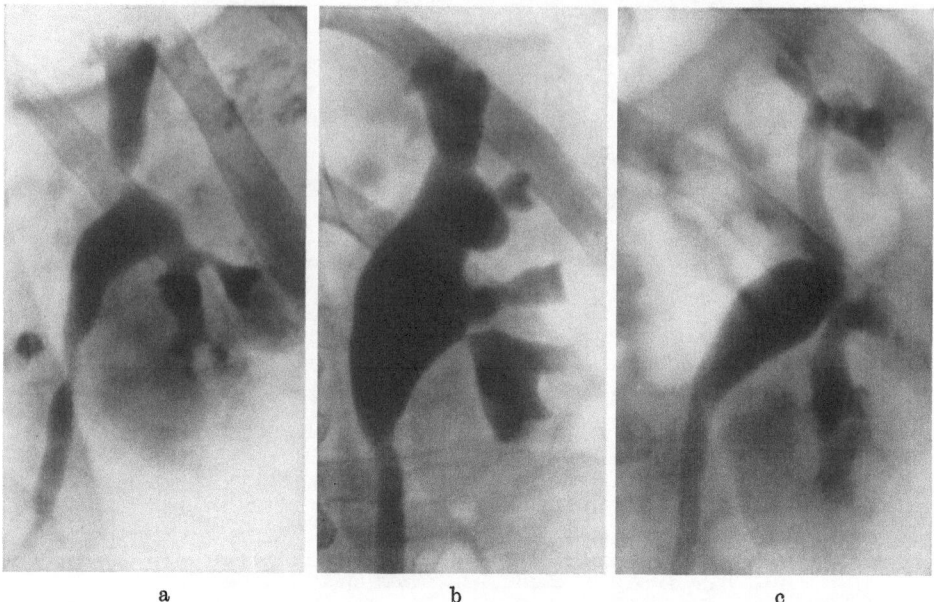

Fig. 197. Examples of marked tendency to shrinkage of kidney pelvis in longstanding chronic tuberculosis. a) Complete exclusion of middle calyces. Distortion of stem of adjacent calyces and almost complete obstruction of base of cranial branch. b) Blocking of small calyx belonging to middle part of kidney and severe obstruction of base of caudal branch. c) Blocking of calyces to middle part of kidney. Cavities in communication with filled calyces. Severe distortion of confluence laterally. Pursing of branches

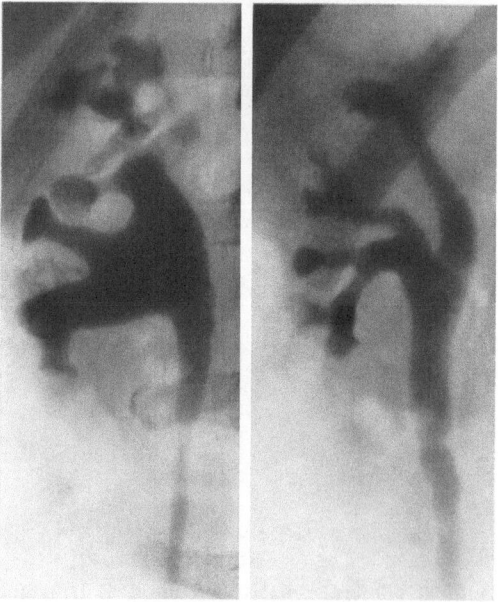

Fig. 198. Different types of tuberculous ureteritis. Slightly irregular outline of kidney pelvis and of part of ureter. Cavities in cranial kidney pole in both cases

the parenchyma. When the stenosis involves an entire branch the latter often terminates in a series of more or less well defined cavities in the parenchyma. The narrowing may make it difficult to obtain a filling and make prolonged ureteric compression necessary during the urographic procedure. Experience has also shown that urography with prolonged compression is a better method than pyelography for obtaining a filling of cavities almost completely occluded.

By severe narrowing one (Fig. 193) or more calyces (Fig. 194) may be occluded or even an entire branch (Figs. 195, 196), so-called auto-amputation of part of the renal pelvis. A calyx or a branch may, as mentioned, be shut off completely in such a way as to prevent demonstration of the lesion in the pyelogram. The films must be carefully compared with those taken previously, particularly at check examination during chemo-therapy, in order to permit detection of any occlusion of a minor part of the renal pelvis.

Distortion of one or more calyces by cicatrization of tuberculous tissue usually produces characteristic pyelographic changes in advanced renal tuberculosis (Fig. 197).

It is important to take films in different planes in order to ascertain in what part of the kidney a tuberculous process is located, in particular whether it is situated in the ventral or dorsal part of the kidney. This is of importance in contemplated partial nephrectomy and can be determined easily during urography by turning the patient in suitable projections. It may be occasionally advisable to examine the patient in the prone position also, in order to obtain a filling of cavities situated in the ventral part of the kidney.

The appearance of a typical pyelogram in renal tuberculosis is often described in the literature as resembling that of a marguerite, a brush, a sod, or some other fanciful object. Such pictorial descriptions based on single cases or projections are dilettantish and their use is unjustified. Roentgendiagnostics with the use of appropriate methods and adaptation of the technique to meet the requirements of the individual case aims at recognizing changes that can be described in patho-anatomic terms.

a) *Ureteric changes*

(Figs. 198—200)

Even relatively small tuberculous foci in the kidney are capable of causing dilatation of the ureter. Such a change has often been regarded as being of functional origin. It is

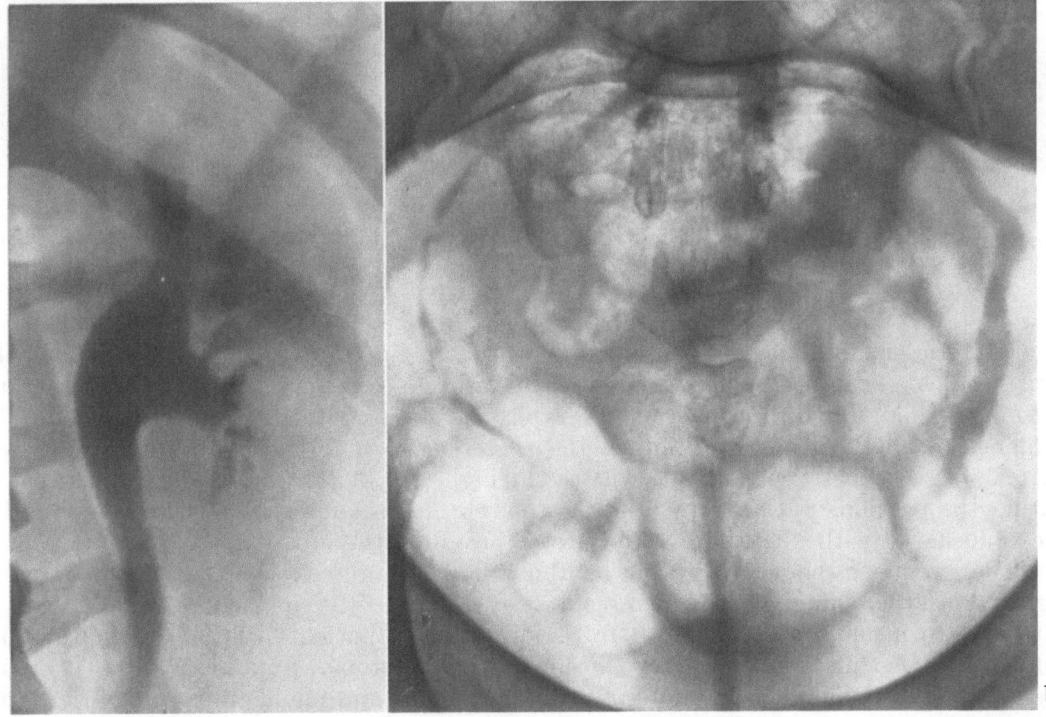

Fig. 199. Renal tuberculosis. a) Solitary papillary ulceration in caudal kidney pole. Narrowing of stem of calyx draining the affected papilla. b) Slight ureteric stenosis due to edema in ureteric orifice and demonstrable in continuous filling of ureter and slight dilatation

usually due, however, to edema around the ureteric orifice with slight obstruction and stasis as a consequence. Early ureteritis, with edema of the mucosa, then, is seen in the roentgenogram as a slight dilatation of the ureter and a slight irregular outline. Strictures are more common causes of dilatation. They are prone to occur at those levels where the ureter is normally narrow, *i. e.* at the pelviureteric junction and in the ureteric orifice in the urinary bladder (Fig. 200). The strictures may be short or long, single or multiple. In the beginning the narrowing is due to edema, later to granulation tissue, and eventually to shrinkage. Changes in the lower part of the ureter and in the bladder around the ureteric orifice particularly, can cause severe ureteric dilatation. Ureteritis may be confined to the actual ureteric orifice, just as it may extend a fair distance up the ureter with marked narrowing of the lumen as a consequence.

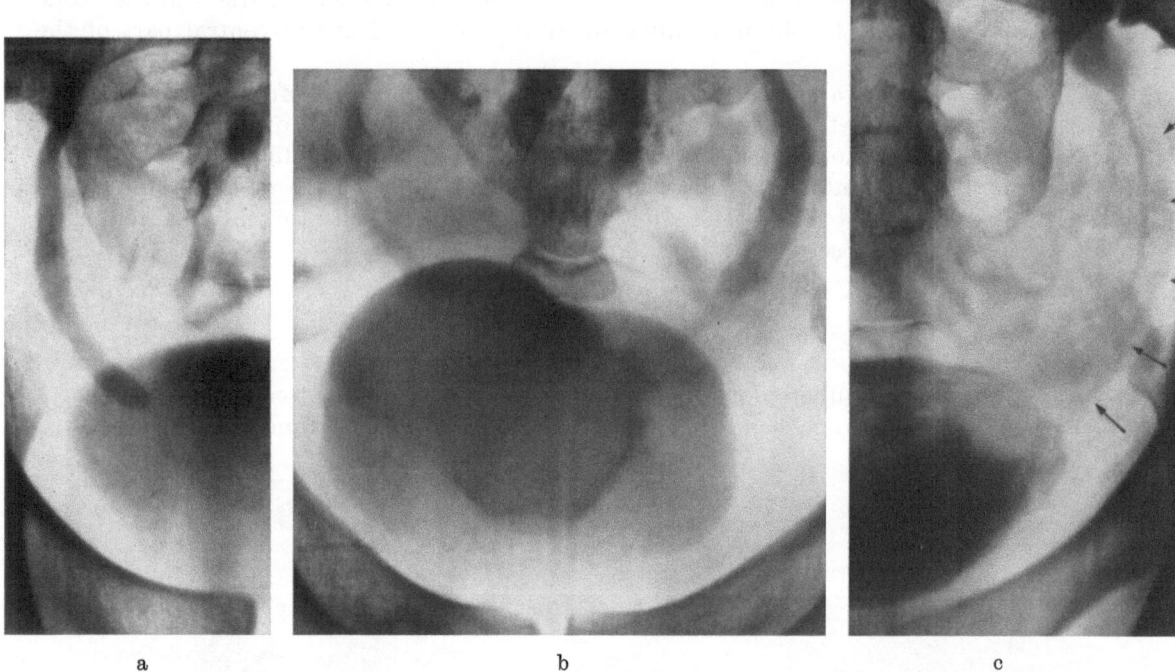

a   b   c

Fig. 200. a) Tuberculous stricture at distal ureteric end. b) and c) Tuberculous cystitis around the ureteric orifice. Note outline of thick wall of ureter (arrows)

Ureteric changes may be caused or accentuated by trauma sustained during catheterization, for example. A very well verified case has been described by ERICSSON and LINDBOM (1950) in which neither at urography nor at subsequent pyelography could any evidence of a pathologic condition in the ureter be seen. Four months later, however, edema was demonstrated at the level to which the tip of the catheter had been passed during the previous pyelography, and another six months later a stricture was found at the same level, with dilatation of the ureter proximal thereto.

The examiner should always be on the watch for ureteric changes, and many urologists are of the opinion that if nephrectomy is indicated the operation should always be extended to include ureterectomy. On review of seven patients who had definite tuberculous involvement of the ureter at the time of nephrectomy, SENGER *et al.* (1947) found the ureter to be sclerotic in five cases and dilated in one, and found empyema of the stump in one case. Inflammation of the lower part of the ureter or the urinary bladder (Figs. 201, 202, 203) can cause destruction in the remaining kidney by increasing the intrapelvic pressure. This mechanism has often been the cause of death in uremia after nephrectomy,

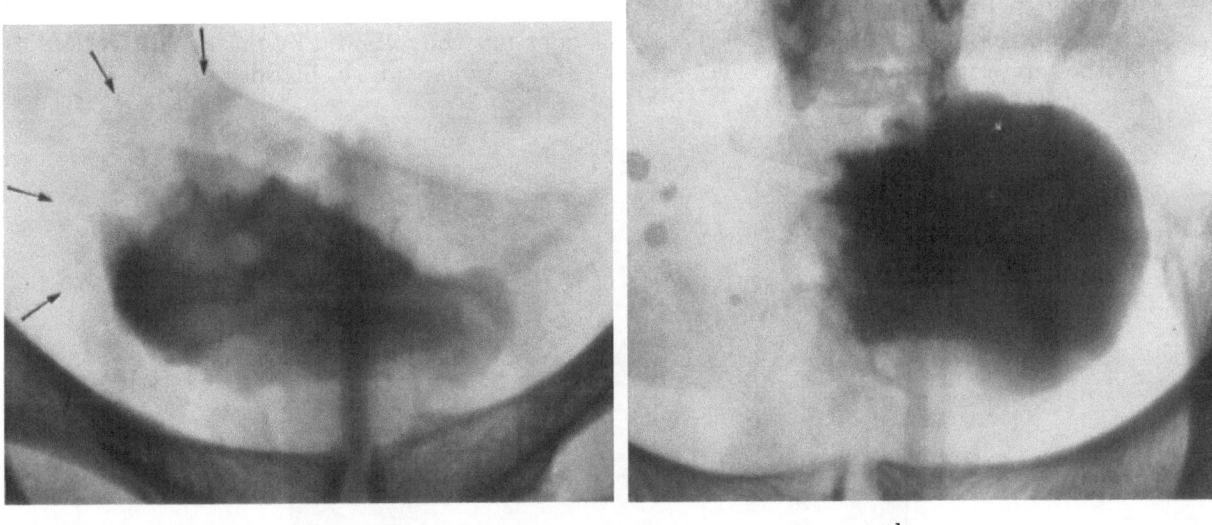

a   b

Fig. 201. Bladder tuberculosis. a) Left-sided, long-standing kidney tuberculosis with marked dilatation of kidney pelvis and ureter on "normal" right side. Marked edema in bladder mucosa except for small part on right side. Thickening of bladder wall. Dilatation on right side caused by bladder changes. b) Left part of bladder free of changes. Right-sided renal tuberculosis

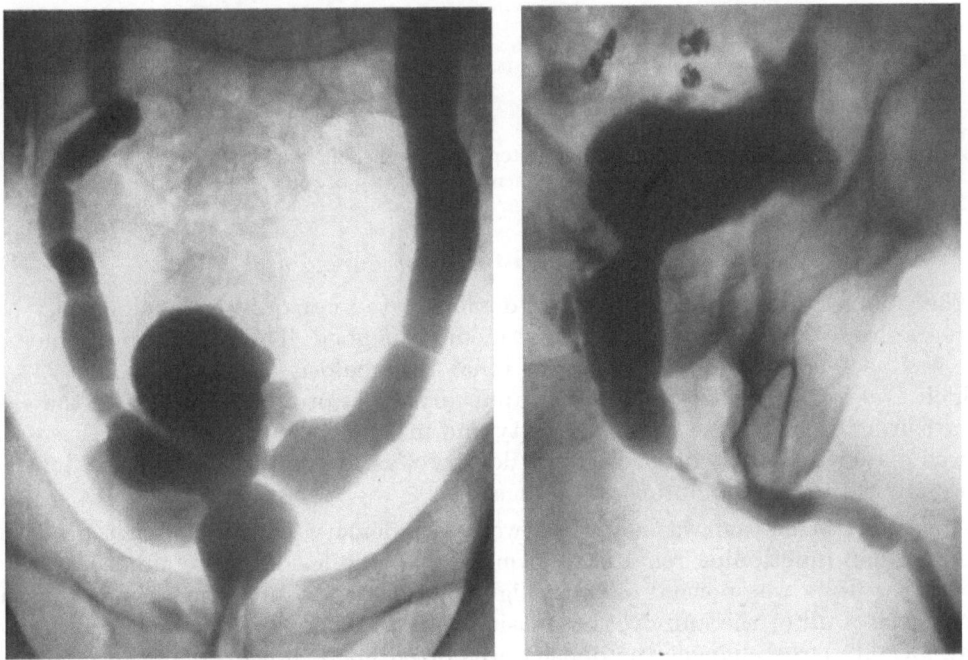

Fig. 202   Fig. 203

Fig. 202. Irregular contracted bladder. Marked dilatation of ureters. Prostatic abscess

Fig. 203. Urethrocystography: irregular, contracted bladder. Prostatic abscesses. Calcified seminal vesicles. Multiple urethral strictures

although the remaining kidney was free of tuberculosis. Note the French expression "la mort du rein restant" (Cibert, 1946).

Nephrectomy in cases with shrunken bladder may be followed by marked dilatation of the ureteric stump which then serves as a supplementary bladder, so to speak (Fig. 204).

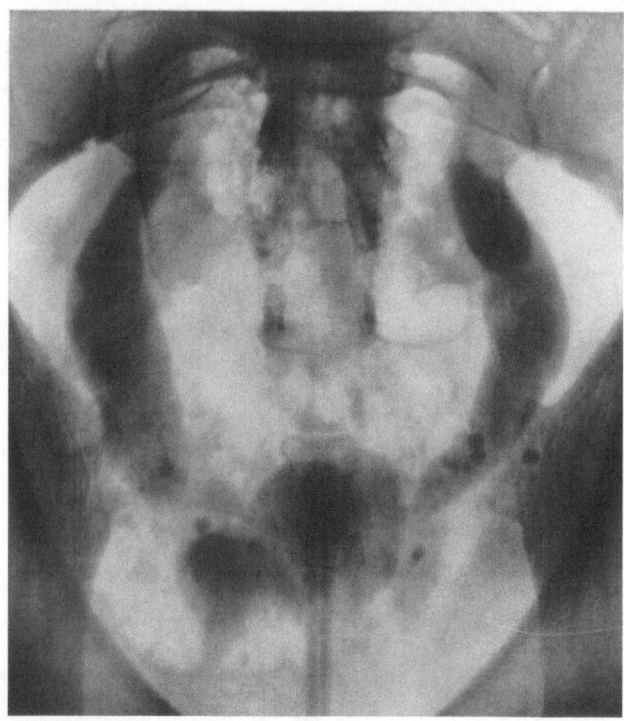

Fig. 204. Contracted bladder with dilatation of ureter to remaining left kidney and of right ureter stump after nephrectomy. Ureter stump increases capacity of contracted bladder

b) Excretion of contrast medium during urography

The changes described above can be demonstrated not only by pyelography but also by urography if the excretion of contrast medium is good. The excretion of contrast medium was as follows in our material of renal tuberculosis (Olle Olsson, 1943, 1946), in which every case was examined urographically: in approximately half of the cases the contrast urine excreted was of good density and in about two-thirds of these cases the density was excellent. In the other half the density was low, and in about one-tenth of the whole material there was no excretion at all.

A certain correlation was found between the density of the contrast urine and the amount of non-functioning renal parechyma. When the lesions were small the density of the contrast urine was normal or only slightly decreased, but when the lesions had involved most or all of the kidney, the density was very poor or no contrast urine was excreted. Despite large changes the density was often good, however, because that part of the renal pelvis draining the affected portion of the kidney was shut off. The pelvis was then filled with urine of ordinary density excreted from unaffected parts of the kidney.

Small lesions can thus, as a rule, be diagnosed under optimal contrast conditions. All of our cases with ulceration of a solitary papilla could be diagnosed urographically. Large lesions, on the other hand, can be observed even when the excretion of contrast medium is severely impaired. In cases with no excretion, pyelography may be useful, but then associated changes in the bladder and/or ureter often make catheterization impossible.

It should be observed that a kidney showing poor excretion of contrast medium may still have some reserve capacity. We have seen a case with widespread tuberculous lesions in one kidney and no demonstrable excretion of contrast medium. The patient had an attack of pain because of stone in the ureter on the "normal" side. There was no excretion at all on this side at urography during the attack, but slight excretion by the tuberculous kidney from which no excretion could previously be demonstrated.

Low density of contrast medium excreted has often been ascribed to some toxic effect involving the whole kidney. It is apparent from the remarks set forth above, however, that the density of the contrast medium is to some extent proportional to the amount of functioning renal parenchyma. An observation arguing against a general toxic effect being responsible for poor concentration of excreted contrast medium is that in double kidney with tuberculous lesions in only one half of the kidney, the density of the contrast urine in that half will be low, but in the other half excellent. This is borne out still more distinctly by the phenomenon described under the name of selective pyelography (OLLE OLSSON, 1943): In films taken immediately after injection of the contrast medium, the latter will be first excreted only in normal calyces draining unaffected renal parenchyma. After these calyces have been filled the renal pelvis will be filled from them in retrograde direction. The entire renal pelvis is thus filled with contrast urine excreted by unaffected parts of the renal parenchyma. Sometimes urine of low contrast density may appear simultaneously in calyces draining affected parts of the renal parenchyma. The contrast density of the urine coming from unaffected parts of the kidney is normal. When this urine is afterwards diluted with urine in the major portion of the renal pelvis the density of all the contrast medium accumulated in the renal pelvis may be low, but the fact that urine of ordinary contrast density can be excreted from one or more unaffected papillae in a kidney harboring widespread tuberculous lesions definitely argues against any general toxic effect on the renal parenchyma influencing the excretion of contrast medium. It should be stressed that the general toxic effect on the renal parenchyma is discussed here only in regard to its influence on the excretion of contrast urine.

c) Renal angiography

In the discussion of angiography it must never be forgotten that urography and especially pyelography have their greatest value in the investigation of open tuberculosis, which sheds bacilli into the urinary tract with the risk of the disease spreading to the ureter and bladder. With these methods lesions can be demonstrated in the renal pelvis and in the ureter and parenchymal changes can be seen only if they are in open communication with, or distort the renal pelvis. They do not yield detailed information on lesions within the actual renal parenchyma shut off from the renal pelvis. Recent therapeutic advances have created an ever—increasing demand for information on parenchymal involvement. Chemotherapy leads to blockage owing to shrinkage of single calyces or major parts of the renal pelvis. The extent of a process can then no longer be judged from the contrast filling of the renal pelvis. Conservative therapy therefore makes information on the kidney parenchyma necessary. If partial nephrectomy is contemplated, knowledge is desirable not only of the anatomy of the vessels but still more of the extent of the disease, particularly within the renal parenchyma. Renal angiography is valuable not only because it demonstrates the vasculature of the kidney and any vascular changes in the region of tuberculous foci, but also because in the nephrogram the state of the renal parenchyma can be studied. (WEYDE, 1952, 1954; FRIMANN-DAHL, 1955; OLLE OLSSON, 1955, 1962).

The arteriograms will make possible demonstration of dislocation of vessels around an inflammatory focus, variation in size or irregularity in outline of vessels, any abrupt termination of vessels by thrombi or by endarteritis and new formation of vessels (Fig. 208). On the basis of autopsy studies AMBROSETTI and SESENNA (1955) have endeavored to refine the diagnosis by means of arteriography. Their investigation is of particular interest in the discussion

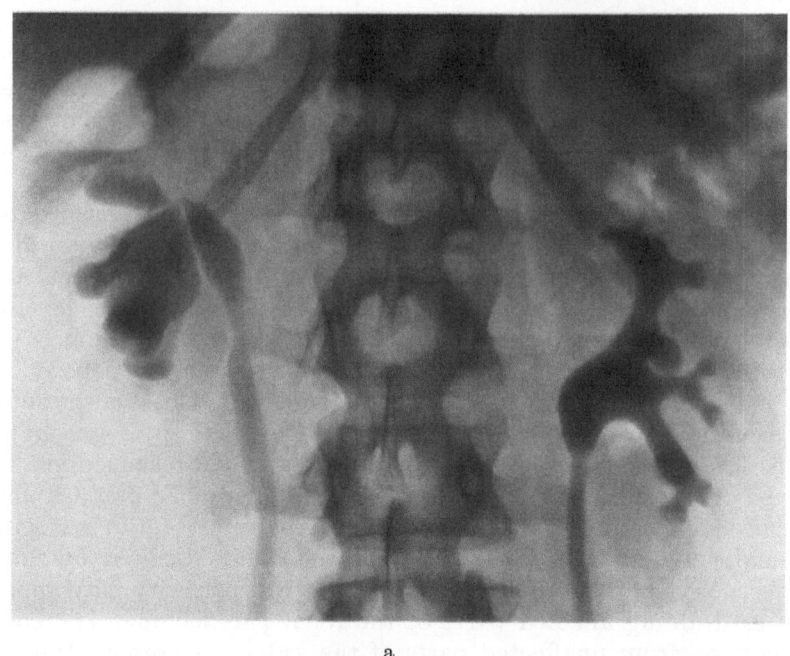

a

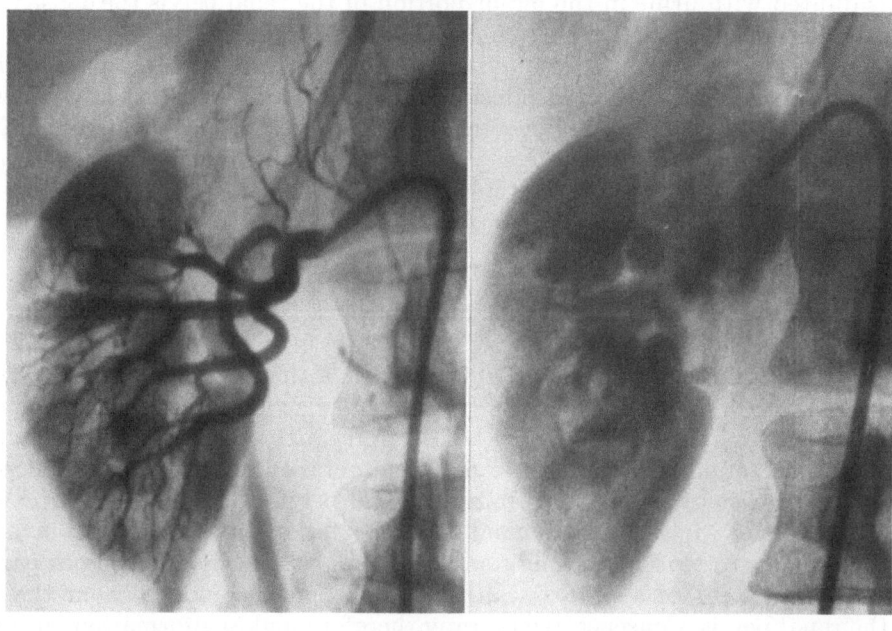

b   c

Fig. 205. Right-sided renal tuberculosis. a) Urography: Marked shrinkage and exclusion of cranial part of kidney pelvis. b) Angiography, arterial phase: Only slight vascularity in cranial kidney pole. c) Nephrographic phase: Fairly well demarcated tuberculous focus in greater part of cranial pole

of so-called tuberculous infarctions in the kidney due to tuberculous endarteritis. They have also contributed to our knowledge of fine vascular changes in tuberculosis. As yet, however, the findings in the nephrogram are in my opinion the most important. The nephrogram yields most information on the extent of the tuberculous process in the kidney and its exact localisation (Fig. 205—207). It must be remembered, however, that because of disturbances in the circulation around the tuberculous focus the nephrogram may suggest that a pathologic process is larger than it really is and in other cases with small changes it may not be possible to assess the full extent of the process because of a relatively thick overlying mass of normal renal tissue. The best information is obtainable from combined angiography and simultaneous multiplane body-section radiography.

Renal angiography will also make possible demonstration of reduction in the caliber of the renal artery and thereby the reduction in amount of functioning renal parenchyma.

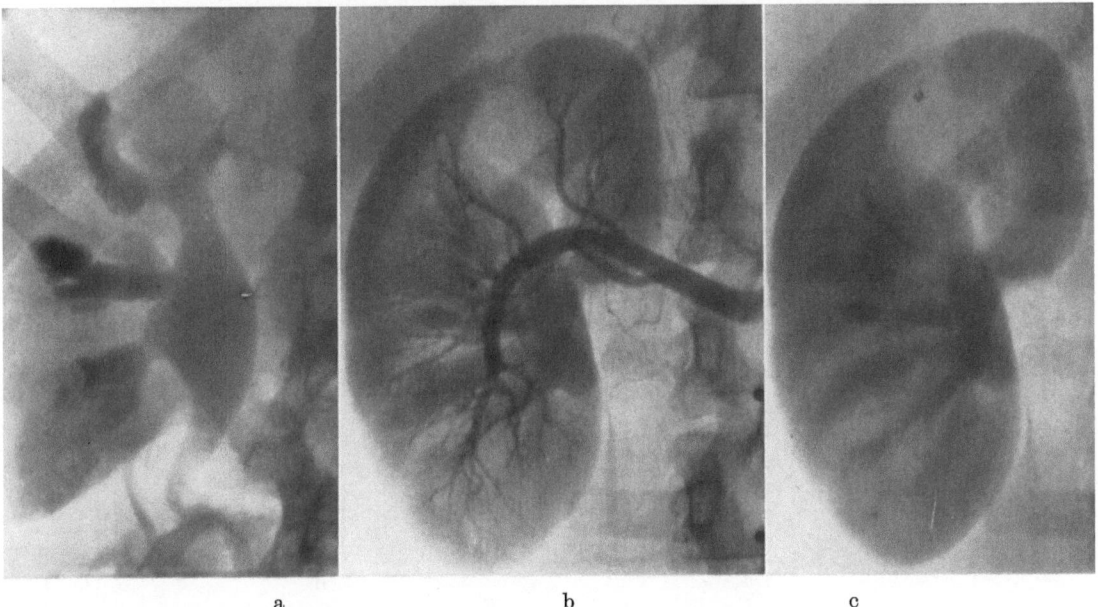

a   b   c

Fig. 206. Right-sided renal tuberculosis with at urography: (a) papillary ulcerations in middle and upper part of kidney and large cavity in cranial pole. b) and c) Angiography, arterial and nephrographic phases: no vascularity in fairly well demarcated parenchymal lesion in cranial kidney pole with diameter of 3 cm. Other changes only papillary

This adds renal tuberculosis to diseases with those fundamental problems related to potential renal function which can be solved by means of renal angiography. These problems are discussed in Chapter E.

3. Differential diagnosis

It cannot be emphasized enough that scarcely any of the roentgen findings in renal tuberculosis are pathognomonic. The wide variation in extent, age and form of tuberculous changes calls for caution in the interpretation of the roentgen findings. On the other hand, this fact stresses the necessity of keeping this disease in mind when encountering changes of the type mentioned, particularly in countries where renal tuberculosis is seldom seen. Many nontuberculous processes can cause changes similar to those seen in different stages of renal tuberculosis. It has also been claimed that the only truly pathognomonic change in renal tuberculosis is that of putty kidney. Marked irregular cicatrization and distortion of the renal pelvis are also fairly characteristic. A diagnosis of renal tuberculosis cannot be made as a rule, however, on the basis of roentgen examination only. Roentgen examination will permit a probable diagnosis, but a firm diagnosis requires demonstration of tubercle bacilli.

If the lesions are small, they must be differentiated from fornix reflux described by OLLE OLSSON (1943, 1948) and LINDBOM (1943). In urograms small sinus refluxes often simulate papillary ulcerations. Should such a change appear during examination, ureteric compression should be prolonged. The reflux will then spread and the contrast medium

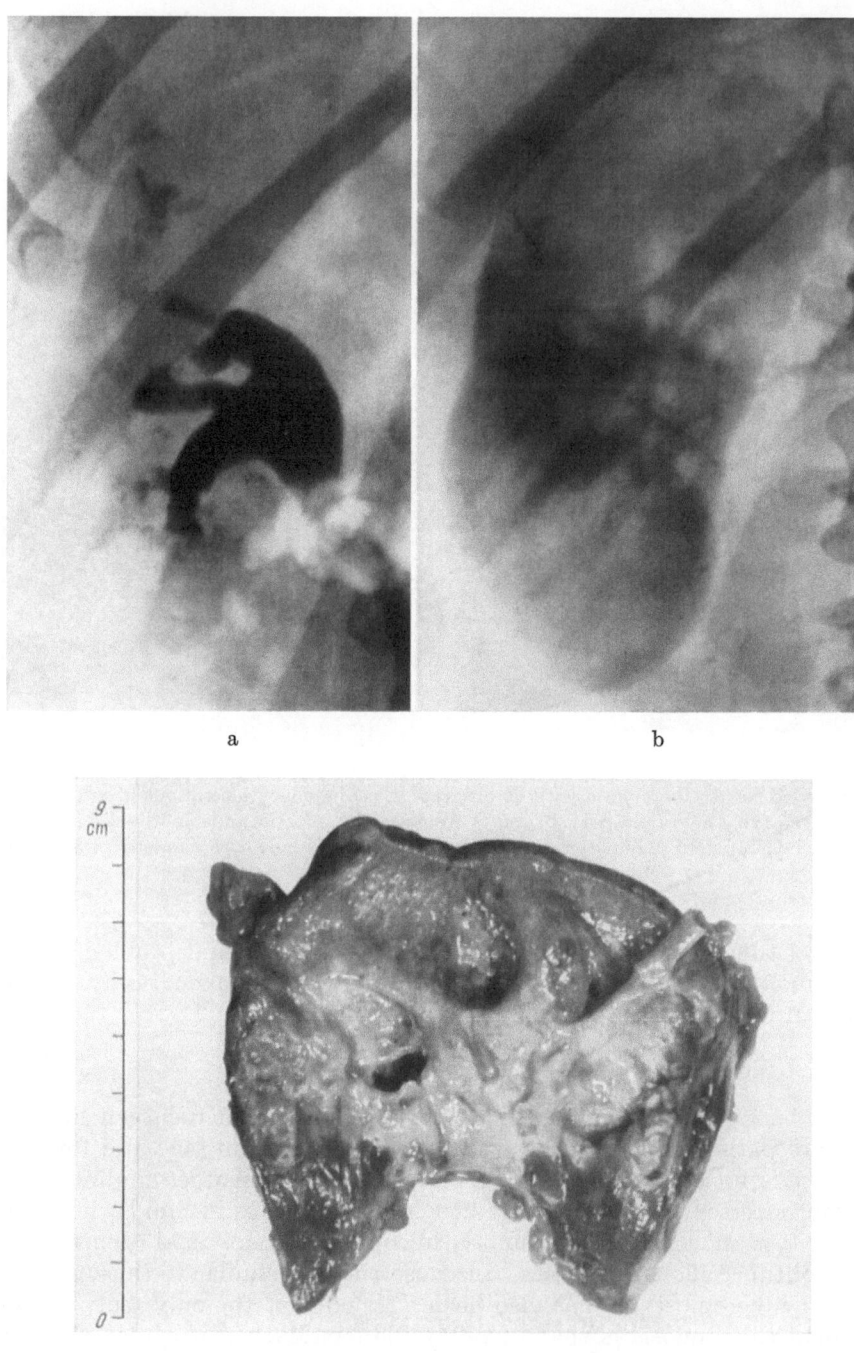

a   b

c

Fig. 207. Long-standing right-sided tuberculosis. a) Urography: Complete blocking of cranial branch. Increased volume of cranial kidney pole. b) Renal angiography, Nephrogram: Large thin-walled cavity in cranial pole. Partial nephrectomy of upper half of right kidney. Specimen. Resected part of kidney is completely cavernous with caseation and wide-spread fresh tuberculous granulation tissue. c) Operative specimen

ooze down along the stems of the calyces and possibly further into the sinus. If the examination cannot be prolonged, the patient may be re-examined after an interval of one to two weeks, by which time the fornical rupture will have healed. The so-called tubular reflux in pyelography, which can also be demonstrated at urography during ureteric compression and is then due to tubular stasis, usually offers no differential-diagnostic difficulties. Pathologic processes of differential diagnostic importance are also papillary necrosis, pyelogenic cyst, calyceal border evagination, calyx hypoplasia with spherical calyces and hydrocalyx caused by calculi, for example. If the process is more advanced, secondary renal changes due to stone and various stages of pyelonephritis may offer

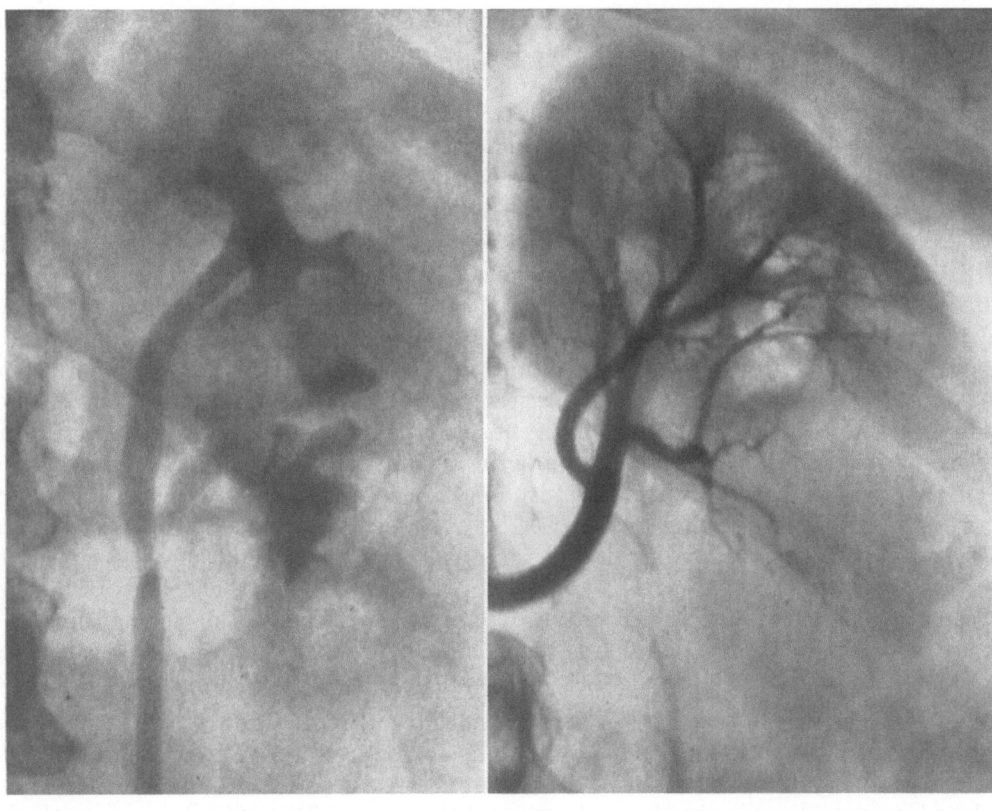

a   b

Fig. 208. a) Urography: deeply split kidney pelvis. Tuberculosis in each papilla of distal half of kidney. b) Angiography, arterial phase: slight displacement, in a curve cranially, of branches at middle of kidney. Low vascularity in caudal half of kidney with marked vasculitis. Arteries and parenchyma corresponding to upper part of kidney pelvis without changes

differential-diagnostic difficulties. The differential diagnosis can ultimately be established by bacteriologic examination. In most cases nowadays, however, the problem is not the differential diagnosis of tuberculosis versus, for example, non-specific pyelonephritis with papillary destruction, but the inclusion of tuberculosis in the differential-diagnostic discussion of changes of the type often seen in pyelonephritis.

The vascular changes caused by renal tuberculosis and demonstrable at angiography are fairly characteristic but not pathognomonic. If the tuberculous process has an expansive character and vascular changes are seen during angiography, with demonstration of an unsharp border between affected parenchyma and normal parenchyma in the nephrographic phase, the changes may be mistaken for tumor. Therefore, also in this respect, the possibility of tuberculosis, although rare, must always be kept in mind.

4. Follow-up examinations

Conservative treatment has made knowledge of the roentgenographic course of renal tuberculosis imperative. The course varies widely. If the vital resistance is low, the process may progress rapidly, while accidentally detected cases such as renal tuberculosis in males discovered in association with epididymitis show that it can run a very slow and insidious course with increasing cavitation or with healing with cicatrization, blockage of the calyces and calcification. Blockage of a single calyx or of a major part of the renal pelvis can run a course of many years. On the other hand, such blockage may occasionally progress rapidly and be complete within three to four months, even without chemotherapy. This variation in the course should be remembered in the roentgenologic evaluation of the effect of conservative treatment, particularly chemotherapy. It should also be borne in mind that renal tuberculosis does not heal with *restitutio ad integrum* but with some type of definite deformation of the renal pelvis (Figs. 209, 210; see also Figs. 193, 195).

A question of great importance formerly was, and to some extent still is, whether the disease is unilateral or bilateral in a given case of renal tuberculosis. Now that it is widely accepted that infection occurs on both sides simultaneously, but that it may develop in different ways in the two kidneys, it appears that the conservative attitude adopted towards renal tuberculosis in recent years is well founded. This provides a possibility of following the course with repeated roentgen examination for a long period. Such repeated control is, of course, necessary — especially for assessment of the effect of therapy, chemotherapy in particular. As a rule, renal tuberculosis thus requires roentgen follow-up. After nephrectomy the patient should be examined at long intervals mainly for checking of any progression of tuberculous lesions known to exist in the remaining kidney, of the development of any lesions in the remaining kidney and of any vesical or ureteric obstruction causing ureteric stenosis with hydronephrosis and impairment of renal function as a consequence. It is, however, largely the use of chemotherapy that has made check examinations so necessary in renal tuberculosis. All check examinations should be performed in the same way as the original examination. Thus, if prolonged ureteric compression was necessary to demonstrate a cavity, it should also be applied at check examination.

At repeat examinations it can be shown that untreated renal tuberculosis runs a variable course and that the process may remain stationary for several years, or it may even regress, with stricture and distortion of part of the renal pelvis. As mentioned, this must be taken into consideration in the evaluation of the effect of therapy. In cases with chemotherapy, scar formation at the pelviureteric junction or in the ureter may develop rapidly and cause complete obstruction. It may also be local in any part of the kidney pelvis (GAY, 1949; CAVAZZANA and MENEGHINE, 1956). Such occlusion, as mentioned, may occur rapidly after institution of therapy with tuberculostatics. HANLEY (1955) stresses the importance of check radiography as early as a few months after the institution of conservative therapy to detect any obstruction of drainage of the renal pelvis.

Pathologically such occlusion is a sign of regression, but clinically it may sometimes be considered a progression. Scar formation and shrinkage may result in a stricture of a calyx or a branch of the renal pelvis. Behind this closure, however, the process may be florid (see Fig. 207). Such shrinkage may also be localized to the pelviureteric junction or to the ureterovesical junction and give rise to hydronephrosis with all the risks thereby entailed.

In some cases the obstruction is not due to scar formation but to edema and specific granulation tissue and should not be mistaken for a sign of healing. Calcifications in the parenchyma demonstrable in plain radiograms, a sharp outline of the process in the nephrogram, or no further changes in the rest of the kidney since the foregoing examination are signs of regression. Any regression of papillary ulceration will be manifested by sharper definition of the previously irregular outlines of the papillae against the renal pelvis and by a smoothing out of the ragged outline of filled cavities.

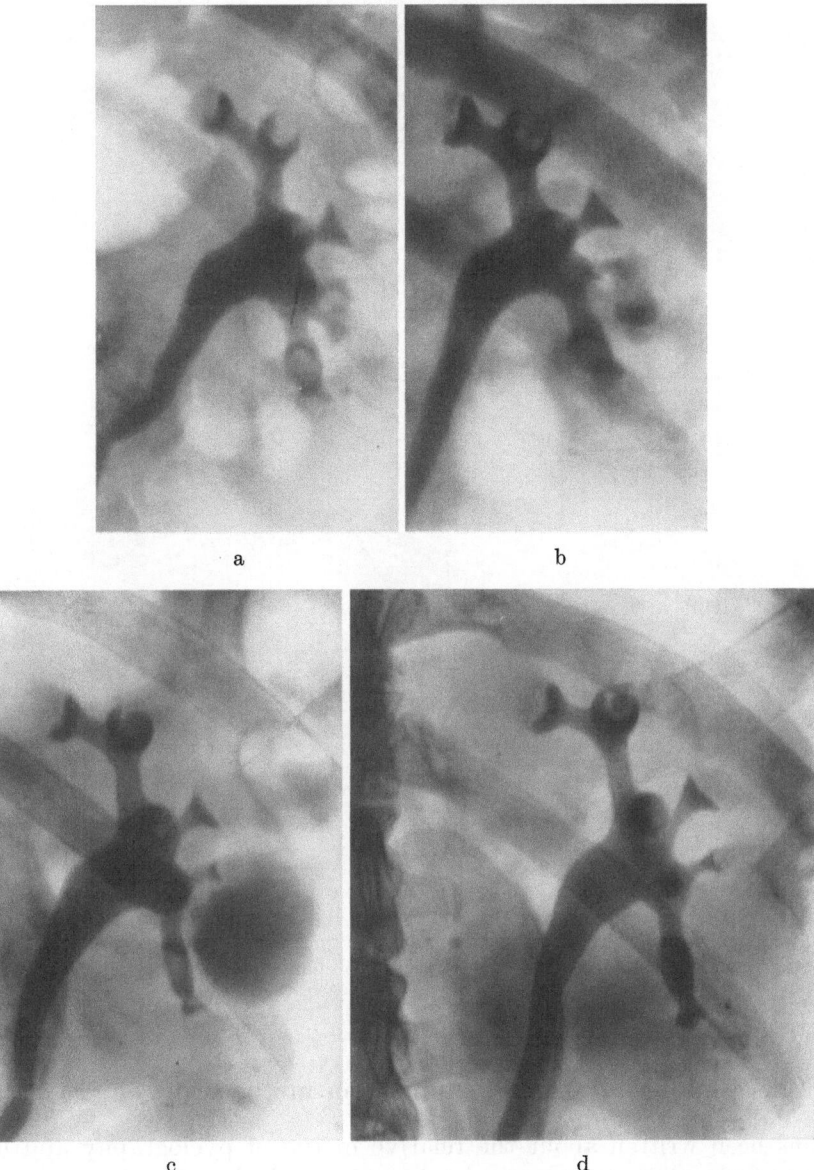

Fig. 209. Check examinations during conservative treatment of left-sided tuberculosis. Patient had many tuberculous lesions in chest, spine, pelvis, etc. and her vital resistance was low. Responded slowly to conservative therapy, now well. a) Slight irregularity of edge of next-to-lowermost calyx. b) One year later: small cavity formation. c) Another three years later: large cavity with displacement of nearby calyces. Cavity wall fairly smooth. d) Five years later: complete exclusion of cavity. Note spondylitis with abscess displacing kidney laterally. Calcifications in abscess

As mentioned, many urologists consider partial nephrectomy to be indicated in the treatment of well defined local lesions, usually located in the poles of the kidney. The appearance of the kidney in check roentgenograms after partial nephrectomy will be the same as after the same type of operation for other diseases.

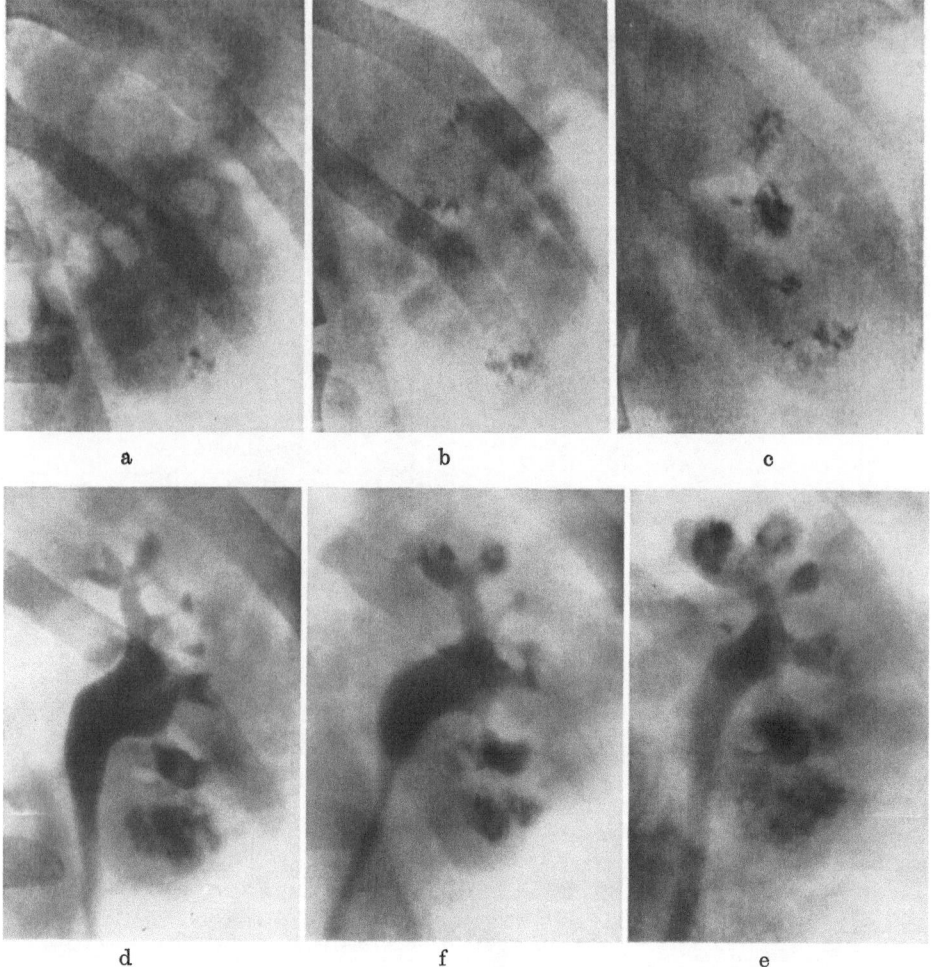

Fig. 210. Bilateral tuberculosis refractory to chemo-therapy with progression in left kidney. Plain roentgeno-grams of left kidney. a) Slight calcifications in caudal pole. b) Five years later: small irregular calcifications in middle of kidney and cranial pole. c) Another three years later: wider-spread calcifications in most pyramids d), e), f) Urography at corresponding intervals: progressive changes with caseation, blocking, and decreased function

III. General observations on examination methods in renal tuberculosis

Much has been written about the relative merits of pyelography and urography in the diagnosis of ulcero-cavernous renal tuberculosis. Both methods are useful and often supplement one another. Pyelography requires catheterization, which is sometimes not possible owing to changes in the urinary bladder or to ureteric stricture, for example. On the other hand, a necessary condition for successful urography is that the kidney still possesses some functional capacity. Urography should first be tried, however, since experience has shown that both cystoscopy and catheterization of the ureter are attended by risks, particularly if these examinations must often be repeated for check examination, such as during chemotherapy. In addition, the injection of contrast medium may cause pyelovenous reflux with spread of tubercle bacilli into the blood stream. A well verified case has been described by LINDBOM (1944) in which such reflux caused fatal miliary tuberculosis. As mentioned, urography may also cause reflux but this is, as a rule, a sinus reflux and extremely seldom a pyelovenous reflux (see chapter P). As pointed out previously, urography will not only permit establishment of the diagnosis but also yield the detailed information required by modern methods of treatment. The importance of urography was brought into sharp focus by OLLE OLSSON (1943) on the basis of a large tuberculosis series. It has been emphasized by CIBERT (1946), ERICSSON and LINDBOM (1950), FRIMANN-DAHL (1955) and others.

The roentgen examination methods used have varied with the advances made in the treatment of tuberculosis. The history of the treatment of renal tuberculosis falls into three periods. The first period is characterized by Albarran's law: Unilateral renal tuberculosis = nephrectomy. For such cases pyelography was a good diagnostic method. Then followed the period of conservative therapy, which required repeated check radiography. After systematic investigations had confirmed the value of urography, that procedure became the method of choice. Urography permits check examinations at fairly short intervals with scarcely any risk and only slight inconvenience to the patient. (During such check examinations proper shielding for ray protection of the patient's gonads is of course imperative.)

The third period is characterized by a combination of conservative and surgical therapy, namely partial nephrectomy or cavernostomy in association with conservative medical treatment. This type of treatment requires knowledge of the extent of the process in the parenchyma. Renal angiography, particularly the nephrogram, yields valuable information on this point and on vascular anatomy and is therefore now an important diagnostic method in renal tuberculosis.

I. Primary vascular lesions

Renal function is intimately related to the blood supply to the kidneys. Investigation of the renal vasculature is therefore important in many situations. Changes occur in the pattern of the renal vessels in a variety of renal diseases and characteristic abnormalities may then be demonstrated by angiography. When this is the case, the appearance of the pathologic findings is described in association with the underlying disease, e.g. vascular atrophy in the chapter on stone and hydronephrosis, pathologic vessels in renal carcinomas in the chapter on renal tumors, etc., usually under the sub-heading of renal angiography. These vascular changes are secondary to or part of a primary renal disease. Certain primary vascular changes are also of great roentgen-diagnostic interest:

I. Arteriosclerosis, fibroplasia, and other types of arterial disease

Of changes in the renal artery, arteriosclerosis is the most common. In plain roentgenograms arteriosclerotic changes can be seen if calcification of the process is present. Often intimal calcifications are present in the lumbar aorta and sometimes these calcifications include the region of the origin of the renal arteries. A calcified complete, or incomplete ring is seen in one or both sides at the mouth of the renal artery. Occasionally, more widespread calcifications are seen in the intrarenal branches. Usually, however, calcifications in most branches of the renal artery are due to medial calcificationsy (Fig. 211, 212).

At angiography, indentations are seen in the aorta and the origin of the renal artery on one or both sides. In the presence of multiple renal arteries all arteries may have corresponding changes. The plaques sometimes stenose the arterial lumen markedly and a post-stenotic dilatation is often present. The stenosis may be complete (Fig. 214). In stenoses varying from marked to complete, a collateral circulation may develop (Fig. 215). Such a development may be very rapid. Thus in acute occlusion of a renal artery, collateral circulation can be demonstrated angiographically within a few hours.

17*

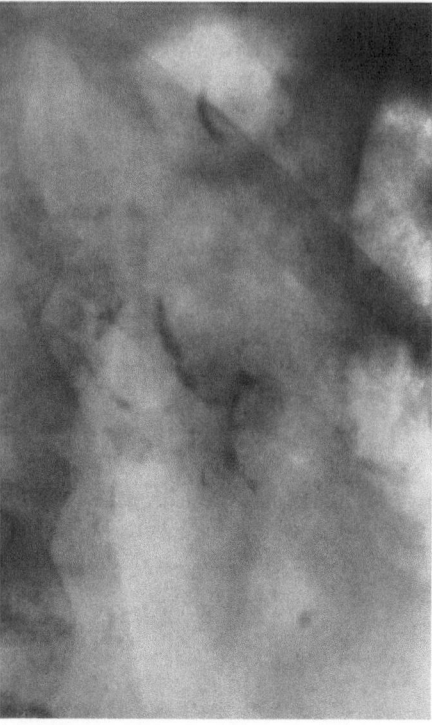

Fig. 211. Intimal calcifications in arteriosclerosis localized to wall of lumbar aorta, main artery, and large intrarenal branches

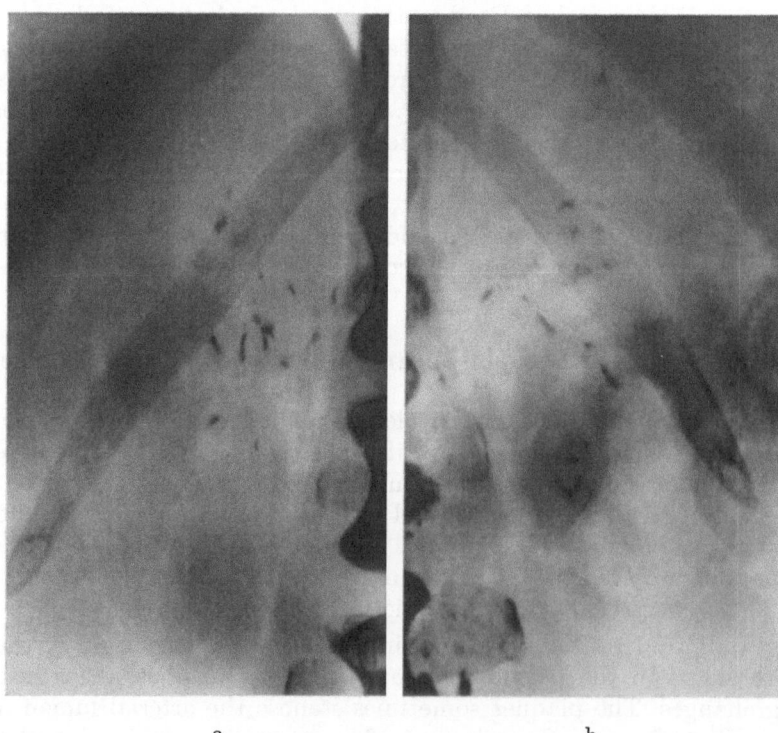

a   b

Fig. 212. Intimal calcifications in arteriosclerosis. a) Plain roentgenograms of both kidneys: calcifications in intrarenal arterial branches. b) Urogram including oblique view, right kidney: calcifications immediately outside kidney pelvis

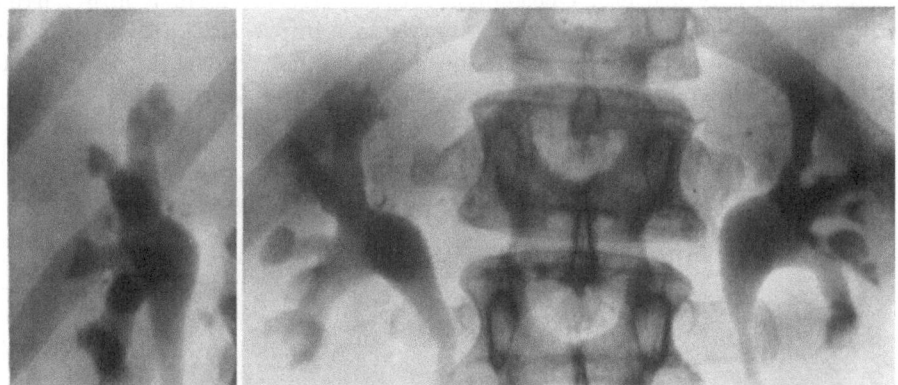

Fig. 212 b

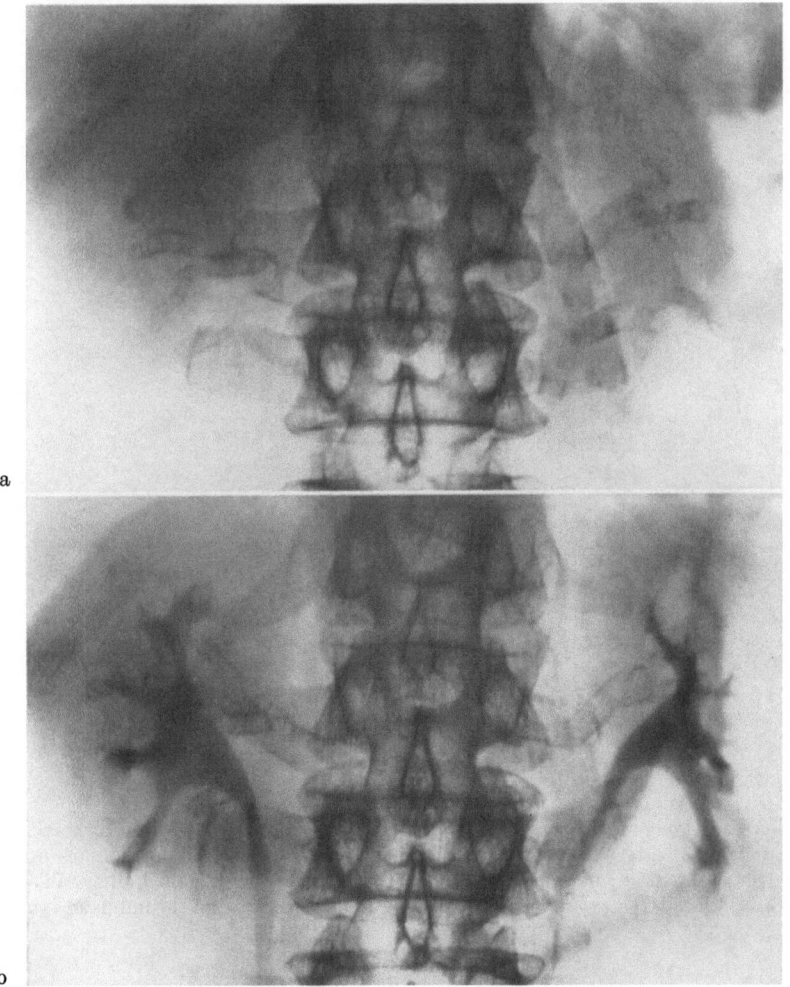

Fig. 213: Calcifications in main renal arteries in intrarenal branches and in supplementary arteries to caudal
pole bilaterally. a) Plain roentgenography. b) Urography

Many arteries can contribute to this collateral circulation: capsular arteries, lumbar arteries, suprarenal arteries, etc. Occasionally these arteries form a large, irregular net of markedly tortuous vessels. Such arteries may cause impressions in the renal pelvis and in the ureter. Slight impressions may also be made in the renal pelvis and the ureter by anatomically ordinary arteries because of wall rigidity and tortuosity.

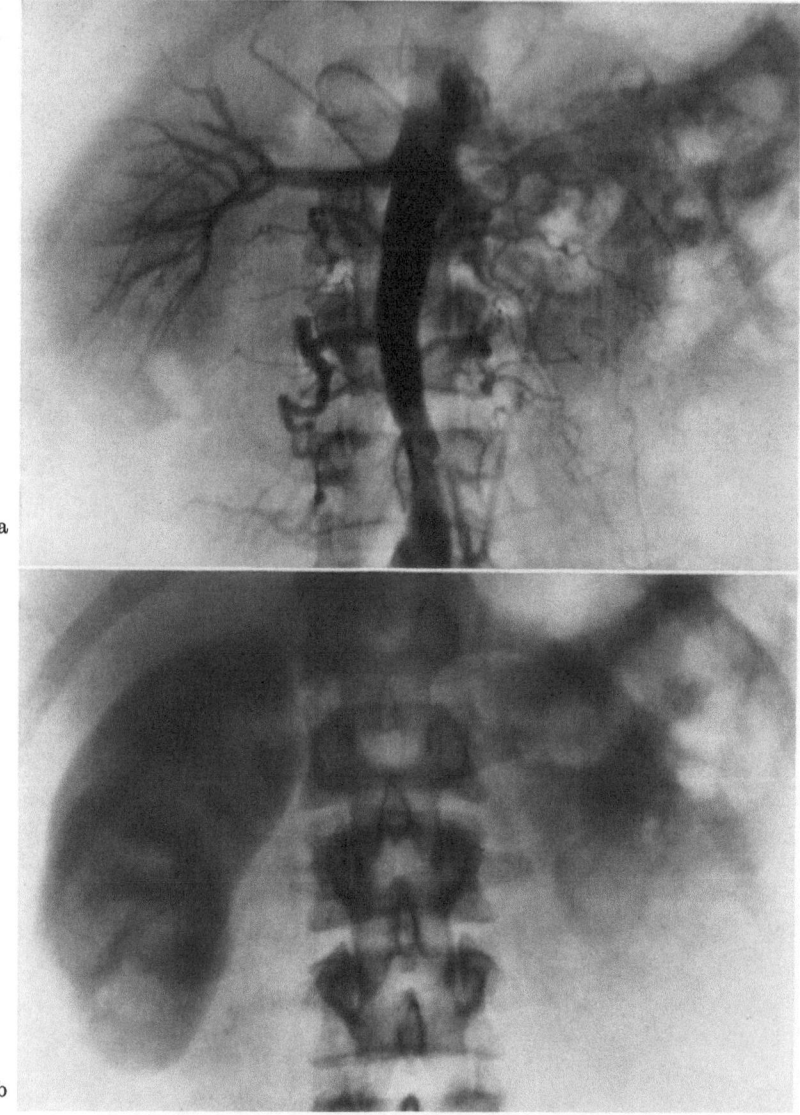

Fig. 214. Arteriosclerosis. Long-standing, severe hypertension. Renal angiography: a) Marked arteriosclerotic changes in aorta. Left renal artery almost completely occluded at origin. Slight changes in proximal part of right renal artery. b) Nephrogram: normal parenchyma in somewhat large right kidney. Very small, irregular, atrophic left kidney. Operation: small contracted kidney. Organized thrombus in renal artery

The arteriosclerotic changes may cause diminished bloodflow to the kidney and thus cause decrease in kidney size (Fig. 216). Mention should be made of the possibility of atheromatous emboli to the kidneys. Single or multiple emboli from arteriosclerotic plaques may pass into the kidneys, either spontaneously or in connection with a catheterization procedure and cause local infarction or generalized shrinkage (CIEVIEWICH, 1969).

Arterial stenosis will also cause delay in the transport of contrast medium to the kidney parenchyma. At urography this will cause changes in excretion time of the kidney and emptying time of the kidney pelvis and the ureter (see chapter on urography). At angiotomography, a kidney with arterial stenosis has lower opacification initially than has an ordinary kidney (LIESE, 1960; RATHE, 1961). Not only parenchymal changes but also vascular changes may be caused by radiation in connection with radio-therapy, where the

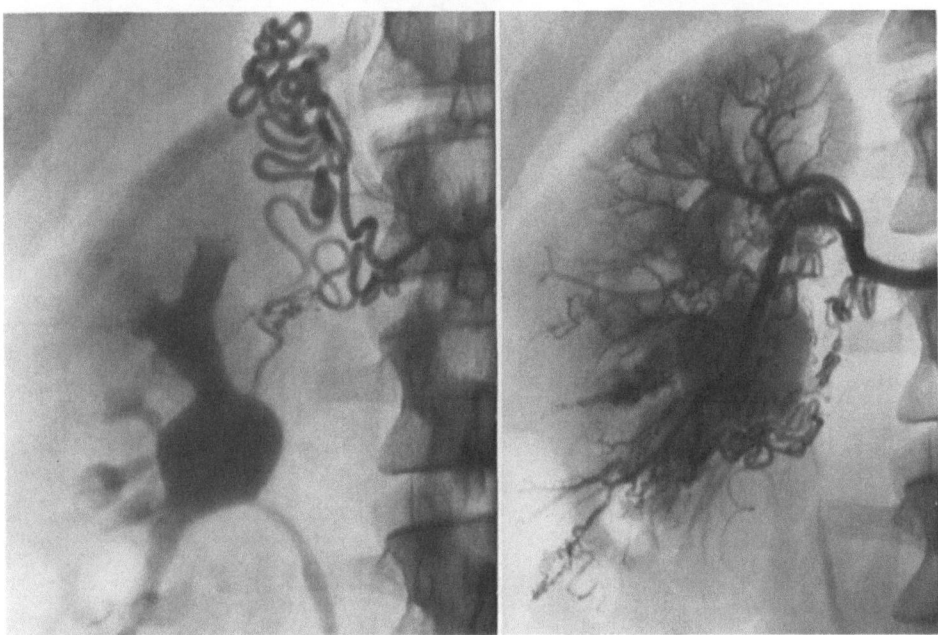

Fig. 215. Collateral arterial circulation

kidneys are in the field of radiation. These changes may consist of more or less marked, single or multiple narrowings of one or both renal arteries which in turn, secondarily, may further affect renal parenchyma. The stenosis caused by the radiation may have the same appearance as a stenosis seen in patients with renal hypertension (Fig. 217).

Periadventitial fibrosis causes an external constriction of the artery, for example by bands from the pleura diaphragmatica (BROLIN, 1967). Such constriction is funnel-shaped, concentric, and has smooth contours. Occasionally it is irregular in outline and cannot be differentiated from an arteriosclerotic stenosis. A combination of the two is also possible.

Fibroplasia may also affect the medial layer, the subadventitial layer and the intimal layer of the arterial wall.

Intimal fibroplasia and so-called fibromuscular hyperplasia (Fig. 218) affect the middle and/or the distal third of the renal artery, contrary to arteriosclerosis in which the proximal part is most commonly involved (PALUBINSKAS, 1961). The artery has several short narrowings and, in between, a slight widening which gives the appearance of a string of beads. Fibromuscular hyperplasia may also be combined with arteriosclerosis. In the early stage the disease gives no definite angiographic changes.

It has been suggested that fibromuscular hyperplasia should be related to alternate stretching and relaxation in cases in which the kidney has an increased, pathologic mobility. Angiographic examination, with the patient in recumbent and upright positions, has been proposed. Experiments in dogs (ROFFIELD, 1969) did not corroborate this view.

GILL and MEANEY (1969), in reviewing a material of 203 patients with medial fibroplasia, found that the disease was more severe on the right side in patients with unilateral

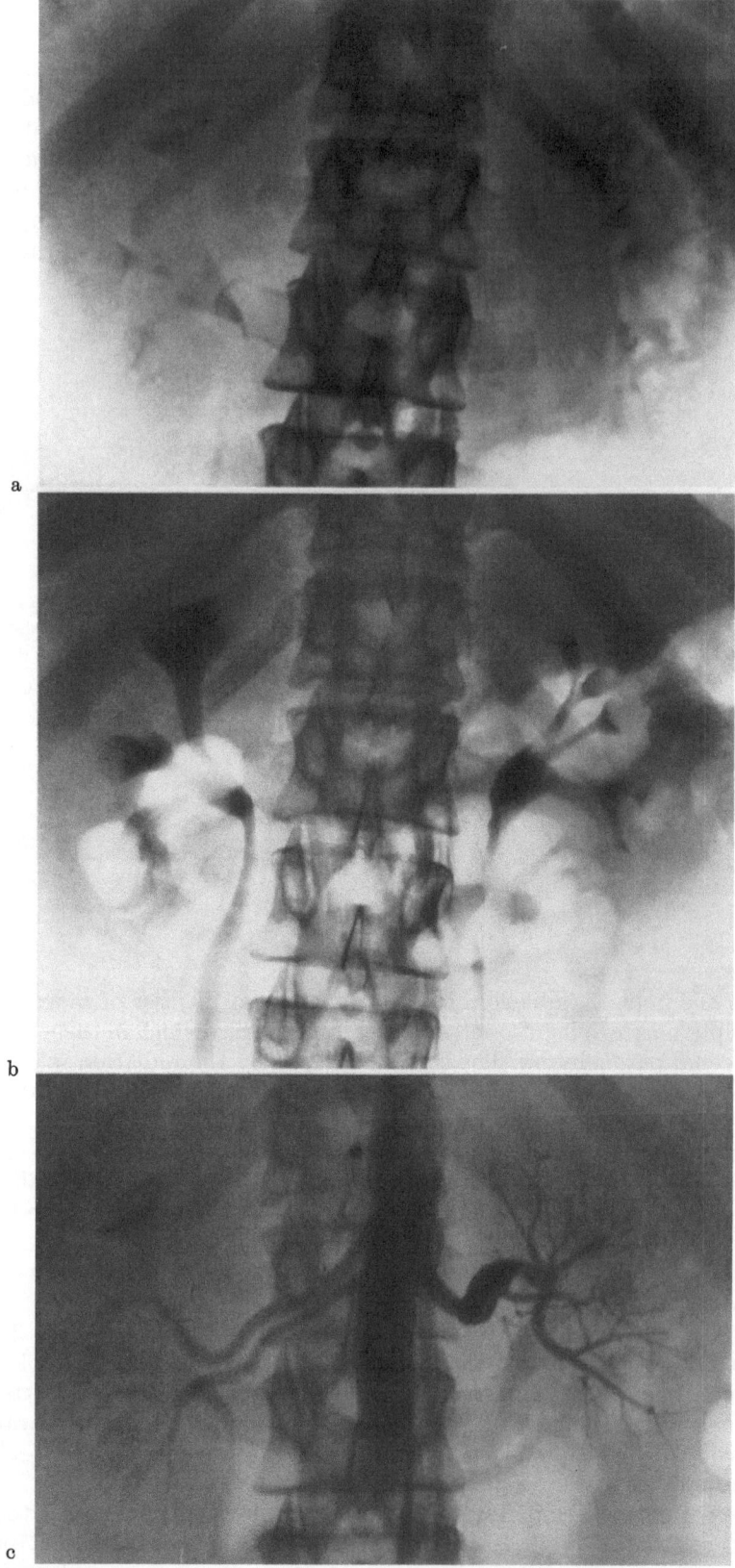

a

b

c

Fig. 216. Renal hypertension, rapid sequence. a) Urography, early phase: excretion on both sides. Filling of calyces, kidney pelvis, and ureter on right side. Filling of only calyces on left side. Left kidney markedly smaller than right kidney. b) Urography, late phase: higher concentration of contrast urine on left side as compared with right side. Notching in upper part of ureter medially. Impression in confluence part of renal pelvis at base of branches. c) Angiography: marked stenosis in left renal artery. Post-stenotic dilatation. Descending ventral branch impresses kidney pelvis laterally. Widened ureteric artery impresses upper part of ureter

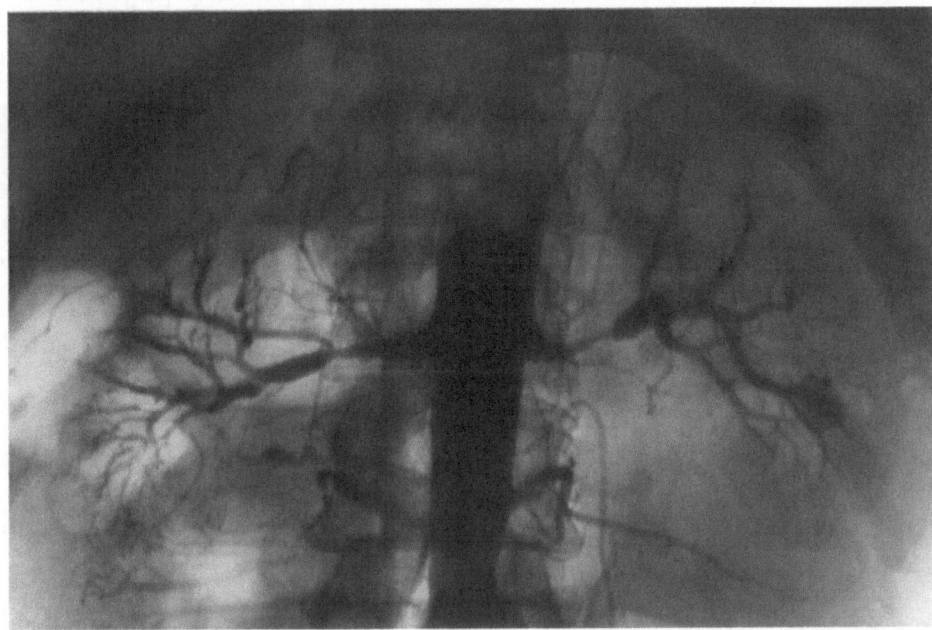

Fig. 217. Radiation therapy because of seminoma with glandular metastases 10 years before actual examination Dose to right kidney = 3,280 Rad, to right renal artery = 3,150 Rad, to left renal artery = 1,050 Rad. Stenosis both renal arteries. In addition, chronic glomerulonephritis

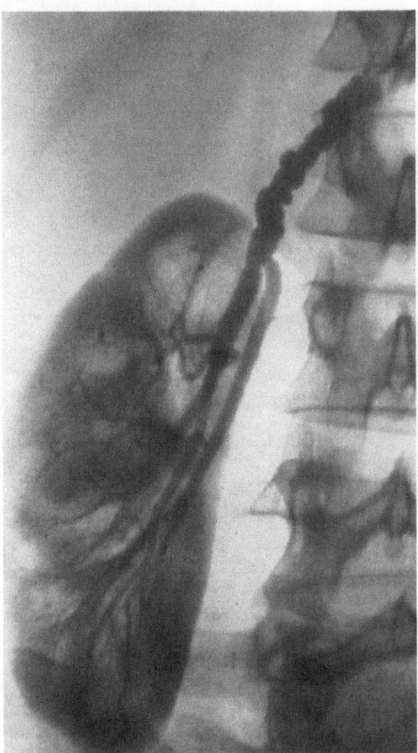

Fig. 218. Fibromuscular hyperplasia in the right renal artery to mobile kidney

disease and that it was commonly of greater severity on the right side than on the left in patients with bilateral disease. The authors suggest that ptosis may play a role in at least aggravating the disease process. KINCAID *et al.* (1968) found that the disease affects predominantly young adults and that it occurs in women more than four times as frequently

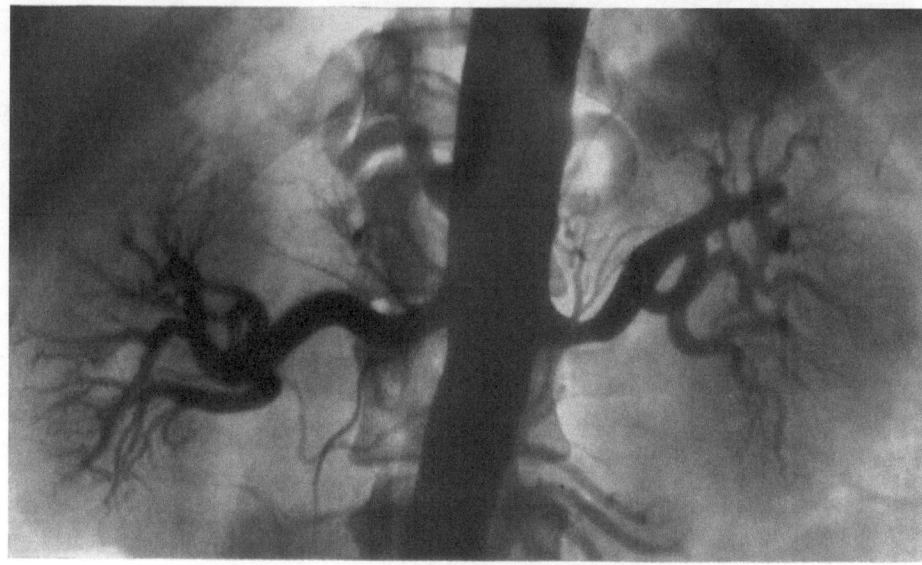

a

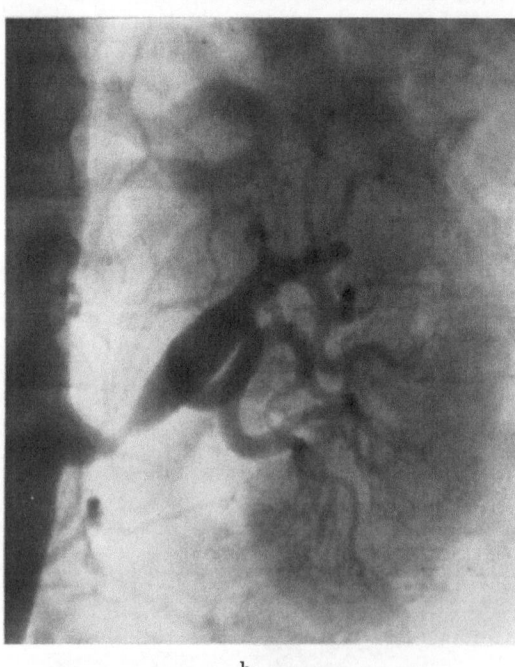

b

Fig. 219. Development of stenosis in renal artery. a) Slight stenosis in main renal artery on left side. b) Thirteen months later: stenosis has markedly increased and post-stenotic dilatation is developing

as in men. The authors classify the lesions as multifocal, focal, and tubular. In 12 out of 84 patients with multifocal disease, aneurysms had formed and renal artery dissection was present in five of a total of 125 patients, renal artery occlusion in five patients, and rena infarction in 13 patients. Involvement of arteries other than the renal arteries is occasionally seen.

Repetitive studies of different types of stenosing arterial lesions have been made by MEANEY et al. (1968) with intervals of six months to ten years in 91 hypertensive patients with arteriosclerotic (39 cases) and non-arteriosclerotic (52 cases) lesions of the renal artery. The non-arteriosclerotic lesions were medial fibroplasia with aneurysms, subadventitial fibroplasia, intimal fibroplasia, and fibromuscular hyperplasia. In 10 of the 39 arteriosclerotic arteries, the stenosis increased and thrombosis occurred in four cases (Fig. 219). In the other group progress occurred in only four cases. KINCAID et al. (1968), however, found lesions develop significantly in six out of 16 repeat examinations in fibroplasia.

Arteriosclerotic changes occur progressively in patients as a result of aging, increasing markedly in very old patients. Alteration in the arcuate arteries is said to express the process of aging more frequently and invariably than other vascular changes, and these alterations appear to progress in a centripetal pattern in the kidney. Smaller peripheral vascular changes thus precede abnormalities in the larger, more central vessels (DAVIDSON et al., 1969).

Dissection of the artery may occasionally be seen in connection with stenosis.

Mention should be made here of lesion in the arterial wall and dissection caused by the tip of the catheter and the contrast injection in renal angiography. Such subintimal injection of contrast medium can cause a slight to complete block of the passage through the artery. The subintimal fluid is usually rapidly absorbed and passage re-established.

II. Arterial aneurysms

Arterial aneurysms may be true or false. The latter are due to rupture of an artery and consist of hematomas in a connective tissue capsule and may assume considerable proportions. True aneurysms consist of local widening involving the entire arterial wall. They are small, usually less than one centimeter in diameter, most frequently rounded, but

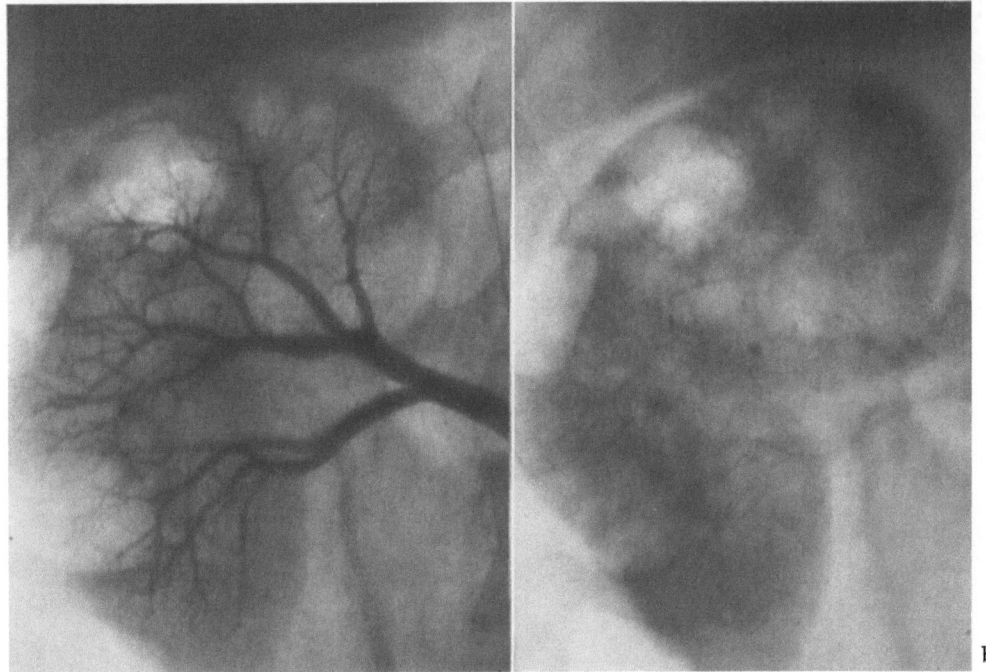

a   b

Fig. 220. Multiple small arterial aneurysms throughout the kidney. a) Arterial phase. b) Late arterial phase: some aneurysms still filled with contrast medium. Clinical diagnosis = polyangiitis nodosa

occasionally fusiform. Sometimes, however, they may be fairly large and irregular. Aneurysms may be single or multiple. Fairly large aneurysms are most often single, but two aneurysms in the same kidney is not a rare phenomenon; cases have been reported with four aneurysms of this type in the same kidney (ACKER *et al.*, 1962). Aneurysms may be bilateral, but this is a rare phenomenon. However, an incidence of five cases of bilateral aneurysms out of seven cases has been reported by EDSMAN (1957). Small aneurysms in great numbers throughout the kidney can be seen in polyangiitis nodosa (FLEMING and STERN, 1965) and in connection with rheumatic disease (Fig. 220).

Aneurysms may arise in the main renal artery and in a supplementary artery. They are usually seen in age groups above 50 years. Renal artery aneurysms are relatively rare and much less common than aneurysms in the splenic artery, for example.

The false aneurysm is often traumatic and consists of a hematoma communicating with an arterial lumen. Small traumatic aneurysms may entirely resemble true aneurysms, however. True aneurysms have the same causes as aneurysms elsewhere. Their incidence, pathologic anatomy, etc., have been described thoroughly by ABESHOUSE (1951). NEWBIT and CRENSHAW (1956) write: "Although renal artery aneurysms are rare, the prognosis of the untreated case is so extremely grave that the practicing urologist should acquaint himself with the entity." Mycotic aneurysms are the result of an infected embolus. CLARK, MCNAMARA and PALUBINSKAS (1972) report a case of mycotic aneurysm due to an infection with staphylococcus aureus in the kidney and review the literature on this lesion.

According to La Place's law, an aneurysm increasing in size and with a corresponding thinning of the wall shows an increasing risk of rupture.

Plain radiography, urography and angiography

Aneurysms often calcify and then appear as irregular, more or less distinct crescent-shaped or circular calcifications 1—3 cm in diameter. The calcifications are seen as a ring, with a small defect corresponding to the neck of the aneurysm, *i.e.* its connection with the renal artery. Other types of fragmentation may also occur, however, since the wall of the

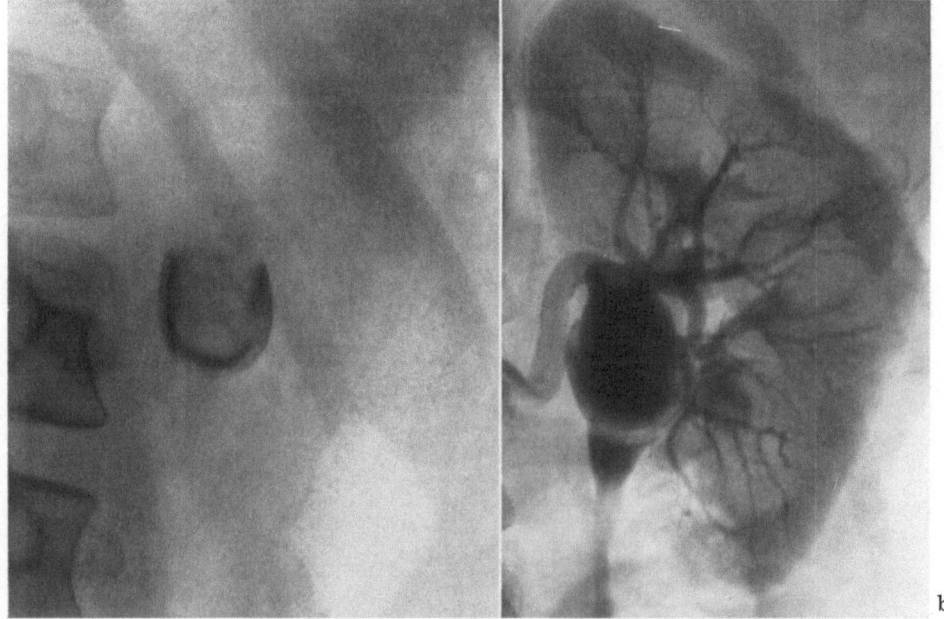

a   b

Fig. 221. Large arterial aneurysm. a) Plain roentgenogram: The calcification is open cranially, corresponding to wide communication with main renal artery. b) Arteriogram: contrast filling of aneurysm

aneurysm is irregularly calcified and calcium plaques lying in different planes can be partly superimposed upon one another. The calcifications, which may be large, are usually situated outside, but close to the kidney (Figs. 221, 222). Occasionally, however, they are seen within the kidney. They may occasionally be fairly long and assume the shape of irregular tubes. A calcified aneurysm in the renal artery has the same appearance as a calcified aneurysm in the splenic artery, which is much more common and therefore well known to the radiologist. Coexistent aneurysm calcifications may be seen in the renal artery and in the splenic artery. In the presence of aneurysm arteriosclerotic calcifications are often seen also in other vessels, usually in the lumbar aorta. On suitable projection, it is always easy to determine the relation of the calcifications to the kidney. Stereoscopy is unnecessary, as is tomography. BOIJSEN and KÖHLER (1963) reported on a material from our department of 12 patients with aneurysms in whom calcifications were seen in four cases. In two of these the entire wall excluding the neck of the aneurysm was calcified. In the third case the

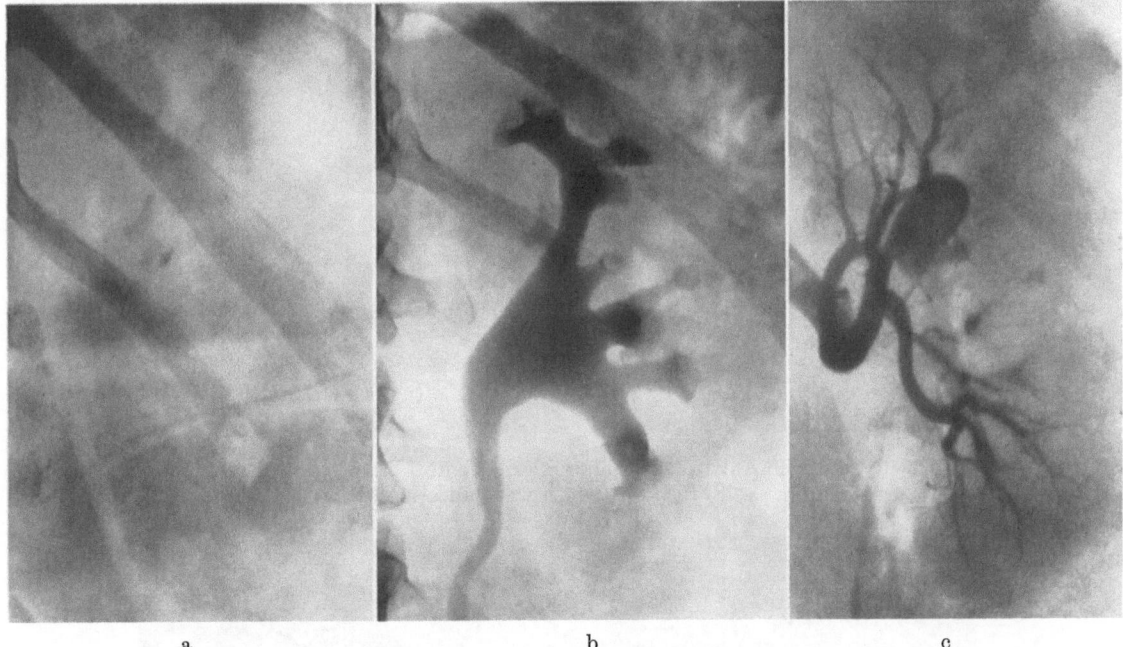

a   b   c

Fig. 222. Arterial aneurysm. a) Plain roentgenogram: Irregular uncharacteristic calcification. b) Urogram: Calcification is localized outside the kidney pelvis. c) Arteriogram: filling of aneurysm corresponding to calcification

calcification was irregular and fairly small, while in the fourth case the mural calcification resembled a renal calculus. Calcification may be seen in an aneurysm on one side, whereas an aneurysm in the other kidney may be uncalcified.

In urography and pyelography the calcifications will be seen adjacent to the renal pelvis and will often cause an indentation in the latter, usually in the upper medial part of the renal pelvis because the renal artery always enters the sinus in this region. The indentation may be of the same type as that caused by a bend in a tortuous artery. In exceptional cases it may be tumor-like, however (MATHE, 1948; TIBKANNAN, 1955). Changes in the renal parenchyma can occasionally be seen concomitant with aneurysm, consisting of a local scar formation or generalized reduction of parenchyma. The parenchymal changes, especially in traumatic aneurysms, may be so marked as to cause complete cessation of excretion of contrast medium.

Angiography is naturally the rational diagnostic procedure to demonstrate aneurysms. The shape and size of the aneurysm can be demonstrated, as well as possible thrombosis in the aneurysm. Usually the aneurysm is of the saccular type, but fusiform aneurysms with a fairly long extension in an arterial branch are not rare. They may be very irregular. Contrast blood may be retained in the aneurysm for a few seconds.

Aneurysm must be distinguished from post-stenotic dilatation, which can occur in the renal artery, as in any other artery. This type of dilatation is occasionally called jet aneurysm.

As mentioned above, aneurysms are often calcified. This is by no means always the case, however. Arterial aneurysms not demonstrable in plain roentgenograms or producing no filling defect in pyelograms are discovered, often accidentally, at renal angiography performed for some specific purpose (Fig. 223).

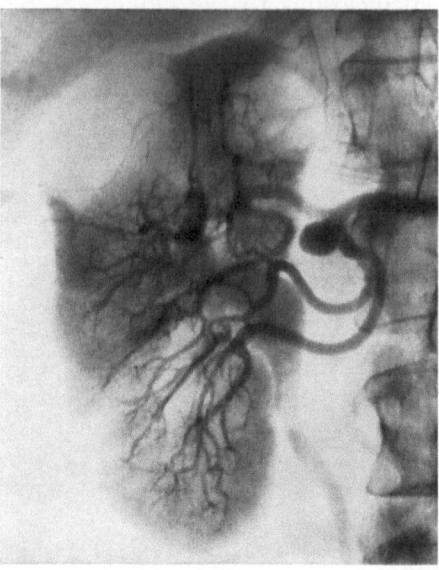

Fig. 223. Arterial aneurysm in bifurcation between dorsal and ventral branches of renal artery (in addition to cysts in upper pole of kidney, which was indication for angiography)

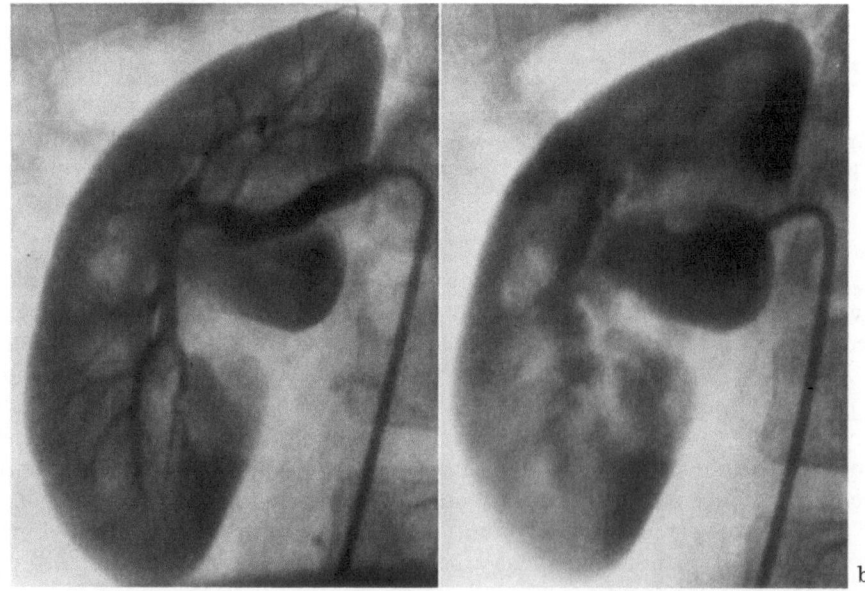

Fig. 224. False aneurysm. Several punctures of right kidney were made. At urography one month later an expansivity in the kidney was noted. At angiography (because of the latter) a large irregular aneurysm was seen corresponding to origin of dorsal branch of renal artery. a) Arterial phase. b) Nephrographic phase: aneurysm still filled with contrast blood

It may be concluded that an aneurysm need not be calcified and that a calcified aneurysm on one side may be accompanied by an uncalcified aneurysm on the other side and that renal angiography is, of course, the most rational diagnostic method. Aortic renal angiography or bilateral selective angiography is thus always indicated if arterial aneurysm is suspected because of pain or hematuria, or if a calcified aneurysm is found on one side.

III. Arteriovenous anastomoses and fistulae

Arteriovenous communications may be congenital or acquired. The congenital arteriovenous aneurysm or hemangioma is a rare phenomenon, usually with small changes

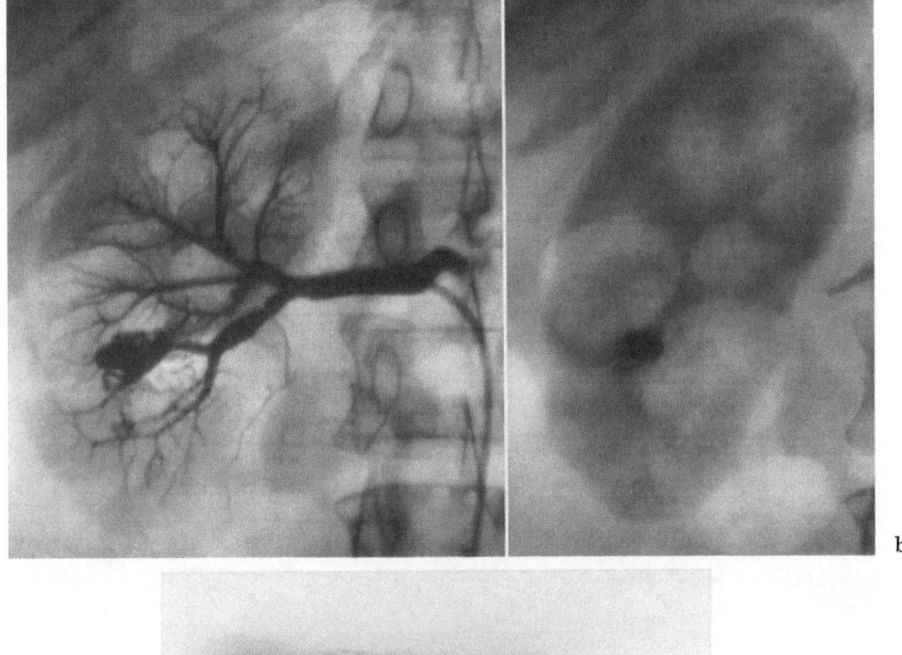

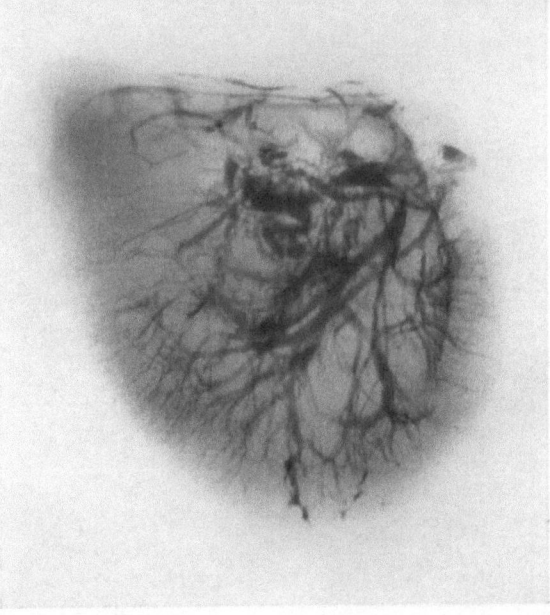

Fig. 225. Arteriovenous aneurysm. At acute urography because of right-sided renal colic and hematuria, stasis on right side was found. Pyelography: blocking of lower branch of kidney pelvis. Suspicion of tumor. Angiography: a) Arterial phase: dorsal branch of renal artery is somewhat widened. Filling of arteriovenous aneurysm.
b) Nephrographic phase: aneurysm still filled. c) Partial nephrectomy. Arteriography of specimen

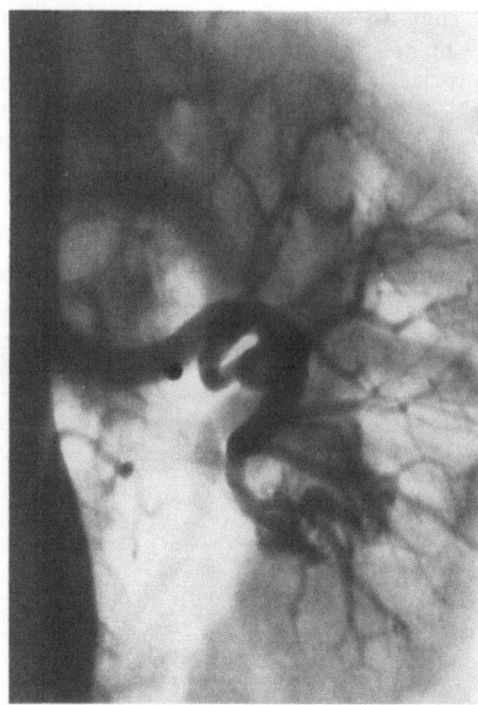

Fig. 226. Arteriovenous aneurysm, 2 cm in diameter, lower pole, left kidney

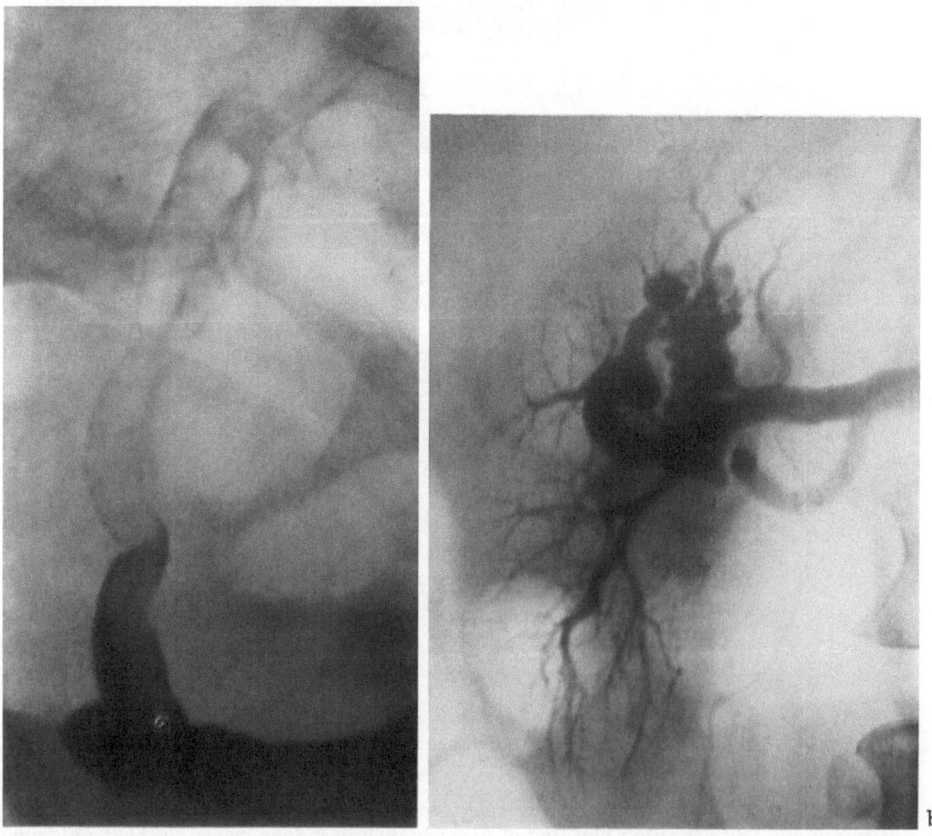

a
b

Fig. 227. Large racemose hemangioma in right kidney. Acute renal colic with marked hematuria. a) At urography: large blood clot in right ureter. b) Angiography performed because of the latter

consisting of a net of thin, irregular arteries, and may be seen in connection with pyelone-phritis (Fig. 225, 226). A hemangioma may be fairly large, however (Fig. 227). We have had a case where at urography a marked displacement laterally of the lower part of the kidney pelvis was seen, with an even impression in the confluence and lower branch, medi-ally. The expansive lesion was assumed to be a tumor or cyst. At renal angiography, however, a large arteriovenous aneurysm, a hemangioma, was found. (The same kidney, as it happened, harbored a small renal carcinoma in the upper pole, which could not be seen in plain films or at urography). The hemangioma may be very small and may be loca-lized at the tip of the papilla. Hemangiomas of this type are difficult to demonstrate angio-graphically. Thus Andersson et al. (1967) described eight cases out of which five could

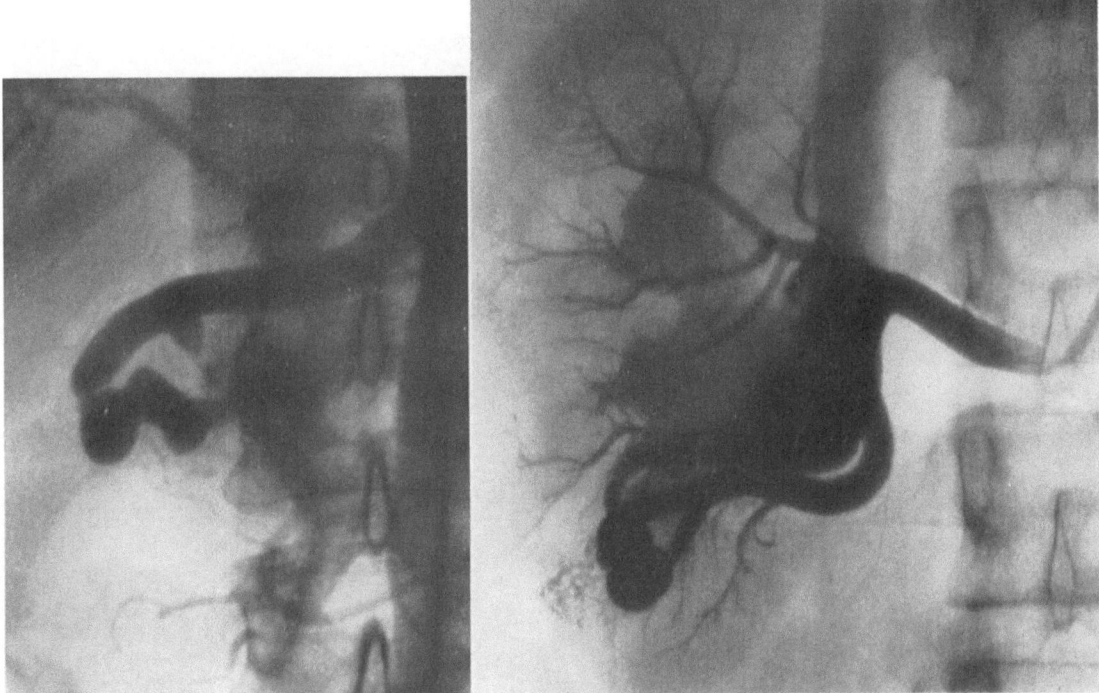

Fig. 228   Fig. 229

Fig. 228. Large arteriovenous fistula after nephrectomy

Fig. 229. Large arteriovenous fistula due to percutaneous needle biopsy 2 years previously

not be demonstrated angiographically. All of these hemangiomas were less than 10 mm in diameter and of the capillary type with very thin vessels.

Acquired arteriovenous fistulae are a common occurrence nowadays. Their origin may be traumatic, the trauma being most commonly iatrogenic, related either to operation or to needle biopsy. They may also be caused by rupture of an arterial aneurysm into a vein, by an organized hematoma connecting artery and vein, or rupture in connection with blunt trauma to the kidney. They may result from a penetrating trauma, for example a bullet wound. A very slight trauma is sufficient to cause arteriovenous fistulae in pathologic renal parenchyma, for example polycystic disease (Chisholm, 1966).

Large arteriovenous fistulae are seen in surgery as a sequela of a nephrectomy (Fig. 228). Schwartz et al. (1955) described a case with an arteriovenous connection between the stump of the renal artery and the renal vein five years after nephrectomy.

The most common cause, however, is needle biopsy (Fig. 229). The first description of angiographic diagnosis of arteriovenous fistulae related to renal biopsy came from our department (BOIJSEN and KÖHLER, 1962) and the same year another report was presented by FERNSTRÖM and LINDBLOM. A large number of reports have followed (see literature survey in EKELUND and LINDHOLM, 1971). The latter authors report on arteriovenous fistulae in eight patients in a material of 1464 renal angiographies. All the patients had been subjected to percutaneous renal biopsy. In an angiographic material consisting of 140 cases where selective renal angiography was performed immediately before and after biopsy LUNDSTRÖM (1971) found arteriovenous fistulae in 22 cases. It is noteworthy that none of these cases had clinical signs, not even murmur or thrill over the kidney. In addition, in several cases, a local disturbance of the blood flow was seen as a small ischemic zone surrounding the puncture site. In a number of cases perirenal hematomas were produced by the biopsy procedure (see chapter on injury to the kidney).

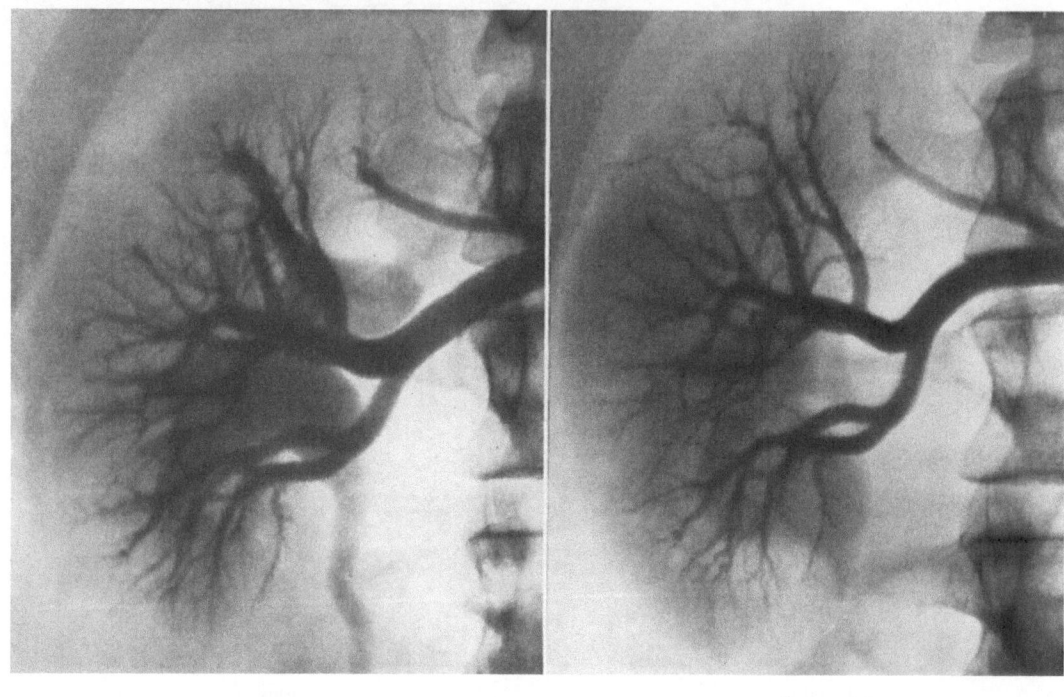

a   b

Fig. 230. a) Arteriovenous fistula in upper part of right kidney 10 days after percutaneous needle biopsy (glomerulonephritis). b) Angiography 16 months later: fistula now closed

There is a relationship between the frequency of fistulae and the time interval between biopsy and angiography, with a great number of fistulae close to the time of biopsy. This means that arteriovenous fistulae may close spontaneously (Fig. 230, 231). Such spontaneous closure has been reported by BENNET and WIENER 1965), NILSON and ROSS (1967), EKELUND and LINDHOLM (1971). HALPERN (1969) has reported five cases of spontaneous closure of fistulae caused by trauma other than biopsy.

EKELUND (1971) has studied the tendency to spontaneous closure of renal arteriovenous fistulae experimentally in rabbits. Repeat angiography two months after kidney puncture in 20 rabbits with proved fistulae revealed closure in 14 cases (70 %), indicating that treatment of such fistulae should be primarily conservative.

EKELUND (1971) suggests a relation between arteriovenous aneurysm and bleeding in connection with biopsy, and therefore recommends prevention of bleeding by the use of fibrinolytic inhibitors given to the patient before biopsy. In an experimental study in

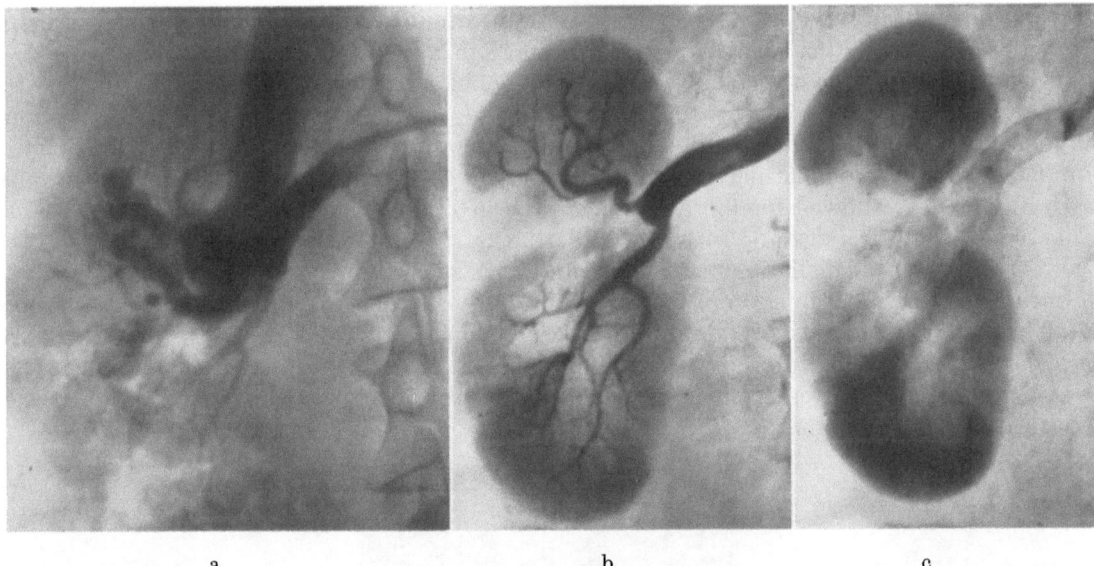

a   b   c

Fig. 231. a) Large arteriovenous fistula after percutaneous needle biopsy. b) and c) Post-operative conditions after extirpation of fistula

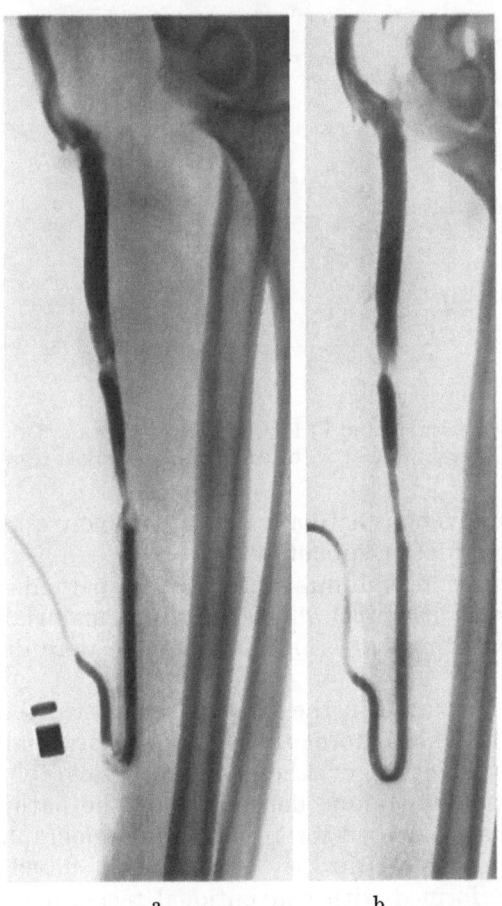

a   b

Fig. 232. Arteriovenous shunt in forearm. Contrast medium injected into the venous half of the shunt. To the left: after conventional de-clotting but before streptokinase infusion, clot obstructing lumen at the teflon tip. To the right: one day later after streptokinase infusion, complete disappearance of clotting

rabbits, anti-fibrinolytic premedication with tranexamic acid (Cyclocaprone) had a significant effect upon fistula formation, with a marked decrease in frequency.

Studies of renal flow in cases with arteriovenous fistulae were made in experimental animals and in human patients by Ekelund et al. (1971). The course of arteriovenous fistulae after biopsy could be studied closely with repeated angiography and dye-dilution examinations, and in older fistulae the shunt flow could be estimated. Pharmaco-angiography with angiotensin allowed for increased accuracy in diagnosing fistulae. The smallest fistulae could be detected only with the dye-dilution technique.

Certain types of malignant renal tumors which may show considerable arteriovenous shunting may be mentioned here from a differential-diagnostic point of view (see chapter O). These may in this respect resemble arteriovenous aneurysms in the brain, which are occasionally difficult to differentiate from malignant tumor, especially glioblastoma multiforme with marked arteriovenous shunting and cerebral metastases from a highly vascularized renal carcinoma.

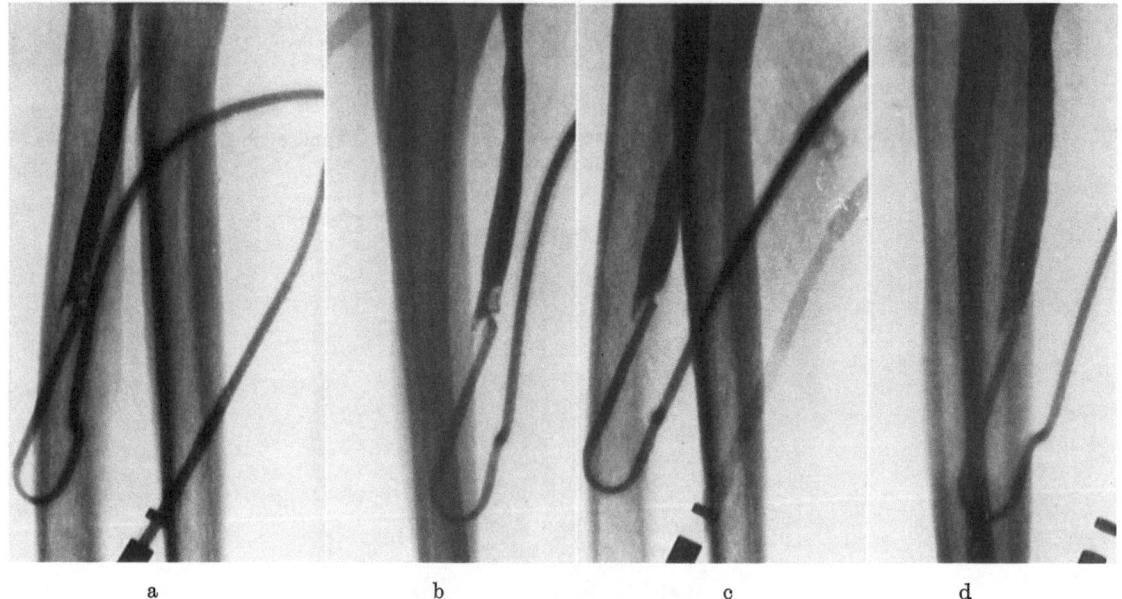

a   b   c   d

Fig. 233. Shunt for dialysis in forearm. a) and b) Frontal and lateral view, local thrombosis. c) and d) Corresponding projection after treatment with streptokinase. Marked regression of thrombosis

A special type of arteriovenous fistula is that operatively established for hemodialysis. Such a fistula may be external or subcutaneous.

Extracorporeal arteriovenous shunts were used in patients by Alwall et al. (1949) but did not come into wider use until all-silastic shunt material was available (Quinton et al., 1960). Subcutaneous direct arteriovenous fistulae were designed by Brescia et al. (1966).

The shunts are usually placed in the forearm, in most cases distally, occasionally in the lower leg. They may be placed more centrally in the brachial or femoral artery, especially in children. Because of clotting or other trouble, angiography may be indicated (Figs. 232, 233). The angiographic technique depends upon the nature of the problem and is mainly of the same type as that used for all kinds of angiography of peripheral vessels.

In open shunts the vessels are directly accessible; in closed shunts arteriography or phlebography may be performed with conventional technique (Hurwich, 1968). In our material the most common indication for shuntography is suspected clotting. If such clotting has been established, control examinations after rinsing or treatment with streptokinase, for example, may be indicated.

IV. Emboli and thrombosis in the renal artery

Autopsy studies have shown that emboli in the renal artery are not uncommon in cardiac disease, primarily rheumatic heart disease with atrial fibrillation and arteriosclerotic cardiovascular disease (HALPERN, 1967). The infarction is usually small and causes only mild clinical symptoms. When the embolus is somewhat larger, especially if it obstructs the entire renal artery, acute symptoms occur. In such cases roentgen examination in the acute stage is occasionally performed because the clinical picture of the patient is that of renal colic or of an acute abdominal attack of unknown origin. The kidney may be enlarged and surrounded by edema. Contrast excretion during urography is impaired or has ceased.

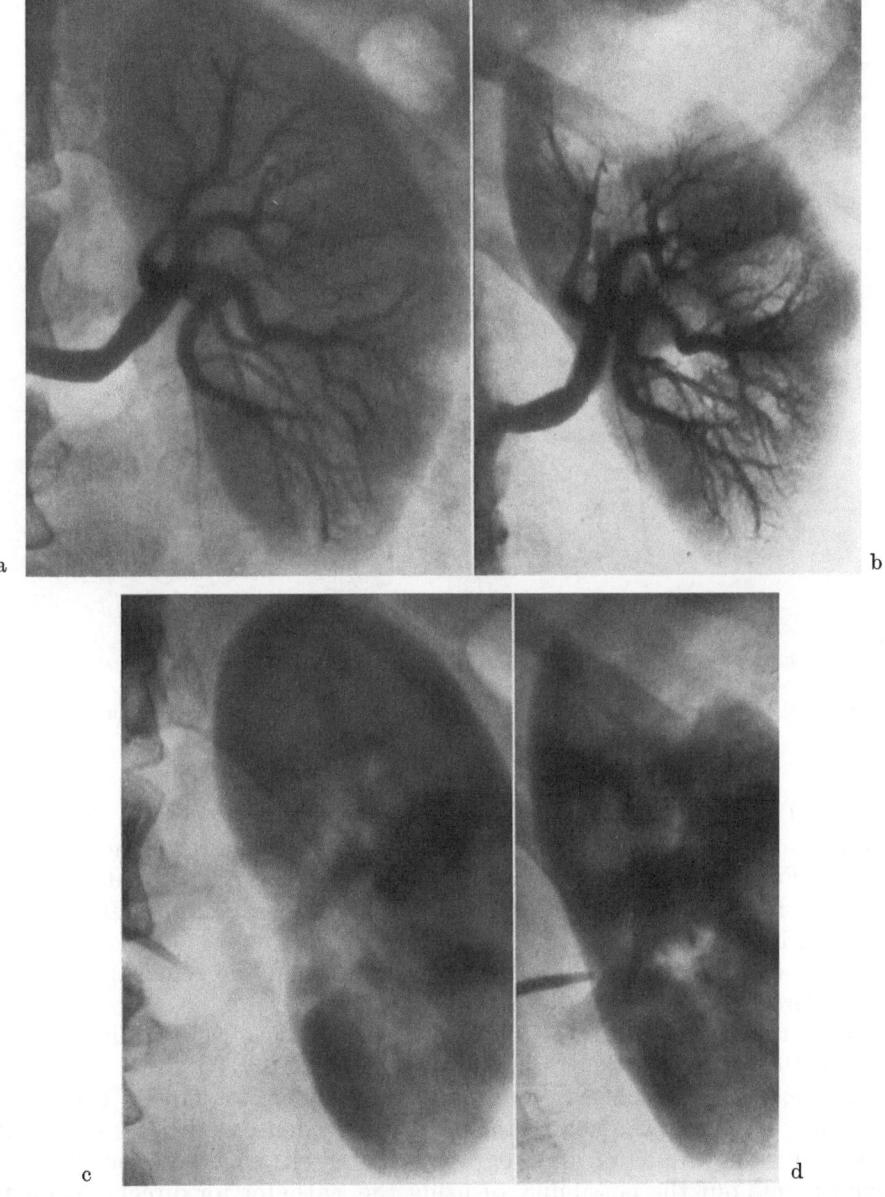

Fig. 234. Embolus in branch of renal artery caused by clot formation in catheter in renal angiography. a) Angiogram, arteriographic phase: first injection: normal conditions; b) second injection: embolus in second branch directed cranially. c) and d) Corresponding nephrographic phases. In d) large filling defect in cranial kidney pole corresponding to field of nutrition by embolized branch

If the infarction is small, the outline of the kidney after the lesion has healed will sometimes show an indentation at the site of the infarction. At renal angiography small indentations in the outline of the kidney are seen in the nephrographic phase due to scarring after the infarctions. If the infarction involves the entire kidney, the roentgenologic course is characteristic: the kidney, which is initially somewhat enlarged, decreases progressively in size and becomes a small, shrunken kidney. At urography the excretion is impaired. At pyelography the renal pelvis is shown to be of ordinary shape and to diminish with the reduction in the size of the kidney. LIEDHOLM (1944) described a pathognomonic triad allowing diagnosis of complete block by embolus of a renal artery, namely no excretion of contrast urine at urography, progressive reduction in the size of the kidney, and normal retrograde pyelogram. It should be pointed out that infection often supervenes and causes considerable change in both the kidney and renal pelvis.

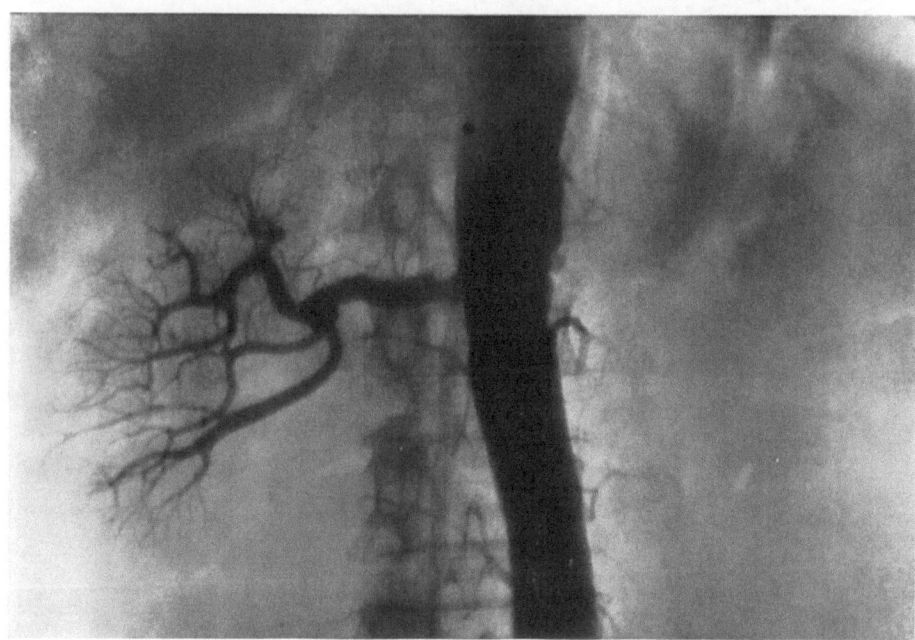

Fig. 235. Complete block by embolus of left renal artery in patient with cardiac arythmia. In addition, marked arteriosclerotic changes

The rational method for diagnosing embolus is renal angiography. This method can be used to demonstrate either complete block of the renal artery or incomplete block of the blood flow (Figs. 234, 235, 236). Marked vascular constriction is usually seen in branches distal to an incomplete block. An embolus or several emboli may also be localized in more peripheral branches.

An embolus is often situated in the ventral branch of the renal artery because this branch is the direct extension of the main renal artery.

A clot formation in or on the catheter may occasionally cause embolization of a branch peripherally in the kidney at renal angiography (Fig. 234).

For instance, in connection with trauma to the kidney, a complete thrombosis of the renal artery may occur. In the acute stage a marked edema is usually seen and there is complete loss of kidney function at urography. Later on, shrinkage occurs.

HALPERN points out the possibility of using the catheter for direct intra-arterial perfusion of the renal artery with heparin in cases of acute renal artery embolus. In addition, a vaso-dilating drug such as papaverine can be used to counteract the effects of renal vasospasm.

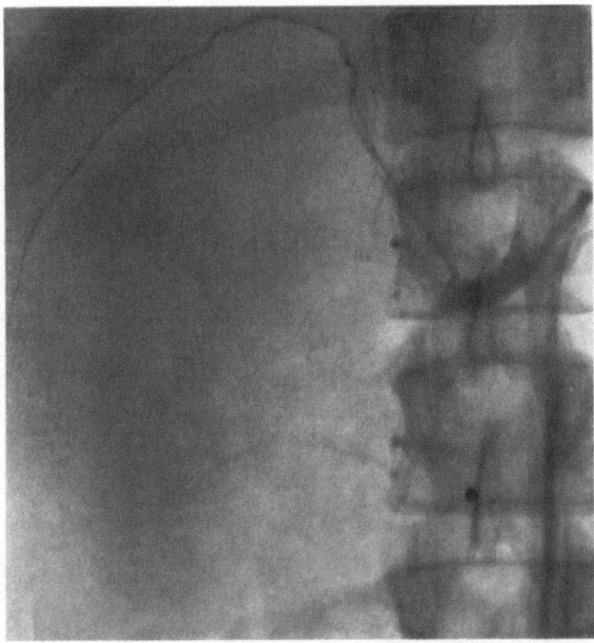

Fig. 236. Complete right-sided arterial stenosis due to blunt trauma to the abdomen

Angiography is valuable not only in the diagnosis of an embolisation of the renal artery or its branches but also as a check procedure after attempted thrombolysis (Böttger et al., 1971).

V. Thrombosis of the renal vein

(Figs. 237—240)

Obstruction of the renal vein by tumor has been described in Chapter O.

Renal vein thrombosis may develop in the same way as thrombosis elsewhere. It is uncommon and when it occurs may be unilateral or bilateral and is usually a serious complication in an already serious disease. It is more common in children than in adults and is associated with infarction of the kidney. The patient experiences severe pain in the flank and runs a temperature. This infarction has sometimes been demonstrated at roentgen examination during an acute attack of pain by the finding that the kidney was enlarged, that at urography the excretion of contrast urine was absent or delayed, and that large filling defects could be seen in the renal pelvis due to blood clots (Eikner and Bobeck, 1956). This type of thrombosis is said to indicate immediate nephrectomy. If nephrectomy is not performed, the kidney will end up as a small atrophic kidney.

Other types of renal thrombosis with a less acute and less serious course have been revealed through angiography. In such cases the thrombosis may give an incomplete block or the thrombosed vein may be recanalized. In many cases collaterals also develop. Normally the kidney is drained by small subcapsular veins to intrarenal veins which drain into the main renal vein. The subcapsular veins anastomose with a venous net in the perirenal fat and this vein net is in communication with the adrenal veins, the gonadal veins, and the ureteric veins. This venous system can take over flow in blockage of the main renal vein. It must be noted that the left kidney has somewhat better collateral conditions than the right kidney because the gonadal and adrenal veins on the left side empty into the renal vein, on the right side, directly into the caval vein.

Hellekant and Kaude (1972) have reported on our material of renal vein thrombosis, 24 cases, three of which had traumatic cause. One was iatrogenic, caused by prolonged catheterization in connection with a clinico-physiologic study.

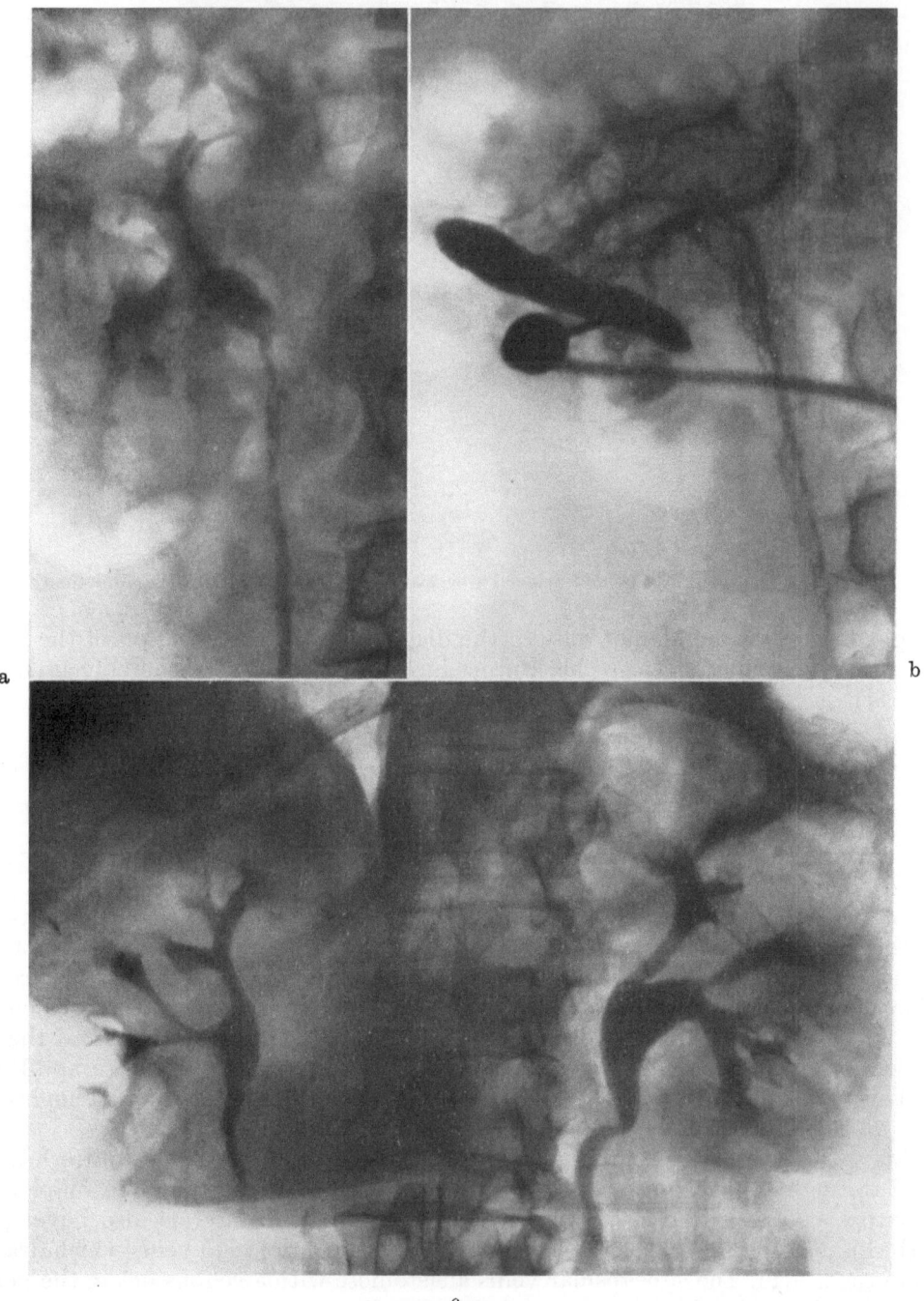

Fig. 237. Renal vein thrombosis. a) Urography: marked indentations in right kidney pelvis and ureter. b) Trans-renal phlebography: complete block of renal vein and marked filling of venous collaterals in kidney and along ureter. c) In another patient: marked indentations in renal pelvis and ureter, right side. d) Phlebography: marked venous collaterals

Transparietal renal phlebography in the left kidney was used by GILSANZ *et al.* (1971) to study conditions of the veins in patients with a nephrotic syndrome and revealed a relative frequency of the association between obstructions of the left renal vein and the nephrotic syndrome due to primary or secondary glomerular lesions.

Thrombosis may also be seen in connection with circulatory decompensation in children.

Acute renal vein thrombosis is known as a serious complication in gastrointestinal infection and dehydration.

The kidney in acute stages is large and plump in plain films; it is of normal size and shape in later stages and is small and irregular in outline in end stages.

The excretion of contrast medium at urography may be normal. However, it is usually absent in serious thrombosis, whereas it may be delayed in partial thrombosis. Inden-

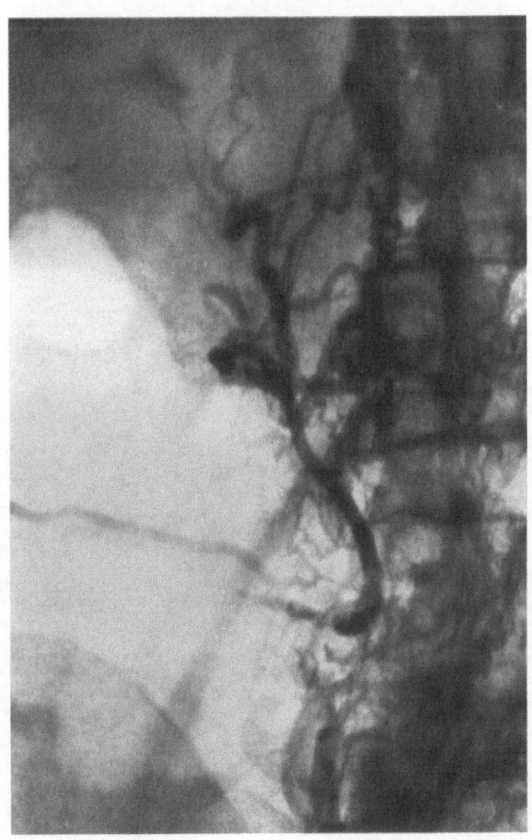

Fig. 237 d

tations on the kidney pelvis and the ureter of wide venous collaterals can be seen (Fig. 239).

A reduction in caliber of the renal artery at renal angiography was seen in 25 % of our cases and together with incomplete filling of peripheral arterial branches, a prolonged arterial phase, decreased concentration in the nephrographic phase, and reflux to the aorta at selective technique, is a sign of increased peripheral resistance in the kidney.

Collateral veins were occasionally filled. The angiographic findings were normal in connection with complete recanalization of the thrombus in two cases.

Recanalization and partial obstruction can be demonstrated at phlebography. Percutaneous transrenal phlebography can be used to demonstrate collaterals and complete block of the renal vein.

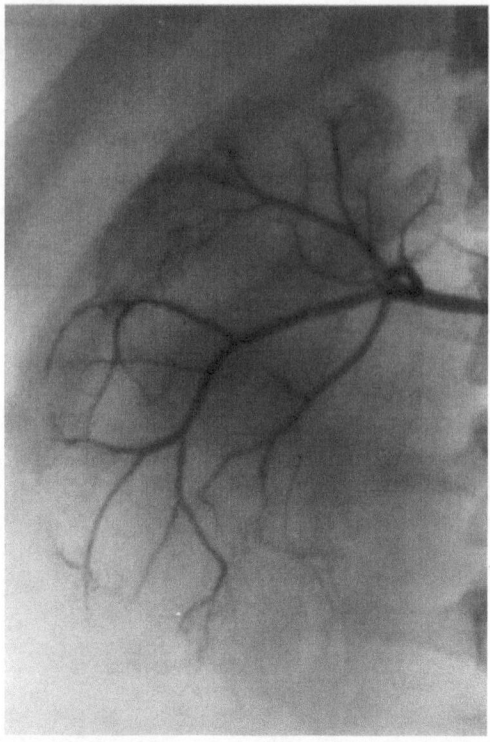

a

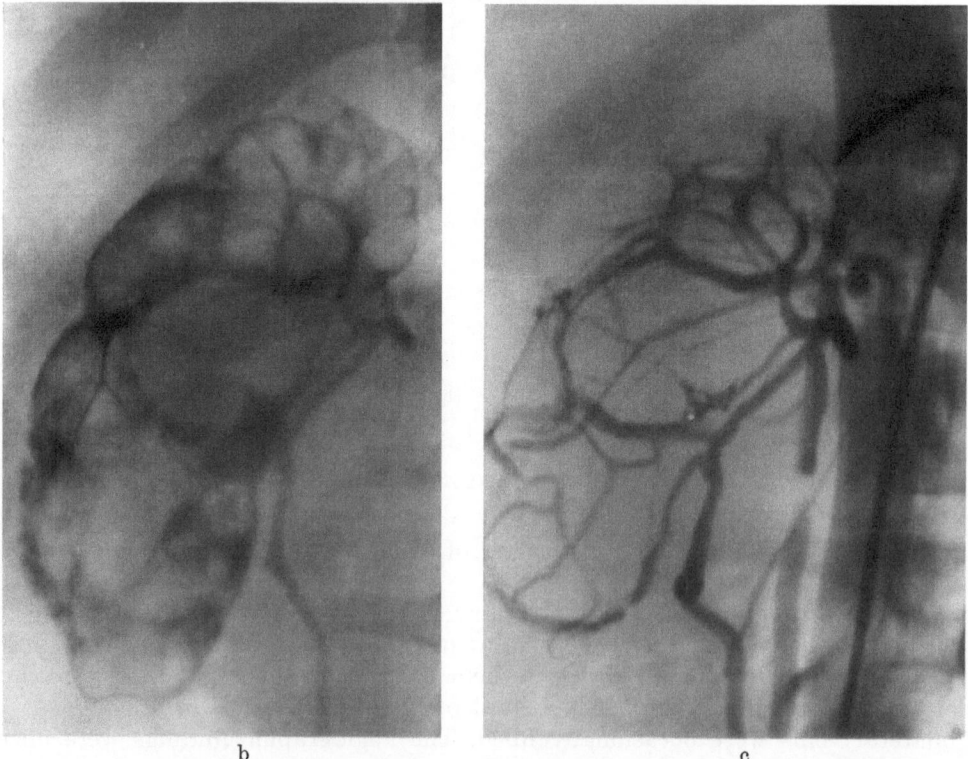

b   c

Fig. 238. Renal vein thrombosis and hydronephrosis. a) and b) Renal angiography, arterial and late nephro-
graphic-early venous phase: practically complete atrophy of parenchyma. Main venous trunk blocked. Intrarenal veins stretched. Filling of spermatic vein. c) Selective phlebography: main renal vein thin and markedly
irregular, recanalized thrombosed vein (patho-anatomically verified). Venous drainage via collaterals

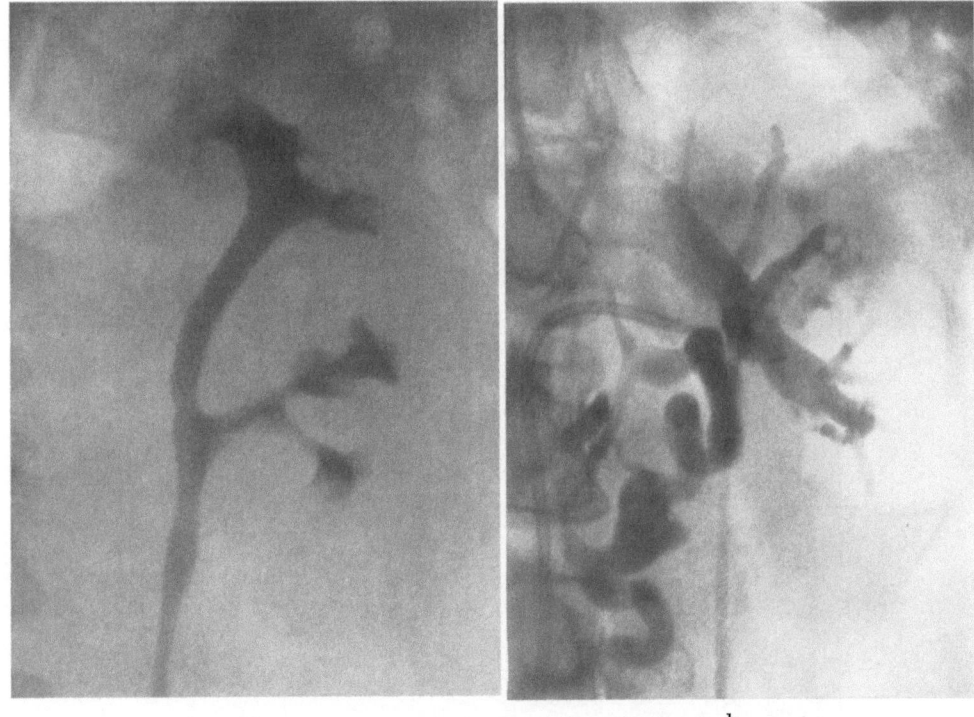

a   b

Fig. 239. Thrombosis of left renal vein. a) Urography: irregular impressions in branches and confluence of left kidney pelvis and in upper part of ureter. b) Phlebography: wide collateral veins

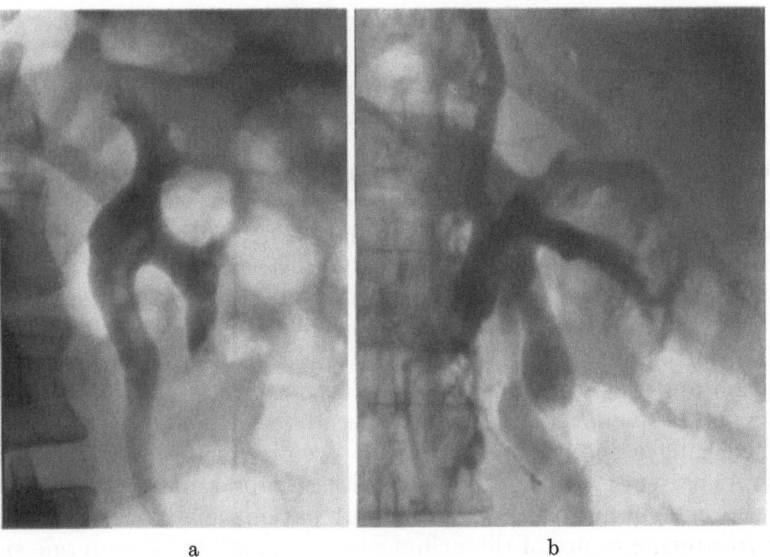

a   b

Fig. 240. Blockage of inferior caval vein. Multitude of venous collaterals. a) Urography: impressions by dilated venous branches in kidney pelvis and proximal part of left ureter. b) Phlebography: corresponding to impressions: wide, tortuous collaterals along left ureter

Varices

Varices may occasionally be seen in the kidneys. Widened veins may at urography be seen to cause filling defects or indentations in the renal pelvis and in the ureter (Fig. 239, 240, 241). The nature of these indentations can be clearly demonstrated at phlebography. Wide tortuous veins are occasionally seen in the wall of a simple cyst.

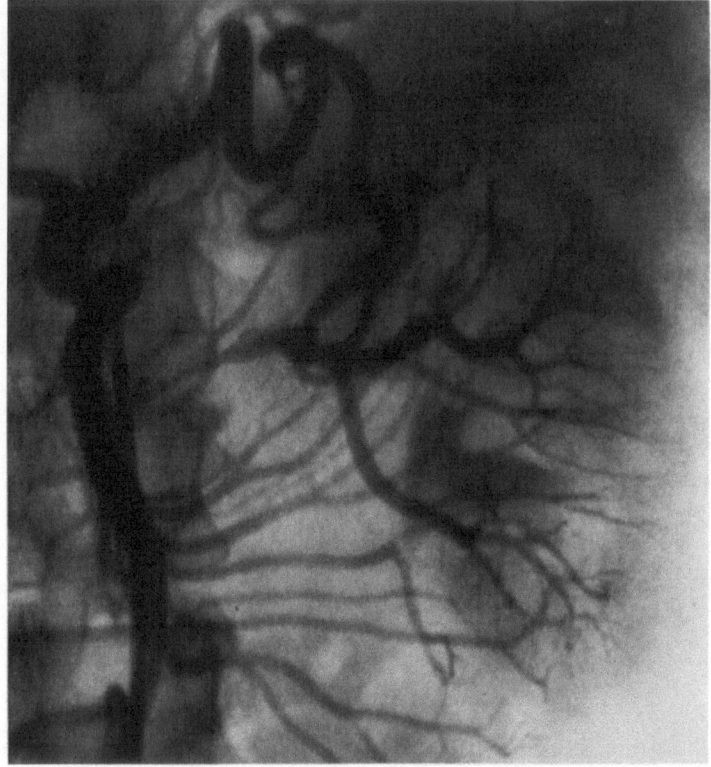

Fig. 241. Operative anastomosis between splenic artery and main renal artery on left side. Complete long stenosis of main renal artery

VI. Roentgen-diagnostics in renal hypertension

In the search for a renal genesis for hypertensive disease, several types of renal lesions may be considered. Chronic pyelonephritis is most common in our material, but other types of generalized parenchymal disease are also common. Polycystic disease, polyangiitis nodosa, healed renal rupture, radiation nephritis, chronic perirenal hematoma may also be found responsible for hypertensive disease.

Renal arterial stenosis is the lesion which attracts particular interest in this connection. It is an uncommon cause of renal hypertension in our material, as compared with chronic pyelonephritis, for example. Surgical therapy is available, however; therefore diagnosis of the condition and study of its relation to hypertensive disease is important.

The type and frequency of stenosing arterial disease have been described in previous chapters. The changes should be diagnosed, preferably and rationally with the use of angiography. As patients with hypertensive disease represent a very large group, screening tests have been used in an attempt to sort out patients with arterial stenosis.

In plain roentgenography of the urinary tract a small kidney on one side may indicate stenosis of the corresponding renal artery. Slight asymmetry in length is a frequent finding normally, but asymmetry in length of one centimeter or more may suggest renal arterial stenosis (Dahn, 1961). Amplatz (1964) reviewed 80 proved cases of renal vascular hypertension caused by unilateral renal artery stenosis and found a discrepancy in kidney size of 1.5 centimeters in only 56 % of the cases. He points out the importance of keeping in mind the fact that both kidneys may be equal in size or that the involved kidney may be even larger if duplication of the collecting system is present.

In patients suffering from arterial hypertension, the right kidney is said to assume a relatively high position (Garti and Salinger, 1969). It has also been shown (Garti *et al.*, 1971) that the level of origin of the renal arteries is significantly higher in hypertensive patients than in normal patients.

Specific modifications may be used at urography to stress a possible difference between a side with stenosis and a side with ordinary flow. The stenosis will cause diminished flow of contrast blood through the kidney. Rapid sequence films after injection of contrast will make it possible to demonstrate a slight delay in appearance of the nephrographic phase and appearance of contrast medium in the kidney pelvis. Induced diuresis with urea and saline or manite will, on the other hand, wash out excreted contrast urine more easily on the side not stenosed (AMPLATZ, 1964). Because of prolonged passage through tubules due to decrease in back pressure and a corresponding increase in reabsorbtion of water the concentration of the contrast urine on the stenotic side will be greater. This is easily seen on occasions, at the end of the urographic examination.

KANEKO (1970) in a comparison of rapid sequence urography with washout urography using manite, found that the relation between a stenotic lesion and a positive finding was better in rapid sequence urography than in washout urography. The former method was positive in 82 % of cases with stenosis of the renal artery, the latter method in 76 %.

Delay in the emptying of the renal pelvis on the stenotic side may be found at urography, because of the slower production of urine on that side, and in sequence urograms the number of ureteric contractions on the stenotic side may be seen to be less than on the other side. At urography collaterals in connection with a severe stenosis may be seen. These collaterals cause indentations in the kidney pelvis and in the ureter (THOMAS and LEVIN, 1961; HALPERN and EVANS, 1962).

WOLFE and WILSON (1971) found in animal experiments that kidneys with a moderate unilateral renal artery stenosis did not respond to renovaso-dilator drugs.

The rational method for the diagnosis of arterial changes is angiography. When angiography is used in the search for arterial stenosis in hypertensive patients, the examination should preferably first, or only, be made with aortic injection, in order to study both renal arteries. The aortic injection guarantees filling also of the part of the renal artery close to the aorta — the origin of the renal artery. A direct comparison of both sides is also possible from aortic injections with films in slight, oblique views. In addition, localized spasm in the renal artery can be avoided through aortic injection. It is well known that the catheter or the injection pressure at selective studies can cause spasm at the site of the tip of the catheter or peripheral to this. Also, an intimal lesion can occur through careless catheterization of a renal artery, causing slight, severe or complete stenosis of the renal artery. WELZER *et al.* (1961) in aortography of 821 patients, found 417 with renal arterial stenosis. Of these cases 276 were found in patients with hypertensive disease. FOLIN (1967), in reviewing a material on changes in the main trunk of the main renal artery, found arteriosclerotic stenosis in 25 patients, periadventitial fibrosis in eight, fibromuscular hyperplasia in four, and arteriitis, intimal fold, and aneurysm in one case each. (For further references, see KINCAID, 1966).

Each stenosis detected is not necessarily responsible for the hypertensive disease. The stenosis must have a hemodynamic significance. This can be evaluated by exchanging the catheter for selective angiography with a thin catheter which can be passed through the stenosis for pressure measurement over the stenotic area (AMPLATZ, 1962). Even a small pressure gradient may be significant but the gradient is usually in excess of 40 mm/Hg. If no pressure gradient is found, a lesion can be considered hemodynamically insignificant, thus indicating that no improvement in blood flow can be expected through surgery (AMPLATZ, 1964).

GÄRSTEN *et al.* (1971) draw attention to the demonstration at angiography of antegrade flow in extrarenal arteries arising distal to a renal arterial stenosis in order to evaluate the degree of hemodynamic significance.

The diminished flow through a kidney with arterial stenosis at renal phlebography causes prolonged washout time of the contrast medium in the vein (ABRAMS, 1971).

Thus it is possible with roentgen-diagnostic methods to arrive at a diagnosis of renal arterial stenosis and to a great extent also to arrive at significant conclusions as to the hemodynamic effects of a stenosis.

In connection with stenosis of the celiac axis, a steal mechanism with diversion of blood for the kidney through various adrenal collaterals to the splanchnic region may be seen (ALFIDI et al., 1972). Renal artery blood flow measurements proximal and distal to the steal have shown significant diversion of arterial bloodflow through the steal. The authors suggest this as a rare cause for renal vascular hypertension.

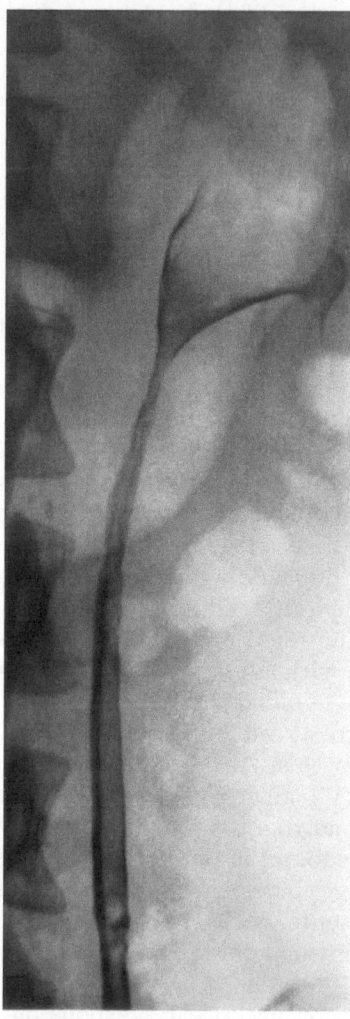

Fig. 242. Hematuria in patient with hemophilia. Kidney pelvis and ureter completely filled with coagulum

Anastomosis operations are occasionally undertaken between, for example, the splenic artery and the renal artery (Fig. 241). Renal angiography is useful in checking results of operative treatment of an arterial stenosis in these as in other procedures.

Addendum

Roentgen examination of patients with hematuria. Most cases of hematuria call for thorough roentgenologic investigation, particularly so if the hematuria is localized as coming from one ureter.

In hematuria, blood clots may form in the kidney pelvis, the ureter, and the bladder. Such blood-clot formation may fill the entire lumen (Fig. 242) and thus make it impossible to study details in the urinary pathways. Blood clot may also mimic expansivities intruding upon the lumen, or they may give a false impression of the size of a tumor in the lumen by adding to the volume of the tumor.

After hematuria has ceased, search must be concentrated on the vaguest details, such as small calcifications with low calcium content, small irregularities in the shape of the kidney and the kidney pelvis, etc. A thorough preparation of the patient is necessary and should never be omitted.

If no changes are seen in plain films with suitable projections, at pyelography or urography, or if changes are seen which do not permit a definite diagnosis, the rational diagnostic procedure in bleeding is examination of the vasculature—renal angiography. At this examination pathologic processes are often found which produce no or vague urographic symptoms. Such lesions may be vascular, for example hemangiomas, arteriovenous fistulae. Diagnosis of these is important because they may be difficult to find at an exploratory operation. If a pre-operative diagnosis is not made, nephrectomy may be necessary instead of a small resection. It must be strictly kept in mind that marked hematuria may be caused by bleeding from superficial hemangiomas smaller in size than can be detected at even a highly qualified angiographic procedure. Thus in a material of eight patients referred to above, all with solitary hemangioma in a kidney, the hemangioma could be demonstrated angiographically in only three cases, whereas the hemangioma was small (below one centimeter in diameter) and localized at the tip of a papilla in five cases.

In the examination of patients with hematuria the following rule should govern all roentgen-diagnostic procedures: Use the method with judgment and for good indications but once a decision is made to use it, it must be used to its full advantage, with every detail of the diagnostic procedure as perfect as possible.

J. Injury to kidney and ureter

The importance of diagnosing possible renal injury in connection with trauma to the trunk has increased greatly, particularly with the increasing number of traffic accidents. Roentgen examination not only plays an important role in the diagnosis, but also acts as a guide in deciding whether treatment should be active or expectant.

Opinions differ on the clinical evaluation of renal damage especially as to whether treatment should be conservative or surgical, the choice of cases for surgery, and the time for such operation. Some authors adopt a very active attitude, while others prefer to try conservative treatment as long as possible. Without assuming any definite attitude regarding these questions, it may be stated that the opinions of all except adherents of most active surgery are based to a large extent on the roentgen findings. There are two points of particular interest in the discussion of roentgen examination, namely the examination method and the time of the examination.

It should be pointed out already here that opinion as to treatment has been given a much better basis for judgment since the introduction of angiography in the examination of patients with suspected renal rupture.

The first question to be decided upon is whether or not pyelography should be performed. Many consider this examination contra-indicated on the grounds that instrumentation can cause a recurrence of hemorrhage by detaching a clot and, secondly, that the examination involves risk of infection. The question then is what information can be obtained by methods not requiring instrumentation.

There is wide agreement that the examination should be performed as soon as possible, in order that the roentgen findings may be included in the data to be considered in the decision as to type of treatment: conservative or active. This opinion is supported by the fact that renal damage often produces few symptoms during the first few hours and that symptoms from the urinary tract may be masked by symptoms from other organs, with the result that valuable time is lost before institution of treatment of possible renal lesions.

I. Classification of renal ruptures

ADAMS (1943) recognized three groups of renal ruptures:
1. contusions and the sub-groups
   a) without subcapsular hematoma and
   b) with subcapsular hematoma;
2. fracture with sub-groups
   a) incomplete and
   b) complete;
3. tears in the renal vessels or ureter.

The third type is usually associated with other severe renal injuries but may occur alone. To the last-mentioned injuries may be added post-traumatic infarction of the kidney, which may occur because of a secondary thrombosis. This consequence of trauma has received increased theoretic interest since the publication of cases in which vascular spasm was assumed to be the cause of the infarcts, and since the work of TRUETA et al. (1947) (compilation by LYNCH and LARGE, 1951). This classification is based on clinical pathological findings. Classifications based partly on roentgen findings are also available. McKAY et al. (1949) distinguishes thus between three types of renal rupture:

1. patients with intact pyelograms and clear renal and psoas contours not requiring exploration;
2. patients with any rupture of the renal collecting system or loss of renal and psoas contours requiring exploration within 72 hours;
3. patients in unresponsive or recurring shock due to rupture of the renal vascular pedicle, requiring operation as an immediate lifesaving measure.

HODGES et al. (1951) recommend the following classification:
1. minor injuries;
2. major injuries;
3. critical injuries.

Urographic or pyelographic demonstration that the pelvis and calcyceal systems are intact is the greatest single criterion for placing injuries in the minor group. To the second group are assigned cases with evidence of urinary extravasation in the retrograde pyelogram. Since perirenal hematoma belongs to the latter group, plain radiography is of importance for classification. In the group "critical injuries" urography is necessary only in order to check that the kidney on the other side is not damaged. Like all other classifications, this one is incomplete in so far as there may be evidence of extravasation without the injury's being classified as major.

The renal rupture may vary from a small capsular rupture or a medullary scratch to small or large fractures of the renal parenchyma and, further, to total contusion of the kidney or laceration of the renal pedicle. In capsular damage, possible in connection with parenchymal damage, a perirenal hematoma may develop, and may enclose the entire kidney, or it may be localized around the actual rupture of the capsule. If the capsule is intact, the hematoma may be intracapsular.

The changes that can be demonstrated roentgenographically thus are: a change in the bed of the kidney and a change in the size, shape and position of the kidney. Extravasation of contrast medium and patency of the ureter can be demonstrated at pyelography and urography. Urography also allows for evaluation of the state of renal function.

Renal angiography is a most important examination method leading to basic conclusions as to the state of the kidney parenchyma and of the kidney vasculature.

II. Plain radiography

The discussion of roentgen examination of patients with renal injury has been centered mainly on the question as to whether pyelography or urography is preferable; it appears that the valuable information available from plain radiography has not received the attention it deserves. This examination is usually made in the acute stage with the patient unprepared, so that intestinal contents may make it difficult to study the anatomy of the retroperitoneal space. Trauma may have caused local or generalized meteorism, which may make the analysis still more difficult.

A reflex skoliosis of the spine, with the concavity facing the injured side, is sometimes present. This must be remembered in the evaluation of the edge of the psoas muscle. A blurring of the edge of the psoas muscle in a case with trauma to the trunk is frequently referred to as a sign of kidney rupture. Even slight skoliosis, true or due to the position of the patient on the examination table, may, however, cause the sharp outline of the psoas muscle to disappear, and this should then not be interpreted as being due to bleeding or edema.

Injury to the tissues around the kidney causes changes that may be misinterpreted as renal damage. Laceration of muscles can, for example, cause perirenal hematoma and displace the kidney. A perirenal hematoma may be so local as to simulate a local bulge in the outline of the kidney. In the presence of a large perirenal hematoma the retroperitoneal soft tissue anatomy is blurred and an increased density is seen. The kidney can be displaced in different ways, depending upon the site and the longest diameter of the hematoma. The kidney is displaced easiest by a hematoma situated dorsally, where the capsular space is broadest and loosest, so that the kidney will be displaced ventrally. This increases the object—film distance and thereby produces an enlargement of the image of the kidney in the film. This should not be interpreted as a true enlargement of the kidney due to intracapsular hemorrhage.

If the hematoma is intrarenal, the kidney will be enlarged and plump, but well defined.

At plain radiography, fractures will also often be seen of one or more of the lower ribs or of the transverse process of one or more lumbar vertebrae. If a transverse process is fractured, a hematoma will often be seen in the psoas muscle. The lateral edge of the muscle is then well defined in its cranial part, for instance, whereas further down a soft tissue density is seen, due to hematoma. The caudal renal pole may then be displaced laterally by the hematoma, and urography is then usually necessary to demonstrate whether or not the kidney is intact.

III. Urography and pyelography

If plain radiography is possible (Figs. 243—251), urography is usually also possible. In recent years more and more authors have realized the diagnostic possibilities of urography in renal injury. It is also now widely believed that urography should be given preference and retrograde pyelography should be resorted to only if information obtained by urography is uncertain (LJUNGGREN, 1936). Critical voices have also been raised against urography, however. In 1951 HODGES et al. wrote: "Moreover, it has become increasingly apparent in this study that excretory urography, while extremely valuable in demonstrating the presence of a normally functioning kidney on the opposite side, is frequently unsatisfactory in delineating the extent of injury on the affected side." I completely agree with this view as will be evident below on discussing renal angiography.

An important advantage of urography is that information is immediately available as to whether or not the contralateral kidney is functioning. Cases are on record in which nephrectomy for renal rupture has been performed on patients with only one kidney.

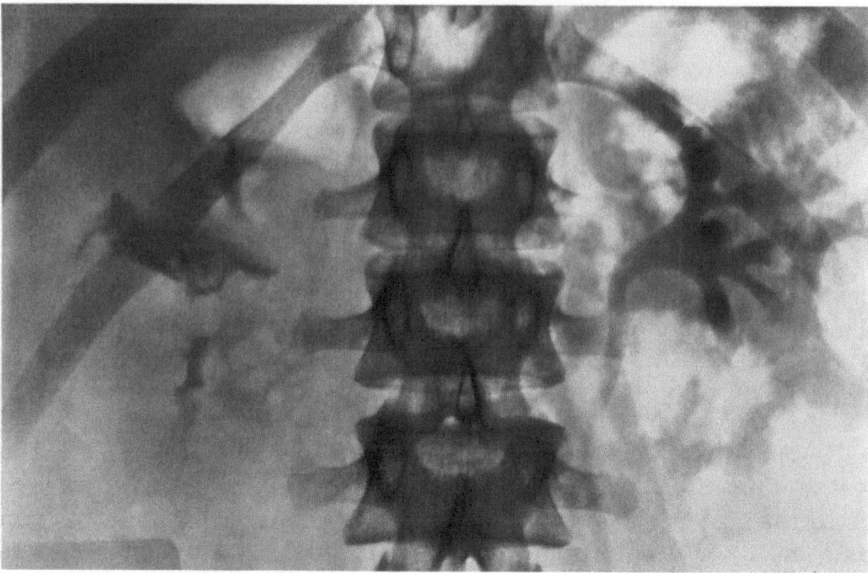

Fig. 243. Trauma to right kidney. Acute urography: from middle calyces, filling of wide rupture through kidney out to capsule

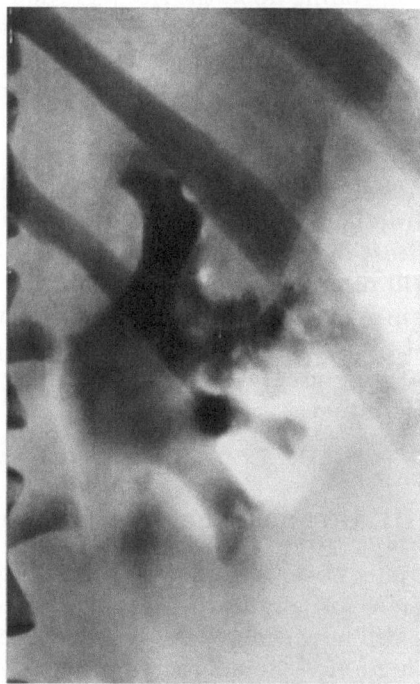

Fig. 244. Kidney fracture. Trauma to back (fall from bar during gymnastics). Hematuria. Urography 33 minutes after injection of contrast medium, no ureteric compression. Straight rupture from middle calyx to surface. Perirenal hematoma. Contrast urine escapes through rupture and spreads in sinus along adjacent parts of kidney pelvis as in sinus backflow

The urographic findings in renal injury may be divided into two groups: 1. cases where excretion is observed; 2. cases where no excretion is observed. In the latter group, which includes few of the cases of renal rupture, a clot may block excretion, or the kidney may be so severely damaged as not to function. It must be stressed in this connection that

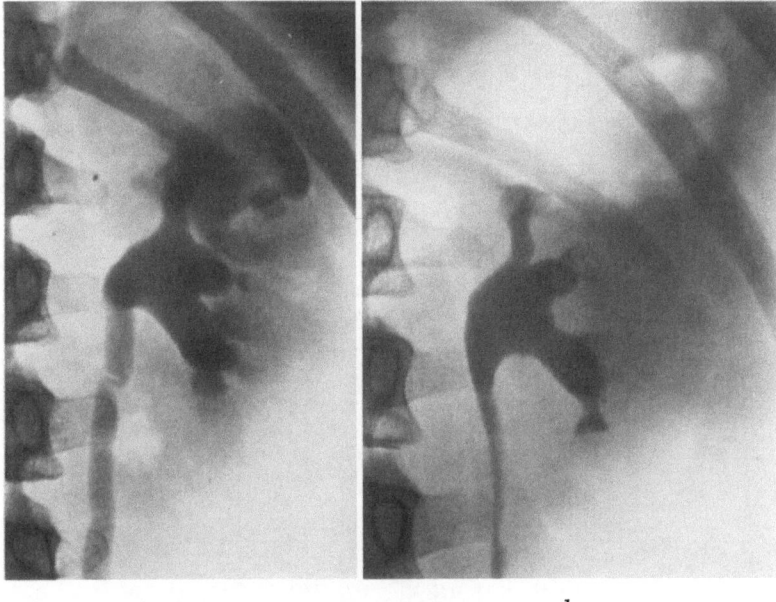

a   b

Fig. 245. 8-year-old girl. Traffic accident. a) Urography two weeks after trauma: from ruptures in cranial calyces, filling of irregular cavity in cranial part of kidney. b) Four years later: marked shrinkage of cranial pole of kidney. Otherwise normal

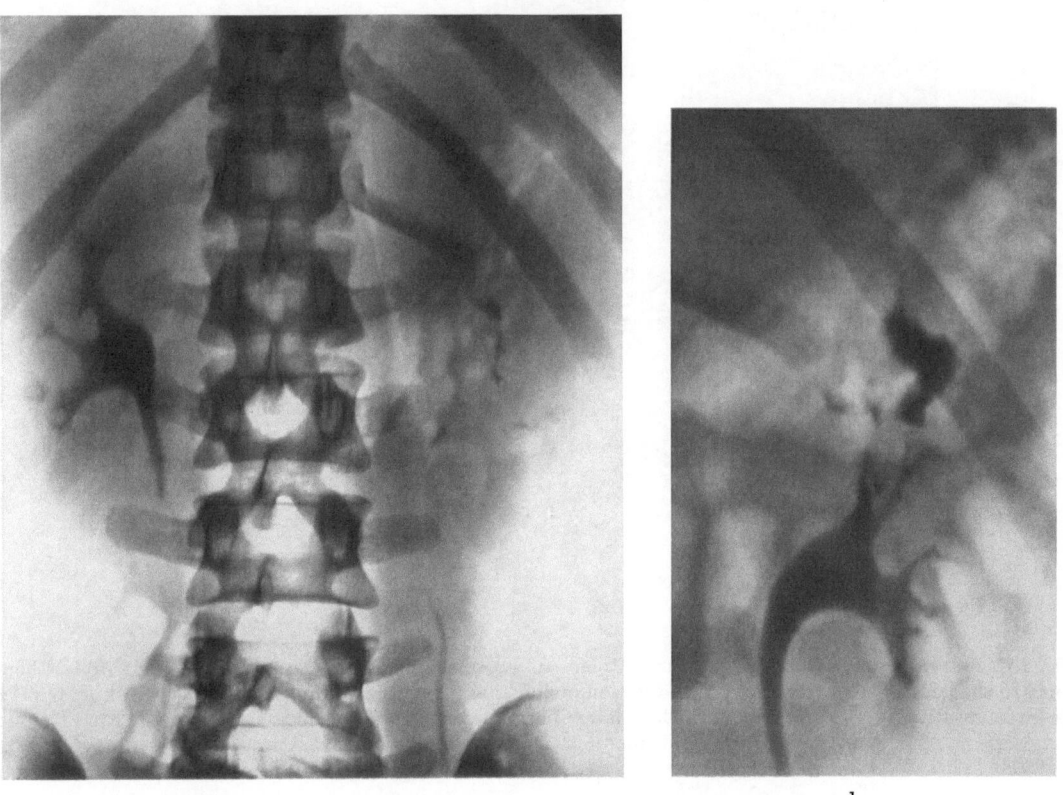

a   b

Fig. 246. Kidney rupture with intra- and extrarenal hematoma. Car accident. Hematuria. a) Urography: enlargement of left kidney; impaired excretion; deformity of kidney pelvis. Ureter normal. Conservative treatment b) 6 weeks later: marked regression of kidney size. Contrast excretion fairly good; ruptured cranial branch and contrast-filled irregular cavity in cranial pole

19*

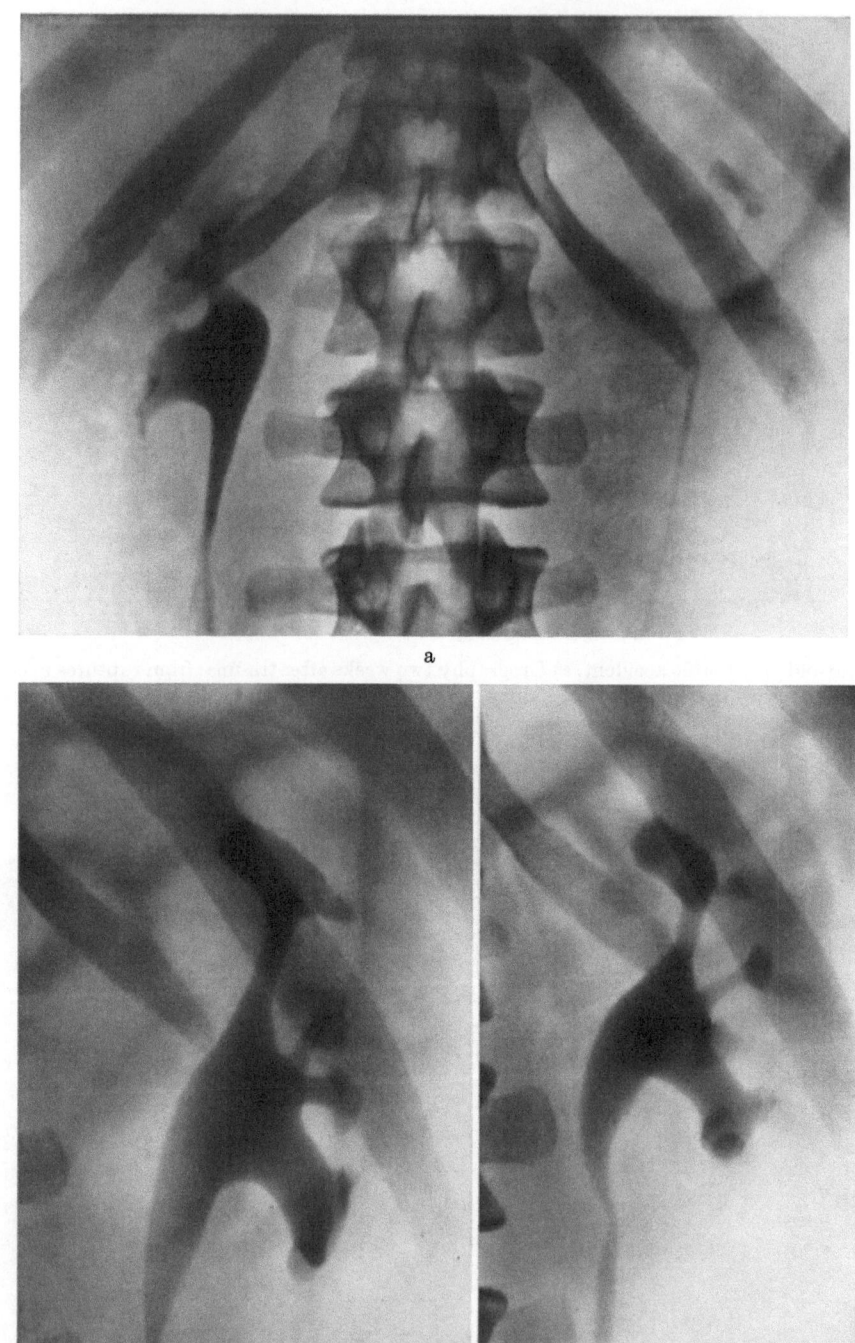

Fig. 247. Fall from horse. Shock. Hematuria. Roentgen examination during acute stage: retroperitoneal hematoma to the left. a) Urography: contrast excretion on left side; incomplete filling; compression of kidney pelvis. No extravasation. Ureter normal. b) 17 days later: normal excretion. No rupture. Kidney flattened by retroperitoneal residual hematoma. c) 1½ years later: normal urogram

there is no evidence of the possibility of shock or reflex anuria being responsible for non-functioning of only one of the kidneys. If, at urography, function is absent on one side only, pyelography may be resorted to. It must be kept in mind that it is of great importance to check whether or not the ureter has been torn. Laceration will cause extravasation of contrast medium and the localization and degree of rupture can be estimated.

Pyelography in cases with suspected renal damage should always be performed under fluoroscopic control in order to avoid refluxes simulating traumatic rupture.

The specific type of rupture called lateral flexion injury should be mentioned here. A trauma may cause such a marked lateral flexion of the body that the contra-lateral ureter may rupture. At urography in such a case, leakage of contrast urine may be seen and no filling of the ureter is obtained (LOPEZ, 1971).

In the group of cases with excretion during urography, the situation can usually be cleared up without the use of pyelography. Pyelography need be employed to check the possibility of ureteric rupture only in those cases in which no contrast medium passes into the ureter. Special attention should be given to those films taken soon after the injection of contrast medium, in order to determine which parts of the kidney are excreting

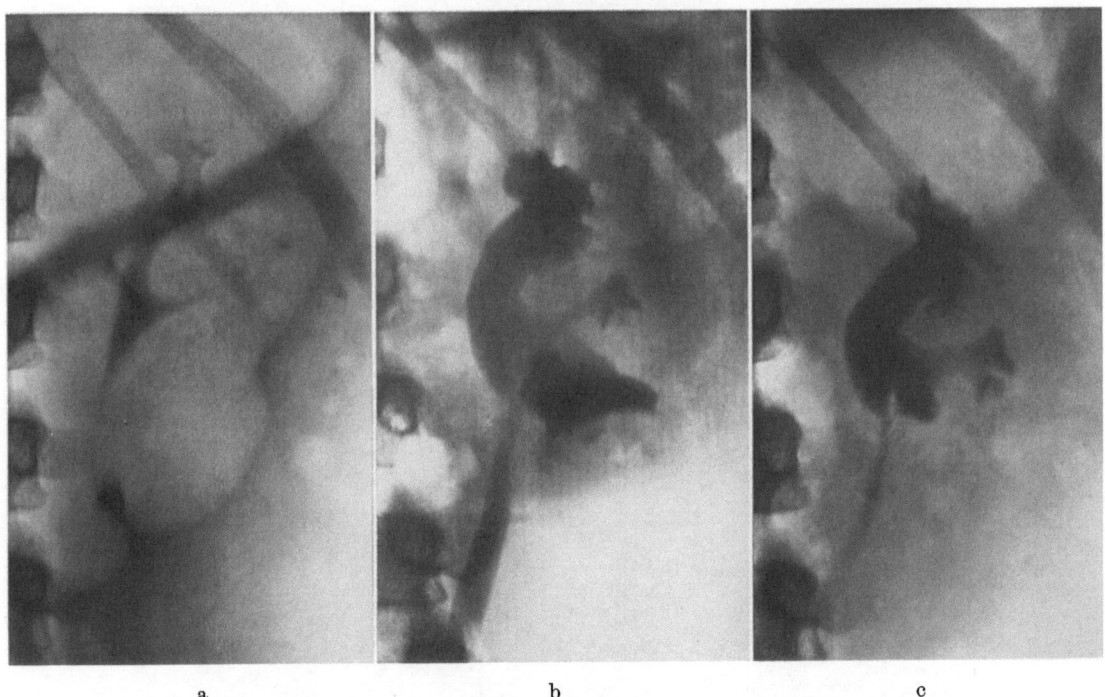

a   b   c

Fig. 248. 7-year-old girl. Traffic accident. a) Acute urography: marked compression of caudal part of left kidney pelvis. b) 5 weeks later: filling of irregular cavity in caudal pole. c) One year later: marked shrinkage of caudal kidney pole

urine. Excretion will occasionally be seen in only one or a few calyces, while the remainder of the renal pelvis contains no contrast medium. A filling will gradually be obtained also of the lacerated parts of the renal pelvis and contrast medium will flow out into the renal tissue or around the kidney. Compression caused by bleeding or edema may also be demonstrated. Calyces into which urine is excreted may be dilated because of compression of the corresponding branch or blockage of the branch by a blood clot. Small ruptures appear as small extravasates of contrast medium along one or more calyces. They may be of the same appearance as a sinus reflux (Fig. 244). In these cases such an extravasation cannot be due to reflux because urography is performed, of course, without the application of ureteric compression.

GYEPES et al. (1971) found at routine urography following percutaneous renal biopsy, that signs were present of bleeding in the kidney as in a local injury. These authors do not find routine performance of post-biopsy urography indicated, but the appearance of any clinical sign or symptom or laboratory data suggesting bleeding should indicate urography.

Findings at urography are only occasionally such as to demonstrate a rupture and its extent completely. The definite demonstration of a rupture is due to the escape of

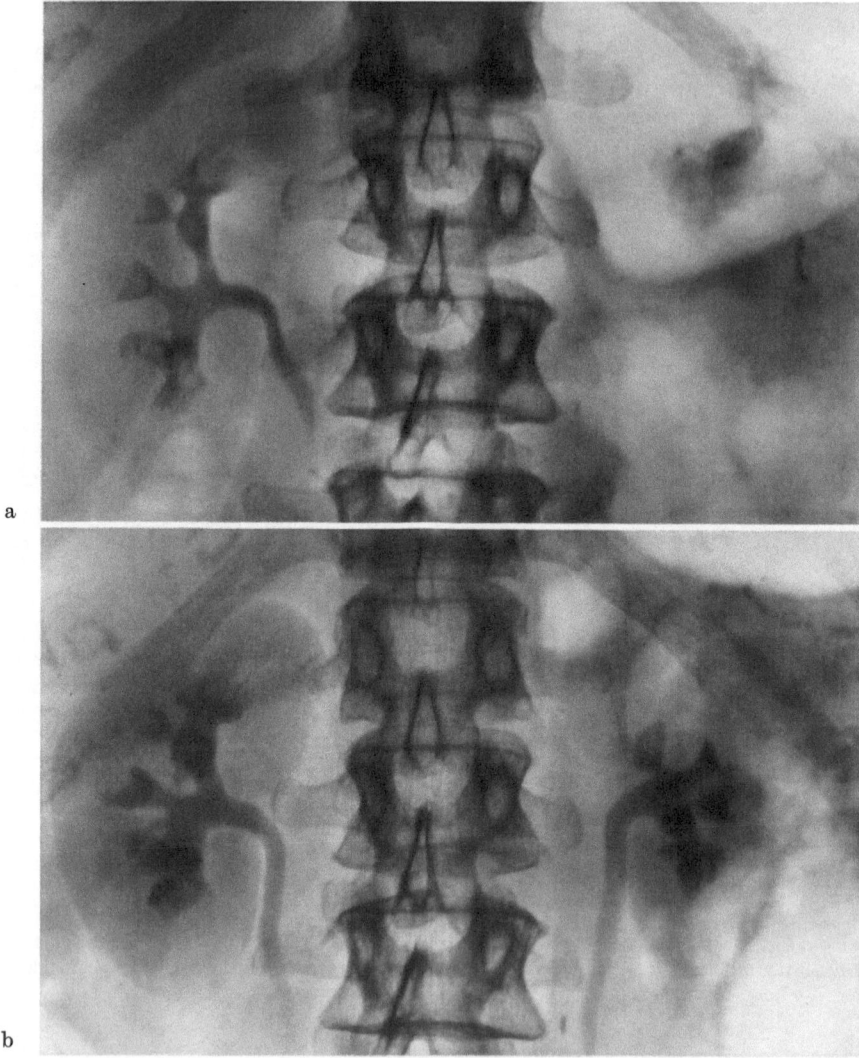

Fig. 249. Kidney rupture. Fall against hard edge. Hematuria. Roentgen examination during acute stage. Left kidney enlarged and ill defined. Roentgen anatomy of retroperitoneal space deranged. Kidney rupture with perirenal hematoma. a) Urography: Large extravasation in cranial part of left kidney. Ureter filled. b) 5 months later: small kidney; cranial branch changed into a small irregular sprout. Residuum after kidney rupture

contrast urine out into the rupture. This direct sign of rupture is, however, fairly rare. A rupture therefore is usually diagnosed through indirect evidence: excretion of contrast medium is delayed or diminished, the kidney pelvis is incompletely filled and more or less markedly deformed.

If the patient is not operated upon, urography may be performed again a few days later, when it may be possible to apply slight ureteric compression in order to obtain a

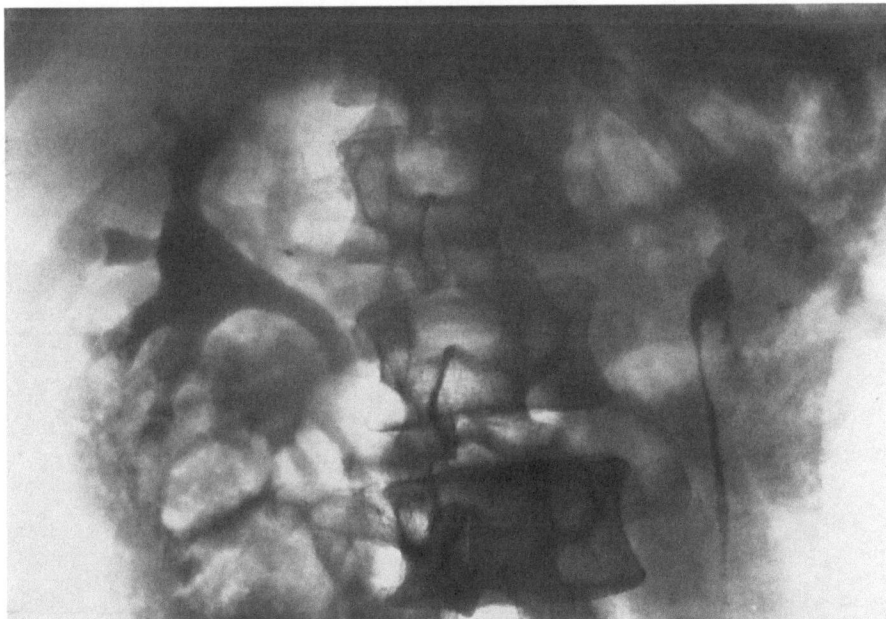

Fig. 250. Residuum after kidney contusion. Trauma to left kidney several years previously. Now at urography: hyperplasia of right kidney; marked shrinkage of left kidney with calcifications in shrunken old hematomas

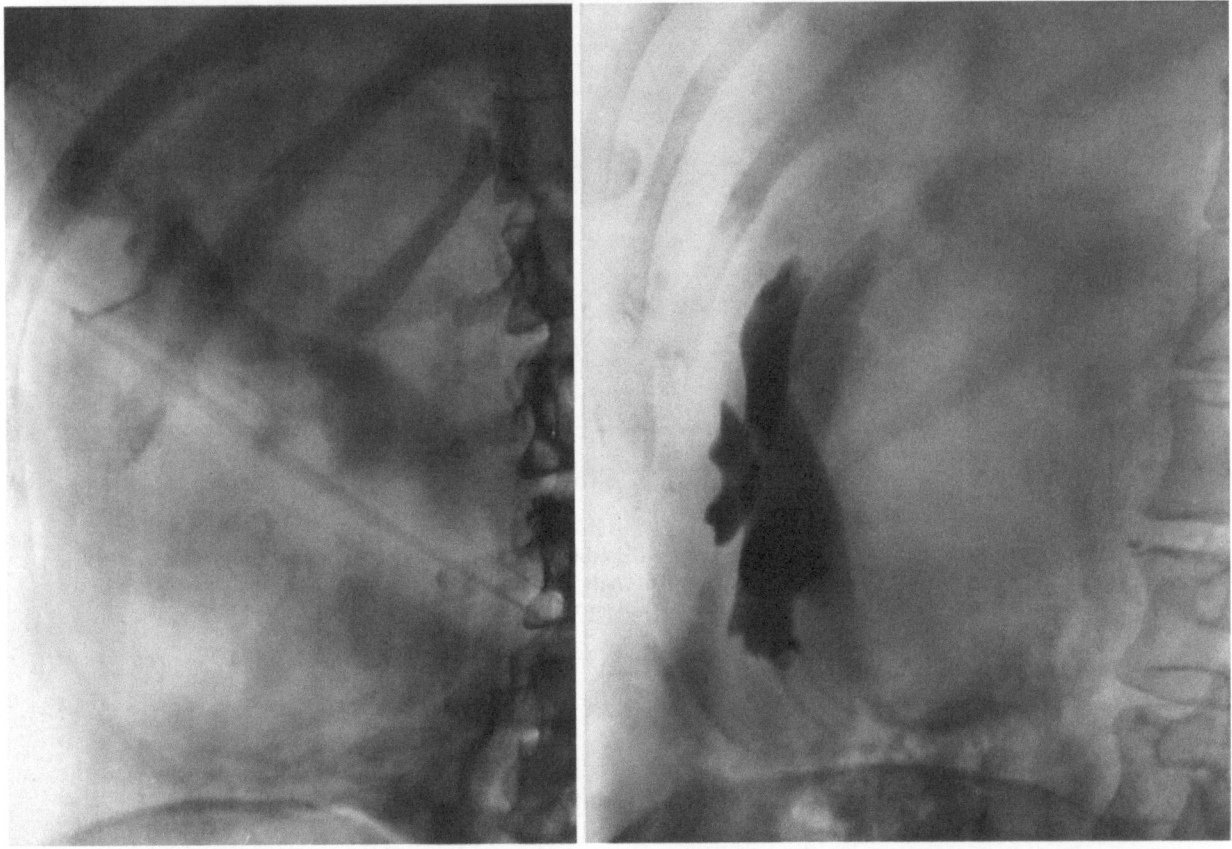

a   b

Fig. 251. Perirenal organized hematoma. Severe trauma to abdomen two years previously. Plain roentgenography: very well defined mass in right kidney region. a) Urography: contrast excretion impaired; kidney pelvis displaced and flattened. b) Pyelography: large extra-renal, well defined space-occupying lesion displacing and flattening kidney. Operation: old encapsulated hematoma containing one liter of fluid

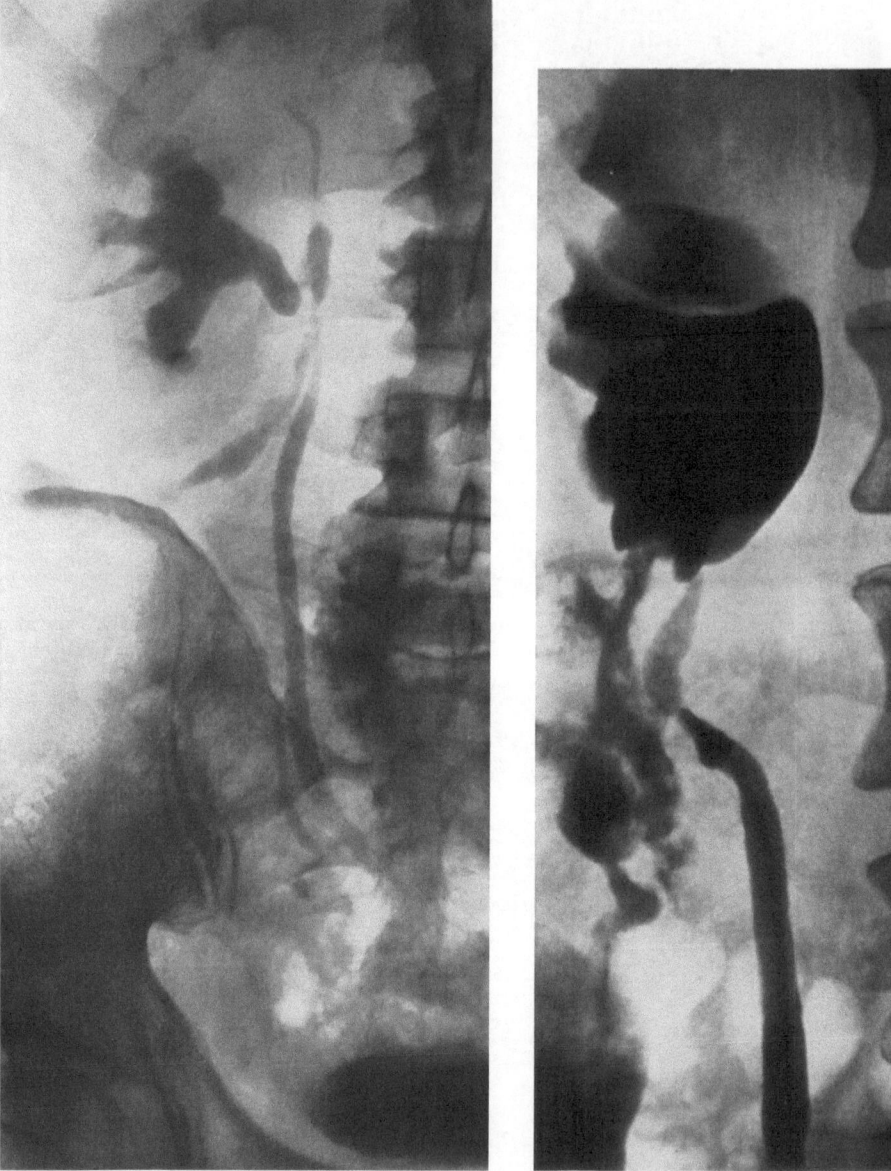

Fig. 252   Fig. 253

Fig. 252. Iatrogenic "trauma". Double kidney and double ureter. Pyelolithotomy in caudal kidney pelvis. Urography some time after operation: leakage through pyelotomy into retroperitoneal space. Pyelotomy kept open because of stone in distal part of corresponding ureter with obstacle to flow

Fig. 253. Iatrogenic "trauma". Retrograde pyelography: leakage through pyelostomy in caudal part of kidney pelvis

better filling of the renal pelvis for a more detailed study of its morphology. It is striking to note, on check examination, how soon roentgenologic signs may disappear.

In children, in whom trauma is common and in whom renal tumors are often symptomless and therefore likely to assume considerable proportions, the injury may occur in a kidney with a tumor. LEVANT and FELDMAN (1952) have described two cases of embryoblastoma which had been symptomless and were discovered at examination in association with trauma.

The renal pelvis may be ruptured also during instrumental examination. It may be perforated by a catheter. STRNAD (1936) has shown that a simple, ordinary ureteric catheter can perforate the renal pelvis, usually at the fornix of the cranial calyx (compare Fig. 264). Check examination of such a case, with consequent injection of contrast medium subcapsularly, showed that the rupture healed very soon (Köhler, 1953).

Injection of contrast medium can rupture a pathologically changed renal pelvis (BARETZ, 1936). Rupture in connection with the reflux or backflow phenomenon is discussed in Chapter P.

More or less acute perforation may also be produced by decubital lesions caused by stone in the renal pelvis. Concrements in a calyx can perforate the renal parenchyma and

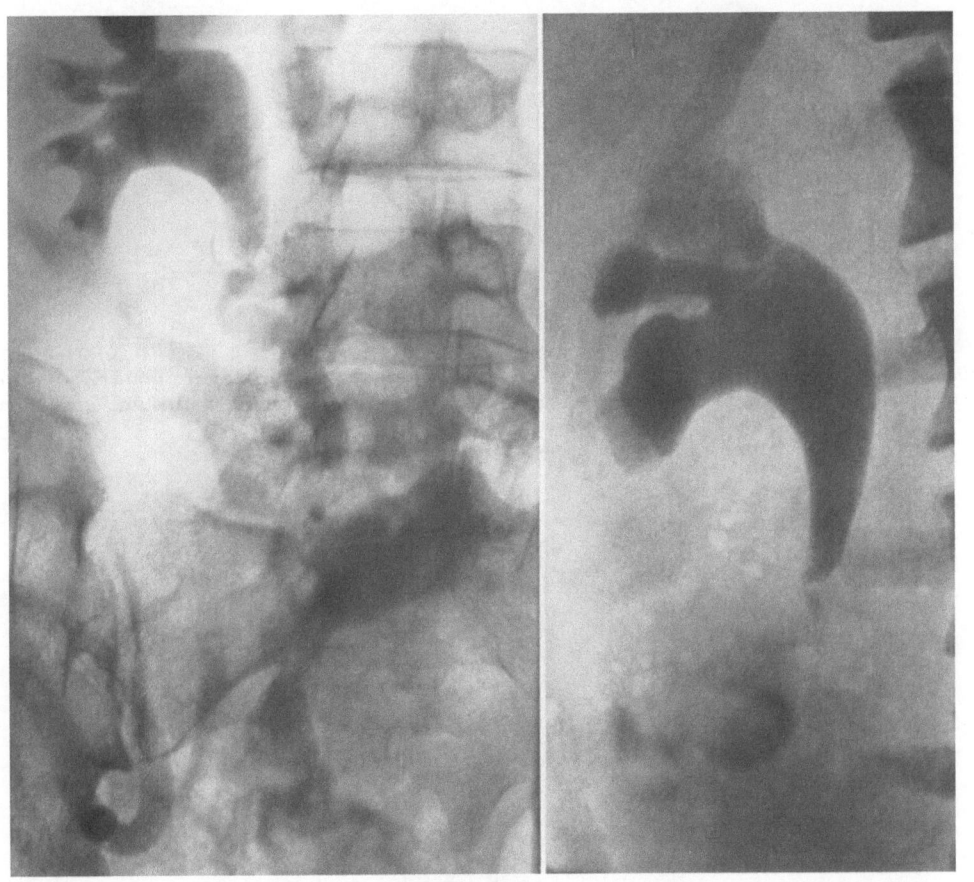

a   b

Fig. 254. Iatrogenic "trauma" with leakage of contrast medium into the retroperitoneal space during urography. a) Lesion of right ureter in connection with gynecologic operation. b) Lesion of right ureter in connection with bowel resection

pass directly out into the perirenal space. One case of bilateral perforation has been described by MARQUART (1958). Spontaneous rupture of the renal pelvis has also been described (RENANDER, 1941).

Ureteric injury may occur in connection with renal lesions but also alone, in which case usually following instrumental examination (Fig. 255, 256). The diagnosis is based on the disturbed flow through the ureter and on the development of extravasation and offers the same problems as those described above in association with injury to the renal pelvis and upper part of the ureter.

Inflation of the balloon of Dourmashkin's special catheter can rupture the ureter (Fig. 256).

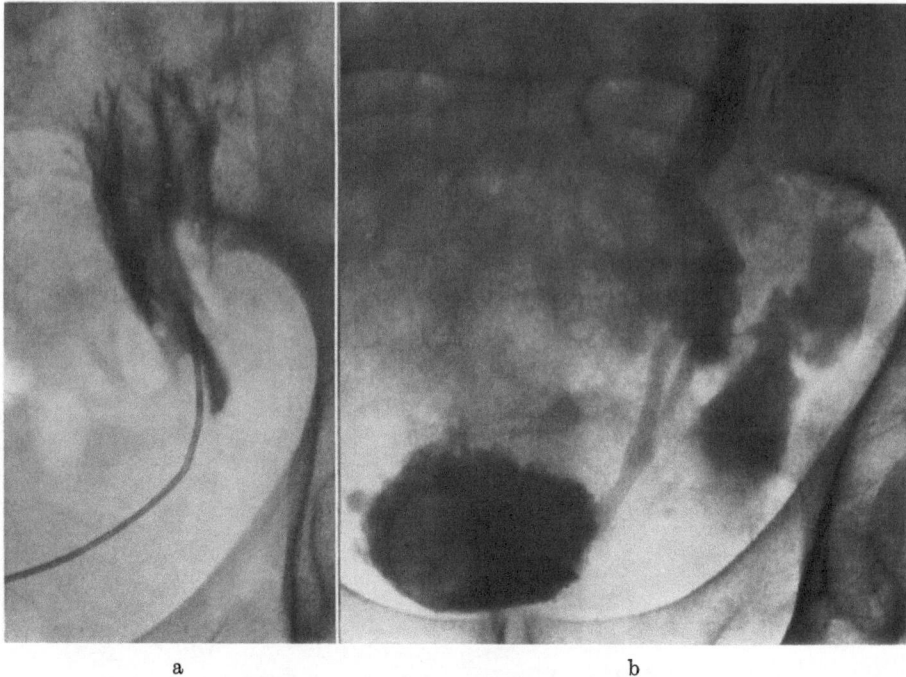

a   b

Fig. 255. Iatrogenic "trauma". a) Perforation of ureter in connection with catheterization. Escape of contrast medium out into periureteric space. b) Perforation of ureter in connection with stone extraction

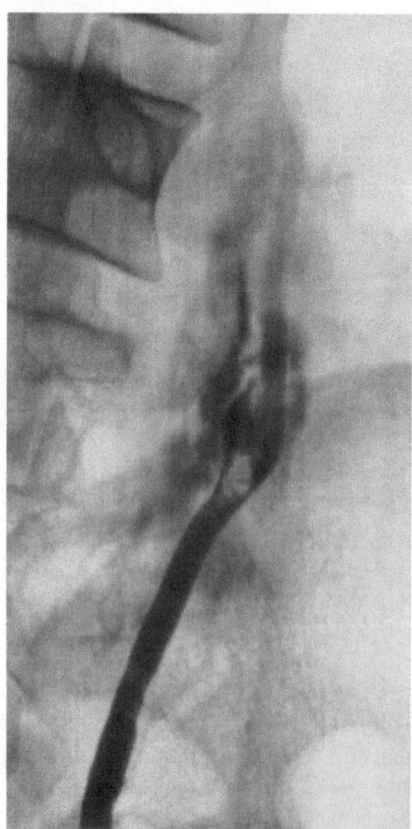

Fig. 256. Rupture of ureter by balloon catheter used for study of kidney pelvis in pyelography. Extravasation of contrast medium around ruptured ureter. Blood clots in ureter

IV. Renal angiography
(Figs. 257—263)

In order to arrive at direct diagnostic evidence in cases of suspected renal rupture, renal angiography is a very useful method. A rupture can be demonstrated to its full extent in the nephrographic phase. It is necessary to use different projections at selective renal angiography because a small rupture may be localized entirely to the ventral and dorsal part of the kidney and may escape detection unless proper projections are used.

Intrarenal hematomas can be demonstrated by displacement of the arterial branches, occasionally very marked displacement. Extrarenal hematomas can be demonstrated by

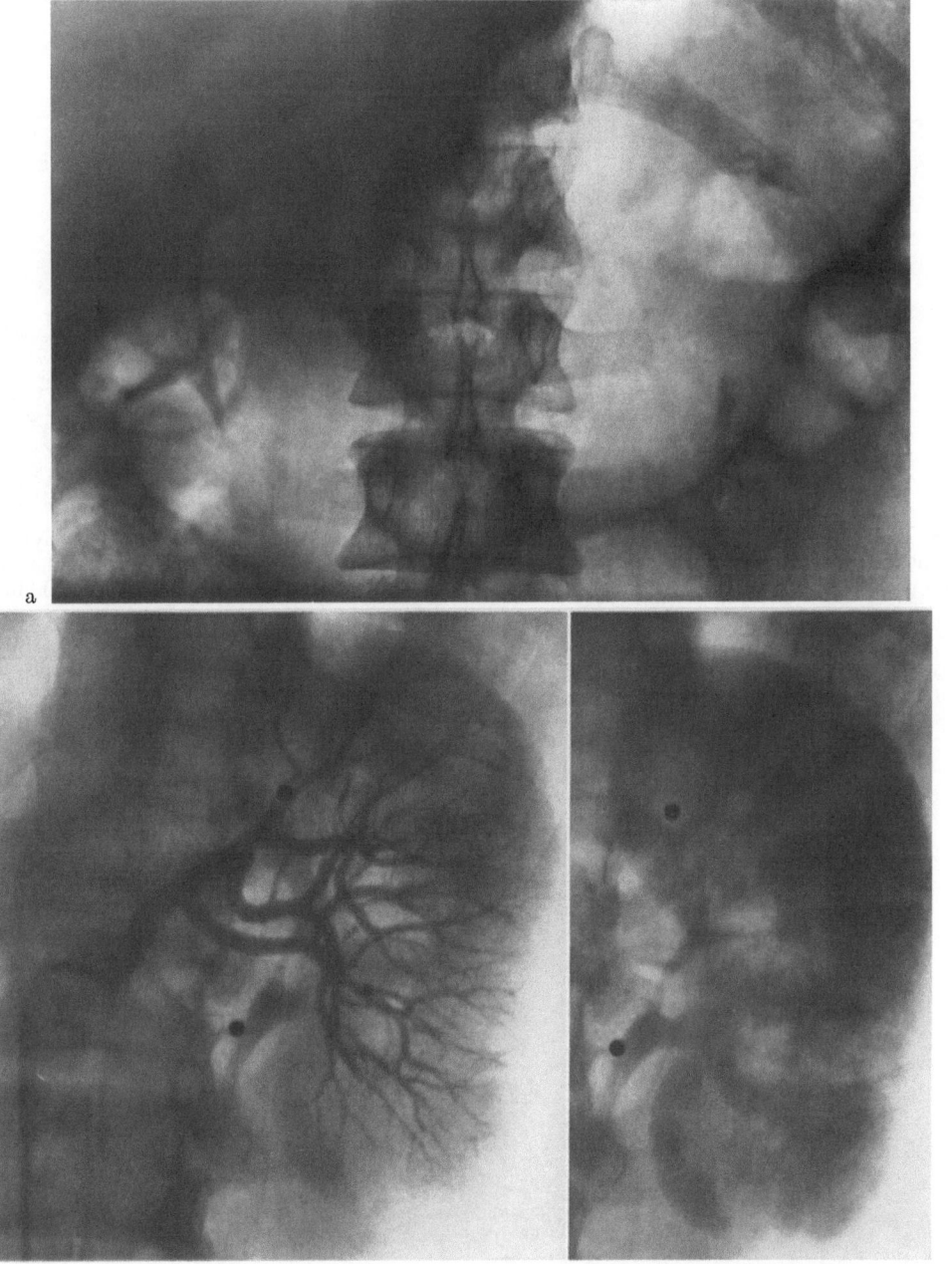

Fig. 257. Renal rupture. a) Urography: marked compression of left kidney pelvis. No extravasation of contrast medium. b) and c) Angiography: ruptures in caudal kidney pole with slight displacement of fragments

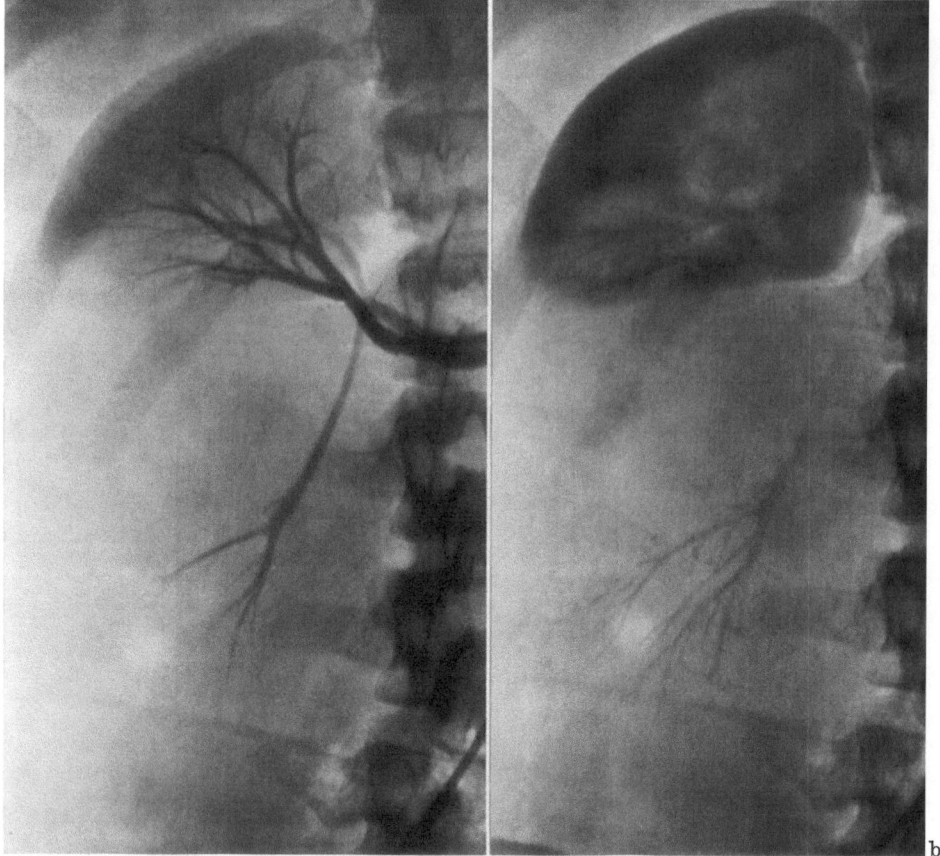

Fig. 258. Renal rupture. Trauma to right kidney. Acute urography: no excretion. Angiography: kidney is divided into two parts. Cranial part is well arterialized a) and well delineated. b) Nephrogram: complete contusion of caudal part. Operation: caudal part crushed. Excision of this part and suture of ruptured edge of kidney pelvis

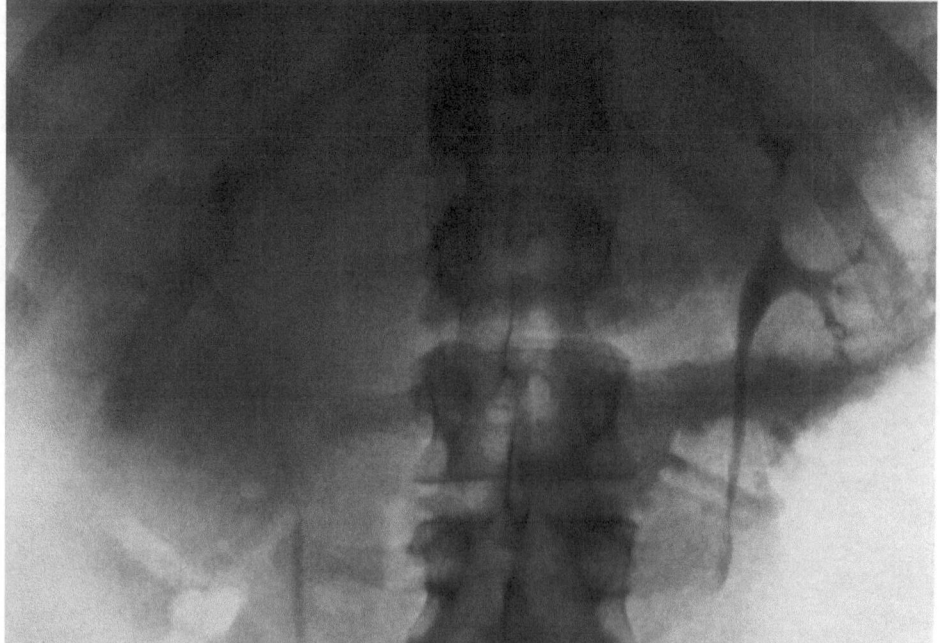

Fig. 259. Trauma to right kidney. a) Acute urography: incomplete filling of right kidney pelvis; marked enlargement of right kidney. b) and c) Acute angiography: no renal rupture; large perirenal hematoma caused by bleeding from small severed artery. d) Urography 6 weeks later: normal conditions

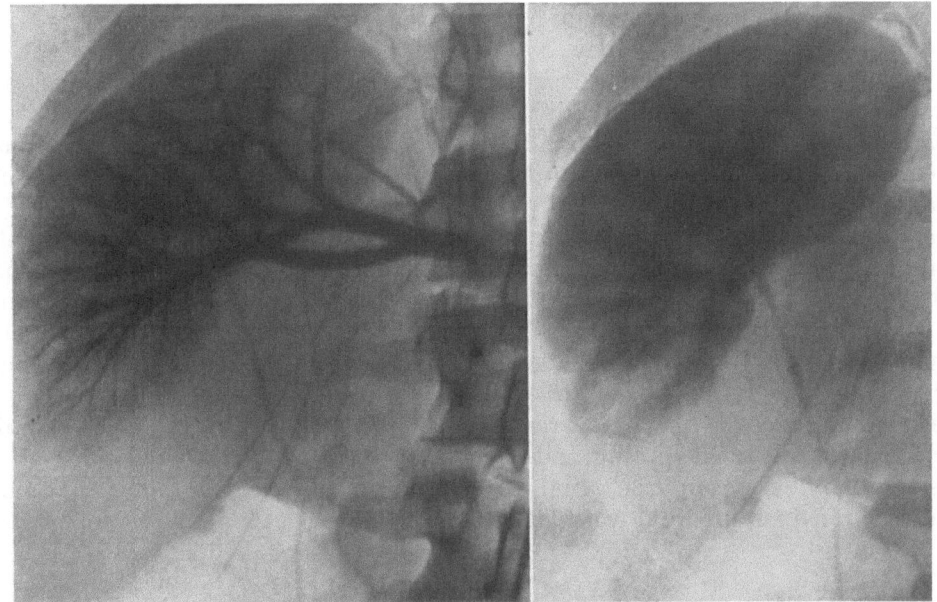

b   c

Fig. 259 b, c

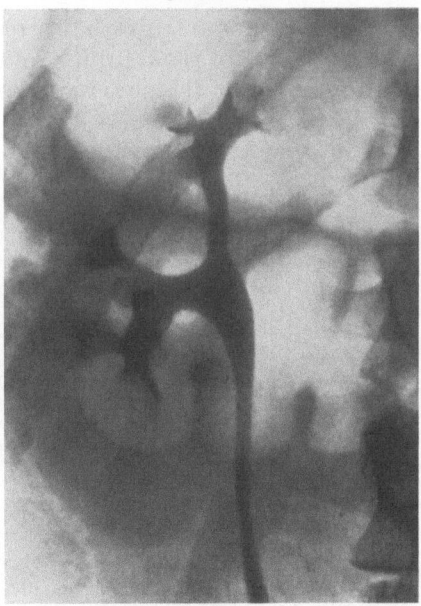

Fig. 259 d

the impression and displacement of the surface of the kidney or of the kidney as a whole. Any vascular rupture with actual, marked bleeding is demonstrable angiographically by extravasation of contrast blood.

The iatrogenic injury due to percutaneous needle biopsy needs special attention. At immediate post-biopsy angiographic studies a high incidence of false aneurysms and extravasation of contrast material was shown, due to damage to large arterial branches (MENG and ELKIN, 1971). Extensive hematoma formation could also be seen in some patients. Further sequelae of percutaneous needle biopsy are arterial aneurysms and arteriovenous fistulae (see Chapter I).

LUNDSTRÖM (1971) has performed angiography five minutes after biopsy. He has often found large perirenal hematomas (without clinical signs!). These have disappeared, probably completely.

True infarction is very uncommon in connection with biopsy. Small indentations may be seen in the surface of the kidney, as a result of biopsy.

A very important observation can be made in the comparison of findings at plain radiography and urography with those at renal angiography. The changes may be due entirely to hematoma without evidence of true renal rupture. Small lesions may cause very large hematomas and thus give the impression of much more serious anatomical changes than are actually present in the renal parenchyma (Olle Olsson, Lunderqvist, 1963).

The formation of arteriovenous fistulae may be observed in the subacute stage of renal injury. They may disappear later. Rupture of arterial branches can be demonstrated through blockage of a branch. Atrophy of the arterial branches and of the main renal artery can be seen. Scar formation and infarctions in the kidney are observable in the nephrographic phase. In some cases large hematomas are well circumscribed and the renal parenchyma may be seen markedly displaced and reduced.

It is evident from the above that renal angiography is most useful in the examination of cases of suspected renal rupture and is superior to any other method available for the demonstration of lesions in the renal parenchyma. It will also enable differentiation between true renal rupture and capsular or completely extrarenal hematoma.

V. Healing of renal ruptures

There is widespread agreement in the literature that a renal rupture has an excellent healing tendency. Upon reviewing 54 cases of renal injury several years after the accidents causing them, Steinbock (1948) found that the shape of the renal pelvis was normal in

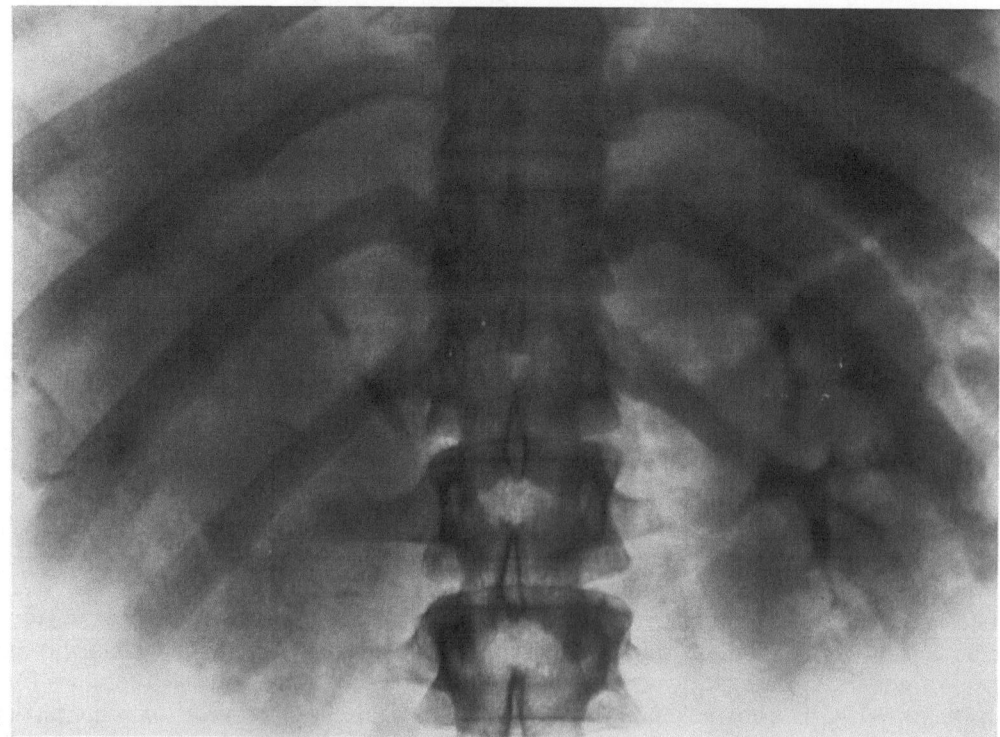

a

Fig. 260. Residuum after trauma. Repeated trauma to right kidney during skiing several months previously. Examination now because of hypertensive crisis. a) Urography: contrast excretion on right side impaired; kidney pelvis markedly displaced and incompletely filled. b) Angiography: marked displacement of intrarenal arterial branches by large cystic expansivities. Operation with emptying of post-traumatic cysts. c) Post-operative urography: right kidney small; kidney pelvis normal

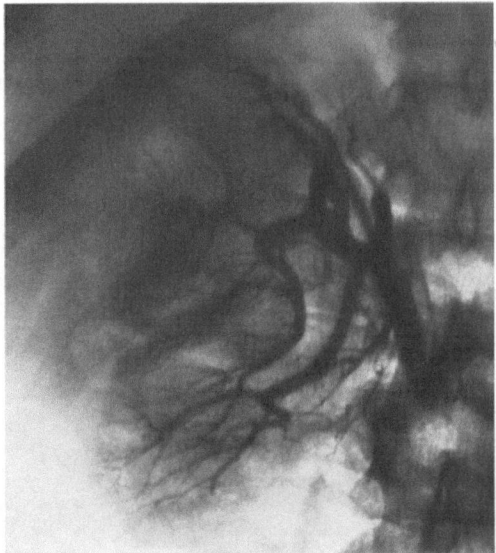

Fig. 260 b

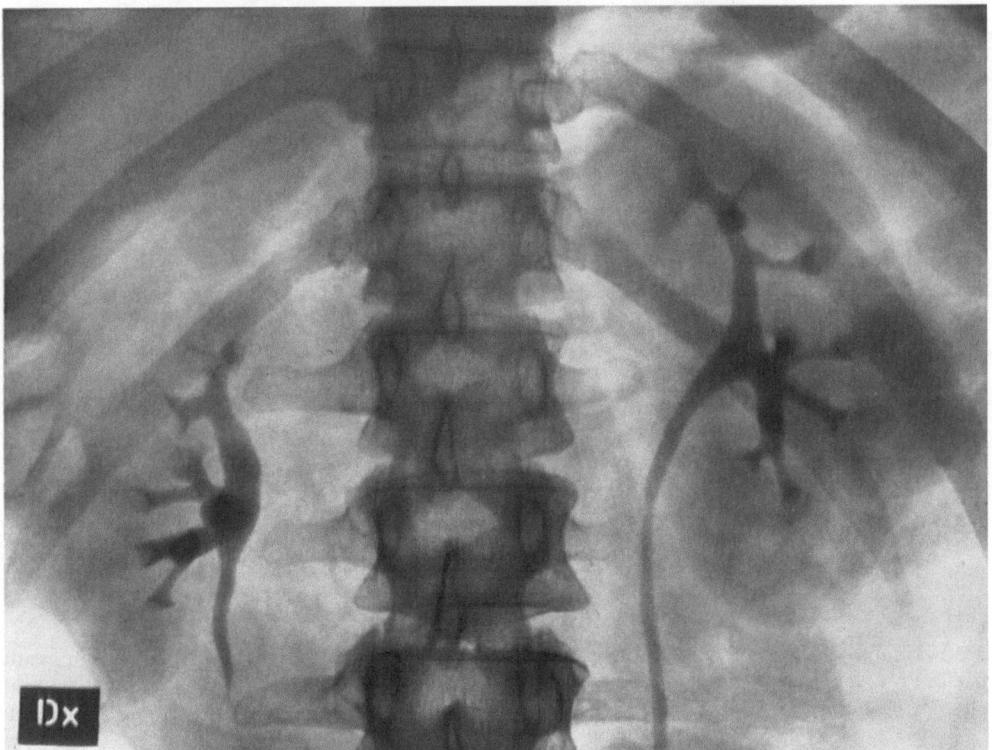

Fig. 260 c

40 cases, the kidney functionless in only two (one case had a hydronephrosis and the other a pyonephrosis with stone), seven cases showed small changes in the renal pelvis due to scar formation. On the other hand, upon reviewing 13 cases at varying intervals after trauma to the region of the kidney, COLSTON and BAKER (1937) found marked pathologic changes in the kidney or in the perirenal tissue. The latter authors claim traumatization of the kidney and hematuria as indicators of immediate examination, and follow-up at regular intervals to avoid any late complications. Old kidney ruptures may show different degrees of deformation of the kidney pelvis upon check examination, depending mainly

on the extent and localization of the damage (Figs. 250, 251). An uncommon late complication is the development of a large intrarenal cyst. I have seen a case in which a cyst of
the size of a child's head and containing clear fluid developed within three months of trauma. In one case the kidney was completely changed into large cysts, with no function.
This patient came for examination because of hypertensive crises (Fig. 260). Arteriovenous
fistulae and arterial aneurysms may also be residuals of trauma (Figs. 261, 263).

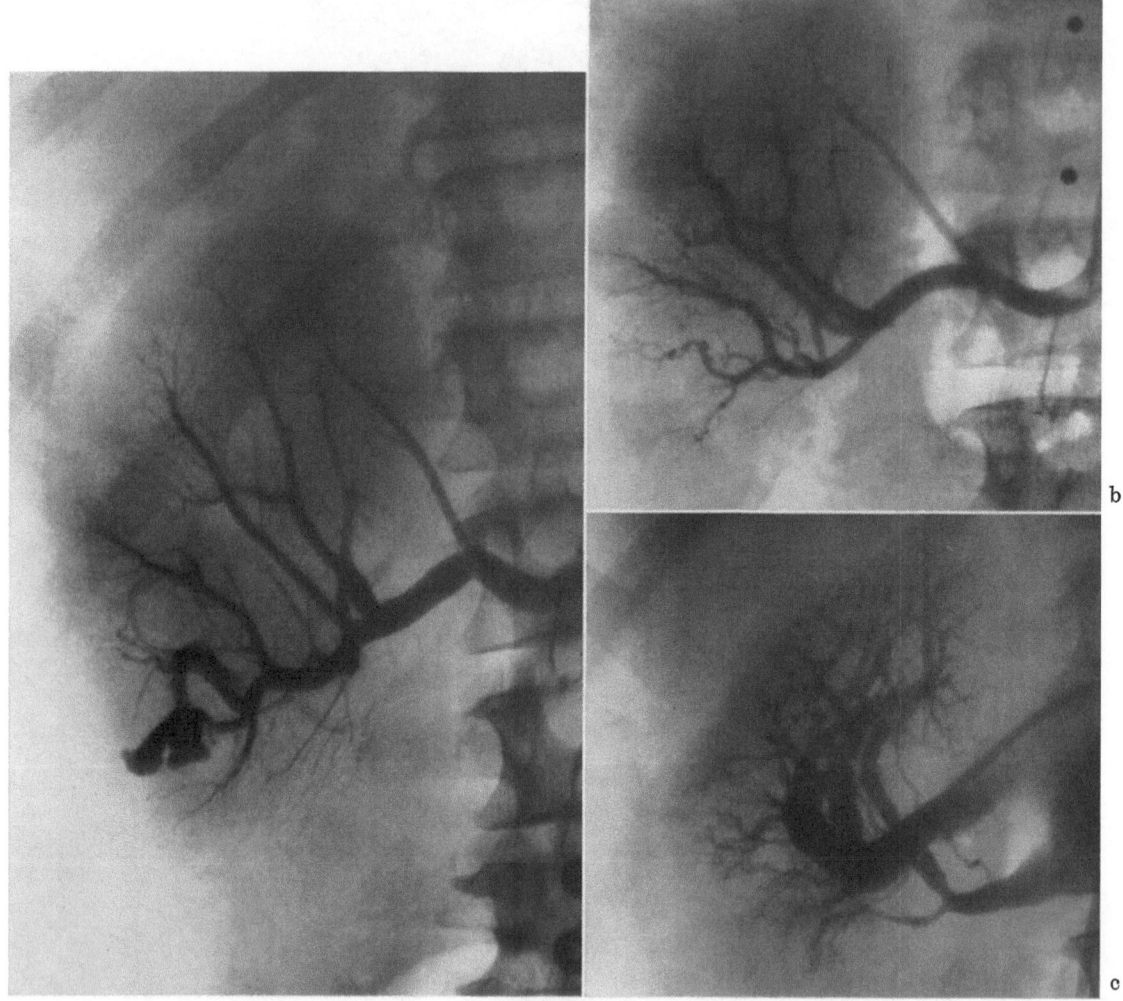

Fig. 261. Residuum after trauma. At acute angiography: extravasation from arterial branches in caudal pole
of right kidney. a) Selective angiography 9 days later: decrease in volume of caudal kidney pole; arteriovenous
fistula in this part of kidney. b) Angiography 6 weeks later: arteriovenous fistula closed. c) Selective phlebography with hypertensin: marked shrinkage of caudal kidney pole.

Upon scrutiny of the possible basis for the common opinion that the healing tendency
of a renal rupture is excellent, it is obvious that it derives from the urographic findings at
examination in connection with the trauma and comparison of these findings with later
urographic check examinations: At the first examination marked changes are seen; at the
check examinations conditions appear to be normal or the changes appear to be considerably diminished. This common opinion may be completely wrong for two reasons:

1. Changes seen at the acute examination, however marked, may not be due to a
rupture — a hematoma may be responsible. Resorption of the hematoma, usually fairly

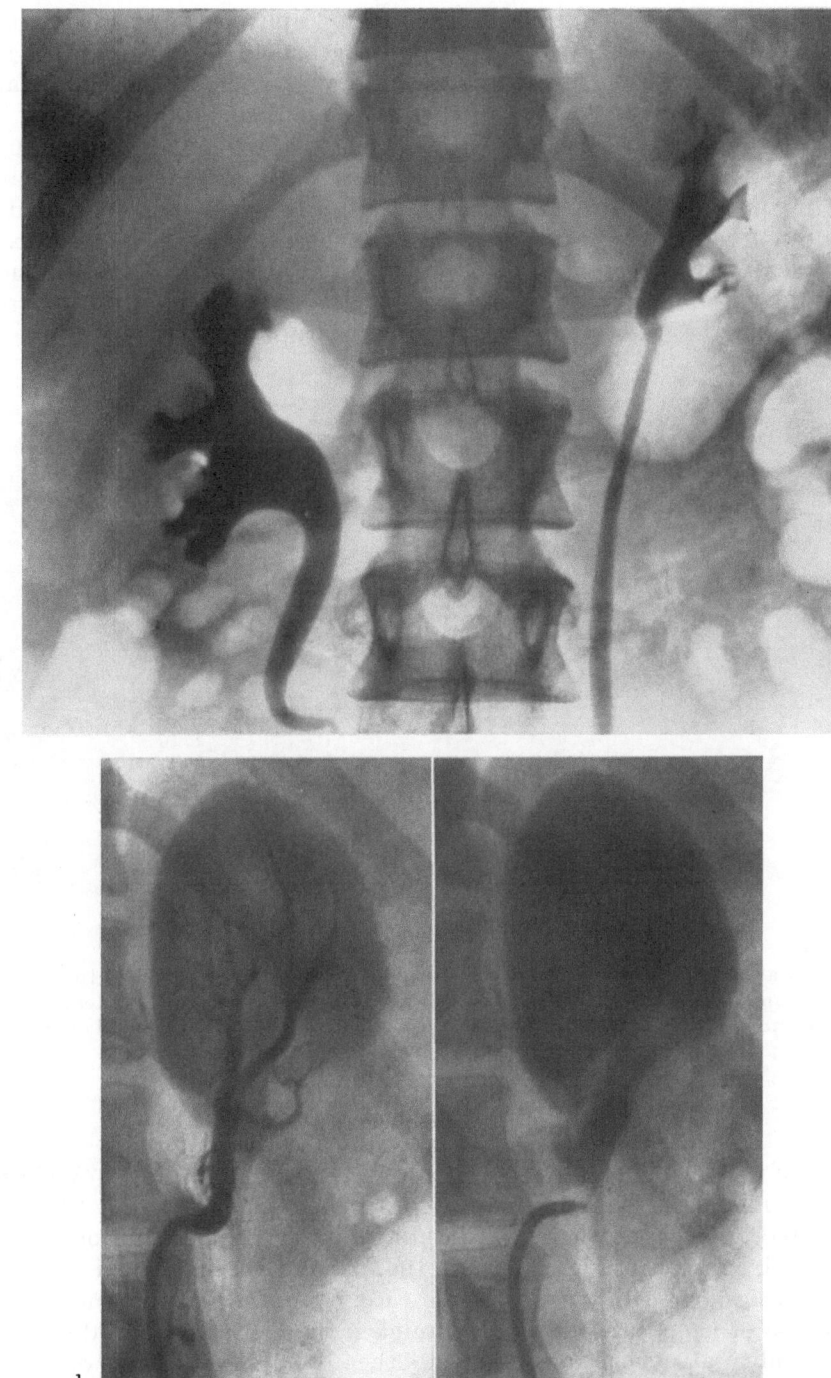

Fig. 262. Residuum after trauma. Accident several years previously with trauma to left kidney. a) Urography: small left kidney; shrinkage of calyces in caudal part of kidney. b) and c) Angiography: cranial half of kidney normal, caudal half completely atrophied

rapid, brings conditions to normal. This cannot be taken as evidence of excellent healing tendency, however. Where there is no rupture, no rupture can heal (OLLE OLSSON, 1970).

2. Normal conditions, or findings of only slight changes, at check examinations cannot exclude marked residual changes due to renal damage. It was demonstrated by OLLE

OLSSON and LUNDERQUIST (1963) that at renal angiography performed in patients of this type, very marked vascular and parenchymal changes incurring considerable risks could be revealed. Thus atrophy of large parts of the kidney parenchyma and vasculature could be seen, together with fragmentation of the kidney and separation of large fragments. Cases have since been examined in which arteriovenous fistulae, arterial aneurysms, etc. have been found. Angiography can therefore definitely demonstrate on one hand that at examination in connection with trauma, marked urographic changes may be due only to hematoma and not to renal laceration and that on the other hand at check examination after trauma, normal conditions or only slight changes at urography do not exclude marked lesions. The conditions found at urography cannot, therefore, be used without reservation for an opinion as to the healing tendency of a renal rupture.

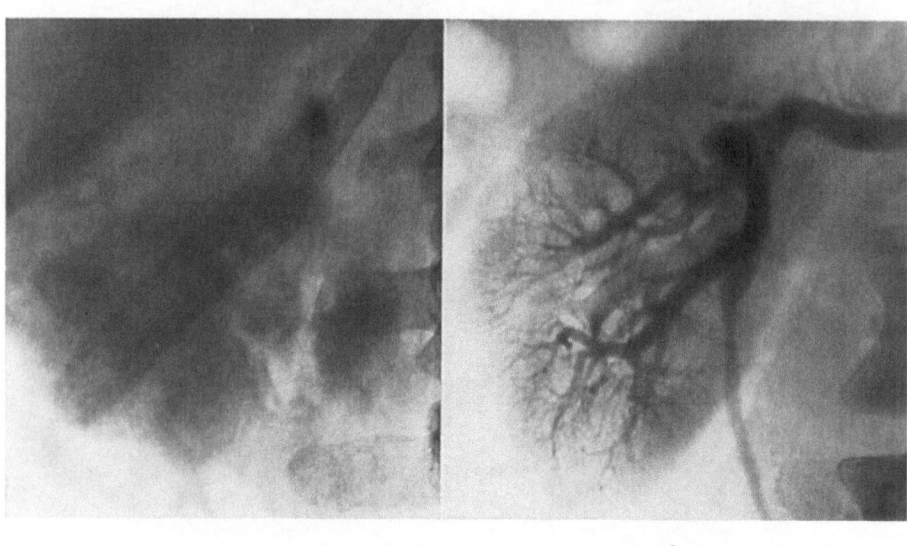

a   b

Fig. 263. Residuum after trauma caused by kick of horse in region of right kidney 15 years previously. a) Plain roentgenography: calcification in cranial pole of right kidney. b) Angiography, arterial phase: complete atrophy of cranial kidney pole; arterial aneurysm. Calcification is localized in wall of aneurysm

VI. Choice of therapy

The choice of treatment is largely decided by the roentgen findings. "Viele stehen auf dem Standpunkt möglichst rein konservativ vorzugehen..." (STAEHLER, 1959). An active attitude was advocated by LOWSLEY and MENNING (1941). Some authors, however (see LYNCH, 1957, and NILSSON and SANDBERG, 1962), have recommended conservative or active therapy according to the merits of the case. Conservative treatment is obviously sufficient in a case of hematuria following trauma if the kidney is normal in size and presents no abnormality at pyelography. On the other hand surgical intervention is necessary in the presence of irresponsive shock or signs of a hematoma that is increasing in size. Most cases lie between these two extremes. It is clear from the analysis of published series of renal injury examined by common methods that both the clinical and the roentgenologic evidence in a given case is often insufficient to decide the extent of damage with any degree of certainty. Since the renal parenchyma and blood vessels are mainly affected the desired information should be obtainable by a method by which these may be demonstrated, i.e. renal angiography. (OLLE OLSSON and LUNDERQUIST, 1963).

Consideration of the therapeutic approach has a much better foundation when renal angiography is used. This also forces the surgeon into a more individualized judgment.

VII. Perirenal hematoma

Hemorrhage around the kidney may develop in association with trauma or may be spontaneous. A possible cause of retroperitoneal hematoma which should be borne in mind is perforation of a vessel by a needle or catheter during the increasingly common arterial and venous punctures and catheterizations for different purposes. An equally important, if not more important, possibility is bleeding into the perirenal space in connection with percutaneous renal biopsy. LUNDSTRÖM (1971) reports on an angiographic material consisting of 140 cases where selective renal angiography was performed immediately before as well as immediately after biopsy. In one case a clinically proven perirenal

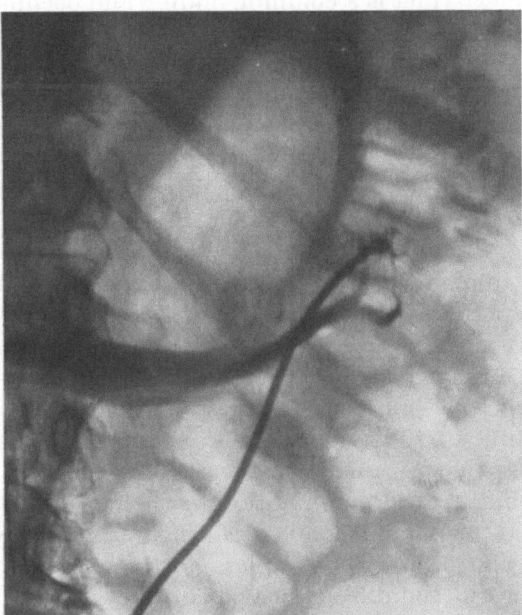

Fig. 264. Iatrogenic "trauma". In connection with catheterization of left kidney pelvis for pyelography the catheter has been forced into the renal parenchyma. On injection of contrast medium, filling of intrarenal venous branches to main renal vein

hematoma occurred. In another case the symptoms and signs of a renal peritoneal hematoma were present. In 111 out of the 140 cases angiographic changes were seen, consisting mainly of leakage of the contrast medium through bleeding in connection with the biopsy channel. In 20 of the 140 cases perirenal bleeding was observed which could be regarded as extensive. Hematoma around the right kidney may also be due to liver biopsy with hemorrhage into the right retroperitoneal space.

Spontaneous perirenal hematoma can occur in association with hemophilia (JASIENSKI, 1937), various other diseases, or from unknown causes. Intrarenal and perirenal hematoma may develop in patients on anticoagulant therapy.

The roentgen findings in these different types of hematoma agree essentially with what is described below in relation to perinephritis of varying extent. No signs of edema will be seen, however. It must be noted that spontaneous subcapsular renal hemorrhage can be caused by a small tumor as pointed out by POLLACK and POPKY (1972). In three patients with spontaneous subcapsular bleeding a small renal tumor was responsible for the bleeding in each patient. WATNICK et al. (1972) also in a case report on subcapsular hematoma, point out the sudden bleeding produced by a small renal carcinoma associated with renal infarction.

Old extrarenal hematomas can be well delineated and simulate a well defined space-occupying lesion (Fig. 251). Severe displacement of the kidney and possible impression in the renal pelvis will then be seen at examination with contrast medium. Such hematomas may also be the cause of large shell-shaped calcifications at the site of the kidney or of irregular perirenal calcifications (MILLER and CORDONNIER, 1949; Engel and PAGE, 1955). Old hematomas can develop into hygromas (KEMM, 1923). Angiography may be helpful in the diagnosis of old hematomas.

K. Dilatation of the urinary tract

Dilatation of the urinary tract is a common finding and occupies an important position in diseases of the kidney requiring surgery.

There is a certain confusion regarding nomenclature. The term hydronephrosis is often used to designate the clinically important entity: obstruction of the pelviureteric junction resulting in dilatation of the kidney pelvis. The same term is also used, however, to describe dilatation of the entire urinary tract unilaterally or bilaterally, regardless of cause. The whole problem of dilatation will be discussed here, but the reader is referred, in addition, to certain other chapters for further discussion of different aspects of dilatation.

The rule should be to diagnose, if possible, the nature and localization of the pathogenetic factor and to report secondary influences on renal drainage. Dilatation may be unilateral or bilateral. It may involve the renal pelvis and the entire ureter, or a part of the latter. If may also be limited to only a part of the renal pelvis. Border-line cases are common and it is difficult to decide in these cases whether or not a dilatation is pathologic. It is also occasionally difficult to decide whether or not a demonstrable local narrowing is truly pathologic and capable of causing obstruction. In addition, the degree of dilatation may vary widely according to the examination method and technique used and the circumstances under which the examination is performed. The kidney pelvis can be markedly dilated on one occasion and have a more or less normal appearance on another.

The roentgen findings in the different types of dilatation of the urinary tract most commonly encountered in routine work are described below. If the dilatation is due to well known changes such as stone, tumor or anomalies, the roentgen findings will be described under sections describing these conditions; otherwise they will be analogically evident under one of the following sections:

I. The obstructed pelviureteric junction

In this book the junction between the renal pelvis and the ureter is called pelviureteric junction instead of ureteropelvic junction. The latter term is probably based on the instrumental pyelographic procedure, whereas the term pelviureteric is consistent with the direction of the urinary flow.

Obstruction of the pelviureteric junction can cause intermittent or permanent dilatation of the renal pelvis. Such dilatation is usually known as hydronephrosis. The name pyelectasis (BRAASCH and EMMETT, 1951) is regarded by some authors as being preferable to hydronephrosis, but the latter term is preferred because it is so deeply rooted. In my opinion, the term hydronephrosis has the advantage that it draws attention to the fact that it is the entire kidney that is affected and not only the renal pelvis. The effect of the obstructed drainage on the kidney is the most important factor.

The normal anatomy of the pelviureteric junction varies widely. The junction between a markedly or only slightly dilated renal pelvis and a ureter of ordinary width will usually show a marked and short narrowing. The upper portion of the ureter may be fixed to the renal pelvis along a length of 1—3 cm by more or less loose adhesions.

These may cause a sharp, more or less rigid bend in that part of the ureter fixed to the renal pelvis. This fixation can be accentuated by a vessel crossing the pelviureteric junction. Such a vessel running in front of the ureter will then press the bent ureter against the dilated renal pelvis. The fixed ureter can also be hooked and strangulated by the vessel.

Another component of the obstruction is diminution of the lumen of the pelviureteric junction by a more or less regular, intrinsic stenosis varying in length from one case to another, sometimes having the shape of a valve.

The different forms of obstructions described above: adhesion, compression by a vessel, and intrinsic stenosis may occur separately, although they more often occur in combination, in varying degrees.

The obstruction caused by these factors is greatest when the renal pelvis is dilated, e.g. in marked diuresis. That part of the ureter adherent to the renal pelvis will then be stretched still more and be compressed, and drainage of the renal pelvis will consequently become gradually poorer or cease altogether.

In the beginning, the obstruction may occur intermittently if for some reason or other the renal pelvis is dilated and drainage impaired. After such an attack of intermittent hydronephrosis, a certain degree of dilatation may persist. It may be accentuated further after repeated attacks, and the dilatation may become permanent. The wider the renal pelvis becomes and the more it expands ventrally, the more it will obstruct drainage. Such urinary stasis leads to atrophy of the renal parenchyma and favors infection.

The purpose of the roentgen examination is to demonstrate the site of the obstruction responsible for the hydronephrosis, its severity and nature, its effect on the renal parenchyma, and any complications such as stone formation. Considerable information can be required from the roentgen examination, and the diagnostic problems it is called upon to solve are important. This necessitates full utilization of all the diagnostic possibilities of the various examination techniques.

The fact that the answers to many important questions cannot be arrived at through the use of conventional methods and that a study of the renal vasculature and of the renal parenchyma is important, markedly increases indications for renal angiography. This type of examination is often not only necessary but should be instituted at an early stage of the diagnostic procedure.

1. Plain radiography

The findings obtained at plain radiography depend upon the degree of the hydronephrosis. If the dilatation is only slight, the examination will reveal no signs of a pathologic condition; if moderate, the kidney will appear enlarged and the hilum wider than usual; if severe, the dilated confluence of the renal pelvis will appear as a soft tissue mass at the hilum of the kidney and the kidney may be displaced laterally and its lower part rotated laterally. Dilatation of the calyces may also manifest itself as an irregular plump bulging of the outline of the kidney. If the dilatation is still greater, a more or less well-defined soft tissue mass will be seen at the site of the kidney (Fig. 265). It may fill half of the abdomen and even extend beyond the midline. A corresponding displacement, particularly of the stomach, small intestine and large intestine, is then demonstrable. I have also seen a uterus towards the end of pregnancy displaced severely to the left by a right-sided hydronephrotic sac containing eight liters of fluid (Fig. 265).

Hydronephrosis may be an hereditary disease. This fact should be borne in mind in every case of unilateral hydronephrosis detected in a child (JEWELL and BOUCHERT, 1962).

Hydronephrosis is an important differential diagnostic possibility, which must be remembered when a retroperitoneal space-occupying lesion is found at the site of the kidney. Thus, when at plain radiography a large, more or less regularly outlined kidney is found while at urography absence of excretion is detected, the possibility of hydronephrosis should always be borne in mind.

Calcifications are occasionally seen, representing single or multiple stones in the renal pelvis. Marked changes in position of such a stone at change of position of the patient make clear its localization in a dilated kidney pelvis.

2. Pyelography and urography

Of the remaining methods available, pyelography is that used most. However, since urography yields largely the same information as pyelography, it is gradually superseding pyelography. The part of the urinary tract on which pyelography will give the most valu-

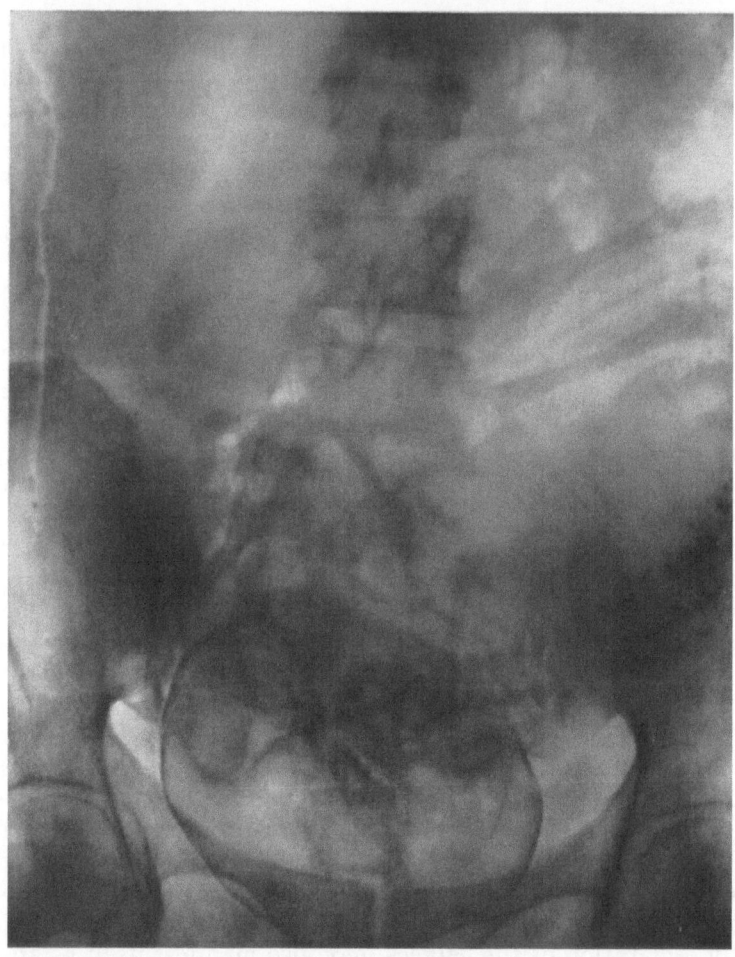

Fig. 265. Giant hydronephrosis. Plain radiography during pregnancy: large soft tissue mass to the right, displacing uterus with foetus and gasfilled large bowel. Post-partum operation disclosed hydronephrotic sac containing 8 liters of fluid

able information is the pelviureteric junction. However, the more the examiner is familiar with the different types of obstructed pelviureteric junction and the more often renal angiography is used in the diagnosis, the more the combination of urography and renal angiography will be used instead of pyelography. From the small field of vision over the pelviureteric junction, the detailed anatomy of which is of minor importance in advanced cases, once the site and severity of the obstruction have been established, the examiner will have widened his interest to embrace the morphology and function of the kidney as a whole. Thus evaluation of indications for operation and choice of surgical method can now be made on a broader anatomic and physiologic basis.

a) Pyelography

Judging from the literature, there is more or less general agreement that pyelography should not be performed on a patient with hydronephrosis, particularly because of the risk of infecting an organ the drainage of which is blocked. If pyelography is performed, the patient should be turned in different directions in order to obtain a filling of all parts of the renal pelvis. Examination in the prone position is important because the heavy contrast medium flows to the declivous parts of the renal pelvis, i.e., in prone position, the ventrally situated region including the pelviureteric junction. This region is most important and at pyelography the anatomy here will be better demonstrated than at urography. It may also be worthwhile to examine the patient in the erect position because an obstruction, e.g. by a supplementary vessel, may be more marked when the patient is standing than when lying. ROLLESTON and RAY (1957) found a horizontal lateral view, with the patient

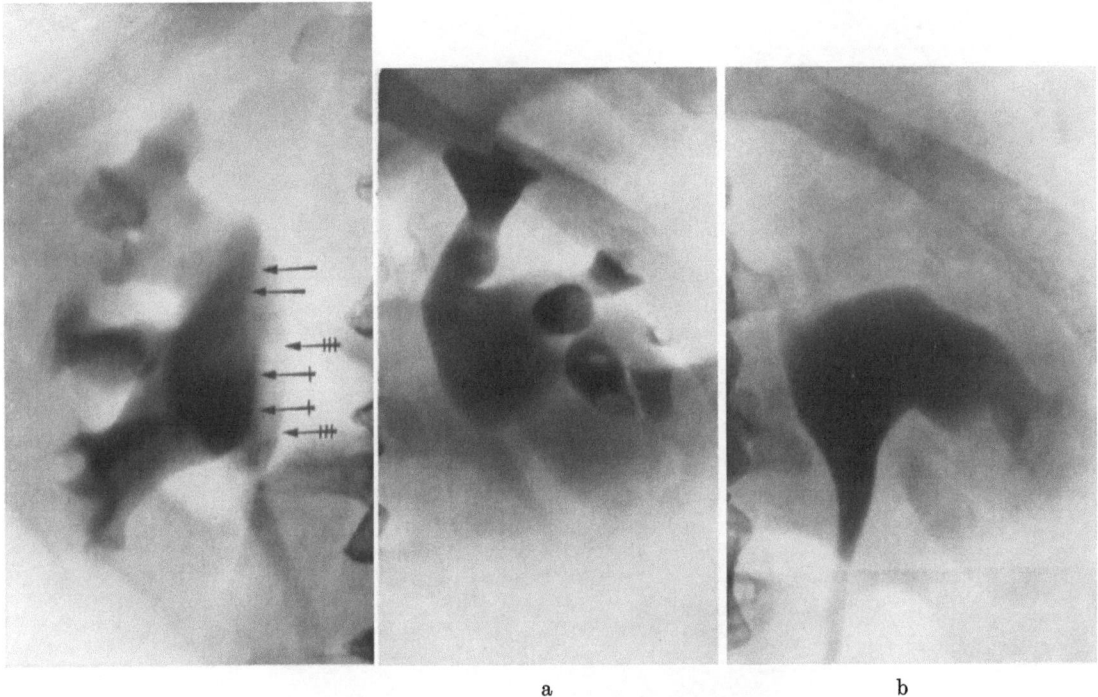

a   b

Fig. 266   Fig. 267

Fig. 266. Layer formation in urography in slightly dilated kidney pelvis. Release of ureteric compression. Three steps of impression into kidney pelvis by oblique lateral part of psoas muscle are seen. Upper branch of most dorsal part is impressed by most lateral part of muscle, which is most dorsal (←). At lower branch, situated somewhat more ventrally, is impressed by middle portion of muscle. At ←⦀ confluence, situated most ventrally, is only slightly impressed

Fig. 267. Layer formation and its influence on examination technique. Slight obstruction of distal part of ureter. a) Supine position: dorsal calyces and dorsal part of confluence filled. No filling of pelviureteric junction. b) Prone position: ventral parts including pelviureteric junction now contain contrast urine

supine, to be particularly important because in that position the kidney is dragged posteriorly, tending to place it on the stretch, with resulting compression of the fixed upper portion of the ureter.

During injection of the contrast medium into the renal pelvis a compensated hydronephrosis may be converted into an acute manifest hydronephrosis. Occasionally a renal pelvis of relatively normal appearance may suddenly expand during retrograde pyelography. If a large amount of contrast medium has been injected into the renal pelvis, the

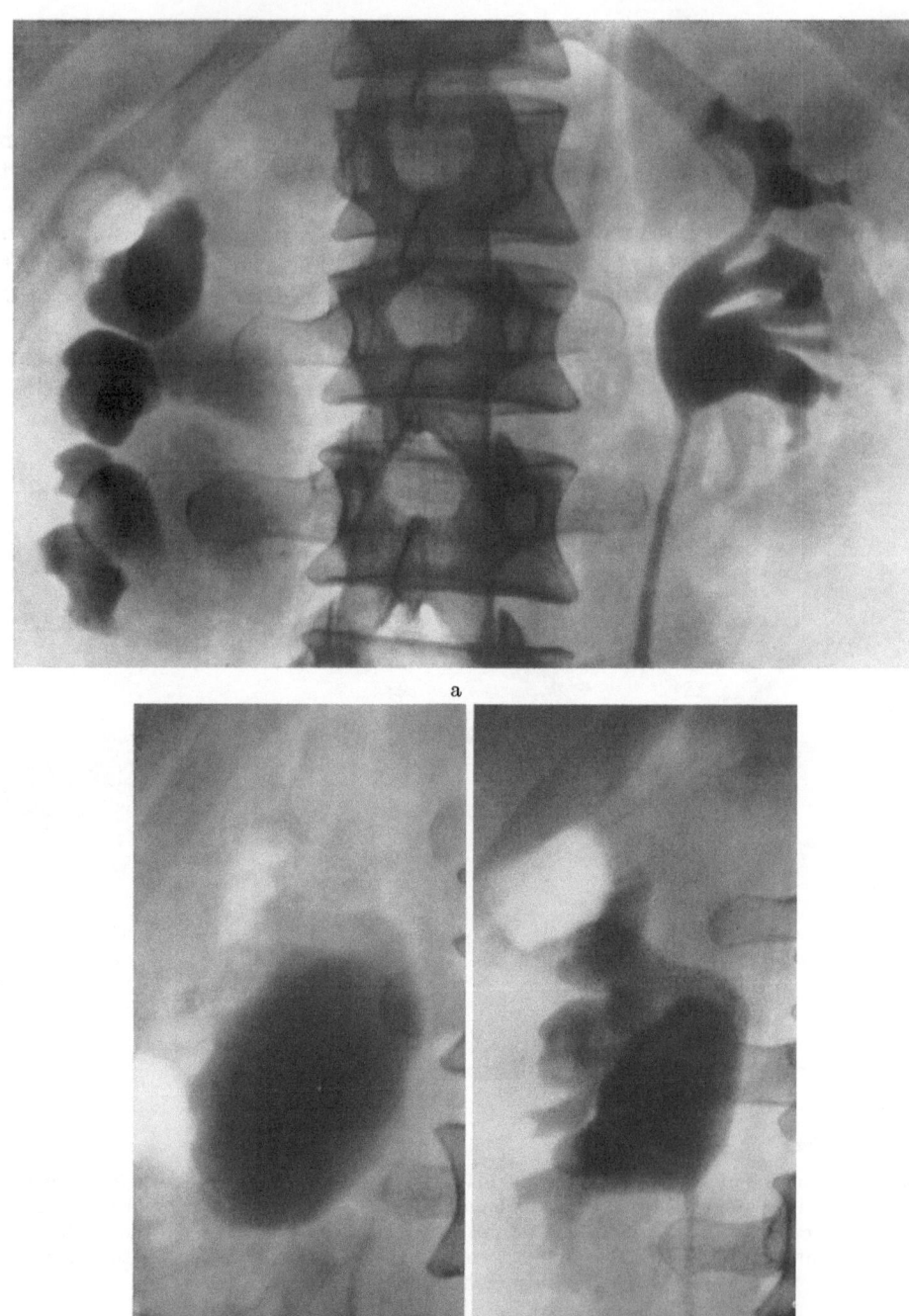

Fig. 268. Hydronephrosis. a) Urography: dilatation of right kidney pelvis by obstructed pelviureteric junction. Marked narrowing of junction on contralateral side but no dilatation. b) Prone position: filling of confluence part of kidney pelvis. Contrast urine runs over into ureter, which is not dilated. Pyeloplasty. c) Postoperative check urography: regression of dilatation. Undisturbed flow over into ureter already in supine position

catheter should be left *in situ* for a while to facilitate drainage after the end of the examination.

Here, too, the findings will vary with the severity of dilatation. If obstruction is intermittent, the finding may be quite normal, although a narrow pelviureteric junction may suggest the possibility of obstruction. Even in slight dilatation and especially in cases with persistent slight dilatation after long standing, fairly marked dilatation, the so-called psoas edge sign (HUTTER, 1930) may be demonstrated. This sign consists of the medial part of the renal pelvis being pressed against the lateral surface of the psoas muscle so as to appear with a sharp, even outline instead of the usual rounded, medial outline. This phenomenon is due to the fact that the renal pelvis is more likely than not to be moulded readily by surrounding tissue and thereby to be deformed by the firmer psoas muscle and, secondly, by the layer formation between the contrast medium in the urine. This phenomenon is discussed in the chapter on retrograde pyelography. This layer formation plays an important role in the examination of hydronephrosis (Fig. 266, 267). Thus, the contrast medium will accumulate in the lowest calyces, i.e. the dorsal and the cranial

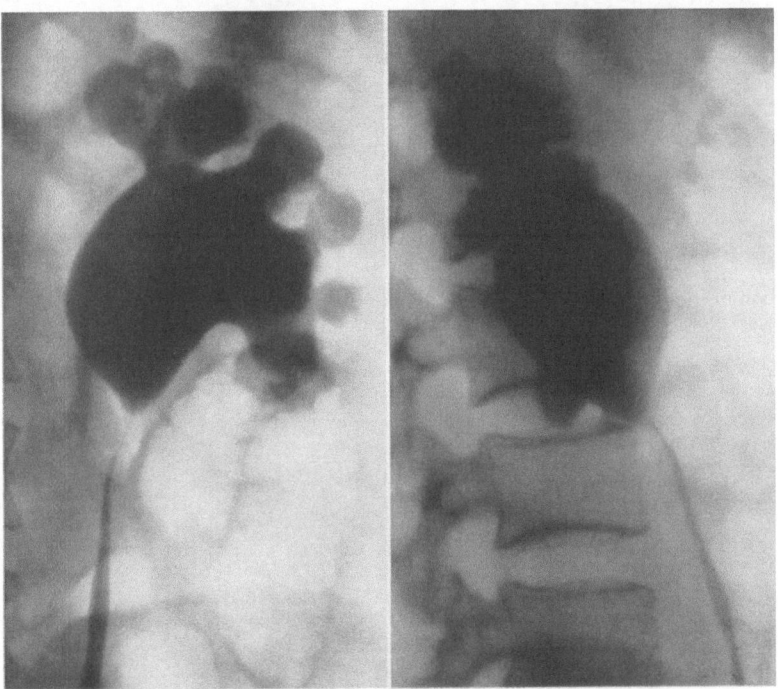

Fig. 269. Hydronephrosis through intrinsic stenosis in pelviureteric junction. Pyelography, extrarenal pelvis: marked atrophy of papillae. Note position of calyces and confluence in lateral view

if the patient is examined in the supine position. In order to form an opinion of the other calyces, and above all of the confluence of the renal pelvis, it is necessary either to use a large amount of contrast medium to secure a filling of the entire renal pelvis or to turn the patient over into a prone position so that the confluence of the renal pelvis, which is directed ventrally, will lie lowermost and thus receive the heavy contrast medium (Fig. 268). Layer formation is also demonstrable on examination of the patient in the erect position.

The renal pelvis becomes wider also in that part bordered by the parenchyma, which results in an increase in size of the renal sinus and a flattening of the papillae, so that the calyces become plumper (Fig. 269). This sign has been utilized for determining whether the kidney should be regarded as hydronephrotic or not. O'CONOR (1954) pointed out that a hydronephrotic kidney always has minor calyces showing distortion from the usual umbilicated outline; thus the papillae are flattened and the calyces blunted.

The renal pelvis empties slower than usually, so that examination at an interval of an hour, so-called delayed picture, may be of value.

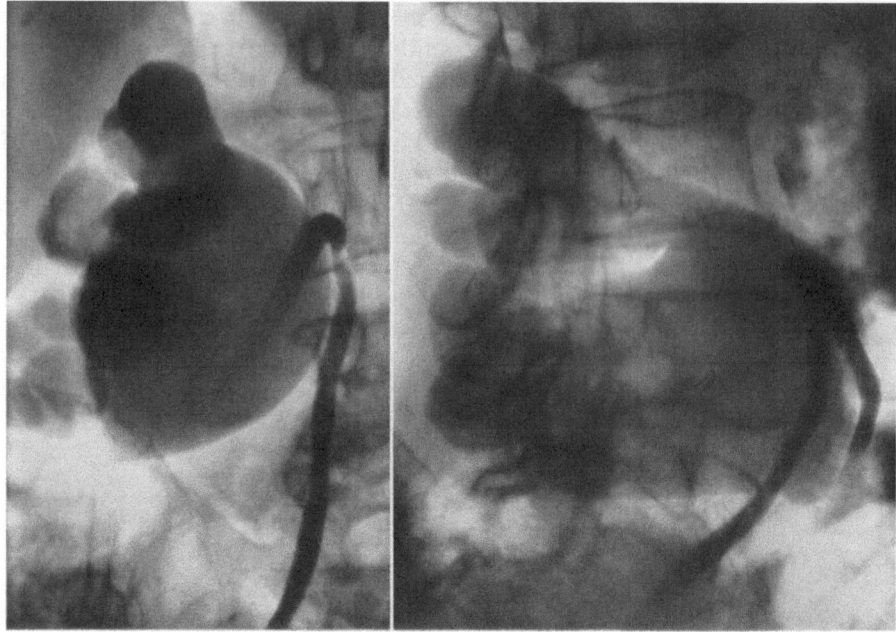

Fig. 270. Dilatation of kidney pelvis and sharp angular fixation of ureter to confluence by adhesions. No vascular anomaly

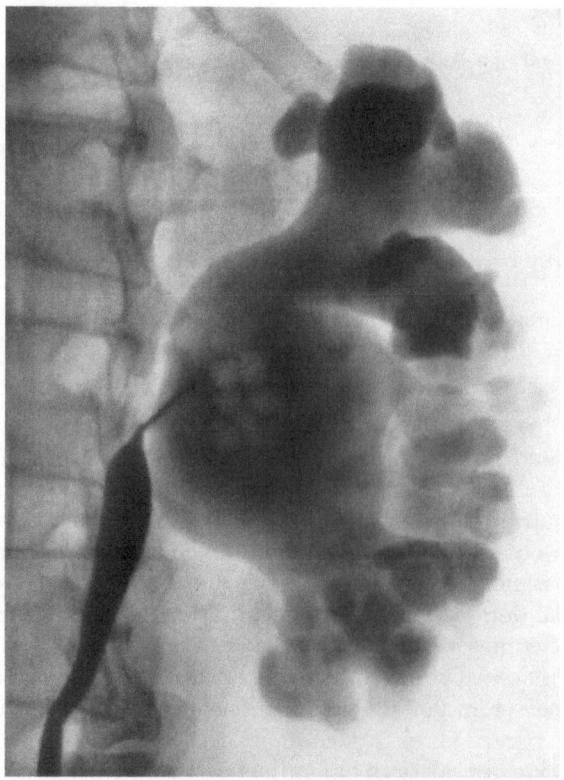

Fig. 271. Hydronephrosis due to short intrinsic stenosis. Pyelography: contrast medium injected into ureter under pressure passes through obstructed pelviureteric junction as a long jet into the confluence, giving impression of long stenosis. Multiple stones. Marked papillary atrophy

Dilatation may be mainly intrarenal or extrarenal. If intrarenal, the effect on the renal parenchyma will appear sooner and be more severe, with striking widening of the sinus. If the dilatation is mainly extrarenal, large extrarenal hydronephrosis may develop, sometimes without appreciably impairing renal function.

At the pelviureteric junction the upper part of the ureter will be situated close to the dilated renal pelvis, which it follows ventrally, cranially before bending off sharply in caudal direction (Figs. 269, 270). The ureter will often show an extra bend or a small transverse band-shaped filling defect caused by the crossing of a vessel. These changes can be recognized best by turning the patient to a varying extent during fluoroscopic check. If the patient is supine, a filling defect due to an obstruction may be confused with layer formation in the ureter owing to a sharp bend so that its ventral, uppermost part does not contain contrast medium but shows a short filling defect. Judging from illustrations in various journals and manuals, such confusion is common. Another common misinterpretation is due to the fact that in a kidney situated somewhat lower than usual, the dilated renal pelvis, even if the dilatation is only slight, will be pressed against the ureter, which will show a gentle kink that will not be filled with contrast medium. When the kink is straightened out by change in position of the kidney e.g. by change in the position of the patient, a good filling will be obtained and no obstruction will be demonstrable. Nor should a transient contraction of the pelviureteric junction be interpreted as a stricture.

Another source of error should be observed: if contrast medium is injected under fairly high pressure near the obstruction, it may be forced through the latter into the fluid in the renal pelvis like a stream (compare the jet phenomenon from a ureteric orific into the bladder). This should not be interpreted as an obstruction of corresponding length (Fig. 271).

If obstruction is complete, making impossible injection of contrast medium into the renal pelvis via a catheter, or if for some reason catheterization is not possible, antegrade pyelography may be resorted to.

b) Urography

If contrast urine is excreted, urography offers largely the same diagnostic possibilities as pyelography and, in addition, gives information on the function of the kidney. For complete filling of the renal pelvis, contrast medium can be injected repeatedly until the renal pelvis flows over into the ureter or the postural position can be changed to the prone position, as above (see Fig. 268). Ureteric compression is unnecessary and often contraindicated. The diuresis produced by the contrast medium, like the contrast injection for pyelography, can be sufficient to convert a case of hydronephrosis from a compensated to an uncompensated condition. It may be mentioned here that in the presence of intermittent hydronephrosis or suspected intermittent hydronephrosis, the examination should be performed preferably during an attack of pain (Fig. 272, 273, 274). While the anatomic conditions may show only slight abnormality during remission, examination during an attack — if this is due to hydronephrosis — will show the renal pelvis to be widened and the contrast excretion to be impaired because of increased intrapelvic pressure.

The examination may also be performed under such conditions as — according to the patient — usually produce pain. If pain occurs when the patient has drunk a large quantity of liquid, he may be given such a quantity to drink before urography. Liquid can also be given by infusion in such cases (OLLE OLSSON, 1962). We call this procedure "water-loaded urography" (see chapter on urography technique). This technique has also been used by KENDALL and KARAFIN (1967). In one case described by COVINGTON and REESER (1950), consumption of 1500 cc of fluid produced pain. Severe hydronephrosis was seen at urography, whereas no signs of a pathologic condition had been found at previous examination.

We have used "water-loaded urography" for evaluation of the pelviureteric junction in doubtful cases. In patients with slight to moderate narrowing, or a narrow pelviureteric junction and data suggesting intermittent hydronephrosis, we have tried to test the function in the narrow junction. The contrast medium is injected when diuresis has started after water loading. At marked diuresis the renal pelvis and the ureter and often also the narrow pelviureteric junction, will be seen to widen.

The junction can often be studied with advantage cineradiographically with an image intensifier. A narrow junction may then sometimes be seen to widen to ordinary caliber for a short time. This part of the urinary tract lends itself well to cineradiography. How-

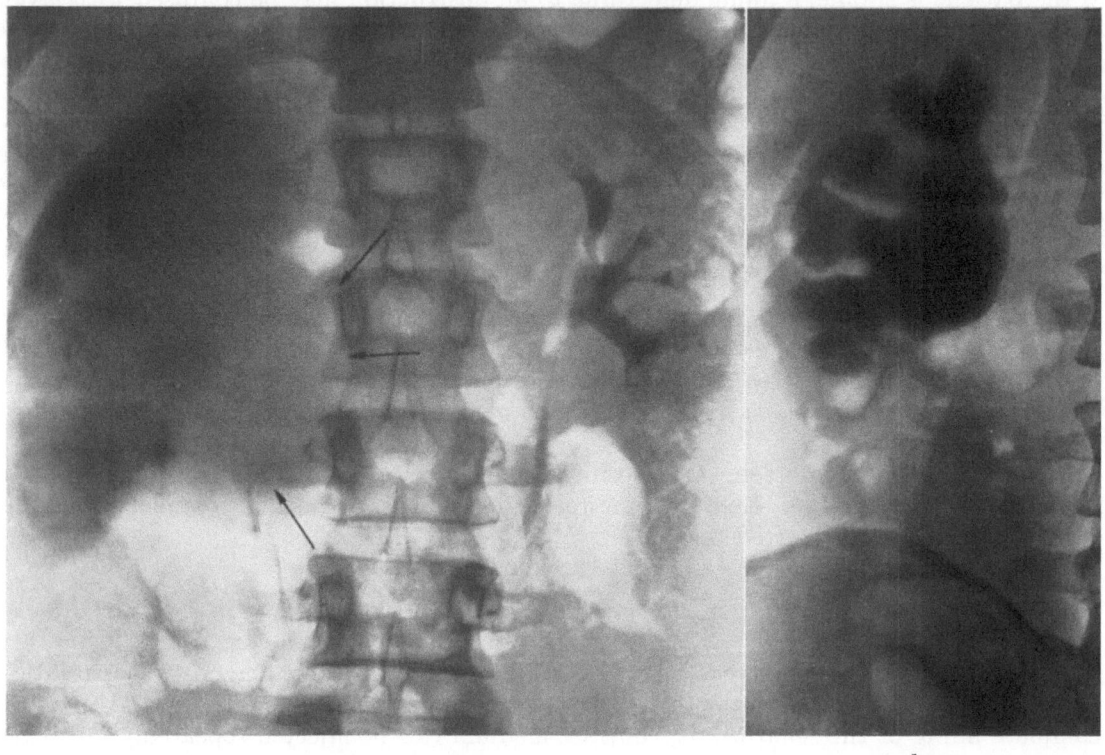

a   b

Fig. 272. Intermittent hydronephrosis in male, 25 years of age. a) Severe right-sided renal colic, acute examination. Urography: ordinary excretion on left side. No contrast excretion on right side. Marked dilatation of kidney pelvis can be seen (see arrows). b) Urography after pain subsided: marked decrease in dilatation of kidney pelvis

ever, neither the normal nor pathologic behavior of the pelviureteric junction has as yet been properly investigated.

It cannot be stressed enough that narrowing of the pelviureteric junction, as demonstrated by pyelography or urography, is often bilateral. The narrowing need not be of the same severity on both sides, however. It may be severe on one side and only slight on the other. In the investigation of a given case, however, it is important to determine whether the changes are unilateral or bilateral.

Urography offers a possibility of judging renal function, including estimation of the rate at which the renal pelvis is drained, and the condition of the renal parenchyma. The drainage rate is influenced by the position of the patient, the concentration of the contrast medium, the size of the dose injected, the degree to which the bladder is filled etc. and must therefore be judged with caution and preferably compared with the contralateral kidney if conditions there are normal.

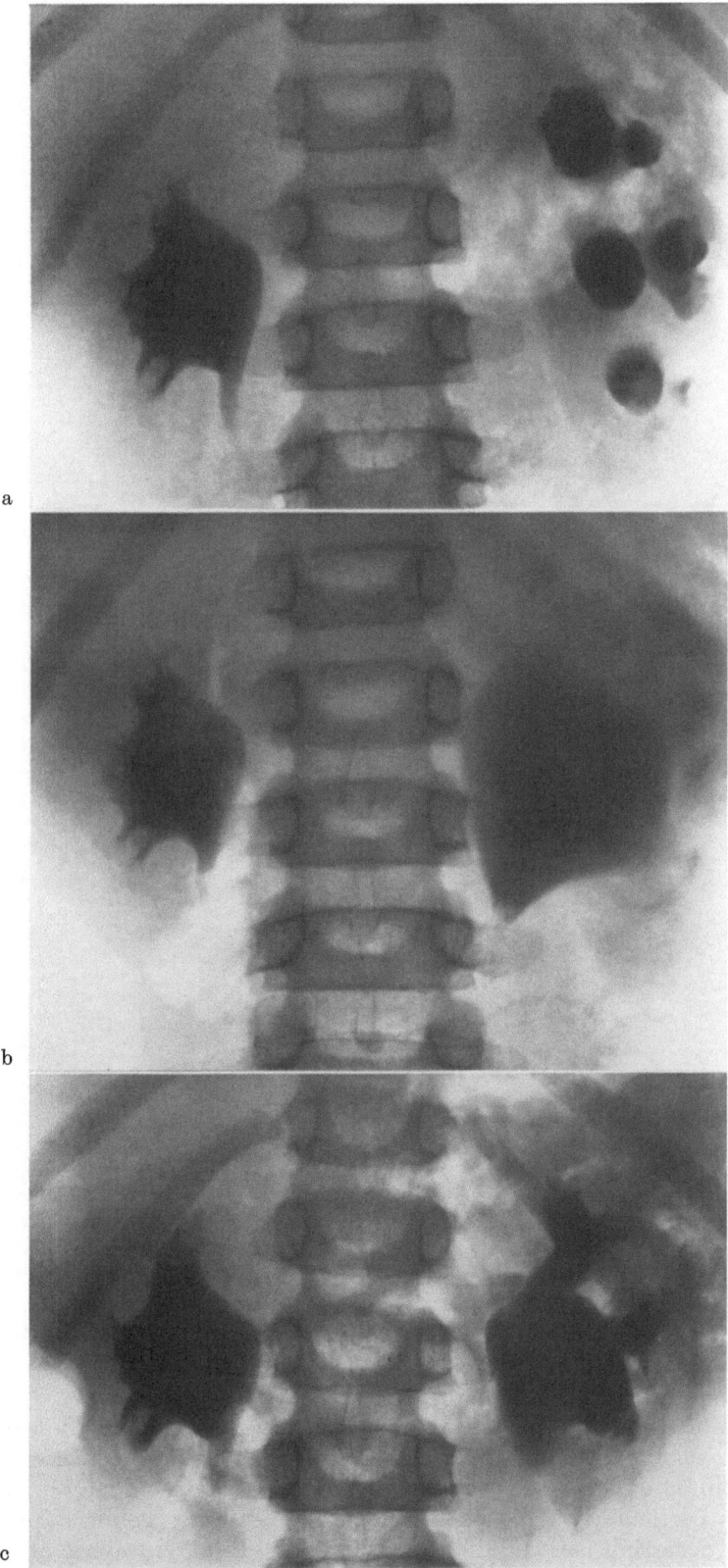

Fig. 273. Intermittent hydronephrosis in child 10 years of age. a) Urography immediately after renal colic attack on left side: marked dilatation of calyces. b) Same examination in prone position: marked dilatation of left kidney pelvis to pelviureteric junction. c) Urography some days later: dilatation and intrapelvic pressure have decreased markedly

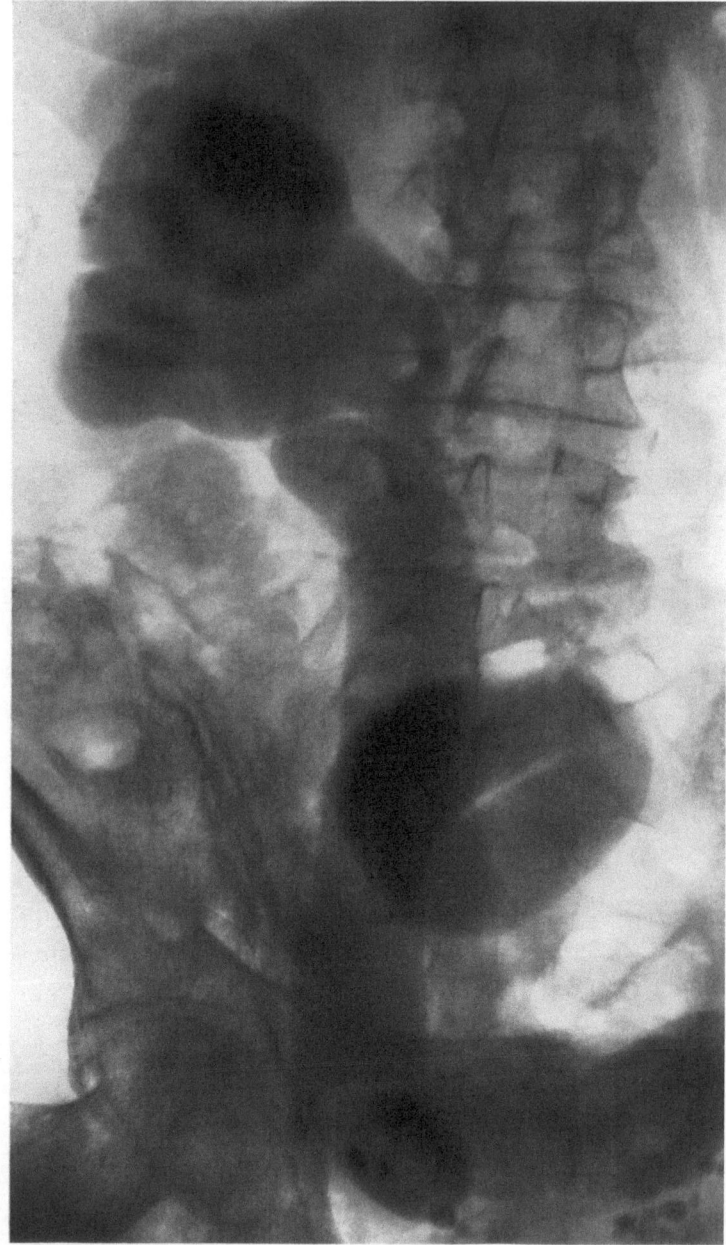

Fig. 274. Dilatation of urinary tract on right side. Urography 24 hours after injection of large amount of contrast medium: enormous increase in length and width of right ureter down to obstructed ureterovesical junction. Tortuosity with complete U-turn at middle of ureter

The state of the renal parenchyma can be crudely judged from the excretion of contrast urine: *i. e.* whether it is ordinary, of low density, or whether excretion has ceased. It should be pointed out that at urography the renal parenchyma may increase in density. This is obvious particularly if no excretion into the kidney pelvis is present. Extreme hydronephrosis occurring early in life and usually due to pelviureteric obstruction can be diagnosed as such if a thin margin of functioning parenchyma is seen in the nephrographic phase of the urographic procedure (ALLEN *et al.*, 1963).

Extreme hydronephrosis can be present at birth. The most common cause of an abdominal swelling from a renal mass at birth is polycystic renal disease. Nephroblastoma may also be the cause. In such cases urography with the observation indicated above is important and the demonstration of a margin of functioning parenchyma is diagnostic of pelvic dilatation.

In the evaluation of the condition of the renal parenchyma, the following considerations merit attention: If the excretion of contrast urine is good, it indicates good, although not necessarily normal, renal function. If the excretion is impaired or not demonstrable, it may be due to temporarily high intrapelvic pressure preventing secretion, the kidney recovering function as soon as the pressure has been released. It may also depend on the renal parenchyma's having suffered loss or impairment of function. In such cases urography will not produce sufficient information for solving the problem. This should also be borne in mind in comparing results at pre-operative and post-operative examination. It cannot be shown by urography whether cessation of function is temporary or permanent. The literature contains many articles in which this dilemma has not been observed. Absence of excretion of contrast urine has been taken as evidence that the kidney is destroyed and nephrectomy has then been performed. It is important to be familiar with the influence of the secretory pressure and of the intrapelvic pressure on the urographic findings if erroneous diagnoses are to be avoided. Definitive evaluation of the amount of functioning parenchyma i. e. potential renal function, requires renal angiography.

c) Renal angiography

In the arterial phase the intrarenal arteries can be seen to be distended and displaced a-round the dilated renal pelvis (Fig. 279). The main renal artery and even the aorta may be pushed aside by a markedly dilated pelvis. The interlobar arteries are displaced in wide arches over the branches of the renal pelvis. The narrowing of the arterial branches may be due not only to their distention but also to atrophy. It can be extremely marked. The findings in the presence of atrophy and the principle of interpretation were described in chapter G XIII. Attention should be given not only to the caliber of the renal artery but also to that of its intrarenal branches and the amount of renal parenchyma, as seen in the nephrogram. Knowledge of the width of the intrarenal branches is essential, particularly because atrophy begins in the renal parenchyma and thus involves the intrarenal branches first. In some cases of acute hydronephrosis delay in filling of secondary and tertiary arterial branches can be noted (SIEGELMAN and BOSNIAK, 1965).

The amount of functioning renal parenchyma can be assessed from the nephrogram (Fig. 276). A generalized or local atrophy of the parenchyma may be seen and a corresponding marked dilatation of the renal sinus. An irregular reduction in the accumulation of contrast medium or irregular hypervascularization and indentation in the surface of the kidney may be seen as signs of pyelonephritis. Proper evaluation of the renal parenchyma requires films taken during the actual nephrographic phase. A single film may be taken at such an unsatisfactory moment in relation to the initial accumulation of contrast medium that no nephrographic effect can be expected to show.

In the venous phase the renal vein may be seen to be displaced in the same way as the renal artery.

It is obvious from what has been said that renal angiography properly performed and critically judged forms a sound basis for assessing potential kidney function. The decision whether conservative therapy should be tried in a given case or whether nephrectomy should be resorted to is facilitated to a great extent by the information obtained from renal angiography.

Renal angiography also offers a possibility of detecting supplementary arteries and veins (Figs. 277—280). Almost half of our series of renal angiograms of patients with hydronephrosis show multiple arteries. This frequency is consistent with that found by others (ANDERSON, 1953, EDSMAN 1954). The importance of a supplementary artery in a given case of hydronephrosis varies. Sometimes its course is such that the possibility of

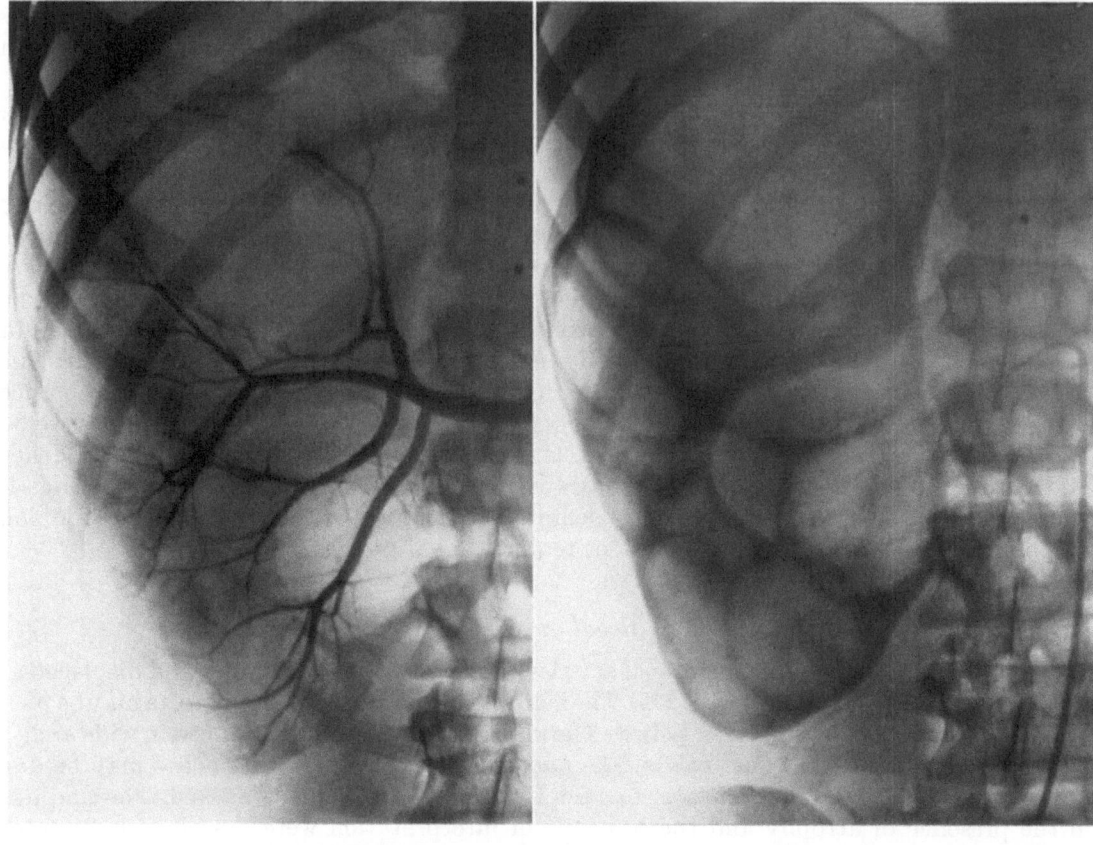

a   b

Fig. 275. Hydronephrosis on right side. Renal angiography: a) arterial phase: slight atrophy and marked stretching of intrarenal branches, which are displaced by dilated calyces. b) Nephrographic phase: narrow brim of functioning renal parenchyma around markedly dilated calyces

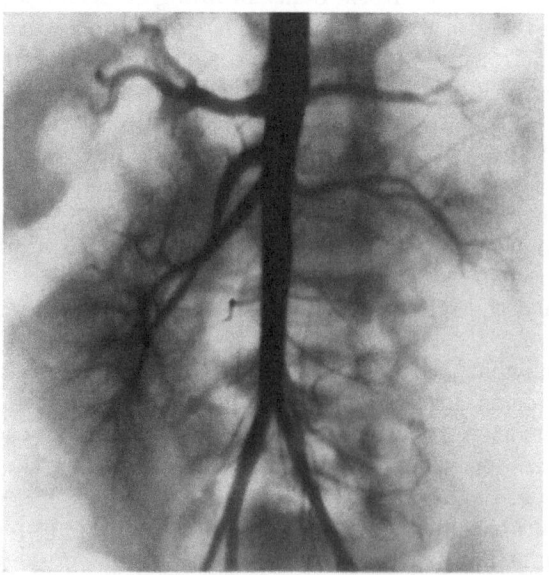

Fig. 276. Hydronephrosis on left side in child 4 months of age. Angiography: marked atrophy and displacement of left renal artery and branches. In nephrographic phase no functioning renal parenchyma could be seen. Nephrectomy: hydronephrosis with complete atrophy of renal parenchyma

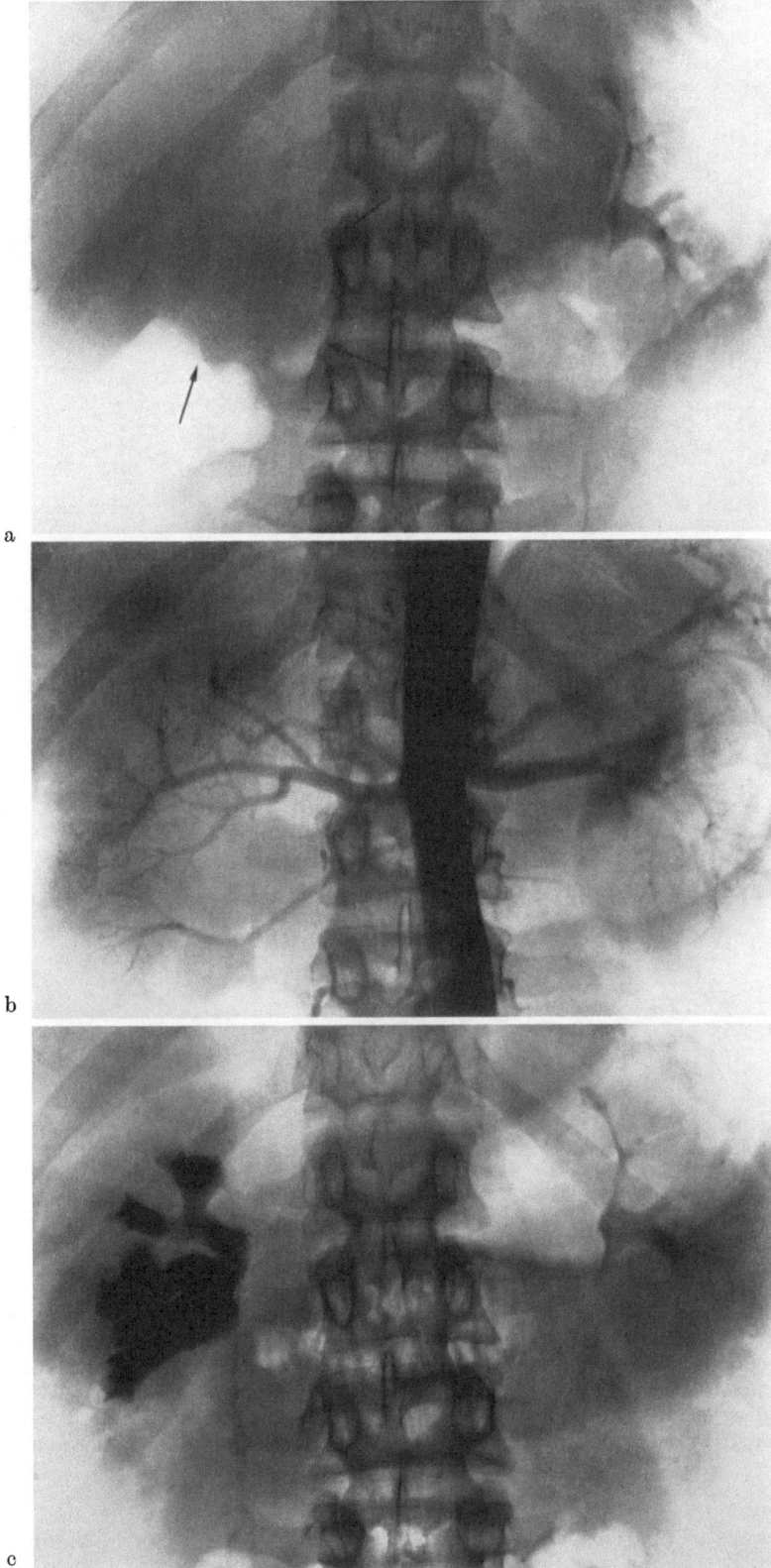

Fig. 277. Right-sided hydronephrosis. a) Urography: palpable mass in right side of abdomen. Ordinary excretion of contrast medium on left side. No excretion on right side. Dilatation of kidney pelvis can be seen as soft tissue mass corresponding to hilus of right kidney and medial to latter (arrows). Long axis of right kidney displaced with caudally open angle to mid-plane of body. b) Angiography: two renal arteries to right kidney with short distance between the arteries. Main renal artery displaced in slight curve cranially. Second artery markedly displaced in curve caudally, corresponding to dilated kidney pelvis (not filled). Operation: lower renal artery partially responsible for dilatation. c) Postoperative urography: Marked regression of dilatation. Free flow in right ureter

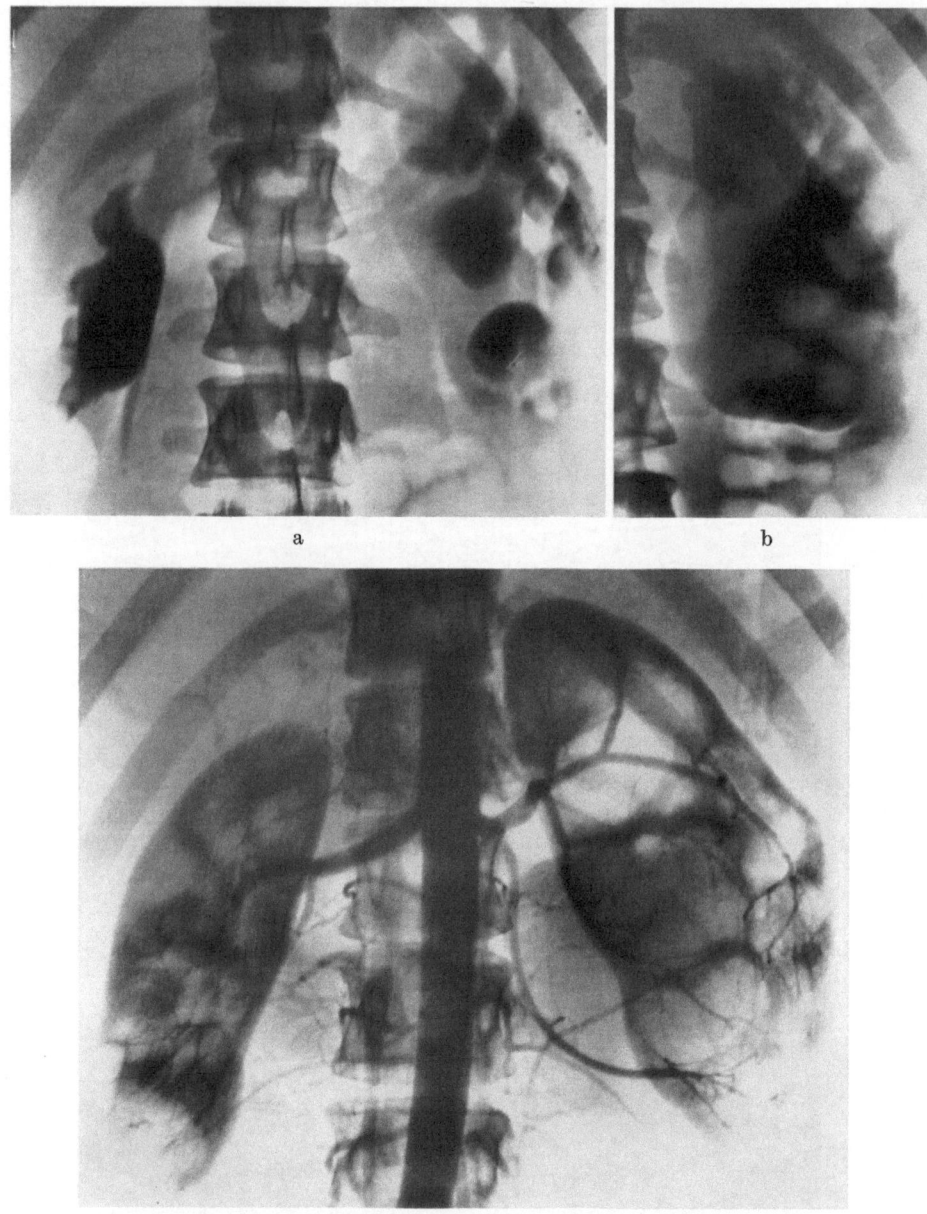

a   b

c

Fig. 278. Hydronephrosis caused by supplementary artery. Urography in a) supine position: marked dilatation of left kidney pelvis. Dorsal calyces filled; b) prone position: severly dilated confluence filled. Renal angiography: c) Arteries displaced by widened renal pelvis. Fairly good caliber of all branches. Supplementary artery to caudal pole stretched around dilated pelvis. Origin of supplementary artery is close to main renal artery. d) Nephrographic phase: kidney enlarged. Sinus markedly enlarged by dilated calyces. Operation with transposition of supplementary artery. e—h) Corresponding examinations: regression of dilatation. Arteries no longer displaced. Normalization of size of kidney and sinus

its being the cause of obstruction of the pelviureteric junction can be dismissed. In other cases the vessel may run close to the site of the narrowing. As a rule in such cases the vessel originates close to the main renal artery, runs in a curve corresponding to the periphery of the dilated renal pelvis, and crosses the junction. The vessel is narrow and distended, and that segment crossing the pelviureteric junction will correspond to a possible transverse filling defect observed in a previous pyelogram. The situation can be more easily

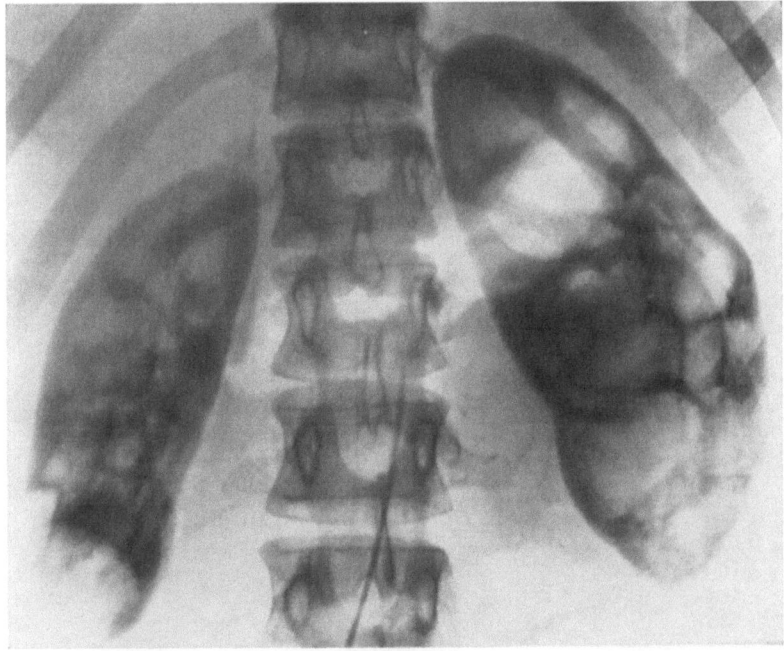

Fig. 278 d

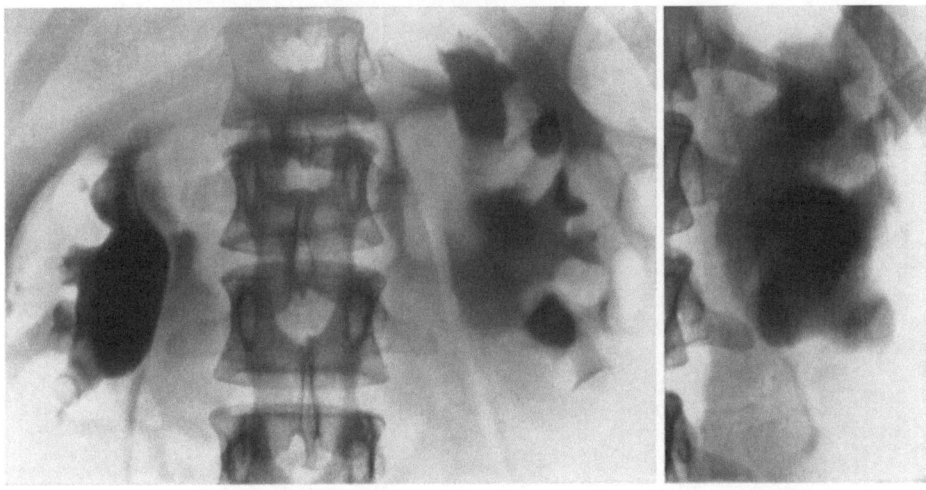

Fig. 278 e   f

judged if renal angiography is followed by urography, with the patient in the same position. It is then possible to form an accurate opinion of the relationship between the artery and the renal pelvis by tracing the arteriogram onto the urogram.

Sometimes the density of the nephrogram will be decreased in that part of the renal parenchyma supplied by the distended supplementary artery.

Even if the artery does run along the border of the dilated renal pelvis, that does not necessarily imply that the vessel is the cause of the hydronephrosis or even partly responsible. Occasionally even a distended artery may not interfere with drainage. More frequently, however, such a vessel may be a contributory factor but not the only cause. In addition to such a vessel, operation reveals, for example, an adhesion outside the renal pelvis and ureter as well as reduction in the lumen of the ureter. It is occasionally not possible to decide to what extent a supplementary artery is responsible for the obstruction until operation is performed, when attempts are made to widen or empty the renal pelvis.

21*

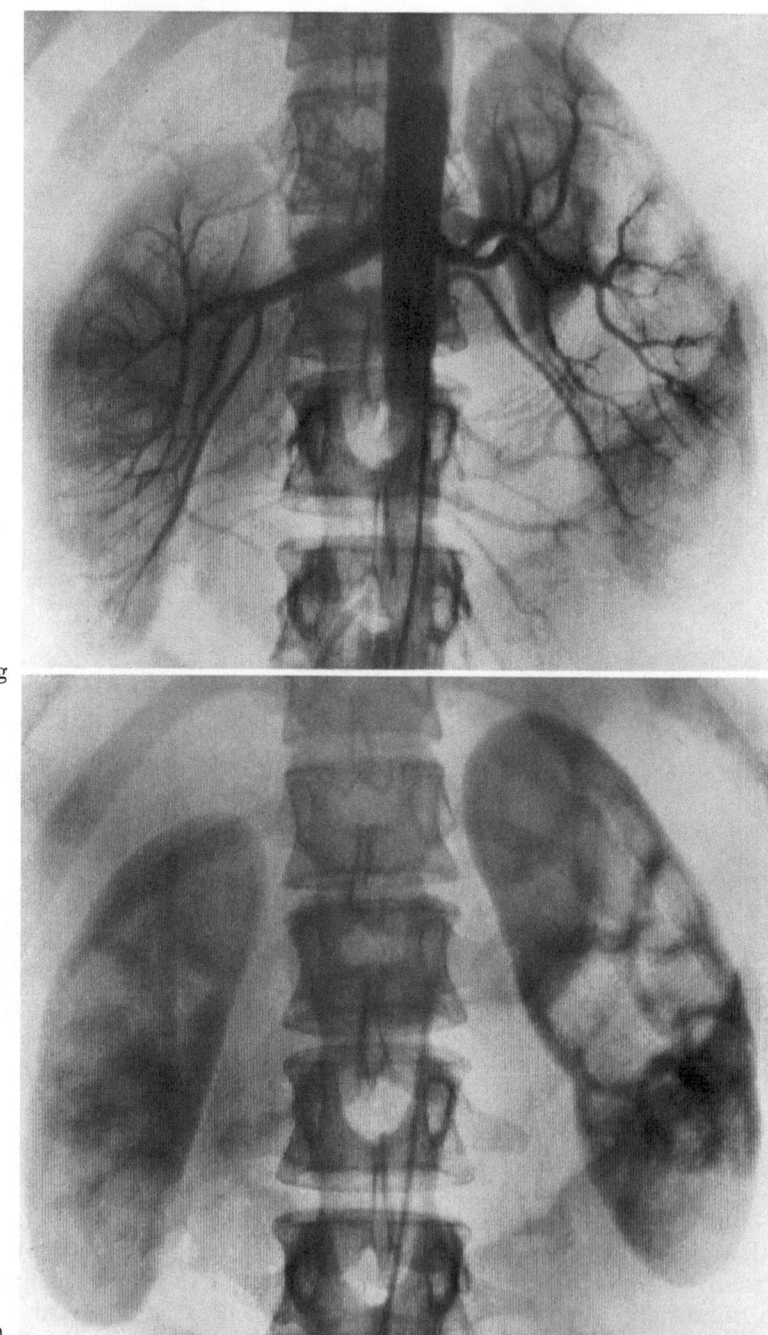

Fig. 278 g, h

Supplementary veins often accompany the arteries and may contribute to such obstruction or be entirely responsible for it, while the supplementary artery may be of no importance, or there may be a supplementary vein and no supplementary artery.

If operation shows a supplementary artery to be responsible for the obstruction, the artery should not be severed as this would result in atrophy of the part of the renal parenchyma supplied by it. Cases are on record in which such resection has resulted in hypertension. The vessel should be transposed in such a way as not to disturb drainage.

The adjusted course of the vessel can be checked by angiography after operation. If the operation is successful, the renal parenchyma supplied by the supplementary artery

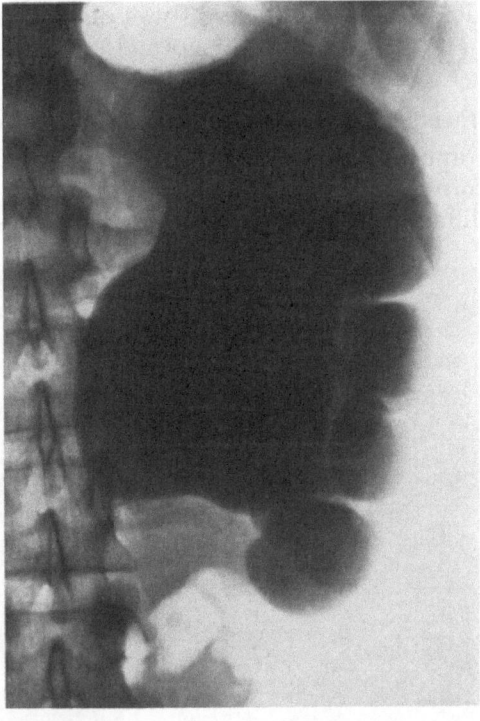

a

b c

Fig. 279. Hydronephrosis due to supplementary vein. a) Urography: marked dilatation of kidney pelvis to pelviureteric junction. b) Angiography, arterial phase: two renal arteries to left kidney. Slight displacement of main renal artery cranially and of supplementary artery caudally. c) Venous phase: vein corresponding to lower part of kidney artery markedly displaced in a curve caudally. At operation this vein was found to cause a sharp kink in the ureter and to be mainly responsible for the hydronephrosis

which was of decreased density when the vessel was distended before operation, can be seen at post-operative angiography to have a normal appearance.

4. Check roentgenography after operation for hydronephrosis

At check roentgenography to assess the result of an operation, it is important that the examination be performed under the same conditions as before the operation, as mentioned above. Any difference between the findings at pre- and post-operative uro-

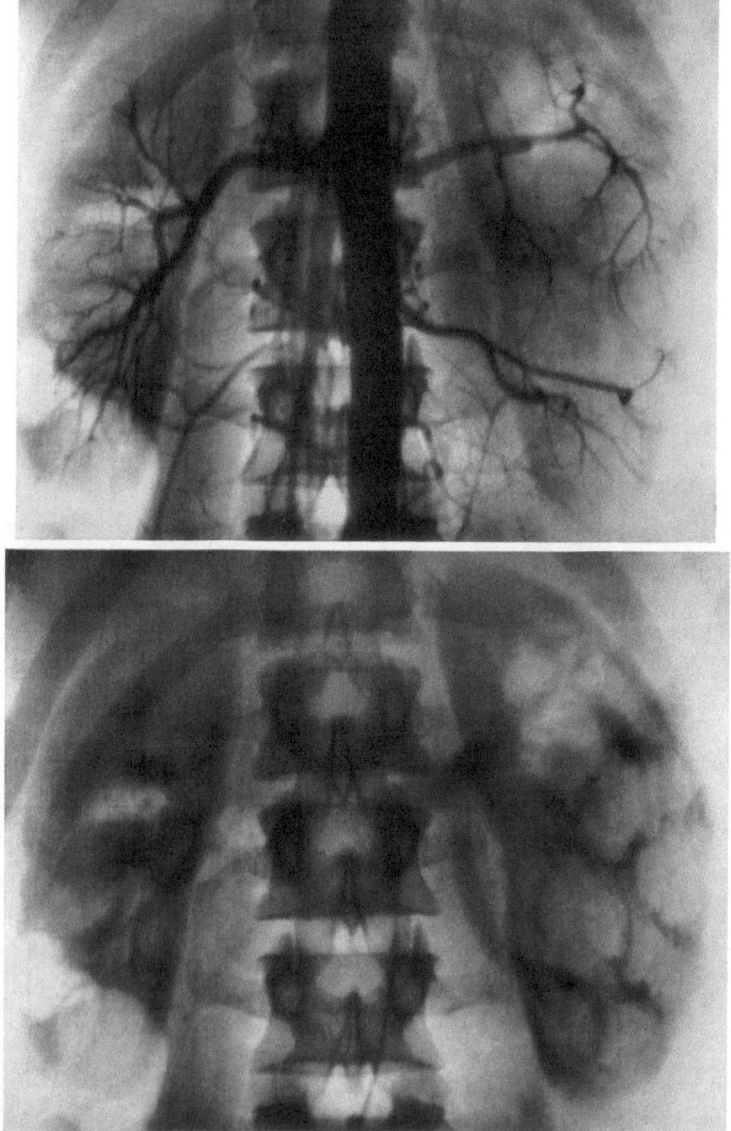

Fig. 280. Hydronephrosis due to supplementary artery and corresponding vein. Urography: scanty excretion on right side and marked dilatation of kidney pelvis. Obstruction at pelviureteric junction. a) Renal angiography: two arteries to left kidney displaced apart. b) Kidney enlarged and sinus widened. Displacement of vein from caudal pole around dilated pelvis. Operation: transposition of obstructing artery and vein. Loosening of adhesions. Urography: marked regression of dilatation. Free flow into ureter. c) and d) Postoperative renal angiography: no displacement of arteries or veins. Kidney size reduced. Urography: Left kidney e) before and f) after operation

graphy can then be ascribed to the operation and the possibility that differences in examination technique are responsible can be dismissed.

Judging from our experience, if any difference occurs, it does so rapidly, so that the situation seen on the first complete examination after operation may usually be regarded as the end-result.

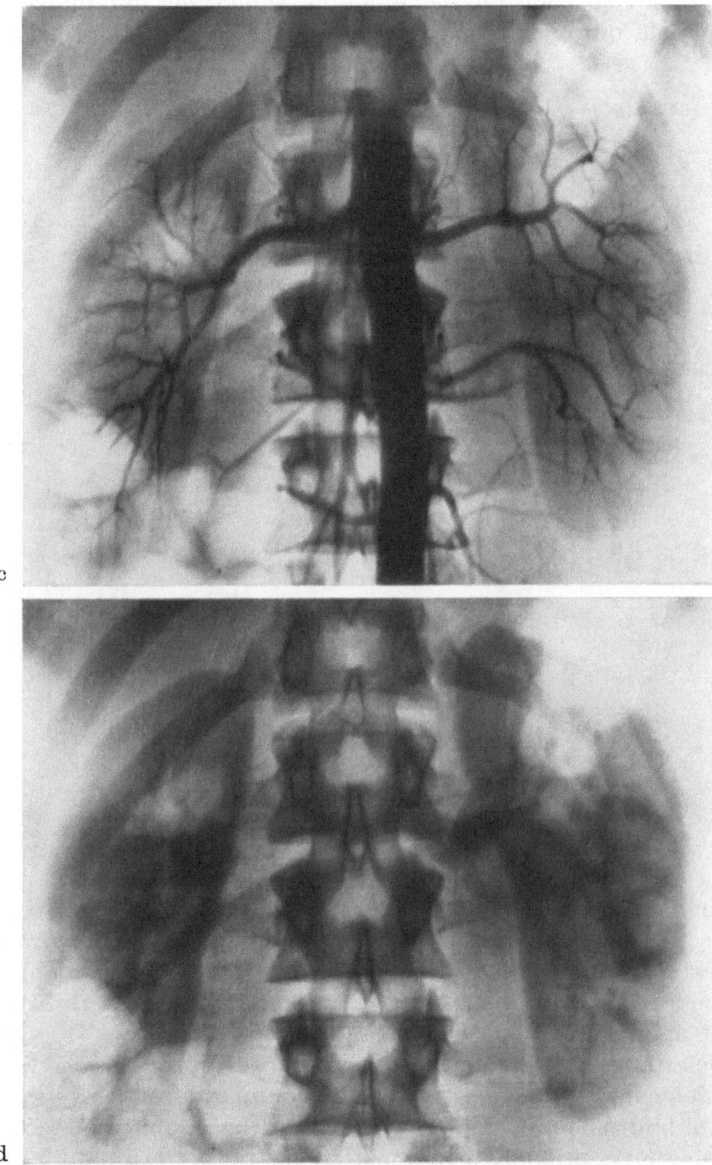

Fig. 280 c, d

We have also found the best anatomic results to be achieved in patients in whom the obstruction was due entirely or mainly to a vessel. The disappearance or regression of the dilatation in such cases is striking. In patients with stenosis, on the other hand, where the vessel was not responsible for the obstruction and where plastic surgery was performed, regression of dilatation after operation was less conspicuous. This discrepancy in the state of the renal pelvis in the two groups suggests that the congenital inhibitory malformation represented by fixation and stenosis is associated with congenital dilatation of the renal pelvis.

Urography and renal angiography in combination yield the best information on obstructed pelviureteric junction. Only on the actual local narrowing of the junction will pyelography give better information. This information is less valuable, however, than all of the important details on morphology and actual and potential function that can be obtained from urography and angiography and from direct comparison of the two sides. The supplementary information on the junction, sometimes obtainable only by pyeolography, can be gained only at the price of considerable risk of infection.

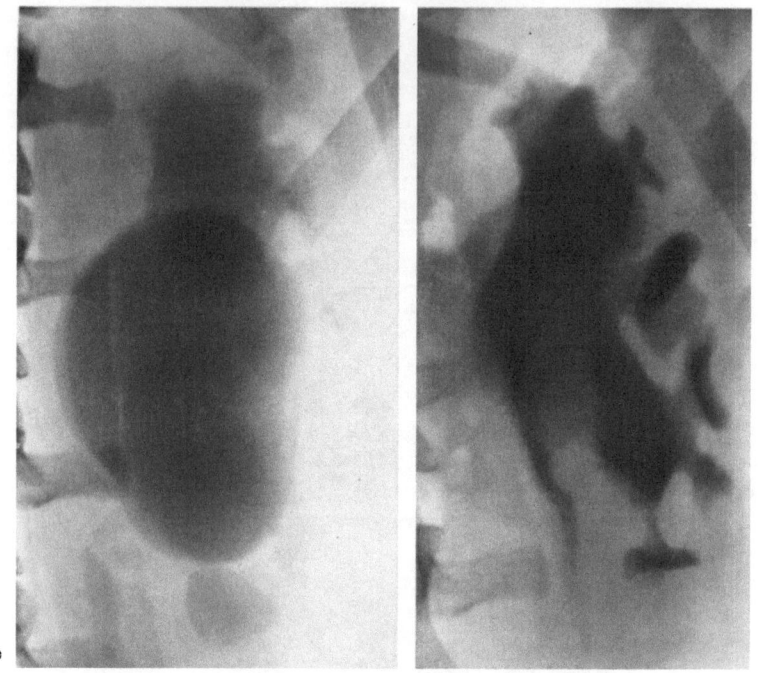

e   f

Fig. 280 e, f

3. Vessels and hydronephrosis

The significance of the vessels occupies a central position in the debate on the cause of hydronephrosis. This applies to supplementary arteries or ordinary branches, especially the lower polar artery. The problem can be successfully attacked roentgenologically by means of renal angiography and by comparison of the findings in this examination with those obtained at urography, at operation, and at post-operative urography. The discovery that multiple arteries are common in patients with hydronephrosis and demonstrable by renal angiography may lead to an overestimation of the role played by the vessels in the pathogenesis of hydronephrosis. A comparison of the findings, in accordance with the principles set forth above, provides a better basis for proper evaluation of the role of the various causal factors in a given case of hydronephrosis. Our material analyzed by BOIJSEN (1959) consisted of 39 cases of hydronephrosis in which supplementary arteries were found at renal angiography, and in which these supplementary arteries were verified at operation. The pelviureteric junction was carefully examined during operation, and urography was performed both before and after surgery. The cause of the obstruction was found to be due to the artery alone in 14 cases, artery + adhesions in two cases, and artery + adhesion + intracanalicular stenosis in one case, adhesions alone in four cases, and stenosis alone in 11. The supplementary artery was a causal factor in 17 cases out of 39, and was the only cause of the obstruction in 14 of these cases. In all of the other cases, i. e. in more than half, the vessel was in no way responsible. In all of the cases in which the vessel was a causal factor it ran ventrally to the renal pelvis. The supplementary artery regularly arose within 40 mm of the origin of the main renal artery from the aorta.

Criteria arguing for a supplementary artery causing hydronephrosis are as follows: the artery runs in caudolateral direction to the lower pole of the kidney and is displaced in a curve, with the convexity facing caudally; the artery arises within 40 mm of the main artery. In the absence of any deformity of the contralateral pelviureteric junction, the vessel may be the cause of obstruction; otherwise it is probable that the obstruction by the vessel is only secondary to a congenital stenosis, or that the vessel has nothing to do with the stenosis. Like other rules, this rule is not without exception.

As mentioned above, an abnormal vein may cause the same changes as an abnormal artery.

On contemplated transposition of a vessel and check examination of the results, renal angiography is, of course, the only acceptable examination method.

II. Dilatation of varying origin

As mentioned in the introduction, a variety of urinary diseases, particularly in childhood, are often associated with dilatation of the urinary pathways. The roentgen findings are largely the same except for differences due to variations in the primary disease.

Dilatation of the urinary tract is seen, for example, in the presence of stone in the ureter, tumor in or encroaching upon the ureter, vesical tumor involving the ureteric orifice, inflammatory edema or skrinkage, as in tuberculosis, retroperitoneal fibrosis, certain vascular anomalies such as anteureteric inferior caval vein, lesions of the ureter such as in association with ureterolithotomy, and in narrow ureterostomies or ureteroenteroanastomoses, post-radiotherapeutic edema, or cicatricious contraction, etc. (Fig. 281). Ureteric dilatation is also likely to occur in a large number of diseases which obstruct flow to the bladder and the emptying of the bladder. In all of these diseases, unilateral or bilateral dilatation of varying degrees occurs, as well as temporary or permanent impairment of renal function.

Direct encroachment of the carcinoma on the ureter in carcinoma of the colon may cause dilatation; pressure on the ureter may have the same effect. Urography should be performed prior to operation on every patient with a colon carcinoma, because of the relation between the ureters and the distal part of the colon.

One or both ureters may be involved in regional enterocolitis (Crohn's disease) usually in connection with abscess formation (ROMINGER et al., 1961). GOLDMAN and GLICKMAN (1962) expressed the opinion that urography should be included as part of the investigation of all patients for whom a diagnosis of regional enterocolitis has been made. The reason is that a slowly developing ureteral obstruction can be silent clinically, masked by the typical symptomathology of ileitis.

Epithelial necrosis may occur in connection with the use of Sendoxan causing blockage of ureters or of the bladder, with consequent delay of contrast excretion and dilatation, as seen at urography.

Broadly speaking, the principal remarks set forth above on the investigation of cases with obstruction of the pelviureteric junction also hold for these types of dilatation. The special investigation of the local obstruction due to the primary disease is added. Renal function should be the center of interest (Figs. 282). It may not be out of place again to stress the value of renal angiography in the evaluation of any impairment of renal function due to stasis and in deciding whether conservative or radical methods should be used if surgery is contemplated.

Mention should here be made of the possibility of a vessel obstructing flow in the distal part of the ureter by compressing the ureter (PRIESTLEY et al., 1954). An artery may thus cross the ureter a few centimeters above the ureterovesical junction (YOUNG and KISER, 1965). The vessel is most probably not the cause of the obstruction but is seen because of

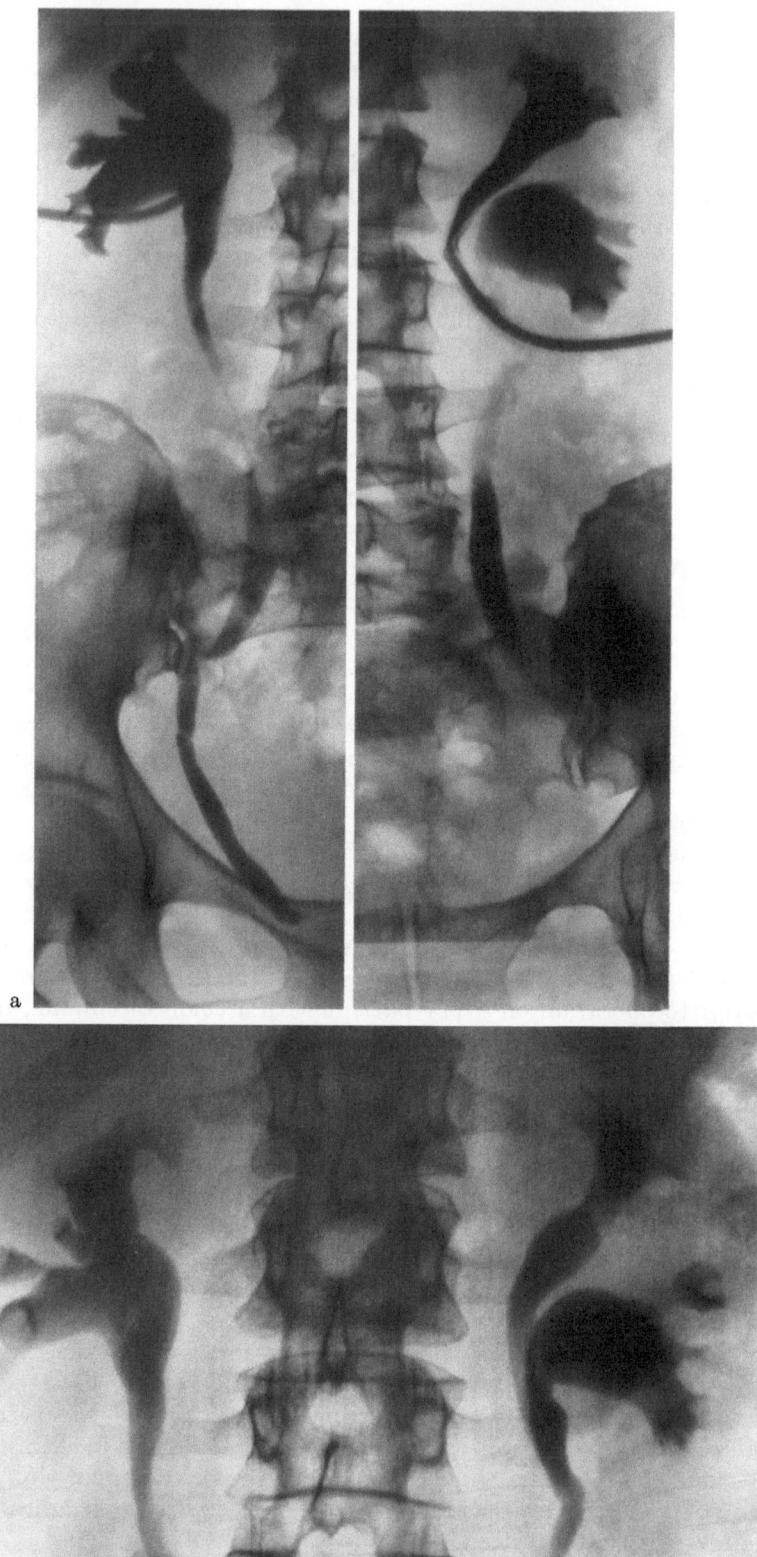

Fig. 281. Pyelostomy and antegrade pyelography bilaterally. Amputation of cervix uteri with accidental bilateral ligation of ureters and consequent anuria. Pyelostomy 2 days later. a) Antegrade pyelography: Complete blocking of caudal end, right ureter; somewhat more cranially, also of left ureter. Operation. b) Postoperative urography: Good excretion. No dilatation

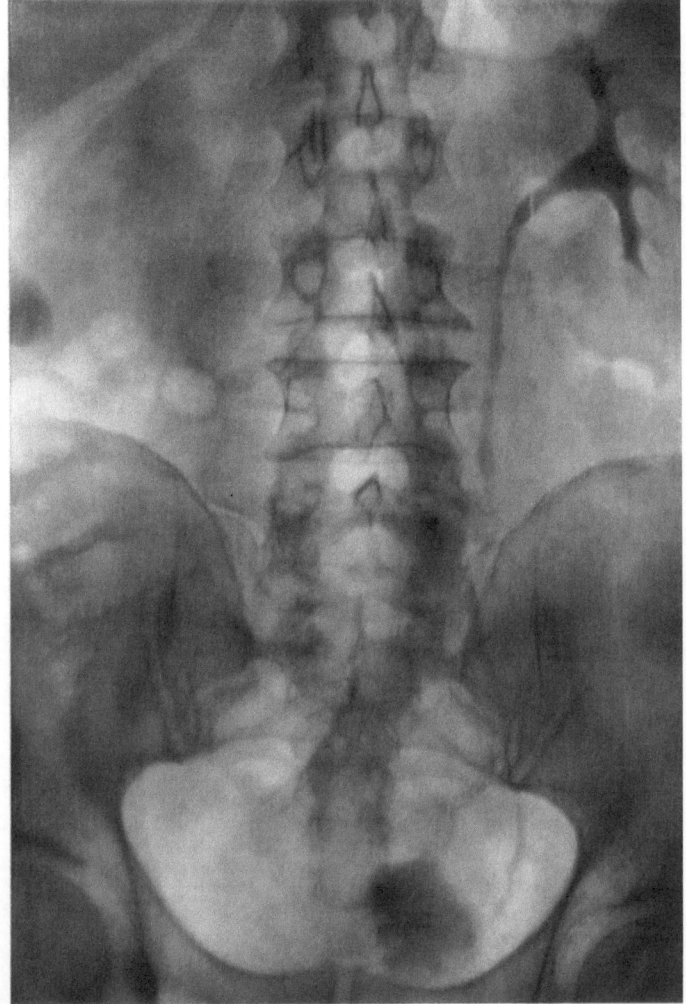

a

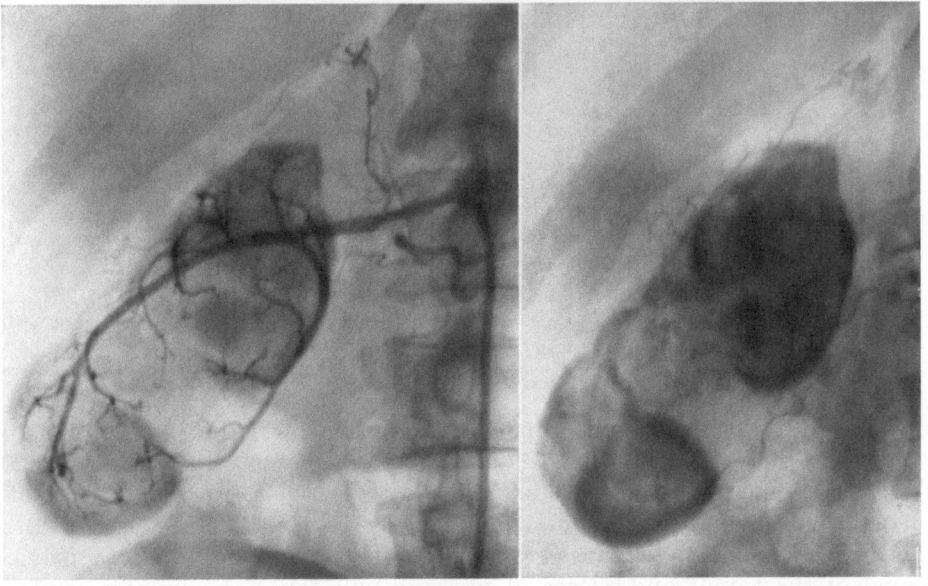

b   c

Fig. 282. Dilatation because of obstruction of right ureter by bladder carcinoma. a) Urography: Very slight
excretion on right side. b) and c) Renal angiography: Marked vascular and parenchymal atrophy. Large sinus
caused by dilated kidney pelvis. Irregular accumulation of contrast medium in kidney parenchyma and irregularity of kidney surface because of pyelonephritis

the dilatation. However, it may contribute to an increase of existing dilatation. (see chapter on Anomalies).

As to the examination technique, it should be borne in mind that the examiner should try to obtain a complete filling of a dilated renal pelvis and of a dilated ureter at urography. This may be secured by utilizing the high specific gravity of the contrast urine. Thus the patient should be placed in the supine position so that the confluence will be the lowest

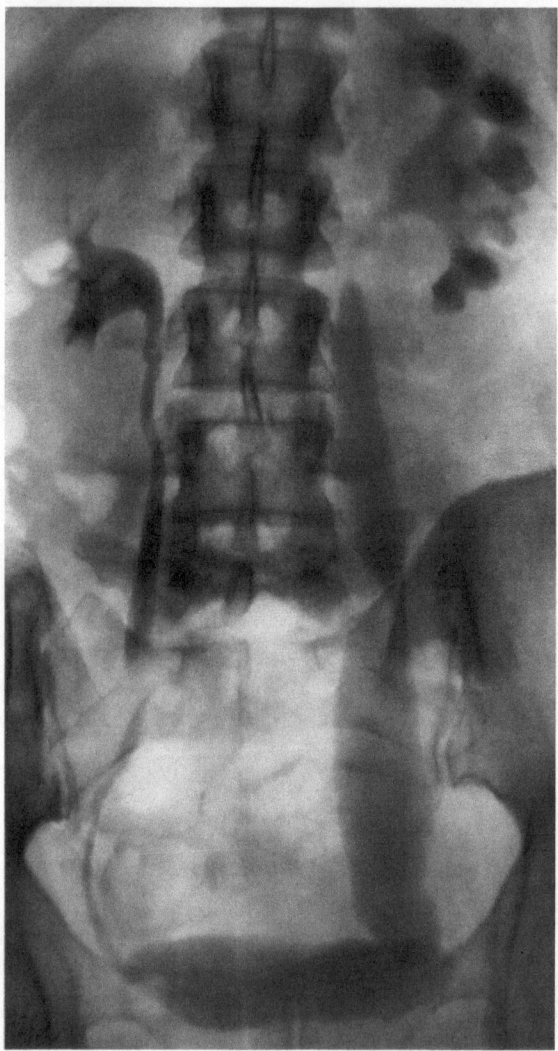

Fig. 283. Pyelonephritis with marked papillary atrophy and hydroureter due to incompetence of vesicoureteric junction

point in the renal pelvis, and the distal part of the ureter lower than the proximal portion. If the caudal part of the ureter is obstructed, the patient may be allowed to get up and walk about for a while (one minute to an hour, depending on the nature and degree of the obstruction) so that the contrast medium may sink to the obstruction (Fig. 283).

When a hydronephrosis is caused by compression of the ureter by a pelvic tumor, the removal of the tumor and release of pressure will cause the kidney pelvis and the ureter to return to ordinary width within one to four weeks after operation, even if the tumor has been present for several years (COKIER and EPSTEIN, 1962).

A few further details on special conditions are given below.

1. Dilatation of the urinary tract in infants

Dilatation of the urinary pathways in childhood is very often due to diseases in the bladder and/or urethra which are dealt with in greater detail in Part II of this volume.

A large number of diseases in childhood can cause dilatation of the urinary tract, such as urethral stenosis through a valve or a tumor, vaginal atresia and hydrocolposis (MUANG-MAN and UEHLING, 1971). CAMPBELL (1951) claims that more than 90% of all serious urologic diseases in childhood are due to urinary stasis in connection with infection. This is the case in meningocele, for example, and in other innervation disorders. ROSE and SMITH (1963) found at urography in 119 patients with myelomeningocele 12 (10 %) show-ing evidence of hydronephrosis. Urography must in these cases be considered as a screen-ing procedure. Cystography with study of possible vesico-ureteric reflux is the important type of examination (Fig. 283). It must be noted that in the majority of cases the urinary lesions are of a silent and progressive nature (GRAF *et al.*, 1964).

Bladder neck obstruction is another common cause of dilatation of the urinary tract, as is ureterocele. The latter condition is common in infants with duplicated renal pelvis (which occurs more often in girls than in boys) and in children with symptoms of disease of the urinary tract (see below).

If urination is difficult, the pressure in the urinary tract will be enhanced by the raised intravesical pressure, partly because the emptying of the ureter into the bladder will be obstructed and partly because an incompetent ureteric orifice does not provide a barrier against the increased intravesical pressure.

The dilatation may affect the urinary pathways on one or both sides. Unilateral dila-tation should draw the examiner's attention to the possibility of the obstruction's being in the distal part of that ureter, such as in the case of a ureterocele. The fact that the di-latation is present on only one side does not necessarily mean, however, that the obstruction must be prevesical. It may simply mean that only one of the ureteric orifices is incompe-tent.

The degree of dilatation varies. It is often considerable, with marked tortuosity of both ureters, so-called mega ureter (see below). Some authors attempt to distinguish a type of ureteric dilatation of mainly functional origin, differing in roentgenologic appear-ance from other types of dilatation. Such a distinction is not possible, as a rule.

Roentgen examination with contrast medium is often simplest in association with urethrocystography, which should always be performed. It cannot be stressed enough that *investigation of the urinary tract in children should, as a rule include urethrocystography because the cause of the disease is often found in the bladder and in the urethra*. In other words the examiner should not rely too much upon urography in the examination of children.

At urethrocystography, reflux of the contrast medium up into the ureters and renal pelves will often occur without special measures. Urethrocystography makes it possible to demonstrate not only the competence of the ureterovesical junction but, in incompe-tence, also the anatomy of the ureter and of the kidney pelvis. The filling may be rapidly transient. This filling can be facilitated by placing the patient with the head low. At incompetence in infants, a filling can be regularly obtained by lifting up the small patient by the feet, with the head down (see chapter on ureteric reflux).

Instrumental pyelography should be resorted to only in exceptional cases. The diagnostic problems can be solved, as a rule, by urethrocystography and urography since (as mentioned above) dilatation of the urinary tract in infants is due largely to changes in the bladder and urethra.

Therefore urethrocystography is almost always a necessary supplementary exami-nation in the investigation of urinary tract dilatation in children or at any rate it makes necessary the careful examination of the bladder during urography. It must be borne in mind, however, that even primary ureteric changes, e. g. ureter valve, unilateral or bi-lateral, may cause hydronephrosis.

2. Dilatation in prostatic hyperplasia

Micturition difficulties in prostatic hyperplasia impair drainage of the renal pelvis and ureter. Drainage may be impaired still more by the angulation of the distal part of the ureters because the base of the bladder is lifted by the enlarged prostatic gland. The common involvement of the urinary tract indicates roentgen examination, particularly if operation is contemplated. Experience has shown that, as far as contraindications for prostatectomy are concerned, the abnormal urogram is of direct positive value (TROELL, 1935; BRAASCH and EMMETT; v. HERMANN and KRAUS; MINDER, 1936; LIEDBERG, 1941).

a) Plain radiography

Since most of the patients are fairly old, it may be difficult to outline the kidneys because the fatty capsule is thin. In addition, the kidneys are often located low because of pulmonary emphysema and senile kyphosis, in which case their caudal poles are projected onto the bony pelvis. The presence of stone must be excluded and calcifications due to stone must be distinguished from vascular calcifications so common in these age groups. If the renal pelvis is markedly dilated, it is often possible to recognize its medial part.

b) Urography

Delayed excretion and dilatation of the renal pelves and ureters are common findings in advanced prostatic enlargement. The patient is placed in prone position for a while to secure a filling of the whole renal pelvis and the ureters, The dilated ureters are often very tortuous and dilatation most marked in their distal parts. The lower parts of the ureters swing more or less sharply medially-cranially before entering the bladder. (Fig. 284).

After establishment of drainage for about a month, the roentgenographic appearance becomes more normal: dilatation is less marked, excretion starts earlier, contrast density increases, and the emptying time of the renal pelves becomes shorter. The bladder and urethra are of course of great diagnostic interest. Changes in these parts of the urinary tract are dealt with in part II.

It should be noted that at urography prior to prostatectomy, a significant number of renal changes can be detected. Some of these renal abnormalities, according to BONA et al. (1961), merit precedence over prostatism for immediate treatment.

3. Dilatation of the urinary tract during pregnancy

Ever since CRUVEILHIER (1842) at autopsy demonstrated that severe dilatation of the upper urinary tract occurs during pregnancy the phenomenon has received much attention and prompted much speculation. Pyelographic and particularly urographic investigations have proved such distention to be common. In fact, it occurs in almost every pregnant woman. Dilatation of the renal pelvis and ureter, often in association with tortuosity, thus also with increase in length of the ureter, occurs in more than 90 % of all cases and is somewhat more common in multiparae than in primigravidae. Dilatation on the right side is more common, occurring twice as often as on the left side. It is also more marked on the right side in bilateral cases. Dilatation involves the renal pelvis (Fig. 285) and ureter, the latter to a considerably less extent or not at all distally. The dilatation usually ceases at the innominate line or at the level where the ureter crosses the iliac artery. The dilatation begins in the tenth week of pregnancy in primigravidae and in the sixth week in multiparae (SENG, 1929) and is more marked and more frequently seen in multiparae. During the first two to four months after its start, dilatation is only moderate but it increases gradually with advancing pregnancy and the ureters are often pushed laterally, including even the segment in the small pelvis (Figs. 285—287).

A certain regression of the dilatation may be seen already during the last part of pregnancy and after parturition the urinary pathways rapidly recover their ordinary width. Thus BRAASCH and EMMETT (1951) stated: "In more than half the cases the urinary tract returns to normal within two weeks after delivery. In almost all cases it will have returned

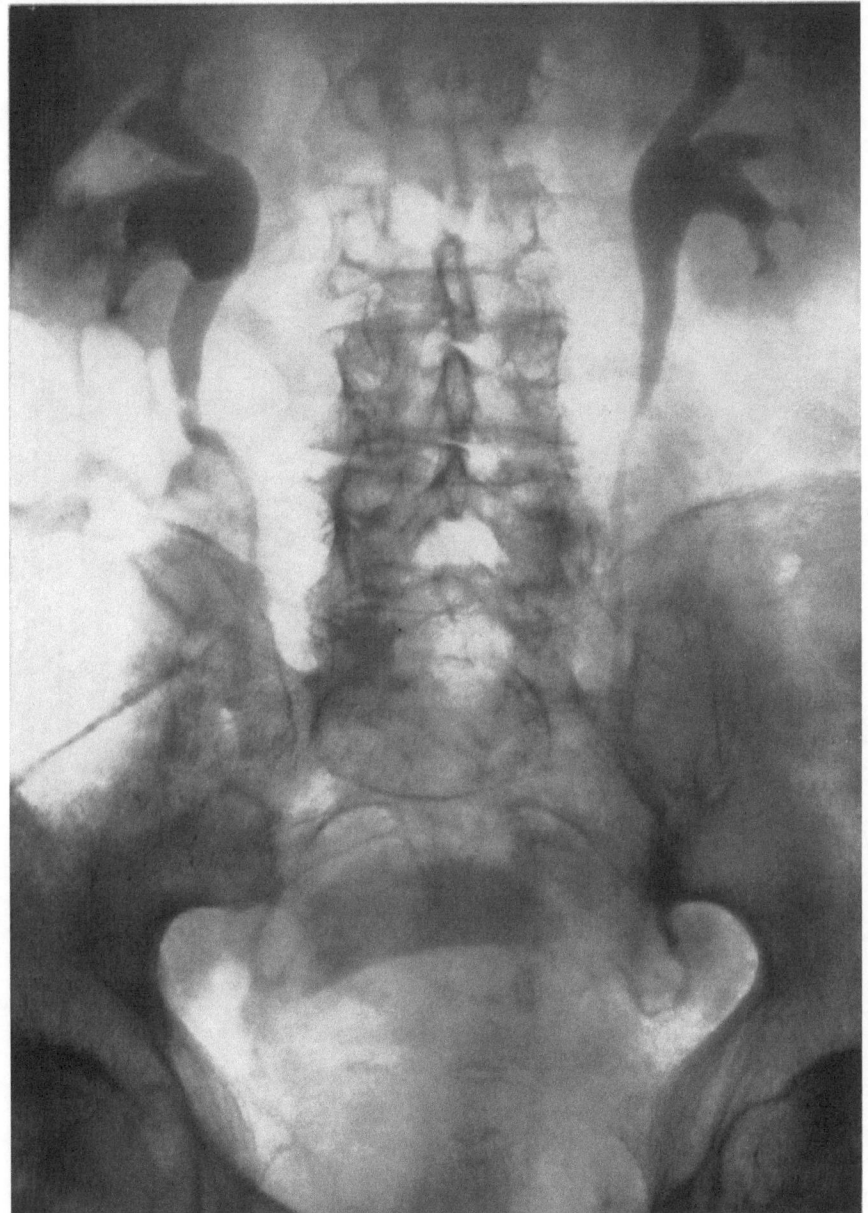

Fig. 284. Prostatic hyperplasia. Urography: slight dilatation of kidney pelvis bilaterally. Continuous filling of ureters. Marked displacement cranially of distal ends of ureters by large prostatic gland impressing upon bladder and displacing roof of bladder

to normal by the end of 12 weeks." However, slight widening may persist for a considerable time and the right renal pelvis will often be permanently widened to a slight degree and the upper part of the ureter may be dilated for the remainder of the patient's lifetime (OLLE OLSSON, 1956) (Fig. 286). This may explain the majority of cases with slight dilatation in which the right renal pelvis is, as a rule, slightly wider than the left. Most conspicuous is the frequently persisting slight dilatation of the right ureter in the part cranial to the crossing of the iliac artery. In cases with such dilatation, fixation to the artery obviously may readily cause dilatation of a ureter, with laxity of its wall. If pregnancy has been complicated by severe pyelitis, a marked widening may persist for a considerable length of time (CRABTREE, PRATHER and PRIEN, 1937; PUHL and JACOBI, 1932; CONTIADES, 1937). It may also be permanent (BRAASCH and MUSSEY, 1945).

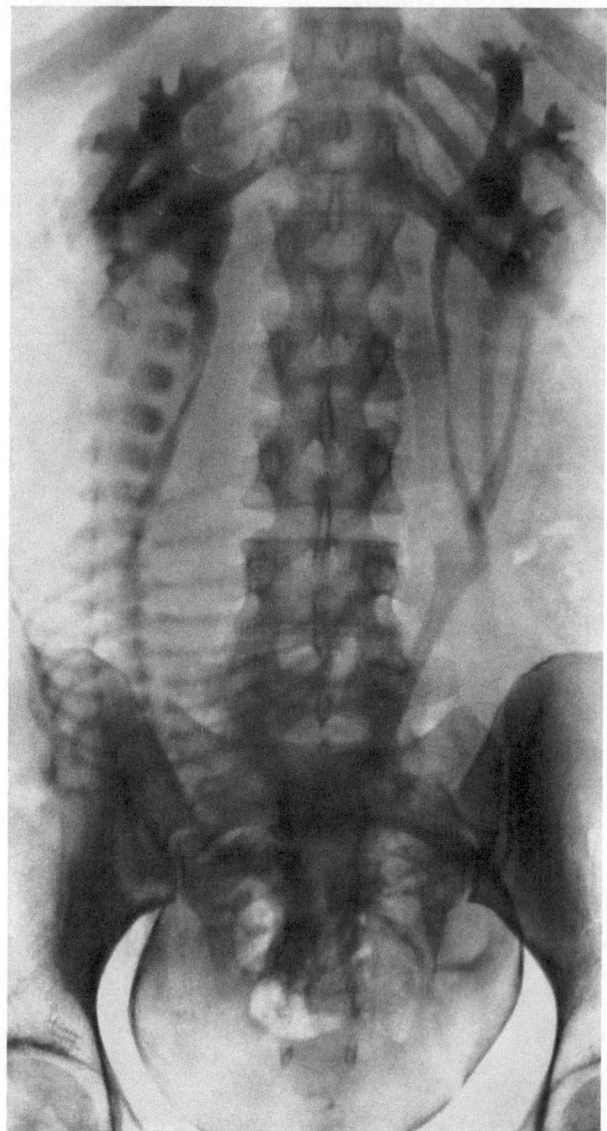

Fig. 285. Dilatation during pregnancy. Urography: slight bilateral dilatation, somewhat more marked on right side

Opinions have differed from one period to another as to the cause of dilatation. In the beginning it was explained on purely mechanical grounds, it being supposed that the dilatation was due to pressure of the enlarged uterus against the ureters on their way across the bony pelvis. With increasing knowledge of hormones, attempts were made to explain the dilatation on purely hormonal grounds and, on the basis of experiments on mice and monkeys, to ascribe the dilatation entirely to a hormonal effect. It is difficult, however, to explain why the pelvic parts of the ureter are not dilated and why dilatation is more common on the right side. Another point arguing against the hormone theory as the only explanation is the fact that in patients receiving estrogen therapy — thus not pregnant patients — the ureter does not become markedly dilated. Further, no such dilatation is seen in quadrupeds (KEATES, 1954). In addition, dilatation of similar type

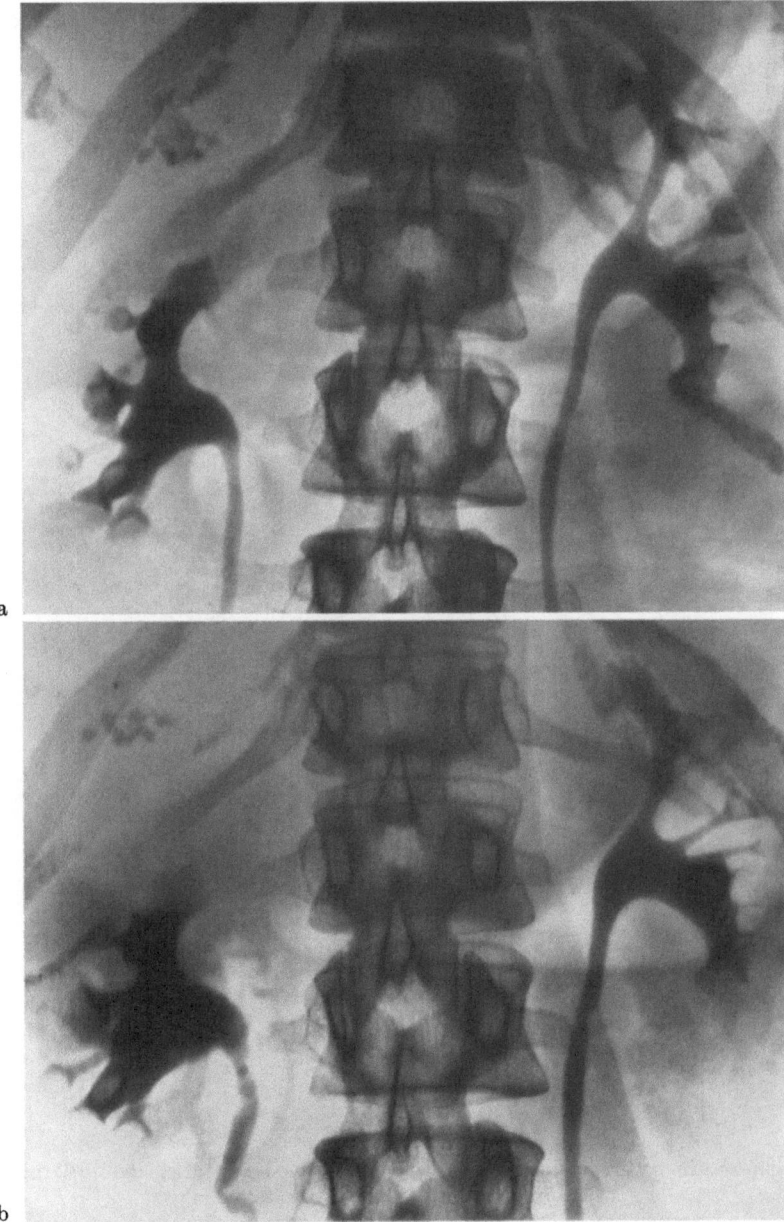

Fig. 286. Persisting slight dilatation of right kidney pelvis and ureter after pregnancy. Urography a) before pregnancy and b) three years later, two years after uncomplicated pregnancy

may be seen in tumor of the small pelvis without estrogen production (Fig. 287). A mechanical factor is undoubtedly mainly responsible. On the other hand, I have observed that in low ureteric stone in gravidae a resulting dilatation of the ureter is much more marked also in the distal part of the ureter than in non-pregnant women. A certain laxity of the ureteric wall is undoubtedly present and is in fact responsible for the severity of dilatation.

Baker and Lewis (1935) offer a simple explanation for the fact that distention is more frequently seen on the right side. In a post mortem study of a pregnant woman they noticed that the sigmoid colon acted as a pressure absorber, absorbing most of the pressure that would otherwise be exerted on the left ureter by the enlarged uterus. With this in mind the authors made colon studies in pregnant women. Their findings suggested that the colon not only functions as a pressure absorber and thereby protects the left ureter, but that it is also responsible for the so-called physiologic dextroposition of the pregnant

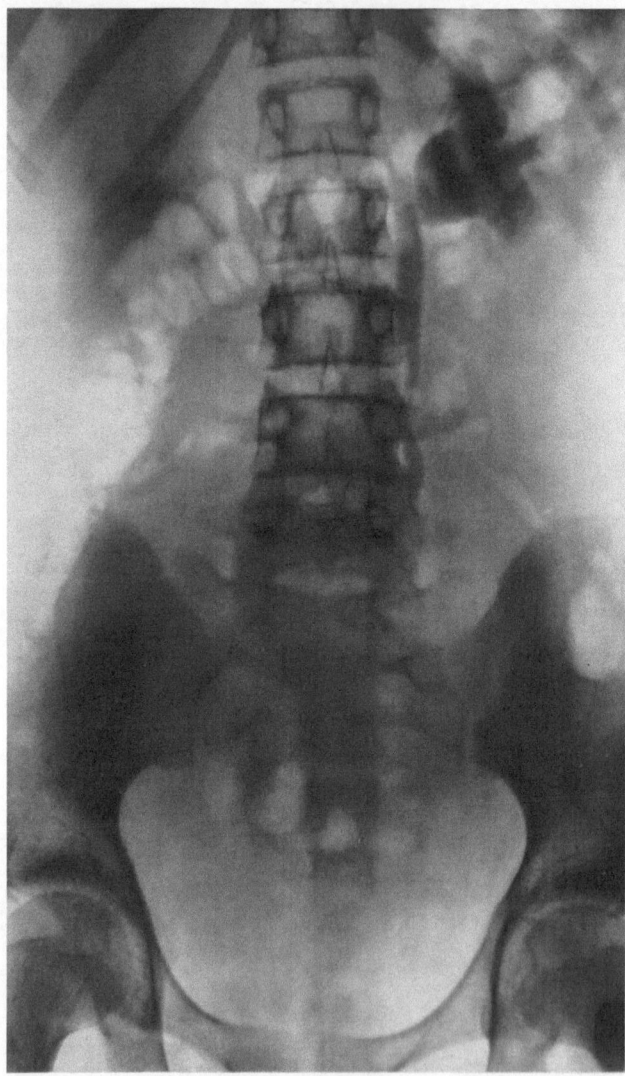

Fig. 287. Dilatation of urinary tract of same type as in pregnancy. Dilatation due to large ovarian dermoid cyst without hormonal disorder

uterus, which exerts a strong pressure against the right ureter. If the ureteric dilatation developing during pregnancy, with decreased tonus of the ureter, does persist to a certain extent for the remainder of the patient's lifetime, there is reason to give more attention to this problem in view of the risks which it may imply.

There is at the same time reason to warn against unnecessary roentgen examination of this condition or of urinary tract disease during pregnancy. This restriction is dictated by the amount of radiation necessary for proper examination of a pregnant woman and the large amount of secondary radiation from the uterus to the ovaries.

4. Ureteric dilatation following pregnancy

A special method for investigating ureteric dilatation following pregnancy is proposed by KAUPPILA *et al.* (1972). This method consists of simultaneous uterine phlebography and retrograde pyelography. The authors believe that by this method it is possible to demonstrate that pressure by a pelvic vein is a factor contributing to the ureteric dilatation. So far convincing results are lacking.

5. Ureteric dilatation following use of oral contraceptives

With the increased use of oral contraceptives containing estrogen and progestogen, a discussion has flared up around possible non-desirable effects of this use, for example an increased tendency towards thrombosis. Another suggestion is that the contraceptives could cause slight ureteral dilatation, which in turn could promote infection with its complications. In 1966 MARSHALL *et al.* reported two cases of ureteral dilatation during the use of oral contraceptives. In 1970 GUYER and DELANY described slight dilatation and over-distensibility of the upper urinary tract seen during urography of six nulliparous patients using oral contraceptives. Of these patients five had persistent or recurrent urinary infections. The dilatation was only slight. In a large material, so far not published, the presence of such dilatation or over-distensibility has not been confirmed.

6. Local dilatation of the urinary tract

A widening of a single calyx or group of calyces is called hydrocalicosis. It is due to a process obstructing the lumen of a branch or a stem of a calyx (Fig. 288). Corresponding

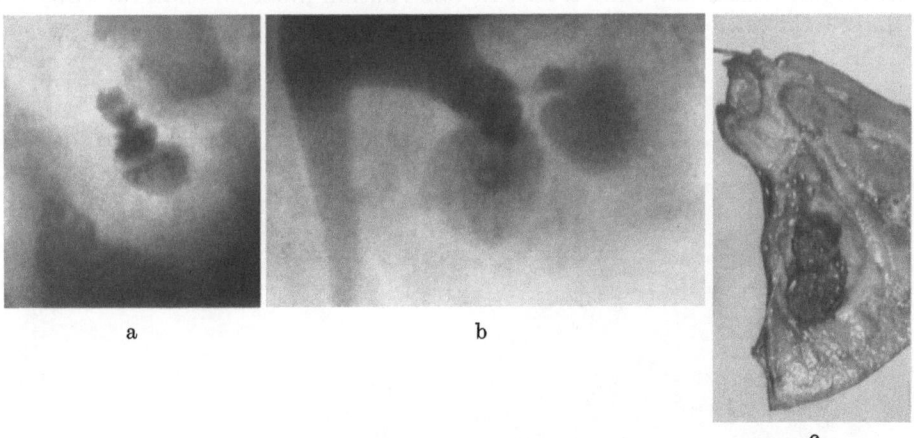

a   b

c

Fig. 288. Plain radiography: a) Stones in caudal part of left kidney. b) Urography: stone obstructs flow from caudal calyces, which are severely dilated. Corresponding papillae are atrophic. c) Operative specimen. Polar nephrectomy

parts of the renal pelvis are widened and the papillae are flattened. The process is often associated with marked atrophy of the papilla, which enlarges the cavity filled with contrast medium.

Hydrocalicosis is always secondary to a pathologic lesion. A stone wedged in a calyceal stem, narrowing of an already narrow part of the renal pelvis by inflammatory edema, or contraction such as in tuberculosis etc. is the cause of hydrocalicosis. The roentgenologic changes in this condition and its differential diagnosis are therefore discussed together with the fundamental diseases.

As described under the sub-heading "calyces" in Chapter F, hydrocalicosis has been regarded as a disease *sui generis*, an assumption devoid of supportive evidence.

22*

7. The Megaureter

A special type of dilatation is represented by the-so-called megaureter. There is much confusion as to the meaning of the word, however. Some authors include every dilated ureter under this classification, regardless of the cause. Some exclude from the classification those cases where dilatation is caused by factors in the bladder or by a pathologic process distally in the ureter, for example a ureterocele. Some authors reserve the name for cases secondary to obstruction at the vesico-ureteral junction or secondary to massive cysto-ureteral reflux. There is some reason for acceptance of the first classification, but no reason for acceptance of the second or third.

Another classification divides megaureters into primary and secondary types. The secondary group would then include every dilated ureter where a patho-anatomic lesion such as stone, stricture, valve, etc., can be found in the urethra, the bladder or the ureteric orifice, causing block of free urinary flow.

Primary megaureter is thus a congenital, dilated ureter without patho-anatomic explanation. The primary megaureter has been assumed to represent a urogenic disorder but an etiology based on anatomic conditions at the ureteric orifice has also been proposed. Radiologically, the primary megaureter or megaureter *per se* is a dilated ureter without pathologic changes directly explaining the dilatation, which may be unilateral or bilateral, may affect the ureter and the kidney pelvis, the ureter alone, or the distal part of the ureter, and which may be only slight or very marked.

The diagnosis of megaureter *per se* should not be made roentgenologically until pathologic changes that could be responsible for ureteric dilatation have been ruled out. It should be stressed again that a peripheral obstruction to urinary flow does not necessarily mean that ureteric dilatation caused by this obstruction must be bilateral. Only one ureter may be dilated, the orifice of the other ureter being competent.

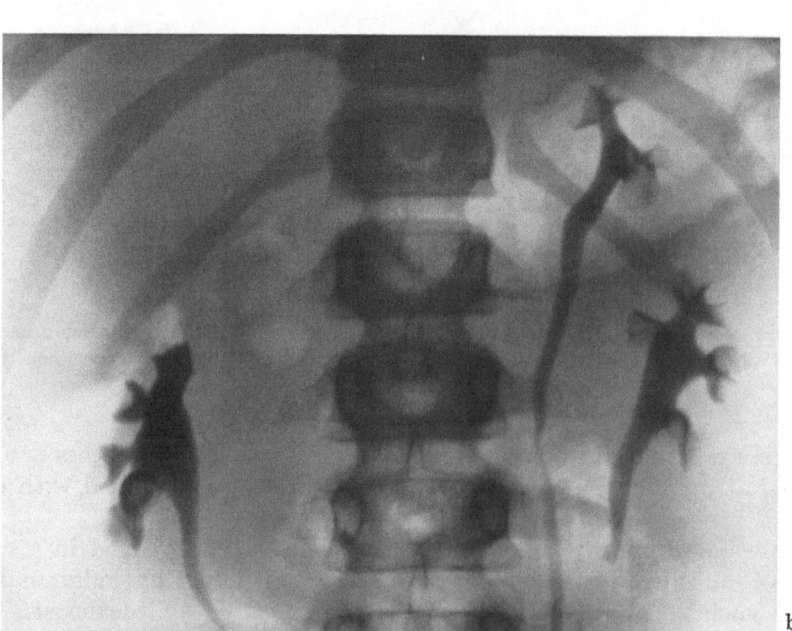
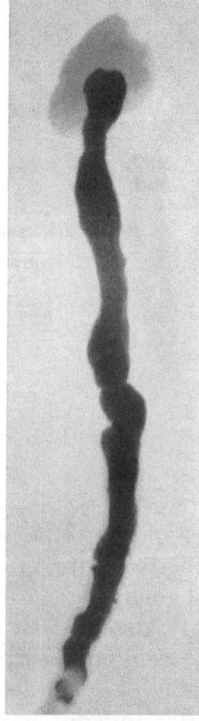

a   b

Fig. 289. Dilatation of cranial pelvis in double kidney. Ureterocele, right. a) Urography: double kidney on left side, single kidney pelvis on right side. Position of pelvis within kidney with large cranial pole definitely argues for presence of another dilated pelvis. Extirpation of cranial pole of kidney and widened ureter. b) Pyelogram of specimen

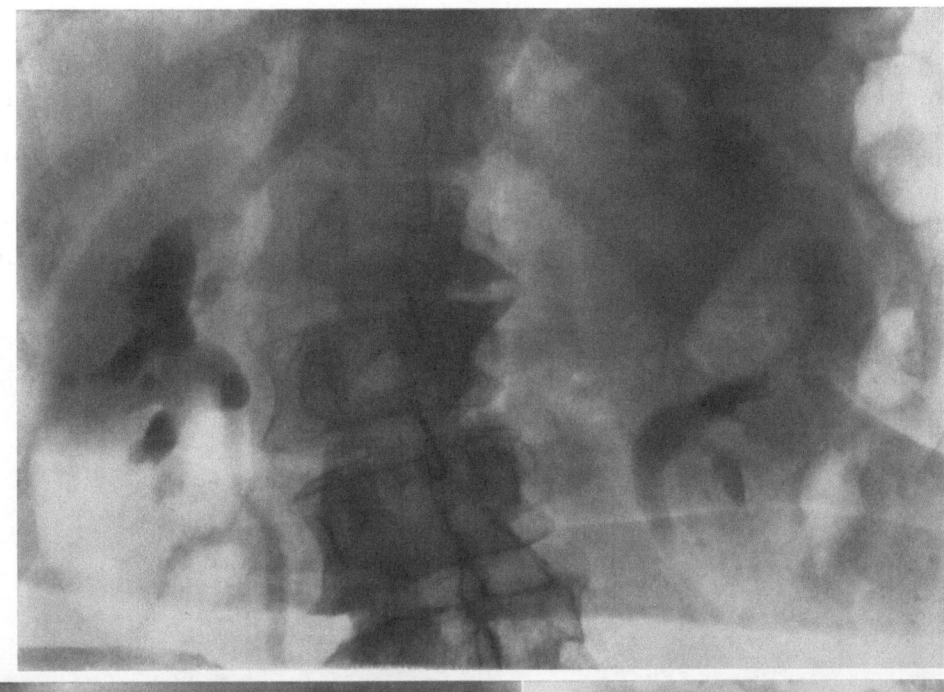

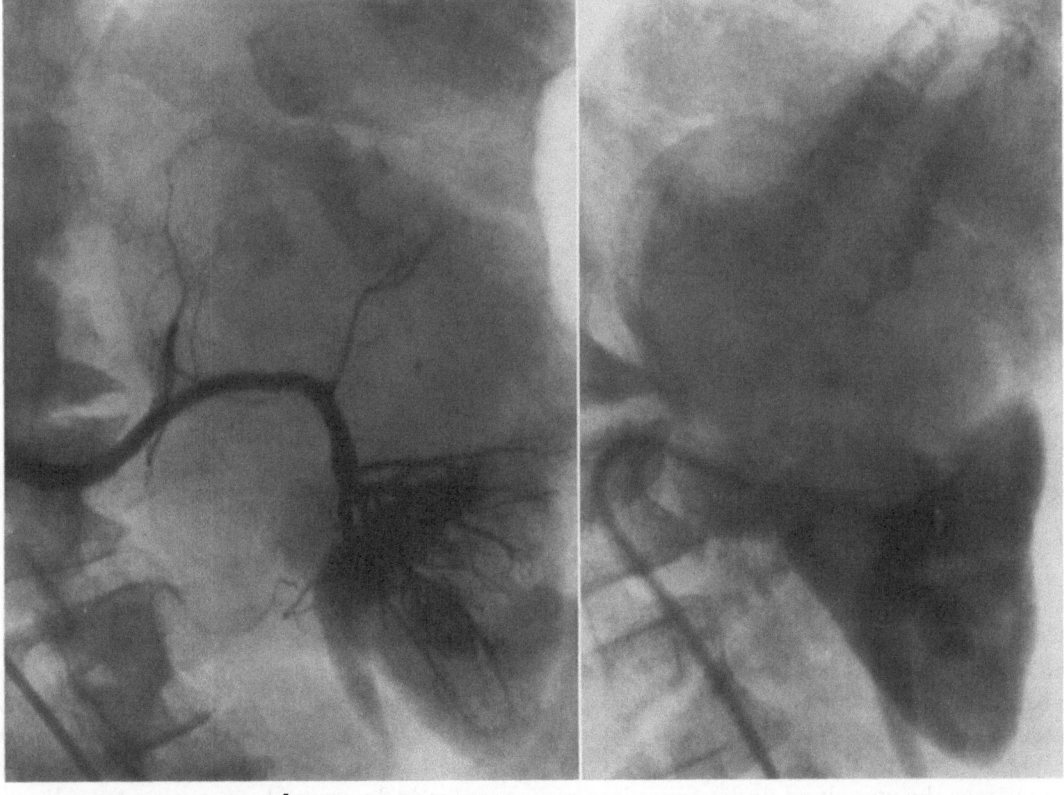

Fig. 290. Dilated cranial renal pelvis in left-sided double kidney. a) Urography: excretion only in caudal kidney pelvis, which is flattened cranially and displaced caudally. Large expansivity cranial to kidney pelvis. b) Renal angiography, arteriographic phase: ordinary conditions in lower pole of kidney corresponding to filled kidney pelvis. Marked atrophy of arterial branches to upper part of kidney, which are stretched and displaced. Displacement of renal pelvic artery in a curve medially. c) Nephrographic phase: no functioning kidney parenchyma corresponding to markedly dilated upper kidney pelvis

8. Dilatation of the urinary tract in double renal pelvis

The conditions described above which are capable of causing a dilatation of the urinary tract can also cause dilatation of one of the renal pelves of a duplicated kidney.

The diagnostic problems are the same as those described above for kidneys with a single pelvis. However, this anomaly offers certain diagnostic difficulties. This is the case when the dilatation is due to an ectopic orifice of one of the ureters and in all cases in which a filling is obtained of only one of the pelves at urography.

It is nearly always the cranial renal pelvis which is problematic, and the examination is usually indicated by urinary incontinence.

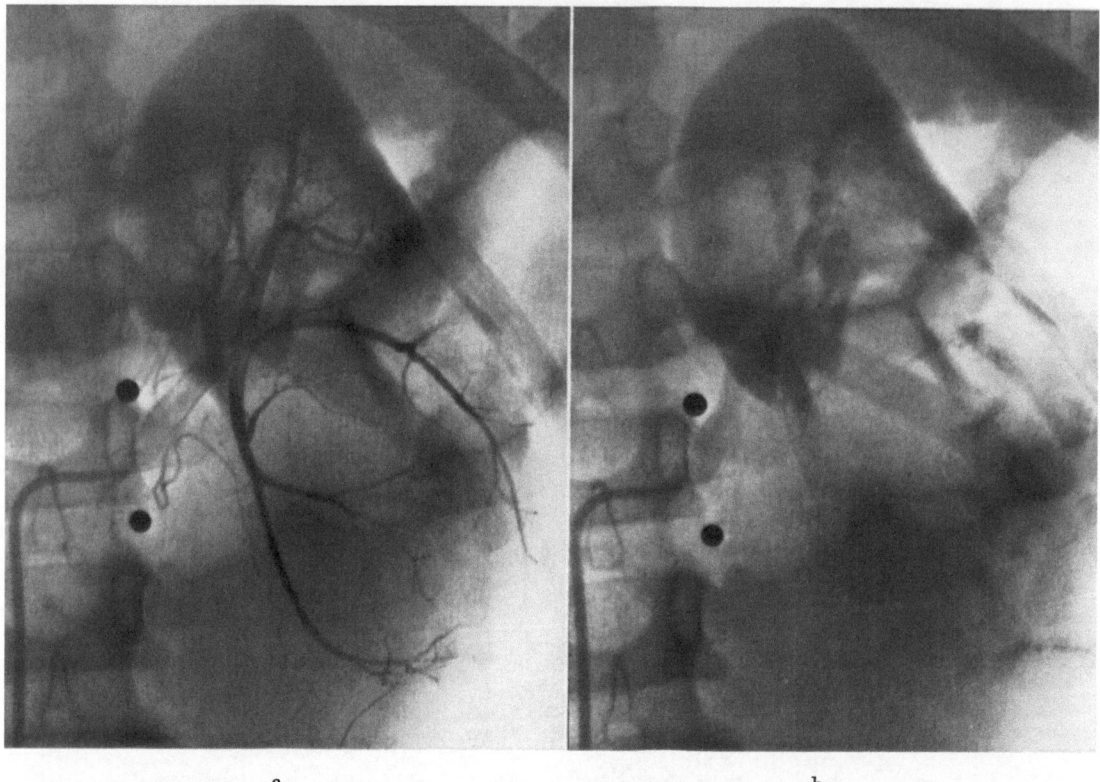

a   b

Fig. 291. Hydronephrosis in caudal kidney pelvis in double kidney. a) Angiography: atrophy, stretching, displacement of branches to caudal half of kidney. b) Nephrographic phase: marked atrophy of parenchyma in distal half of kidney

The purpose of the examination is to demonstrate whether a double kidney is present. If excretion of contrast medium can be demonstrated in both pelves in the double kidney, the diagnosis is, of course, simple. As a rule, however, stasis in the upper renal pelvis has existed for such a long time that no excretion will be seen in this part. In some of these cases, at plain radiography and urography the shape of the kidney and of the renal pelvis will be seen to be such as to indicate the existence of a second renal pelvis (Fig. 289—292). Sometimes the combined findings in plain radiography and urography permit a firm diagnosis, since a large cranial renal pole will be seen with a long distance between the outline of the pole and the cranial calyx. The cranial part of the renal pelvis of the lower kidney may then be compressed and flattened.

In some of these cases, especially in adults, differentiation from tumor and cyst may be difficult. Despite dilatation of a cranial renal pelvis, which can originally be very small,

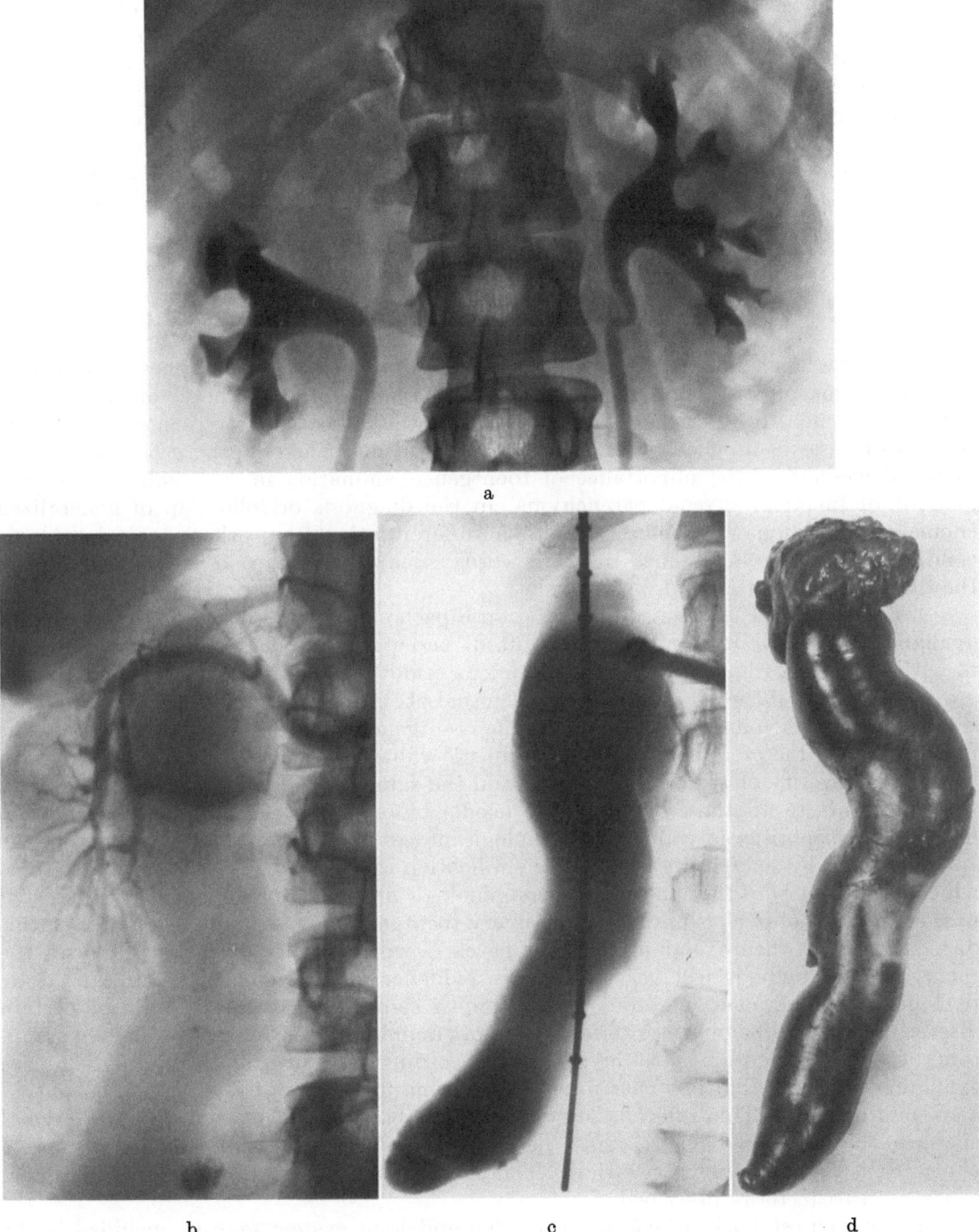

Fig. 292. Dilatation of kidney pelvis and ureter in double kidney, right side. a) Urography: displacement of caudal kidney pelvis and impression in its cranial part by dilated upper kidney pelvis; b) angiography: marked displacement cranially of renal artery; excretion in markedly dilated upper kidney pelvis and corresponding ureter; c) antegrade pyelography by percutaneous puncture of dilated kidney pelvis and filling of ureter; d) operation specimen

the diagnosis may sometimes be difficult if the renal pole is only slightly enlarged and the contrast-filled renal pelvis of ordinary shape.

Renal angiography may be valuable. In the nephrogram, atrophy of the renal parenchyma will be seen in the area corresponding to the dilated renal pelvis (ECKERBOM and LILJEQUIST, 1952; IDBOHRN and SJÖSTEDT, 1954) (Fig. 291). In some of these cases a ureterocele can be found at urography (Fig. 289). If roentgen examination has given reason to suspect a double renal pelvis with hydronephrosis of the cranial pelvis, a thorough search must be made for a ureter with an ectopic orifice. The ectopic ureter often has a ureterocele extending down into the bladder neck and posterior part of the urethra. In a monograph ERICSSON (1954) described 20 cases of ureterocele. In 14 of these the orifice was ectopic. For study of ureterocele see Chapter R.

I. Generalized diseases of the renal parenchyma

The term "generalized diseases of the renal parenchyma" embraces such conditions as pyelonephritis, glomerulonephritis and tubular nephritis. These conditions have much in common roentgen-diagnostically, such as the indications for roentgen examination. Most cases of uremia belong to this group and may therefore be grouped together in the discussion of the importance of roentgen examination in the evaluation of the amount of functioning renal parenchyma, in the diagnosis or follow-up of generalized edema and pulmonary edema, and in their differentiation from other surgical urologic conditions resulting in uremia. In other words, such cases occupy a central position in the discussion of acute renal insufficiency.

A firm diagnosis is often difficult because patho-anatomic verification is often not available. Operative biopsy and, more often, percutaneous needle biopsy are resorted to with increasing frequency. Biopsy specimens removed by this or any other technique are of value only if they are taken from the actual site of changes. Unless performed under sight control or in connection with a suitable roentgenologic procedure, the percutaneous technique may therefore be of limited diagnostic value, particularly in pyelonephritis, in which the severity of the changes in one and the same kidney is known to vary widely from one part to another. Percutaneous needle biopsy may yield reliable information in glomerulonephritis, in which the pathologic process is roughly even throughout the entire kidney. Pyelonephritis is often a complication in some other disease such as stone, which dominates both the clinical and roentgenologic findings. Roentgenologists interested in the diagnosis of pyelonephritis — and every roentgenologist certainly should have this disease in mind when examining urologic cases — will find that in various diseases the roentgenologic findings will very often give evidence of additional changes caused by pyelonephritis. However, in order to distinguish signs more or less specific of certain diseases and to give diagnostic criteria satisfactory definitions, the diseases producing symptoms under investigation must be grouped according to a firm and definite diagnosis, excluding other possibilities. Therefore this grouping must be based, as a rule, on patho-anatomic evidence. This rule has often not been observed in generalized parenchymal changes, the roentgen-diagnostic signs having been related to diseases diagnosed merely clinically, occasionally not very strictly. Therefore the roentgen symptomatology is sometimes not satisfactorily described.

It is a well established fact that the bone and joint system may be included in the disease pattern of certain infectious diseases of the urogenital system. Thus metastatic gonococcal arthritis is very well known, as is the relationship between pelvospondylitis, prostatovesiculitis and so-called uro-arthritis, those rheumatic conditions developing in association with urogenital infections. It has been found that rational treatment of urogenital infection favorably influences the development of the diseases mentioned (ROSENTHAL et al., 1971).

The diseases referred to above have a common roentgen-diagnostic baseline, where the differential diagnosis is of less importance in the acute stage. It is represented by acute renal insufficiency. In this clinical entity, roentgen examination is of importance from several points of view which will be discussed below.

I. Acute renal insufficiency

1. General considerations

The general considerations in the roentgen examination of patients with acute renal insufficiency, as they have developed in cooperation with the units for urology and nephrology at our hospital, are set forth below.

Patients with acute renal insufficiency, as a rule, are in a poor general condition, often moribund, which makes roentgen examination difficult and requires well planned, quick and reliable examination with the aid of proficient assistance.

The first point to decide is whether the renal insufficiency is due to changes in the renal parenchyma such as generalized parenchymatous changes, toxic damage, tumor, etc., or to obstructed drainage such as by stone, tumor, post-radiotherapeutic edema, periureteritis obliterans, etc. It should be observed that a retroperitoneal tumor extending from the intestines or the bladder, or from the female genital organs may obstruct both ureters. In addition to performing instrumental examination to check the patency of the ureters, the examiner must be on the watch for any signs suggesting stone or any other obstacle obstructing urinary flow. The roentgenologist should therefore pay special attention to the size of the kidneys and to the width of the renal pelvis. Dilatation of the renal pelvis can occasionally be detected in plain roentgenograms. The possibility that the patient may have only one kidney should regularly be considered.

The next step is to assess the amount of renal parenchyma. If the kidneys can be outlined (zonography or tomography may be helpful) the mass of renal parenchyma — with certain reservations — can be estimated in plain roentgenograms, in accordance with the principles given in Chapter C. Such estimation is important not only in the general evaluation but particularly in the choice of therapy. This is influenced by the types of changes in the kidneys causing the acute insufficiency: for example if any enlargement of the kidneys can be demonstrated and ascribed to an acute disease from which the patient can probably make a complete recovery, or if severely contracted kidneys are found to be the cause.

The size of the kidneys is of prognostic importance. This point will be discussed below.

2. Edema

Edema in connection with renal disease is a very complex phenomenon with varying pathogenetic aspects operating in combination with basic differences in various renal diseases. In some diseases the renal insufficiency is the decisive factor. In anuria, for example, edema may develop a few days after onset of the anuric state. In acute diseases, for example acute glomerulonephritis, the edema develops much more rapidly from extrarenal factors. It must be noted also that in some types of edema a hypervolemia is part of the process, whereas edema in nephrosis, for instance, is characterized by hypovolemia.

Examination of patients in a state of acute renal insufficiency brings into sharp focus the importance of roentgen examination in checking edema. Examination of the lungs is of great value. This is apparent from the fact that, as pointed out by several workers in this field, even in severe pulmonary edema the findings at physical examination of the patients are often scanty and contrast sharply with the lung changes seen roentgenologically. This makes the roentgen examination of these patients essential because pulmonary edema is a serious and life-threatening complication. In pulmonary edema of this type the changes are usually bilateral but may differ markedly in extent, from side to side, and may occasionally be unilateral. The changes usually involve the major portion of the lungs. The peripheral parts of the lungs are free, as pointed out above all by HERRN-HEISER (1958). The changes are thus localized to the central part of each lung and each lobe (Fig. 293). The terms "butterfly edema" or "bat wing shadows" are often met in the literature. These terms are related to a non-roentgenologic method of studying roent-

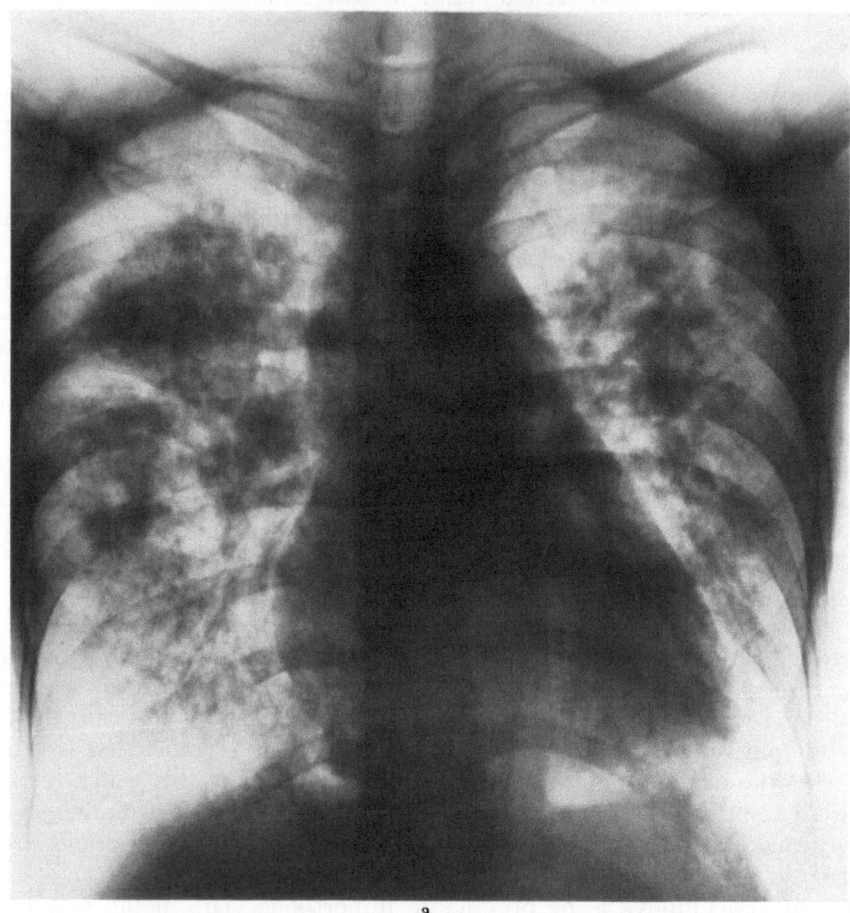

a

Fig. 293. Pulmonary edema: a) bedside examination: severe edema localized centrally in pulmonary lobes. b) and c) Two days later, after successful treatment: edema has diminished markedly. Slight changes are seen centrally in lungs

genologic changes and relate to an impression given in a frontal view of the chest in some cases. Such terms are non-roentgenologic and should be abandoned.

A differential diagnosis is naturally of importance in the planning of treatment. It is sometimes difficult to distinguish between this type of pulmonary edema and cardiac edema, certain types of pneumonia, or atelectases, particularly since a combination of these lesions is not unusual (Fig. 293). As mentioned, this pulmonary edema is characterized by the fact that the changes are bilateral and localized mainly to the center of the lungs, the margin of the lungs being entirely free from changes. Experimental investigations at our department on dogs with various types of pulmonary edema, induced by different methods and in different vascular regions, have shown this most distinctly (BORGSTRÖM et al., 1960). These investigations have also shown that the characteristic localization of the changes may be due to their relation to the regions of supply of the bronchial arteries.

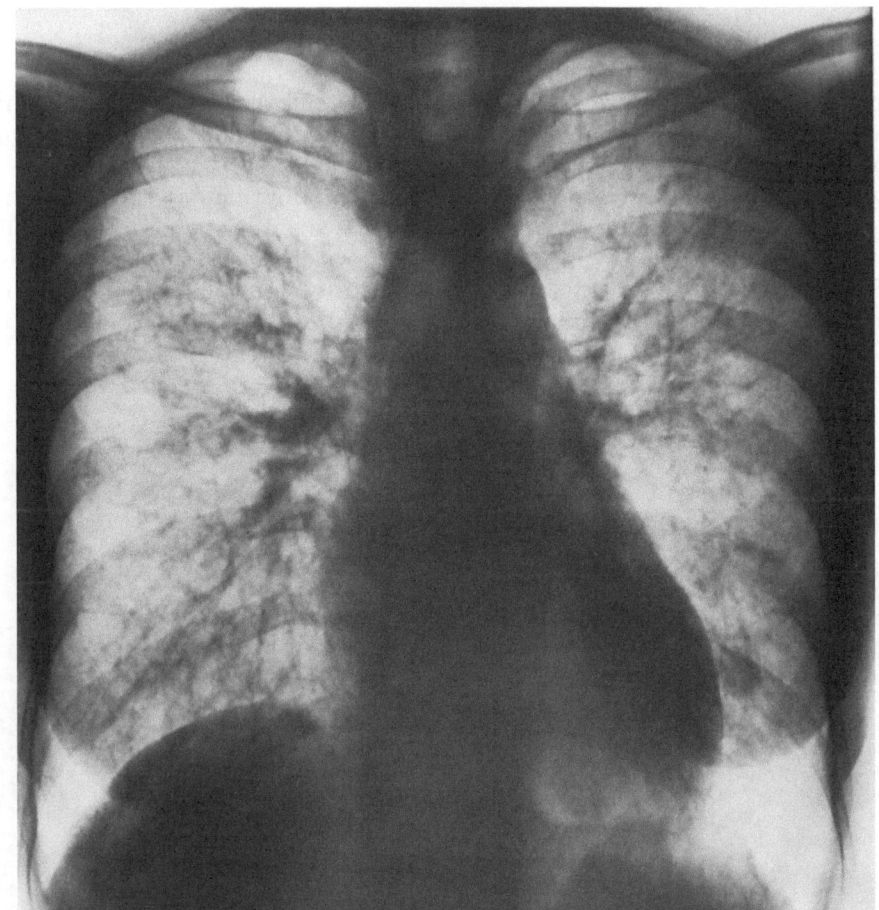

Fig. 293b

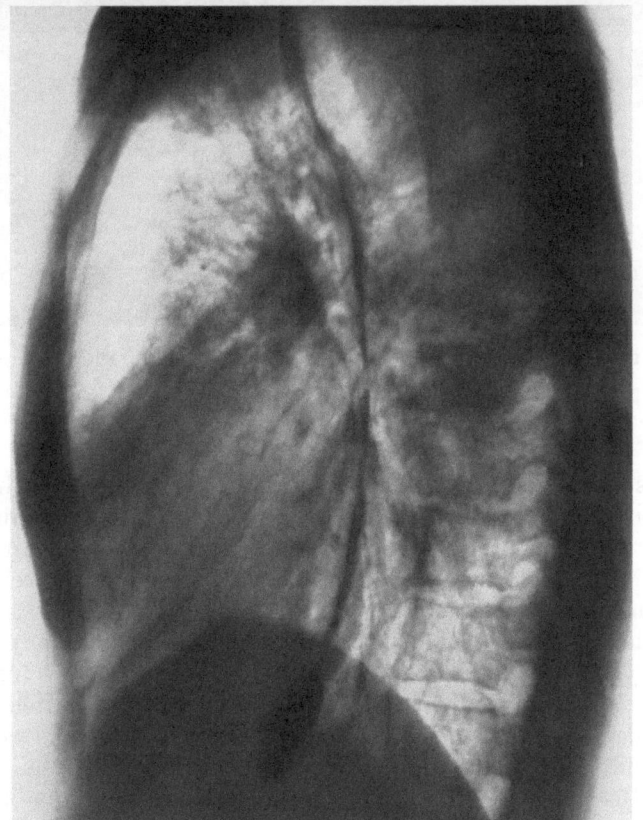

Fig. 293c

The changes consist essentially of marked edema in the wall of the large bronchi in contrast to the cardiac edema and different types of pneumonia in which the filling of the alveoli is the main feature.

The pulmonary changes are reversible. Check examinations of the chest are therefore of great value in the management of acute renal insufficiency. In early pulmonary edema and in the healing stage of edema, the only changes consist of an increased amount of fluid in the pleural cavity. To demonstrate small amounts of pleural fluid, the patient must be examined in lateral decubitus with horizontal direction of the roentgen

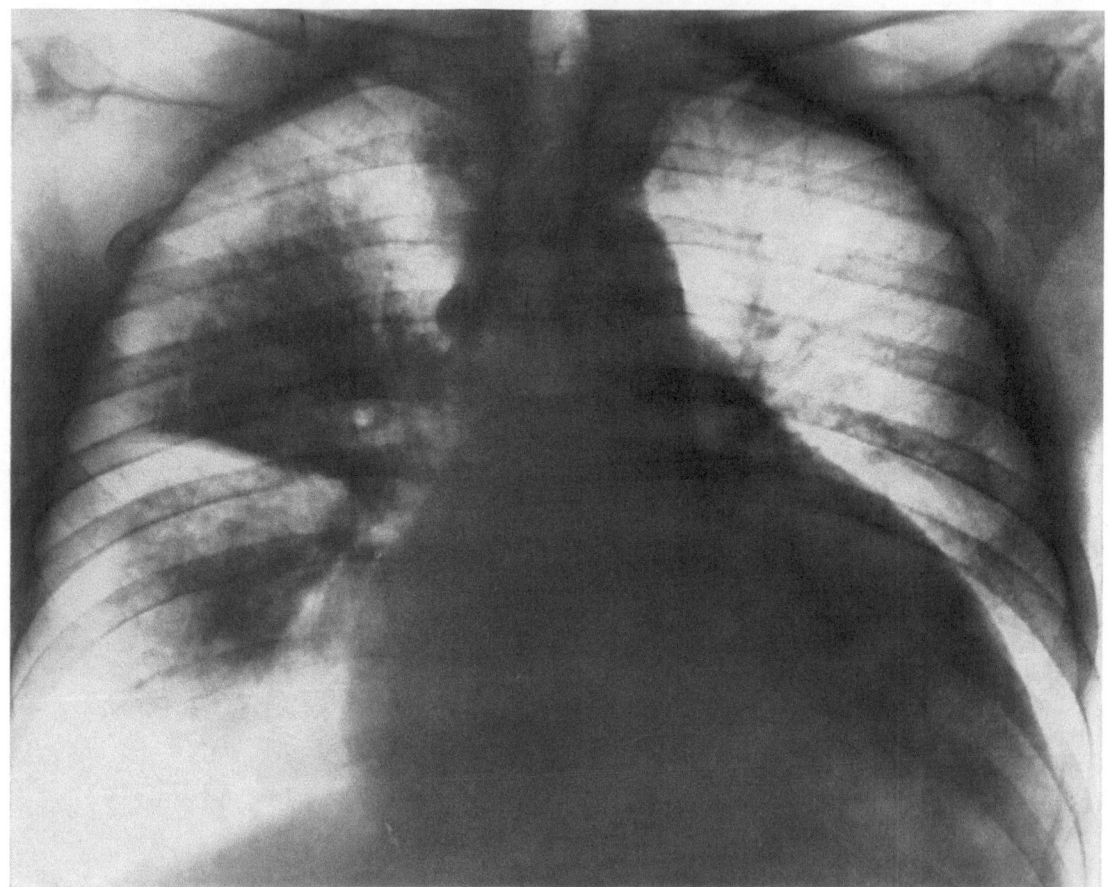

Fig. 294. Pulmonary edema with unilateral engagement: only central parts of the lobes in right lung are engaged (bedside examination)

rays. The patient is placed on the side to be examined, with one cushion in the armpit and one under the hip. The X-ray tube with horizontal direction is behind the patient and a cassette is placed standing at the patient's frontal side. The patient should be rotated about 10° with the upper side forward and the head somewhat lowered. Even very small amounts of fluid can be demonstrated in this way, as the fluid floats along the chest wall.

In this connection mention should be made of the so-called Goodpasture's syndrome with initial hemoptysis in a young person followed by pulmonary infiltration, anemia, renal failure, and a short fatal course. The pathologic findings limited to lungs and kidneys include pulmonary hemorrhage and an alveolar septal lesion as well as glomerulonephritis, first focal and later disseminated. LARSSON *et al.* doubt the necessity of using this syndrome in the medical literature as the syndrome probably coincides with malignant glomerulonephritis with pulmonary hemorrhage (see also MORTENSSON *et al.*, 1967).

The presence of any edema can also usually be detected at plain roentgenography of the urinary tract. In the examination of the patient in the acute stage it is often difficult to recognize the outline of the kidneys, mainly because of the conditions under which the examination is performed. The patient is often unable to co-operate during the examination: he is not prepared for the examination, and uremia is often accompanied by considerable meteorism. Ascites and retroperitoneal edema also often add to the difficulty

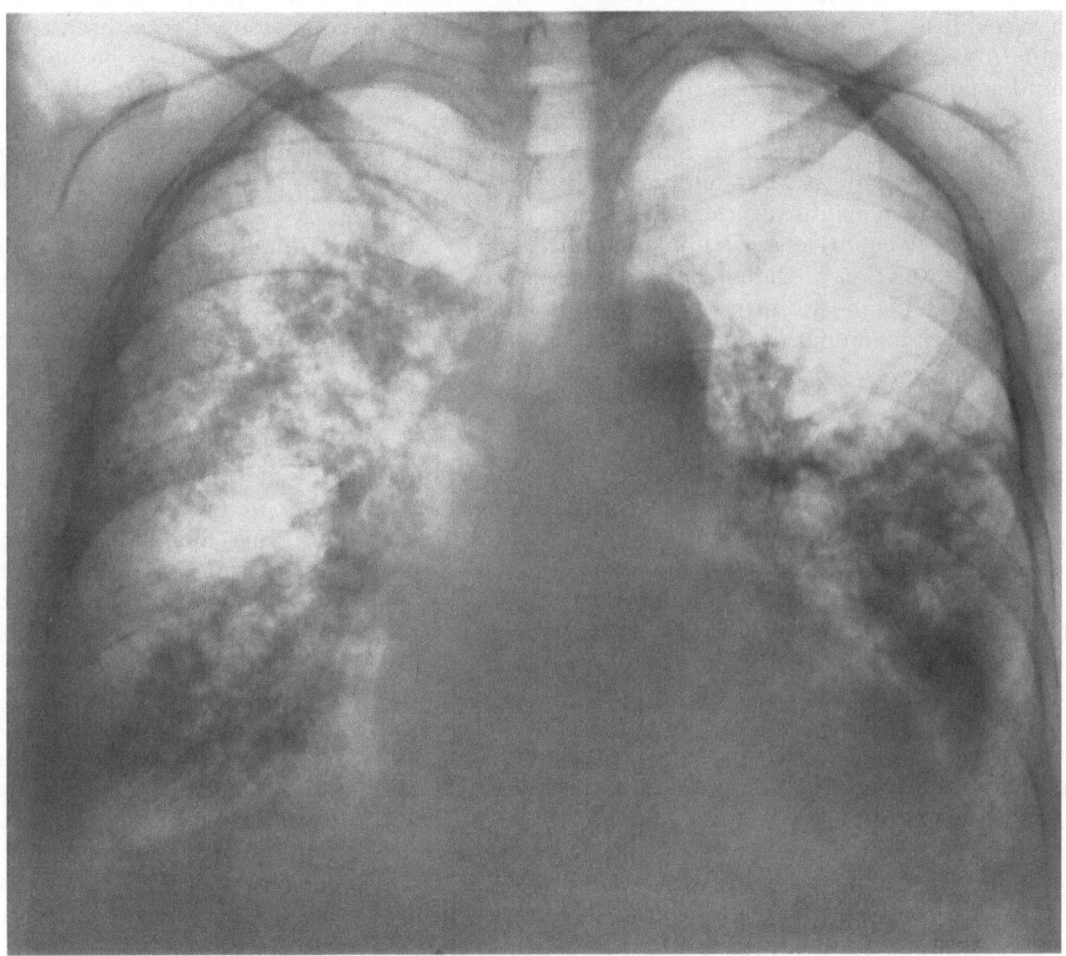

Fig. 295. Acute glomerulonephritis with hemoptysis and hemosiderosis. Bedside chest examination: widespread bilateral parenchymal changes with more generalized engagement of different lobes than in changes characteristic of uremic pulmonary edema

in recognizing the outline of the kidneys, but, on the other hand, these conditions add to the diagnostic information of the examination the fact that edema is present. (It is assumed that the reader is familiar with the roentgen diagnosis of ascites.) Retroperitoneal edema has been described in the chapter on perinephritis. In these cases the edema is more generalized, with a marked increase in density of the entire retroperitoneal space. This increase abolishes the difference in contrast between organs and tissues in the retroperitoneal space, and it is often not possible to define the psoas muscles, kidneys etc. In the treatment of the fluid retention, with regression of the edema as a consequence, the kidneys gradually become distinct.

3. Estimation of the size of the kidneys

Estimation of the size of the kidneys during the course of the disease is important. If the kidneys are enlarged, it may be due not only to stasis, which has been dismissed from the differential diagnosis by this stage of the disease, but to generalized parenchymatous changes such as glomerulonephritis, tubular nephritis, pyelonephritis, etc. General enlargement of the kidneys may also be due to amyloidosis and other types of nephrosis before the kidney has begun to shrink, infiltration of the kidney by leukemic tissue, for example, and infarction of the kidney. Extensive granuloma formation in the kidneys in sarcoidosis, for example, also belongs to this group of conditions. These diseases can lead to a considerable enlargement of both kidneys. Another condition to be borne in mind is polycystic kidney (described in Chapter G). In the stage of acute renal insufficiency, polycystic kidneys are usually so large and irregular as to offer no diagnostic difficulties.

If the kidneys are small, glomerulonephritis and pyelonephritis are prevalent, together with hypoplasia, but many diseases may have a final stage of kidney contraction such as collagenous disease, arthritis urica, etc.

Glomerulonephritis and tubular nephritis are of roentgen-diagnostic interest mainly in the investigation of the effect of the disease on the size of the kidney. Pyelonephritis is of greater diagnostic interest because it is the most common renal disease.

At check examination soon after the acute stage the following points should be borne in mind:

a) Enlarged kidneys

The kidneys may be enlarged in acute and sub-acute glomerulonephritis, tubular nephritis and acute pyelonephritis, in the nephrotic syndrome, in gross bilateral renal cortical necrosis, and in the early stages of certain other conditions. The enlargement is occasionally considerable. Both kidneys are enlarged to the same extent except in pyelonephritis, in which only one kidney may be affected, or sometimes only part of one kidney. The kidneys are plump but have a smooth surface. Occasionally they cannot be completely outlined because of edema. Oblique views facilitate recognition of their borders. Zonography or tomography may sometimes be useful.

It is important to follow the course of the disease. If there is any doubt about the size of the kidney, check examination should be performed as soon as the edema has abated. Repeated check examinations for any further change in the size of the kidney should be performed preferably at intervals of two weeks, later at longer intervals. During such roentgen follow-up, persistence of the kidney enlargement shows that the pathologic process is still active. In some cases the kidney may assume and then retain normal size, while in other cases the kidney may continue to decrease in size, i. e. to develop into a contracted kidney.

In cases of uremia, bleeding in the mucuous membranes of the gastrointestinal tract, esophagus, stomach, small bowel, and colon may occasionally occur. Small bowel changes are not uncommon during long-term hemodialysis mainly due to edema in the bowel wall (King et al., 1971). The roentgenologist should be familiar with the roentgen symptomatology of such lesions.

b) Kidneys smaller than normal

Chronic glomerulonephritis and pyelonephritis, as well as late stages of tubular nephritis, renal cortical necrosis, and certain other diseases may be accompanied by marked shrinkage of the kidneys. In pyelonephritis the change is usually more severe on one side than on the other. In patients with a small solitary kidney the question arises whether this condition is congenital or due to shrinkage. It is often not possible to answer this question. What is described in the literature as a hypoplastic kidney due to an embryologic disorder may in reality be a contracted kidney due to early pyelonephritis, emboli, etc. (see chapter on Anomalies).

Variations in the size of the kidney will be discussed below, against the background of two diseases, namely glomerulonephritis and tubular nephritis.

4. Glomerulonephritis

At examination of patients acutely ill, the examiner must first ascertain the stage of the disease, as patients not infrequently have glomerulonephritic shrunken kidneys without any earlier history. In patients acutely ill the kidneys are often normal in size but are sometimes enlarged, occasionally markedly so. On the other hand, the kidneys may be smaller than normal. This means that the uremia is not due to acute glomerulonephritis and, if the kidneys are very small, that the uremia represents a final stage of renal insufficiency.

In anuria, recognition of the stage of the disease is of paramount importance. Extremely active therapy is available and must be applied, especially in cases of acute glomerulonephritis with anuria. It has been demonstrated by RUDEBECK (1946) that the mortality from acute glomerulonephritis (diagnosed clinically) is highest when the clinical picture at the onset of the disease is very intense. On the other hand — if these patients survive the initial stage — the prospects are not worse than for those in whom the clinical picture was moderate in the beginning. Therefore every effort must be taken to carry the patient over the acute stage.

The rate at which the disease progesses from an acute to a chronic stage seems to vary widely from one case to another. According to VOLHARD and FAHR (1914), acute nephritis occasionally reaches the stage of a contracted kidney within a few months. On the other hand, one case was reported in which glomerulonephritis was still in the subchronic stage after 3½ years. The possibilities enabling the pathologist to obtain a clear idea of the general course of glomerulonephritis are limited, of course, as fortunately the percentage of cases coming to post-mortem examination is relatively small. Here roentgen examination can contribute considerably to our knowledge of the patho-anatomic course of the disease because it is practically always possible, by repeated check examination, to follow the gross anatomic changes as judged by the size of the kidney. The general views in the course of the diseases are also influenced by the diagnostic advantages of needle biopsy.

In a given case the routine roentgen examination plays another role: by assessing the size of the kidney in the course of the disease it is often possible to evaluate the actual condition as well as the prognosis because the size of the kidney reflects the amount of surviving parenchyma. At check examination it may be shown how enlarged kidneys reassume a normal size or how enlarged or ordinary-sized kidneys become smaller and continue to decrease in size until the stage of contracted kidney is reached.

Advances in immunology and certain results in treatment of glomuleronephritis with immuno-suppressive drugs have stressed the need for more specific diagnostic possibilities in this disease. To increase roentgen-diagnostic acumen, we have tried renal angiography (EKELUND et al., 1971) (Fig. 296). In a material of 66 patients with glomuleronephritis in different stages (all cases were verified at biopsy) angiography was performed with the following results: In the acute group of eight patients the kidney size was slightly increased in five cases and was normal in three. All eight patients had angiographic changes consisting of stretching of intrarenal branches, poor definition of cortical branches, and slightly widened or ill-defined cortex. In the chronic stage with normal kidney function, of 43 patients all except one had normal kidney size and normal conditions at urography. Eighteen of these patients had slightly pathologic angiograms with widening and increased tortuosity of the intrarenal branches and slight cortical changes as above. In 30 patients with chronic glomuleronephritis with decreased kidney function, kidney

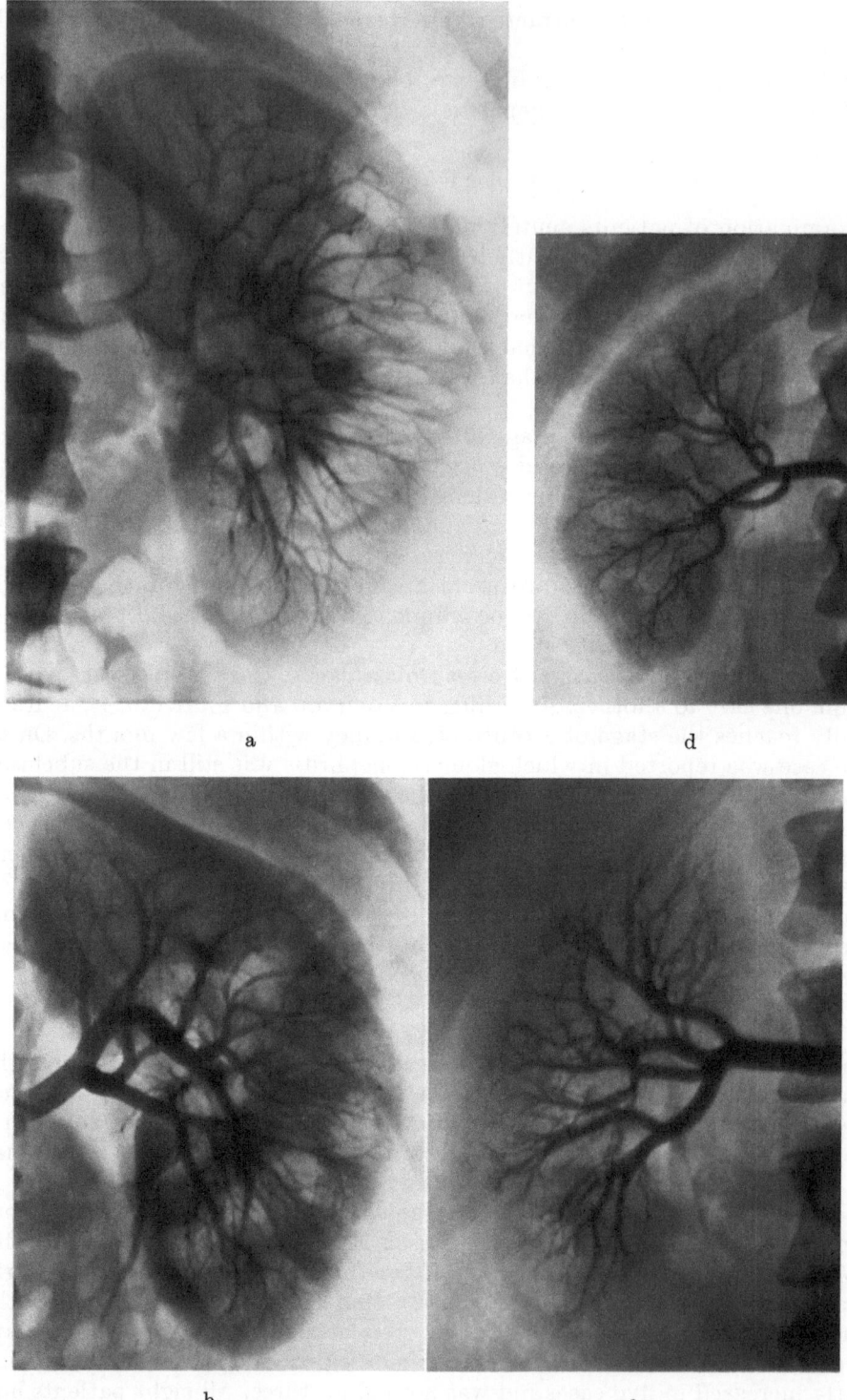

Fig. 296. a) Glomerulonephritis, acute stage: kidney markedly enlarged; only very slight filling of branches to cortex. b) later stage, same patient: regression of swelling of kidney; somewhat better filling of cortical branches, especially in caudal kidney pole. c) Glomerulonephritis, male 22 years of age: Chronic glomerulonephritis with normal kidney function; kidney of ordinary size and shape with wide intrarenal branches but no peripheral branches. d) Glomerulonephritis, female, 37 years of age: Advanced chronic glomerulonephritis: kidneys small but of ordinary shape, with fairly even surface; cortex very thin

size and urography were normal; 11 of the 30 patients had slight angiographic changes, as in the previous group. In advanced chronic cases with contracted kidney, it was not possible angiographically to differentiate between the final stage of a glomerulonephritis and of a pyelonephritis. Thus, although angiographically demonstrable changes are slight, they may add to the diagnosis of this disease.

Mention should be made here of a research project by HABIGHORST et al. (1970) on angiographic differential diagnosis of different types of contracted kidney. This is an arteriographic examination on autopsy kidneys where attempts have been made to collect angiographic data for various types of renal contraction, for example through infarction, pyelonephritis, hydronephrosis, glomerulonephritis, arteriosclerosis. No clinically decisive differentiation could be made, but research along this line must be continued.

In experiments on rats, LJUNGQUIST et al. (1971) found that induced radiation nephritis resulted regularly in development of hypertension after removal of the non-irradiated kidney. At micro-angiography a reduction of the cortical vasculature was found, whereas the medullary vasculature showed nothing pathologic. This project also belongs to fields of research where gains to clinical angiography can be expected.

In this connection reference is made to an experimental study with induction of unilateral acute renal failure by intra-arterial Norepinephrine infusion in the dog by KNAPP et al. (1972). The authors believe that there is definite evidence of an intrarenal mechanism for the maintenance of the extreme renal vasoconstriction found in acute renal failure.

Another promising diagnostic possibility common to generalized renal diseases giving an opportunity for selecting cases with very slight pathology, is estimation of cortical volume (HEGEDÜS and FAARUP, see above). This method has been used by HEGEDÜS and RAVNSKOV (1971) in a pathologic group of 36 patients with 49 apparently normal kidneys. The patients had clinical signs or suspicion of generalized kidney disease or hypertension, or had abnormalities commonly associated with generalized kidney disease in the contralateral kidney, such as papillary necrosis or local scarring. In these apparently normal kidneys the superficial cortical volume expressed in percent of total kidney volume showed a great and statistically significant difference from a normal group. This easy and practical method also appears to add some diagnostic possibilities in an obscure field.

Mention should be made again of Goodpasture's syndrome, which is a rapidly progressive glomerulonephritis associated with intrapulmonary hemorrhage and pulmonary hemosiderosis. The pulmonary changes are supposed to constitute an antibody — antigen process. These changes may vary from slight to extensive. Resolution of the changes is seen after nephrectomy (SIEGEL, 1970).

5. Tubular nephritis

Acute renal failure is characterized by rapid development of renal insufficiency with onset of acute uremia. The etiology is varying; a common cause is shock, for instance in connection with bleeding or a postoperative state. Other causes are intoxication of many different kinds, for example from mushrooms, snakebites, drugs, etc.; infection, for example in peritonitis, pneumonia, sepsis. Renal disease such as glomerulonephritis, pyelonephritis, blockage of drainage from the kidney of many types represent other causes.

Patients with tubular nephritis usually come for roentgen examination in the stage of acute renal failure. What is said above about acute renal insufficiency is applicable to this stage.

At roentgen examination of a patient with tubular nephritis it may be well to remember the following more or less widely accepted stages: the initial stage during which the injury takes place, the anuric-oliguric stage, which is defined as the period during which the daily urinary volume is 400 ml or less and which is said to last about 10—12 days, the diuretic stage, defined as beginning when the daily urinary volume exceeds 400 ml and with still reduced renal function, and the late diuretic stage when the kidney function gradually improves and in most cases becomes normal.

Roentgenologically, the initial stage is a diagnostic stage, in which at plain roentgenography of the abdomen, equal enlargement of both kidneys can be demonstrated, with a contour varying in distinctness with the severity of retroperitoneal edema.

In the anuric-oliguric stage, the purpose of the examination is often to decide whether the patient has edema, especially pulmonary edema, and to check the effect of therapeutic procedures. In the diuretic stages, the question is mainly to assess the prognosis by the rate at which the kidney returns to normal size or shrinks still further. As a rule the kidneys return to normal size within one or a few months, but occasionally a slight enlargement persists for a considerable time (Fig. 297). Sometimes the kidneys shrink. It should be observed that gross bilateral renal cortical necrosis may be the final stage of grave tubular nephritis.

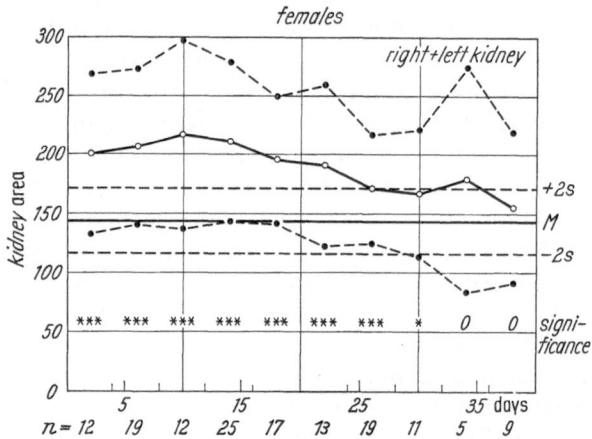

Fig. 297. The area of both kidneys in acute renal failure in a material of 66 cases. The straight lines represent the mean value and the standard deviation in 100 cases with "healthy" kidneys. (After Moëll)

6. Gross bilateral cortical necrosis

Gross bilateral cortical necrosis occurs most frequently in association with concealed accidental hemorrhage (Sheehan and Moore, 1952) and since oliguria—anuria is a predominant clinical feature, what was said above about acute renal insufficiency also applies to this disease. Formerly the disease was of less interest from a roentgen-diagnostic point of view because it often runs a rapid and fatal course. By means of rational conservative therapy and, when indicated, by the use of artificial kidney (dialysis, ultrafiltration), it has become possible to keep patients with renal insufficiency alive for a long time. Moëll (1957) has reported two cases of gross bilateral cortical necrosis, one with 70, the other with 116 days of oliguria—anuria. Both patients contracted acute renal failure in connection with the birth process. In the early stage of the disease the size of the kidneys was distinctly increased. Shrinkage was rapid afterwards, however, and the kidney surface became irregular. Cortical calcifications appeared in one case after two months. In the other case cortical calcifications could be seen in post-mortem films of the kidneys.

Judging from observations made by Moëll, renal cortical necrosis is obviously more common than is widely assumed. He has found cortical calcifications in some cases of advanced tubular nephritis. Obviously there are two types of cortical necrosis, one generalized and one focal.

7. Pyelonephritis

Pyelonephritis is a focal, non-specific bacterial infection affecting, primarily, the interstitial renal tissue and the mucuous membranes and, secondarily, the specific renal parenchyma and the vasculature. It is of chronic nature, causing focal or generalized scar formation.

Pyelonephritis is the most common of all renal diseases, either as a primary lesion or as a complication of other types of renal disease such as stone, stasis of all kinds, gouty kidney, and other types of metabolic renal disorders. In renal hypertension pyelonephritis is the most common cause and in renal insufficiency pyelonephritis is also a factor of great importance.

The roentgen diagnosis of pyelonephritis has been difficult so far because the disease varies in extent and course from case to case and because many of the roentgen-diagnostic findings are not specific. When collecting diagnostic signs characteristic of a disease, the important search for invariants must be strictly limited to cases with the diagnosis established as firmly as possible, in other words patho-anatomically. The abundant literature on the roentgen findings in pyelonephritis is based mainly on examination of cases in which the disease was diagnosed on clinical grounds but not confirmed by patho-anatomic examination. In addition, information on the motility, tonus, etc., of the urinary tract in pyelonephritis is often founded on less satisfactory examination methods and described in terms for which the examination technique does not furnish complete cover. Nevertheless some publications on the roentgen diagnosis of pyelonephritis deserve due consideration (WULFF, 1936; PREVOT and BERNING, 1950; BRAASCH and EMMETT, 1951; DEJDAR and PRAT, 1958; BOIJSEN, DEJDAR, 1959 etc.). DEJDAR and PRAT (1958) stressed the importance of roentgen examination in the investigation of pyelonephritis. Although their illustrations are not convincing in all respects and their material consisted of cases diagnosed only clinically, their results are interesting.

The roentgenologic understanding of pyelonephritis has been given a new dimension by the use of angiography in the examination of suspected chronic pyelonephritis. The disease was formerly called "pyelitis." This name stressed changes in the renal pelvis, the pyelon. The renal pelvis can be examined by pyelography or urography. Patho-anatomic examination, however, found pyelonephritis to be characterized mainly by changes in the renal parenchyma and the term "pyelonephritis" was coined on the basis of these observations. This forced the roentgenologist to focus his interest on the renal parenchyma. This could be studied in plain films when the size and shape of the kidney could be estimated and any irregularities through scar formation noted. At pyelography or urography, the borderline elements between the kidney pelvis and the kidney parenchyma, the papillae, can be studied and have attracted much interest, particularly so when papillary necrosis is found to be combined with, or a representative part of, pyelonephritis in a great number of patients. Many lesions give no or inconclusive changes when studied in this way, however. The rational method for studying the renal parenchyma is through angiography, and this examination method has increasing importance in the investigation of cases of chronic pyelonephritis.

a) Plain roentgenography

In the acute stage of the disease, one or both kidneys are enlarged. The enlargement is seldom marked. As the disease heals, the kidney assumes normal size, but the decrease in size may continue and within some months result in unilateral, bilateral or locally contracted kidney. If shrinkage is generalized, the length of the kidney may be reduced to 4—7 cm and the breadth to 3—4 cm. The kidney may then have an irregular surface and it may increase in density due to deposition of calcium in the renal parenchyma appearing as small, irregular, opaque, multiple, scattered calcifications. I cannot confirm DEJDAR's (1959) statement that the kidneys decrease in density. Only in the very few cases with severe changes and replacement lipomatosis (see below) in which the parenchyma is replaced to a large extent by fatty connective tissue, can the sinus increase in size and the central part of the kidney then appear less dense.

On clinical exacerbation of lesions in a pyelonephritic contracted kidney, even if extremely small, the kidney will often increase in size. If the pyelonephritic process affects only one kidney pole, for example, this will shrink. The remainder of the kidney may increase in size through hyperplasia, often markedly. The kidney may therefore retain its ordinary size in spite of marked local shrinkage. Occasionally the hyperplasia may be localized to only one part of the kidney. This hyperplastic part may then give a tumorlike protrusion in the surface of the kidney.

In double kidneys, pyelonephritis is very often localized to only one part of the kidney, usually the caudal part. If double kidneys are bilateral, changes may sometimes be seen in the caudal kidney pelvis on both sides, often with varying degrees between the two sides.

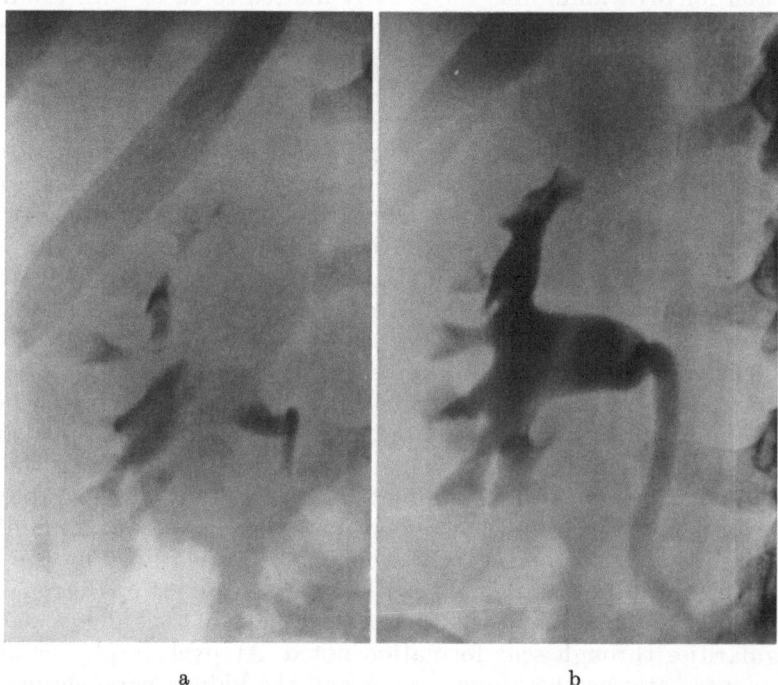

a   b

Fig. 298. Pyelonephritis. a) Urography: multiple impressions in kidney pelvis because of high plasticity of pelvic wall. b) Impressions diminish and disappear during ureteric compression. c) Renal angiography, arterial phase: impressions in kidney pelvis coincide largely with intrarenal arterial branches

b) Urography

Urography is the most gentle examination method and, in addition to demonstration of morphologic changes, it yields information on renal function. In the differential diagnosis between acute pyelonephritis, acute abdominal disease or renal and ureteric stone, we have found that in most of the patients in the acute stage examined at our department, excretion is ordinary (WULFF, 1936), i.e. time of onset of excretion, density of contrast urine and drainage. Occasionally, however, excretion may be somewhat delayed, the contrast density may be somewhat low, and drainage slow because of slight stasis caused by inflammatory edema of the ureteric mucosa. In chronic cases the roentgen findings will vary with the extent of the process. Excretion may be ordinary, have decreased, or be absent. As a rule, the density of the contrast urine is somewhat decreased. It should be observed that urography performed for assessing renal function is a crude

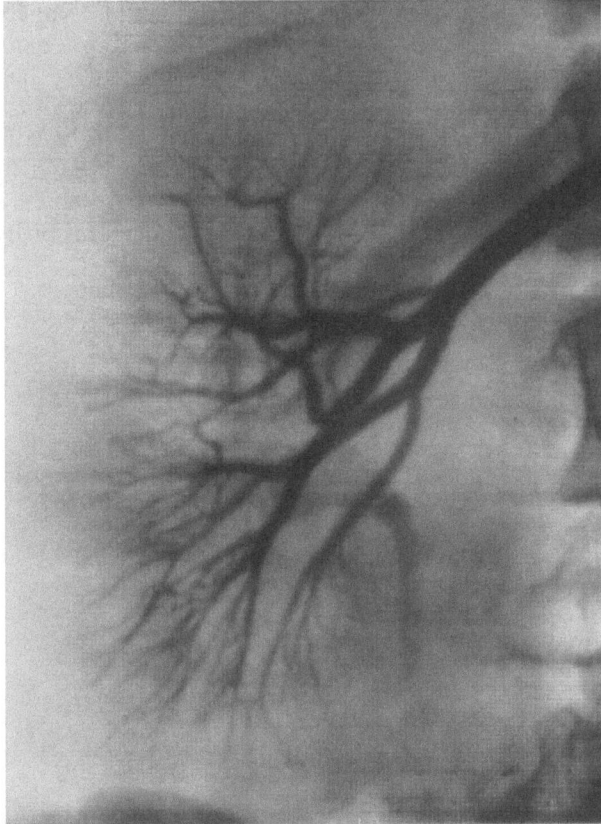

Fig. 298 c

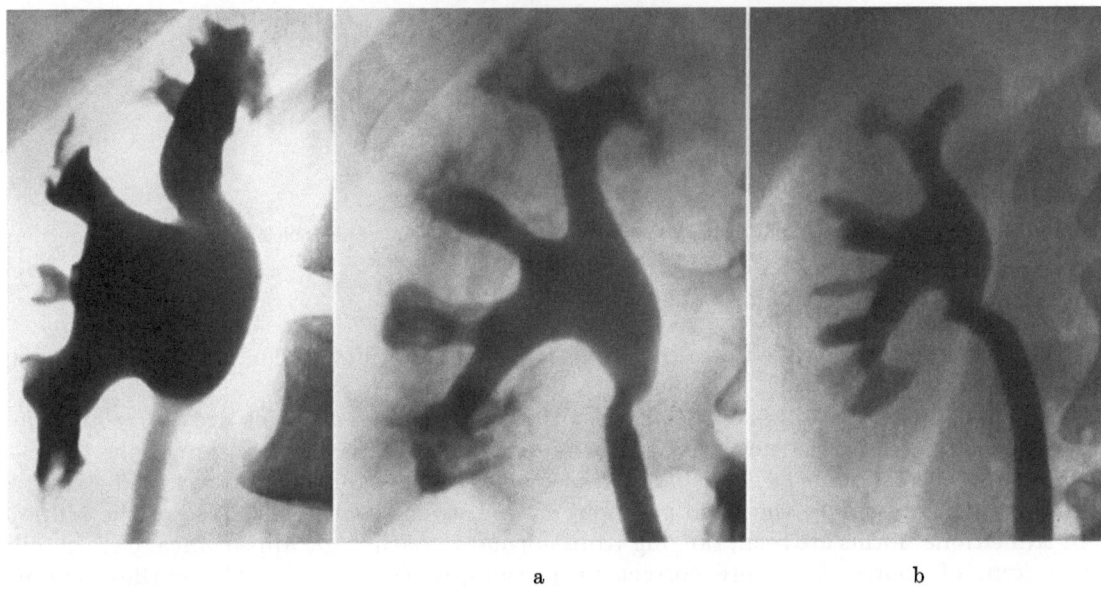

Fig. 299   a   Fig. 300   b

Fig. 299. Pyelonephritis with papillary necrosis, early stage: superficial changes in a few papillae

Fig. 300. Pyelonephritis with papillary necrosis. a) Early stage: contrast medium penetrates into necrotic zones at base of all papillae; b) four years later: marked shrinkage of kidney; necrotic papillae are shed

method (see Chapter C III, 2b). The renal morphology will also vary widely with the severity and extent of the process. In the early stage and in an acute exacerbation of a chronic process, the filling of the stems of the calyces is often defective because of a swelling of the mucosa, and contraction of the renal pelvis and the pelvis wall is markedly mouldable. (Fig. 298). On occasion it may be difficult to obtain sharp films because of marked contractions in rapid succession. These contractions can be demonstrated by cineradiography.

It should be observed here that the motility of the kidney pelvis should not be studied with the aid of pyelography because it is influenced considerably by catheterization and

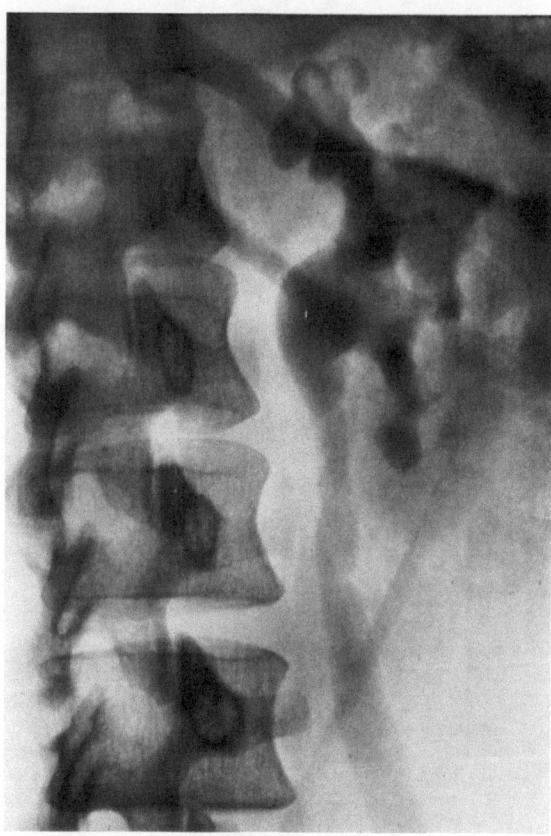

Fig. 301. Pyelonephritis with papillary necrosis: changes in all papillae in cranial pole of kidney. Contrast medium surrounds shed papillae still in place

injection of the contrast medium. Investigation of the motility under such conditions will give misleading results.

In more advanced stages of the disease other changes appear which are due to affection of the parenchyma. Destruction of one or more papillae leads to dilatation of the calyces, when they become more or less spherical (see chapter on papillary necrosis). The calyces may extend far out into the renal parenchyma and even reach the surface of the kidney. All transitional forms are seen, ranging from normal to pathologic appearance. Care should be taken, of course, to secure correct projections of the calyces. The earliest change consists simply of a flattening of the papillae. In local or generalized hypoplasia, it is often not possible to decide whether anomalies or pyelonephritis, or perhaps both, are responsible for the changes seen (see Chapter D). With our present knowledge of the roentgen features of pyelonephritis, the scope of the term "hypoplasia" is in sore need of revision (Figs. 299—308).

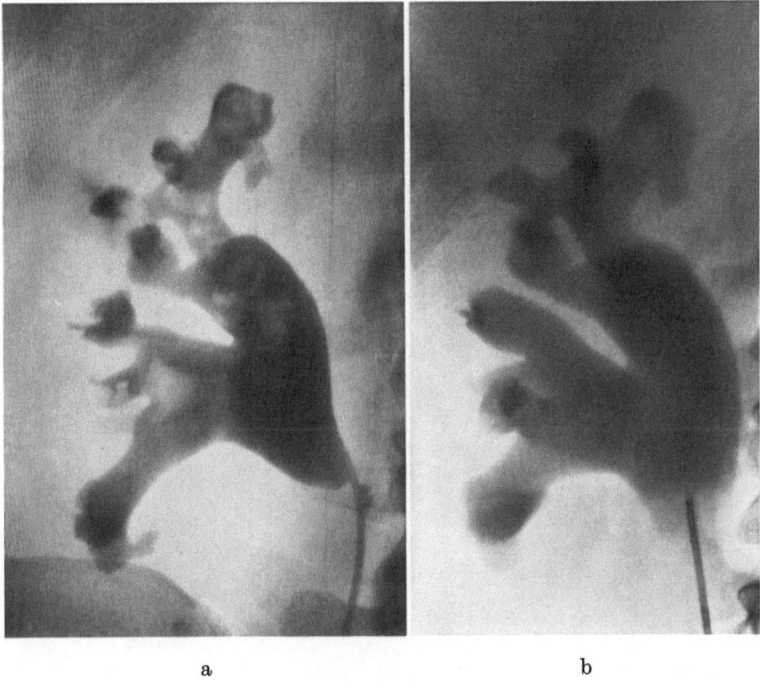

Fig. 302. Papillary necrosis: a) necrotic papillae are partly in place, mainly dislodged out into kidney pelvis; b) half a year later: most papillae are shed

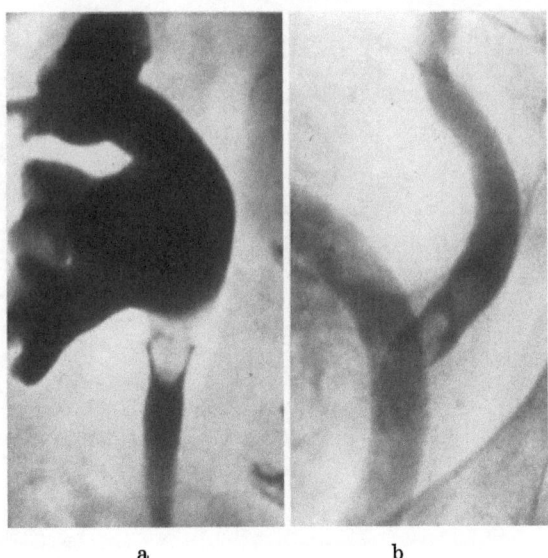

Fig. 303. Shedding of necrotic papillae in papillary necrosis: a) papilla is stuck in the cranial part of ureter; b) several papillary fragments are stuck in distal part of ureter

All stages of papillary necrosis are observed with the details described below (see Fig. 309, 310). Often only the final stages are seen with deformed calyces extending to the surface of the kidney.

In very advanced stages with pyonephrosis the same roentgen findings can be made as in stone pyonephrosis, described in chapter E.

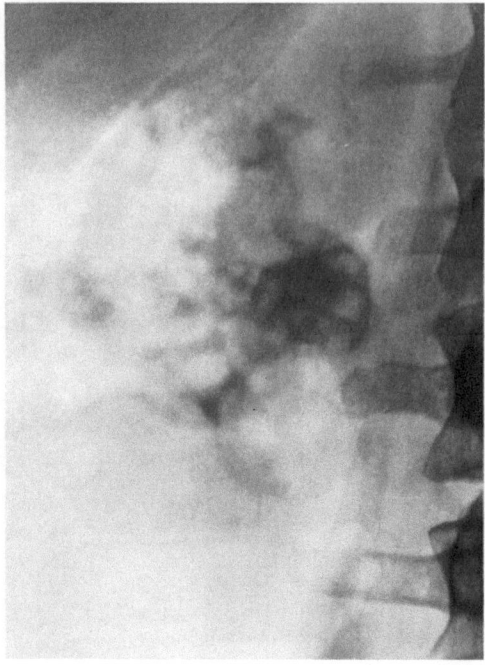

a

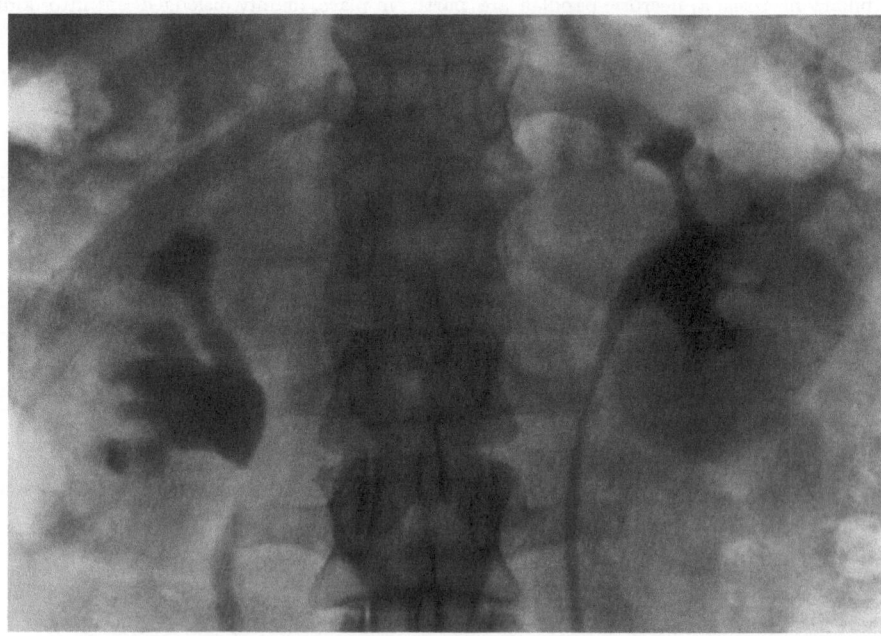

b

Fig. 304. Acute papillary necrosis: kidney pelvis full of shed papillae; b) a few months later: papillae are
shed; remarkably slight changes in shape of calyces

Of greatest interest is, of course, the early diagnosis, particularly since effective
therapy is now available for this stage of the disease. Slight changes in the calyces and in
the motility and plasticity of the renal pelvis in combination seem to be sufficient to permit
a firm diagnosis. Pyelonephritis is often responsible for the changes, with distinct indentations in the renal pelvis by vessels and by the edge of the parenchyma. as described in
Chapter CIII. This point requires further research, however. Findings of urinary infec-

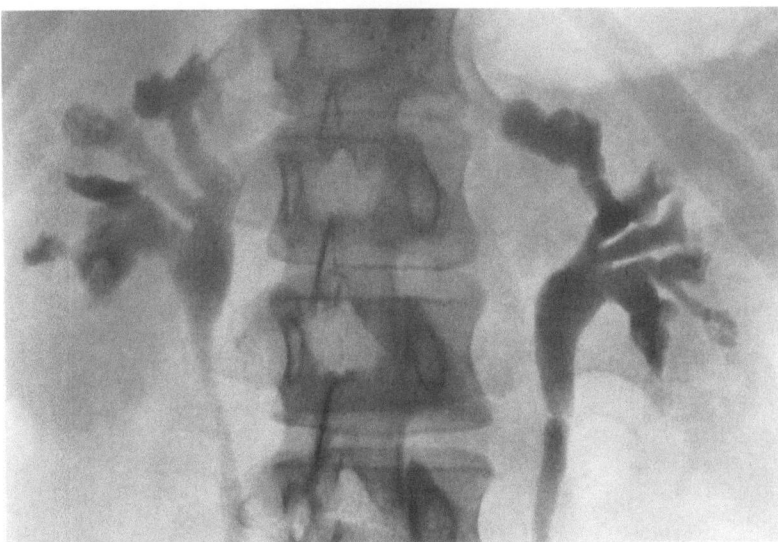

Fig. 305. Bilateral pyelonephritis with papillary necrosis, intermediate stage

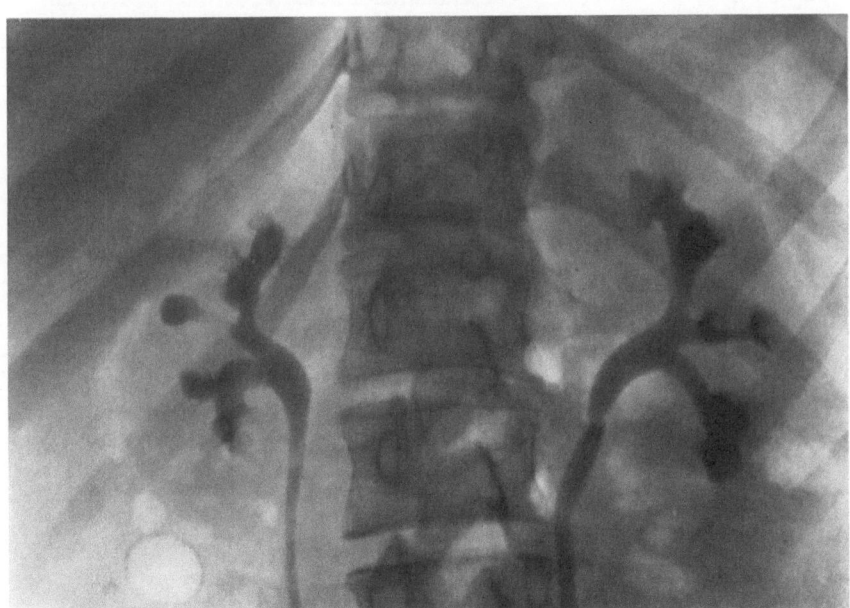

Fig. 306. Pyelonephritis on right side with papillary necrosis: marked shrinkage of kidney; multiple well delineated papillary and medullary cavities

tion are often made in connection with widespread health-check examinations. Urography is often indicated in patients thus selected and will in many instances help in the detection of pyelonephritis with papillary necrosis.

Because renal lesions are fairly common and often important, we have made it a rule in our department in connection with all examinations in which contrast medium is injected, for example in angiography of different types, to take a film of the kidneys at the end of the examination. This urogram will help reveal pathologic changes of different kinds, mostly unexpected (OLLE OLSSON, 1973).

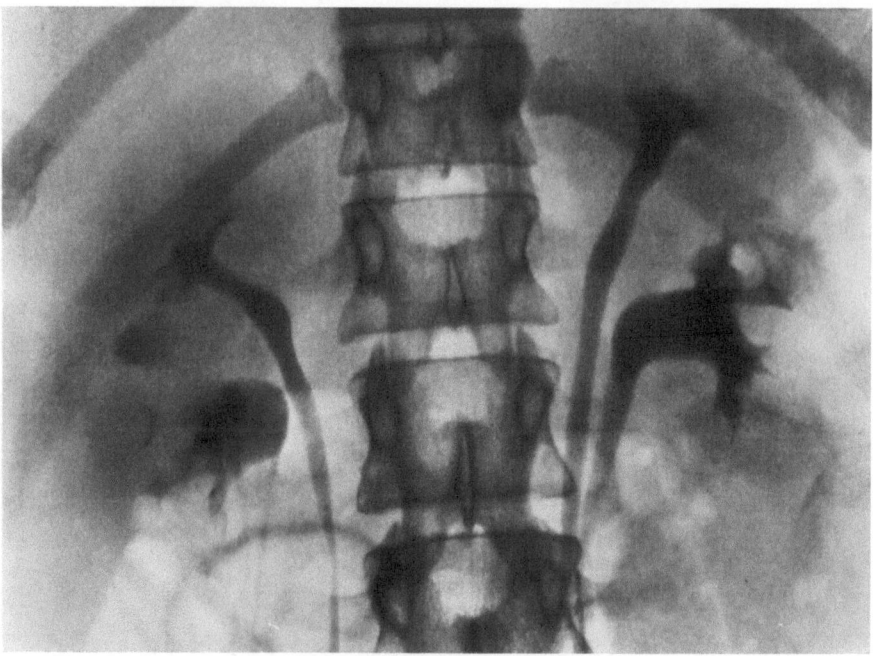

Fig. 307. Double kidneys bilaterally: Marked pyelonephritic changes in caudal part of right kidney

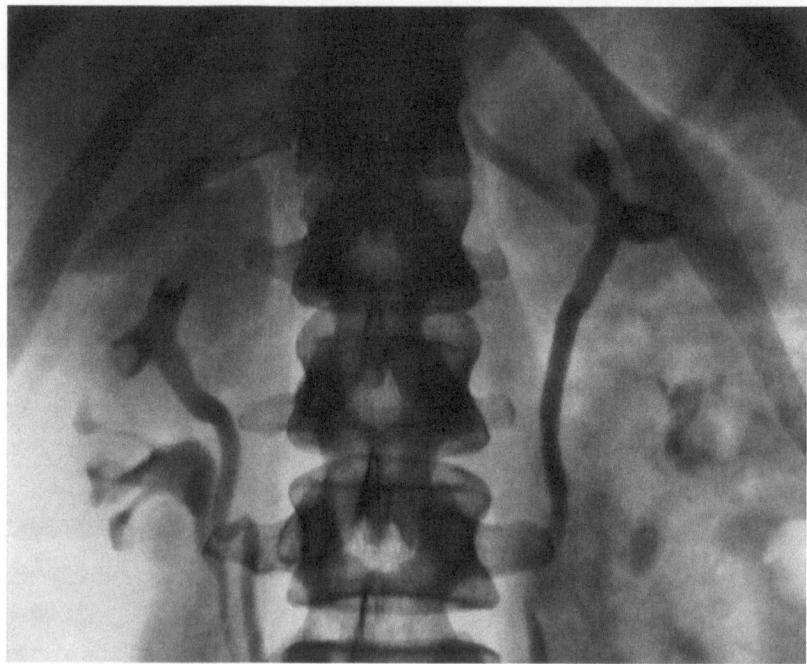

Fig. 308. Chronic pyelonephritis in caudal parts of double kidneys. Operation on left side showed marked pyelo-nephritic atrophy. Note compensatory hyperplasia of cranial part of both kidneys, with marked nephrographic effect during urography

c) Renal angiography

The important changes in the pyelonephritic process are localized mainly in the renal parenchyma. Through renal angiography, means are provided for studying the parenchyma and the vasculature (Figs. 311—315).

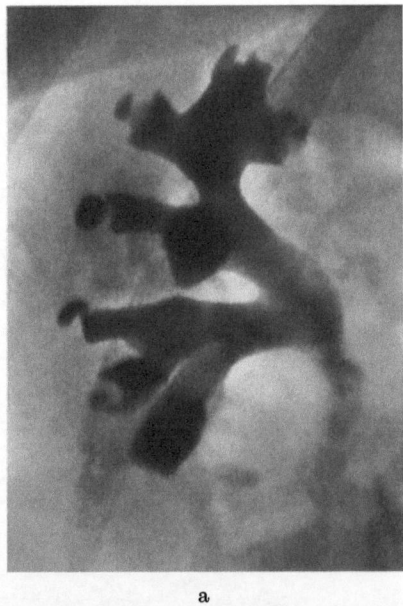

a

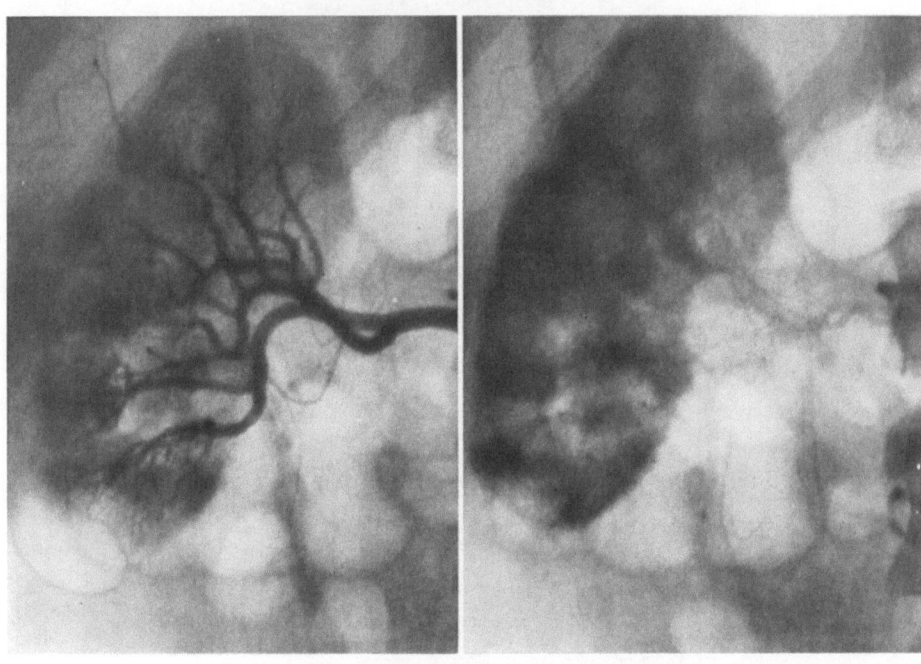

b   c

Fig. 309. Pyelonephritis with papillary necrosis: a) small necrotic cavities in most papillae; b) and c) angiography, arteriographic and nephrographic phases: marked generalized changes with destruction of cortex and marked generalized scar formation

Generalized or localized changes can be seen in the late stages of the disease. The localized changes may be single or multiple. The angiographic changes may be unilateral or bilateral and the extent of the changes may vary considerably in the two kidneys.

Late generalized changes consist of decrease in the size of the kidney, the surface of which is slightly irregular. More marked local scar formation can be seen in a kidney with otherwise generalized changes. The cortex is thin, the arterial branches somewhat widened. The main renal artery has a decreased caliber. In local changes at one or several places, a complete disappearance of functional parenchyma has caused a deep scar forma-

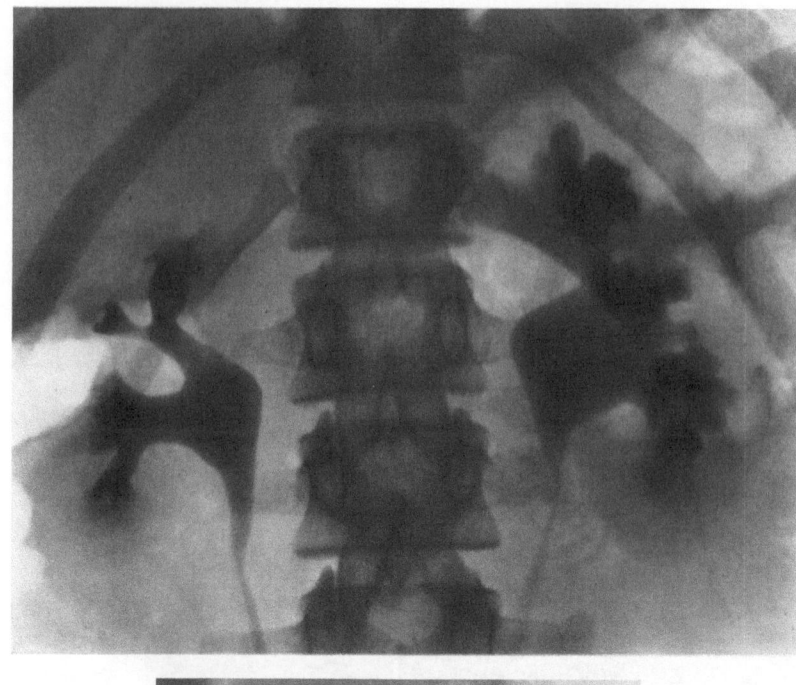

a

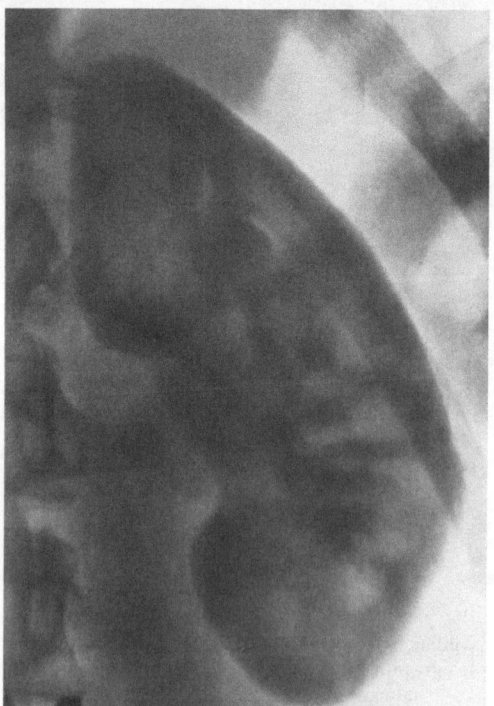

b

Fig. 310. Papillary necrosis with large cavities in all papillae in left kidney; b) angiography, nephrographic
phase: changes are exclusively localized to papillae; no cortical changes

tion from the surface into the sinus. The deep scars can divide the kidney into different
parts, or can exclude a pole of the kidney. Parts of the kidney between the scars increase
in size and have ordninary structure in the nephographic phase.

The local changes may be very small; in completely normal urography, angiography
may demonstrate a single peripheral pyelonephritic lesion.

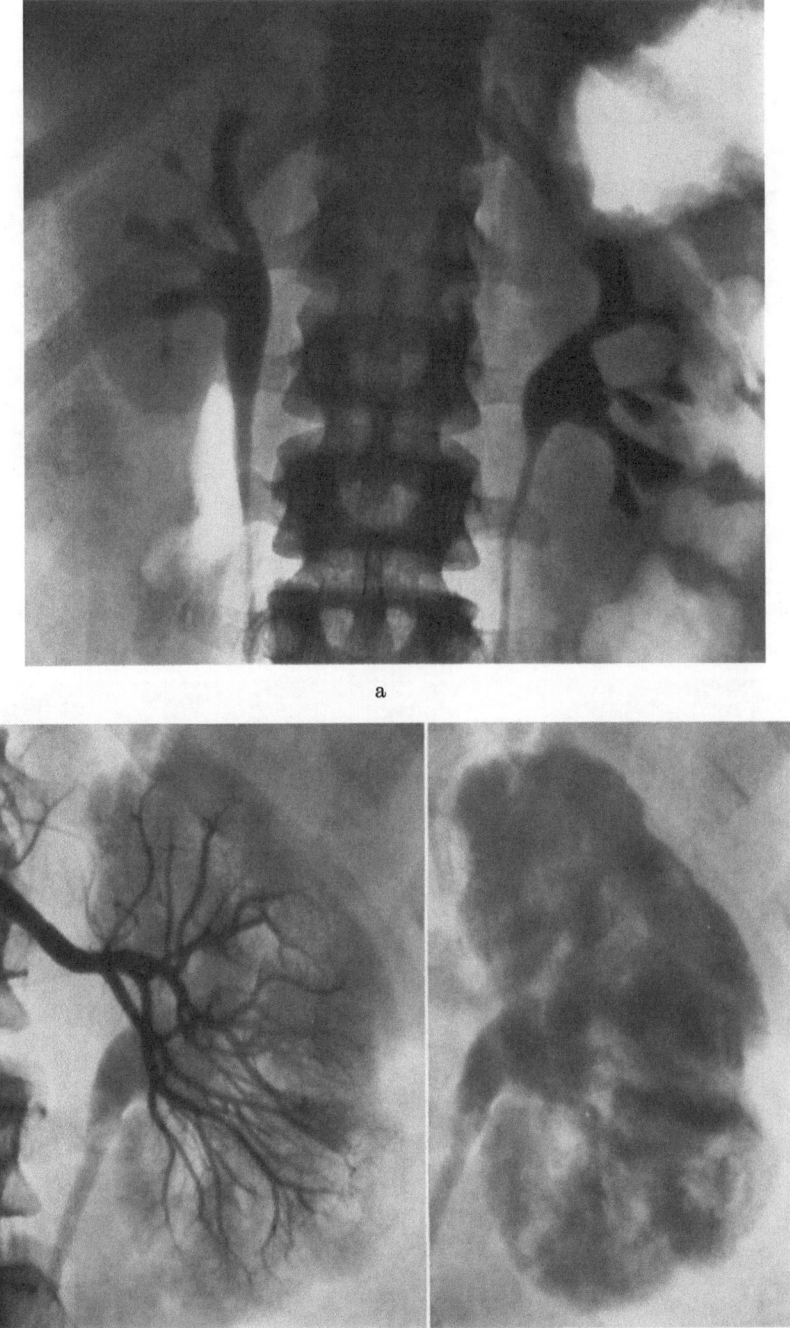

a

b   c

Fig. 311. Chronic pyelonephritis a) urography: marked changes in right kidney; very slight changes in left kidney; b) and c) angiography, arterial and nephrographic phases: left kidney: marked generalized changes with cortical shrinkage and scar formations throughout kidney

At earlier stages the lesion in a local florid process may produce irregular areas with abundant delicate vessels and a diffuse increase in contrast, as a sign of an inflammatory focus.

Changes may occasionally be found on one side, normal conditions on the other, at urography. Bilateral changes may be demonstrated at angiography.

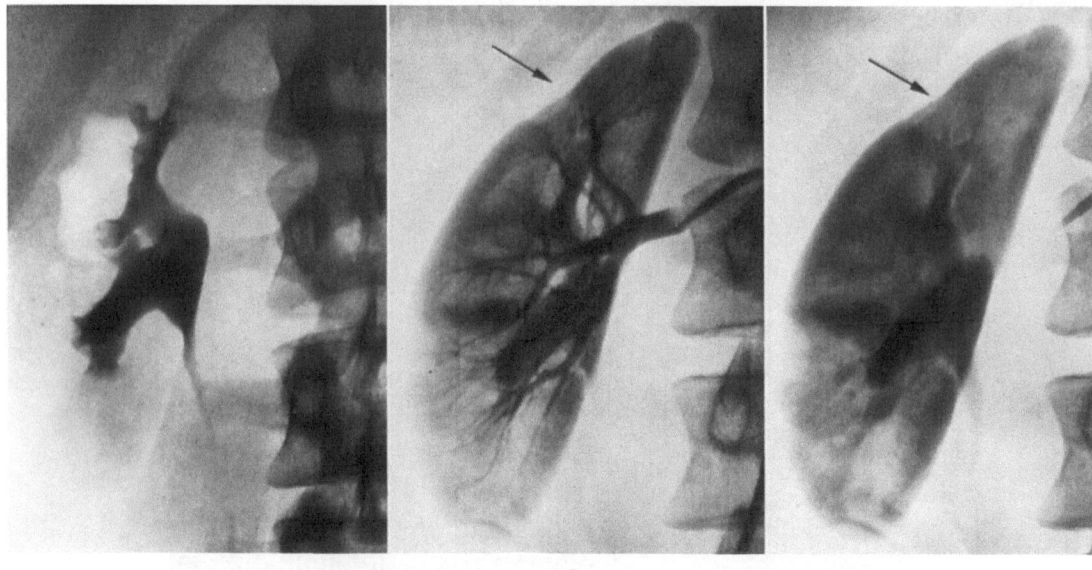

Fig. 312. Chronic pyelonephritis. a) Urography: no changes to be seen; b) and c) angiography, arterial and nephrographic phases: local scar formation cranially-laterally (arrow)

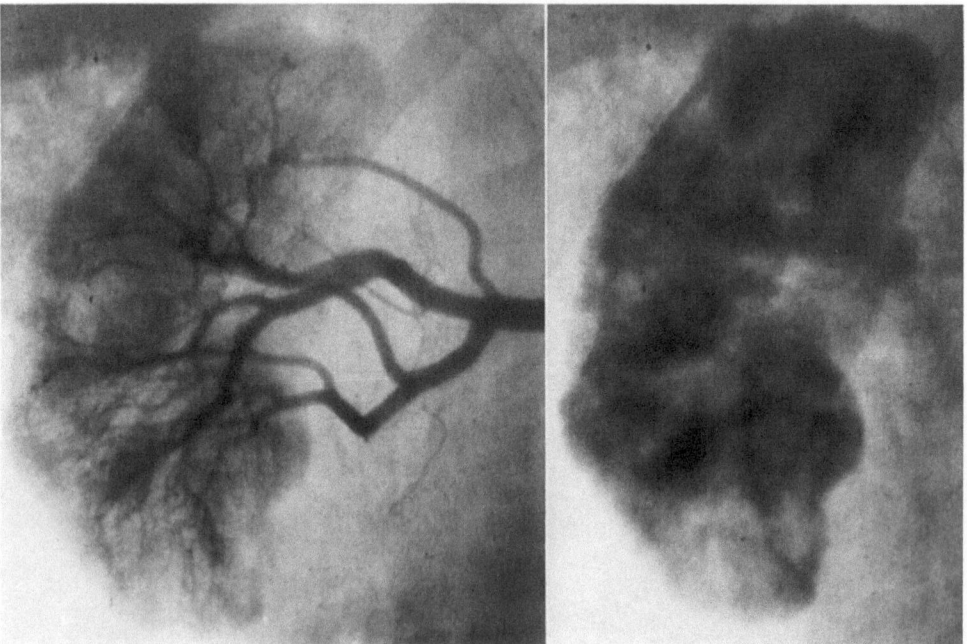

Fig. 313. Chronic renal shrinkage in phenacitin abuse. Angiography, arterial and nephrographic phases: marked irregular shrinkage of kidney; hypertrophy of renal pelvic and ureteric arteries

A local calyceal lesion can be demonstrated at urography. Generalized changes may be found at angiography, in addition to the local process.

It is obvious from the above that angiography is an indispensable method for examining patients with chronic pyelonephritis. Knowledge of the angiographic signs of pyelonephritis is also important in examining patients with localized renal disease, for example scar formation after renal rupture, arterial aneurysms, arterio-venous fistulae, etc., in which pyelonephritic changes are present in addition to the original disease.

d) Pyelonephritis and the lower urinary tract

Pyelonephritis is often seen in connection with stasis, as discussed above. This may be caused by lesions of the bladder and the urethra. Chronic pyelonephritis seen in connection with vesico-ureteric reflux should be mentioned specifically here.

HODSON and EDWARDS (1960) have found that vesico-ureteric reflux is very common in cases of chronic pyelonephritis. The changes associated with reflux are radiologic evidence of chronic pyelonephritis based on the demonstration of localized diminution in thick-

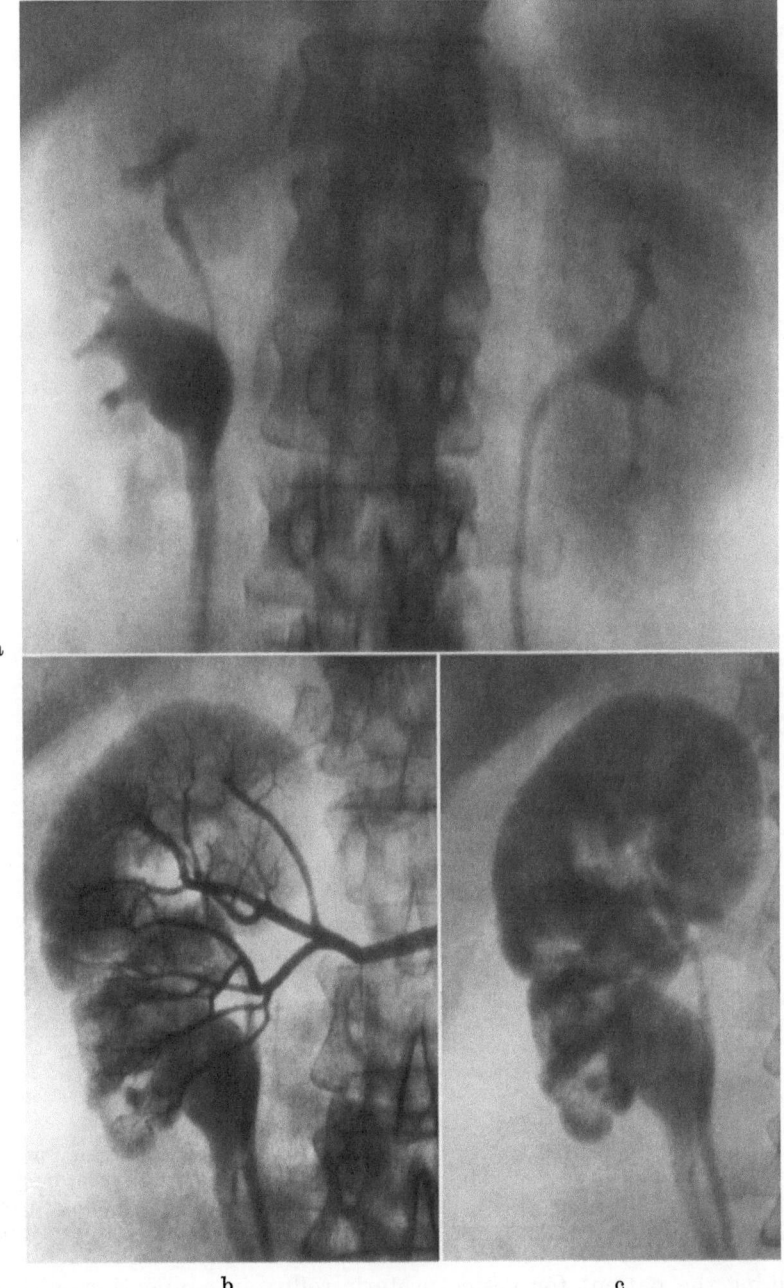

Fig. 314. Double kidney on right side. Pyelonephritis in caudal kidney pelvis. a) Zonography: dilatation of caudal kidney pelvis; slight papillary changes; b) and c) angiography, arterial and nephrographic phases: marked irregular shrinkage of caudal part of kidney corresponding to caudal kidney pelvis; marked hyperplasia of cranial part of kidney

ness of the renal substance, accompanied by shrinkage of the pyramids. Very small kidneys with generalized widening of the calyces can be seen, together with non-obstructive dilatation of the upper urinary tract. If the reflux is unilateral, the changes in the kidney may also be unilateral. Reflux in double kidneys is more common in the caudal kidney pelvis and ureter because of the shorter submucous course of the distal part of that ureter.

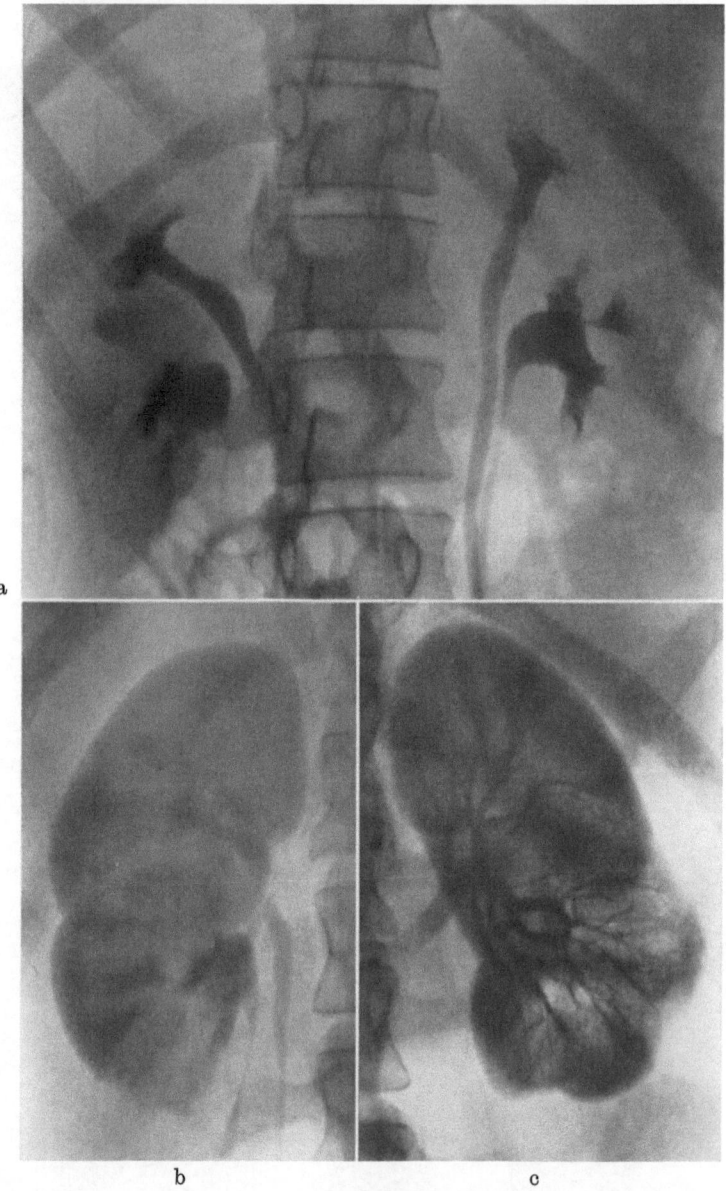

Fig. 315. Double kidney bilaterally. a) Marked pyelonephritic changes in caudal kidney pelvis on right side; b) angiography, nephrographic phase: right kidney: irregular shrinkage of caudal pole; moderate hyperplasia of other parts of kidney; c) left kidney, arteriographic phase: marked changes in kidney parenchyma corresponding to caudal kidney pelvis with cortical shrinkage and large scar formation

In examining the patient for vesico-ureteric reflux in connection with cystography, films should be taken of the ureters and the kidney, with the patient in supine position, head lowered; otherwise observations must be made during fluoroscopy. The phenomenon of reflux may be temporary and disappear rapidly. The kidney pelvis may have ordinary size at urography. A very marked distensibility may be noted, however, at filling of the renal pelvis during reflux. Decrease in concentration and excretion capacity from a pyelonephritic kidney can be masked by reflux from the bladder of urine excreted from the other kidney, if only one kidney is engaged. Thus, reflux should be suspected in every case of pyelonephritis when the renal pelvis is filled better in later films in the urographic study (AMAR, 1971).

8. Papillary necrosis

Papillary necrosis was long regarded as rare and the diagnosis as remarkable. Separation of one or more of the renal papillae is not uncommon, however, as has been shown in recent years. An exhaustive survey of the literature on this disease is given in a monograph "Renal papillary necrosis" by LINDVALL (1960). The disease has been described under the name of papillary necrosis, papillitis necroticans renalis, renal papillary necrosis, necrotizing renal papillitis, renal medullary necrosis, etc.

The changes are characterized patho-anatomically by necrotic destruction usually of several papillae, which are partly or entirely separated. All forms from partial to total demarcation are seen which affect an entire papilla, only its tip, or both the papilla and the pyramid. The disease may be unilateral but is usually bilateral, affecting several papillae, although the changes may involve only one papilla. In LINDVALL's series of 155 patients, 132 cases were bilateral, 23 unilateral. All the papillae were affected in more than one-half of the patients, and single papillae in only one-sixth. In the bilateral cases, the changes were usually similar in distribution on both sides. The necrosis may heal by epithelialization, giving the cavity a smooth surface. The necrosis may affect the papilla, or only a part of it. It may also be deeper and invade the whole pyramid out to the surface of the kidney, and healing scar formation, with local or generalized shrinkage, may result.

Separated parts of a papilla or entire papillae may be excreted with the urine, often in association with renal colic. These may also persist in the renal pelvis and have a tendency to collect calcium and form concrements.

The disease is more common in females than in males and shows the highest incidence in age groups above 40 years. It is most common in diabetics (GÜNTHER, 1937). EDMONDSON et al. (1947), at autopsy of 859 diabetics found 107 (12.4 %) with urinary tract infection and 222 (27.1 %) with papillary necrosis. Of 31,141 non-diabetic patients 1,023 had urinary tract infection and of these 21 had papillary necrosis. Several other autopsy and clinical series have shown that the disease is more common among diabetics and patients with pyelonephritis. Diabetes is by no means a prerequisite for papillary necrosis, however. In LINDVALL's series of 155 cases 19 patients were diabetics. Use of phenacitin was recorded in 89 cases. Specific attention should be given to patients showing abuse of phenacitin. Interstitial nephritis related to large doses of phenacitin was reported by ZOLLINGER in 1955. In these cases papillary necrosis is very frequent. Urinary obstruction also favors papillary necrosis.

The disease has an insidious course. This fact together with progress in therapy in pyelonephritis has made papillary necrosis a more benign disease than in the past. The disease is usually seen in connection with pyelonephritis, which represents part of the patho-anatomic changes in the disease (see below).

a) Plain radiography

Enlargement of the kidney is often seen at plain radiography. Stone — calcified papillae or fragments — may occasionally be seen in the renal pelvis, ureter, or bladder. The concrements are often multiple. They increase in density from one examination to the other, at intervals of weeks, and often have the shape of papillae. Occasionally a defined papilla-shaped part of a stone may be seen as the nucleus of an irregular concrement. Micro-radiography of a stone removed from such a kidney has also shown such a papilla to be the core of the concrement (ENGFELDT and LAGERGREN, 1958). Parenchymal calcifications are occasionally observed which correspond to one or more necrotic papillae that have not been separated. These calcifications are rounded or oval and are less radiopaque; they resemble a shell because of the collection of calcium on the outer surface of necrotic papillae (LUSTED *et al.*, 1957). Gas may occasionally be seen in the renal pelvis at plain radiography, produced by Bact. coli in the urine in diabetics. This gas may fill the entire cavity formed upon the separation of the papillae. Papillary necrosis can then be diagnosed from such a spontaneous gas pyelogram (OLLE OLSSON, 1939).

b) *Urography and pyelography*

The characteristic pyelographic appearance of papillary necrosis was first described by GÜNTHER (1937) and ALKEN (1938) and the first case diagnosed by urography was described by OLLE OLSSON (1939). Some authors claim that pyelography is the only roentgenologic method that can be used. In reality, the choice of examination method depends on the functional capacity of the kidneys. If function is good, urography is preferable. A case described by ESKELUND (1945) in which he claims pyelography to be responsible for papillary necrosis with a fatal issue, can hardly be used as an argument against pyelography, however. Instrumentation in cases of diabetes must be carried out under strictly aseptic conditions in order to prevent the introduction of new bacteria (WALL, 1956).

Papillary necrosis will be manifested in the contrast-filled renal pelvis by an accumulation of contrast medium at the site of a papilla. The changes may resemble those in papillary destruction in other diseases, e.g. tuberculous papillary ulceration. The appearance varies widely with the extent and stage of the process. Papillary necrosis cannot be diagnosed until the papilla has changed in such a way as to permit the entrance of contrast medium into a demarcation zone. If the entire papilla is separated, or if only a fragment has been shed from the side or middle of a papilla, the defect thus produced will be filled with contrast medium. If the process is florid, the persistent papillary surface may be irregular and, in fact, the earliest finding is an irregularity of a papillary tip. In long-standing processes the surface is smooth and the affected calyx assumes a more or less spherical shape. If the papilla or pyramid is not separated entirely, a varying amount of the contrast medium can enter the demarcation zone (Fig. 300, 301), which may then resemble certain forms of sinus reflux. If the entire pyramid is outlined but not separated, a large irregular ring of contrast medium will be seen round a calyx or a group of calyces, where the separated papilla or pyramid is responsible for the contrast defect in the center of the ring. This type of change is very characteristic of papillary necrosis (Fig. 302).

One or more filling defects are often seen in the renal pelvis, usually in a calyx, due to separation of one or more papillae. The defects may be distinctly papilla-shaped, they calcify easily, and generally show more or less marked increase in density. Completely uncalcified papillae or fragments of papillae may also be seen, single or multiple, sometimes together with calcified papillae, sometimes not. All papillae may necrotize and separate at the same time and a large number of papilla-shaped filling defects are seen in the contrast-filled kidney pelvis and the ureter. Calcified or non-calcified papillae occasionally pass over into the ureter and cause blockage, with resulting acute renal colic (Fig. 303). Shed papillae may often pass without symptoms, however. It is surprising how discreet final changes in the shape of the calyces may be in certain instances in spite of the destruction of all papillae (Fig. 304).

Papillary necrosis embraces several problems. The number of cases observed has increased with increasing knowledge of its roentgenologic appearance. It was formerly believed that papillary necrosis was a dramatic acute disease with a fatal issue. Not all cases of papillary necrosis run a dramatic course, however, and not all cases are fatal. THELEN (1947) made a distinction between local and diffuse types, both types with an acute, a subacute, and a chronic course.

Changes will more frequently be found due to destruction of papillae, the more the examiner is interested in pyelonephritis and the more he performs urography with ureteric compression in order to obtain detailed information of the morphology of the renal pelvis, particularly of the calyces. It is surprising, also in connection with diagnosis of renal stone, how often changes are seen at urography which are due to papillary necrosis in single or multiple papillae. The possibility of papillary necrosis must also be considered in all chronic cases with papillary changes of an obscure nature.

It is important to bear the diagnostic criteria in mind, since papillary necrosis may represent a very severe acute situation and since energetic therapy can control necrotizing pyelonephritis. It can arrest necrosis and prevent the formation of concrements.

Papillary necrosis has been regarded as related to and as being an accompaniment of pyelonephritis in diabetics as well as in non-diabetics. Renal function studies by EDVALL (1958) in cases of chronic pyelonephritis on the one hand and of papillary necrosis on the other hand, suggest that it is a question of two independent diseases. This view is supported by the finding of papillary necrosis without infection (HULTENGREN, 1958), which gives reason to doubt the existence of a relationship between papillary necrosis and pyelonephritis. It is of interest to note that in 31 patients with papillary necrosis, HULTENGREN found as many as 29 to have a history of severe headache or migraine. A combination of papillary necrosis and pyelonephritis is very common, on the other hand. In LINDVALL's series all patients examined histologically had signs of chronic pyelonephritis, some with elements of acute pyelonephritis. The histologic type of changes was the same whether the patient had diabetes, urinary obstruction, or phenacitin abuse, and did not differ from that in patients belonging to other pathogenetic groups. LINDVALL concludes: "There is much to suggest that the papillary necrosis is caused by pyelonephritis, instead of the reverse. It is then to be regarded as a symptom and not as a disease entity. The common association of renal papillary necrosis with diabetes mellitus, chronic urinary obstruction, and a history of phenacitin abuse is consequently attributable to the fact that those factors predispose to nephritis or aggravate that condition when already present. The predominance of women in the series may be accounted for by their greater susceptibility to infection in the urinary tract and to their more frequent abuse of phenacitin."

Knowledge of roentgenologic changes after recovery from papillary necrosis is important. As mentioned above, in some cases rounded defects or rounded cavities are seen at the site of an entire papilla or part of it. Some of the changes known as hypoplasia coincide in appearance with those seen after generalized papillary necrosis. As mentioned earlier, papillary necrosis can also produce some of the changes characteristic of pyelonephritis. Certain so-called calyceal diverticula also fall within this group. In addition, changes due to shrinkage and scar formation are common. Such changes may be the same as in pyelonephritis without papillary necrosis. Very often, however, one or more pyramids have completely disappeared, and the corresponding part of the kidney pelvis has widened, with cavities reaching the surface of the kidney, which is usually contracted in that region.

As pyelonephritis is a chronic disease, a combination of changes of different duration is common, from long-standing to fresh changes. Alterations in appearance are common, through shedding of papillae, calcification of shed papillae, disappearance of calcifications, and development of non-calcified papillae into staghorn calculi of calcified papillae. Shrinkage of the parenchyma or part of it, may occur very rapidly. The course of the disease, and thus also the roentgenologic changes, is influenced to a great extent by rationality in therapeutic measures.

c) Renal angiography

The changes in the papillae have so far not been diagnosed by renal angiography. This is easily understood since papillary necrosis is thought to occur because the arterial supply to the papillae is normally poor. The marked changes often seen in other parts of the kidney are the same as those seen in pyelonephritis and are described under that heading.

9. Fibrolipomatosis of the kidney

In decrease in the volume of parenchyma, fibrosis or fatty replacement of the destroyed tissue is sometimes seen in association with diseases causing destruction of the renal parenchyma. This condition is called replacement lipomatosis, renal lipomatosis, fibrolipomatosis, fibrosis, fatty replacement of destroyed renal cortex, fatty replacement of kidney, etc. (KUTZMANN, 1931; PEACOCK and BALLE, 1936; ROTH and DAVIDSON, 1938; PRIESTLY, 1938; FRUMKIN, 1947; SIMRIL and ROSE, 1950; HAMRE, 1957). The condition is generally due to pyelonephritis. The accumulation of fat is always intra-capsular and should be distinguished from the rare lipoma in or adjacent to a kidney. In fibrolipomatosis, the fat is not incapsulated and histologically does not contain smooth muscle, vascular elements, and cartilage, as do lipomas and hamartomas. The fatty connective tissue is most abundant in the renal sinus around the renal pelvis, which may be dilated.

The packing material for the renal pelvis, the arteries, veins, and lymphatics in the sinus of the kidney consist of fat, which makes the sinus easily accessible for roentgen examination. Thus the anatomy is well demonstrated in the nephrographic phase at urography, especially if stasis is present. Fat can also be seen in plain films, particularly when supplemented by zonography or tomography. The sinus is well demonstrable in this way, especially in obese patients.

Replacement lipomatosis may be extensive and become a source of error to be borne in mind in the evaluation of the amount of renal parenchyma, judged by the size of the kidney. A kidney may thus appear to be only slightly decreased or even increased in size but nevertheless have only a small amount of parenchyma remaining, the intracapsular content consisting of fibrous or fatty tissue.

The kidney may be slightly enlarged or of normal size, or a small kidney may have a more or less widened sinus. The changes may be bilateral. Characteristic narrowing and lengthening of the branches of the kidney pelvis may be demonstrated at urography. The distance between the branches may also have increased, the calyces may show lateral displacement and are often slightly and characteristically indented from the sinus side. This slight displacement and deformation of the calyceal system is most marked in the early phases of urography when there is only slight calyceal filling (OLLE OLSSON and WEILAND 1963). The fatty tissue in the sinus of the kidney may be markedly compressible. Thus the characteristic shape of the kidney pelvis due to fibrolipomatosis may be seen only when the intrapelvic pressure is low. During urinary compression or marked excretion, for example in connection with angiography, the width of the renal pelvis may increase and the pelvis with branches may then attain ordinary configuration. At angiography very characteristic changes can be found (OLLE OLSSON and WEILAND, 1963) (Fig. 316, 317). The intra-arterial branches of the renal artery are narrower than normal and the distance between them is increased in cases of fibrolipomatosis. The vessels are sometimes arched and stretched and an increased distance between the ventral and dorsal arteries is often evident. This combination of atrophy and displacement is also characteristic of hydronephrosis with atrophy of the parenchyma. The basic mechanism for the appearance is the same in the two conditions. In fibrolipomatosis it is fat and in hydronephrosis the distended kidney pelvis containing fluid that fills out the widened sinus.

It is generally stated that fibrolipomatosis is rare, that it is always unilateral, and that a pre-operative diagnosis has never been made. In our experience (OLLE OLSSON and WEILAND, 1963) fibrolipomatosis is not uncommon and is often bilateral and, if cases of pyelonephritis are examined closely and tomography is employed to evaluate the sinus,

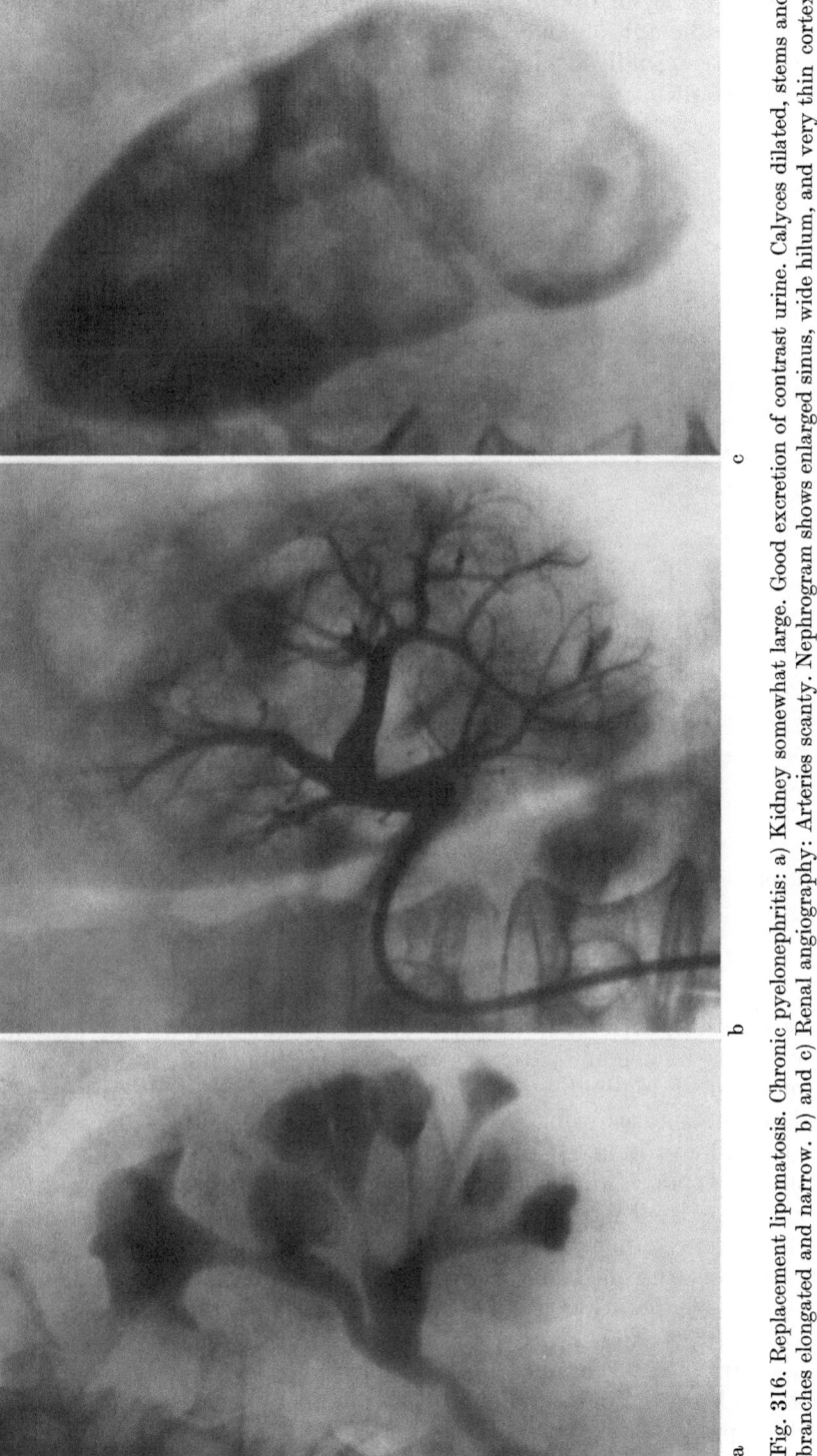

Fig. 316. Replacement lipomatosis. Chronic pyelonephritis: a) Kidney somewhat large. Good excretion of contrast urine. Calyces dilated, stems and branches elongated and narrow. b) and c) Renal angiography: Arteries scanty. Nephrogram shows enlarged sinus, wide hilum, and very thin cortex

these points will be confirmed. In suspicion of tumor, renal angiography is conclusive as to the positive diagnosis of fibrolipomatosis and exclusion of tumor.

VOEGELI (1971), in reviewing our material on fibrolipomatosis, found it to be most common in middle and old age, and especially in prostatic cases. It is also seen in chronic pyelonephritis, especially in cases with concomitant nephro- or ureterolithiasis. Other causes are less important.

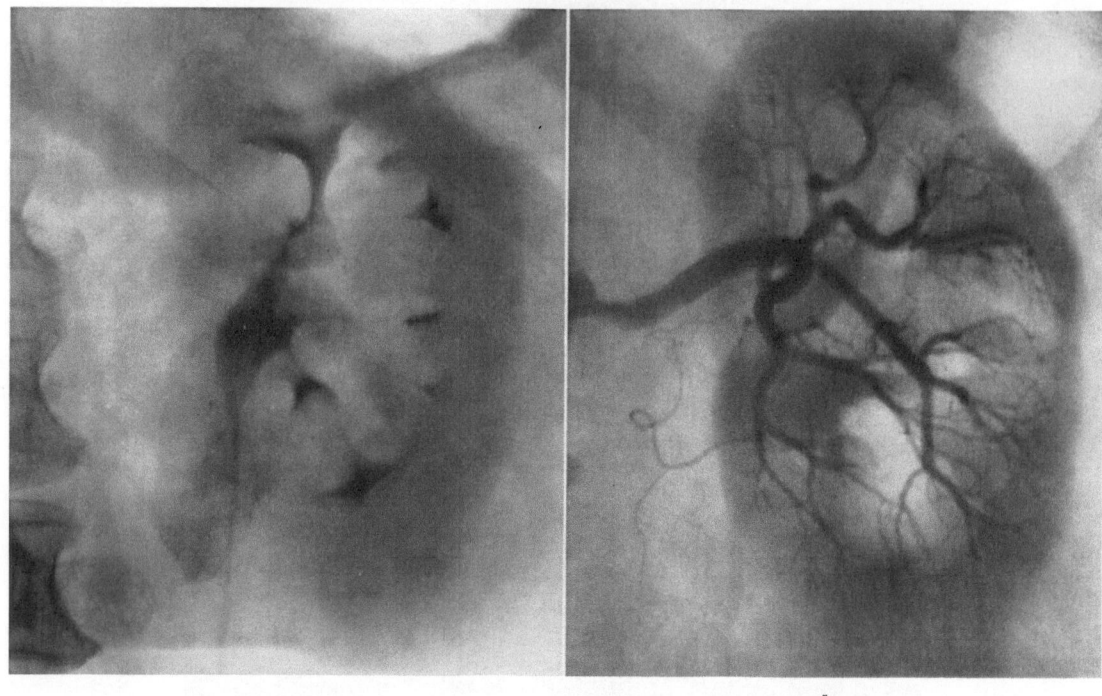

a   b

Fig. 317. Replacement fibrolipomatosis. a) urography: wide sinus, necks of calices stretched. b) angiography: stretching of intrarenal arterial branches

10. Radiation nephritis

In connection with radiotherapy of malignant lesions outside the urinary tract, the kidneys and the urinary pathways may be partly included in the radiation beam. Thus in treatment of abdominal lymph glands in, for example, lymphogranulomatosis, or in lymph gland metastases from, for example, malignant testes tumors, one or both ureters, one or both kidneys or parts of them may be irradiated.

In 1950 ZUELZER et al. reported on three young patients in whom after radiation treatment for retroperitoneal tumors, the kidneys, normal in structure and function, one to two months after completion of treatment showed changes resembling glomerulonephritis but with necrosis and degeneration of the endothelium. In this type of change at a later stage, tubular degeneration, interstitial scarring, and glomerular hyalinization are seen (DAVEY et al., 1952). Marked shrinkage will eventually occur. This shrinkage may affect a kidney or part thereof, for example, then usually the caudal pole, as the field of radiation is supposed to keep the kidneys outside the beam. In such cases a marked atrophy is seen in the kidney pole, whereas the rest of the kidney is hyperplastic (Fig. 318, 319). The kidney changes may cause hypertensive disease and may make nephrectomy necessary (LEVITT and ORAM, 1956).

In 1970 SCANLON, using microangiography to study both the early and late irradiation changes in the kidney of the rabbit, found intense spiraling of arterioles with obliteration

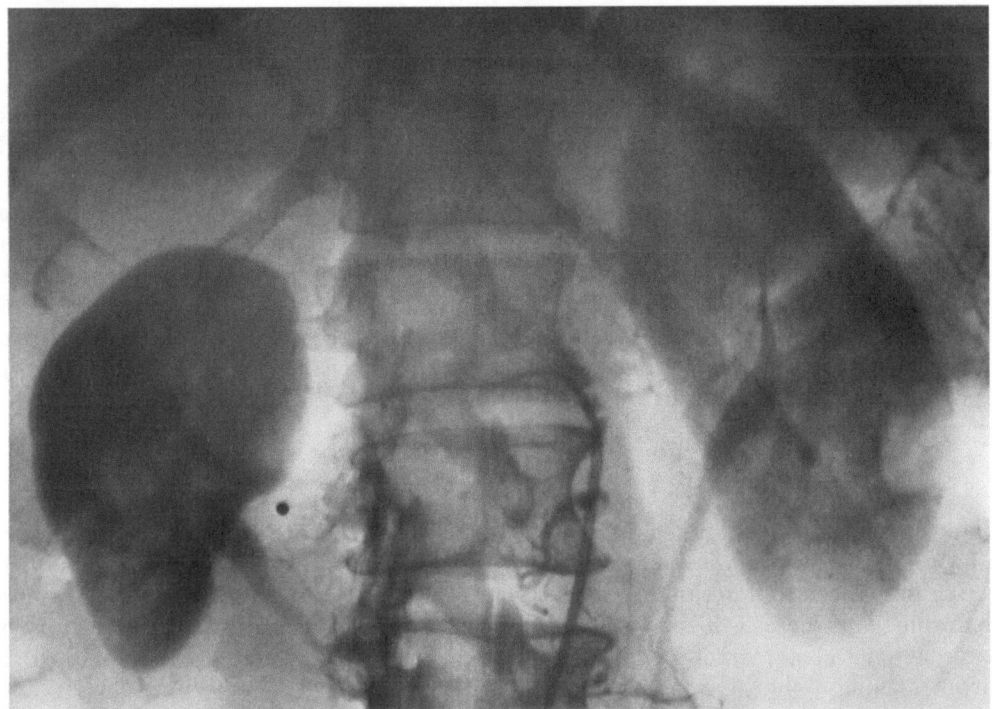

Fig. 318. Radiation nephritis. Radiation treatment for papillary adenocarcinoma in right testis with metastases to lymph glands to the right in the abdomen. Caudal half of right kidney included in the beam. Semi-selective abdominal angiography 20 years after treatment (patient now has hypertensive disease): Marked shrinkage of caudal half of right kidney and hyperplasia of cranial part

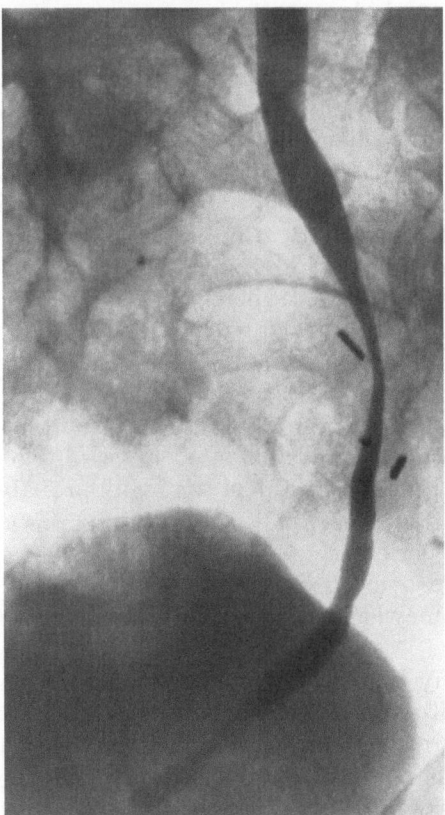

Fig. 319. Residuum after radiotherapy for cancer of the collum of the uterus: Irregular stenosis in distal part of left ureter with dilatation proximally

of most of the glomeruli. The contrast material passed through the kidney without passing through glomeruli. LJUNGQVIST *et al.* (1971) induced radiation nephritis in rats, which resulted in the development of hypertension but only after removal of the non-irradiated kidney.

In local treatment of, for example, carcinoma of the collum of the uterus, parts of the ureter or of one ureter may be within the field of radiation. This can cause marked localized edema, later followed by shrinkage causing a short, occasionally marked, stenosis of the ureteric lumen, which will affect passage of urine and thus cause hydronephrosis and secondary shrinkage of the corresponding kidney. Fig. 319 illustrates a patient of this type, where the shrinkage made necessary anastomosis between the unaffected proximal part of the ureter and the small bowel.

11. Renal hyperplasia

The one kidney will increase in size, as a rule, if the other kidney is missing, as in aplasia, or if the function is poor, as in severe hypoplasia, or if one kidney has been removed or has ceased to function because of such conditions as stasis, infection, degeneration, for example. This increase in size is called compensatory hypertrophy or renal hyperplasia. There is a general agreement that this increase is due to growth of different parts of the nephron, although the number of nephrons does not increase, or at most only slightly.

A marked increase in the size of the kidney will be found in plain roentgenography of the urinary tract, particularly on comparison with films taken before development of the disease causing hypertrophy of the kidney. The increase in size is generalized as a rule, and the kidney becomes plump. The remainder of the kidney may also show compensatory hypertrophy if any part of the kidney is the seat of a pathologic process, while the pathologically changed part will retain its original size. This explains the varying appearance of the kidney in some cases of local hypoplasia of one kidney, in which the other kidney shows marked generalized hypoplasia. Preserved parts of the locally hypoplastic kidney may become hypertrophic to such an extent as to suggest the presence of a space-occupying lesion.

The healthy or residual kidney does not always increase in size. In a series of nephrectomized patients examined before and after nephrectomy, SCHROEDER (1944) found an increase in the size of the remaining kidney in two thirds of the cases. The increase was less marked in the higher age groups. Hypertrophy can occur in patients somewhat over 50 years of age, as shown by HANLEY (1940).

The increase in area in SCHROEDER's material was, on the average, 30 %, was somewhat larger in females than in males, and larger in young patients than in elderly. WIDÉN (1958), in an experimental investigation in dogs, found that on total obstruction of a ureter for 30 days at most, the other kidney increased in size by 20 %. After a ligation period of more than 30 days, the kidney showed a statistically probable further increase of 15 %.

The kidney size usually increases rapidly and then remains at a certain level, although a continuous increase over a period of 2—3 years has also been noted (BRAASCH and MERRICKS, 1938). These authors pointed out that the large single kidney (with agenesia on the other side) is situated somewhat more caudally than the usual position of a normal kidney.

It is shown at urography that in the so-called compensatory enlargement of the kidney, the width of the renal pelvis is also slightly increased. This is most readily demonstrated in cases in which urograms are available from the pre-nephrectomy period.

It is also shown at renal angiography in these cases that the renal artery is wider than is normal. IDBOHRN (1956) found that, on unilateral ligation of the ureter in rabbits, the caliber of the renal artery on the other side rapidly increased to a moderate extent. WIDÉN (1958) made the same observations in dogs.

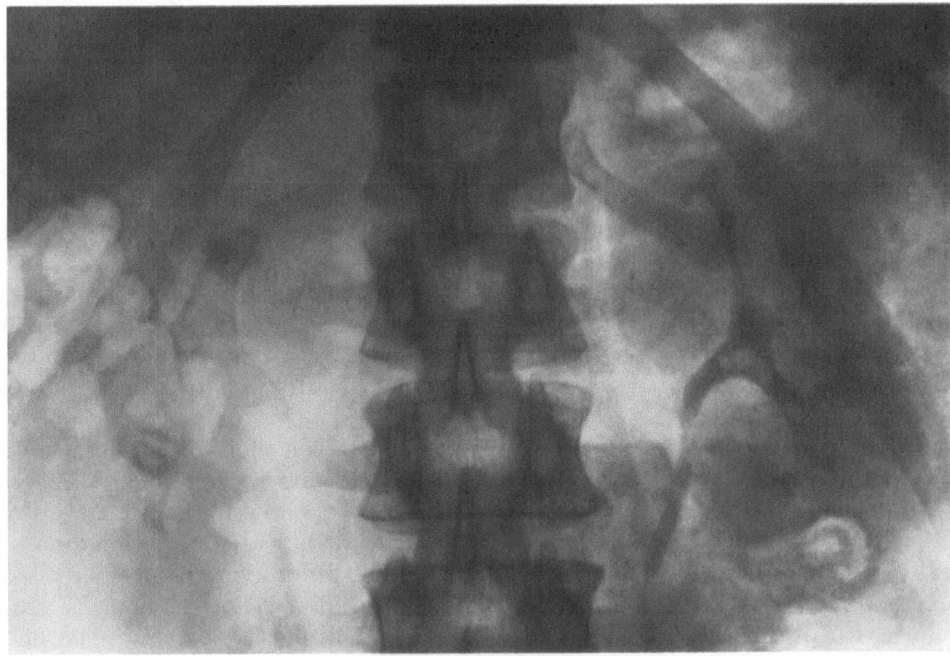

a

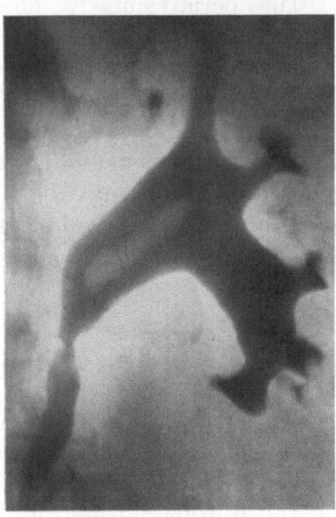

b

Fig. 320. Mycosis in both kidney pelves, Candida albicans, in patient treated with antibiotics because of urosepsis: a) Right kidney pelvis filled with mycotic masses. In left kidney pelvis, small balls of mycotic material. b) After pyelotomy with emptying of masses on right side: ordinary conditions. On left side, two months later: still mycotic material in kidney pelvis

12. Mycosis

A specific type of infection which can occur in the kidney pelvis is mycosis. It was recently discovered that large amounts of fungi could be found forming lumps in the stomach. We have seen one such case of infection bilaterally in the kidney pelvis. On one side the kidney pelvis was completely filled with fungi; on the other side, a large polyp-like mass was found (Fig. 320).

Fungus balls may also be seen in the urinary bladder (MacDonald and Fagan, 1972).

Renal candidiasis is common in systemic candidiasis and may result from prolonged use of in-dwelling catheters, chemotherapy, and immuno-suppressive agents (CLARK *et al.*, 1971).

II. Problems in connection with hemodialysis

The specific roentgenologic problems met with at examination of patients under hemodialysis are treated in different sections of this book. For the sake of an over-all study they will be summarized here:

Kidneys. Diseases causing renal insufficiency and necessitating hemodialysis represent a broad scale of usually generalized renal pathology, for example chronic glomerulonephritis, pyelonephritis, polycystic disease. A combination of diseases is common and a combination of chronic renal disease with a residuum after acute trauma may also be encountered.

The roentgenology of these diseases is described under their respective headings.

Chest. Pulmonary edema, acute and chronic, represents an important problem. The changes in connection with acute pulmonary edema of different degrees are described under the heading "Generalized renal disease." Other types of lung lesions may also be important, for example acute and chronic pneumonia, pulmonary hemosiderosis, etc.

Bone and soft tissues. In chronic hemodialysis decalcification of bone is a common occurrence with fractures of, for example, vertebrae and ribs as common complications. Changes of the type renal osteodystrophy may also be seen. Depositions of calcium phosphate are often seen in the soft tissues periarticularly. These calcifications may be confined to one or a few joints but may also be very widespread, engaging most joints.

The arteriovenous shunt. The different types of arteriovenous shunts used in hemodialysis may cause problems, usually because of thrombosis. These complications are described in the chapter on vascular disease.

Renal transplantation. Most patients under hemodialysis represent candidates for renal transplantation. Therefore renal angiography may be necessary to define the vascular anatomy. Conditions and complications after transplantation are described in the chapter on renal transplantation.

M. Perinephritis, renal abscess and carbuncle

A local inflammatory process in the perirenal tissue is known as perinephritis. Other names used for this condition are perinephritic abscess, paranephritis, epinephritis, etc. According to ISRAEL (1901) the two last-mentioned names should be reserved for inflammation of the fatty capsule and the fibrous capsule of the kidney, respectively. The inflammatory process usually involves all the soft tissues around the kidney, however, and the name perinephritis, which simply indicates the presence of inflammation around that organ, is therefore satisfactory.

The inflammation may be due to an intrarenal lesion. In renal carbuncle, one or more renal abscesses can perforate the capsule out into the space enclosed by the renal fascia (see Chapter CII, 2., Retroperitoneal pneumography). An inflammatory process may also involve the perirenal tissue via the lymphatics. The hilum is particularly rich in lymphatics, as is obvious from pyelolymphatic reflux (see chapter on backflow) and the possibility of spreading through the hilum to the perirenal space is obvious from conditions in connection with backflow.

Perinephritis, however, may also be secondary to inflammatory lesions in tissues adjacent to the kidney, such as osteitis of the ribs or spine, pancreatitis, perforated duodenal ulcer, diverticulitis of the colon, etc. It may be a metastatic process due to spread of material from a septic process such as furunculosis, directly to the bed of the kidney.

Perinephritis can break through the renal fascia or can propagate through the open caudal part of the latter. It does not usually spread from one side to the other, however. The spine and large vessels form a barrier against such spread but the main reason that the condition does not spread in this direction is that the renal fascia is closed medially. This has been shown in autopsy studies by MITCHELL (1939) who injected contrast medium post mortem and observed that the passage of the opaque medium from the bed of the kidney on one side to that on the other, occurred only via the pelvis. This is known also from wide experience with retroperitoneal pneumography.

Perinephritis may extend around the entire kidney but, as a rule, it is most marked dorsally to the kidney and caudally towards the opening of the renal fascia. This is due to the basic local anatomy, e.g. the fatty capsule is thickest dorsally and the infection spreads along the path offering the least resistance. It is also in part due to the fact that the patient has usually been lying on his back for a long period. The outline of the lesion may be indistinct but it may also be sharp, like that of a well defined, small or large abscess. Upon examination, the disease may be in the acute or chronic stage, or may be healing with fibrosis.

The roentgen findings vary considerably with the patho-anatomic type and stage of the disease. The course of the disease may be followed by repeated examinations at various intervals.

I. Role of roentgen examination

It is not uncommon for perinephritis to remain concealed until post mortem examination (CAMPBELL, 1930; HIGGINS, 1932 and others). Roentgen examination is therefore indicated in all cases of obscure fever, and on examination of patients for a dubious abdominal or urinary tract disease, the possibility of perinephritis should be considered. It is often noted in the literature that roentgen examination is of but little value in the diagnosis of perinephritis. As a mater of fact, however, the roentgen findings are abundant. Perinephritis is not infrequently diagnosed as an accidental finding. In our series from 1943 (WELIN), roentgen diagnosis was made in 9 patients in whom the disease had been clinically suspected and in 8 in whom the disease had not been suspected and who had been examined radiologically for urinary tract disease.

RIGLER and MANSON (1931) claimed that the roentgen findings are uncertain within 10 days after onset of symptoms and that the absence of roentgen findings after a period of 14 days should throw grave doubt upon the diagnosis of perinephritic abscess. In view of the varying clinical symptomatology of perinephritis, inclusion of such a time factor in the roentgen examination is fruitless. If the examination is properly performed, the roentgen findings are so valuable that, practically speaking, negative findings exclude the possibility of perinephritis despite the length of the history, provided that the examination is performed under favorable conditions: If the history is short and strongly suggestive of perinephritis, and roentgenography negative, the examination should, of course, be repeated after a time.

II. Roentgen findings
(Figs. 321—325)

In the discussion of the roentgen findings it should be pointed out that some of them, by themselves or in combination, may be fairly characteristic but that the findings are, as a rule, non-specific since each may be due to some other disease. Yet in combination and together with the clinical findings they usually permit a diagnosis. Therefore roentgen examination is a valuable adjunct in the diagnosis.

The roentgen findings were first exhaustively described by LAURELL in 1921; since then only details have been added.

1. Plain radiography

Sometimes one of the kidneys is enlarged. Edema, however, is often present in the renal capsule or around the kidney, which prevents the kidney or part of it from being outlined. Owing to the extent of the pathologic process, which may vary widely, and owing to the degree of edema, which may likewise vary considerably, the anatomy of the retroperitoneal space may be deranged in such a way as to mask the lateral outline of the psoas muscle or part of it. If the process extends far laterally, the anatomy of the soft tissues of the flank may also be changed.

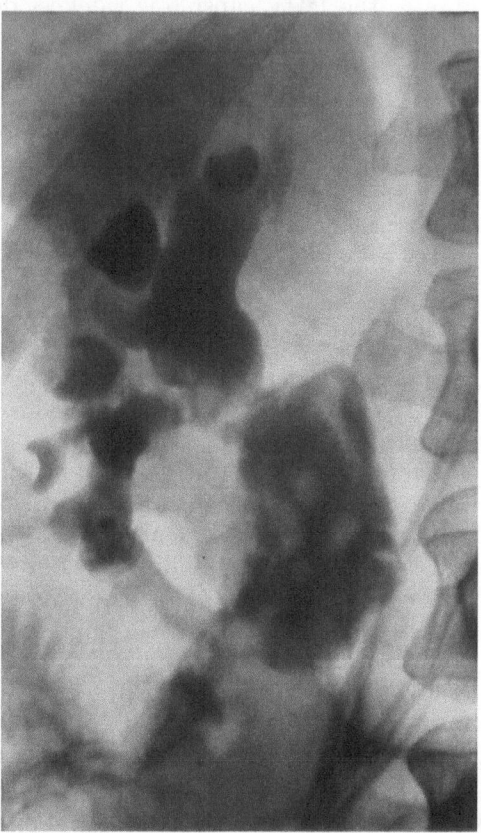

Fig. 321. Perirenal abscess. Pyelolithotomy. Infection and fistulation postoperatively. Antegrade pyelography via fistula. Filling of irregular fistula and large irregular abscess cavity adjacent to kidney

The abscess may vary in size, with consequent variation in the roentgen findings. The findings also vary with the severity of the inflammatory edema. If the process is very acute, the edema marked, and the outline diffuse, the roentgen findings will be dominated by a blurring of the normal roentgen anatomy of the soft tissues. If the process is long-standing and well defined, the findings may be the same as those produced by a local space-occupying lesion.

The kidney may be displaced, often laterally and caudally, and its mobility may be diminished, as may be seen by the limitation of its movements in the respiratory cycle. The kidney may also be displaced ventrally. Because of the examination conditions (increased object—film distance on examination in supine position) the kidney may then appear larger than it really is.

The outline of various organs and muscle layers, which is often very distinct because of the difference between the density of fat and other soft tissues, is blurred by edema because the increased amount of fluid decreases the difference in density of the various tissues. This implies a more or less general increase in the density of the retroperitoneal space, which may be striking.

Meteorism is often generalized, but it may be more or less limited to the local inflammatory process.

Muscle contracture often causes skoliosis, with the concavity facing the side involved by the perinephritis. Gas in the colon and stomach often makes it possible to observe displacement of, or impressions in, these organs.

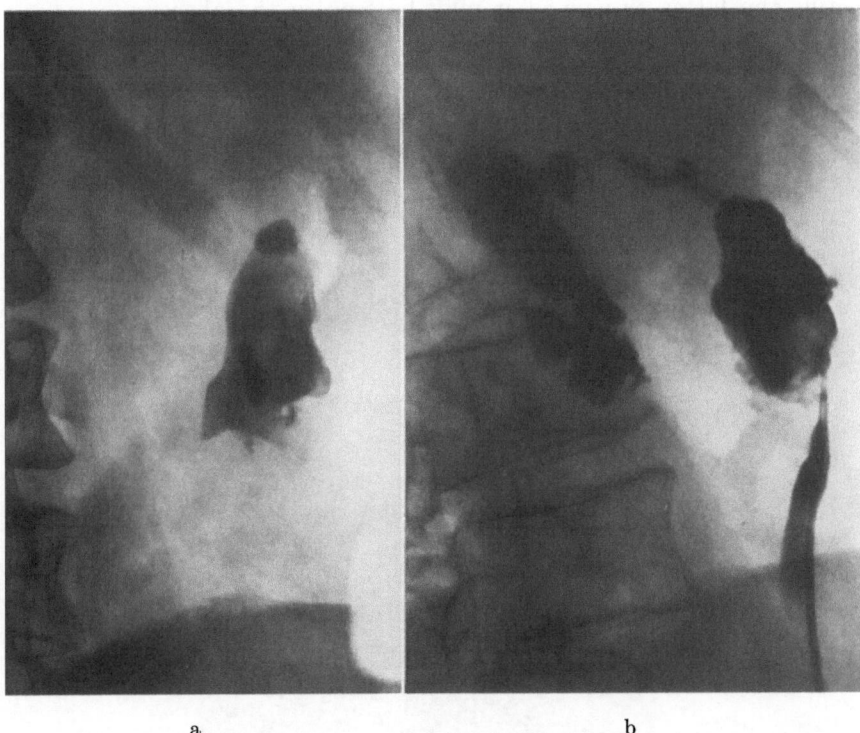

a   b

Fig. 322. Perirenal abscess through fistula in infected stone kidney. a) Large stone in left kidney which is enlarged and not well outlined. During urography: no excretion b) Pyelography: contrast medium escapes from cranial part of kidney pelvis via an irregular fistula into the retroperitoneal space

The findings are not pathognomonic; they may be caused by all types of inflammatory processes in the retroperitoneal space. Acute pancreatitis may thus cause roentgen changes of the same nature as unilateral perinephritis.

All of the findings mentioned must be judged with caution and with due allowance for the influence of the examination technique on the results. Thus in emaciated patients the soft tissue markings may be absent because of lack of retroperitoneal fat, and thus not because of edema. Skoliosis may be due to the unsatisfactory positioning of the patient on the examination table, or it may be due to spinal deformity. Skoliosis as such can also prevent the lateral border of the psoas muscle from appearing in the usual way (this has been described in detail by SKARBY 1946). In the presence of skoliosis the kidney may be tilted less than otherwise and therefore appear wider. A kidney may also — as mentioned — appear larger than it is in reality if it is lifted ventrally by a dorsal abscess. Intestinal contents may also make it difficult to judge the state of the retroperitoneal space. Since the patient may have been bed-ridden for a long time, considerable fecal matter and meteorism are common.

To the findings described above, direct changes may be added. Sometimes gas is seen in the abscess; sometimes it is abundant as in a case of a diabetic described by BRAMAN and CROSS (1956). Otherwise the amount of gas is usually small, and if the pus is thick, the gas will be seen as small bubbles. On examination with the horizontal beam with the patient standing or lying, fluid levels will form against the gas.

An old process may calcify and then be surrounded by an irregular calcium shell, or irregular calcium deposits may be seen in the abscess. This is very common in tuberculous perinephritis. Sometimes a stone may be seen in the abscess e. g. a renal or ureteric stone that has perforated and caused the abscess in which it is embedded. If the abscess is due to a projectile, the latter or part of it may be seen in the abscess.

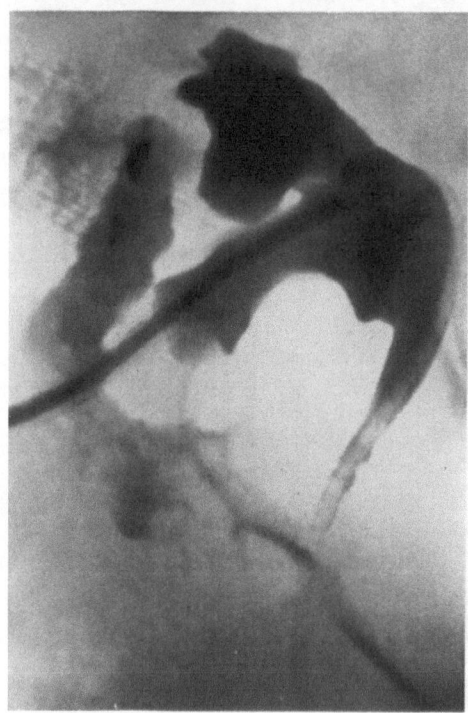

Fig. 323. Perirenal abscess in connection with bowel resection in regional enterocolitis. Lesion in right ureter. Antegrade pyelography: through lesion in ureter contrast medium escapes into irregular cavity surrounding part of right kidney

2. Examination with contrast medium

Since the abscess presses against the kidney, at pyelography or at urography deformation of the renal pelvis and displacement of the ureter will often be shown. If the abscess is small and well defined, the deformation of the renal pelvis may resemble that seen in the presence of an intrarenal space-occupying lesion near the surface of the kidney. The abscess and the edema more often cause a more generalized compression, however. The pyelographic findings vary with the direction of the pressure and the position of the patient and the extent to which the renal pelvis is filled. Therefore, during the examination the technical conditions, e. g. the density of the contrast medium, the degree of filling, and the position of the patient, should be varied in order to decide which factors are constant. Since the space-occupying lesion is often situated behind the kidney, lateral projections are usually informative.

With due consideration to the pathologic anatomy, it is, as a rule, not difficult to decide whether the lesion is extrarenal or intrarenal (DEUTICKE, 1940; OVERGAARD, 1942). PREHN (1946) reported a case in which rotation of 90° of the upper calyx in a kidney was described by the author as a new sign of perinephritis. In reality the accompanying reproduction of a pyelogram shows a lateral and caudal displacement of the renal pelvis and a large bow-shaped impression in the medial part, as well as an impression laterally in the gas-filled stomach, thus a large expanding process which, judging from the pyelogram, was well defined and located mediodorsally. Undoubtedly perirenal abscess has often

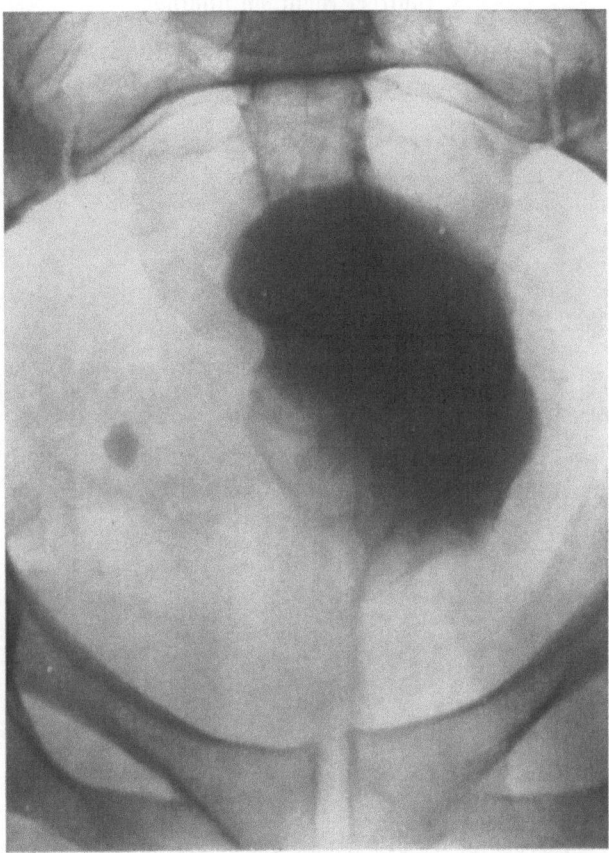

Fig. 324. Abscess around distal part of ureter with fairly large stone. The abscess displaces bladder, impresses its right part and causes inflammatory edema in bladder mucosa

been mis-diagnosed as an expanding process in the kidney. On the other hand, it must be remembered that renal carbuncle and perinephritis in combination are so common that in the presence of a local expanding process and a perirenal component the possibility of renal carbuncle must always be considered.

If the lesion has perforated into the renal pelvis, contrast medium can flow into the abscess at retrograde pyelography (Figs. 321, 322) (ALKEN, 1937; WELIN, 1943). If the abscess is due, for example, to a perforated diverticulum of the colon, on examination of the colon with contrast medium the fistula may be filled with the contrast medium, which may enter the abscess cavity (Figs. 321—325).

On perforation of the surface of the skin, fistulography may be performed. Water-soluble contrast medium is injected into the fistula, possibly via a catheter. With suitable injection pressure and suitable positioning of the patient, contrast medium may fill the entire cavity. The abscess may also be filled by percutaneous puncture of the abscess and injection of gas (LAURELL, 1931) or by positive contrast (FECI, 1927).

The roentgen-diagnostic signs described above also hold true for abscess formation around the ureter in perforation by stone, for example. An abscess around the distal end of the ureter may impress or encroach upon the bladder (Fig. 324). The bladder mucosa then shows edema of the type not seldom seen in diverticulitis of the colon, with abscess formation involving the bladder wall.

3. Indirect roentgen findings

In addition to the signs described above, the examination may show a number of indirect signs. The diaphragm on the diseased side is often higher due to the space-occupy-

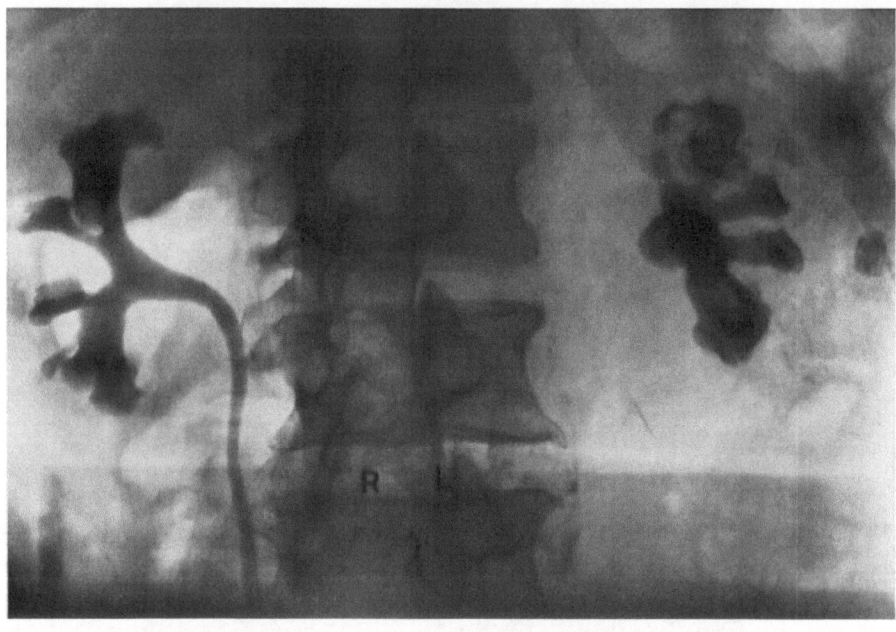

a

Fig. 325. Non-functioning stone kidney on the left with fistula to skin. Urography: a) Kidney pelvis on left side filled with staghorn calculus. Two calculi laterally, one outside kidney. No excretion. b) Fistulography: Filling of irregular fistula system with connection to descending colon

ing nature of the process or to interference with the motility of the diaphragm, the abscess often being situated directly on the dorsal part of the diaphragmatic musculature, which extends far caudally. The diaphragmatic excursions are often limited on the diseased side. Therefore lamellar atelectases are seen in the basal part of the lung on the side involved. The pleural cavity on that side often contains fluid. NESBIT and DICK (1940) stated that of 85 patients with perinephritic abscesses, 14 (16,5 %) were found to have supraphrenic complications. The frequency varies with the examination technique, of course. If the patient can be examined only at the bed-side, the frequency of pathologic findings will be lower than otherwise. At examination in the lateral decubitus position with the beam horizontal — this is the only way to demonstrate small amounts of pleural effusion — pleural involvement will very often be shown. Judging from the above-mentioned publication, the examination of the chest was incomplete and included only frontal views.

An abscess can perforate the diaphragm and cause empyema, or it may perforate to the pericardium and cause pyopericarditis.

As mentioned above, gas in the intestines and colon is occasionally sufficient to allow for the diagnosis of displacement of these organs. Upon examination with contrast medium, the displacement can often be shown more clearly, however, and narrowing of the lumen and mucosal edema can be demonstrated. If the process is on the left side, the changes are often striking in the descending colon, or, if it is on the right side, in the duodenum, which is close to the right kidney.

An osteitis in the form of spondylitis, for example, or osteomyelitis of the ribs, or of one or more transverse processes of the vertebrae, can also be diagnosed roentgenologically. Such osteitis may be the primary cause of the abscess formation. It may, however, be secondary, an erosion of skeletal parts being produced by an abscess lying in direct contact with the skeleton.

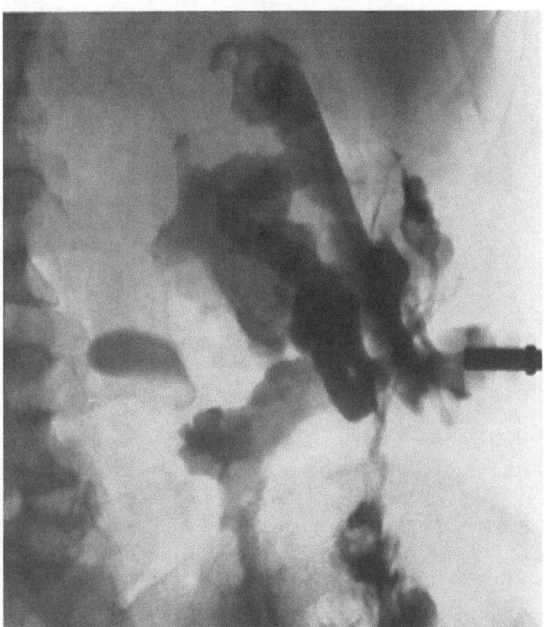

Fig. 325 b

It is clear from what has been set forth above that the roentgen findings in perinephritis are abundant and often permit diagnosis, and occasionally also demonstration of the origin of the perinephritic abscess. The frequency of different components given by different authors varies. These frequencies are of less importance, however. Here, as in all cases, roentgen diagnosis should not consist of a list of various components of very different degrees of importance, but in integrating the various roentgen-diagnostic observations into a general picture that can be described in terms of clinical pathology.

III. Carbuncle and abscess of the kidney

(Figs. 326—331)

Carbuncle and renal abscess are local inflammatory processes in the kidney. The former is also called furuncle and anthrax. As to the latter designation, it should be observed that in the Romance languages anthrax (French) and antrace (Italian) mean carbuncle in general, while in English the term anthrax means a carbuncle caused by the bacillus anthracis. Renal carbuncle should be regarded as the tumor-like multilocular inflammatory process in the parenchyma .The fact that it is multilocular indicates that it is composed of several larger or smaller abscesses. In addition, it consists of more or less firm granulation tissue. The cut surface may resemble that of a well defined renal carcinoma. The renal abscess differs from a carbuncle in being unilocular.

Renal infection is often a manifestation of a pyemia and one may therefore occasionally see a renal carbuncle in one kidney, for example, and a solitary renal abscess or multiple cortical abscesses in the other kidney. The disease may occur at all ages from childhood. It has always been very rare in our clientele. Renal carbuncle can break through the fibrous capsule of the kidney, or infection may be carried via the lymphatics out into the surround-

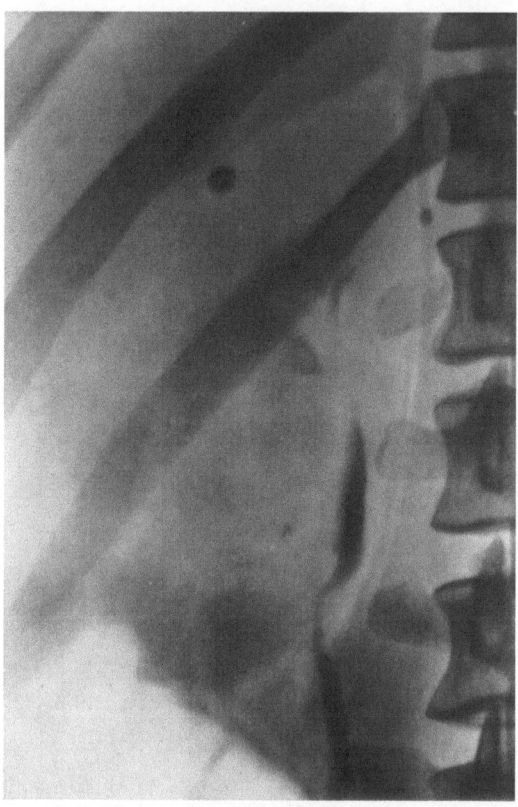

Fig. 326. Renal carbuncle in anterior part of kidney. Elevated temperature. Pain on right side. Tenderness. Right kidney moderately enlarged and plump. Outline sharp cranially but blurred laterally. Urography: good excretion of contrast medium. Kidney pelvis compressed

ing areas. This results in perinephritis. The carbuncle is thus often not diagnosed as such but as perinephritis.

The findings at plain roentgenography are therefore often dominated by signs of perinephritis, as described above. If the perinephritic changes are mild, the carbuncle may be seen as a local, large or small bulge in the outline of the kidney, or as a general enlargement of the kidney. In this respect the findings resemble those described for renal tumor.

A bulge in the outline of the kidney due to a carbuncle may be combined with changes in the capsule and the pararenal tissue. The findings at plain radiography may then resemble those seen in tumors infiltrating perirenally.

Examination with contrast medium

Renal carbuncles and renal abscesses are rare and experience with pyelography and urography is therefore limited. It was formerly widely believed that pyelography was of little diagnostic help. A case described by LJUNGGREN (1931) showed that both pyelography and urography gave definite information about the expansion, which together with the clinical findings gave the preoperative diagnosis of renal carbuncle. A compilation by SPENCE and JOHNSTON (1939) also shows the value of examination with contrast medium. In 36 cases of renal carbuncle, roentgen examination had been performed in 30 and urography or pyelography in 26. At pyelography in four of these cases no signs of a pathologic condition were revealed, while in 22 cases some abnormality or another was shown. In a compilation by GRAVES and PARKINS (1936) of 66 cases, only 15 gave positive findings

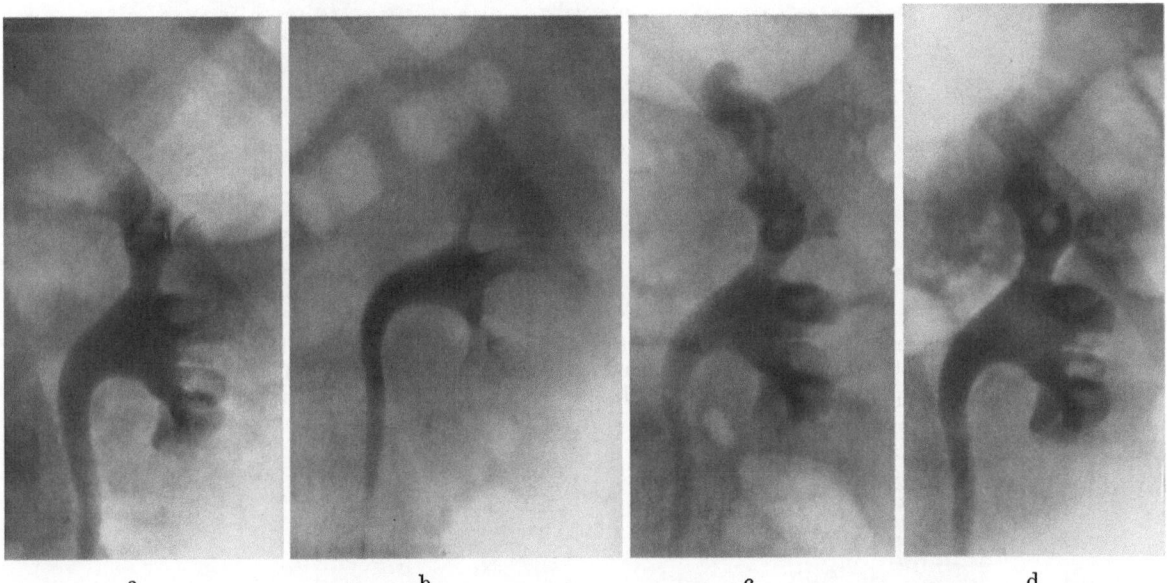

a   b   c   d

Fig. 327. Renal abscess. Fever, pains on left side. Small stones in left ureter passing spontaneously a) Urography prior to this attack (examination because of stone): normal conditions. b) Present urography: cranial pole left kidney enlarged, ill-defined. Kidney pelvis displaced downwards, cranial branch compressed. Several days later: pus in urine. Temperature returns to normal. c) Urography: expanding lesion in cranial pole diminishing. Kidney pelvis of normal shape. Communicating with uppermost calyx is an irregular cavity corresponding to lumen in thick-walled abscess with fistula to kidney pelvis. d) Urography two months later: no signs of pathologic condition

at pyelography. It may be presumed that the examination in some of these cases was not complete. Detection of an expanding process by pyelography often requires projections at different angles.

Signs of expansion will be exhibited at pyelography and urography; the comments given above on deformation of the renal pelvis and ureter in the presence of solid tumor or cyst also apply here (Figs. 326—331).

A renal carbuncle may fistulate into the renal pelvis and empty via the latter (Fig. 327).

In view of the fact that the patient is often referred for examination because of an acute infection, perinephritis is an important differential diagnosis. On the other hand, one must always have in mind in perinephritis the possibility that the process may be of intrarenal origin.

Not only will signs of an expanding process occasionally be seen at pyelography, but also contractions with rapid filling and emptying of the renal pelvis which are not

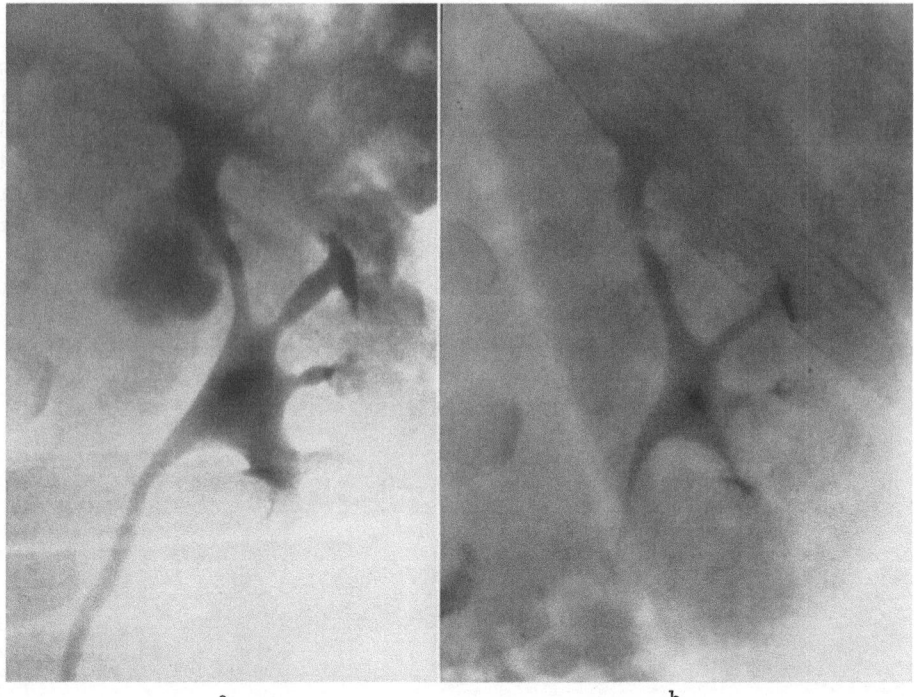

Fig. 328. Abscess in left kidney. a) Urography: escape of contrast medium from kidney pelvis into irregular abscess. Moderate displacement of upper branch and medial part of kidney pelvis. b) After six weeks of conservative therapy, abscess has healed. No displacement of kidney pelvis. Kidney well outlined

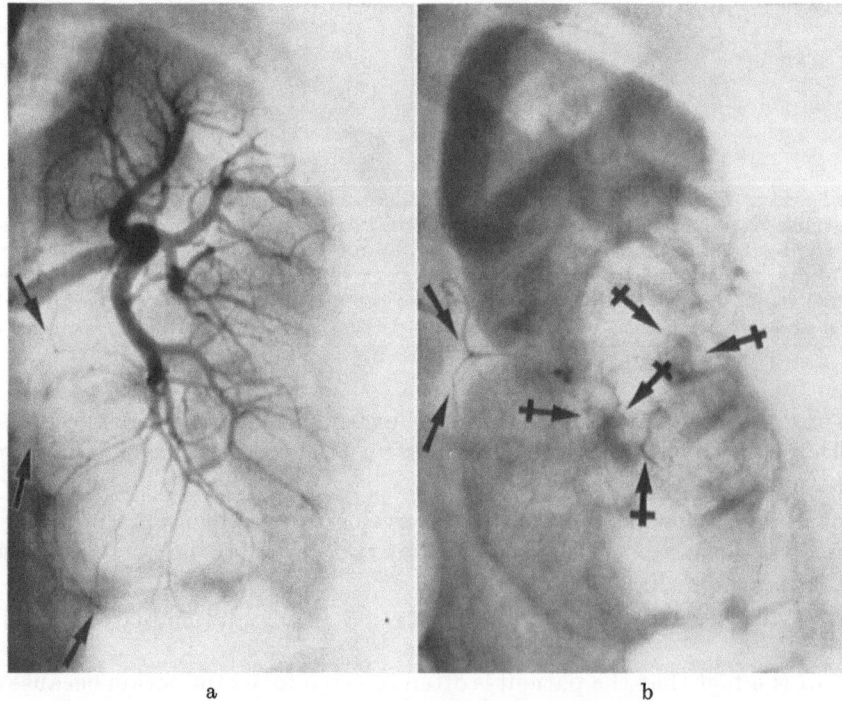

Fig. 329. Chronic renal abscess. Urography: sign of expansivity in caudal part of left kidney. Angiography a) arterial phase: marked displacement of arterial branches. Anastomoses between intrarenal arteries and capsular arteries (arrows). b) nephrographic phase: irregular filling defect in caudal half of left kidney. Multitude of irregular arteries and veins with blush (⊹→). Changes definitely do not represent cyst. As arterial changes were of inflammatory type, diagnosis was abscess. Diagnosis was confirmed by operation and histologically

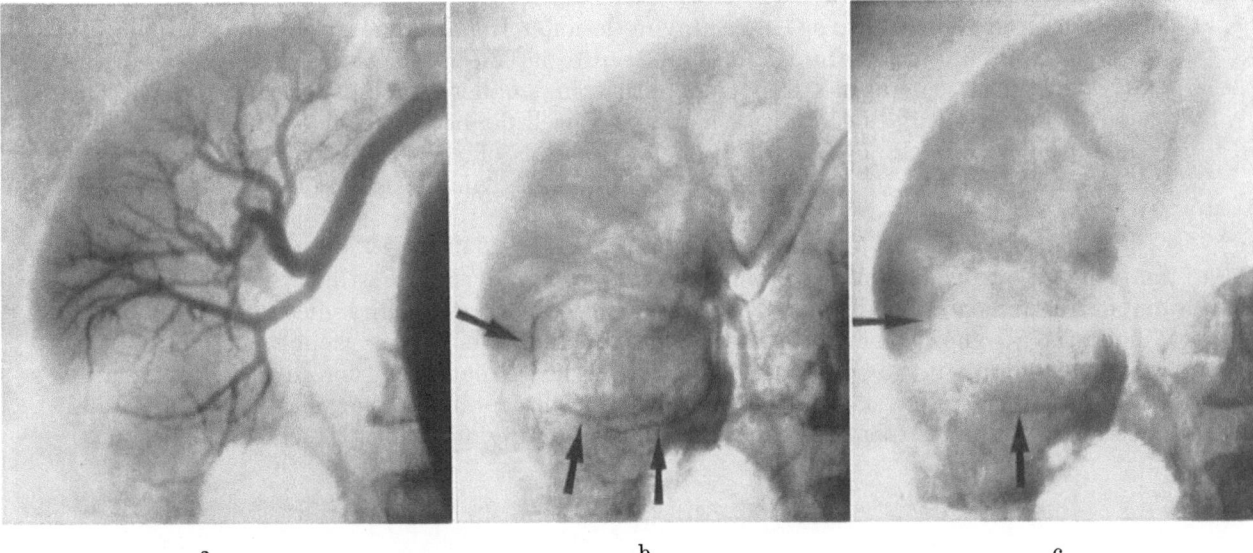

a b c

Fig. 330. Abscess in caudal part of right kidney. Urography: expansivity in caudal part of kidney. Angiography: no pathologic vasculature. Ill defined expansivity corresponding to finding at urography. Definitely not cyst but papillary renal carcinoma cannot be excluded. Tumor was diagnosed at operation, microscopically and by palpation, and nephrectomy performed. At pathologic anatomic examination chronic pyelonephritis was found with marked inflammatory changes in wall of cyst. a) Arterial phase; b) Capillary phase; c) Nephrographic phase

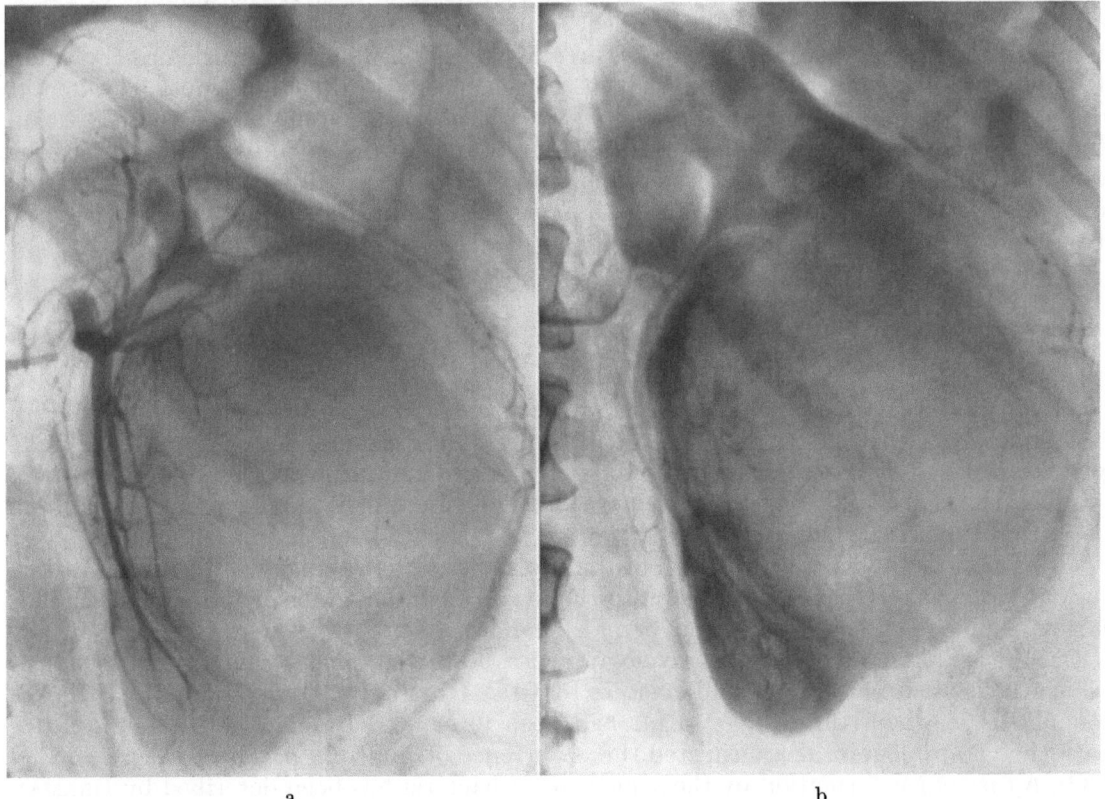

a b

Fig. 331. Large renal carbuncle. Angiography: a) arterial phase: marked displacement of intrarenal branches. Hyperplasia of capsular arterial branches surrounding expansivity; b) capillary phase: expansivity not well outlined towards normal renal parenchyma. Puncture with emptying of 400 cc of pus. Later operation: renal carbuncle

seen in non-inflammatory, space-occupying lesions. Renal angiography may be helpful. At angiography a renal carbuncle may be seen to have a hypervascularized region of the type sometimes seen in florid pyelonephritis in smaller portions of the kidney. The hypervascularity may be localized in a large, well defined portion of the kidney. This hypervascularity does not include pathologic vessels of the type occurring in malignant renal tumor. It should be remembered in the differential diagnosis of renal tumor, however, (De Vries, 1959).

It has been pointed out by Voegeli (1971) (Fig. 329, fig. 330), on the basis of our material of angiographically examined cases of renal abscess, that the lesion can be diagnosed angiographically as such in many cases, but that in some cases the definite differential diagnosis versus papillary carcinoma of the kidney is not possible. Percutaneous puncture of the angiographically established expansive lesion must then be made.

Syphilitic gumma should be mentioned in this connection as, like a chronic renal abscess, it resembles roentgenologically a space-occupying lesion (Hunter, 1939).

N. Gas in the urinary tract and fistula formation

A wide variety of conditions are accompanied by gas in the urinary tract, in varying amounts, particularly in the renal pelvis. The examiner must therefore be familiar with the roentgen findings.

Gas in the urinary tract may be masked by intestinal gas. If the amount of gas is large, the entire renal pelvis will be filled, as in a gas pyelogram. Thanks to the typical form of such an accumulation of gas, it is readily recognized as such in the urinary tract. If only a small amount of gas is present in the renal pelvis, projections must be taken at different angles in order to ascertain that the gas observed is actually situated within the kidney. The outline of such gas is then often found to correspond to some part of the renal pelvis, such as a calyx. Gas usually migrates upon change of position of the patient; upon examination in the standing position, it will be seen in the cranial group of calyces. However, it may be entrapped in a cavity formed in a pathologic process.

Gas in the urinary tract may be of intrarenal or extrarenal origin.

Development of gas in the urinary tract

Gas may occur in the urinary tract in the presence of gas-producing bacteria in an inflammatory renal lesion. In urine in diabetics, for example, fermentation can take place, with the formation of carbon dioxide. In sugar-free urine which contains protein, gas may be produced by Bact. coli or Bact. aerogenes. Bact. coli can also produce sulphuric acid from the urinary sulphates.

Gas may be produced in the wall of the urinary tract and bullae can be formed which may rupture, with escape of the gas into the lumen of the bladder or kidney pelvis. This is what happens in emphysematous or phlegmonous cystitis.

One case of spontaneous gas pyelogram has been described by Nogueira (1935) in which the cause is not known, and one case by Olle Olsson (1939) in a diabetic with pyelonephritis in whom the urinary sugar had been fermented by Bact. coli. In the latter case the gas pyelogram demonstrated the occurrence of multiple papillary necroses (Fig. 332). A case of gas formation by the same type of bacteria has been described by Braman and Cross (1956) in a patient with a coexistent perinephritic abscess which also contained gas.

Several reports on emphysematous pyelonephritis have since appeared in the literature. A review is given by Turman and Rutherford (1971) in which they point out that em-

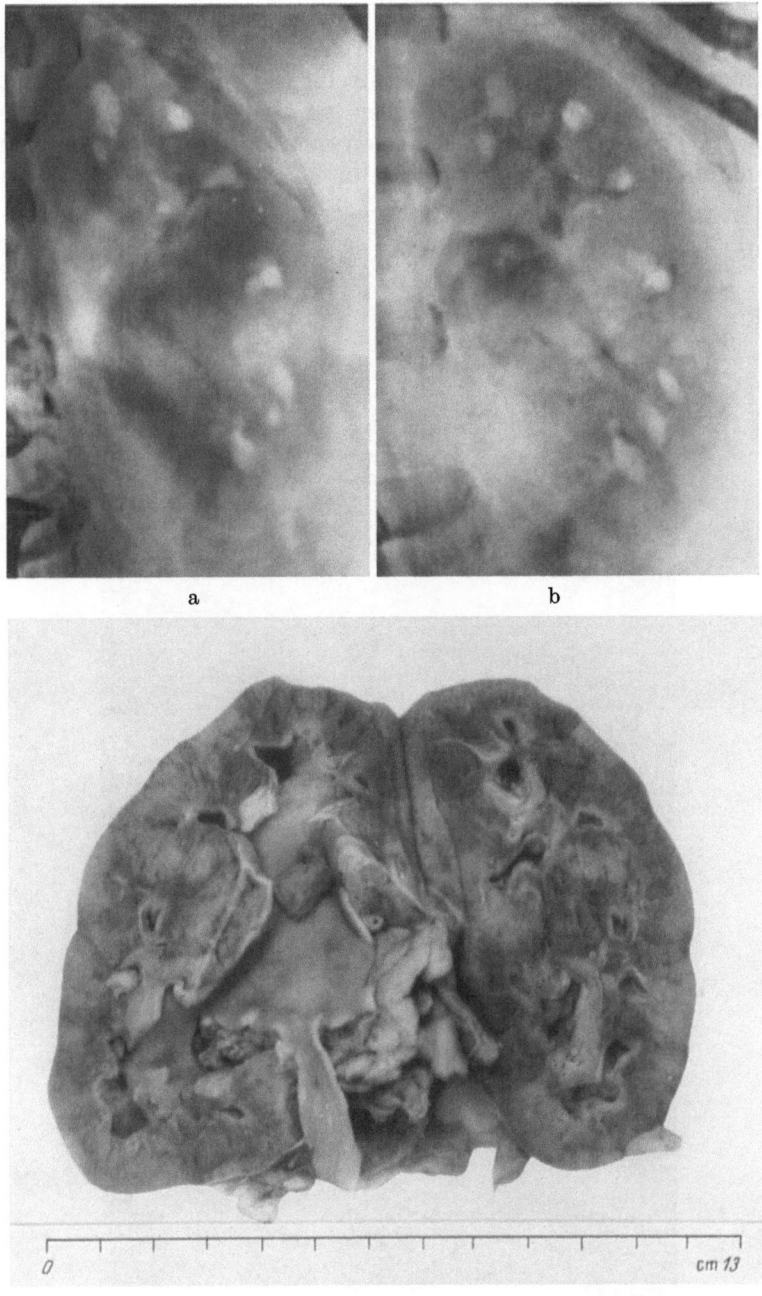

a   b

c

Fig. 332. Gas in kidney pelvis and in cavities caused by papillary necrosis. Diabetic woman, 69 years of age, with glucosuria and pyuria. Gas formed by fermentation delineates kidney pelvis and cavities at site of papillae. Papillary necrosis. a) Plain roentgenogram. b) Urogram. c) Specimen

physematous pyelonephritis is a fulminating renal infection which is usually marked by sepsis, renal necrosis, abscesses and gas formation in the renal and perirenal tissues.

Gas may also enter the urinary tract from without. This may occur through direct exposure to the external environments, and is common in association with catheterization of the ureter.

Gas can also enter via a cutaneous ureterostomy and via perforating lesions, caused either from without (by a weapon, for example) or from within (by *fistulation* from a concrement, for example). Gas may also enter via a direct communication between the urinary pathways and a cavity which normally contains gas. This is the case upon transplantation of the ureter to the intestine, e. g. ureterosigmoideostomy (Fig. 333). A patient with an incompetent ureteroenteroanastomosis may continuously have gas in the renal pelvis. Gas may also enter the urinary tract upon spontaneous fistulation with the digestive tract and in inflammatory processes, tumors, or necroses. The fistula may communicate

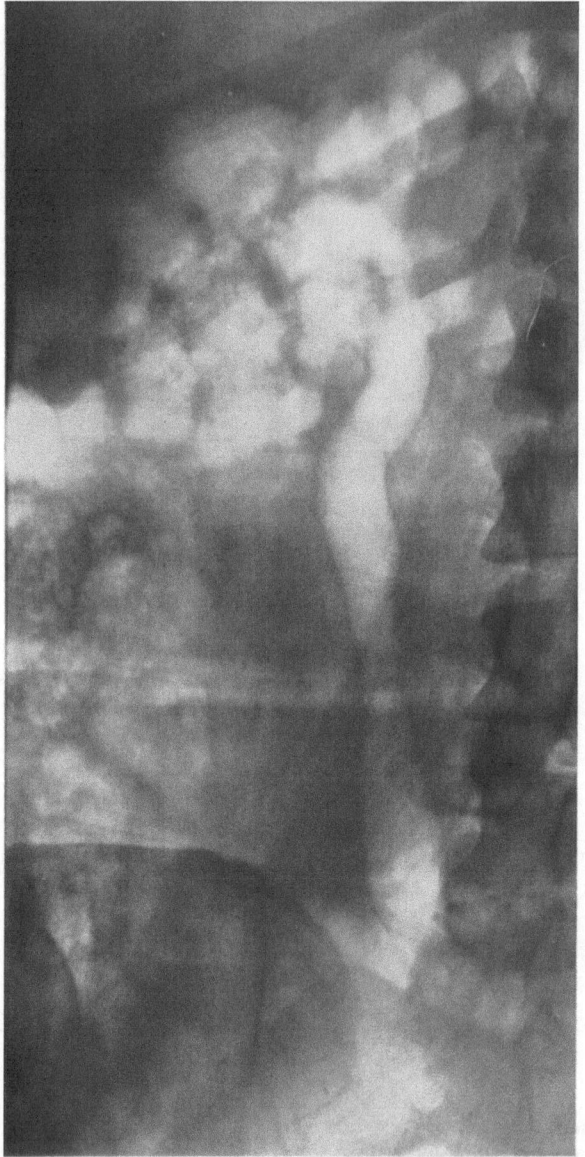

Fig. 333. Ureterosigmoidostomy: Complete filling of the kidney pelvis and the ureter by gas, with slight dilatation

with the stomach, small intestine, or large intestine. It may be primary in the urinary tract, the gastro-intestinal tract, or in the tissues outside these organs.

A glandular process of inflammatory or neoplastic nature may infiltrate both the urinary tract and the gastro-intestinal canal and form a fistula between them. One case has been described by Narins and Segal (1959) in which a large staghorn concrement migrated via a fistula into the intestines and was passed per rectum.

Upon fistulation between the urinary and the gastro-intestinal tract, spontaneous or surgical infection is likely to occur, with concrement formation or renal damage of the type described in the chapter on pyelonephritis. In the presence of such fistulation into the colon, barium contrast can flow into the urinary tract on examination of the colon with contrast (see. fig. 325). This can give rise to barium concrements. Contrast medium may also pass in the opposite way, from the ureters over into the large intestine, in urography, for example, Here the contrast medium may spread over the major part of the large intestine. At urography in patients with ureteroenteroanastomosis, contrast excretion by the kidneys can be observed to continue much longer than normally is the case. This can hardly imply anything but that the contrast medium excreted and transported to the colon is absorbed to some extent by the intestine and re-excreted.

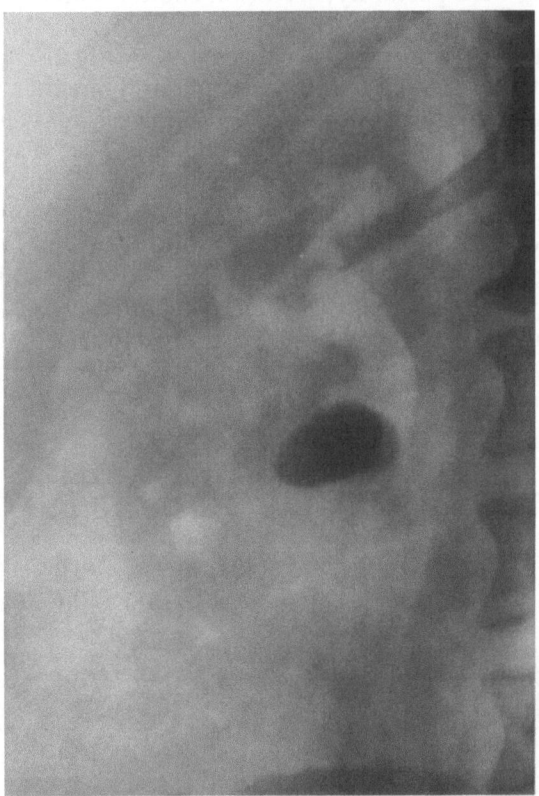

Fig. 334. Spontaneous gas pyelogram after ureterosigmoidostomy. Extirpation of bladder because of tumor. Repeated attacks of acute pyelonephritis and stone formation. Plain roentgenogram: Kidney pelvis filled with gas. Large stone in confluence and caudal branch. Calyceal deformation caused by pyelonephritis

O. Medullary sponge kidney (benign renal tubular ectasia)

LENARDUZZI in 1939 reported on a disease entity which he named medullary sponge kidney (rena a spugna medollare) and described it as characterized mainly by ectasia of the tubuli. "Renal tubular ectasia" would therefore be a better name. PALUBINSKAS (1969) has proposed the name "benign tubular ectasia." VESPIGNANI (1957) proposed the name "cystic dsyplasia of the renal pyramids" and ANDWAN et al. (1964) "l'ectasie canaliculère precalcienne." In the history of the literature there is a lapse of 10 years between the original publication concerning the disease and the next report of a case. This is interesting to note since the disease has been found to be fairly common. A large number of cases have been reported since and a great and well studied material of 35 patients was reported by Lindvall in 1959.

The disease represents a congenital malformation based possibly upon a genetic defect or a toxic factor causing a disturbance in the zone where the nephrogenic tissue and the Wolffian ducts unite (Cacchi and Ricci, 1949) Many other explanations have been presented (see Di Sieno and Guareschi, 1956). The disease may be familial. Kerr *et al.* (1962) classify as congenital cystic kidneys the classical polycystic disease of the adult, the medullary sponge kidney without liver disease, and congenital hepatic fibrosis with renal lesions. In the latter group nearly half of the cases are familial. The above authors recommend that patients with a diagnosis of medullary sponge kidney who are below the age of 40 years should have further examinations of the liver, and that children and young adults presenting with portal hypertension should undergo kidney examination by urography.

The connection between renal tubular ectasia and cystic disease of the liver is stressed by Reilly and Neuhauser (1960). Here too it is pointed out that the condition is heredofamilial and that portal hypertension and portal cirrhosis may be the presenting symptoms.

Patho-anatomically the disease is characterized by changes in the pyramids. No changes are seen in the cortex. The kidney may be slightly enlarged with generalized changes. The medulla of one or more or of all pyramids in one or both kidneys contains cystic cavities causing an increase in size of the pyramid and of the corresponding calyces. Microscopically in an increased stroma of connective tissue are found generally widened tubules or tubules with irregular diverticular-like widenings together with tubuli of ordinary caliber. Signs of infection and of calculus formation are common (see exhaustive literature survey in Ebeshaus, 1960).

1. Plain radiography

(Figs. 335—338)

Lindvall (1959), on the basis of 35 cases gives a thorough description of the roentgenologic changes. In plain roentgenograms the kidneys may be seen to be

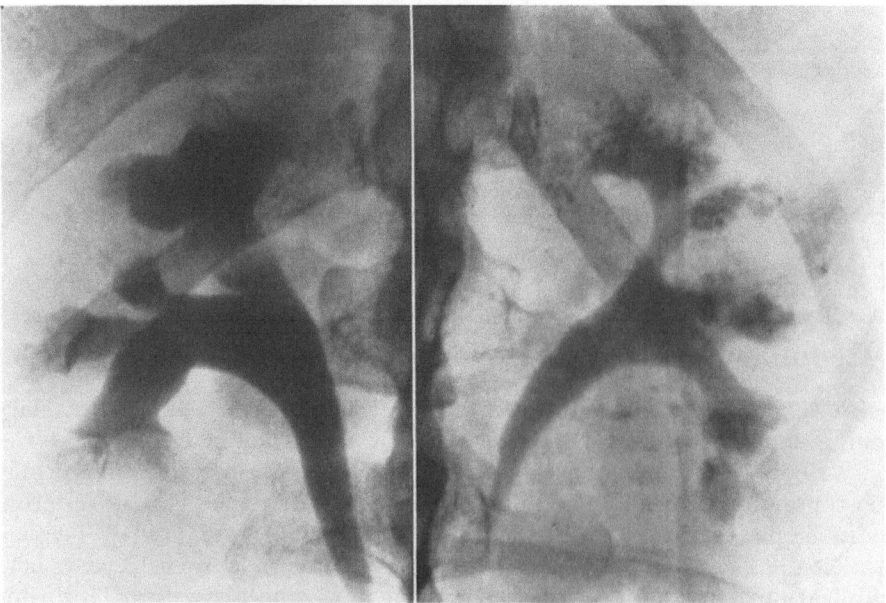

Fig. 335. Tubular ectasia with generalized changes and moderate hypertrophy of some papillae

slightly enlarged. They are usually of ordinary size but may be diminished and often have an irregular surface. Small, rounded, single or multiple calculi, usually in a very great number and of high calcium content, are seen corresponding to the papillae. They may be scattered throughout the kidney or localized to a part of the organ and may occur on one or both sides. Occasionally only one papilla or part of it shows calcifications. The changes vary in severity from one part of the kidney to another. If only one papilla or group of papillae is involved, a local accumulation of small calcifications may be seen. They are of fairly characteristic appearance and even when less numerous and small, their appearance in plain roentgenograms would suggest medullary sponge kidney.

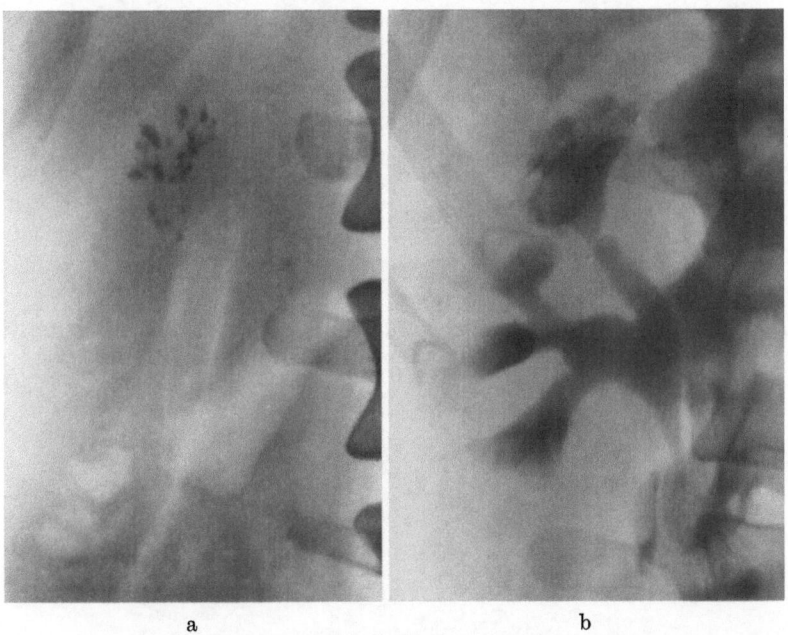

a   b

Fig. 336. Localized tubular ectasia, cranial pole right side. a) Plain roentgenogram: characteristic small calculi. b) Urography: calculi in dilated ducts

2. Urography

Urography is the method of choice for further examination; at pyelography the changes are often not demonstrable. At urography the excretion of the contrast urine is usually normal. The renal pelvis and the calyces may be of ordinary outline. Papillary hypertrophy is common, however, and occasionally grotesque. One or a pair of papillae may be hypertrophic, while others which also have changes may be of ordinary size. The calyces corresponding to enlarged papillae are widened and often flattened. More or less well defined widened tubuli are seen in the pyramids. They often form a striation in the papillae and occasionally cause an irregular increase in density. Parts of the pyramid may not be filled because of non-communicating cysts.

Renal tubular ectasia may be complicated by infection, as mentioned above. In that case signs of pyelonephritis may overlap the signs referred to.

The characteristic changes are more readily demonstrable by urography than by pyelography. Only in exceptional cases are they more distinct in pyelograms. This is because at pyelography the contrast medium cannot force its way up through the narrow mouth of the widened ducts. This may help to explain why the condition was discovered so late, although it is not uncommon. During urography the contrast filling comes from the parenchyma, thus providing a much better possibility of obtaining a contrast filling of the dilated collecting tubules.

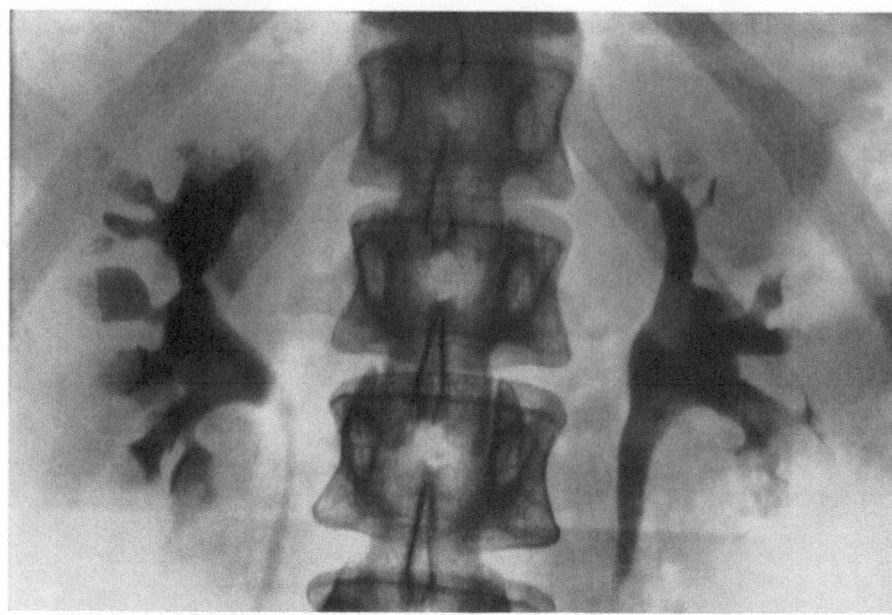

Fig. 337. Tubular ectasia bilaterally. Urography: widened ducts in most papillae, at some places resembling ordinary tubular stasis, some with slight cystic dilatation

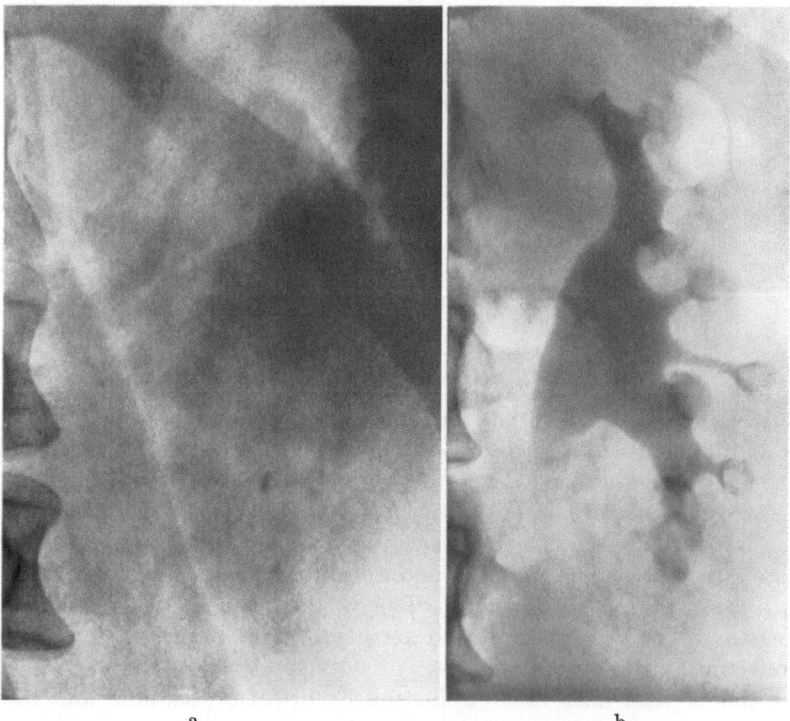

a   b

Fig. 338. Tubular ectasia localized in caudal pole. a) Plain radiography: small scattered calcifications in caudal kidney pole. b) Urography: markedly widened ducts around calcifications

A large number of lesions have been mentioned differential-diagnostically in the literature, such as renal tuberculosis, papillary necrosis, nephrocalcinosis. The difficulties in diagnosis are represented mainly by borderline cases with tubular stasis in connection with compression at urography.

The lesions usually remain unchanged during years of control, with the exception of changes in the number of stones. Changes when present are due to added pyelonephritis or dilatation of the urinary pathways. Renal colic is naturally a common phenomenon in patients with renal tubular ectasisa with stone formation.

According to our present knowledge, as can be expected, renal angiography does not contribute to the diagnosis. Ordinary vascular anatomy is seen, however (ALKEN *et al.*, 1951), when renal angiography is performed.

P. The backflow phenomenon

The backflow or reflux phenomenon has received much space in the literature and has been the subject of experimental, anatomic and clinical investigation. In some of the clinical studies its importance from the points of view discussed has undoubtedly been overrated. The phenomenon is of particular interest from a purely roentgen-diagnostic point of view and here it will be discussed only from this angle.

It is generally agreed that reflux is due to a rupture of the fornix of one or more calyces with overflow of the renal pelvic contents into the sinus and then into the perivascular spaces, which extend from the main part of the sinus into the renal parenchyma. When the extravasate dissects along veins in this stage, ruptures occur in the walls of the veins with passage of contrast medium into their lumina. Such ruptures readily occur when the pressure in the veins is low, while relatively high pressure in the veins tends to prevent reflux (MINDER, 1930). The refluxes may be tentatively divided into the following groups:

1. Reflux into the renal parenchyma, such as tubular reflux and interstitial reflux varying in severity up to subcapsular reflux.

2. Reflux into the blood stream, so-called pyelovenous reflux.

3. Reflux into the lymphatics.

4. Reflux into the sinus with sub-groups: fornix-reflux, peripelvic reflux, perirenal reflux, and reflux further into the retroperitoneal space.

These groups occasionally occur in combination and often represent different stages of one and the same sequence of events.

The reflux phenomenon was first observed by anatomists in connection with the production of casts of the renal pelvis. They found that fluid injected into the ureter escaped through the renal vein (GIGON, 1856). However, the phenomenon did not arouse wide interest until after the advent of pyelography, when these anatomic experiments were reproduced clinically. Many years elapsed, however, after the introduction of pyelography before the phenomenon received systematic attention. HINMAN and LEE-BROWN (1924) and FUCHS (1925) studied the phenomen anatomically, experimentally, and to a certain extent clinically. In recent years reflux in association with urography (see literature OLLE OLSSON, 1948, 1962, 1972) has received wide attention. Reflux has been focused mainly on reflux to the blood stream, i. e. pyelovenous backflow. On the basis of autopsy studies and of certain animal experiments, far-reaching conclusions have been drawn and accepted as holding for human patients. It was presumed that experiments on the above-mentioned material furnished sufficient evidence to attach clinical significance to backflow with regard to features of the patho-physiology of hydronephrosis, for example, as well as to most accidents in retrograde pyelography. It must be observed that when definite and far-reaching assertions were made in this respect, they were not supported by a single correlated clinical observation. A perusal of the literature shows that the term pyelovenous backflow has been used for practically any extravasation beyond the border of the renal pelvis.

It is important from a roentgen-diagnostic point of view to remember that refluxes can occur in connection with both pyelography and urography. The majority of publications on reflux deal with pyelography and many authors claim that reflux is observed only in connection with pyelography. An extensive study of reflux during urography (OLLE OLSSON, 1948) has shown, however, that the phenomenon is not uncommon even during urography, although frequently only in early stages. The roentgen findings in the various types of reflux are outlined below.

I. Tubular backflow

(Fig. 339)

From the middle of a calyx a fairly homogeneous, wedge-shaped area of increased density is seen to extend out into the corresponding papilla, widening towards the cor-

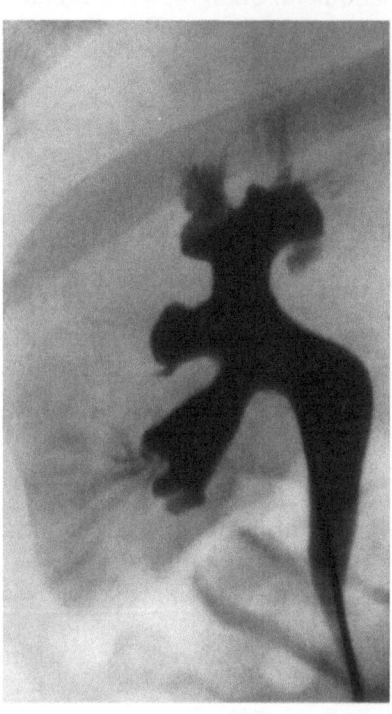

Fig. 339. Tubular and tubulo-interstitial backflow in kidney poles. Small fornical extravasations medial part, cranial calyx, and caudal part of middle calyx

tex. Sometimes the increased density is streaky, with the streaks converging towards the calyx. This type of backflow is due to contrast medium from the renal pelvis flowing into the collecting tubules, which are thus more or less filled with contrast medium. These changes can be observed as a streaky accumulation of contrast medium in a large portion of the kidney e. g. a renal pole or a single pyramid, and continue right out to the periphery of the kidney, sometimes involving large portions of the kidney (KÖHLER, 1953). When an entire pyramid or more than one pyramid is involved, it is, in my opinion, not always due to canalicular backflow but to contrast medium situated interstitially, a tubulo-interstitial backflow. Sometimes the contrast medium in this type of reflux during pyelography is forced through the renal parenchyma out into the subcapsular space, where it spreads to a varying degree in a thin layer.

Tubular backflow can be seen during urography as an increase in density of the papillae (see Fig. 343). It may be considerable and be seen in all or only some of the papillae. In urography it is obviously not a question of backflow but rather of stasis, the increased intrapelvic pressure occurring on ureteric compression, making it difficult for the contrast medium excreted by the kidney to flow to the renal pelvis. Tubular backflow occurs readily in patients with particularly wide ducts (HINKEL, 1957).

II. Reflux to blood-stream. Pyelovenous backflow

The contrast medium runs as one or several fairly broad bands via the renal hilum towards the spine. Perusal of the literature will show that most cases presented as evidence of pyelovenous backflow are not accompanied by illustrations showing contrast filling of veins. KÖHLER (1953) reported that he had never succeeded in finding a single illustration in the literature of a retrograde pyelography in which it would be possible to identify a contrast-filled renal vein. OLLE OLSSON (1948) has described a case seen during urography, which most probably shows a true contrast filling of a vein, thus an illustration of pyelovenous reflux.

The possibility of pyelo-arterial backflow was suggested by BAUER (1957) on the basis of a very incomplete and inconclusive examination of autopsy specimens.

III. Reflux to sinus
(Figs. 340—345)

This is the most common type of reflux. The extravasate is generally seen in the form of a horn-shaped projection protruding a few millimeters from the boundary of a calyx.

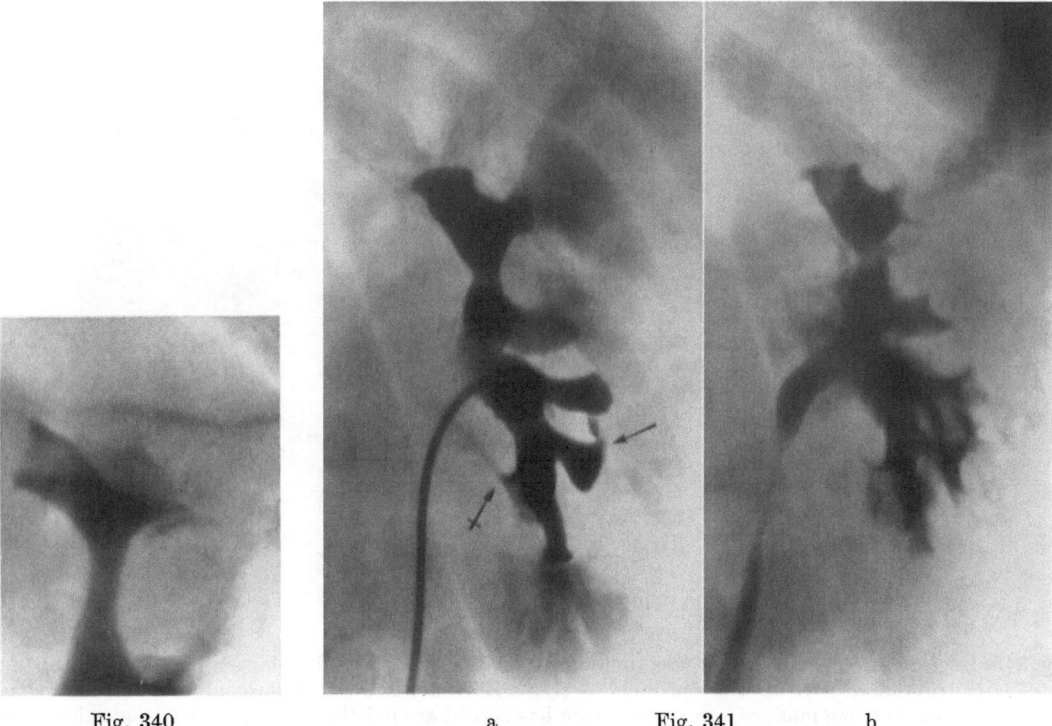

Fig. 340   a   Fig. 341   b

Fig. 340. Fornix reflux. Urography: small extravasate outside calyx. Calyceal wall appears as filling defect between contrast medium inside and outside calyx

Fig. 341. Backflow of different types in same patient. Blind pyelography: a) Tubular and tubulo-interstitial backflow into several pyramids. At ↗ fornix rupture with small extravasate to sinus. At ↗ fornix rupture with extravasate from sinus into perivascular space. b) Later stage of examination: tubular backflow has disappeared. Widespread extravasation into sinus surrounding most calyces and branches and reaching hilum. Catheter withdrawn

The projection may be directed laterally towards the renal parenchyma or substantially medially, towards the sinus. The extravasate is often less distinctly defined, at least laterally. When the calyx is studied in axial projection, the extravasate can generally be seen surrounding a part of the circumference of the calyx. In the upper or lower portion of the

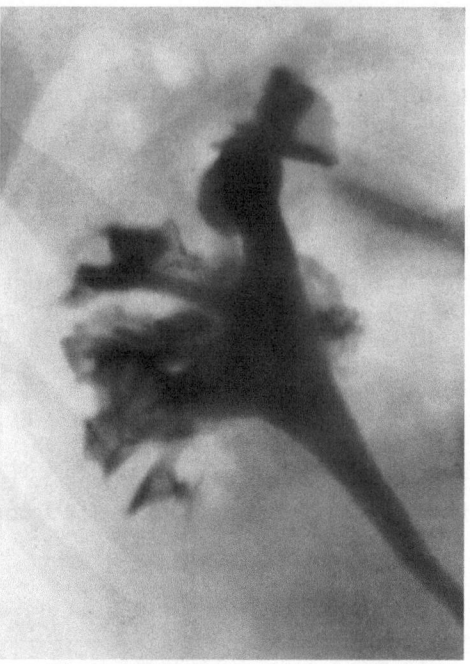

Fig. 342. Large sinus backflow. Blind pyelography: from ruptures at edge of most calyces, contrast medium flows into sinus and out through hilum

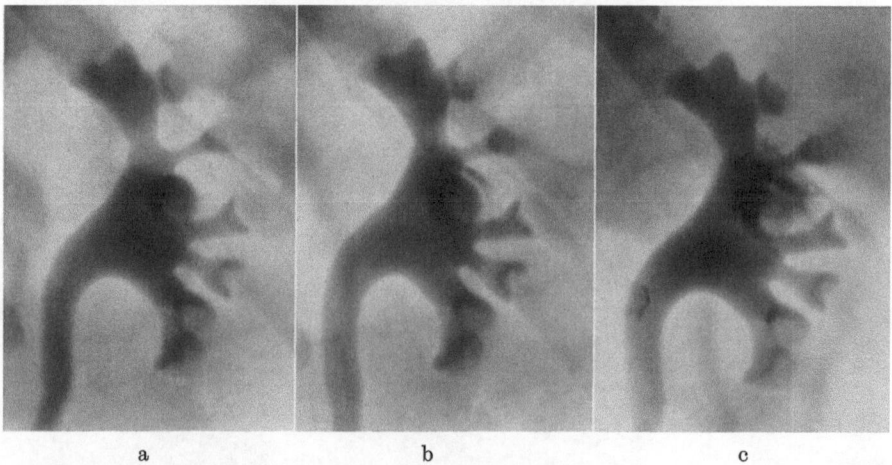

a   b   c

Fig. 343. Development of sinus reflux. Urography a) 10 minutes after ureteric compression: no reflux. b) 14 minutes later: rupture of part of fornix of middle calyx with small extravasate around cranial half of axially projected calyx. c) Some minutes later: extravasate has spread around the stem of the adjacent calyces. Note increased contrast density in papillae caused by tubular stasis

renal pelvis these extravasates often assume a characteristic form resembling an overflow from the boundary of the uppermost or lowermost calyx. In the majority of cases the extravasates — whether they are solitary or multiple — are of this type.

In addition to the small extravasate at the calyceal border, contrast medium is often demonstrable around the stem of that calyx from which the extravasate springs. Medial to the calyx, this medium is well outlined and is separated from the contrast medium in the calyx by a non-opaque zone, about 1 mm wide. This zone corresponds to the thickness of the calyx wall. The lateral outline of the extravasated contrast urine is usually ill-defined. In some cases medium is visible as an irregular accumulation further medially around the confluences of the pelvis or adjacent to or surrounding the stem of neighboring calyces.

In some cases with very extensive extravasation of this type the opaque medium escapes via the hilum along the ureter or around the kidney (Fig. 344). It can spread out into the retroperitoneal space and far down the ureter especially in association with renal colic (OLLE OLSSON, 1948; 1953, 1962, 1972) (Figs. 347—350).

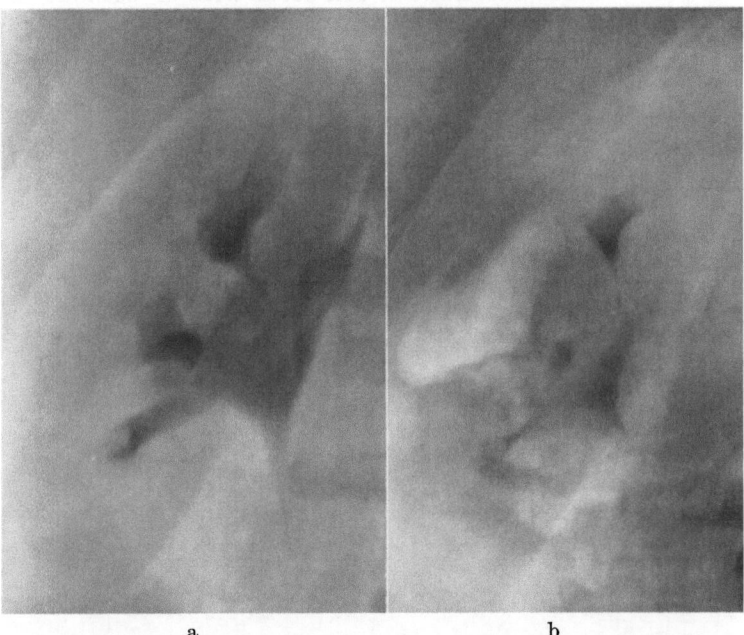

a   b

Fig. 344. Extensive sinus-perihilar backflow. Urography. After 15 minutes of ureteric compression, patient felt pain in right side. a) Sinus extravasate passing through hilum to medial surface of kidney. b) Release of compression. Rapid absorption of extravasate

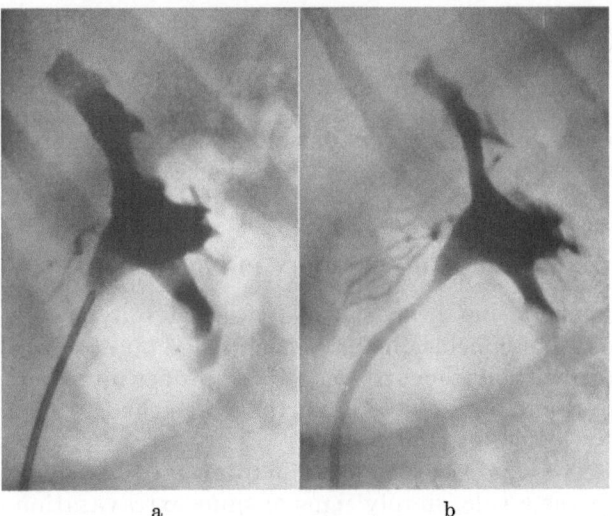

a   b

Fig. 345. Pyelolymphatic backflow. Pyelography. a) Rupture of fornices in middle of kidney. b) Increasing filling of lymphatics

IV. Pyelolymphatic backflow

From one or more fornices, which often show sinus reflux of varying extent spreading along the calyces, well defined, thin, somewhat irregular, single or multiple lymphatics may be seen extending towards the renal hilum, whence they often distinctly bend along the ureter.

Pyelolymphatic extravasation has been considered a rare phenomenon. Perusal of the literature shows, however, that several of the cases said to illustrate pyelovenous contrast filling undeniably belong to the group pyelolymphatic backflow. The frequency of these must therefore be considered higher than was hitherto thought. Often pyelolymphatic backflow is part of sinus backflow. It can occur with or without chyluria. In cases

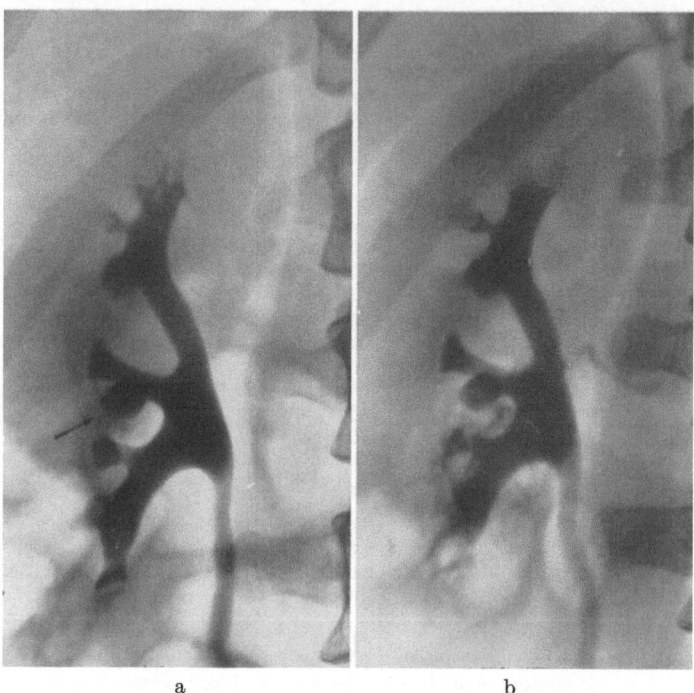

a   b

Fig. 346. Development of reflux. Urography: a) after 20 minutes of ureteric compression: slight extravasation at brim of middle calyx (arrow). b) A few minutes later: spreading of extravasation in sinus and filling of lymphatics

of chyluria at lymph-angiographic examination, retrograde flow of lymph to the renal lymphatics and calices with fistulous communication can often be demonstrated (CHEN, 1971).

V. Relation of reflux to bloodstream

The reflux phenomenon has been considered above only from a roentgen-diagnostic point of view. Far-reaching conclusions have been made on observed or assumed signs of backflow in pyelograms without due attention to, or proper interpretation of, the findings. In addition, the clinical and physiologic importance attached to backflow has not always been based on strictly logical grounds.

The changes observed at roentgen examination and described in the literature as pyelovenous reflux are, as a rule, simply signs of sinus extravasation or mostly pyelolymphatic backflow. Illustrations unequivocally showing flow of contrast medium into a vein on clinical examination are rare.

Fluorescent sodium gives a fluorescence detectable in the skin and mucosa when examined under long-wave ultraviolet illumination. OLLE OLSSON (1948) carried out experiments with fluorescent sodium incorporated in the contrast medium for retrograde pyelography and could demonstrate absence of passage to veins in small sinus refluxes. When, after abruptly raised pressure, fluorescence was noted as a result of venous escape, no venous filling was seen but sinus extravasation was marked in these cases.

Backflow thus occurs readily at retrograde pyelography. It can usually be avoided by the use of a proper technique guided by fluoroscopy. Pyelography under manometric control does not exclude reflux. The escape is limited to a sinus reflux but it can assume the character of a pyelovenous reflux without escape into the vein being demonstrable in the films. This is probably because the contrast medium is rapidly carried off by the blood. This has long been known: contrast excretion has been seen in the contralateral kidney at unilateral pyelography, which must imply that the contrast medium has passed into the blood stream and that the patient has received an intravenous injection producing excretory urograms with contrast excretion in the other kidney also.

KÖHLER (1953) has also examined this phenomenon and found that a pressure of 80—100 mm/Hg is, on the average, sufficient to produce reflux in normal human kidneys. Much lower values have been found by RISHOLM and ÖBRINK (1958) in an investigation in which a very small volume of albumin marked with ^{131}J was injected into the renal pelvis in association with routine cystoscopy. Immediately after the injection the ureter was blocked and the pressure was measured. The radioactivity in the blood was checked by collection of samples at short intervals and preliminary experiments showed that it increased rapidly when the intrapelvic pressure exceeded 15—20 cm water. Since the albumin molecules are too large to pass from the renal pelvis to the bloodstream under normal conditions, it is assumed that reflux may occur at this pressure in the renal pelvis.

The final evidence has been produced by anatomic examinations by STAUBESAND (1956). He has shown good agreement between the anatomic and the roentgen findings described above. In corrosion preparations of normal human kidneys he found that the presence of an open communication between the calyx and the renal sinus is always preceded by rupture of the mucosa. Sinus extravasates often flow along the calyceal wall into the sinus. They often also follow the perivascular spaces into the renal parenchyma. Then — though rarely — they may enter the venous blood. More frequently the fluid emanating from the renal pelvis hugs the vessel walls.

These observations underline how important it is to use a gentle technique in the performance of pyelography and how necessary it is to perform the examination under fluoroscopic control, as mentioned in the chapter on retrograde pyelography.

VI. Frequency of reflux

The frequency of reflux varies widely with the technique used. Pyelography by the conventional technique, as stressed above, should always be performed under fluoroscopic control, if reflux is to be avoided. If this precaution is not observed, refluxes of various types will be common. In a series of pyelograms of 207 kidneys KÖHLER (1953) found sinus reflux in 65, pyelolymphatic in 56, pyelovenous in one kidney, tubular in 66, and both tubular and sinus reflux in 19.

During urography refluxes occur after application of ureteric compression but the compression must have been applied for a few minutes, the renal pelvis must be well filled, and the pressure must have increased so that fornix rupture may occur. As a rule, the refluxes are therefore seen after prolonged compression and at the end of the compression period. During the course of an examination it is possible sometimes to follow the development of the reflux from one film to another and its growth from a small contrast extravasate in the edge of a calyx to a large one spreading along a calyceal stem to the adjacent calyx, then along the confluence and occasionally out through the renal hilum. The extravasated contrast urine rapidly disappears after release of compression.

LINDBOM (1943) found sinus reflux in 15 cases out of 900 in which ureteric compression had been applied. OLLE OLSSON (1948) found the phenomenon in 37 out of 988 similar cases, and BOYARSKY *et al.* (1955) gave a frequency of 2.9 % in association with urography.

VII. Backflow in acute renal colic

(Figs. 347—350)

Small refluxes attributable to renal colic and seen during the actual attack have been described by FUCHS (1931), HENDRIOK (1934), and LINDBOM (1943). During such attacks,

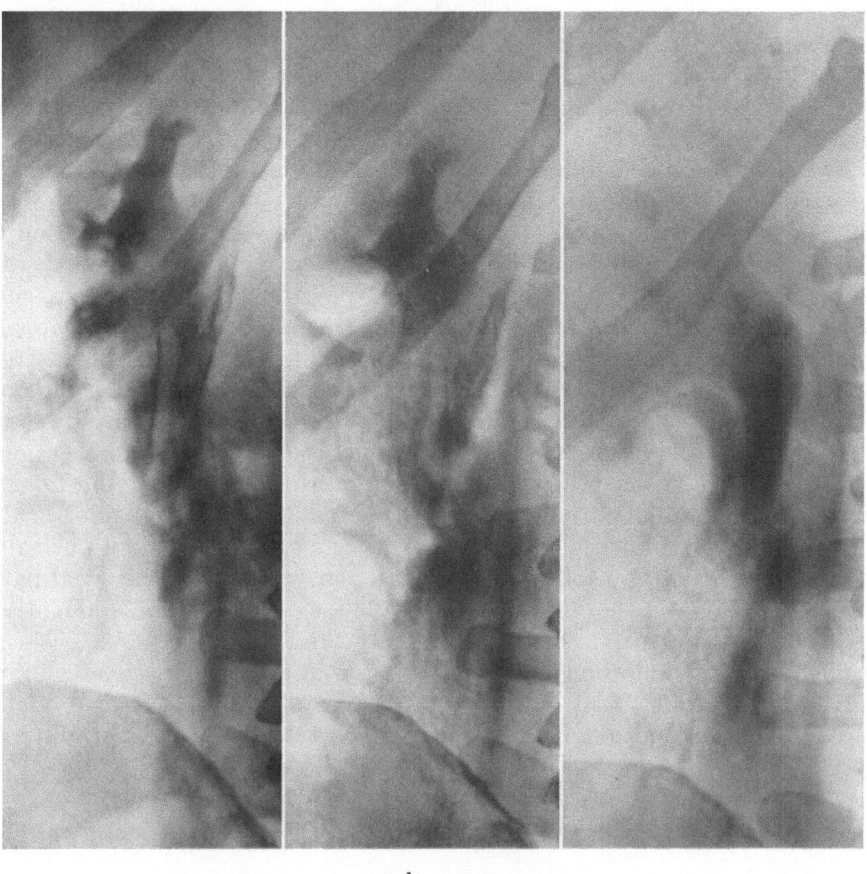

a   b   c

Fig. 347. Backflow to retroperitoneal space in renal colic. Urography (acute examination during pain and 5 hours after onset of pain. No ureteric compression): a) 19 minutes after contrast injection: extravasation from calyces in middle part of kidney into sinus, through hilum and out into retroperitoneal space along ureter. No contrast filling of dilated ureter, which appears as filling defect in extravasate. b) 25 minutes later: extravasate has spread even more. c) Another 5 minutes later (prone position): filling of dilated ureter. Extravasate around ureter has begun to decrease

however, widespread refluxes can be seen in which contrast medium, via ruptures in the fornix, continues through the sinus and renal hilum out into the retroperitoneal space, often far down along the ureter. In 1948 OLLE OLSSON, in a monograph on backflow in urography, reported six cases of backflow in connection with acute renal colic. In a paper from 1953 the same author reported seven more cases, and in 1972 the problem was again studied. A large number of reports on the basis of a large material have appeared continuously in the roentgenologic and urologic and surgical literature.

The most characteristic backflow is that in which at one or several calices a rupture at the fornix allows the escape of contrast urine from the kidney pelvis out into the sinus of the kidney and through the hilum into the retroperitoneal space around the kidney,

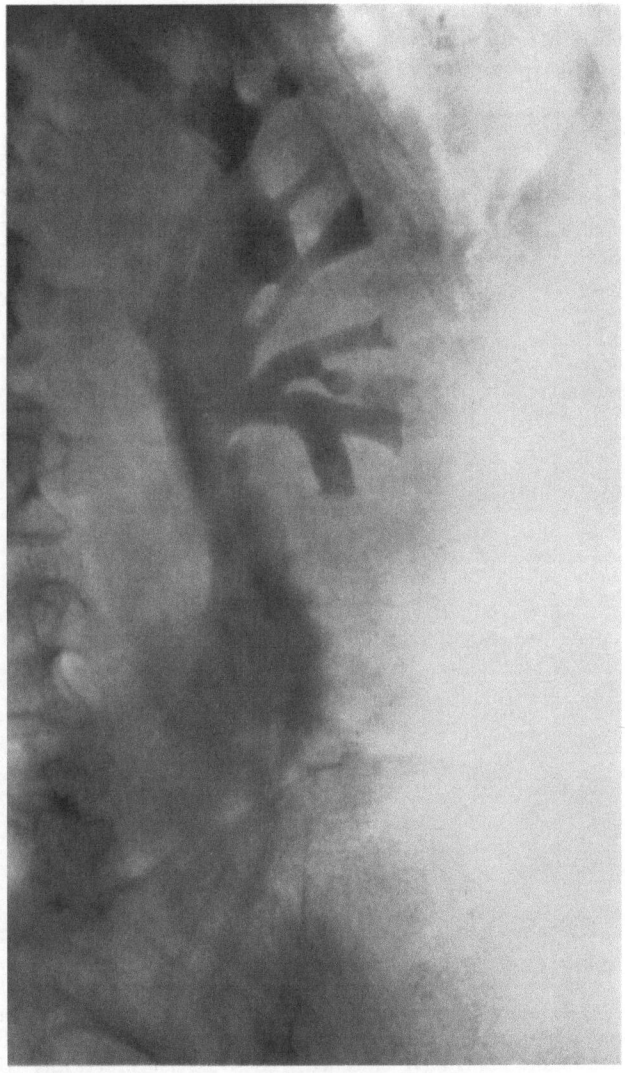

Fig. 348. Backflow to retroperitoneal space in acute renal colic. At plain roentgenography of abdomen caudal part of left kidney was blurred, as was retroperitoneal space from middle of edge of iliopsoas muscle. Urography: large extravasation from rupture at cranial calyces along confluence of kidney pelvis and down along ureter. This extravasation was rapidly absorbed during examination

its lower pole, and down around the ureter. The backflow may, however, be confined to the vicinity of one or two calyces and in some instances, usually at a late stage of a reflux, lymphatics may fill. In exceptional cases a large extravasation may start at an unusual place and take an unusual course. Thus OLLE OLSSON in 1972 reports on a rupture from a large, old scar of papillary necrosis in the upper lateral part of the kidney with perirenal extravasation laterally from the kidney.

Usually, however, the blackflow in acute renal colic has the same character as back-flow seen at ordinary urography where the ureteric passage is hampered by ureteric compression. The most striking difference is the large extravasation in the majority of cases of reflux in acute renal colic, which illustrates the difference in pressure gradient in the two groups.

The extravasation may be limited, as mentioned above. A small extravasation does not mean, however, that the leakage is small. The extravasation may be absorbed very rapidly so that, within a few minutes, a large extravasation may to a great extent diminish or completely disappear (OLLE OLSSON, 1972).

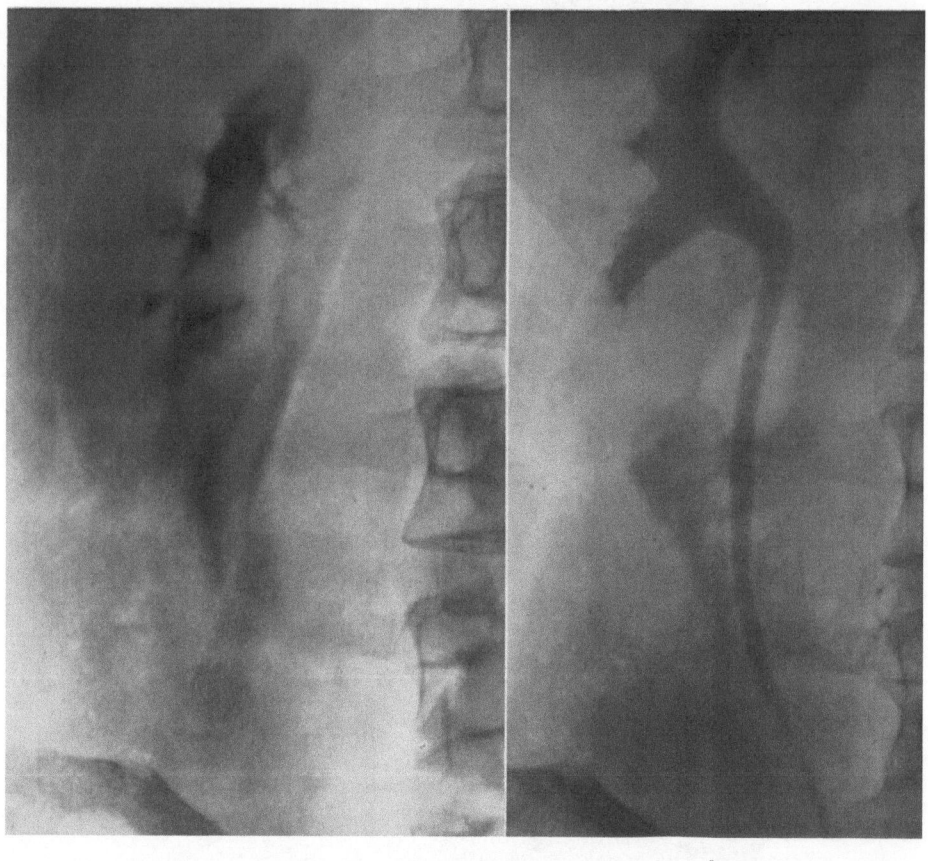

a   b

Fig. 349. Acute renal colic. a) Backflow to retroperitoneal space seen at early stage of examination. Extravasated contrast urine spreads along ureter, which can be seen as filling defect along edge of iliopsoas muscle. b) Same examination 15 minutes later. Pains have subsided. Extravasation practically completely absorbed.

The rupture closes fairly rapidly and only in exceptional cases can an extravasation be demonstrated in check urography a short time after an acute examination with a large extravasation. Such cases have been described by OLLE OLSSON (1953), HARROW, SCHWARTZ et al., BONK et al. (1966).

It is characteristic of the rupture that the intrapelvic pressure at the time of examination is fairly low, demonstrated by the fact that delay of contrast excretion is only slight or moderate, that the dilatation of the kidney pelvis also is only slight or moderate, and that the density of the excreted contrast urine is good. Actually in several instances one has the impression that the rupture is already present at the time of the examination and that the extravasated contrast urine only demonstrates the path the urine already has taken during the attack.

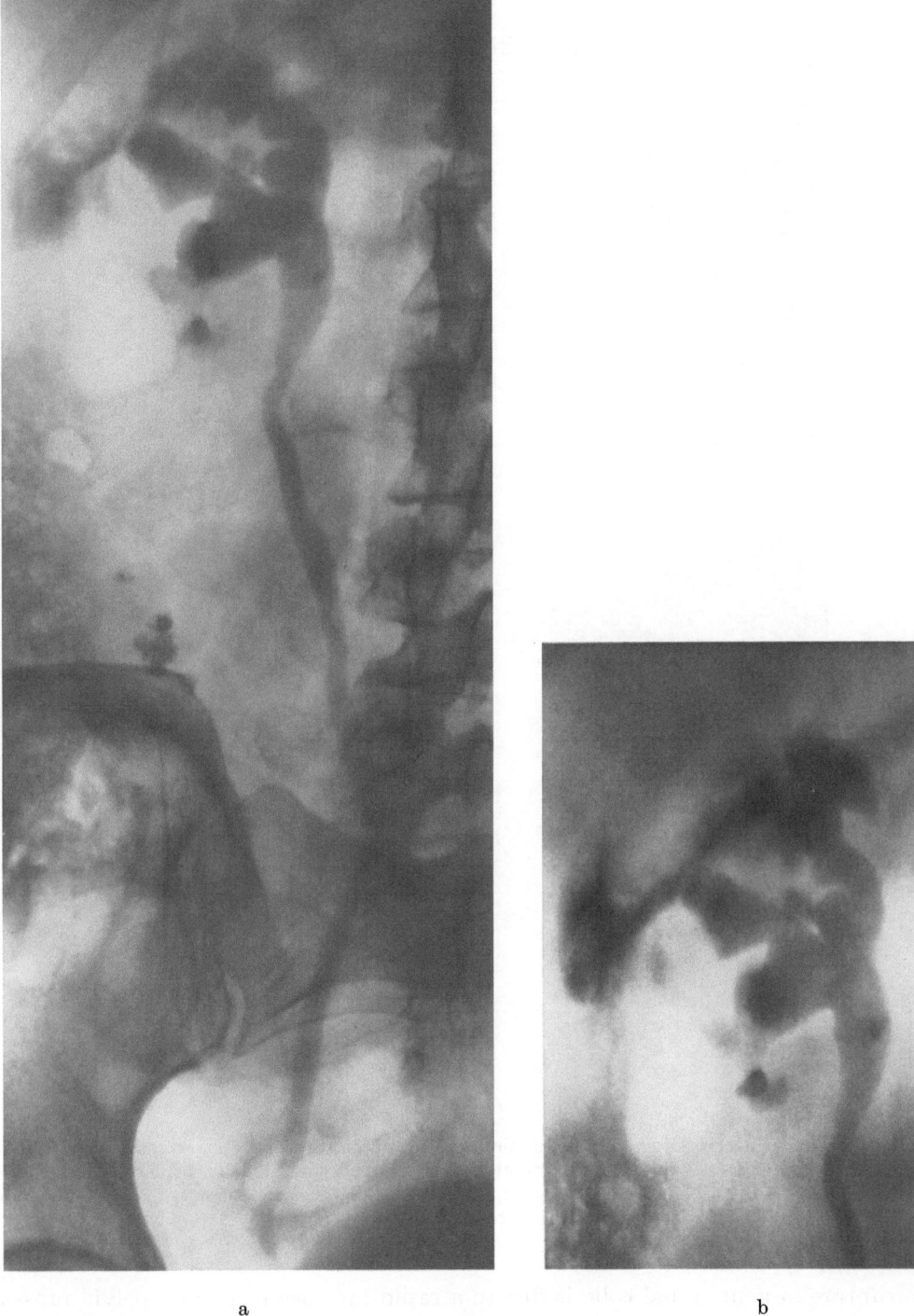

a   b

Fig. 350. Backflow in acute renal colic. Urography with tomography: small right kidney with marked pyelone-phritic changes. Extensive extravasation *laterally* from a cranial calyx spreading extrarenally to caudal pole of kidney

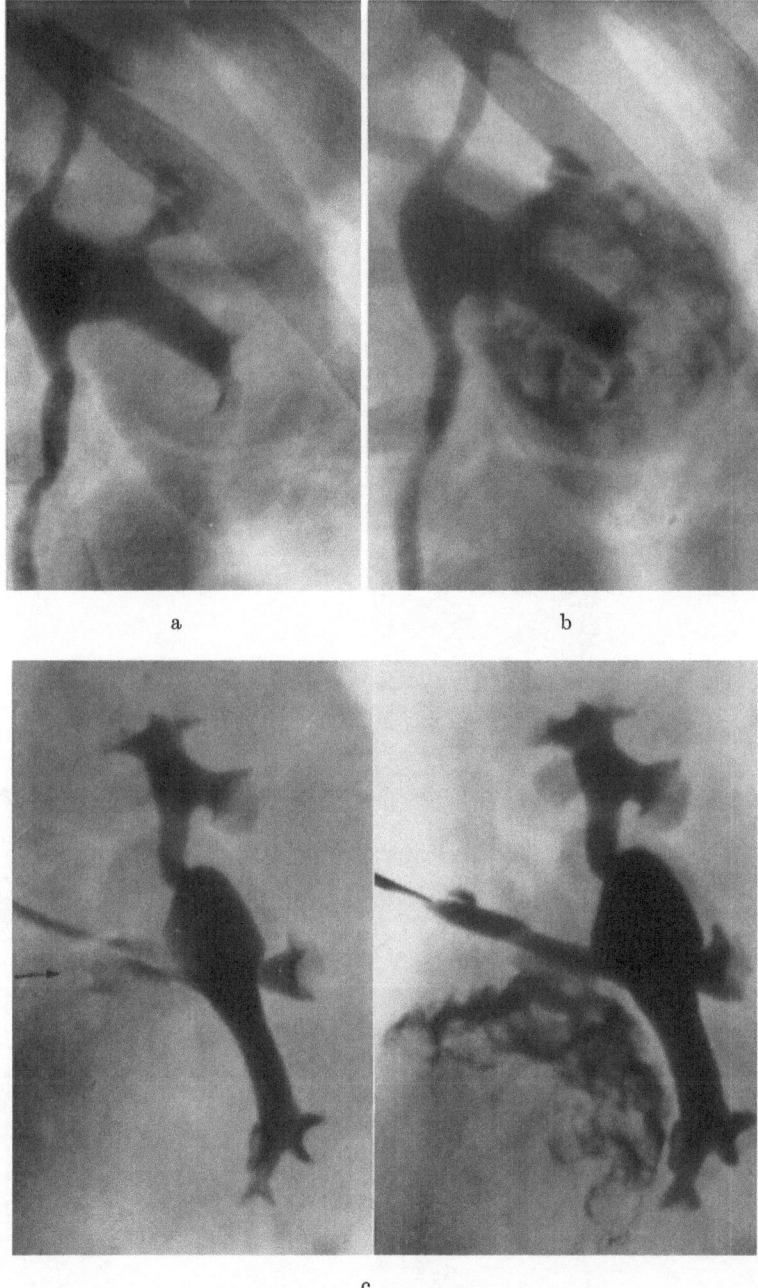

a   b

c

Fig. 351. Backflow into a tumor. Urography a) 10 minutes after application of ureteric compression: flattening and slight displacement of caudal branch. b) 10 minutes later: from edge of cranially displaced calyx backflow into superficial part of tumor. Nephrectomy. Renal carcinoma. c) Pyelograms of operative specimen. Note rupture at edge (arrow) of displaced calyx

The rupture in acute renal colic is due to a rapid increase in kidney pelvic pressure. It has been demonstrated that diuresis can cause rapid rise in pressure at blockage of a ureter. The pain is related to pressure, although with great individual variation. Rapid rise in pressure causes great pain (RISHOLM, 1955). Rapid rise in pressure in this type of backflow is illustrated by several factors: backflow of this type as a rule is seen in patients with a short history of a very sharp attack of pain; the phenomenon is seen mainly in patients examined in the morning hours when the urine production rapidly increases. A ureter blockage established during this part of the day will therefore cause a build-up of pressure much more rapidly than that occurring at any other time of the day. Cases have been reported (OLLE OLSSON, 1972) in which, after the subsidence of an attack of renal colic and after the injection of contrast medium (probably acting as a strong diuretic) a new sharp attack began, combined with extravasation.

Extravasation demonstrated roentgenologically during urography in acute renal colic is not a rare phenomenon. Its frequency is difficult to estimate, however. HARROW (1966) in a discussion on the frequency of spontaneous urinary extravasation associated with renal colic, expresses the opinion that "there can be no doubt about the common occurrence of perirenal extravasation, even if not demonstrated on roentgenograms."

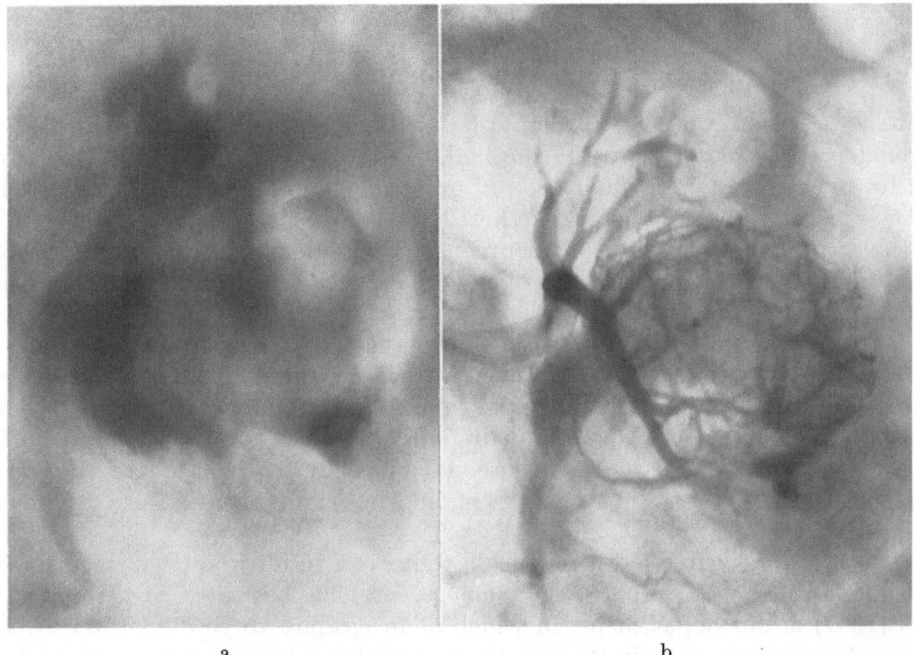

a   b

Fig. 352. Backflow around renal carcinoma. a) Urography: large extravasation of contrast urine around expansive lesion below middle of left kidney. b) Renal angiogram: renal carcinoma. Size and site correspond to shape and site of backflow

He argues that before the last decade such incidences of urinary extravasation outside the renal pelvis were not diagnosed because of lack of knowledge of the roentgenographic characteristics, the smaller number of excretory urographies performed in renal colic, the decreased density of urographic media, the tendency less often to take delayed roentgenograms, and inadequate amounts of injected contrast agent. Several of Harrow's arguments are not valid and other facts support the impression that reflux in acute renal colic is an isolated occurrence and the product of several concomitant factors. There is, however, one additional roentgenologic fact that lends support to the opinion that backflow may be more common than is believed: the frequency of fibrolipomatosis. It has been reported (OLLE OLSSON, 1953, 1962; VOEGELI, 1971) that backflow, by causing proliferation of connective tissue and fat in the sinus, can lead to angiographically demonstrable late changes. At check examination of patients after an attack of renal colic we have in some instances noticed changes of the fibrolipomatosis type on the side of previous stasis (OLLE OLSSON, 1972) (Fig. 353), from which the conclusion can be drawn that, in connection with an attack of renal colic, backflow has occurred. The extravasation may have occurred, however, outside the time covered by the roentgenologic observation or may have been too small to have been noted under prevailing examination conditions. The basic prerequisite for its observation is namely contrast excretion of satisfactory density. In many instances of acute renal colic the contrast excretion is completely blocked or markedly delayed and contrast density is often very low. This, in connection with the fact that no bowel preparation of the patient can be made in the acute stage, that the patient because of pain is uncooperative, and that the extravasation may be small, undoubtedly cause some ruptures to remain undetected. The frequency of radiologically observable backflow at the acute examination appears to be approximately 5 % (Schwartz et al., 1966; Olle Olsson, 1972). This type of backflow may be the explanation for slight temperature reaction, increase in white blood count, and a marked tenderness over the kidney in some patients during and after acute renal colic.

VIII. Significance of reflux from a roentgen-diagnostic point of view

Refluxes are usually roentgen-diagnostic artifacts caused by the increased pressure in the renal pelvis produced by the method, i. e. injection of contrast medium via a catheter for pyelography and application of ureteric compression for urography. Features of this type of reflux were given in further detail above.

In one situation, however, the roentgenologically demonstrable reflux phenomenon is part of a patho-physiologic sequence of events, namely when reflux is seen in connection with acute renal colic.

The pathologist Hamperl (1949) has shown that gross jelly-like masses may be seen in the fat tissue of the renal hilum and even in retroperitoneal fat tissue along the ureters at post-mortem examination of cases with urinary stasis. The spread of the jelly-like mass showed that it was due to some kind of infiltration, as may be expected of a fluid substance that spares the tissue structure. It was definitely related to ruptures of the fornix. It is surprising that such changes should not have been noticed by pathologists earlier, for they are not rare.

The extravasate occurring during such a reflux can result in a tissue reaction of differential roentgen-diagnostic importance. Such a case has been described by Fajers and Idbohrn (1957) in our department, in which at urography three days after an attack of renal colic, changes were seen in the renal pelvis, and in which at follow-up, findings were seen that could be interpreted as renal pelvic tumor but which were considered to be due to tissue reaction after backflow. Explorative surgery in another hospital revealed that the right kidney was embedded in firm adhesions. The hilum was edematous and was felt to contain a small obscure lump. Nephrectomy was performed. Histologically widespread peripelvic refluxes with old hemorrhages were seen (Fig. 354). We have since seen further cases of this type.

Fibrolipomatosis may also result in "chronic" reflux. On the basis of our material Voegeli (1971) has shown that fibrolipomatosis is common in middle-aged and elderly men and is seen mainly in patients with signs of prostatic hyperplasia. The pathogenetically decisive factor seems to be recurrent pyelosineous backflow.

Refluxes are also important from a diagnostic and particularly a differential-diagnostic point of view. From a diagnostic point of view, those few cases may be mentioned here in which contrast medium had escaped into a tumor at retrograde pyelography (Bitschai, 1927; Fuchs, 1930; v. Illyes, 1932; Schubert, 1933; Herrnheiser and Strnad, 1936; Meuser, 1943) or during urography (Olle Olsson, 1948) (Fig. 352). In another case the latter author reported reflux around a small calcified space-occupying lesion and, in addition, I have seen reflux around a renal carcinoma (Fig. 352).

Refluxes are also important diagnostically in retrograde pyelography because if the reflux is large, small anatomic changes may escape detection. In the event of extensive backflow, pyelography is therefore unreliable.

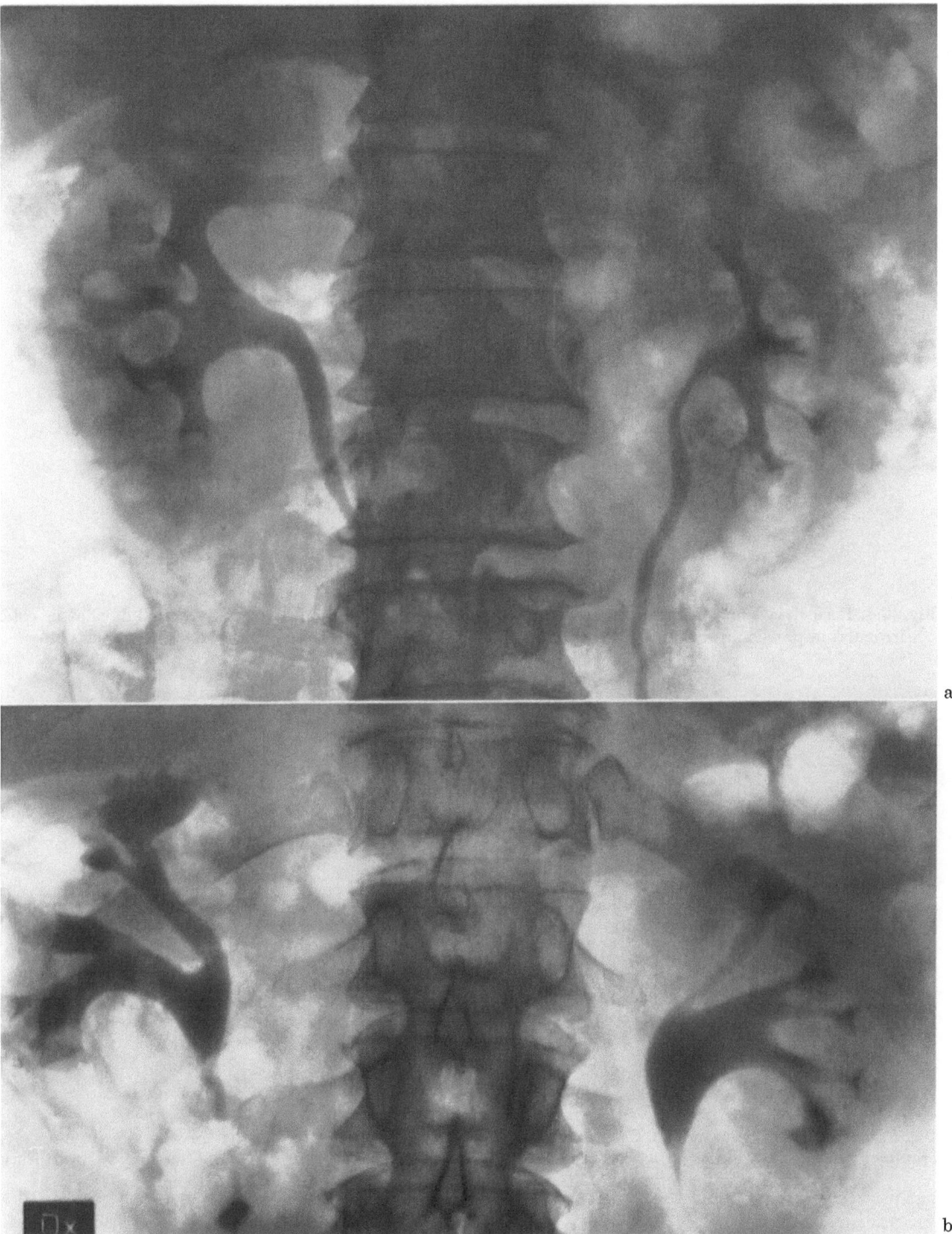

a

b

Fig. 353. a) Fibrolipomatosis after attack of renal colic. Urography 8 days after attack of renal colic without excretion on left side: marked changes in shape of left renal pelvis suggesting fibrolipomatosis. b) Left-side renal colic several years earlier. Actual urography: marked fibrolipomatosis in left kidney

When pyelography has been performed with thorotrast, contrast medium can have escaped into the renal tissue or renal sinus. Thorotrast residue may then remain in the tissues for the rest of life. At roentgen examination it can be seen as thin linings of single calyces or parts of the renal pelvis, the contrast lying in the sinus along the renal pelvis

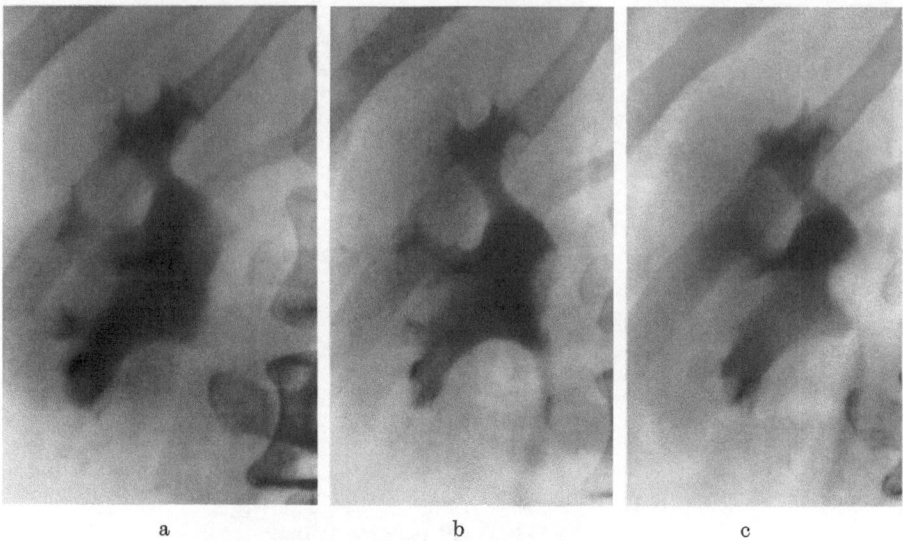

a   b   c

Fig. 354. Peripelvic reflux in renal colic causing expanding tissue reaction. Urography: a) 10 days after colic: irregular impression from hilum into medial part of confluence. Regression b) one and c) three weeks later

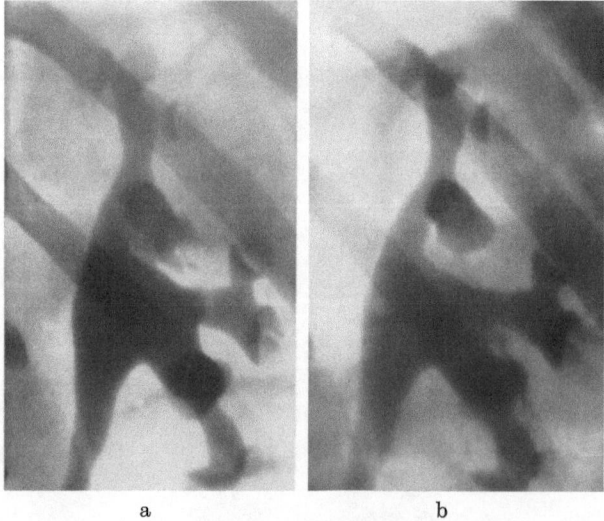

a   b

Fig. 355. Healing of sinus reflux. Urography (tuberculosis suspected): Irregular extravasation around calyx cranial to middle of kidney (probably backflow, but papillary destruction cannot be excluded). b) 19 days later: no reflux. No pathologic changes. Edge of calyx sharp

(SVOBODA, 1954). It may also be seen as radial streaks of contrast medium running from one or more papillae out towards the periphery of the kidney.

From a differential-diagnostic point of view, refluxes are important in the presence of papillary destruction, particularly papillary ulceration in renal tuberculosis. The earlier literature contains several reports in which a reflux was obviously interpreted as a destructive process and nephrectomy had been performed unnecessarily (OSSINSKAYA, 1937; RENANDER, 1939). The importance of considering fornix reflux in the differential diagnosis of papillary ulceration has been stressed (LINDBOM; OLLE OLSSON; STEINERT, 1943). The differential-diagnosis is established by the following procedure: if, during the course of urography, a change is seen that may be a fornix reflux, compression is maintained, the reflux will develop, and the contrast medium will spread out along the calyceal stem. On occasion this is not possible. The differential-diagnosis can then be established by re-examination a few days later. Experience has shown that ruptures causing refluxes rapidly

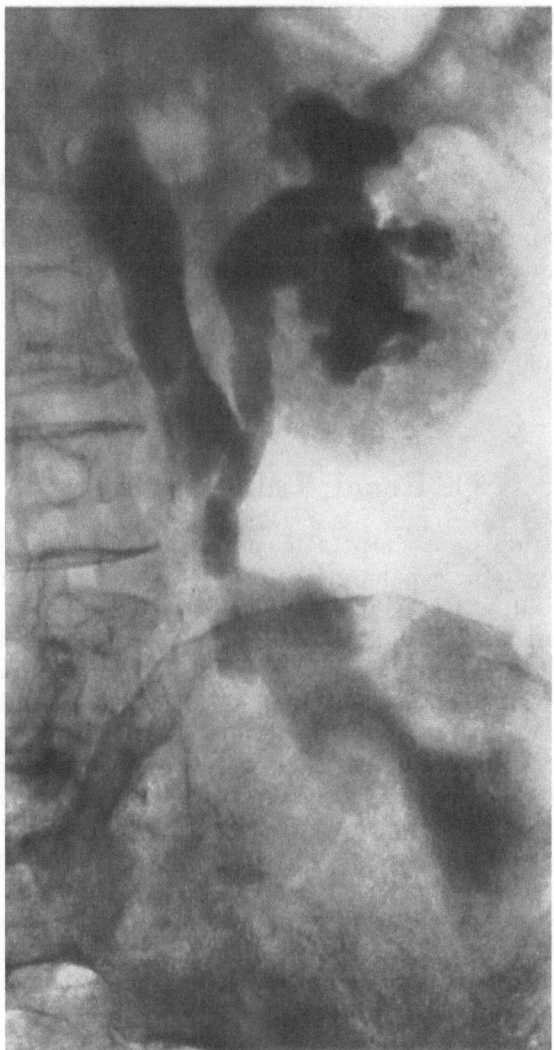

Fig. 356. Chronic reflux in patient with retroperitoneal metastases from carcinoma of coecum; continuous leakage of urine out into retroperitoneal space along psoas muscle

close (Fig. 355). The reflux phenomenon may also be more or less chronic, however (Fig. 356).

Reflux may also be of differential-diagnostic importance in traumatic renal rupture because the roentgen findings in small ruptures are the same as in reflux. This must be kept in mind at retrograde pyelography for suspected renal rupture. Urography in the acute stage of the disease does not give rise to this differential-diagnostic difficulty because urography in the acute stage of suspected renal rupture is performed without the application of ureteric compression.

IX. Risks associated with reflux

The most important risks from a roentgen-diagnostic point of view are those mentioned above, namely the backflow may mask anatomic changes and, secondly, it may be misinterpreted as some pathologic process. Another risk is that, as mentioned, in retrograde pyelography reflux may occur with "injection" of a large amount of contrast medium into the blood stream and consequent excretion. Retrograde pyelography is sometimes used instead of urography in order to avoid the strain placed on the kidneys by the excretion of contrast medium. In such cases the technique used for pyelography should be so gentle as not to cause reflux. Cederlund (1942) stressed that pyelography entails a great risk of large amounts of contrast medium being inadvertently injected into the bloodstream and Politano (1957) writes in a discussion of retrograde pyelography: "Obviously any substance unsuitable for intravenous use should not be used or used only with great care."

As to other risks, many authors claim that reflux is important because it favors spread of infection in the kidneys and blood-stream, introduction into the blood-stream of depressants and of other substances secreted with the urine, etc. Much of the discussion is based on more or less unfounded assumptions. It falls beyond the scope of this presentation of the roentgen-diagnosis of reflux.

Q. Renal Transplantation

Renal transplantation poses important problems for the roentgenologist. In living donors the roentgen examination has the purpose of showing that the proposed donor has two normal kidneys, that the arterial supply to the kidney to be transplanted is normal, i.e. that there is only one renal artery. Importance should also be attached to the anatomy of the main renal artery regarding caliber, length, level of bifurcation, etc.

It is pointed out (Pokieser, 1971) that an angiogram of the donor may also be valuable for comparison if angiography is performed after transplantation. A positioning of a donor kidney on the contralateral side in the recipient patient will make necessary a rotation of 180° of the transplanted kidney, with the ventral surface at the dorsal side of the recipient. This should be borne in mind at comparison.

The donor patient should have a roentgen examination of the chest. It is recommended that an upper-GI-tract examination also be made, in order to exclude ulcer (Starzl, 1964), as a safety measure related to postoperative cortisone therapy.

Alfidi and Magnusson (1972) propose angiography of removed kidneys before transplantation in order to detect thrombi and to study whether or not perfusion of the kidney is complete.

The indication for roentgen examination after transplantation in the recipient is usually oliguria or anuria. This can be due to stenosis or thrombosis in the arterial supply to the transplanted kidney, to abnormalities in the kidney parenchyma itself associated with immunologic rejection or ischemic tubular necrosis, or to disturbances in the outflow from the kidney on the venous side or in the drainage of urine. Several other possibilities for complications can occur with fistula formation and leakage, rejection of the ureteric anastomosis, etc. (Fletcher and Lecky, 1969).

The findings to be expected or suspected in examination of patients who have been the subjects of renal transplantation are thus many. Specific changes are those caused by rejection. Many papers cover these complications and their roentgenology (see, for example, Raphael et al., 1969; Kaude et al., 1970; Samuel, 1970; Navani et al., 1971).

The basic roentgenologic procedure is plain films with estimation of renal size. Any type of postoperative complication usually means an increase in the kidney size. In order to facilitate the estimation of size, it has been the praxis in certain transplantation centers to mark the kidney poles with silver clips during operation.

The next procedure is urography. We usually prefer to perform angiography, however, as the expected changes are in most cases vascular. At the end stage of the angiographic procedures, a urographic examination is automatically offered by using the contrast medium injected for angiography and now excreted through the kidney.

At angiography, ordinary conditions in the transplanted kidney do not differ from those in the normal kidney (Fig. 357). At examination because of oliguria or anuria, the changes to be looked for are those in rejection and in tubular necrosis. The most common changes

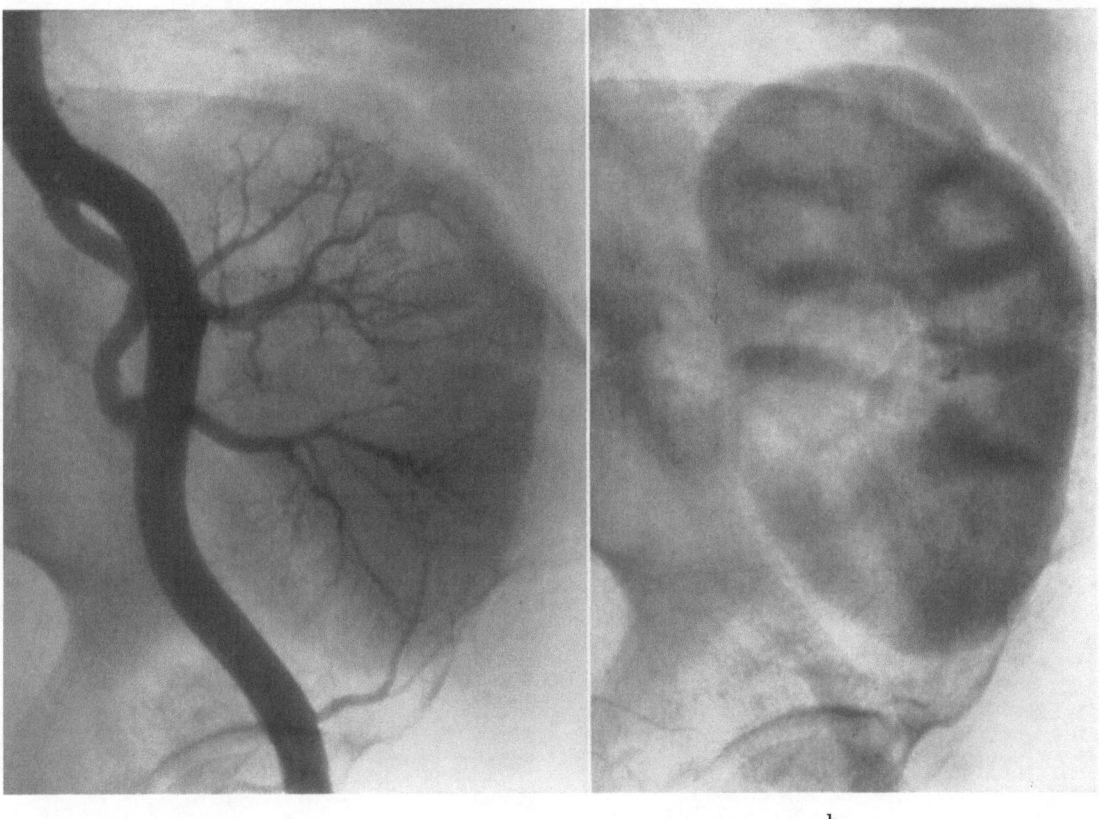

a   b

Fig. 357. Transplantation 5 months previously. Slight irregularity of proximal part of renal artery. Intrarenal arterial branches of ordinary caliber and shape. a) Arterial phase. b) Nephrographic phase. Kidney size and shape normal. Cortex well outlined

are those in rejection. The primary site of immunologic rejection is the vascular endothelium (CALNE et al., 1963), with subintimal, round-cell infiltration and fibrin deposits resulting in mural thrombosis with obliteration. In a material of 35 patients with transplantation SAMUEL (1970) found acute rejection of the transplanted kidney to occur at two main time periods: the first in the early postoperative period (7 days), and the second, between 32—37 days.

No vascular changes are found at the very early stage of rejection. In later stages the changes, as found in clinical examinations and in experiments in dogs (KNUDSEN et al., 1967), are as follows: narrowing and stretching of the segmental and interlobar arteries with irregularities and obliteration in the arterial lumen; non-filling of the peripheral arterial branches and marked decrease in density in the nephrographic phase. In early stages, the circulation time is ordinary, whereas in later stages a marked decrease in flow can be noted, with persistent filling of the arteries from 10 to 15 seconds and no increase in density in the nephrographic phase (POKIESER, 1971) (Fig. 358—361).

At repeat angiography following intensification of immunosuppressive therapy in such cases, a decrease in the edema of the kidney will be demonstrated, with decrease in size and diminished stretching and narrowing of the arteries, but the vascular changes may otherwise persist (KAUDE et al., 1970). In KAUDE's et al. material of clear-cut rejection, the arterial phase varied from 2.5 to 6 seconds. The arterial phase was normal in

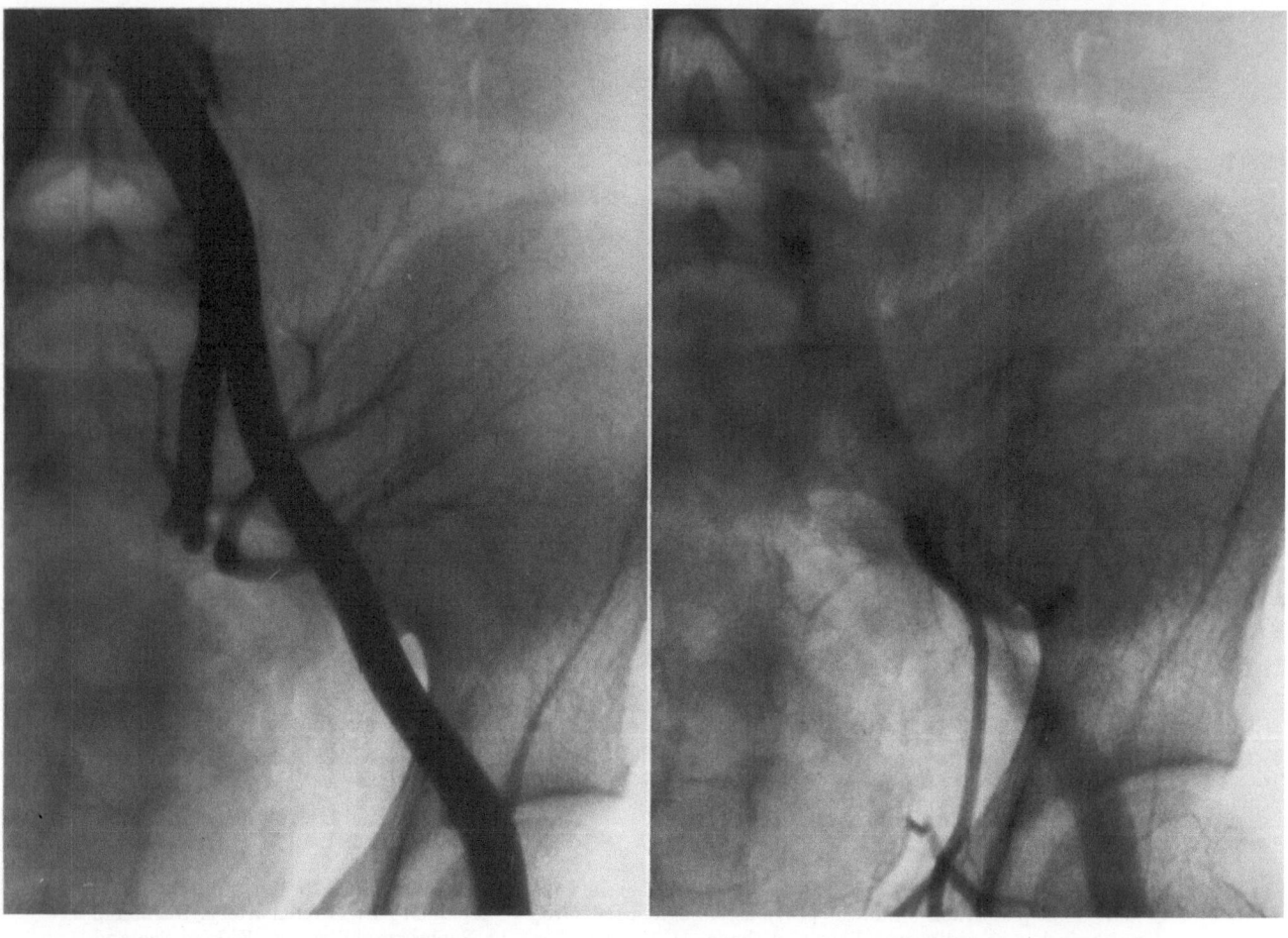

a   b

Fig. 358. Transplantation two weeks previously. Decreasing urinary output. At angiography a) arterial phase: slight stenosis at anastomosis between iliac artery and main renal artery. Intrarenal branches moderately stretched. Cortical arteries not filled. b) Capillary phase: concentration of contrast medium in kidney low. No border between cortex and medulla. Beginning of rejection

three patients with mild rejection, which means one to two seconds determined by the interval between the appearance of the last portion of the contrast medium in the main renal artery and the emptying of the peripheral arteries.

Marked progress of rejection causes occlusion of the peripheral branches of the interlobar arteries, including branches descending into the medulla as well as the primary interlobar vessels themselves, resulting in cortical necrosis. In the material of KAUDE et al. the response to immunosuppressive therapy was seen to result in conversion of the angiographic findings of acute rejection to those of healed or chronic rejection, with reduction of caliber of the renal artery and irregular arterial lumina due to organized sub-intimal infiltration and interstitial fibrosis. In addition, the number of interlobar arteries was reduced because of obliteration of vessels.

The second cause of oliguria-anuria is ischemic tubular necrosis due to prolonged renal ischemia before or during grafting or to vascular changes during rejection. The combination of rejection and ischemic tubular necrosis is thus common.

In ischemic acute tubular necrosis KAUDE et al. found the circulation time to be only slightly prolonged. Focal irregularities could be noted in some smaller vessels as a result

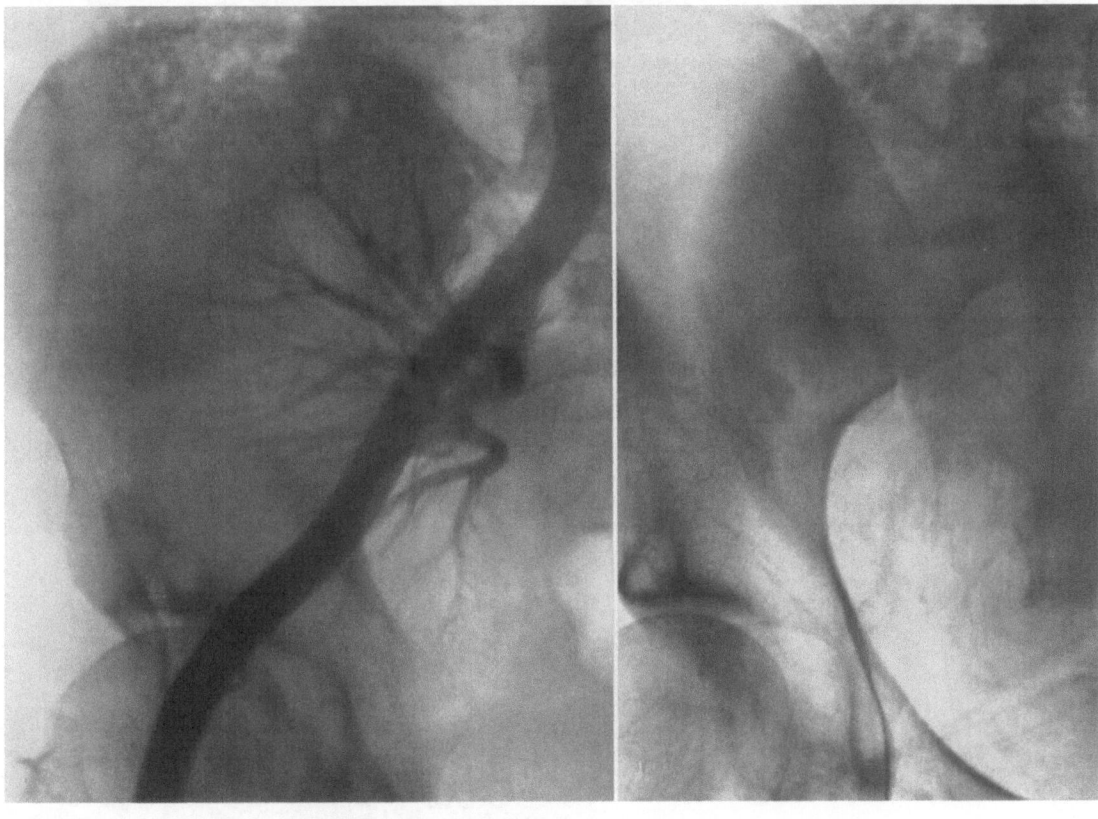

a   b

Fig. 359. Chronic glomerulonephritis and interstitial nephritis for 10 years. Hemodialysis for past two years. Transplantation six weeks previously with A-match kidney which had been perfused during the night prior to operation. Angiography: a) arterial phase: kidney moderately enlarged. Intrarenal branches stretched. No filling of arcuate arteries. b) Nephrographic phase: charging of kidney parenchyma with contrast medium lower than normally. No distinct border between cortex and medulla. No venous filling. Only slight excretion. — Rejection

of localized vasculitis. These were the only arterial changes present. The nephrographic effect was fairly good, although the borderline between the cortex and the medulla was hard to define. Filling of the renal veins was observed, actually with increased concentration of the contrast medium in the veins as a result of the absence of kidney function.

The non-function of the transplanted kidney at the angiographic procedure is found in some instances to be due to occlusion of the artery by thrombosis and in later stages to stenosis at the area of the anastomosis. SAMUEL (1970) points out that some degree of arterial narrowing invariably occurs at the site of the arterial anastomosis and can be demonstrated in the arteriogram. WHITE et al. (1972) in 9 patients with early postoperative kidney transplant dysfunction demonstrated the cause of transplant failure in seven cases to be

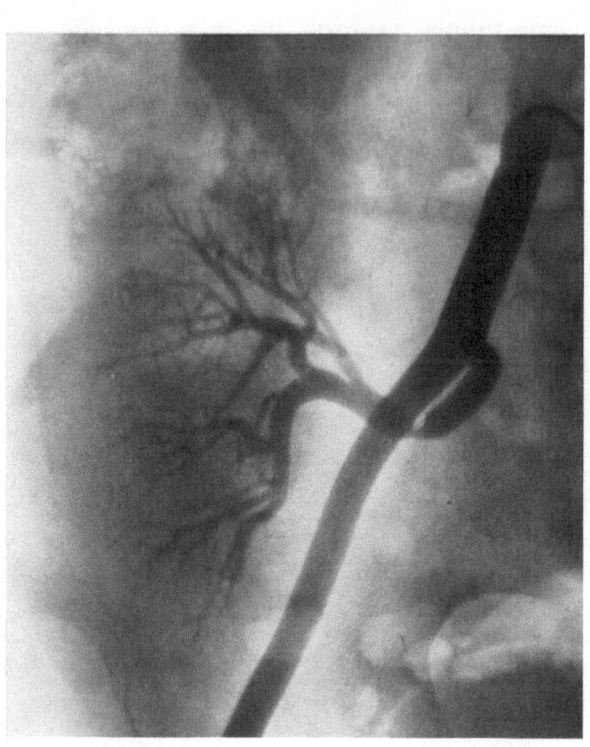

a

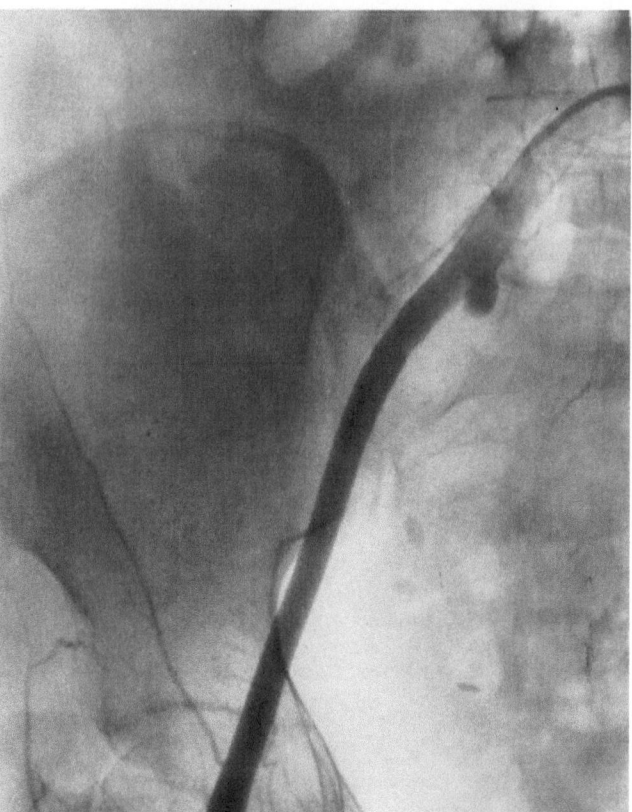

b

c

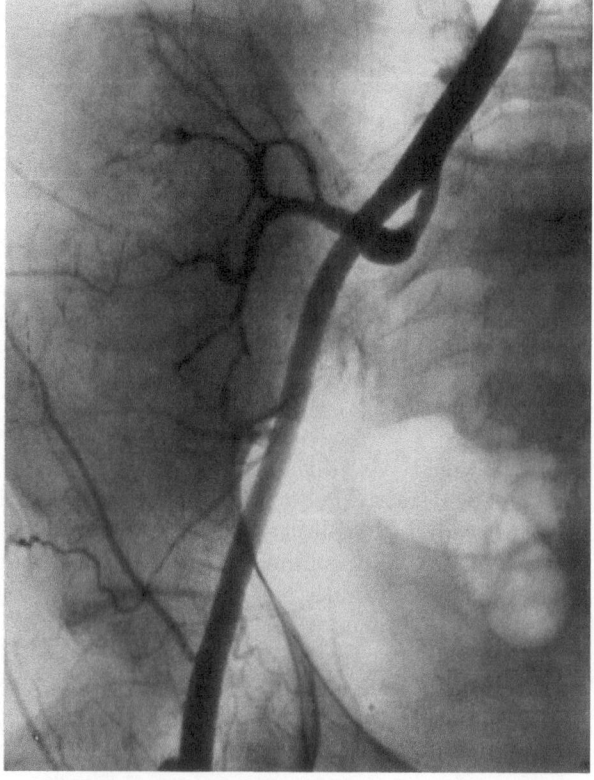

Fig. 360. Renal artery in connection with transplantation. Patient with interstitial nephritis, hypertensive disease, and rapidly progressing renal insufficiency. Renal transplantation. a) Angiography because of increase in hypertension three months after transplantation: marked stenosis in main renal artery. b) Re-operation with complications. Complete occlusion of renal artery. Two-centimeter-long venous graft was inserted and circulation restored. c) Angiography one week later: kidney size diminished. Marked irregular stenosis in several intrarenal branches. Decrease in caliber of branches generally. Multiple arterial occlusions in periphery. In later phase: marked shunting to veins was seen. No excretion into kidney pelvis. Conclusion: marked arterial intrarenal damage

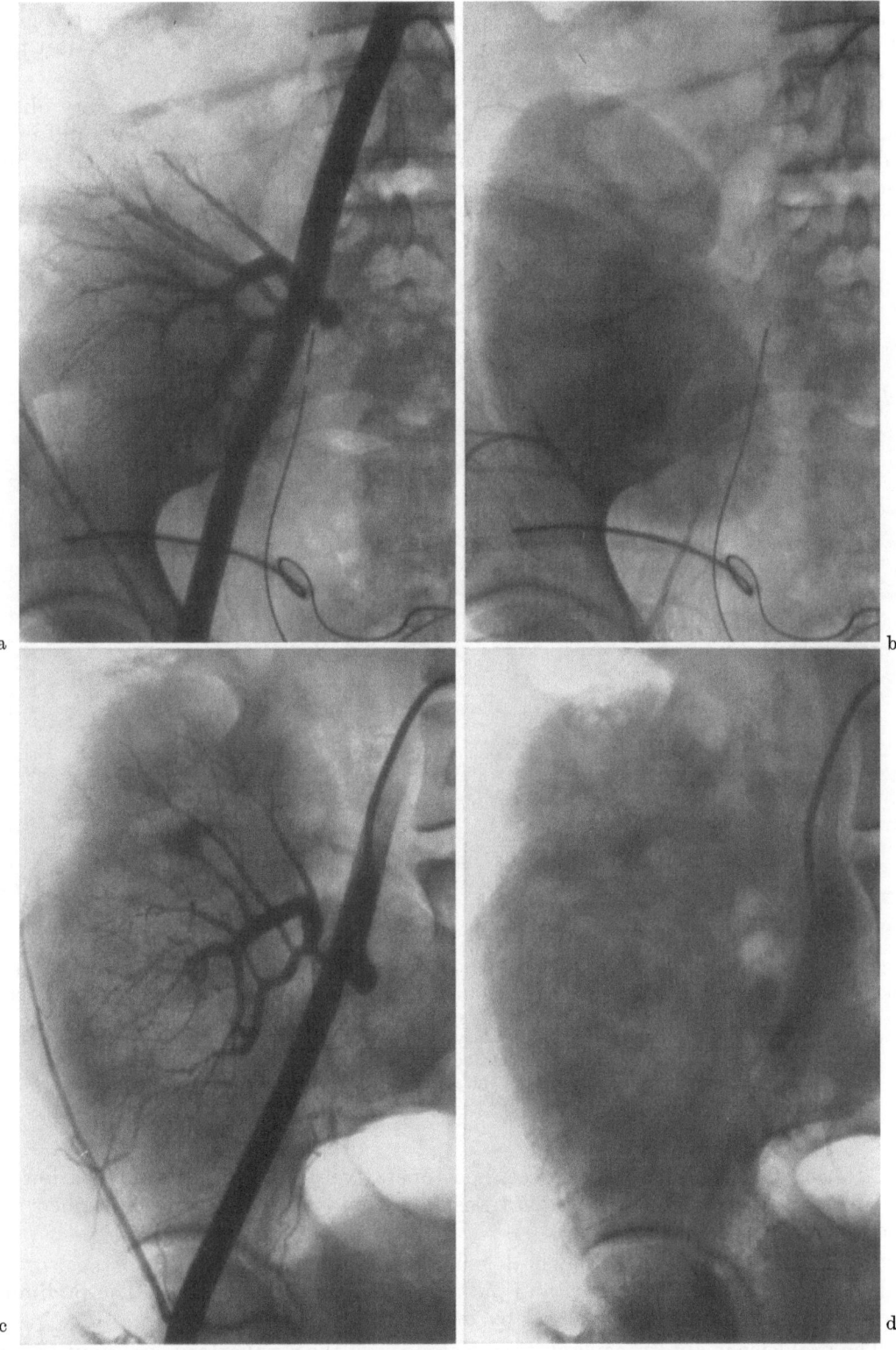

Fig. 361. Transplantation two days previously. Markedly diminished diuresis. Angiography, a) arterial phase; b) nephrographic phase: slight irregularity at anastomosis. Intrarenal arteries normal. Good charging of kidney parenchyma with contrast medium: Delineation of border between cortex and medulla slightly less marked At pyelography normal conditions were found. Diuresis increased. Angiography was again performed nine months later because of decrease in renal function. c) Arterial phase: 5 mm-long stenosis at anastomosis between iliac artery and main renal artery. Intrarenal arteries moderately stretched and irregular. Lack of filling in peripheral part of kidney. d) Nephrographic phase: decrease in charging of kidney parenchyma with contrast medium. No border between cortex and medulla. Moderate increase in kidney size. Chronic rejection

arterial stenosis, renal vein thrombosis, or massive pelvic hematoma. Prompt recognition and correction of these complications led to prolonged survival of the renal transplants in four of the nine patients.

Other causes of oliguria or anuria may be renal failure secondary to urinary obstruction. In the latter case the nephrographic effect is persistent for several seconds and a marked delay in filling of the kidney pelvis or a complete delay of excretion can be noted. In some cases dilatation of the kidney pelvis and filling defects in the kidney pelvis due to coagula can be seen.

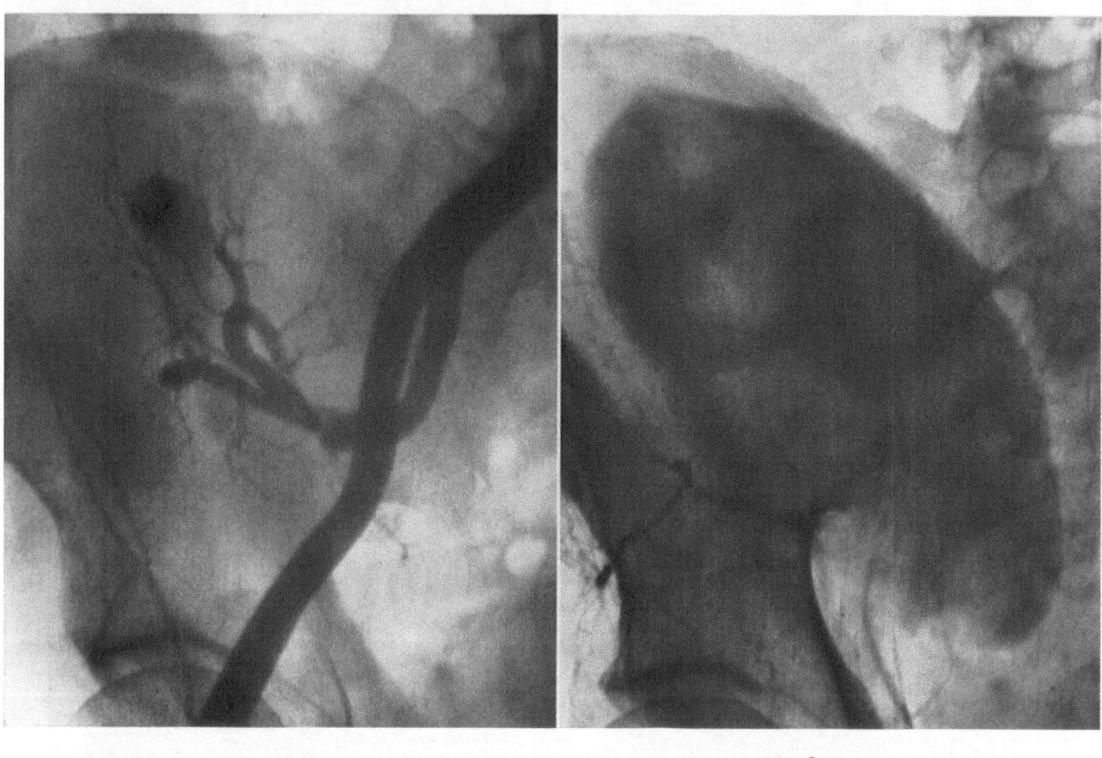

a   b

Fig. 362. Transplantation six months previously, after one year of dialysis. Now decrease in kidney function. Angiography: a) arterial phase: moderate stenosis at anastomosis between right iliac artery and main renal artery. Arteriovenous fistula at middle of kidney. b) Nephrographic phase: large irregular infarction in caudal lateral part of transplanted kidney; otherwise kidney size and shape are normal. Border between cortex and medulla well marked. No signs of rejection

At angiography seven months later, the arteriovenous fistula was found to be closed

Arteriovenous fistula may be seen postoperatively as another complication (Fig. 362). In a patient who has undergone transplantation lymphocele may be formed in the region of the operation site.

Roentgen examination of the chest is important in the postoperative stage, in order to check for bronchial pneumonia and pulmonary edema due to anuria. The preliminary changes may be markedly influenced by immunosuppressive therapy.

The problems in autotransplantation in stenosis of the renal artery are about the same as in other types of transplantation.

R. Miscellaneous changes particularly of the ureter

Since the ureter is exposed to essentially the same injurious agents as the kidney and the renal pelvis, a large number of diseases can occur simultaneously or successively in the kidney pelvis, the ureter, and the bladder, with primary or secondary involvement of the ureter. Therefore the normal roentgen anatomy and physiology of the ureter was described in the section on examination methods. For the same reason, the pathology of the ureter has been included in special chapters on tumor, tuberculosis, stone, anomalies, trauma, urinary tract dilatation, etc. The ureters, however, can be affected by a wide variety of other pathologic changes calling for supplementary consideration.

Since the ureter is simply a duct for transporting the urine formed in the kidneys and accumulated in the renal pelvis to the bladder, and since this pathway is long and narrow, most of the pathologic changes of the ureter obstruct drainage. Some of these changes have been described in detail in the chapter on urinary tract dilatation. Others have been mentioned but call for further description, while still others have not been included in previous chapters.

I. Ureterocele

A ureterocele is a widening of the distal part of the ureter ballooning into the bladder (Fig. 363). It is also called ureteric cyst or ureteric phimosis. The nomenclature is not strictly correct. As pointed out by Bétoulières *et al.* (1959), the name ureterocele means

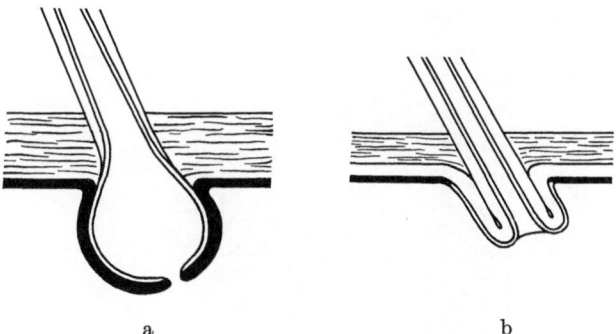

Fig. 363. Schematic drawing: a) Ureterocele. b) Ureteric prolapse. (After Staehler 1959)

literally a prolapse of the ureter into the bladder. Ureter cyst or cystic dilatation of the ureter, on the other hand, should mean a closed formation. Therefore in the French literature the term "dilatation pseudo-cystique de l'uretere terminal" has been used. In English the condition is usually referred to as ureterocele.

The distal end of the ureter shows a round or, in most cases, oval widening (Fig. 364). Since this end bulges into the bladder under the mucosa, it will appear in the cystogram as a filling defect at either or both of the ureteric orifices. Upon simultaneous filling of the ureter and bladder, as often in urography, the dilated end of the ureter will be filled with contrast medium which is separated from the contrast medium in the bladder by a defect a few millimeters wide. This defect corresponds to the wall of the ureter and the bladder mucosa.

The size of a ureterocele varies widely, depending in part on whether or not the ureteric orifice is obstructed. It may consist of such a slight widening of the end of the ureter that it may not be demonstrated in the urogram unless films are taken in proper projection with suitable contrast filling around the ureteric orifice. The filling of a small ureterocele

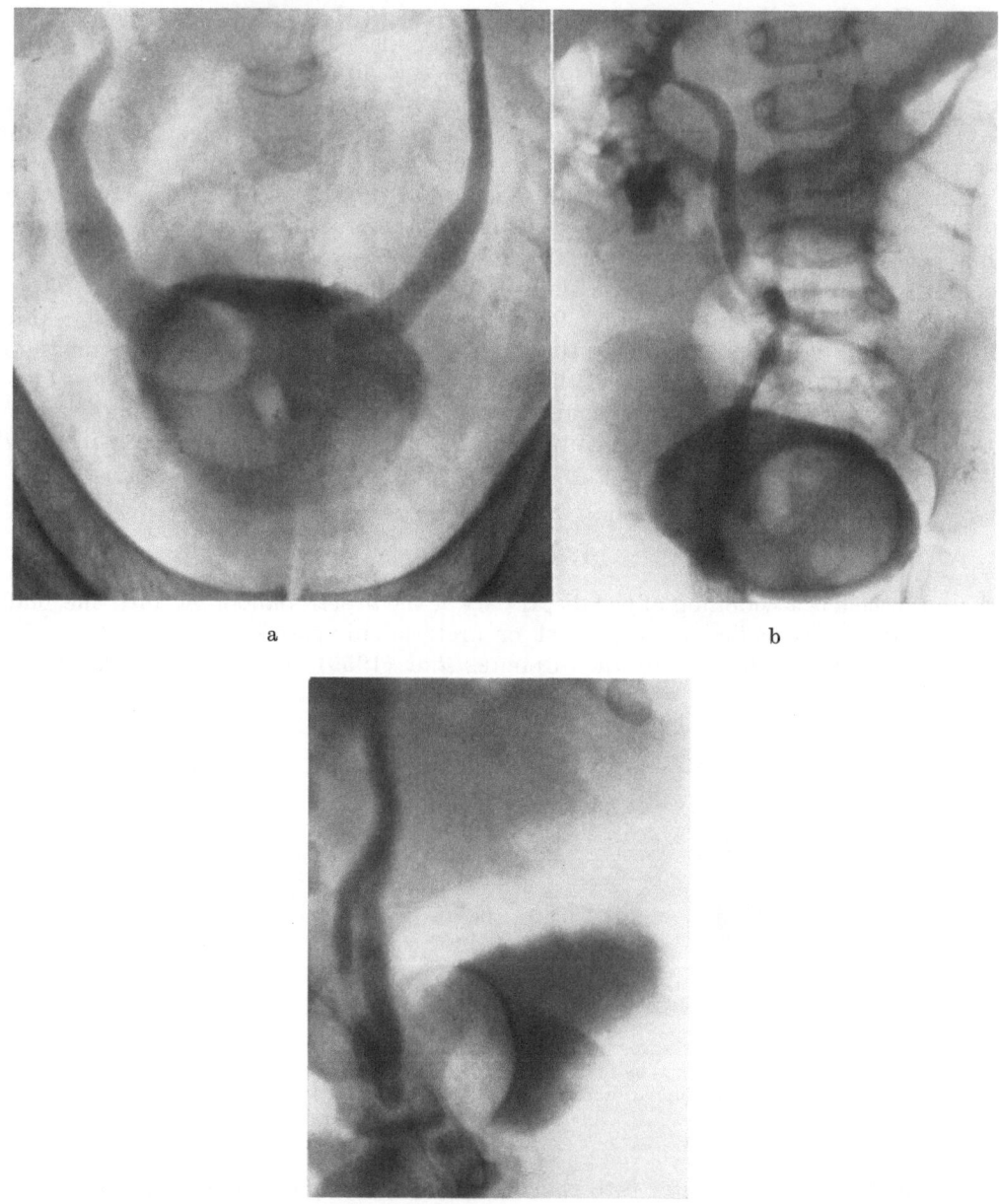

Fig. 364. a) Bilateral ureterocele, small on left side, larger on right side. Moderate dilatation of distal parts of ureters (in addition, catheter with air-filled balloon in bladder). b) Large ureterocele filling great part of bladder. Ureterocele originates at distal end of ureter to left kidney. No excretion on this side (later examination demonstrated marked hydronephrosis and hydro-ureter on this side). Slight dilatation of double ureter on right side. Frontal view. c) Lateral view

may also be intermittent, depending on the flow of urine in the ureter. It may also vary with the extent to which the bladder is filled and disappear on distention of the bladder.

Ureteroceles can also assume considerable proportions, however, and can fill almost the entire bladder (RUHDE, 1948) (Fig. 364). A large, round, symmetric or asymmetric, well-defined formation is then seen, surrounded by a layer of contrast medium in the bladder. The ureterocele itself is not filled with contrast. In such cases urination is difficult simply because the ureterocele obstructs the internal vesical orifice (GUTIERREZ, 1939).

When a ureterocele of this type occurs in a man of middle or old age, differentiation from prostatic hyperplasia is important.

As mentioned earlier, dilatation of the ureter draining the cranial renal pelvis is common (see chapter on urinary tract dilatation). At urography in such cases, the renal pelvis and the ureter will be shown to be widened. A ureterocele of varying size will be seen in the bladder. The ureteric orifice is often ectopic. The ureterocele is then usually situated near the midline in the base of the bladder and near the bladder neck (Fig. 365). In females, if the ureteric orifice is ectopic, the ureterocele can prolapse out through the urethral orifice. On straining, a ureterocele in the bladder at the internal orifice can be pressed out into the urethra. When a ureterocele causes stasis, only one of the ureters may

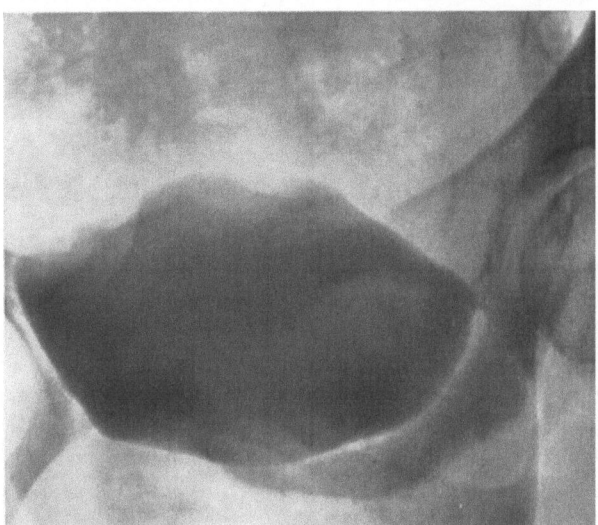

Fig. 365. Ureterocele at distal end of one of two left ureters. This ureter, corresponding to a markedly dilated cranial renal pelvis in double kidney, runs around left and caudal part of the bladder and opens at the bladder neck

be widened, i. e. that which has a ureterocele. It may also involve the other ipsilateral ureter and occasionally the ureters on both sides according to the position and size of the ureterocele.

If the ureterocele has developed in the posterior part of the urethra, urethrocystography will give more detailed information than urography. Occasionally, unilaterally or bilaterally, a ureterocele may lie within a vesical diverticulum (McCALL, 1972). Stasis in the ureter favors stone formation, and the finding of one or more concrements in or above a ureterocele is not uncommon. A concrement situated at the ureteric orifice and seen in the cystogram, separated from the contrast filling of the bladder by a contrast-free zone, is pathognomonic of concrement in a ureterocele (ÅKERLUND, 1935). The finding is thus the same as contrast in the ureterocele, with simultaneous filling of the bladder, as described above. Sometimes, however, a stone of ordinary appearance may be seen above a ureterocele or several concrements moving freely in the ureter (PETROVČIĆ and DUGAN, 1955).

II. Ureteric prolapse

Ureteric prolapse is rare. It consists of an invagination of the ureter through the ureteric orifice (Fig. 363). The formation bulging into the bladder thus has the ureteric lumen in the middle surrounded by a wall of ureteric mucosa. It appears in the contrast-filled bladder as an oblong filling defect in the direction of the ureter (WEMEAU, LEMAITRE and DEFRANCE, 1959).

III. Ureteric endometriosis

In endometriosis of the adnexa and peritoneum, the ureters may become involved. Bladder endometriosis can also affect the ureters if it is situated near the ureteric orifice. Endometriosis localized to the ureter is rare. Cases have been described by RANDALL (1941) and by KAIRIS (1958). Most authors have reported only a single case. A narrowing is seen in the distal part of the ureter. Its appearance is not characteristic. Endometriosis should be suspected if urinary symptoms are found to be due to a narrowing of the distal third of the ureter in a woman who reports that the symptoms usually increase in severity in connection with menstruation.

IV. Herniation of the ureter

A case has been described by LINDBOM (1947) in which at urography in a patient with repeated left-sided attacks of renal colic over a period of eight years, hydronephrosis was revealed on the left side, and at retrograde ureterography with a bulb catheter a loop of the ureter was shown which resembled a hernia protruding in the direction of the sciatic foramen. The loop was constricted at the neck and the ureter was dilated above the constriction. Thus the diagnosis was ureteric herniation in the sciatic foramen, obstructing flow. Operation verified this finding.

More such cases have since been described in the literature (BOLIVERT, 1971). This lesion may be unilateral or bilateral and may or may not be associated with obstruction of the ureter.

The ureter can also herniate down into a scrotal hernia (JEWETT and HARRIS, 1953).

V. Ureteric diverticula

Small diverticula have been described, but not verified, in the presence of ureteric changes (HOLLY and SUMCAD, 1957). Small and large congentital diverticula have been reported in a few cases (see Fig. 51 in chapter on anomalies). They may calcify (MC GRAW and CULP, 1952) and become so large as to contain one liter of fluid. As a rule, however, they are smaller and may occur anywhere along the ureter. They are usually diagnosed as strictures because the neck of the diverticulum is narrow and it is therefore difficult to obtain a filling of the diverticulum.

VI. Ureteric involvement by aortic aneurysm and other pathologic processes

Cases have been described (CRANE, 1958, for example) in which an aneurysm in the lumbar aorta caused hydronephrosis by pressing against or through extensive collagenous connective tissue formations encasing the ureter. An aneurysm may also displace one or both of the ureters (Fig. 366. See also Fig. 29 in chapter on examination methods). Such a displacement can also be caused by marked tortuosity of the aorta with aneurysm formation. The cause of the displacement is easily demonstrated when calcifications, if only slight, are present in the aorta wall. Other pathologic processes may cause displacement of the ureter, such as enlarged lymph glands (see Fig. 30 in chapter on examination methods). A bladder diverticulum may also cause ureteric displacement (Fig. 367).

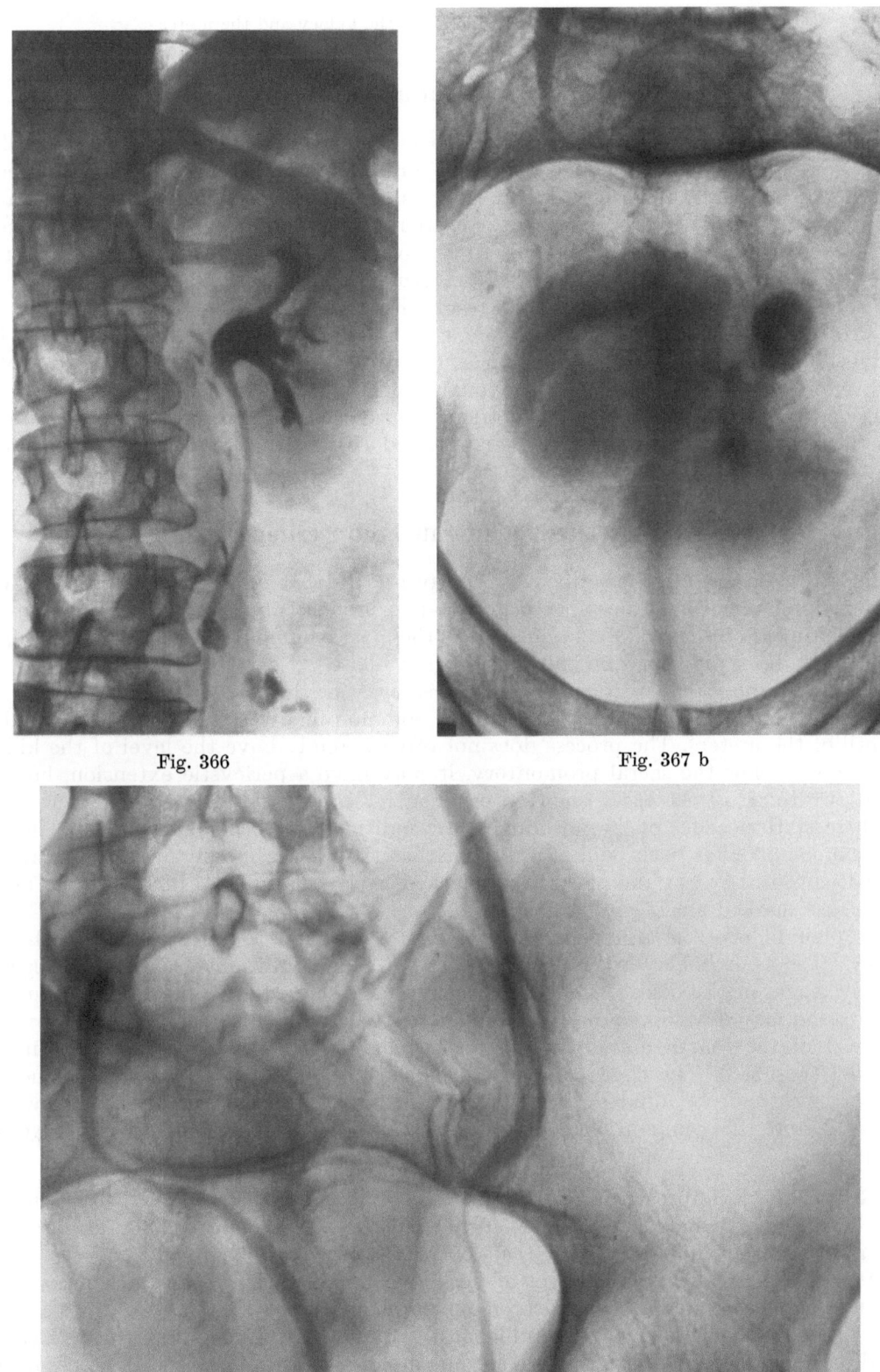

Fig. 366

Fig. 367 b

Fig. 367 a

Fig. 366. Displacement of cranial part of left ureter by moderately dilated tortuous lumbar aorta with wall calcifications

Fig. 367. Urography: a) displacement of left ureter markedly medially by b) large bladder diverticulum

VII. Regional ureteritis

Ureteritis is common in inflammatory processes of the urinary tract, such as pyelone-phritis, or secondary to processes above the ureter, e.g. pyonephrosis, or in processes located immediately outside the ureter such as appendicitis, salpingitis, regional entero-colitis. It may also be secondary to a condition within the ureter, e.g. stone. Stones in such cases can occasionally be difficult to discover; they may be situated in a decubital lesion in the ureteric wall and later cause formation of scars and mucosal hyperplasia with long, severe ureteric stenosis as a result (ELLEGAST and SCHIMATZEK, 1957).

Primary inflammatory infiltration along a few centimeters of the ureter has been described as causing moderate dilatation of the urinary tract (DREYFUSS and GOODSITT, 1958; NORING, 1958). This so-called regional ureteritis has no special characteristics. Ure-teric changes with irregular narrowing along considerable lengths of the ureter can occur in periarteriitis (polyangiitis nodosa) (FISHER and HOWARD, 1948).

VIII. Peri-ureteritis obliterans, retroperitoneal fibrosis

This disease was first described by ORMOND (1948). It is also called primary retro-peritoneal inflammatory process, or primitive peri-ureteritis but the name retroperitoneal fibrosis, proposed by DINEEN et al. in 1960, is the most commonly used. A large number of papers have been published on this subject (see KAUDE et al., 1964).

Patho-anatomically, retroperitoneal fibrosis may be diffuse, local, or segmental, and involve the aorta, the inferior caval vein, the common iliac vessels, the kidneys, and one or both of the ureters. The process does not often extend above the level of the kidneys and seldom below the sacral promontory. lt may have a pericystic extension, however. About two-thirds of the cases reported occur in males and there is a prevalence in the fourth to sixth decades of life, although the condition may occur at any age. The most common complaint is back pain of a dull character but occasionally with acute attacks. The patient loses weight and often has a marked sense of fatigue. If bilateral, the process may cause marked stasis ending in anuria.

In plain films of the urinary tract it may not be possible to outline one or both of the kidneys. The same holds for the psoas muscle. Ordinary conditions are seen at urography in early stages of the disease. In later stages, a cone-shaped stenosis caused by ureteric compression may develop, ending in complete obstruction. This obstruction is usually at the level of the fourth and fifth lumbar vertebrae but any part of the ureter may be involved (Fig. 368). The engagement may be short or long, and the ureter and the renal pelvis above may be dilated. Pyelonephritic changes are often present. Narrowing of the aorta and the common iliac arteries at angiography has been reported (HACKETT, 1958).

Retroperitoneal fibrosis may be "idiopathic" or it may be secondary to other inflamma-tory conditions such as pancreatitis and spondylitis. Peripelvic urinary extravasation may also be responsible for fibrous reaction of the retroperitoneal space.

It must be stressed that changes of this type can be caused by malignant conditions such as lymphosarcoma and adenocarcinoma primary in the kidney.

Plastic perinephritis may be seen higher up around the entire kidney. It has also been called perirenal fascitis, representing a chronic inflammation in Gerota's fascia, resulting in a stricture of the ureter with anuria.

It has been discussed whether or not these two diseases may represent one and the same clinical entity. HUTCH et al. (1959) believe that although these two diseases have some features in common and may ultimately prove to be related, they should be considered separate entities. The authors claim that the plastic periureteritis may be unilateral and

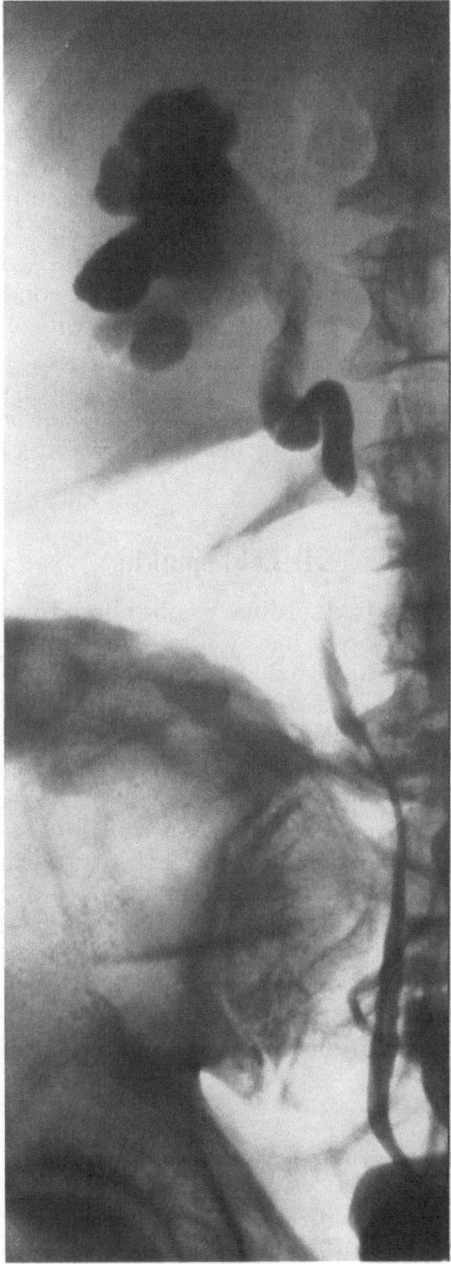

Fig. 368. Retroperitoneal fibrosis. Marked stenosis of ureter at the level of the lumbar vertebra nr. 4. Moderate dilatation cranially to stenosis.

that the ureter can also be changed in its pelvic parts, which is not the case in plastic perinephritis.

IX. Bilharziosis

In cases of infection with Bilharzia, changes of a hyperplastic type can occur in the ureter with abundant small papillomatous formations which may calcify. The changes may also be of a hypoplastic type, however, with mucosal atrophy. In both types the lumen of the ureter is irregularly narrowed and may be obstructed (MAKAR, 1948).

X. Amyloidosis

In amyloidosis, primary or secondary, the kidneys and urinary pathways may occasionally be involved. It is usually the bladder that is the seat of amyloidosis. Cases of this disease in the renal pelvis and ureter have also been reported, however, although mostly in the patho-anatomic literature (AKIMATO, 1927, etc.). Such cases have also been described from a clinical point of view and it has been stressed that on involvement of the ureter the lumen may be narrow and the length of the ureter involved may appear rigid (GILBERT and MC DONALD, 1952; HIGBEE and MILLETT, 1956; ANDREAS and OOSTING, 1958). It has been shown that the narrowing is a progressive condition and in the course of several years can come to block the ureter entirely, with hydronephrosis as a result (HIGHBEE and MILLET, 1956).

The changes described above have no common features which may be described as characteristic of the condition, but amyloidosis should be borne in mind as a possible cause of ureteric stricture and in differentiating between ureteritis and tumor.

XI. Leukoplakia

Leukoplakia means a change from ordinary epithelium to squamous epithelium characterized by keratinization. It may occur in any part of the urinary tract, such as in the renal pelvis and/or in the ureter. It is regarded as a pre-cancerous lesion. The disease is rare.

Leukoplakia may be so severe as to cause complete stenosis of the ureter or widespread mural changes with multiple, moderately irregular strictures. It may involve only a part of the ureter wall or of the renal pelvis and cause slight narrowing, or it may cause a slight rigidity of a minor part of the wall of the renal pelvis. It can also manifest itself as filling defects in the renal pelvis or as a high mucosa demonstrable in part of the renal pelvis and resembling papillomatosis. Neither this type of change nor total obstruction is characteristic of the disease, however. Therefore, as a rule, specific diagnosis cannot be made roentgenologically. Roentgen examination may give a clue but the diagnosis must be established by other methods. It has been stressed (FALK, 1954) that squamous epithelium in large amounts can be found in the urinary sediment. If leukoplakia in the bladder has been diagnosed by roentgenology and cystoscopy, any changes in the ureter and renal pelvis of the type described above may be diagnosed as leukoplakia.

XII. Pyelourteritis cystica

Multiple inflammatory cysts occur in the wall of the urinary tract in pyelitis, ureteritis, and cystitis cystica. They are often seen in the entire urinary pathways, but may be localized only to the renal pelvis or the ureter or, more usually, only to the bladder. The cysts may be single or numerous (Fig. 369).

Changes may be bilateral, but they are more frequently unilateral. They vary in size from large cysts obstructing flow in the ureter, to small and single mural excrescenses. They are more common in the proximal part of the ureter in contrast to papilloma, which is usually located in the distal portion of the ureter.

Roentgenologically diagnosed pyelourteritis cystica was first described in 1929 (JACOBY; JOELSON). The cysts produce filling defects in urograms and pyelograms (Fig. 368). If the cysts are numerous, some of them will always be seen along the margin as outgrowths from the ureteric wall. This gives the ureter a very irregular outline. If the cysts are numerous and if some of them are large, the diagnosis is thus made easy. Upon detection of a single cyst, the roentgenologist should try to demonstrate it in suitable projections and show that the defect is projecting from the wall and is of fixed localization.

It has been stated that a dilatation of the ends of the major calyces, with narrowing of the stems of the calyces and a cystic dilatation at the pelviureteric junction and of the ends of the major calyces, are characteristic of the disease (HINMAN et al., 1936). These are, however, neither obligatory nor typical of this disease.

Instead of being cystic, the pelvic and ureteric mucosa may be granular, so-called granular pyelitis, which resembles pyelitis cystica roentgenologically. The defects are smaller than those produced by cysts.

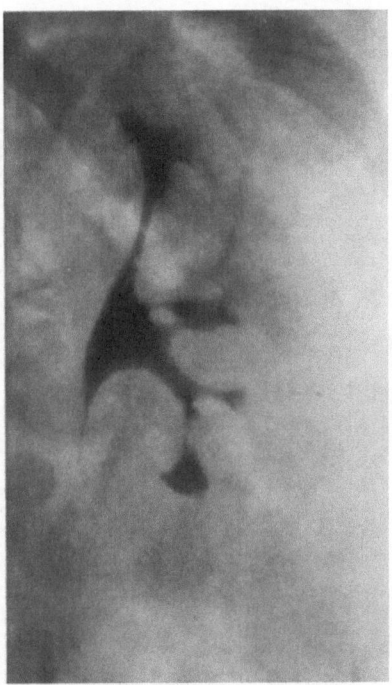

Fig. 369. Pyeloureteritis cystica

XIII. Ureteric stump after nephrectomy

After nephrectomy has left behind part of the ureter, there is the possibility of the maintainence or development of a pathologic process in the stump. A tuberculous or unspecific ureteritis can thus cause persistent pyuria and bacilluria (Fig. 370). Even where the ureter is not involved at the time of operation, infected material can be transported and deposited in it via reflux from the bladder. Cases have been described in which py-oureter has flared up after several years of normal urinary findings after operation for stone pyonephrosis, whether or not stones were left in the ureter (DAVISON, 1942 LIVERMORE, 1950; BENNETTS et al., 1955). In cases of shrunken bladder, the stump of the ureter may develop into a supplementary bladder and thereby increase the urinary reservoir.

It is also known that carcinoma can develop in the ureteric stump, even in patients in whom nephrectomy was performed, although not because of tumor (LOEF and CASELLA, 1952).

The question whether or not primary ureterectomy is indicated is debatable and indications vary. RIESER (1950) recommends that retrograde pyelography be performed regularly with contrast filling of the ureter, the drainage of which should be checked. A film taken about one to two hours after retrograde injection of the contrast medium will indicate whether or not the contents of the ureter will be voided after nephrectomy. The information thus obtained should prove to be of crucial importance and of material assistance in arriving at a definite decision concerning the indications for ureterectomy. Although such a procedure may be of great importance in some instances, it cannot be accepted as a necessary routine measure.

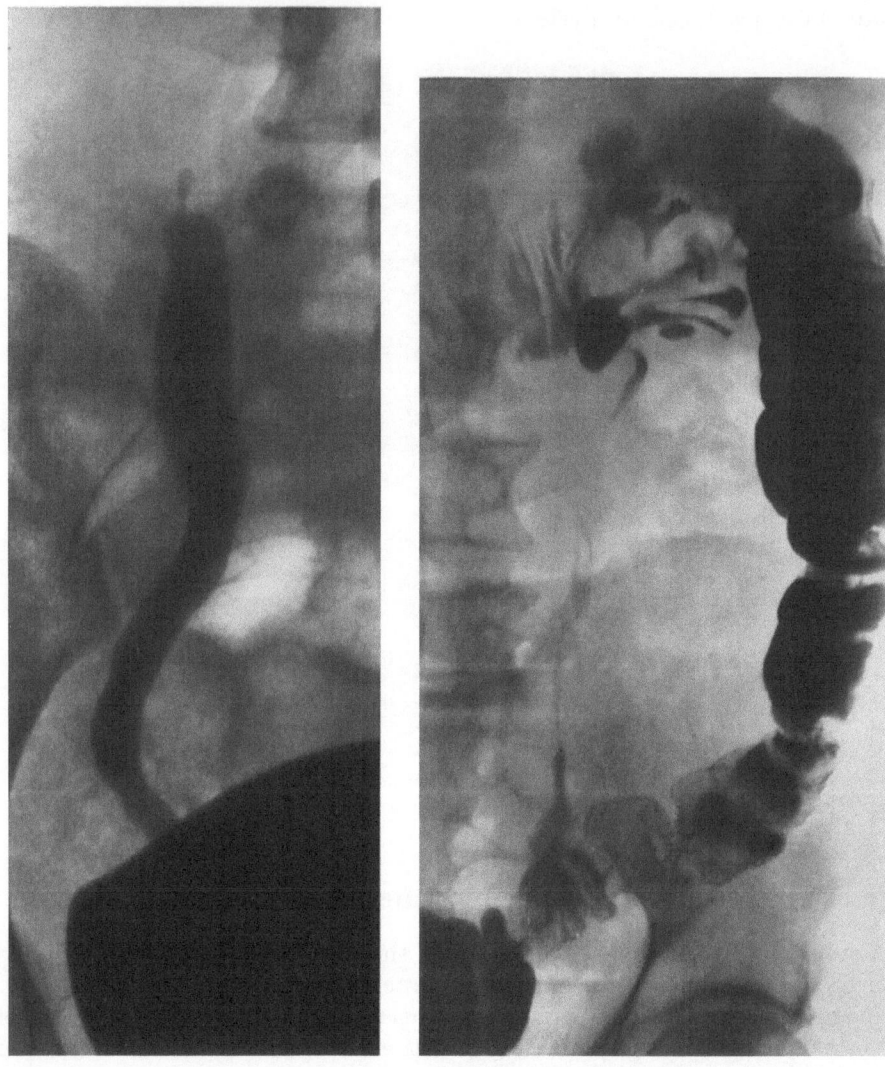

Fig. 370   Fig. 371

Fig. 370. Ureteral stump after heminephrectomy in double kidney with pyelonephritis. Ureteric stump dilated. Persistent urinary infection

Fig. 371. Ureterosigmoidostomy after extirpation of bladder two months previously. Passage of barium from rectum to urinary tract during examination of colon

XIV. Ureteric fistulae

In connection with bladder extirpation, operative fistulae may be formed between one or both ureters and the bowel. During urography contrast medium is seen to pass from the ureter into the bowel. When a fistula is formed between a ureter and the colon, the passage of barium contrast medium during colon examination can be seen in retrograde direction into the ureter and the kidney pelvis (Fig. 371). In patients with operative fistula between urinary pathways and the bowel at urography or pyelography, different stages of stasis can be seen on one or both sides because of edema or shrinkage of the anastomosis (Fig. 372). From the bowel gas can pass in retrograde direction up into one or both of the renal pelves.

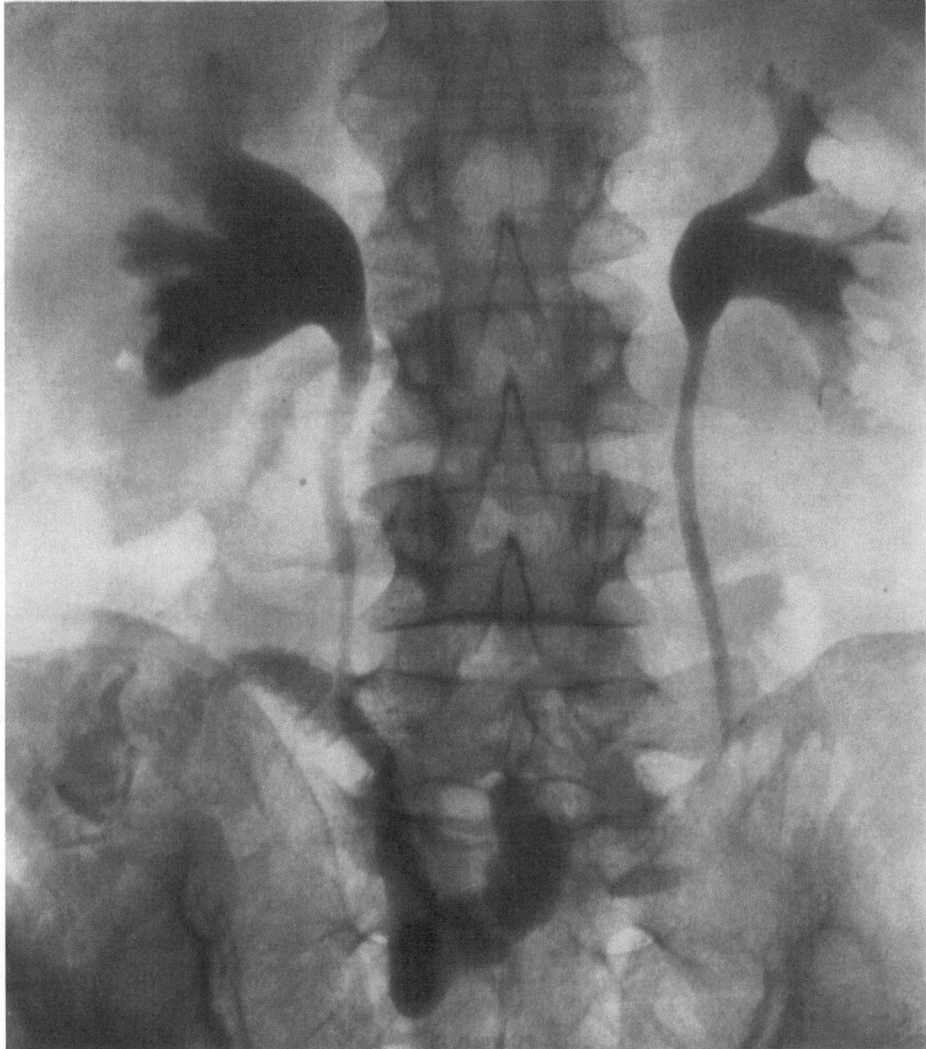

Fig. 372. Anastomosis between both ureters and small bowel after extirpation of bladder. Slight dilatation of distal part of left ureter. Right kidney pelvis and ureter moderately dilated

Fistula formation may also be caused by an operative procedure unintentionally, mainly in operations on the rectum or sigmoid colon or in connection with gynecologic operations. Fig. 373 demonstrates a short fistula between the dilatated part of the ureter above a ureteric scar formation in the left horn of the vagina and Fig. 374 shows a fistula between both ureters and the corresponding lateral walls of the vagina.

In inflammatory lesion, tumor and trauma fistula may be found between ureters and adjacent organs or out in the retroperitoneal space or on the skin surface.

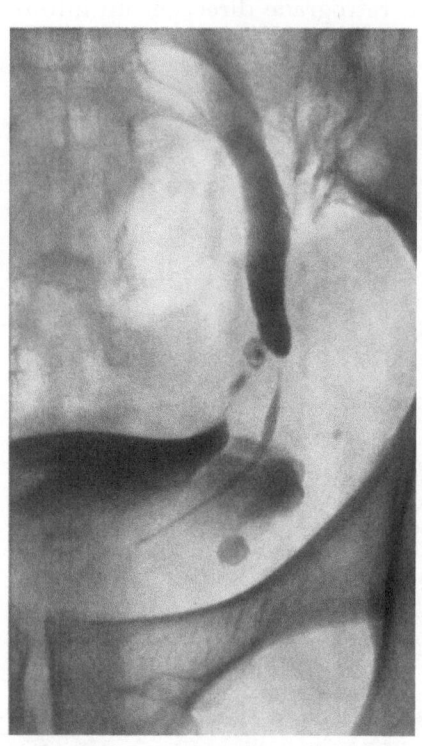

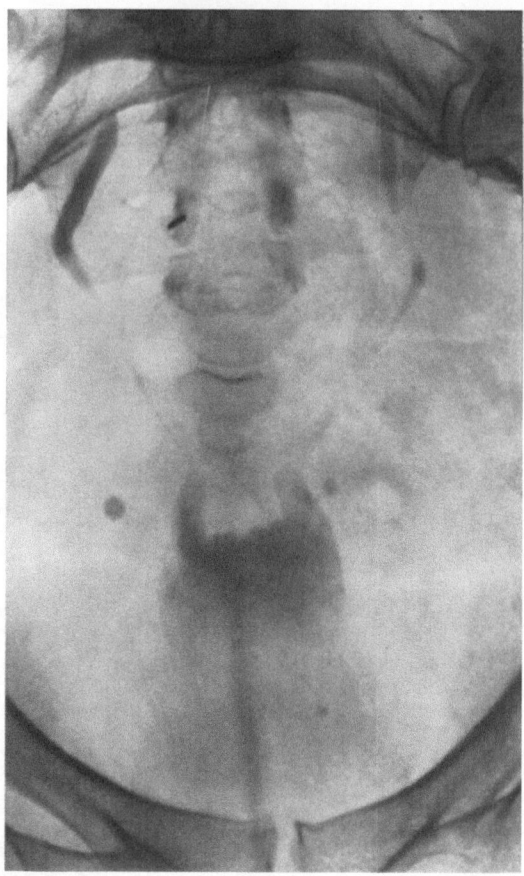

Fig. 373   Fig. 374

Fig. 373. Short thin fistula between distal part of dilated ureter above short ureteric stenosis. Fistula ends in left horn of vagina

Fig. 374. Fistula between both ureters and corresponding horns of vagina as complication after gynecologic operation

Part II:
Roentgen diagnosis of the distal part of the urinary tract

By

Olle Olsson

A. Introduction

In the examination of the distal part of the urinary tract, basic conditions are the same as described in the introduction to the earlier part of this volume "Roentgen examination of the kidneys and the ureters." One point should be stressed specifically: radiation protection. As the genital organs are within the beam at roentgen examination of the bladder and the urethra, special care should be taken to avoid radiation to ovaries and testes.

The same importance should be attached to the proper preparation of the patient as is stressed in the previous chapters. The patient should be informed correctly and thoroughly as to the nature of the examination since there may be discomfort and embarrassment in some cases. The informational preparation of the patient also facilitates that cooperation with physician and staff which is essential in the performance of certain types of examinations.

Strict adherence to precautions for the avoidance of infection is also necessary.

Finally it should be pointed out that although cystoscopic methods may provide important information in many cases of bladder disease or suspicion of such, the roentgenologic method has nevertheless a very important role.

B. Examination methods

I. Plain radiography

Survey films of the bladder should be made in a projection with the tube angulated to direct the beam along the long axis of the small pelvis, with the patient in supine position. This projection will give exposure of the distal parts of the ureters and of the bladder without overprojection of the pelvic skeleton. A great part of the circumference of the bladder, mainly the cranial part, can be seen because of the fat layer on the outer surface of the bladder (Fig. 375).

In females the corpus of the uterus can often be seen, usually forming an impression in the bladder.

The boundaries of the bladder may be difficult to outline at bladder distention. Instead, a large soft tissue mass is seen, filling out the small pelvis and continuing cranially, with displacement of the bowel.

Calcifications can be seen in the soft tissues of the small pelvis. Most common are the so-called phleboliths, which represent calcified thrombi in vein branches (Fig. 376). They can vary in size from hardly perceptible to several millimeters in diameter. They may be single or multiple, unilateral or bilateral. They may be numerous on one side, single or entirely absent on the other. They usually have a fairly high calcium content and often have a concentric layer formation with less density centrally. It may sometimes be difficult to differentiate a ureteric stone from a phlebolith.

Calcifications are often seen in the prostatic gland in adults. These calcifications are irregular and may vary in size from very small to large conglomerates. The calcium content may vary and the size may be different on both sides. Sometimes prostatic calcifications are unilateral. Calcifications can sometimes be seen unilaterally or bilaterally in the vas deferens, the ampulla, and the seminal vesicle.

In adult females, calcifications of different size, calcium content, shape and number may be seen in the uterus, representing calcified necrotic myomas. Occasionally tooth-shaped calcifications can be seen, representing tooth anlage in a dermoid cyst. Such a cyst may also be so diagnosed because of a fat content which makes it absorb less radiation than does the surrounding area. The fluid content is occasionally partly fat, partly detritus with globulin and albumin fractions. In such cases a layer formation may be seen within the cyst at examination with horizontal beam (HELLMER, 1937). The dermoid cyst may also contain wall calcifications.

Calcifications in the walls of the pelvic arteries are common and present no diagnostic difficulties.

Calcified lymph glands may occasionally be seen.

Calcified appendices epiploicae from the bowel are not infrequently seen, and are usually single.

After lymphography, contrast filling of pelvic lymph glands may persist for a considerable length of time. Contrast filling of the appendix or part thereof and of single or multiple colon diverticula, small to very large in size, may be seen as residue after a barium examination of the GI tract.

Diagnostically important changes in the parts of the skeleton exposed in films of the bladder may be seen, changes such as metastases of prostatic carcinoma, changes in the sacro-iliac joints indicating ossifying pelvospondylitis, fresh and healed fractures, etc.

II. Urethrocystography

Urography in many instances is a very important examination in diseases of the bladder and the urethra because many pathological processes occur concomitantly in the upper and lower urinary tracts. Another reason is that disease in the lower urinary tract may affect the kidneys and the ureters secondarily through blockage of urinary flow, for example. Urography is often therefore the basic method in lesions of the lower urinary tract. The examination includes close study of the bladder in suitable projections, with suitable penetration of the radiation, and suitable degree of filling of the bladder. Micturition urethrography may also be performed in connection with urography.

The most common method of examination of the bladder and the urethra, however, is contrast filling, usually by the injection of contrast medium through the external urethral orifice. As the bladder and the urethra are usually examined in the same session, the method is most often called urethrocystography or cystourethrography.

The first publication on roentgenologic examination of the urethra was written by CUNNINGHAM in 1910. He used a 50% argyrol solution as a contrast medium in order to demonstrate strictures in the anterior part of the urethra.

Detailed anatomic studies of the entire urethra were made in the years 1921 (HOWDIECK et al.) and 1922 (BECLAIR and HENRY, JANSSEN). Since that time a very large number of papers and monographs on urethrocystography have appeared with the introduction of new contrast media, presentation of new observations, and attempts to define techniques and indications (see, for example, monographs by KNUTSSON, 1935 and EDLING 1945). This has led to adoption, in this field also, of basic roentgenologic principles with the roentgenologist taking full responsibility for the examination, the application of examination techniques with variations necessary to the study and demonstration of normal anatomy and physiology and the use of this knowledge in the study and documentation of pathologic conditions.

New recording techniques have come into wide use in this process, such as fluoroscopy using image intensification, cine-radiography, and rapid sequence image intensifying fluorography. The use of image intensification permits considerable reduction of the radiation dose, which is of particular importance in the examination of organs directly related to the genital glands. The genital glands may be directly exposed to radiation, or at least to a large amount of scattered radiation, in spite of close collimation, practically always in females and very often in males. The fluoroscopic dose can generally be reduced by a factor of 10 through the use of image intensification, as compared to conventional fluoroscopy. Recording with image intensifying fluorography, as demonstrated by KAUDE et al. (1969) can reduce dose to 10—30 % of that used in conventional radiography.

The least suitable method seems to be cine recording. High radiation dose in combination with poor resolution is the reason. This method should therefore be used only exceptionally, as should videotape recording.

Technique of examination

a) Instrumentation

The contrast medium is injected into the external urethral orifice through a cannula with a cone-shaped mouthpiece. This mouthpiece is introduced into the urethra and secured by a penis clamp (KNUTSSON, 1929, 1935).

A special appliance originally intended for urethrography in females was devised by KJELLMAN in 1952. This instrument is constructed on the principle of suction for adherence to the mucuous membrane surrounding the orifice of the urethra in the female. A catheter may be used instead in patients with hypospadia. An instrument designed by GULLMO in 1956 has been found to be very useful in cases of hypospadia and of urethral fistula. It contains a set of syringe cannulae with a terminal cone ranging in diameter from 2.5 to 11 mm. The cannulae are chosen to fit firmly the opening of the urethra. Occasionally, especially in children, the contrast medium may be introduced into the bladder through a thin catheter.

A special method to expand the posterior urethra has been designed by GULLMO and SUNDBERG (1957) They use a three-channel catheter with an inflatable balloon which cuts off the posterior part of the urethra. The anterior part is occluded by tying a thin rubber tubing around the root of the penis. One of the channels in the catheter is used for draining the urinary bladder, one is used to inflate the balloon, and the third for the injection of the contrast medium. A good filling of the posterior part of the urethra may be obtained with this method. In addition, a good filling of the prostatic utricle can be secured, as can a good filling of the prostatic ducts.

Antegrade cystourethrography can be performed through injection of contrast medium often through percutaneous puncture of a dilated bladder, or via a bladder fistula or a cystostomy.

b) Contrast medium

Iodized oil was used for many years as contrast medium for injection into the urethra. This type of contrast medium is now completely abandoned because of the risk of fat embolism through urethro-cavernous reflux. Thorotrast has also been used. The risk of spreading this medium via the blood stream is obvious, with the danger of storage in reticulo-endothelial elements and other types of retention of this radio-active substance in the body.

Some authors recommend barium suspension as a contrast medium in order to obtain high absorption. The disadvantages of this type of medium are obvious for many reasons. STENSTRÖM and ELO (1971), for example, report on three cases of nephrobarinosis observed after urethrocystography with a barium sulphate suspension. The reflux to the kidneys of the barium sulphate suspension could cause deposition of barium in the renal parenchyma out under the capsule. In one case the reflux contributed to a serious episode of infection which after one year led to renal atrophy.

The commonly used contrast media are water-soluble media of the type used in urography, occasionally slightly modified for this specific use. The medium is often marketed in instillation bottles, the contents of which should be used for only one patient.

General reactions and counter-indications are the same as those described in the earlier chapter on contrast media in urography.

As some water-soluble media may have a slightly irritating effect on the mucosa, the injection of such a medium should be preceded by application of a local surface anesthetic. KJELLBERG et al. recommend the use of an injection of 5—10 cc of Xylocain gel (Astra, Sweden) into the urethra in order to prevent the discomfort caused by the introduction of the catheter in boy patients. The medium also acts as a lubricant for the catheter.

MORALES and HEIWINKEL (1948) designed a medium using carboxy-methyl-cellulose, in order to increase the viscosity of water-soluble media. The medium, Umbradil Viscous U (Astra, Sweden), was a development of Vasco-Reopaque (Hoffmann-Laroche, Switzerland) in which a combination of the contrast medium with polyvinyl alcohol caused increased viscosity. One of the advantages of increased viscosity is considered to be a distention of the posterior part of the urethra because in injection the turbulence of the contrast fluid is eliminated. However, the resistance is great, and the injection pressure high. As the velocity is nevertheless low, the pressure against the urethral wall will be high, causing expansion of the lumen (MORALES and ROMANUS, 1952).

c) Roentgen anatomy of the bladder

The base of the bladder has a triangular surface between the ureteric openings laterally and the urethral orifice caudally. Between the ureteric orifices the interureteric ridge projects into the bladder. The vertex of the bladder is connected with the fibrous remainder of the urachus. The part between the fundus and the vertex is called the corpus of the bladder.

The bladder is localized in the small pelvis but upon filling rises into the abdomen. The greater part of the bladder is in contact with the pelvic floor and the anterior abdominal wall. Muscle fascicles continue from the bladder to adjacent structures. The bladder is only cranially and posteriorly covered by the peritoneum and by a subperitoneal fatty layer.

As described above, in plain films of the small pelvis the upper part of the bladder is usually well seen because of its delineation through the subperitoneal fatty layer. In females the corpus of the uterus can usually be seen also, together with the connection between it and the bladder.

Phleboliths are often seen, single or multiple, large or small, unilateral or bilateral, in all variations.

Prostatic calcifications, large or small, usually irregular and bilateral but occasionally unilateral, are often seen, and are seen regularly in elderly patients.

Calcification in the vasa deferentia is common in diabetic patients. It has been shown by KING and ROSENBAUM (1971) that the onset of radiographically visible calcium deposition in the vasa occur usually ten years later in non-diabetic men than in patients with diabetes.

When the bladder is covered by extraperitoneal fat, the thickness of the bladder wall can be estimated, as it can also when perivesical pneumography is performed. The normal bladder wall thickness is approximately 3 mm at moderate distention.

With the method designed by KJELLBERG et al. (1957) for urethrocystography during voiding, it is possible to study the shape of the bladder and the change in shape and size when the detrusor function is in operation.

A thorough study of micturition in normal women, using urethrocystography and simultaneous pressure flow measurements, was made by PALM (1971). He found that the bladder changed its shape during the transition from resting to activity, becoming more circular. At the same time a serrated mucosal relief appeared from the inter-ureteric crest upwards to the vertex. The descent of the bladder during micturition was expressed by the urethral inclination angle in relation to the horizontal plane. It decreased averagely from 40^0 at rest to 28^0 during maximum flow. In cases of urinary tract disease fractionated micturition was often found, with obstructions of functional nature, presumably due to deficiency in or absence of relaxation of the external sphincter. The most characteristic hydrodynamic and radiographic features were found when an organic obstruction was present in the urethra. This was very rare, however.

At cystography, the bladder when moderately filled has an oval shape and a slightly irregular contour caused by the normal bladder mucosa. The uterus, the rectum, and other parts of the bowel may cause impressions in the normal bladder wall.

d) Roentgen anatomy of the urethra

The posterior part of the urethra is related to the pelvic musculature consisting of the musculi levatores ani and the musculus coccygeus. The levator ani is above the urogenital diaphragm which stretches across the pubic arch.

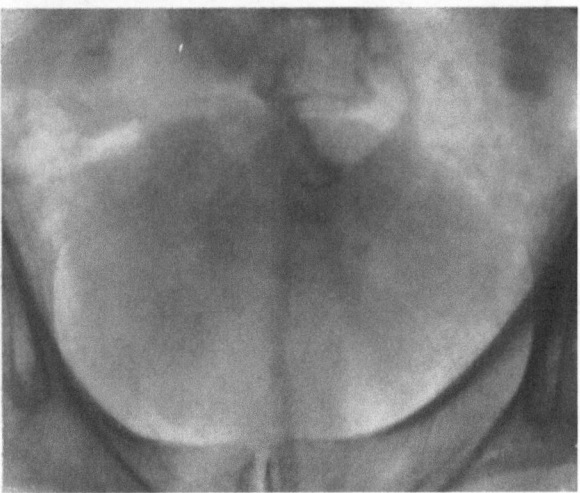

Fig. 375. Plain roentgenogram illustrating the urinary bladder with approximately 200 ml of residual urine

The male urethra has its bladder orifice behind and slightly below the upper part of the pubic symphysis. It is located slightly anterior to the center of the base plate of the bladder, the posterior part of which is the trigon. The muscle layers in the base of the bladder are intimately connected with the layers in the posterior part of the urethra, forming a single anatomical unit. The relationship of smooth and striated musculature is described in detail by MORALES and ROMANUS (1953) and by SHOPFNER (1967) and HUTCH (1968).

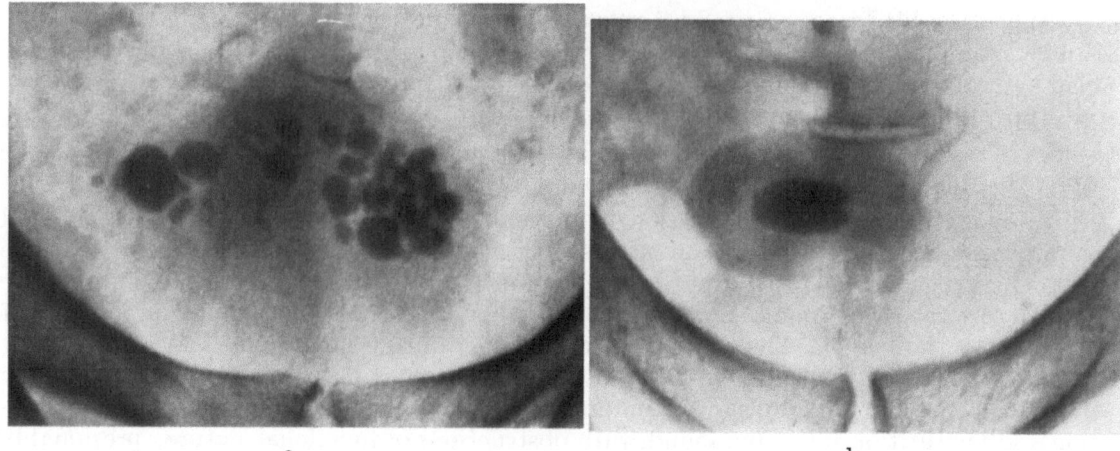

a   b

Fig. 376. a) Multiple phosphate stones in the bladder. b) Bladder stone with a center of calcium oxalate and a
periphery of trippelphosphate

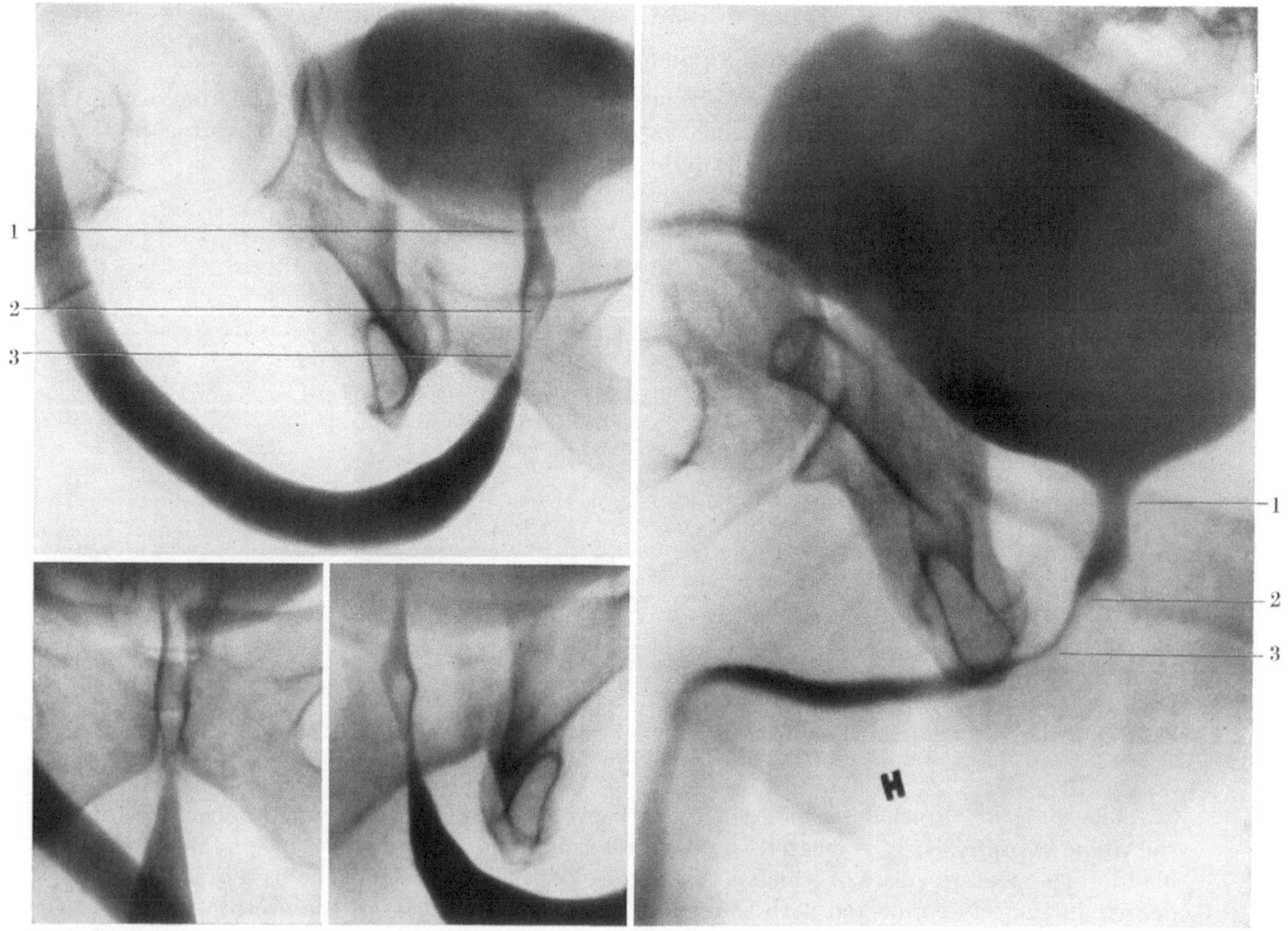

Fig. 377. Normal urethrocystography in man (1 Uro-genital internal sphincter, 2 Colliculus, 3 External sphinkter)

Upon micturition, near the end of the voiding period a trigonal canal is often created by the base of the bladder and its continuation in the urethra. The cysto-urethral junction has a diameter varying in relation to several factors, such as age, sex, stage of voiding, etc. The diameter is wider in girls than in boys.

From the internal sphincter the prostatic urethra, approximately 3—3$^1/_2$ cm in length and slightly concave anteriorly, descends through the anterior part of the prostatic gland. In the posterior part, the verumontanum or the seminal collicle projects into the lumen with a length of 10—12 mm and a width of 3—4 mm, with a groove (the prostatic sinus) at each side. The prostatic urethra is usually divided into the supracollicular, the collicular, and the infracollicular portions.

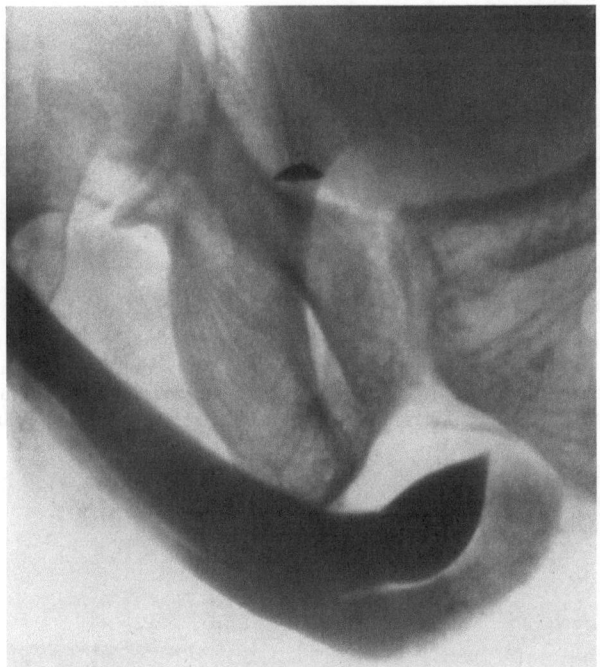

Fig. 378. Urethrocavernous reflux from a rupture at the external orifice

The openings of the ejaculatory ducts from the seminal vesicles are localized on the seminal colliculus, immediately above the posterior part of the prostatic gland. The portion of the prostate between the supracollicular urethra and the ejaculatory ducts is called the middle lobe and the part in the area under the ducts is called the posterior lobe. The remaining part of the prostate is composed of two lateral lobes.

The prostatic gland is composed of tubular glands with ducts — 20 to 30 in number — opening laterally to the colliculus in the prostatic sinus. Where the smooth muscles from the bladder onto the urethra above the urogenital diaphragm unite with the striated muscles from below, an incisure is formed, usually only anteriorly but occasionally circular and of varying depth and position.

Distal to the prostatic urethra, the membranaceous part continues, piercing the urogenital diaphragm as a short and narrow segment. In the midline behind and above the collicle, contrast filling may be seen of an oval, regular, shallow cavity which represents the utriculus prostaticus (See Fig. 380b). This may dilate, a phenomenon often seen in patients with chronic prostatovesiculitis.

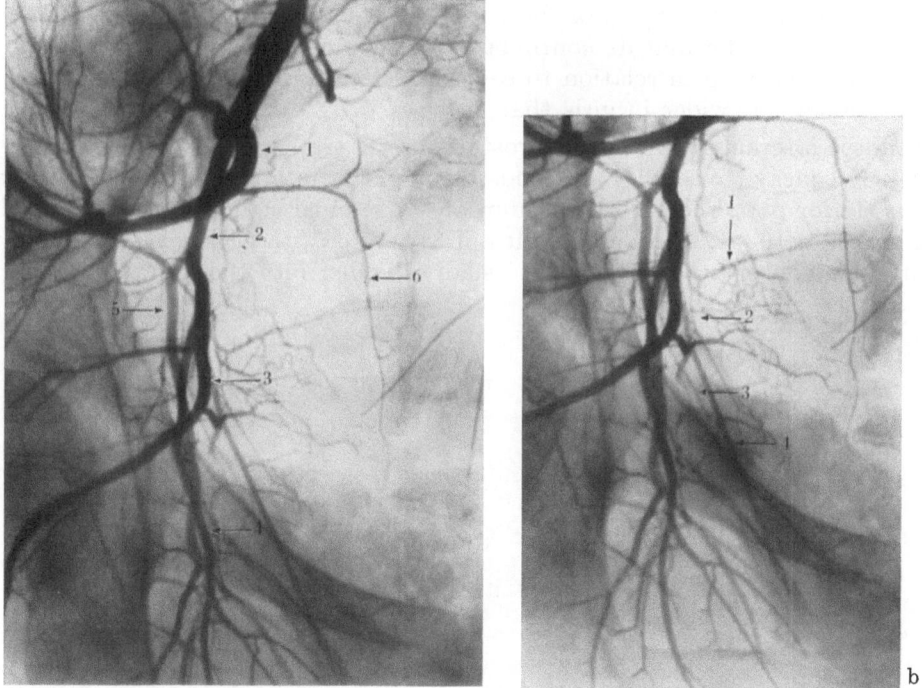

Fig. 379. Angiography with barium sulphate during autopsy demonstrating normal roentgen anatomy of iliac arteries and branches. a) 1) superior gluteal artery. 2) Truncus pudendo glutealis which divides in the inferior gluteal artery and the internal pudendal artery 3) and 4). b) Same preparation. 1) Superior vesical artery with a caudally directed branch (2). 3) Distal part of inferior vesical artery. 4) Distal part of hemorrhoidal artery

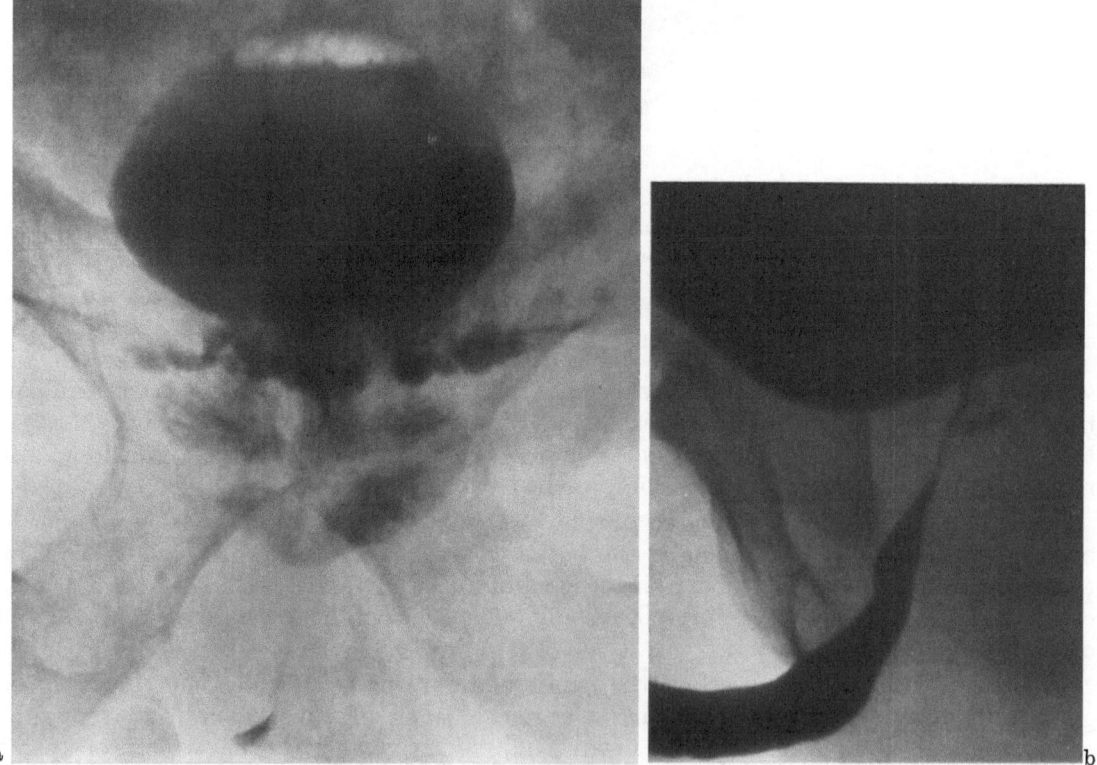

Fig. 380. a) Filling of prostatic ducts and ejaculatory ducts during urethrocystography. b) Filling of prostatic utricle

The cavernous part, 12—15 cm in length, follows and ends in the fossa navicularis. It consists in the pars bulbosa and the pars pendula. Ligamentum suspensorium penis may cause an angulation of the pars pendula urethrae.

The urethra is closed except during the passage of fluid.

A great number of small Littrés' glands open into the urethral lumen in the membranous part and the posterior and anterior parts of the cavernous urethra, where the urethral lacunae of Morgagni also open.

Two small bodies, the Cowperian glands or the bulbo-urethral glands, are localized laterally to and behind the membranous part of the urethra, with 2—3 cm-long excretory ducts opening into the urethra (see Fig. 391). Sometimes the sinus de Guèrin is filled as a thin canal in the dorsal aspect of the anterior part of the urethra.

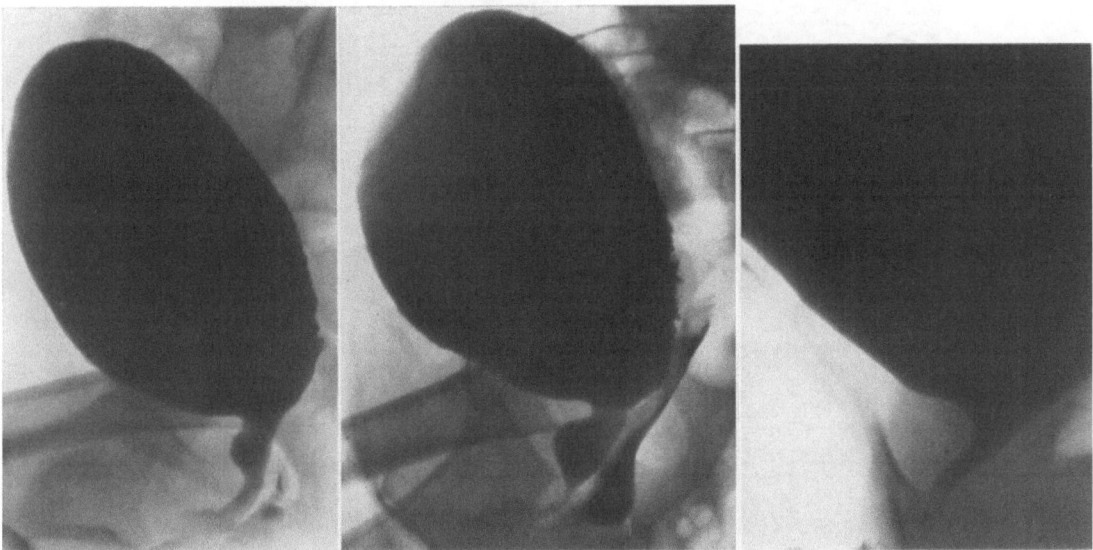

Fig. 381. Different shapes of normal urethra in young girls

During the injection of contrast medium, if this takes place through a cannula attached to the external orifice, the anterior and membranaceous parts of the urethra open and are to some extent distended by the resistance caused by the contracted musculature surrounding the prostatic urethra. This part thus has a narrow lumen. Therefore examination during voiding is very important in order to study, in addition, the normal conditions in this part.

At the proximal end of the cavernous part of the urethra, the bulbocavernosus (or bulbospongiosus) muscle may cause transient narrowing of the urethral lumen by contraction. Such contractions are normal and last usually only a short moment (CURANINO, 1970). There are great variations in the anatomic landmarks mentioned above. These are absent in some patients and the urethra is a straight, tapered tube. The landmarks are only partly influenced by the degree of distention.

The width of the urethra varies greatly and can be considerable without the presence of distal obstruction (SHOPFNER and HUTCH).

The female urethra has a close similarity to the prostatic and membranaceous urethra in the male, except of course for anatomic details such as the verumontanum. It has a length of 3 to 4 cm and is slightly concave anteriorly. It has several urethral lacunae in its proximal part. It is very short from the urogenital diaphragm to its opening, forming the distal urethral segment. The close relation between the distal opening and vagina makes urethrovaginal reflux of contrast medium a common occurrence during urethrocystography (Figs. 381 and 382).

A local widening can occasionally be seen in the distal part of the urethra in girls, immediately inside the meatus. Here the urethra can be fairly wide, indicating a stenosis of the meatus. In these cases an increased pressure is often found in the bladder. During micturition, however, the meatus is seen to widen considerably and this anatomic variation usually disappears spontaneously.

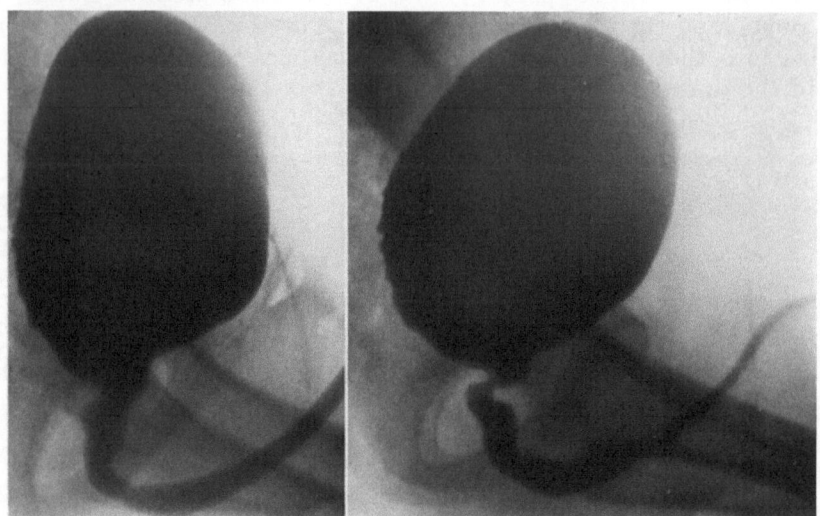

Fig. 382. Different shapes of normal urethra in young boys

e) Performance of the examination

The patient's rectum is first emptied by enema or by other useful means. The patient is told to empty his bladder; otherwise catheterization is employed, with subsequent emptying. Plain films are taken of the bladder and in some cases also of the penis. The area of the urethral orifice is rinsed and the instrument is adjusted as described above. The surface anesthetic is injected into the anterior part of the urethra. Contrast medium is injected after a few minutes, preferably under fluoroscopic control. We usually inject 300 ml of contrast medium of moderate density and after this 20 ml of viscous contrast medium to fill the urethra. The patient is told to relax completely and not to strain. Films are taken in suitable projections when the contrast medium has filled the urethral lumen. Further injection of contrast medium is made, followed by sterilized water to fill the bladder and produce micturition, or to facilitate it. The patient is then told to urinate. During micturition recording in suitable projections is made of the bladder and the urethra.

Specific problems call for modifications of this procedure in order to facilitate close study of certain anatomic and physiologic details.

Before urethrocystography for demonstration of the prostatic gland, massage of this gland may be useful to empty the gland of mucus and pus.

Some patients have difficulty in starting micturition because of psychological inhibitions. To help the patient overcome this difficulty he should be left alone in the examination room and well screened in the room, with the lights dimmed and a water faucet running, if possible. During micturition recording is made with multiple films or, better still, with photofluorography over an image intensifier. Videotape recording or cinefluorography may occasionally be used.

In the study of the bladder, a suitable concentration of the contrast medium is necessary and the penetration of the radiation should be chosen to match the contrast density. Compression of the type dosed compression can be used by inserting a palpator into the rectum (OLLE OLSSON, 1948).

In order to study the patency of the ureteric orifices and to be able to diagnose possible reflux from the bladder into one or both ureters, the patient should be examined in supine position, preferably, with the upper part of the body lowered. Fluoroscopic observation and filming should be made during micturition. Fluoroscopic monitoring of the procedure makes it possible to obtain complete filling of the bladder in order to observe vesico-ureteral reflux and to choose correct projections for documentation of normal and pathologic conditions.

It is important to perform the examination with relation to existing clinical problems. The procedure should be limited to this consideration, particularly in checking results of therapy.

A detailed description of urethrocystographic techniques is given by KNUTSSON, 1935; EDLING, 1945; LINDBLOM and ROMANUS, 1962).

f) Supplementary methods

1. Double contrast cystography

In order to demonstrate more clearly tumors bulging into the lumen of the bladder, the use of double contrast cystography has been advocated (KNEISE and SCHOBER, 1941; BARTLEY and HELÁNDER, 1960, etc.). A small amount (8—10 cc) of a viscous water-soluble contrast medium is injected into the emptied bladder, with the patient in supine position. The contrast medium will coat the bladder mucosa when the injection is followed by an injection of 200—300 cc of CO_2 via a catheter into the bladder. Recording is made with suitable projections for the study of the base of the bladder. BARTLEY and HELANDER recommend a special projection: an axial view of the pelvic inlet is taken perpendicularly to the base, since the plane of the base is roughly parallel with the pelvic inlet. The patient is semi-recumbent and the beam vertical.

2. Perivesical pneumography

In order to study the thickness of the bladder wall and possible perivesical tumor growth, injection of water-soluble contrast medium into the perivesical space has been used in a few instances (FRANKSSON and LINDBLOM, 1952). Injection of gas into this space is more common (for example: TRUK et al., 1951; BARTLEY and ECKERBOM, 1960). An injection needle is introduced above the symphysis, directed caudally and dorsally. Its tip should lie approximately 1 cm behind and below the upper border of the symphysis and its position should be checked. After it has been made clear that the needle has not entered a blood vessel, 700—800 ml of CO_2 is injected and the patient is placed in various positions in order to let the gas penetrate around the bladder. Carbon dioxide is then injected into the bladder until the patient experiences a desire to void, and at that point recording is made.

3. Chain urethrocystography

A special modification of cystourethrography represents the method for chain cystourethrography. A beaded metal chain is used in this modification. The chain is about 20 cm long and lubricated and is passed into the bladder. It is placed in the bottom of the bladder and in the urethra. The posterior urethrovesical angle can then be measured in suitable projections and the descent of the bladder during straining can be appreciated. STOLZ and FOGEL (1972) describe two significant urethro-vesical abnormalities associated with stress incontinence. In Type I the posterior urethro-vesical angle is greater than 100° and the upper urethral angle is normal, with minimum descent of the bladder. In Type II the angle, the upper urethral axis angle, and the descent of the bladder are all normal.

g) Urethrocystography in children

Urethrocystography is often indicated in children. A comprehensive description of the urethrocystographic technique in child patients is given by KJELLBERG *et al.* (1957) and in great detail by SHOPFNER (1971). The main points include skill in performance in order to eliminate technical faults which can otherwise make repeat examinations necessary. An important aspect of the examination technique is immobilization of the patient. According to SHOPFNER this can be accomplished by bandaging the child to a specially designed board. With the help of trained personnel (observe the rules for radiation protection!) the small patient fixed to this board can easily be brought into positions suitable for recording.

A special technique for micturition cystography in children has been devised by BRÜNDORF *et al.* (1960), applicable mainly to children in the post-natal period and early infancy. The patient is made to urinate during the examination by continuous filling of the bladder with contrast medium through a catheter inserted into the bladder by the suprapubic route. This suprapubic catheterization also makes it possible to combine the roentgenologic examination with micturition cystometry (BRÜNDORF and SANDÖE, 1960).

It can occasionally be useful to inject doryl or prostigmin subcutaneously in order to obtain micturition films in newborn children. A sufficient dose during the first months of life is 0.3 cc = 0.08 mg carbacholum or 0.17 mg neostigmin bromide (JORUP and KJELLBERG, 1948).

Handling of children by trained personnel and provision of quiet and comfortable surroundings usually make it possible to perform the examination without great difficulty and without resort to procedures of the type described above.

h) Complications

Upon injection of contrast medium, a tear may develop in the mucosa and the contrast medium may pass through the submucosal veins of the corpus cavernosum and further into the venous system. Such urethro-cavernous reflux may vary in volume from very little to great and may markedly impair study of the recordings. The reflux usually causes no subjective symptoms. Occasionally, however, a slight rise in temperature may be observed some hours after the procedure and may persist for a few hours. Symptoms of hypersensitivity to the constrast medium may also be seen.

It is pointed out by MORALES and ROMANUS (1953) that between the mucosa in the urethra and the cavernous tissue there is an interposed layer of an easily compressible venous vasculature, the so-called pseudocavernous tissue. Bleeding from this tissue easily occurs in connection with mucosal lesions; this phenomenon may also explain the fact that venous reflux can also easily occur in association with urethrocystography.

EDLING (1945) has given close consideration to the possibility of stricture formation in the urethra after urethrocystography but has found no case in which the procedure, as such, caused or increased existing strictures.

III. Angiography of the bladder

A close study of the anatomy and the roentgen anatomy in cadaveric specimens and in clinical angiographic examinations of the arterial supply of the bladder was made by NILSSON (1967) in our department. In his monograph NILSSON also reviews previous studies. The following represents a summary of his observations.

1. Roentgen anatomy of the arterial supply of the bladder
(Fig. 379)

The internal iliac artery has its origin between 10 and 16 cm above the upper border of the symphysis, as measured in the films. The individual variations are great but the difference between the sides in a given patient is smaller than that between patients.

The superior gluteal artery is the largest of the branches given off by the internal iliac artery. It divides into a large number of branches running to the gluteal region. One branch is of importance in angiography of the bladder, viz. one branch situated in the pelvis running in caudal direction and called the lateral sacral artery.

The inferior gluteal artery arises from the pudendal gluteal trunk or a gluteal trunk of varying length. This artery is of significance in angiography of the bladder because the artery or its branches supplying muscles can be projected over the bladder, making it difficult to study bladder arteries. From the inferior gluteal artery no vesical arteries arise. The internal pudendal artery starts most frequently in a common trunk together with the inferior gluteal artery, the pudendal gluteal trunk. These three arteries as well as the two trunks can be readily identified. They are of varying length and have marked differences in their courses, from one patient to another, as well as between the two sides in patients examined bilaterally.

After leaving the pelvic cavity, the inferior gluteal artery continues on a lateral, caudal course, with the internal pudendal artery running anteriorly, caudally and medially. It then returns to the inside of the pelvic wall through the lesser sciatic foramen. This part of the artery is situated on the inside of the pelvic wall but outside the pelvic cavity.

The iliolumbar and the lateral sacral arteries are also readily identifiable, as is the obturator artery. The lateral sacral artery regularly anastomoses with the middle sacral artery and with the lateral sacral artery of the other side. The obturator artery running to the obturator canal is best seen in oblique projections because of its anteriorly directed course.

The superior and inferior vesical arteries are usually easily recognizable. They run a downward course along the lateral pelvic wall with the superior vesical artery usually more medially.

The bladder arteries are best seen in the bladder wall if the bladder is moderately distended, which is best brought about by injection of carbon dioxide into the bladder.

A close study of the pelvic veins has been made by BARTLEY (1958), who advocates the use of flebography in the diagnosis of pelvic tumors. Only occasionally, however, do tumors of the bladder call for this type of study. A case has been described by CARLSSON and GARSTEN (1960) in which the femoral vein was compressed by a markedly dilated bladder.

2. Technique

The best technique for angiography of the bladder is percutaneous transfemoral catheterization with selective catheterization of the internal iliac artery, possibly bilaterally. A non-selective examination may be performed only if this technique proves impossible, for example in the presence of advanced atheromatosis with tortuosity of the arteries and decreasing caliber locally.

(For details of technique see chapter on Renal Angiography).

C. Pathologic changes of the bladder, prostate and urethra

I. The Bladder

A combination of one or more of the types of pathological changes described below is not uncommon in the same patient at the same examination.

1. Anomalies

The bulges described above as variations in the normal shape of the bladder may be so marked as to indicate diverticula (Fig. 383). In congenital diverticula, as opposed to acquired diverticula, the bulges contain all the normal tissue layers of the bladder in their wall. (Lateral and bilateral diverticula give the bladder in frontal projection a shape

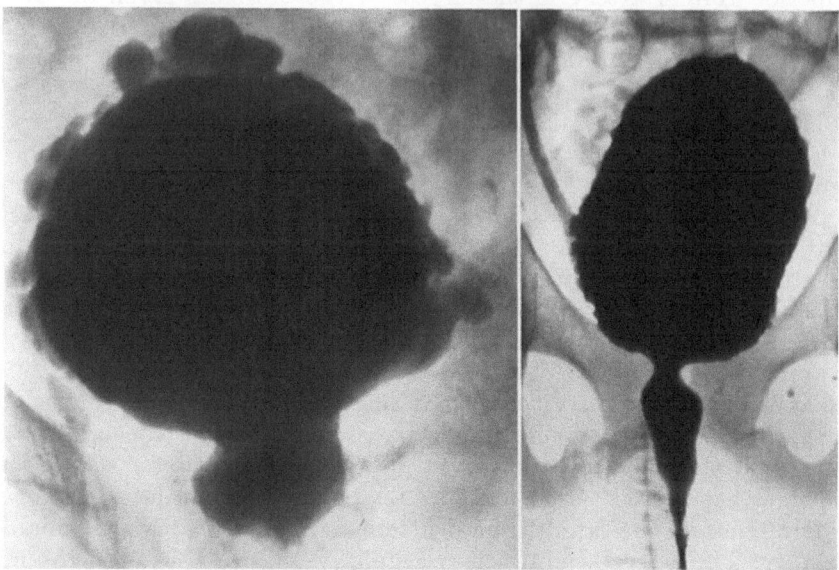

Fig. 383   Fig. 384

Fig. 383. Marked trabeculation of bladder with formation of multiple diverticula. Cause: hyperplasia of the prostatic gland. Prostatectomy performed

Fig. 384. Trabeculation of bladder and ureteric reflux on right side (girl nine years of age with recurrent urinary infection)

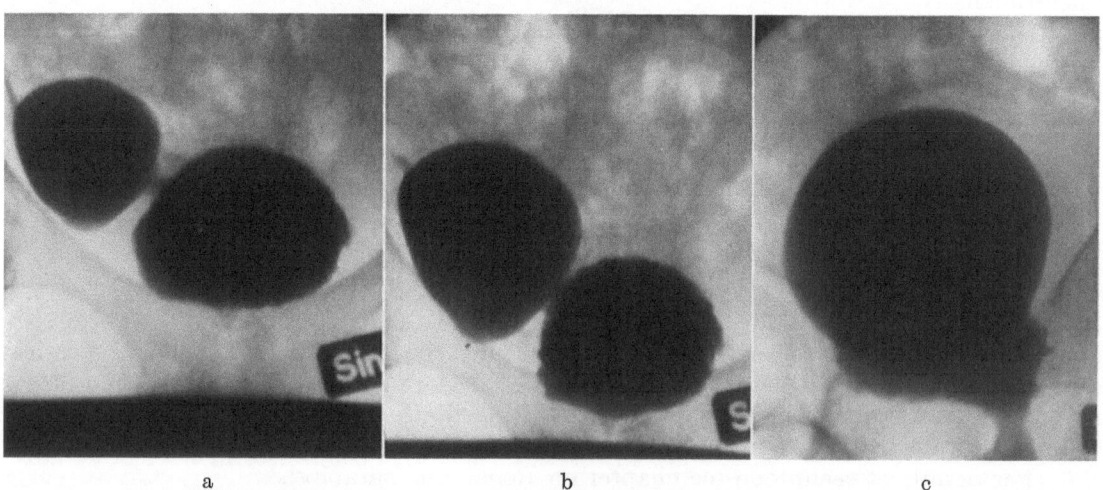

a   b   c

Fig. 385. a) Single bladder diverticulum to the right during micturition. b) and c) Marked increase in filling of diverticulum

which has caused roentgenologists lacking the basic sense of three-dimensional roentgenology to name the bladder "dog-eared bladder," "Mickey Mouse bladder," and other stupidities.) Sometimes there is no sharp division between diverticulosis and so-called trabeculation of the bladder wall (Fig. 384).

The diverticulum may change considerably in size during voiding (Fig. 385). A fibrous septum in the midline may divide the bladder into two compartments of approximately the same size, so-called bipartite bladder. Close to the ureters the bladder wall may bulge locally, causing para-ureteric diverticula.

a) Ectopia or extrophia vesicae

Ectopia or extrophia vesicae, also called inversio vesicae, is an inhibitory malformation in which the anterior part of the bladder and the anterior abdominal wall have not developed. The posterior part of the bladder opens therefore in the abdominal wall, the ureteric orifices lying free. Urethra is also often, in this malformation, an open groove on the dorsal side of the penis or the clitoris, so-called epispadia. The bony pelvis may be characteristically deformed, with a wider and malformed symphysis. Spina bifida may also be present.

b) Megalo bladder

Megalo bladder is often described as an anomaly. Enlargement of the bladder is usually due, however, to drainage difficulties or to neurogenic disorders.

c) Malposition

The bladder may be situated at a great depth or may be displaced downwards at straining (for example at micturition), occasionally to a marked degree, in cases of insufficiency of the floor of the small pelvis. An angulation of the urethra is seen in this connection. The condition is best demonstrable at examination of the patient in a standing position. The displacement may also be a partial herniation through an opening in the pelvic floor. The edge of this floor causes an indentation in the bladder. The part of the bladder distal to this narrowing must be regarded as a cystocele.

2. Displacement of the bladder

The bladder, when moderately filled, fills out the small pelvis to a great extent. Any expansive process engaging this space can impress or displace the bladder to some extent. Filling of the rectum with feces displaces the bladder ventrally and impresses its dorsal part, as do certain pathologic lesions in the sacrum, for example chordoma.

The bladder may be partly displaced into a hernia, laterally or caudally. The herniated part may be mobile and a reposition may follow a change in the patient's position.

The genital organs in females have a close relationship to the bladder and the normal uterus almost always impresses the bladder in its upper part, as can easily be seen on plain films. In tumors, marked impressions or displacement may be seen (Fig. 388). In pregnancy or when the uterus harbors myoma, for example, the impression is marked and can in the latter case be very irregular.

Edema or tumor in the pelvic floor may lift the bladder, as may hematoma, which can also cause marked compression locally or totally. A displacement downward is common in multiparae and a cystocele of part of the bladder may occur downwards in a separation between muscles forming the pelvic floor.

A cystocele of part of the bladder may also be caused by a suprapubic separation of the abdominal rectus muscles or, to a marked degree, by aplasia of these muscles (Fig. 387).

Skeletal changes in the pelvis may impress the bladder if they are expansive, for example in osteogenic tumor (Fig. 389). Displaced fractures, callus in such fractures, and protrusion in connection with hip-joint disease may also cause impressions. WATSON and OCHSNER (1966) report a case with marked compression of the bladder by large cysts emanating from the acetabulum as a result of chronic inflammation in rheumatoid arthritis of the hip joints. Wide and tortuous arteries may also impress the bladder (Fig. 386).

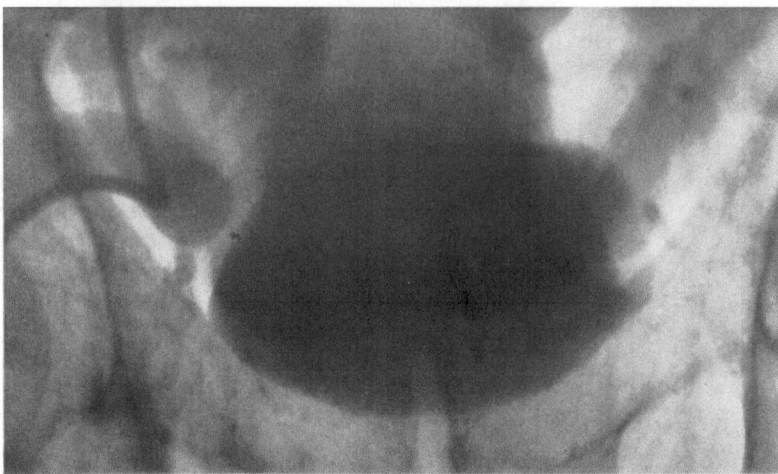

Fig. 386. Impression in bladder by markedly tortuous right iliac artery (with catheter and contrast medium in artery during angiography)

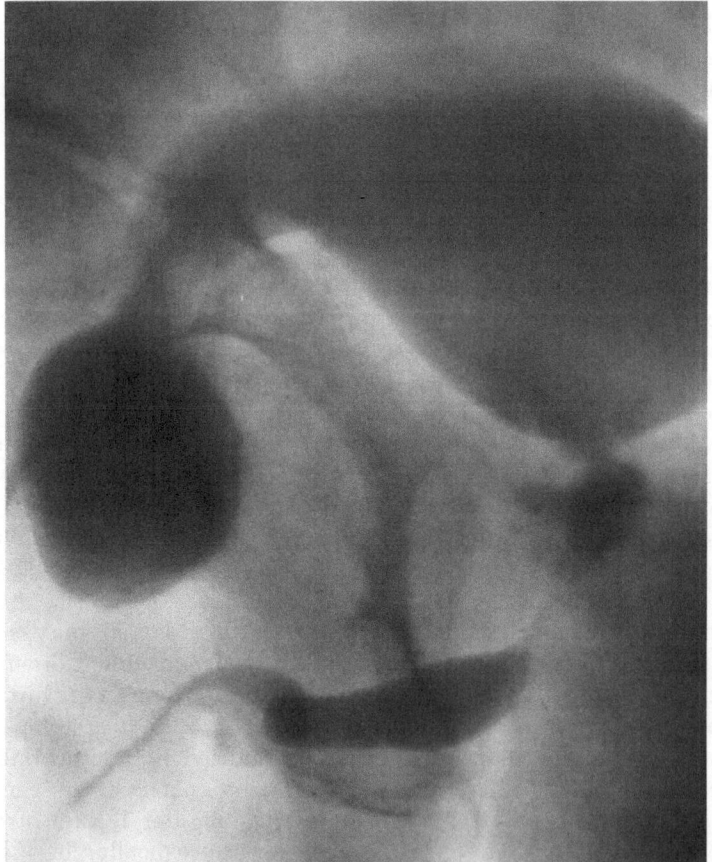

Fig. 387. Urethrocystography: cystocele of anterior part of bladder through gap in abdominal rectus muscles

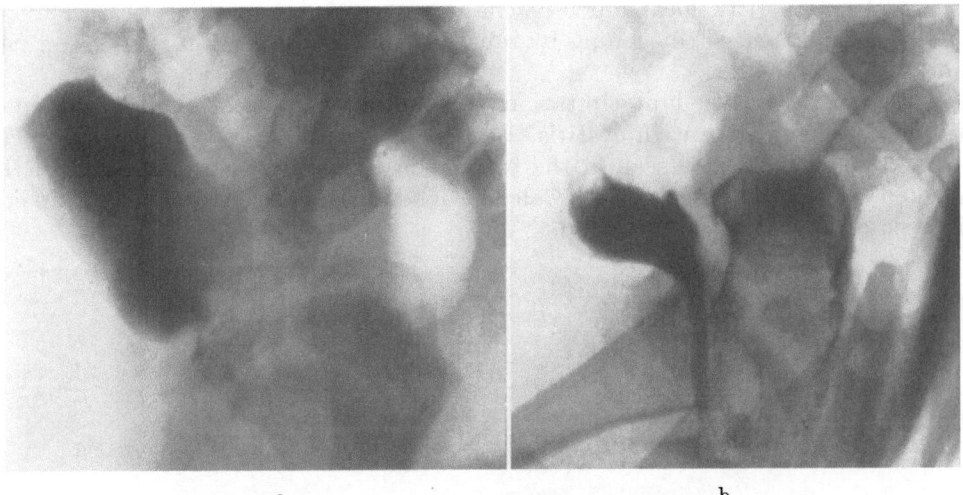

a   b

Fig. 388. a) Displacement of bladder and impression in posterior part by botryoid sarcoma in vagina. b) Contrast filling of bladder, urethra and vagina with tumor

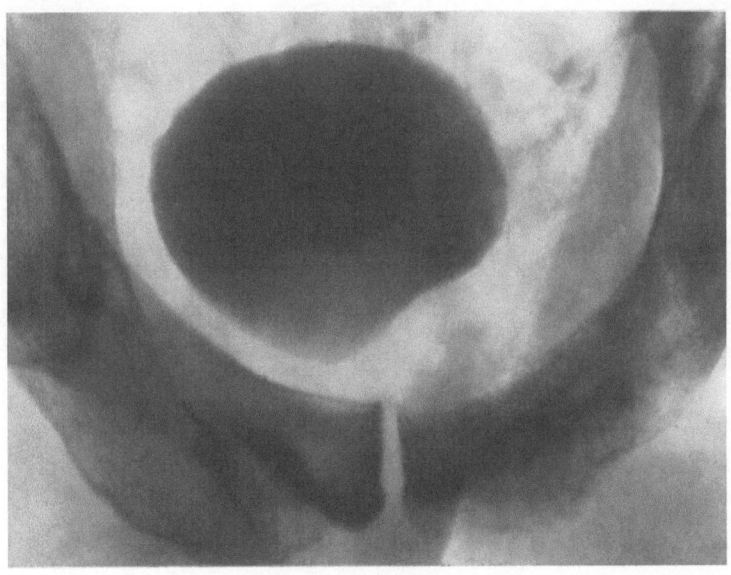

Fig. 389. Impression in left side of bladder base by non-calcified part of metastases in left part of pelvic bone by prostatic carcinoma

3. Infection

In acute cystitis the bladder mucosa may thicken and the contour of the contrast-filled bladder may be irregular (Fig. 390). In chronic cystitis a marked atrophy of the mucosa may, on the contrary, give the bladder a completely even outline. In cystitis, specific or non-specific, the size of the bladder may diminish, occasionally to a very marked degree. The wall of the bladder can increase in thickness very markedly. The contracted bladder may be very small and usually has a spherical shape. No distention of the lumen is obtainable at injection of contrast medium.

A marked asymmetry of the bladder may result from localized changes, for example in the case of tuberculous cystitis around a ureteric orifice. In specific and non-specific chronic localized cystitis, local mucosal changes may cause swelling of the mucosa by edema or locally increased thickening by inflammatory tissue, making the lesion resemble a tumor.

Generalized or localized precipitation of calcium may occasionally be seen in the bladder wall in connection with cystitis.

Marked changes may be seen in the bladder in bilharzia, with thickening of the wall and marked diminution of the lumen. Calcifications in the entire bladder wall are common in this type of infection.

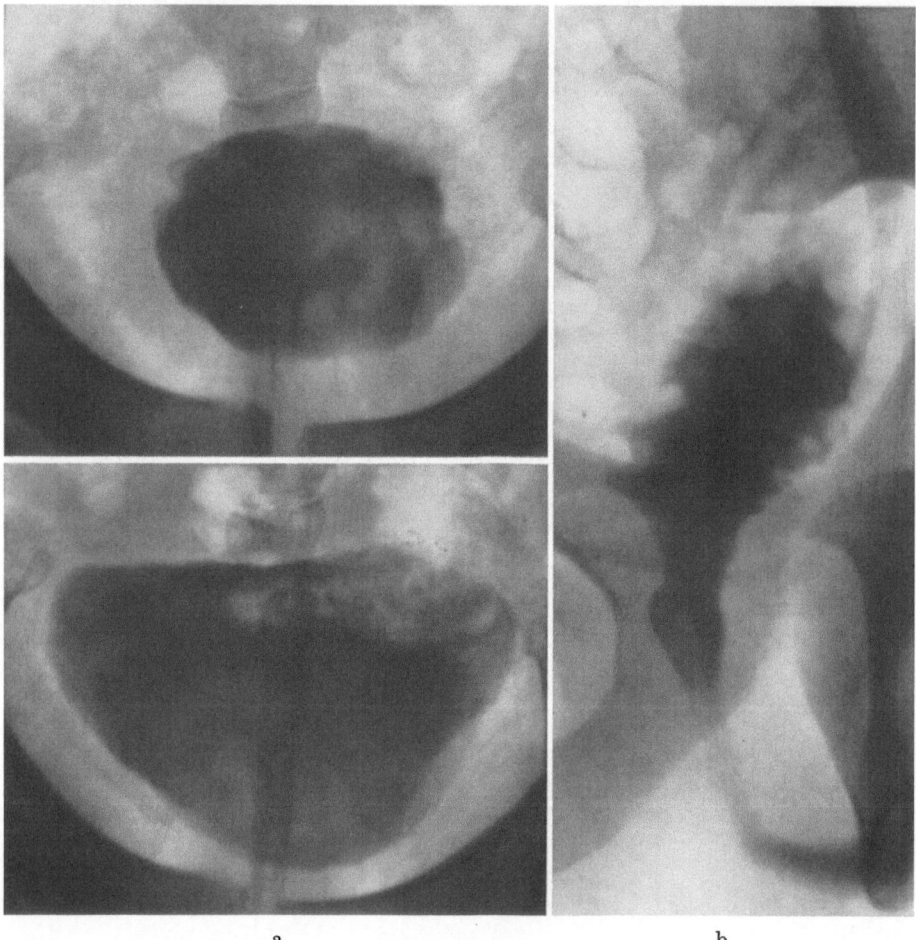

a   b

Fig. 390. Case of acute urogenital infection and Reiter's syndrome, appearing as a severe cystitis with hematuria. a) and b) during acute phase: marked swelling of bladder mucosa

Corresponding changes may be seen in so-called aseptic cystitis.

Irregular contractions in the bladder wall may occasionally be seen in connection with cystitis. KJELLBERG et al. (1957) report formation of a waist in the lower part of the bladder in the end stage of micturition in children suffering from cystitis, caused probably by an increased contraction of the bladder floor. An insufficient widening of the internal urethral orifice was also occasionally seen.

A special type of cystitis is represented by so-called *emphysematous cystitis*, in which gas is formed in the bladder wall (Fig. 391). This condition was first observed by EISEN-LOHR (1888) at autopsy. The first clinical observation was not made until 1932, when RAVICH and KATZEN reported on the observation of gas-filled vesicles in the bladder

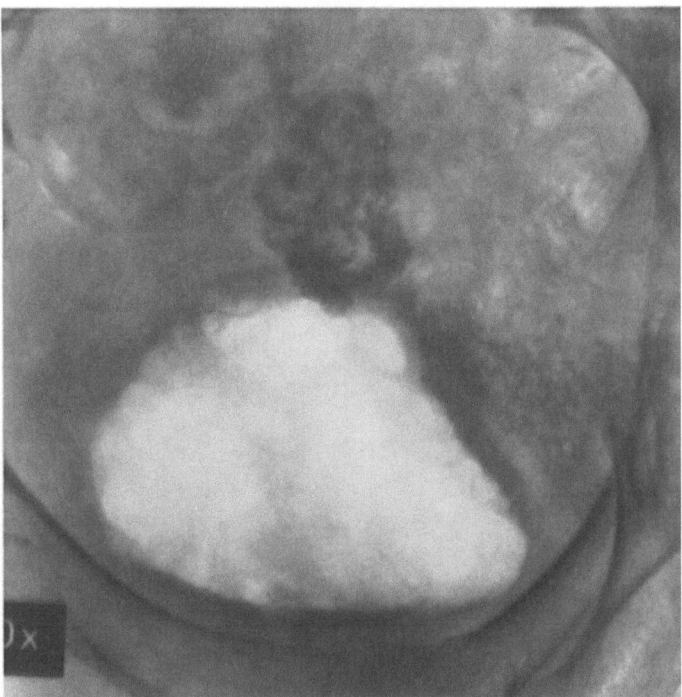

Fig. 391. Emphysematous cystitis. Gas-containing bullae throughout bladder mucosa; thickened bladder wall (above bladder: irregular, calcified necrotic myoma in uterus).

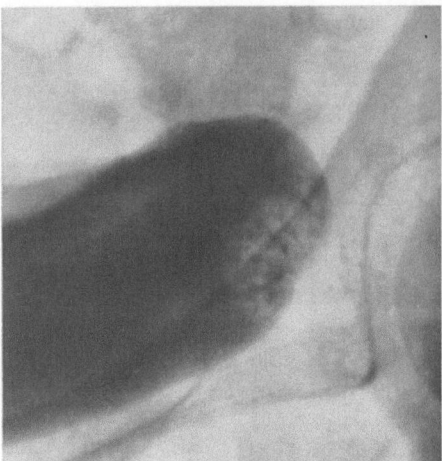

Fig. 392. Benign bladder papilloma without thickening of the wall at the base of the tumor

mucosa at cystotomy. The first report on roentgenologic diagnosis of emphysematous cystitis is that of LUND *et al.* in 1939. A comprehensive review was made by BOIJSEN and LEWIS-JONSSON (1954).

The cause of emphysematous cystitis is gas-forming bacteria. The vesicles are seen at plain roentgenography as gas bubbles in the bladder wall, the appearance corresponding to the stage of the disease at the time of examination. Gas appears in the early stage in a millimeter-wide zone in the bladder wall. The wall later becomes thick and a great number of gas-filled vesicles can be seen intramurally. These vesicles may rupture and freed gas in the lumen of the bladder can then be seen best with the patient in lateral decubitus with horizontal ray, or in a standing position with horizontal ray.

4. Tumors

Bladder tumors are the most common among tumors of the urinary tract. The indication for roentgen examination is hematuria. Cystoscopy has often been performed before the roentgen examination because of this hematuria, and a bladder tumor has been

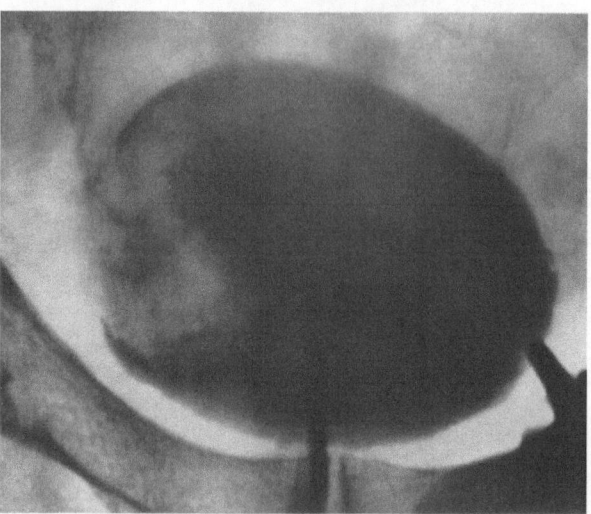

Fig. 393. Broadly based tumor with a nodular surface and thickened wall at base of tumor as sign of malignancy

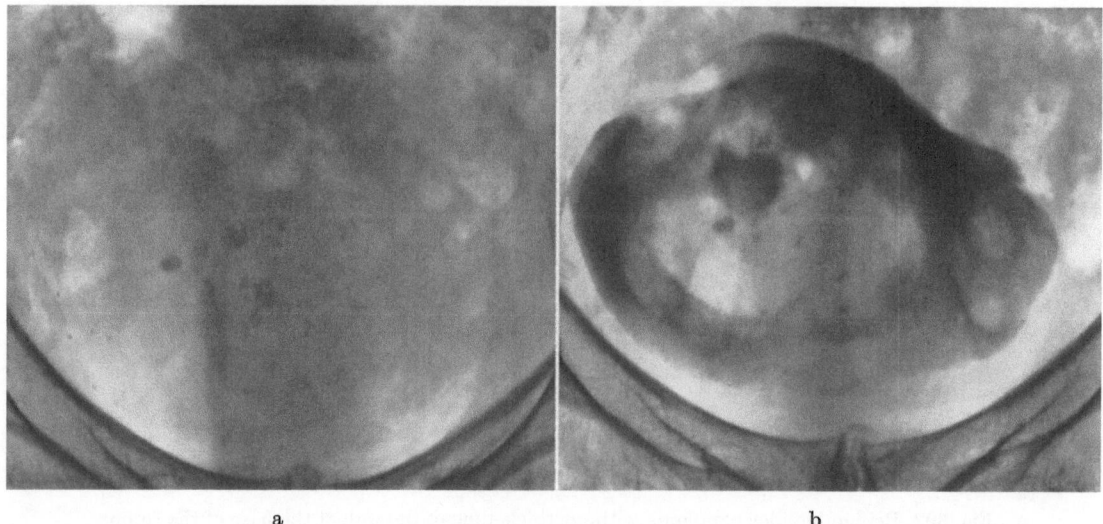

a   b

Fig. 394. Bladder tumor, mucus producing adenocarcinoma, with calcifications a) Plain roentgenogram, b) urography: irregular tumor filling great part of bladder. Cranially to the right, broad attachment of tumor to bladder wall

seen or suspected. The cystoscopist is sometimes in doubt as to whether an infiltrating carcinoma or a marked localized cystitis is present.

The important tumors of the bladder are the benign or malignant papilloma and the solid carcinoma.

As a general rule tumors of the urinary tract are often multiple, with sites in the different parts of the urinary tract, for example in the kidney pelvis and/or the ureter and in the bladder. It is necessary to keep in mind also that the tumors seen in the bladder wall may represent a secondary invasion onto the bladder from a tumor originating outside the bladder, for example a carcinoma of the colon.

Another feature that it is necessary that the roentgenologist be aware of is that dilatation of the urinary tract, unilateral or bilateral, may be secondary to a bladder tumor.

A tumor is seldom observed in plain films of the bladder, Calcifications in bladder tumors are very rare (see. Fig. 394).

A papillomatous tumor is seen at cystography, usually in connection with urography, as a local bulge from the bladder wall (Fig. 392). It is necessary to secure tangential projections of the tumor to demonstrate size and attachment to the bladder wall. It must be remembered that tumors of this type may be multiple. In papillary tumors the papillomatous surface is often well demonstrable as a more or less regular radiation of the surface. A stalk may occasionally be demonstrable.

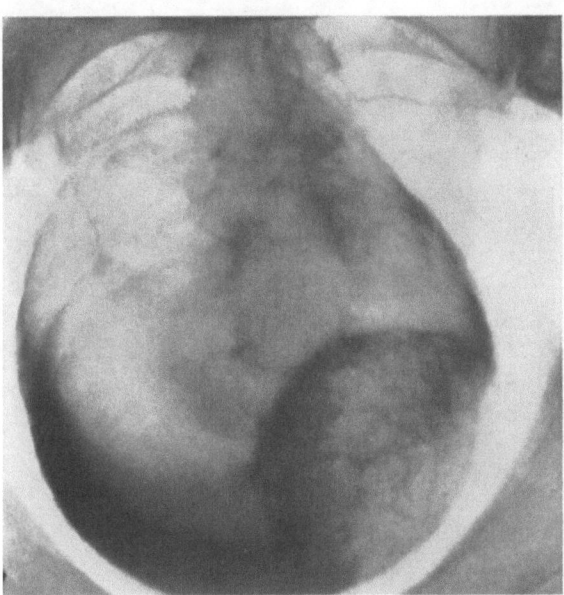

Fig. 395. Tumor and coagulum in bladder. Broadly based tumor with nodular surface basally to the left in bladder. Large coagulum fills rest of bladder

The intraluminal tumor may be well demonstrable, particularly at double-contrast examination. It must be remembered that hematuria is common in connection with tumor. A coagulum in the bladder may mimic a tumor, give the impression that a tumor is larger than it actually is, or occasionally completely cover a tumor (Figs. 395, 396).

If a papillomatous tumor is malignant and infiltrates the bladder wall, a local thickening of the wall can be seen in tangential projections (see Fig. 396). The solid carcinoma may protrude only inconspicuously into the bladder lumen. It may cause asymmetry of the shape of the bladder and a local thickening of its wall. BARTLEY and ECKERBOM (1960) were able to determine the extent of perivesical infiltration of the tumor with a considerable degree of accuracy by using perivesical inflation of gas.

A tumor may be localized in a diverticulum and fill this more or less completely or infiltrate part of its wall (Figs. 398 and 399).

Partly successful attempts have been made by FRANKSSON et al. (1956) to relate the grade of malignancy of a bladder tumor to its appearance at cystography. Tumors of low-grade malignancy have a narrow base and no thickening of the bladder wall, whereas tumors of

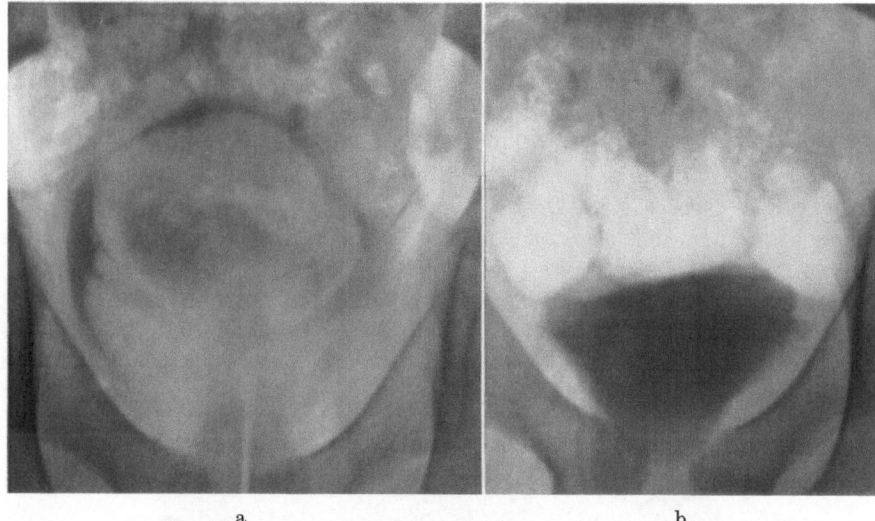

a   b

Fig. 396. Coagulum. a) Urography in association with hematuria: large coagula distending bladder; b) urography after hematuria has subsided: bladder normal

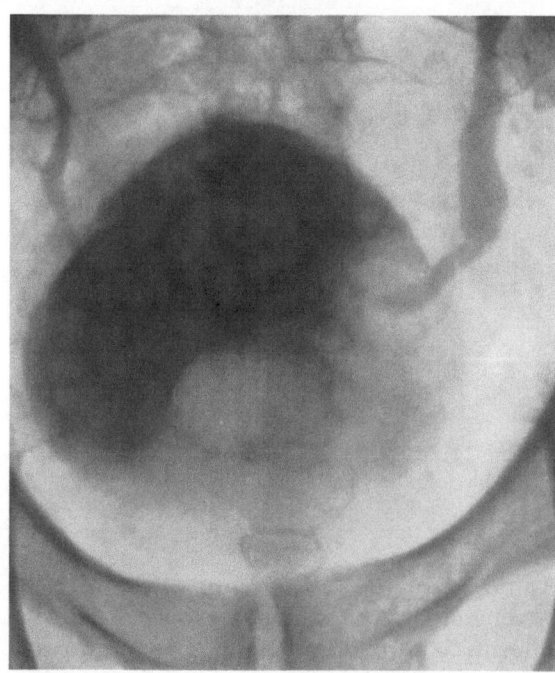

Fig. 397. Tumor at left side in bladder causing slight obstacle to flow from left ureter. In addition, marked enlargement of prostatic gland. Great number of small concrements in bladder

high-grade malignancy are broadly based and show signs of infiltration of the bladder wall, which is thickened.

Impairment of flow through one or both ureteric orifices caused by tumor is seen at urography. This may cause unilateral or bilateral hydronephrosis and may differ in degree between the two sides, if bilateral. The stasis may have been total and long-standing, causing complete and definite cessation of the function of one kidney. Mention must be made here of hydronephrosis caused by kidney pelvis tumor and the possibility of the spread of such a tumor to the bladder (see chapter on dilatation of the urinary tract).

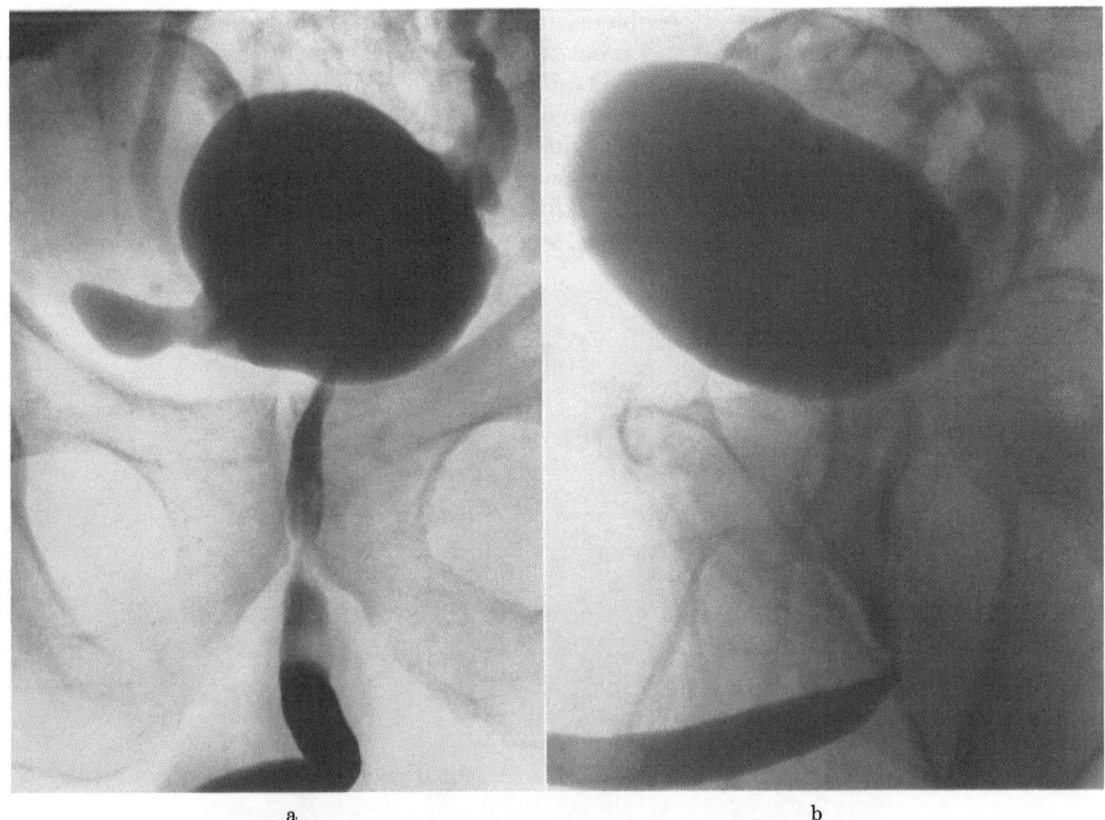

a   b

Fig. 398. Tumor in bladder diverticulum. Multiple diverticula in bladder. Large diverticulum to right and posteriorly is filled with large tumor with irregular surface. a) Left oblique projection. b) Right oblique projection

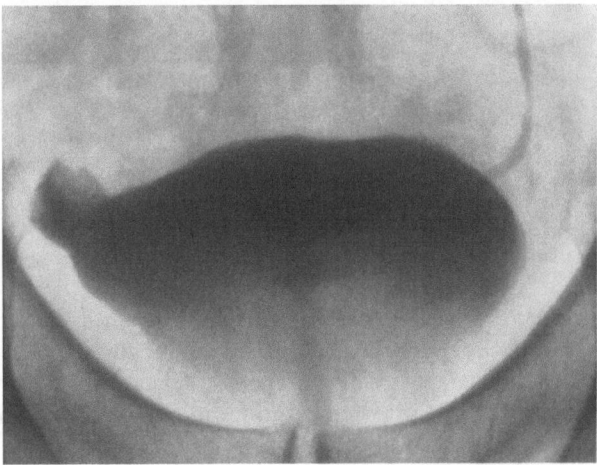

Fig. 399. Tumor in bladder diverticulum. To the right, small diverticulum with infiltration in wall with polypous mass bulging into the diverticulum

There are certain important problems in the diagnosis of bladder tumor which call for further attempts at refining the roentgenologic diagnosis. One such problem is the differential diagnosis between carcinoma and local inflammatory lesion. Another is the involvement of the bladder wall and extravesical tissue by a tumor. Angiography of the bladder has been used in an attempt to sharpen diagnostic criteria

A comprehensive survey of previous work in this field, together with a report of results of anatomic studies and of angiography in a clinical material of 152 patients from our department has been presented by NILSSON (1967). His results are as follows:

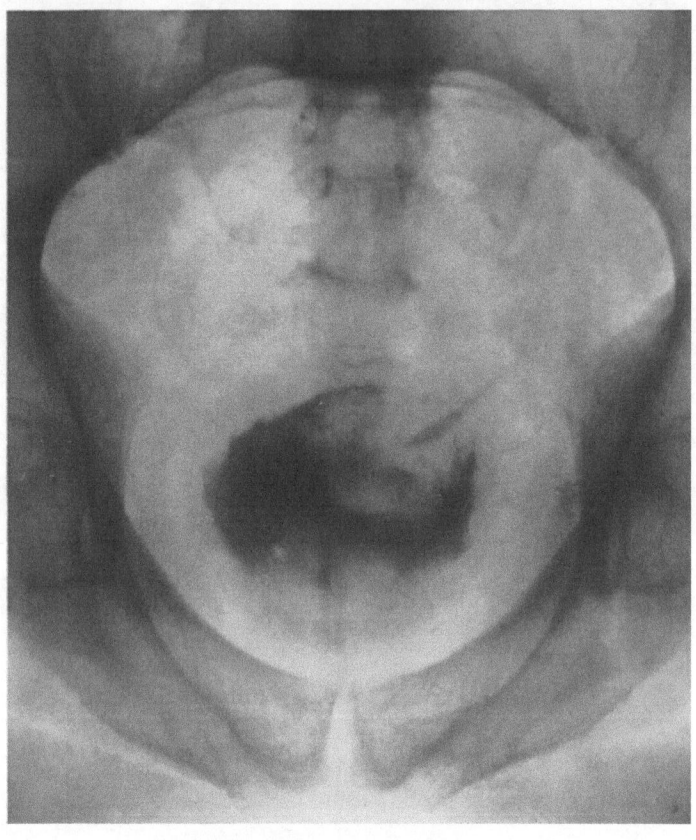

a

Fig. 400. Large papilloma in left side of bladder. a) Urography. b) Angiography, arterial phase: large number of wide, irregular vessels in tumor. c) Angiography, venous phase: wide veins drain tumor

All bladder tumors are supplied by bladder arteries and frequently also by extra-vesical arteries. The supply by extravesical arteries is related to tumor growth and is marked in tumors infiltrating the perivesical tissues. This extravesical supply originates from the obturator artery, the internal pudendal artery, the middle hemorrhoidal artery, and, in exceptional cases, from the inferior gluteal artery, the uterine artery, and the superior gluteal artery. Anastomoses are often seen in the tumor between the varying supplying arteries. Displacement of the large branches of the internal iliac artery is never seen. The tumor growth may cause different degrees of arterial stenosis in large tumors (Fig. 400).

The most important finding is that of tumor vessels, which in NILSSON's material were seen in all tumors with a diameter of one centimeter or more, with the exception of two cases, one with a cluster of small, non-malignant papillomas. Most tumor vessels were seen in malignant tumors, particularly in tumors with extravesical growth. It was

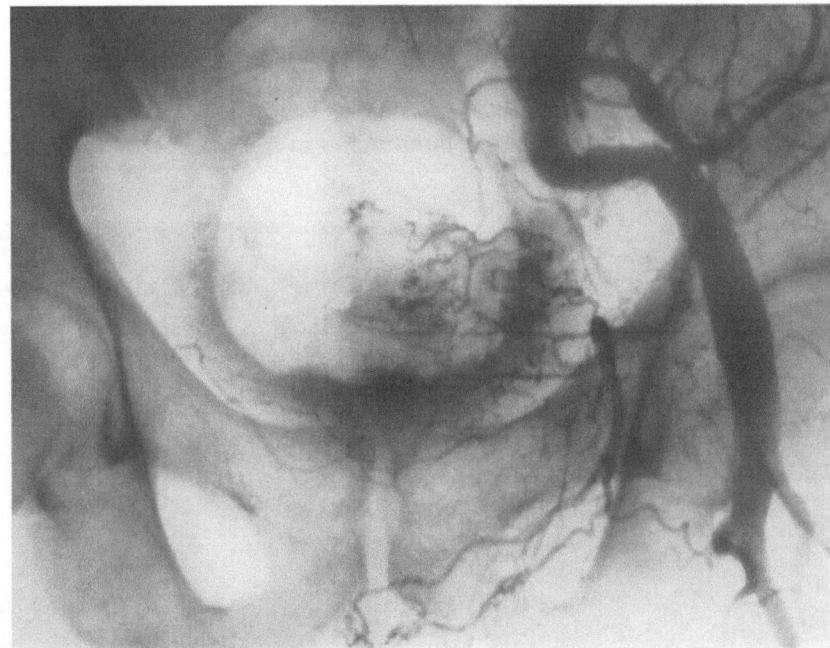

Fig. 400 b

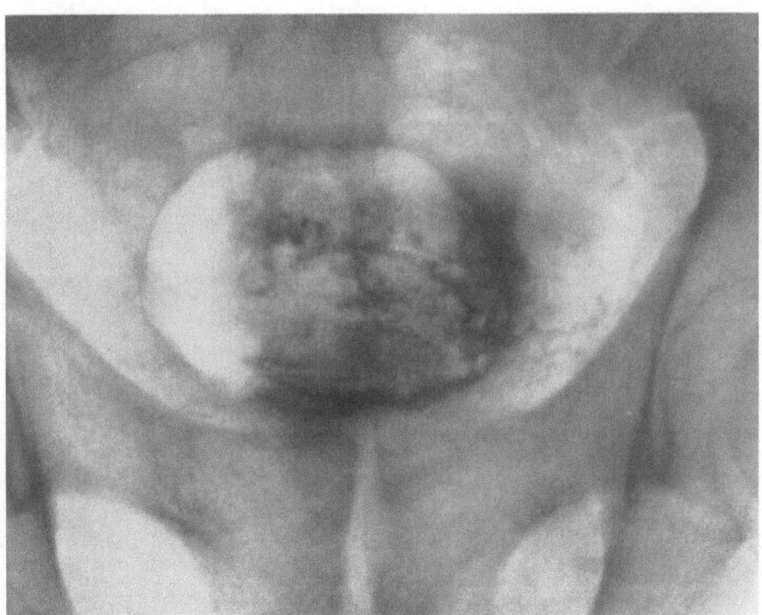

Fig. 400 c

not possible to find a correlation between the number of tumor vessels and the degree of differentiation of the tumors. The tumor vessels in benign papillomas could not be distinguished from those in malignant tumors.

In the capillary phase it is possible to study the thickness of the bladder wall, and the confinement of the tumors to the bladder wall or outside it can be estimated by the distribution of the tumor vessels and the accumulation of contrast medium. In his material of pelvic angiography NILSSON could demonstrate extravesical growth in more than 95 %

of the patients with subsequently clinically verified tumors growing extravesically. In patients with tumors confined to the bladder wall, angiography could exclude extravesical growth in more than 90 %. A definite sign as to confinement of the tumor to the mucosa is the demonstration of a tumor stalk.

Venous changes with wide and tortuous veins are often seen, but their diagnostic importance is limited.

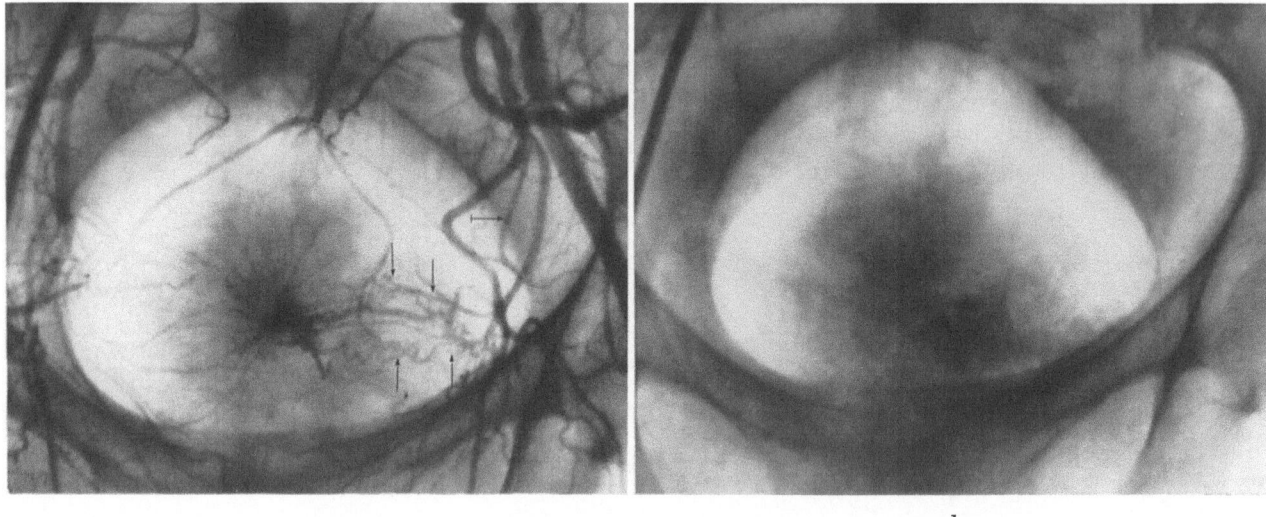

a   b

Fig. 401. Papillary carcinoma with thin stalk. a) Arterial phase: superior vesical artery is wide (wide arteries in stalk of tumor). b) Venous phase: widened veins in stalk of tumor

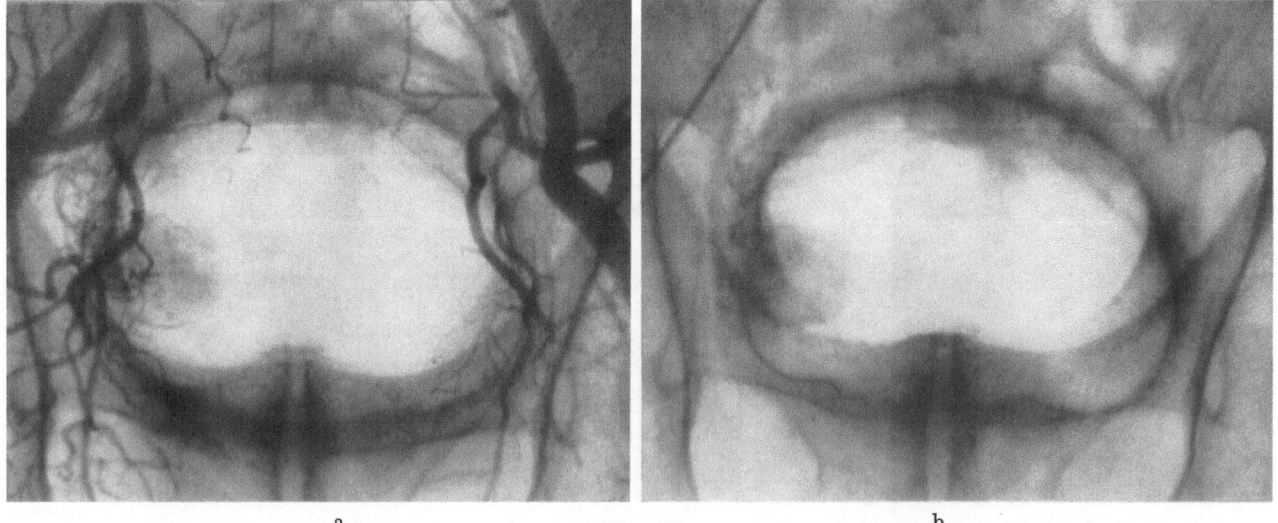

a   b

Fig. 402 Carcinoma at right ureteric orifice. No infiltration of tumor in muscular layer. a) Arterial phase: great number of arteries outside bladder, pathologic vessels in tumor. b) Capillary phase: bladder wall well delineated

Mean circulation time of contrast medium in tumors was definitely shorter than in normal cases and in cases of cystitis. This difference is statistically significant.

A combination of cystitis and tissue reaction to radiation therapy makes it impossible to differentiate the vascular changes from tumor vessels. There are occasionally also difficulties in differentiating inflammatory vessels from tumor vessels.

The effect of radio therapy (betatron or cobalt 60, 6, 400—7,000 R during a treatment period of 40—50 days) on the vascular pattern was studied by HIATALA (1971). At angiographic examination performed two to six months after completion of radiotherapy, a marked decrease down to complete disappearance of the tumors was seen in half of the cases. No tumor vessels were seen but a hypervascularity of the bladder wall was observed at the tumor site.

The regression of the tumor, as seen angiographically, has no direct relation to tumor staging but in tumors of a low degree of differentiation there was a more marked tendency toward regression.

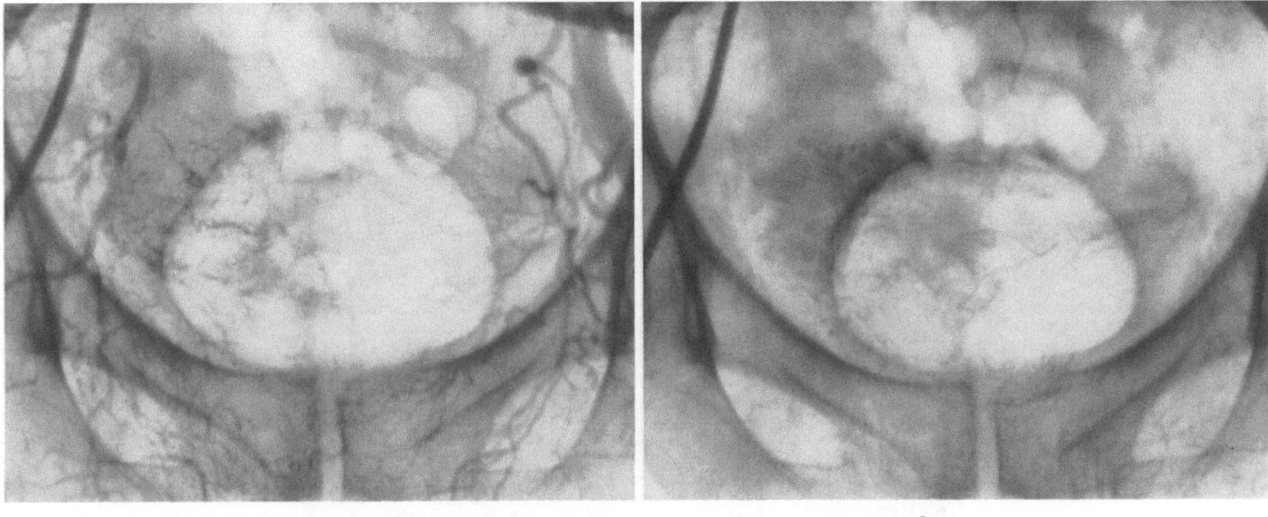

a   b

Fig. 403. Large carcinoma in right side of bladder. Tumor infiltration in perivesical tissue. a) Arterial phase. b) Capillary phase: pathologic vessels and contrast medium in capillaries outside bladder wall

In some cases a later recurrence of tumor growth could be demonstrated angiographically and occasionally both tumor remains and recurrences could be demonstrated angiographically where no cystoscopic findings were present, but where histologic examination verified the diagnosis.

In cases of generalized bladder changes in the post-radiotherapeutic period, vascular changes were found at angiography of a type making differential diagnosis impossible between tumor, radiation reaction, and inflammatory lesions.

Bladder tumors have been classified according to the so-called TNN system, representing a combination of findings at cystoscopy and palpation and of patho-anatomic diagnosis. Angiography may be helpful in this classification, for example in defining infiltration in the bladder wall.

It has been found that there is a fairly strict relationship between the patho-anatomic characteristics of a tumor and the prognosis. Highly differentiated tumors, grade 0—1, are benign, whereas in tumors of grade 2—4 with a lesser degree of differentiation, the malignancy dominates and is represented by a higher mortality. Roentgendiagnostic methods, including angiography, have not so far offered possibilities for tumor grading of this type.

In therapy using increase in intravesical pressure to kill tumor tissue, the effect can be studied angiographically (Fig. 404).

Rare tumors of the bladder. Pheochromocytoma represents a very rare type of tumor in the bladder wall. The tumor itself is very rare. Reference is made in a case report by

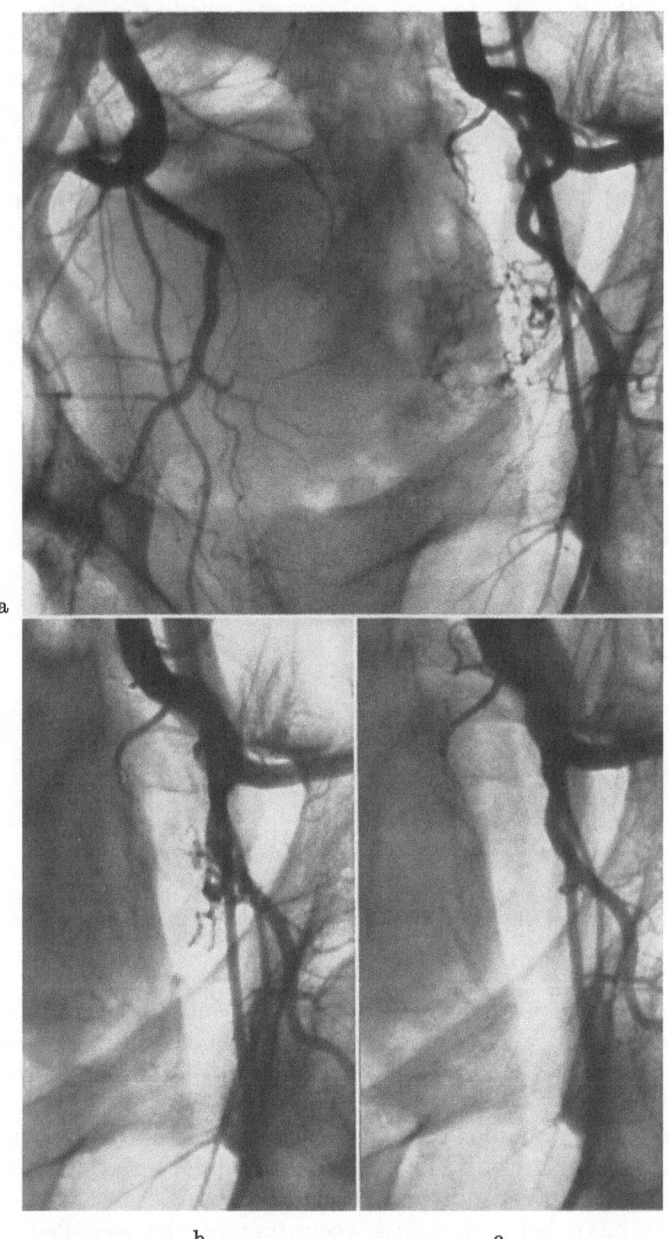

Fig. 404. Large, highly vascularized tumor in left side of bladder. No extra vesical extension. b) Marked reduction of vascularity after increase of intravesical pressure to 60 mm Mercury. c) All vascularity in tumor suppressed at 80 mm Mercury

SIVAK (1961) to ten previously observed cases. Pheochromocytomas in the bladder usually come to be examined because of intermittent hematuria. In one case voiding caused symptoms of marked elevation in blood pressure. Pheochromocytoma in the bladder may bulge into the bladder lumen, as may any other tumor. However, it may also be localized entirely in the bladder wall.

Another rare bladder tumor is myoma. We have seen a patient with suspicion cysto-scopically of a recurrence after operation for bladder carcinoma. At cystography a well outlined tumor with broad base was seen protruding into the bladder. At angiography no tumor vessels were seen. Operation and patho-anatomic examination revealed a myoma (Fig. 405).

Endometriosis of the uterus can affect the colon and can likewise affect the bladder. Usually at cystography a slight rigidity in part of the bladder wall may be seen, or endometriotic tissue may be seen to bulge into the bladder lumen. There are no especially characteristic features in this bulging, which can resemble a primary bladder tumor.

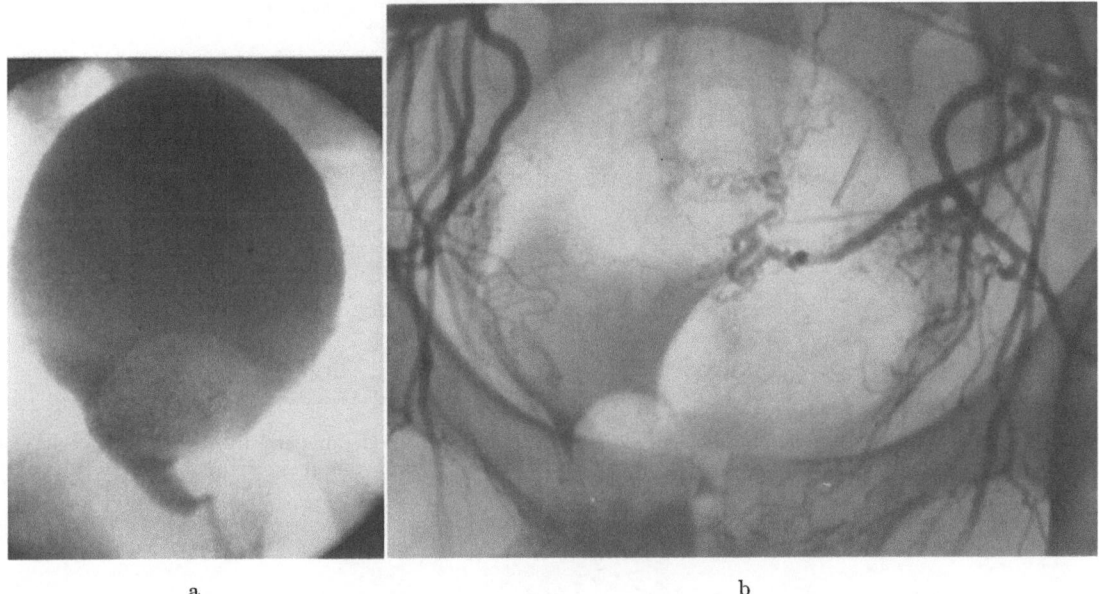

a   b

Fig. 405. Myoma of bladder. Bladder carcinoma several years previously, now healed. Now well defined tumor in base of bladder to the left. a) Cystography (photo-fluorogram): tumor well defined, surface even; b) double-contrast cystography plus angiography: no tumor vessels

5. Trauma

Perforation of the bladder wall can be caused by bone fragments in fracture of the pelvis. Perforations are seen mainly in connection with fractures in the anterior part of the pelvis, the pubic region. The perforations are accordingly localized in the anterior lower part of the bladder. Instruments may pierce the bladder wall, for example from the urethral lumen. Such perforations are localized in the base of the bladder.

Lesions from bayonet wounds and similar lesions such as those caused in automobile accidents may cause laceration, chiefly anteriorly. Gunshot may severely damage the bladder. In such lesions localized edema can be seen at plain roentgenography and fluid blood and urine may cause increased density in the lower pelvis. Free fluid may also be seen in the peritoneal cavity. Gas may be seen in the bladder and in the perivesical tissues. Possible defects in the bladder wall can be seen at cystography, with escape of contrast medium outside the boundaries of the bladder.

A sometimes marked displacement of the bladder may be seen with or without passage of contrast medium outside the bladder wall (Fig. 406, 407). This is also seen in hematoma close to the bladder but without lesion in the bladder itself.

Genuine ruptures of the bladder are rare. HOLM (1943) reported three cases and gave a short survey of incidence. A full bladder must be hit violently for a rupture to occur. Rupture may be combined with pelvic fractures. Such ruptures are extraperitoneal in $^2/_3$ of the cases and intra-peritoneal in $^1/_3$, whereas ruptures without fracture are all intraperitoneal.

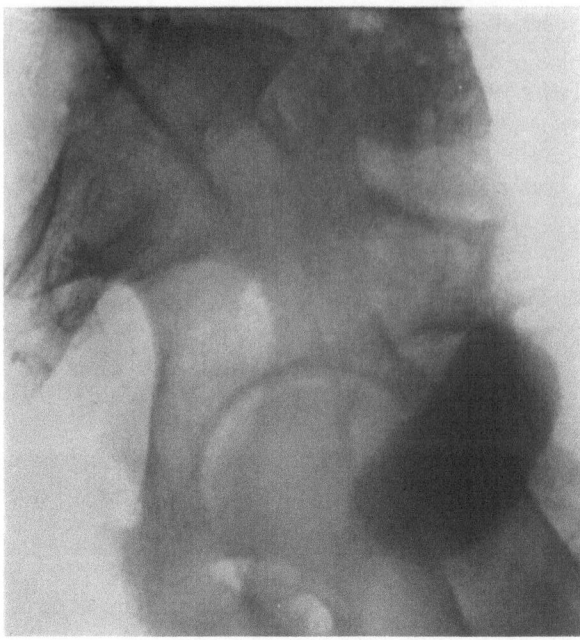

Fig. 406. Retrocystic hematoma (automobile crash, ruptures of duodenum and liver with retroperitoneal hematoma). Marked displacement of bladder anteriorly and compression from behind

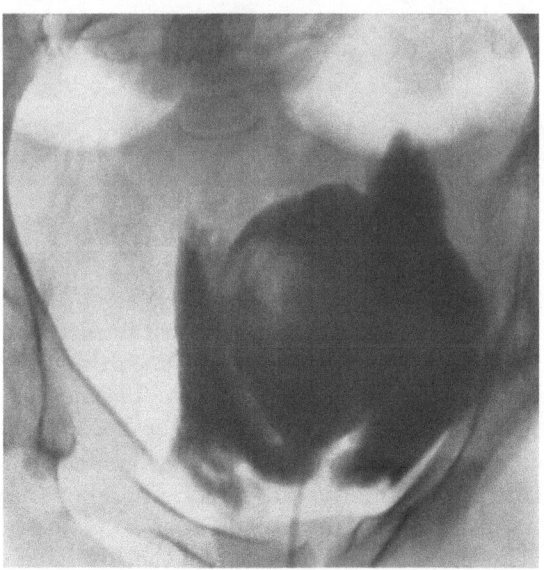

Fig. 407. Rupture of base of bladder from trauma causing fractures in anterior part of pelvis. Marked escape of contrast medium into extravesical space

If the bladder is markedly distended, the trauma-causing rupture may be minimal. This type of rupture may be seen in connection with severe intoxication, for example in cases of alcohol abuse. As long as urine continues to flow into the bladder, La Place's law is applicable to the degree of resistance of the bladder wall: the bladder increases in size in spheric shape, with increasing thinning of the wall and consistent pressure. Then, at marked distention, only a very slight trauma may be sufficient to cause rupture.

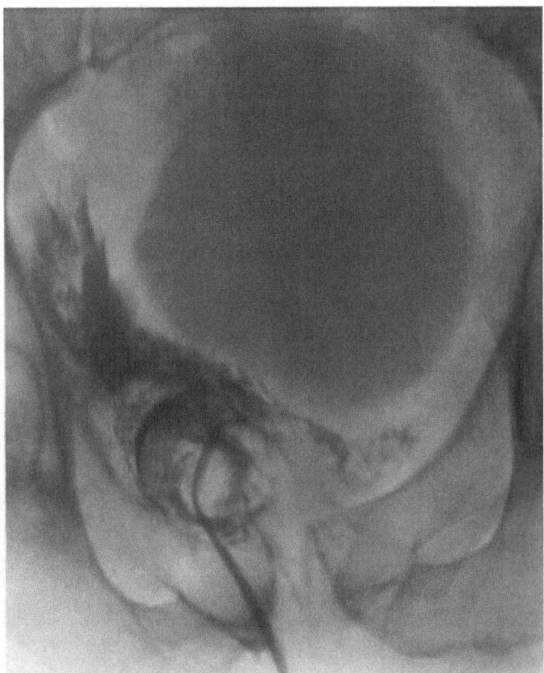

Fig. 408. Traumatic rupture of posterior part of urethra. Catheter has passed through lesion. Contrast medium injected around base of bladder

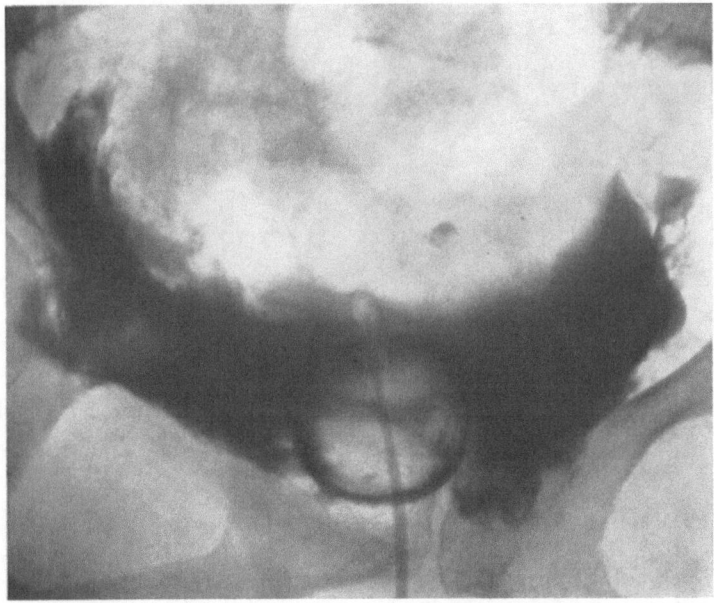

Fig. 409. Unintentional extirpation of bladder. From urethra filling into extraperitoneal space (patient operated in other hospital for large gynecological tumor and because of postoperative anuria referred to us)

During otherwise uncomplicated urethrocystography leakage of contrast medium through a lesion in the bladder wall may be seen. Occasionally marked leakage can occur if during fluoroscopy the escape of contrast medium outside the bladder is not observed immediately (Fig. 410).

Fistula formation may be seen between the bladder and adjacent organs in connection with trauma due to accidents occurring during operation, or as a residuum or complication of radiotherapy. Such fistulae may also be caused by inflammatory lesions, for example, cystitis or diverticulitis in the colon. In Fig. 411 a fistula is seen between the bladder and the vagina formed unintentionally during hysterectomy six weeks previously. Figs. 412 and 413 illustrate fistula formation in connection with radiotherapy for carcinoma of the collum of the uterus.

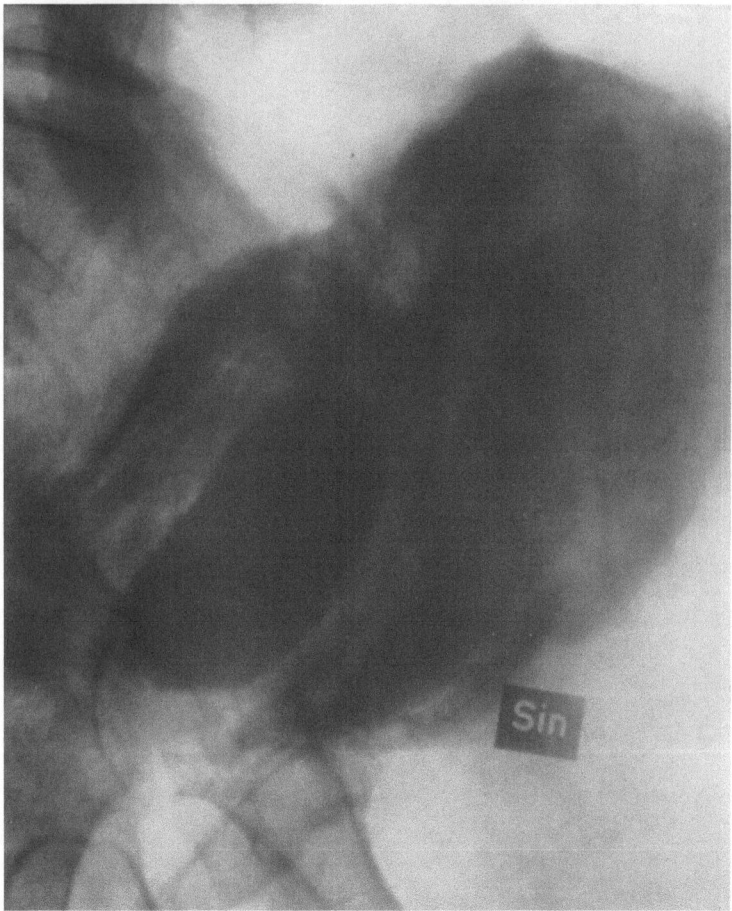

Fig. 410. Lesion in bladder in connection with otherwise uncomplicated urethrocystography. Leakage of contrast medium in wide space around bladder

6. The bladder in urinary obstruction

In acute urinary obstruction a very marked increase in size of the bladder may be seen at plain roentgenography, with displacement of the bowel. In differential diagnosis expansivity in the female genital organs, for example ovarian cyst, is particularly pertinent.

In chronic obstruction to bladder drainage, the bladder wall increases in thickness, with attendant hypertrophy of musculature. This causes trabeculation of the wall. Prolapse of mucosa through openings between muscle bundles very often causes formation of diverticula. As such a false diverticulum has no musculature in its wall, it cannot contract during micturition, in contrast to bulges caused by anatomical variations and bipartite bladder (see above). A diverticulum increases in size at micturition since urine

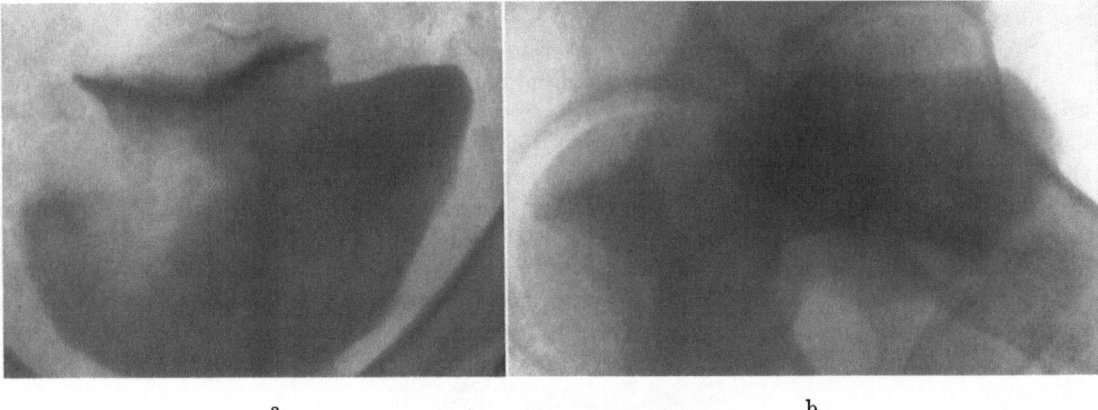

a   b

Fig. 411. Fistula between bladder and vagina (hysterectomy six weeks previously). a) Frontal view: fornical part of vagina seen at top of bladder; b) laterial view: contrast-filled vagina behind bladder

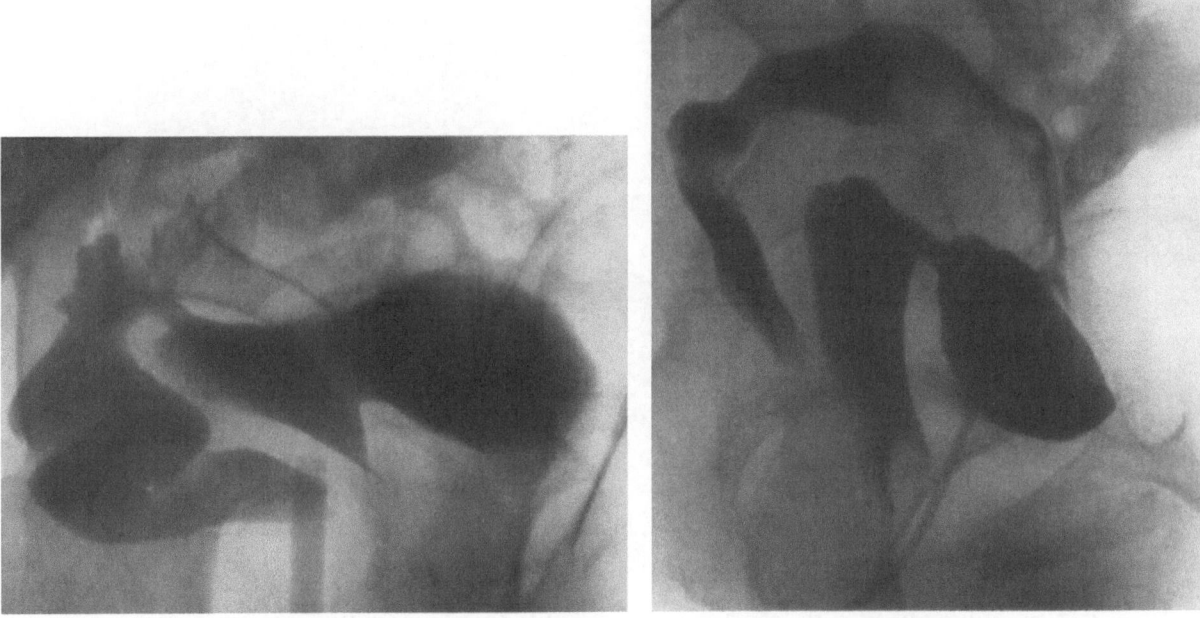

Fig. 412   Fig. 413

Fig. 412. Fistula between posterior part of bladder and upper part of rectum. Marked sclerosis with shrinkage of posterior part of bladder (radiotheraphy for carcinoma of the collum of the uterus two years previously)

Fig. 413. Fistula from bladder cranially — anteriorly to sigmoid colon and cranially — posteriorly to the vagina (post radiotherapy for carcinoma of the collum of the uterus three years previously)

flows into the diverticulum more easily than through the urethra, at contraction of the bladder. This increase in size of the diverticulum may be very marked.

As mentioned above, a diverticulum may also be congenital, in which case it has all the tissue layers in its wall. Periureteric position of a diverticulum may cause displacement of the distal part of the ureter.

A diverticulum may be the site of a tumor, or it may contain stone.

7. Stone

Stone formation in the bladder is a common occurrence.

There is a significant difference in chemical composition between stone primary in the kidney and stone primary in the bladder (LAGERGREN, 1956). Thus pure calcium oxalate and calcium oxalate — apatite mixture comprise the main component in nearly 60% of the kidney — ureter group in LAGERGREN's material, as opposed to only approximately 20% of the bladder stones. The principal components of bladder stones were magnesium, ammonia, phosphate, apatite in mixtures in 40%, and uric acid mixed with urates in 27%. The latter group comprised less than 4% of the kidney — ureter group. Thus bladder stones often have a low calcium content and are accordingly less well demonstrable at plain roentgenography, even when of considerable size.

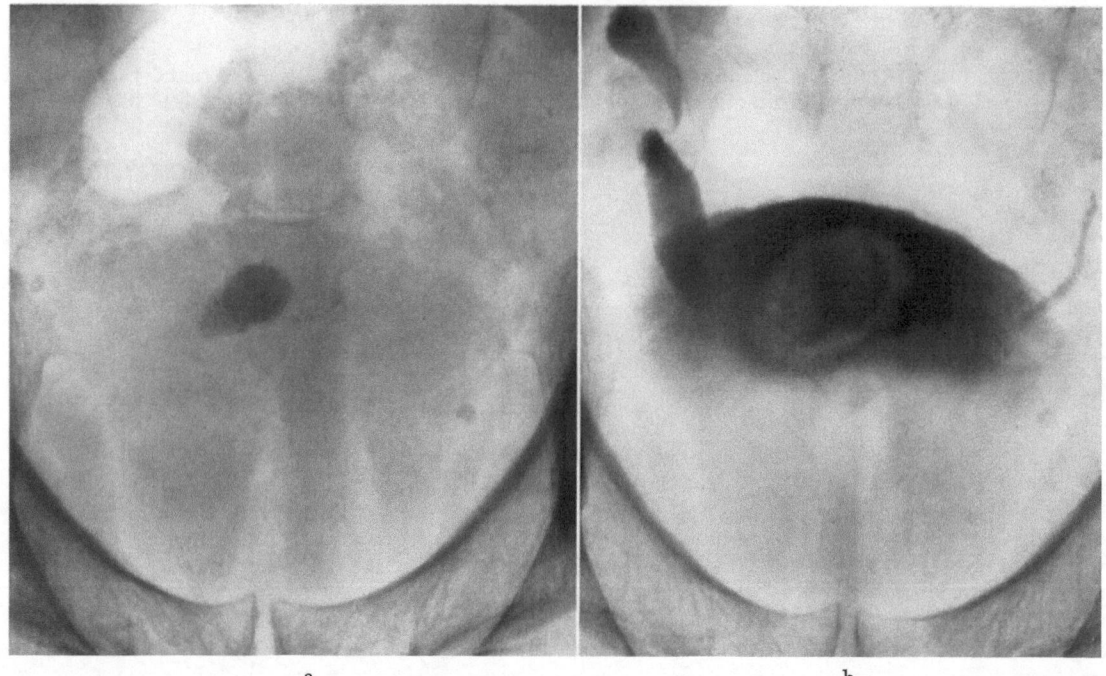

a   b

Fig. 414. Stone in bladder. a) Plain roentgenogram; b) urography: note peripheral zone of stone not containing calcium

Calcium deposits on the catheter in the bladder, especially on the balloon-type catheters, are common in patients with catheter à demeure. The calcium shell may break and increasing calcium deposits will cause increase in stone formation around the fragments.

Formation of stone is common in impeded urinary flow with infection. A large amount of small stones, often of low density, may be seen lining the cranial part of an enlarged prostatic gland.

Solitary or multiple stones are often seen with marked layer formation. The stones may also have a very irregular shape. This shape often represents only the shape of the core of the stone, whereas material of little calcium content surrounds this core, giving the actual stone a smooth surface.

Stones can change position with change in the position of the patient. Stones are occasionally lodged in a diverticulum, however, and retain their localization despite marked change in the position of the patient. Such stones are sometimes difficult to differentiate from extravesical calcifications for example calcified sloughed appendices epiploici, etc.

Stones in the bladder may be stones passed from the kidney.

As bladder stones often have low calcium content, they are occasionally best seen at cystography, usually in connection with urography (Fig. 414).

8. The neurogenic bladder

The neurogenic bladder is usually defined as being related to a supranuclear, nuclear, infranuclear, or peripheral nervous lesion. These lesions cause inhibited reflex bladder, automatic bladder, autonomous bladder and atonic bladder, respectively. A combination of types is very often present, however, and a clear-cut division between these different types and localizations is not possible. Certain trends may dominate. Thus in the supra-

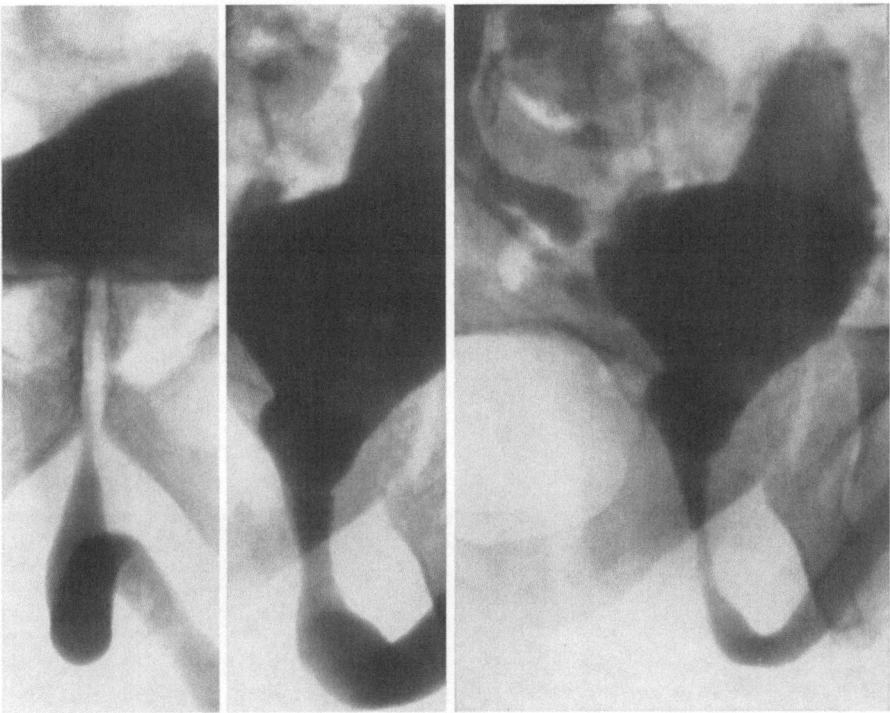

Fig. 415. Neurogenic bladder of supranuclear type with cystitis in a case of paraplegia following fracture of C 5. Left and middle figure during injection; right figure during voiding. Note no external sphincter spasm

nuclear lesion the patient cannot urinate spontaneously but can be trained to start micturition by certain kinds of peripheral stimulation. The posterior part of the urethra then dilates. The filled bladder has a special shape as a result of increased tonus in the wall.

The most characteristic type of neurogenic bladder roentgenologically is that representing a lesion below the spinal center at the level of TH-12 in the conus terminalis. The bladder is large in this infranuclear type of neurogenic bladder and is raised as during micturition. It has often an abundance of diverticula of different sizes and the wall is markedly trabeculated. The external sphincter is closed at attempts at micturition and no micturition takes place. Reflux to the ureters is often seen in these patients. The incompetence of the ureteric orifices may cause marked dilatation of the kidney pelves and the ureters.

The atonic bladder has a great capacity; it is wide and has a thin and even wall without trabeculation.

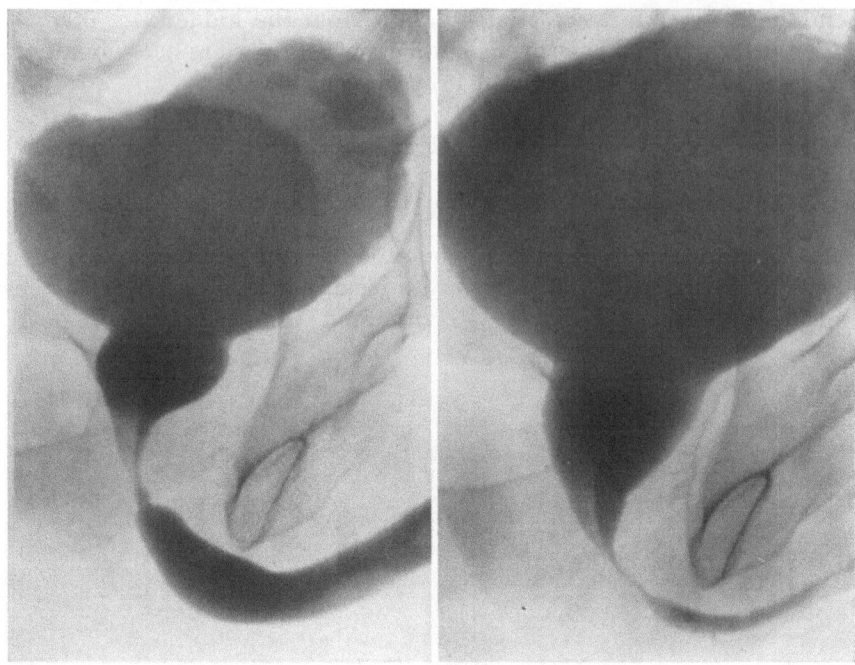

Fig. 416. Neurogenic bladder of infranuclear type in a case of paraplegia after fracture of L 1. Left figure during injection; right figure during voiding. External sphincter spasm and constantly open bladder neck as well as raised bladder are the typical features.

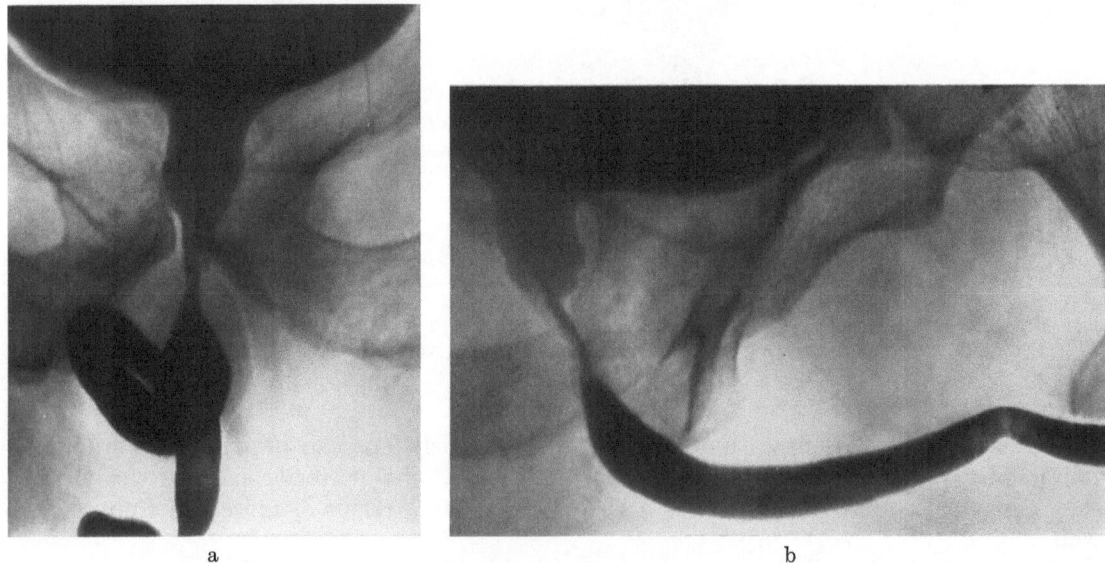

a   b

Fig. 417. Neurogenic bladder and urethra (multiple sclerosis)

The different types of neurogenic bladder are not clear-cut in every instance. KJELL-BERG *et al.* (1957) in a large series of examinations of children with neurologic disorders, found no direct correlation between the type of bladder changes and the localization of the nerve lesion. In most cases of infranuclear lesion the bladder changes were of the type described above, however, with an abnormally raised bladder, increased trabeculation in the wall, a wide bladder neck, and, during micturition, a closed external sphincter (Fig.

415, 416). Infection superimposed upon the neurogenic changes also influences roentgenologic features. Spasm in the external sphincter, cysto-ureteric reflux, for example, may be related to infection. Another common complication is stone formation in the upper urinary tract or in the bladder.

9. Enuresis

Enuresis is the diagnosis of patients with involuntary discharge of urine after an age at which control of micturition should have been attained, usually age three to four years. Pathologic features can be observed at urethrocystography in several instances of nocturnal and/or diurnal enuresis. The opinion as to incidence of such changes varies considerably, however. A survey of the literature is given by KJELLBERG et al. (1957). The authors also present a material of their own of 598 patients, with a moderate predominance of boys.

Urethral valves were found in 22 cases. A slight change in the shape of the bladder, with a waist during micturition, and narrowing of the external sphincter was noted in approximately 10% of nocturnal, and 20% of diurnal enuretics and was considered a sign of bladder irritation in connection with infection. An angular indentation in the ventral urethral wall opposite the collicle was found in 25% of the cases. The authors considered this indentation in different degrees a transition to urethral valves, but the normal intermuscular incisure must be kept in mind. A small number of other, non-specific changes was observed and it was concluded that patients with enuresis appear to present no specific organic changes observable at urethrocystography. The authors point out, however, that anomalies, infection and urologic disease may present symptoms simulating simple enuresis. For this reason, urologic and urethrocystographic investigation is essential in all children who have not gained control of urination by the age of four years. Since the incidence of anomalies and pathologic conditions of the urinary tract is almost twice as high in patients with diurnal enuresis as in normal cases, this specific group of patients need thorough examination. The authors also express the opinion that once organic cause is found, the patient should not be considered an enuretic in the usual sense of the word.

10. Bladder fistulae

Spontaneous fistulae can be present from the bladder to the skin or to neighbor organs. They may be caused by bladder disease or by disease in the neighbor organs.

In inflammatory disease of the bladder, for example tuberculosis, fistulation may occur, particularly if the disease has produced urethral stricture.

In carcinoma of the colon the tumor may infiltrate the bladder and, upon ulceration, cause fistula formation. In regional enterocolitis, Crohn's disease, inflammatory adhesions may be found between loops of bowel with fistulation. In such a lesion part of the bladder wall may be involved. A corresponding type of fistula formation is secondary to disease in the female genitals (Figs. 411, 412).

The presence of a fistula between the bladder and the bowel may be anticipated by findings of gas in the bladder. Unless gas-producing bacteria can be detected and there has been no instrumentation, this is indication of fistula formation.

The fistula can be demonstrated by direct injection of contrast medium into the fistula itself, so-called fistulography. In inner fistulae a passage between the bladder and the bowel can be seen at cystography or at bowel examination. Occasionally the passage through the fistula is obtainable in only one direction and a marked edema in the walls of the fistula may prevent passage temporarily. In some cases the fistula cannot be filled at either cystography or at colon examination and direct catheterization during cystoscopy may then be necessary in order to demonstrate the fistula.

II. The Prostate

1. Hyperplasia of the prostatic gland

The first systematic use of urethrocystography in prostatic hyperplasia was made by KNUTSSON in 1935. He pointed out the basic feature that the increase in size of the pros-

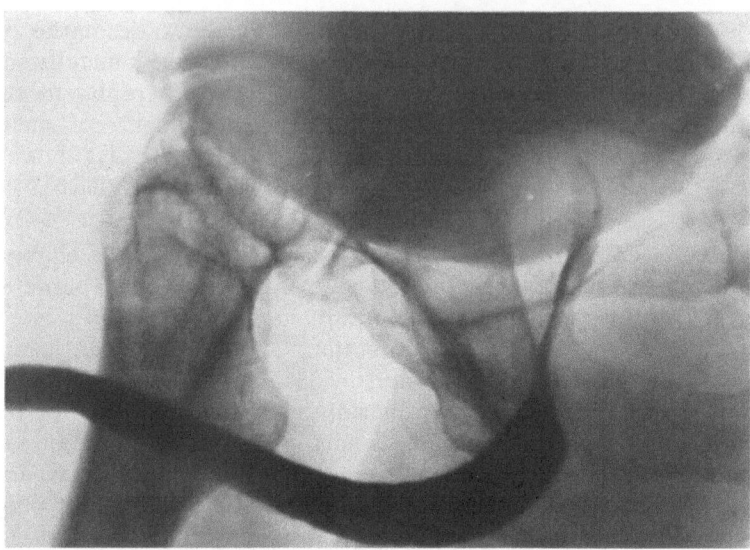

Fig. 418. Hyperplasia of prostatic gland. Even displacement and compression of pars prostatica with corresponding elevation by enlarged gland of floor of bladder

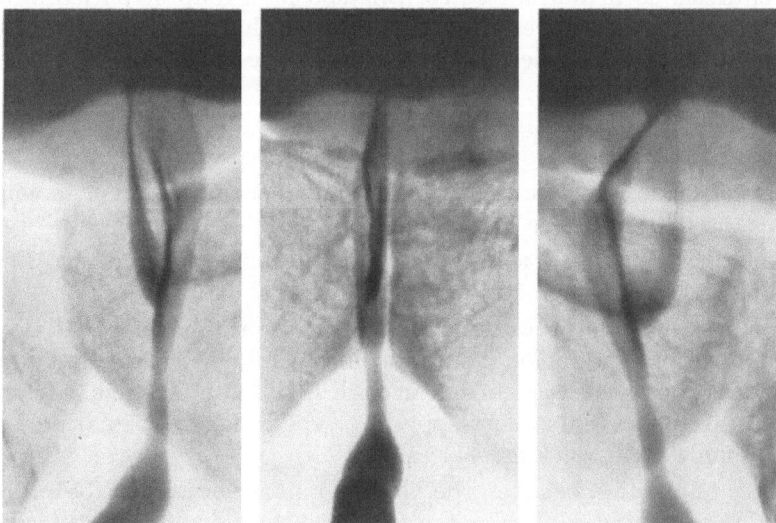

Fig. 419. Prostatic hyperplasia. The ventro-lateral expansion in the supracollicular region makes the urethra lumen Y-shaped in cross sections

tatic gland is limited to the region between the collicle and the bladder orifice. The urethral wall is intimately attached to the adenomatous growth in this region. This growth is localized posteriorly, which causes a displacement of the supracollicular part of the urethra anteriorly. The supracollicular part may also be markedly elongated. The orifice is displaced upwards and anteriorly and the lumen of the urethra is compressed sidewise to form a deep sagittal cleft. In this compressed part of the urethra the collicle disappears and parts of the adenoma may, instead, influence the inner shape of the urethra (Figs. 418, 419). The adenomatous mass may be somewhat asymmetric and a displacement sidewise of the urethra can result accordingly.

Occasionally a lobus tertius, a third lobe in the midline, bulges into the base of the bladder and this third lobe may be the only sign of prostatic hyperplasia (EDLING, 1945)

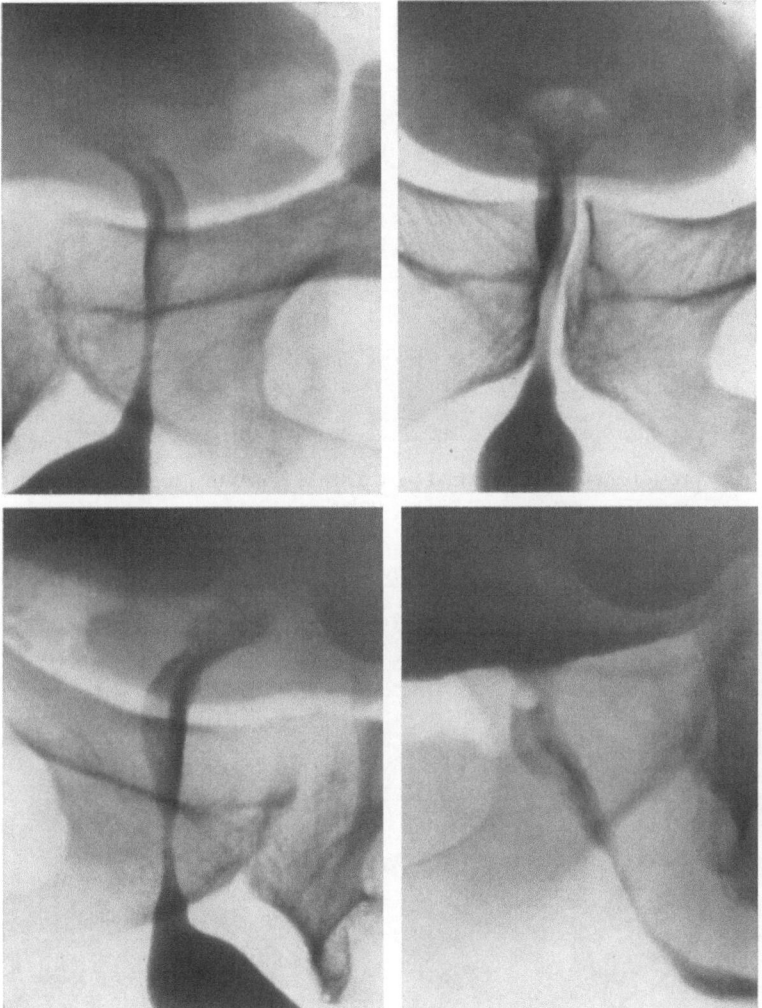

Fig. 420. Prostatic hyperplasia with a posterior lobe prolabating during micturition

(Fig. 420). The posterior part of the internal urethral orifice may bulge forward markedly, forming a broad bar.

The changes in the supra-collicular part of the urethra may be more clearly demonstrable at micturition urethrocystography.

2. Changes post-prostatectomiam

After prostatectomy a cavity may be found representing a more or less marked widening of the prostatic part of the urethra, which may include the internal orifice

(Fig. 421). The cavity is usually supracollicular. The remaining parts of the adenoma or, in later stages, recurring adenoma, may cause local bulging into the cavity (Fig. 422). Occasionally only a slight widening of the prostatic urethra is seen, demonstrable best during micturition at urethrocystography. Scar formation may cause stricture in the

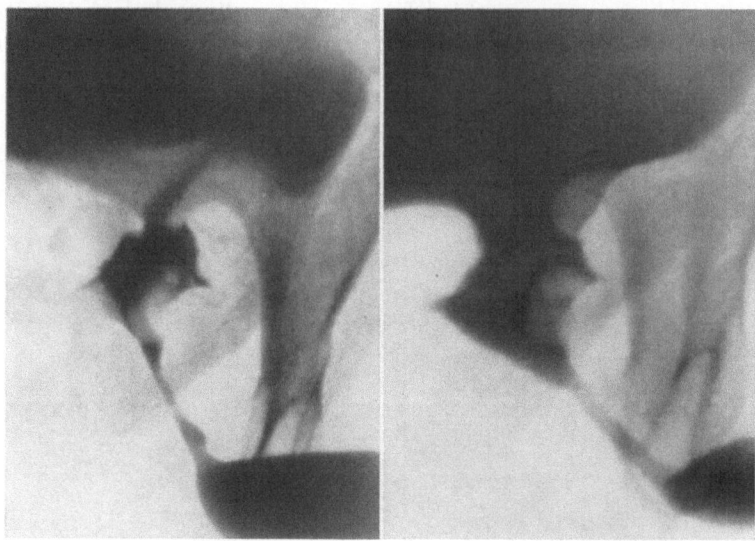

Fig. 421. Status post prostatectomiam. Proximal part of pars prostatica markedly widened and slightly irregular

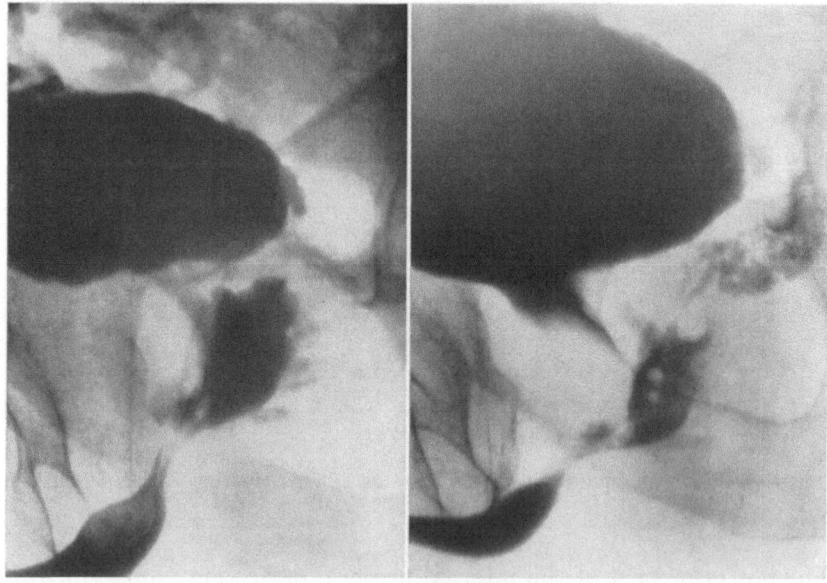

Fig. 422. Status after prostatectomy with naked adenomas bulging into the irregular operation cavity

posterior part of the urethra or of the internal orifice (Fig. 423). It is indicated by MITTY (1971) that when the internal sphincter is damaged the prostatic urethra is constantly exposed to the pressure of urine in the bladder, for example after prostatectomy. Reflux into the vas deferens and seminal vesicle is then common because the ejaculatory ducts often remain patent after prostatectomy.

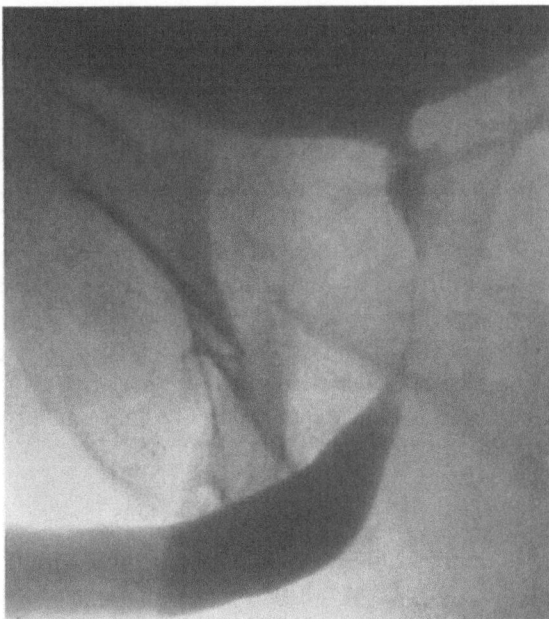

Fig. 423. Status post prostatectomiam. Patient has again difficulty in emptying bladder. Marked short stenosis at internal orifice

3. Carcinoma

Prostatic carcinoma may engage an already hyperplastic prostatic gland, or it may represent a small tumor in an otherwise normal prostatic gland. The former type of tumor shows at urethrocystography changes basically of a type encountered in prostatic hyperplasia. Diagnostic trends representing carcinoma in these cases are signs of infiltration of the urethral lumen, which may be rigid and irregular (Fig. 424). The changes may also

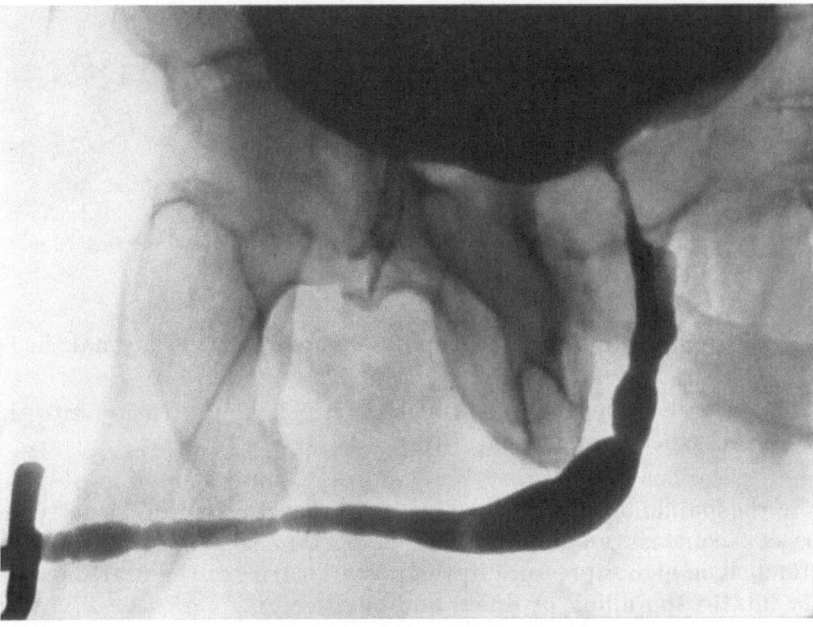

Fig. 424. Prostatic carcinoma and urethral stricture. Irregular infiltration and marked stenosis of pars prostatica. Long irregular stricture in pars pendula with moderate decrease in width of lumen

involve distal parts of the prostatic urethra, whereas the changes at hyperplasia, as indicated above, are limited to the supracollicular part. Asymmetrical displacement of the urethra may occur in hyperplasia and in carcinoma, and is no specific sign of carcinoma. In cases without hyperplasia of the prostatic gland, only slight changes due to infiltration may be seen in the posterior urethra. Slight carcinomatous changes in a hyperplastic prostatic gland very often cannot be detected as such at urethrocystography. The same holds true for a small carcinoma in an otherwise normal prostatic gland.

It should be pointed out that the carcinomatous changes develop on the posterior lobe as a rule, and that an infiltration anteriorly and into the urethra is a late phase of this development of the carcinoma.

At examination of the prostatic region, parts of the pelvic skeleton are seen in the films. Metastases may then be seen and are usually markedly osteosclerotic. The small tumor is said to produce early and widespread metastases, whereas the tumor based in hyperplasia gives off metastases late in its development.

4. Inflammatory lesions

Prostatitis may affect a previously normal gland or a gland with different degrees of hyperplasia. The changes may be small or localized without affecting the anatomy of

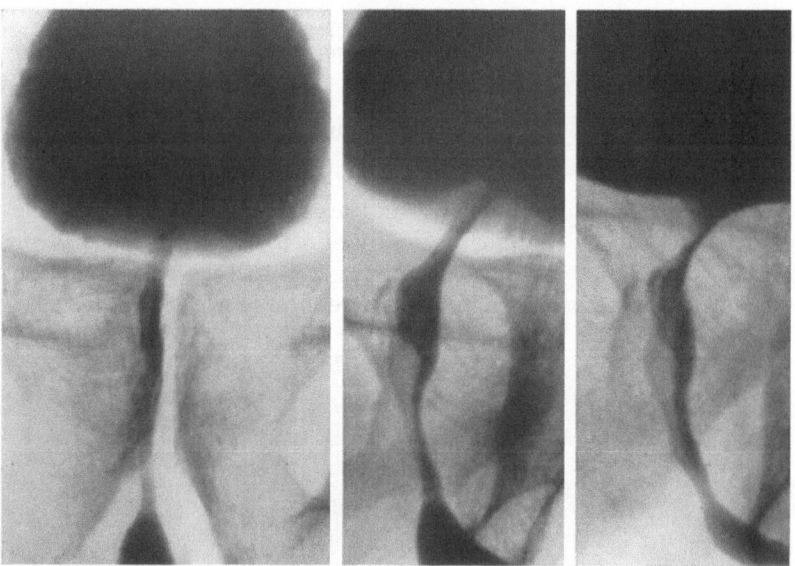

Fig. 425. Chronic prostato-vesiculitis with bladder neck sclerosis

the urethra and thus the urethrocystographic changes may be normal, in spite of florid prostatitis.

The gland is usually enlarged in prostatitis, with slight protrusion into the base of the bladder. The bladder neck may shrink (Figs. 425, 426).

Inflammatory lesions in the prostatic gland may cause formation of cavities, and filling of ducts in the gland may be obtained at urethrocystography. The advantage of using a highly viscous contrast medium in this connection is pointed out by MORALES and ROMANUS (1952). The higher pressure in the posterior part of the urethra when using such a medium facilitates the filling of ducts and cavities in some cases.

The cavities may be small or large, single or multiple. The lumen is often irregular. The ducts may be very small and single but may also occupy the entire glandular tissue.

Occasionally both cavities and ducts fill better during micturition urethrocystography or only during that examination.

Ossifying pelvispondylitis may be suspected or diagnosed in connection with prostatitis. Roentgen examination of the pelvis is then indicated, especially of the sacro-iliac joints and the spinal column. The reader is referred to the monograph by ROMANUS (1953) and to current textbooks for further descriptions of the skeletal changes. In every case of suspected prostatitis it is advisable to give attention to the sacro-iliac joints and to the symphysis in studying films at urography or urethrocystography.

Calcifications of unusual size and shape may be seen in the prostatic gland as a result of inflammatory lesions.

The prostatic gland may diminish in size (so-called prostatic atrophy) as a result of shrinkage in connection with prostatitis, but also in other types of pathogenesis (congenital

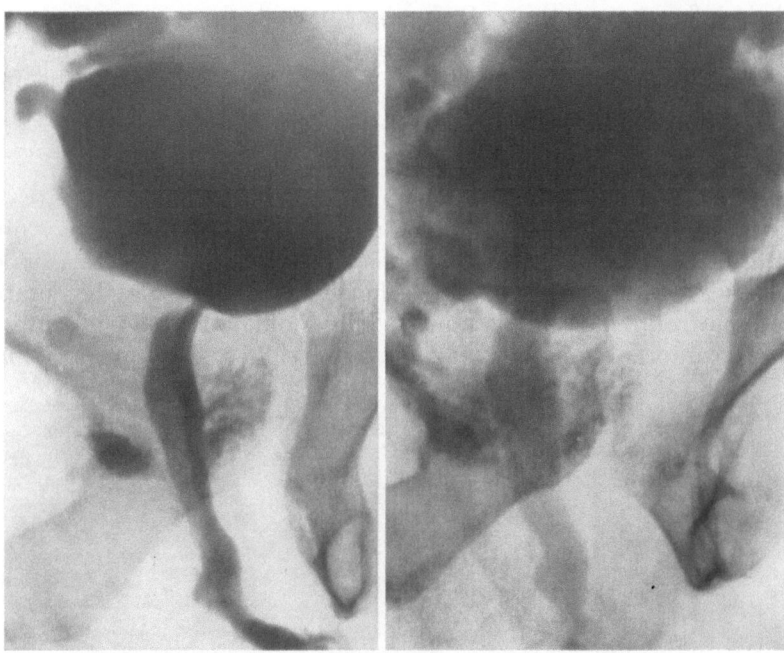

Fig. 426. Chronic prostatitis with bladder neck sclerosis and urethral stricture

hyperplasia, senility, etc.). There may be no changes present at urethrocystography, or the lumen may be more or less regularly dilated.

5. Contraction of the bladder neck

The neck of the bladder may contract and sclerose in atrophy of the prostatic gland, hyperplasia, neurogenic disturbances, inflammatory lesions, etc. This causes a rigidity of the internal orifice, with functional derangement and difficulty in emptying the bladder. As pointed out by EDLING, the process may be of two types: contraction of the bladder neck with bar formation, representing an enlargement of the third lobe of the prostatic gland or contraction of the bladder neck with circular contracture, characterized by a short, circular stenosis. The changes are demonstrable best at micturition. SCHOPFNER (1971) points out that in many cases, however, especially in children, the diagnosis of a bladder neck contracture represents overdiagnosis.

III. The Urethra

1. Anomalies

a) Hypospadia

Hypospadia, the most common anomaly, represents a non-closure of the floor of the urethra. The orifice may open dorsally close to the normal position of the orifice urethra brevis virilis or more proximally between the glans and the perineum.

b) Epispadia

In epispadia there is an incomplete closure of the urethra dorsally. In ectopia of the bladder this anomaly has its most complete form.

These types of anomaly have their main interest, from a roentgen-diagnostic point of view, in their influence on the entire urinary tract, for example in connection with other anomalies and with infection. Locally they may represent problems in the technique of urethrocystography, from the point of view of application of the instrument for examination.

c) Double urethra

In double urethra, constrast medium can be injected through an extra orifice on the glans, in the sulcus coronarius, or in the dorsal part of the penis. It may fill a blind duct of varying length. This incomplete urethra may be close to complete, thus ending in the normal urethra near the bladder (Fig. 427). The double urethra may be complete, however with two urethras from the bladder lumen. The anomalous extra urethra may take its course outside the internal sphincter and in this case gives symptoms of incontinence.

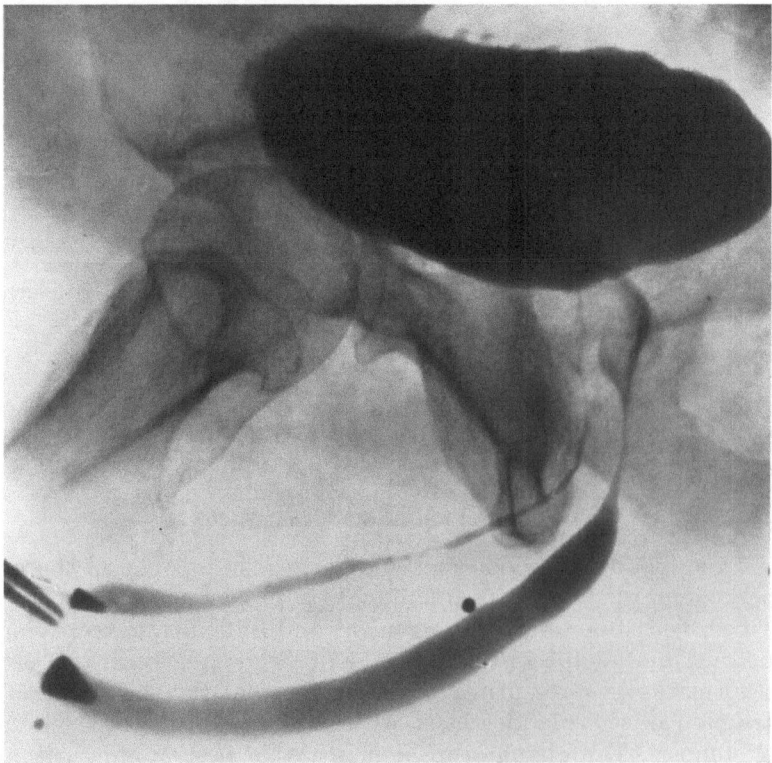

Fig. 427. Double urethra. Dorsal urethra starts in proximal part of pars prostatica of "conventional" urethra, thus incomplete double urethra

d) Diverticula

Diverticula, small or large, single or multiple, are usually localized in the lower part of the urethra and most commonly, in male patients, anteriorly in the cavernous part. They may be oval and flat and have an even contour (Fig. 428). Diverticula may, although rarely, contain stone (Fig. 428).

A related type of anomaly is represented by partial divisions of the lumen by a mucosal fold (EDLING) separating small portions of the urethral lumen from the main lumen.

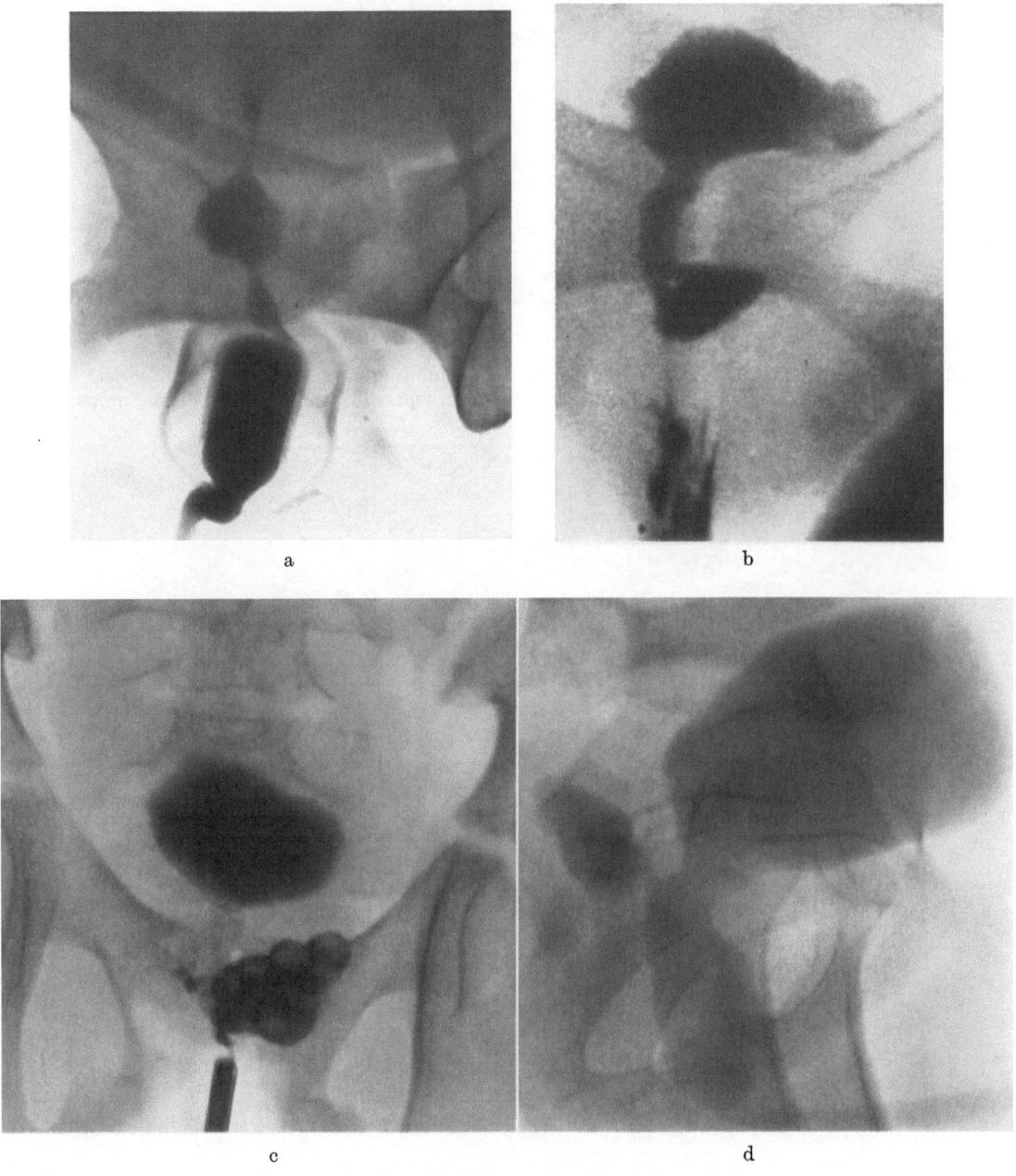

a

b

c

d

Fig. 428. Diverticulosis in female urethra. a) At middle of urethra, b) (photofluorography) in distal part of urethra Diverticulum with stone formation. c) Urethrocystography during voiding. Moderate dilatation of prostatic and membranaceous part of urethra. Filling dorsal to verumontanum of cavity containing stone. d) Urethrography during urethroscopy. Filling, from opening on verumontanum, of cavity containing multitude of stones

e) Urethral valves

Urethral valves represent an important anomaly in children. They are seen almost exclusively in boys and have been referred to in the literature in relation to the intricate embryology of the posterior part of the urethra or in connection with the sexual differentiation of this part.

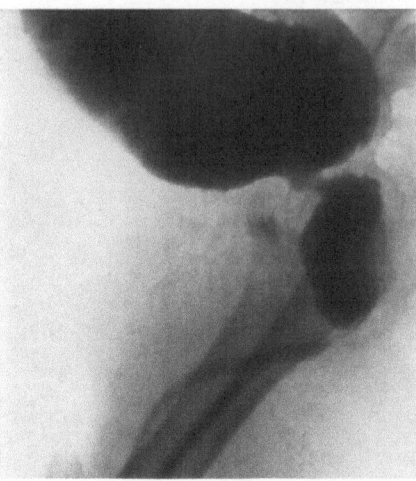

Fig. 429. Sail-like valve formation in posterior part of membranous urethra. At micturition, marked dilatation of urethra proximal to valve. Trabeculation of bladder and reflux into markedly dilated ureters

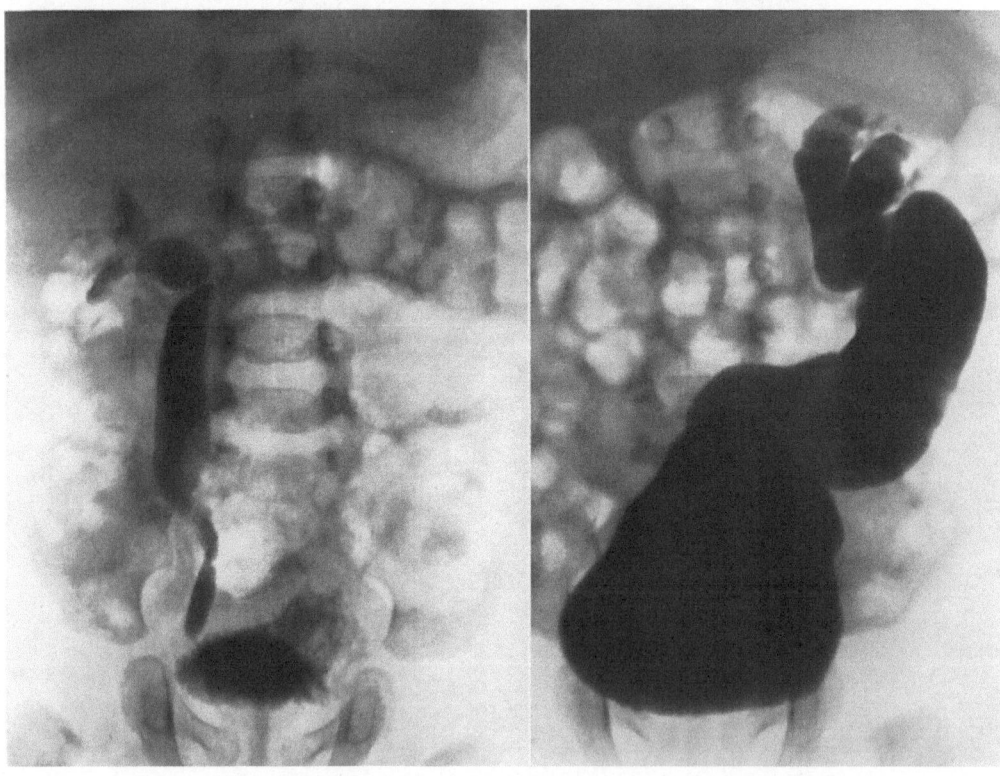

a   b

Fig. 430. Urethral valve. a) Urography: slight dilatation of ureter on right side. No excretion on left side. b) Urethrocystography: marked cysto-ureteric reflux into widened ureter and wide, deformed kidney pelvis corresponding to markedly hypoplastic kidney. c) Urethrocystography: circular membrane in posterior part of membranous urethra. Filling of small colliculus

In general, the literature describes three types of urethral valves: 1) a prominent fold from the region of the collicle runs distally and forms one or, in most cases, two thin sails fixed to the urethral wall, 2) the same type but extending proximally to the interior orifice, 3) a more or less marked, thin diaphragm blocks the urethral lumen anywhere in the posterior part of the urethra. It must be pointed out that a valve formation can vary

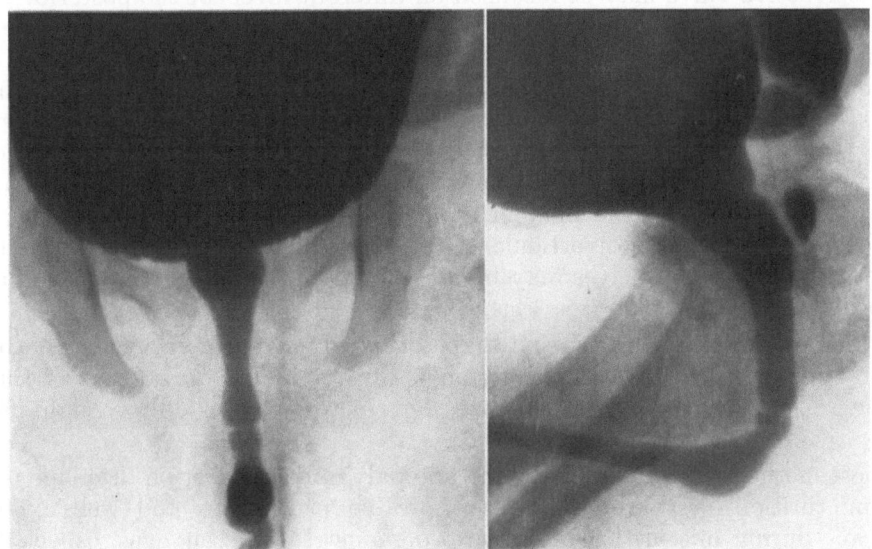

Fig. 430 c

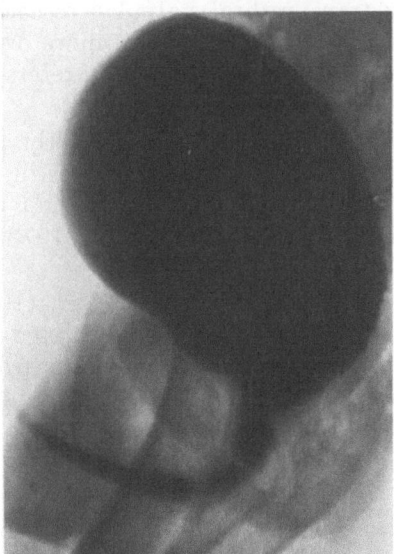

Fig. 431. Urethrocystography: thin fold formation opposite colliculus in pars prostatica urethræ

considerably in shape and size, and borderline cases can be seen where it is impossible definitely to decide if a small plica represents a sail formation or is a normal variation (Figs. 429—431).

A thorough description of the roentgenology of urethral valves is given by KJELL-BERG et al. (1957). These authors have observed two types of valves: a sail-shaped valve and one resembling a diaphragm (corresponding to 1) and 3) above), both with great variations in extension and effect upon urinary drainage. The authors stress that in some instances sail-like, hypertrophic, "normal" folds may be present without causing any obstruction.

The obstructive effect is the important one and can cause marked hydronephrosis and severe renal damage.

The obstructive valve may be localized on different levels of the posterior part of the urethra and affects mainly the ventral part. Valves are usually found at the level of the verumontanum and, accordingly, opposite this anatomic landmark. Reference should be made here to the normal anatomy of the posterior part of the urethra. The intermuscular incisura (see above) must not be mistaken for valves. This incisura is usually localized ventrally, but can occasionally be circular. It does not affect urinary drainage, as does the valve, which more or less markedly causes blockage of the passage of urine at voiding.

In severe obstructions, the bladder wall is markedly hypertrophic, with increased trabeculae and formation of diverticulae. Cysto-ureteral reflux is often present and one or both ureters and kidney pelves may be greatly dilated, as is, of course, the part of the urethra proximal to the lesion (see Figs. 429, 430).

The thickness of the sail in the sail-shaped type of valve can vary considerably. In the diaphragm type of valve, the orifice, which is always in the dorsal part of the urethra, can in severe cases have a pin-point size, but in some cases only a slight fold marks the valve.

The best method of demonstrating the anomaly and its effect on drainage is of course through micturition cystourethrography. Suitable projections and well exposed films are necessary during micturition in order to demonstrate the changes, especially in thin sails or diaphragms.

After treatment (usually transurethral valvular resection), the obstruction can be shown at micturition cystourethrography to have more or less completely disappeared, and secondary obstructive changes in the bladder, ureters, and kidney pelves to have decreased.

Sail-shaped valve formations may also be found in the anterior part of the urethra. HOPE et al. (1970) report the occurrence of such valves in two boy patients. The valve caused no obstruction to the retrograde flow in one of these cases, but produced considerable obstruction during voiding. TEXTER and ENGEL (1972) point out the rarity of this anomaly.

Urine ascites has been reported by MONCADE et al. (1968) in connection with urinary outlet obstruction. A rupture can occur in the dilated collective system. Three cases are described where at cystourethrography reflux was seen from the bladder into markedly dilated ureters and kidney pelves and where from a tear in the superior fornix contrast medium escaped perirenally and into the peritoneal cavity.

2. Inflammatory lesions

There is seldom cause to perform urethrocystography in acute inflammatory lesions of the urethra. The lesions of importance in chronic stages are mainly strictures, fistulae, and diverticula (see above). In less marked stages of an acute or chronic infection, the mucosa is thickened and the floor of the bladder is raised by inflammatory enlargement of the prostatic gland. Passage of contrast medium into the prostatic ducts, and occasionally into the cowperian ducts, can be seen. Swelling of the cowperian glands may cause a slight indentation in the urethral wall. The utriculus may be dilated. The bladder may have a thick wall and trabeculation may be present. The internal orifice may be narrow and a narrowing may also be seen at the external sphincter, which is contracted (Fig. 432).

3. Strictures

Strictures of the urethra may be caused by infection, for example gonorrhea localized mainly in the anterior part of the urethra, tuberculosis (very rare), or by trauma, for example in connection with catheterization or cystoscopy (iatrogenic strictures). The trauma may also be direct or caused by a laceration in fracture of the pelvis. Strictures may also be congenital (see above) (Figs. 433, 434).

A stricture may be localized in any part of the urethra. It may be short or long. Inflammatory strictures are usually long, whereas traumatic strictures are short. A stric-

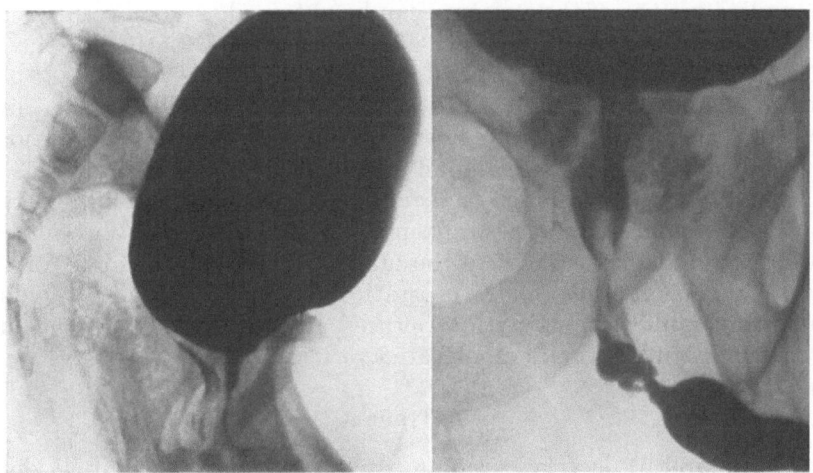

Fig. 432   Fig. 433

Fig. 432. Urethritis in girl five years of age. Swelling of mucosa causing narrowing of lumen

Fig. 433. Marked irregular stricture in pars membranacea (as residuum of gonorrhoic urethritis). Filling of ditated prostatic ducts

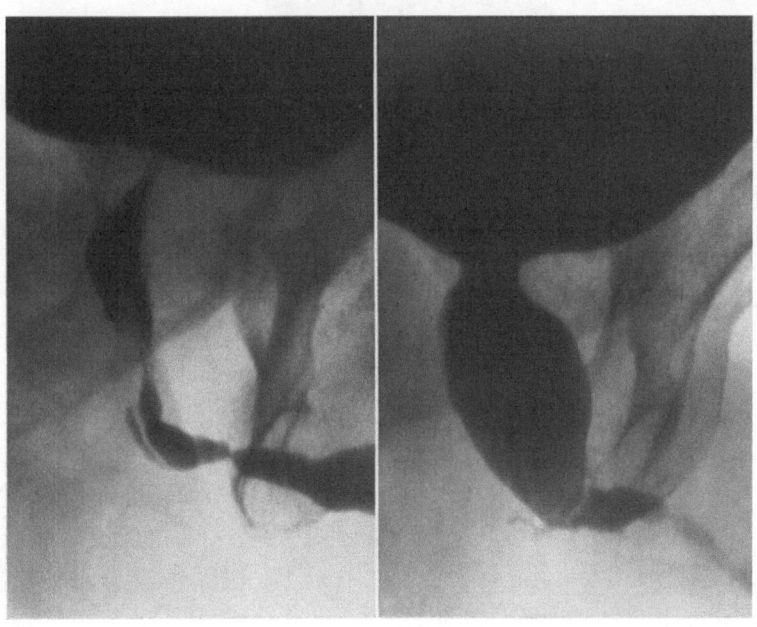

a   b

Fig. 434. a) Marked stricture in pars membranacea. b) Dilatation of urethra proximal to stricture at micturition. Filling of a cowperian gland

ture has occasionally the character of a thin diaphragm. Occasionally long parts of the urethral lumen may be involved. This involvement may be very irregular. Strictures are often multiple. It must be borne in mind that strictures affect the urethral lumen differently. Strictures in the posterior part of the urethra, because of the anatomy of this part, cause prestenotic dilatation at micturition, at a late stage, whereas in the anterior part of the urethra with its pliable wall, a prestenotic dilatation is seen at a very early stage. With the use of in-dwelling catheters in the urethra, strictures are occasionally seen at the penoscrotal angle.

Strictures can be studied at injection of contrast medium and at different degrees of filling a complete picture of the stricture can be obtained. A good result is often secured by the use of micturition urethrography, which can give a picture of the effect of the stricture on urinary flow. It has been pointed out by MORALES and ROMANUS (1954) that during micturition under ordinary conditions, the maximal width of the urethra is not used. Therefore, a very slight stricture, demonstrated at maximal distention of the urethra during urethrography, may not at all affect the passage of urine.

Fistula formation may be seen in connection with strictures and filling of para-urethral cavities may be obtained. They may be from a few millimeters to one centimeter in diameter, usually forming a line parallel to the lumen along the dorsal part of the urethra.

Filling may also be obtained of the prostatic ducts and of Cowper's ducts and glands.

In catheterization of patients with strictures, false passages may be found which at urethrocystography can well be demonstrated.

4. Trauma

Trauma to the urethra is very common. At direct trauma, usually a short laceration may be caused, from which a short stricture may develop. More severe lacerations can cause complete rupture of the urethra and, in some cases, fistula formation (Figs. 435—438).

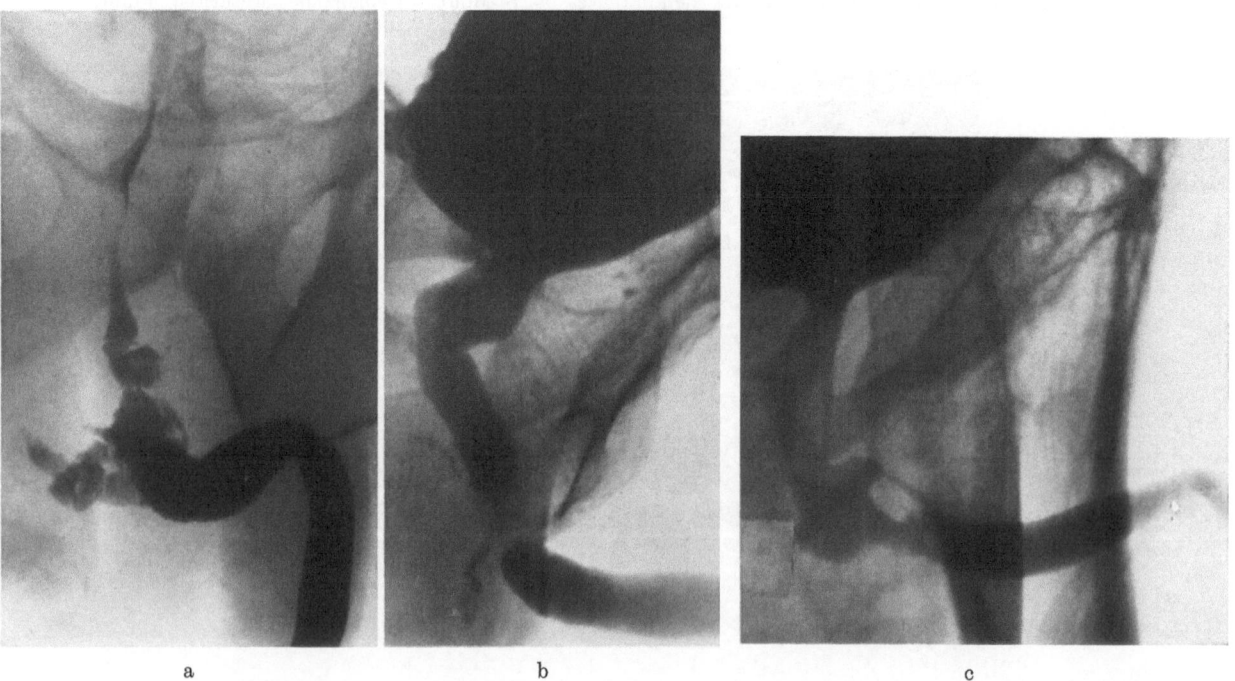

a   b   c

Fig. 435. Trauma with rupture of urethra. a) Urethrocystography: marked extravasation two weeks after trauma. b) Three months later: marked stricture and thin irregular fistulae. c) Post operation: fistulae closed, lumen irregular but wide

Because of the anatomic relationship between the urethra, the pelvic muscles and the bony pelvis, fractures in the anterior part of the pelvis may directly or indirectly cause laceration, with rupture in the posterior part of the urethra.

The most common trauma is the iatrogenic trauma in connection with cystoscopy, catheterization, etc. (Comments have been made above on the anatomic conditions which

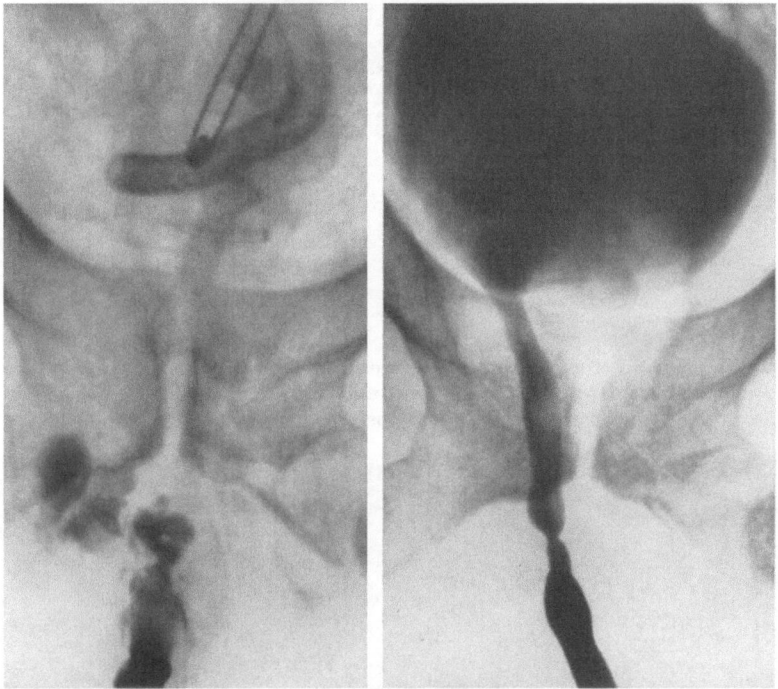

Fig. 436. Complete rupture of the urethra in a case of pelvic fracture (left figure). Non-successful suture, and healing with a false passage outside the external sphincter, consequently with incontinence (right figure)

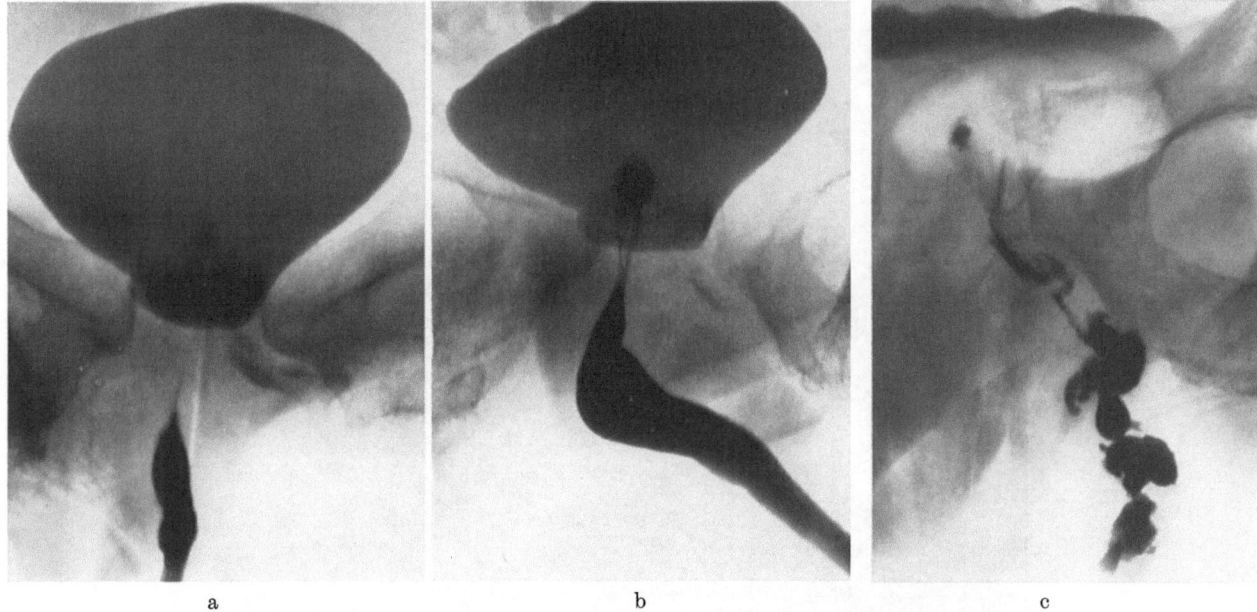

a   b   c

Fig. 437. Trauma with fracture of pelvis, lysis in symphysis and rupture of bladder eight months previously, now fistula to skin a) and b) Urethro-cystography: slight filling of fistula from pars prostatica urethrae. c) Fistulography: long, very irregular fistula to proximal part of urethra

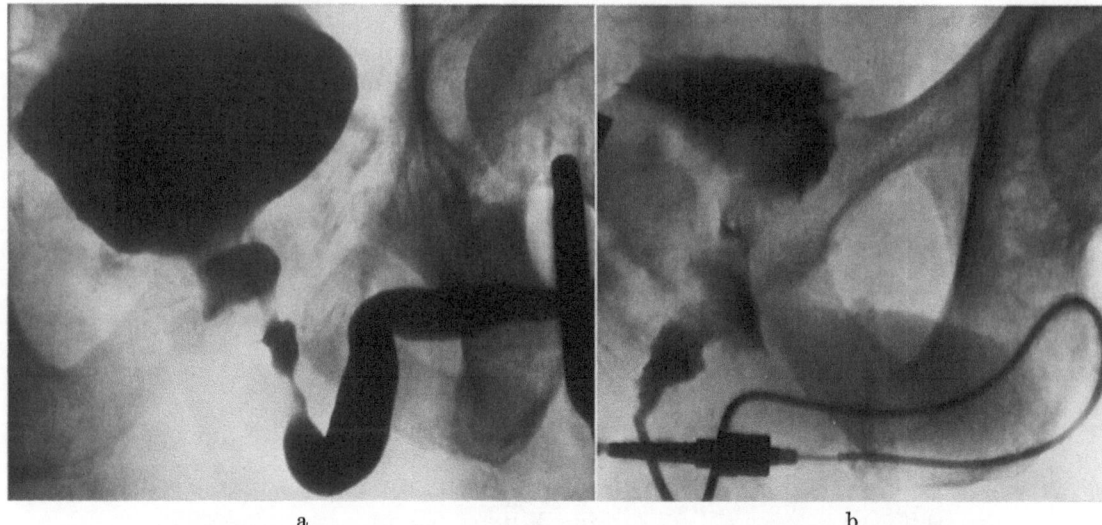

a   b

Fig. 438. Trauma with pelvic fracture and rupture of urethra one year previously. a) Urethro-cystography. b) Retrograde filling via catheter introduced through orificium externum to stricture: marked irregularity by scar formation of pars prostatica and posterior part of pars membranacea

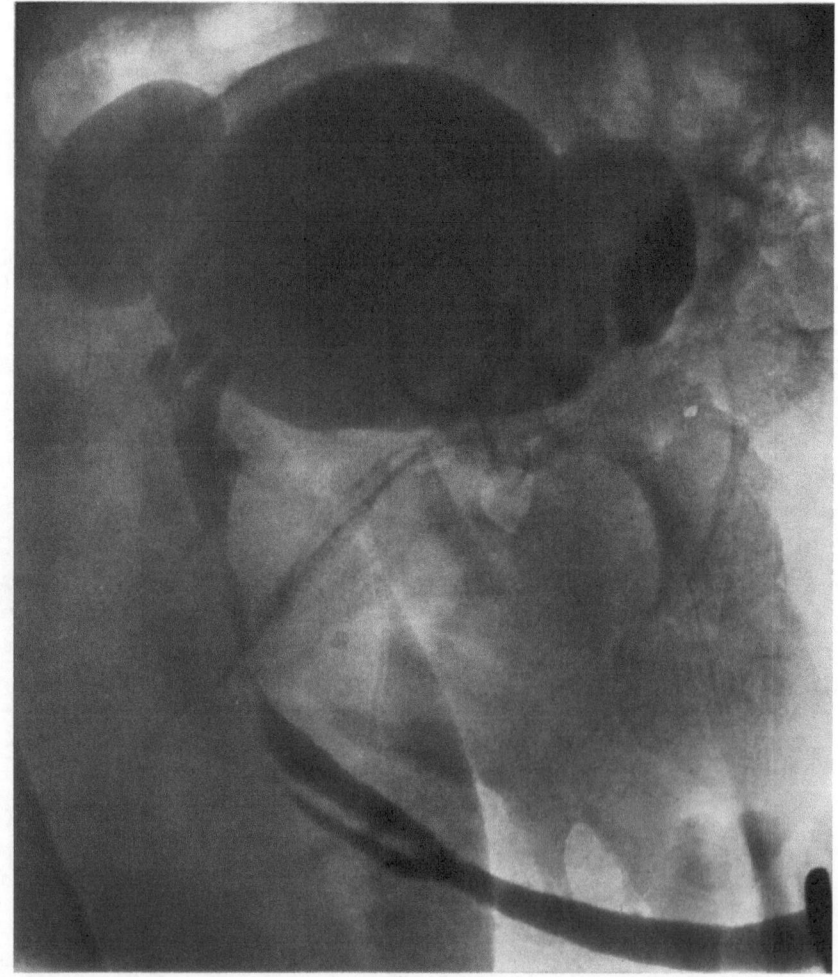

Fig. 439. False passage. Short stricture in posterior part of pars pendula. False passage from stricture along ventral aspect of urethra

make venous reflux easy. This makes the choice of water-soluble contrast agents for urethrocystography necessary). Lesions caused by such procedures may in turn cause local scar formation, with more or less marked stricture.

A so-called false passage may occasionally be detected at urethrocystography (Fig. 439). This may be seen as a double canal of a shorter or longer distance. The two canals unite posteriorly and anteriorly. A dead-end canal may result occasionally when an instrument is forced through the urethral wall and then withdrawn.

5. Urethral tumor

The most common type of tumor engaging the urethra is prostatic carcinoma (see above). A bladder tumor may also encroach upon the adjacent part of the urethra or a papillomatous bladder tumor may continue into the urethra.

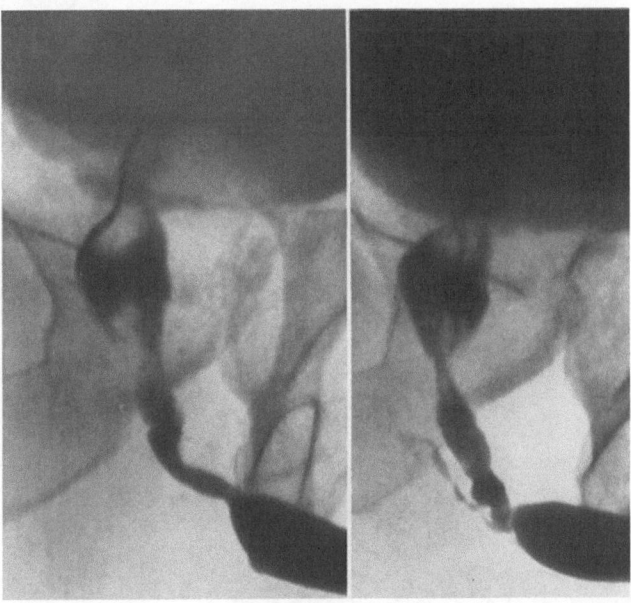

Fig. 440. Primary papillomatous carcinoma of the urethra localized in prostatic and membranaceous parts. (In addition, short irregular, marked stricture and filling of cowperian duct at borderline pars membranacea — pars prostatica)

Malignant tumors primary in the urethra are very rare. Urethral carcinoma is usually of the squamous cell type and located proximally in the anterior part of the urethra, in the bulbous part (Figs. 440—443). In chronic strictures, squamous cell carcinoma may develop. It is difficult to detect at urethrocystography a carcinomatous part of an otherwise very irregular stricture.

Benign tumors of the urethra are more common, but are still rare. The best known type is polyp or papilloma. DOWNS in 1970 found only 29 cases in a review of the literature. The tumor is localized in the posterior part of the urethra, usually at the level of the verumontanum, but it may be found in the anterior part of the urethra and in the most proximal part, at the internal orifice. This type of tumor is found in children and is believed to be congenital because the growth does not follow the general growth of the child (Fig. 444). The earliest detected case of a tumor by urethrocystography was reported by HEGE-DÜS and OKMIAN (1971) in our department, in a girl, on the fourth day after birth. A well

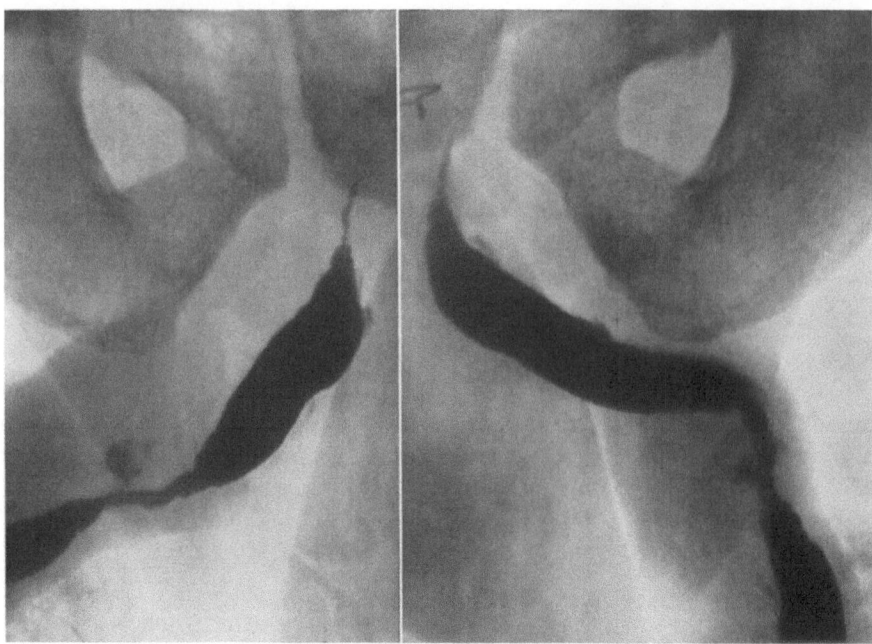

Fig. 441. Primary carcinoma of urethra. Slightly irregular infiltration, 2 cm long, with moderate decrease in width of urethra lumen, in posterior part of pars pendula

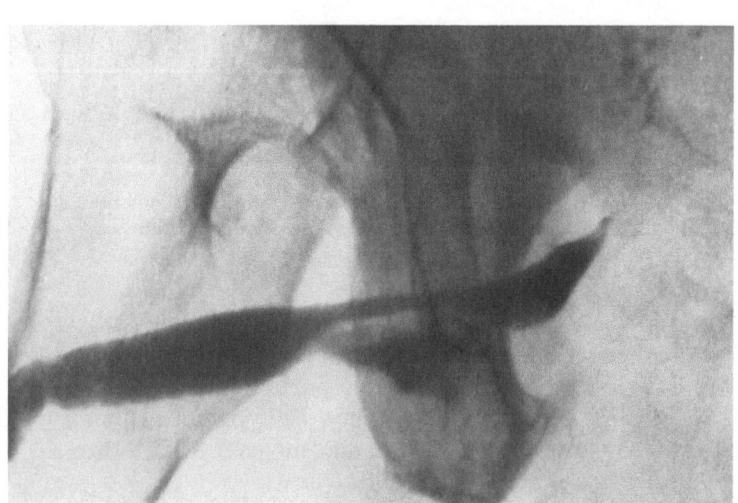

Fig. 442. Primary carcinoma of urethra. Filling of slightly irregular shallow ulceration in carcinoma in posterior part of pars pendula

Fig. 443. Tumor in long part of urethra, mainly pars prostatica, distal part of pars membranacea, and proximal part of pars pendula. Irregular infiltration of wall and some polypous masses. Tumor originated in bladder mucosa at base of bladder with internal orifice

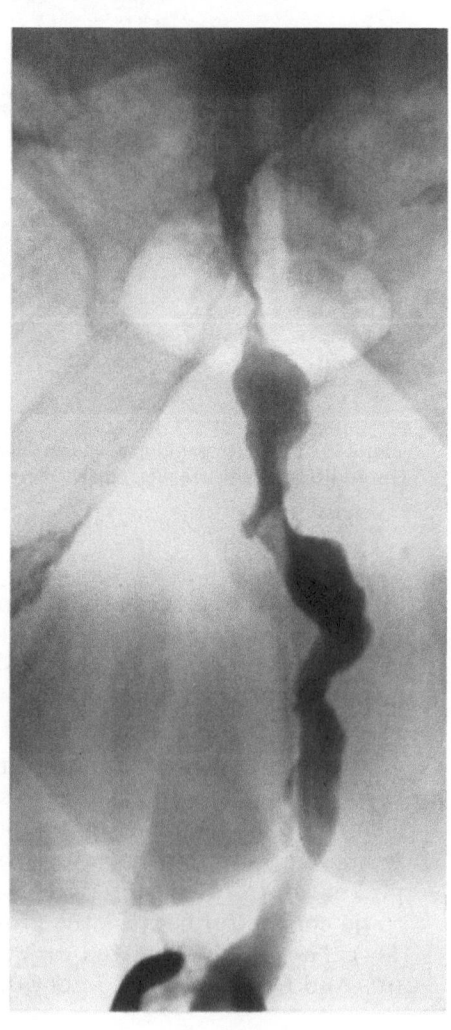

defined, rounded tumor is seen at urethrocystography. The tumor may be slightly moveable within the urethra and, if localized in the proximal part, can pass partly into the bladder and cause urinary obstruction; otherwise polyps are usually detected at examination because of hematuria.

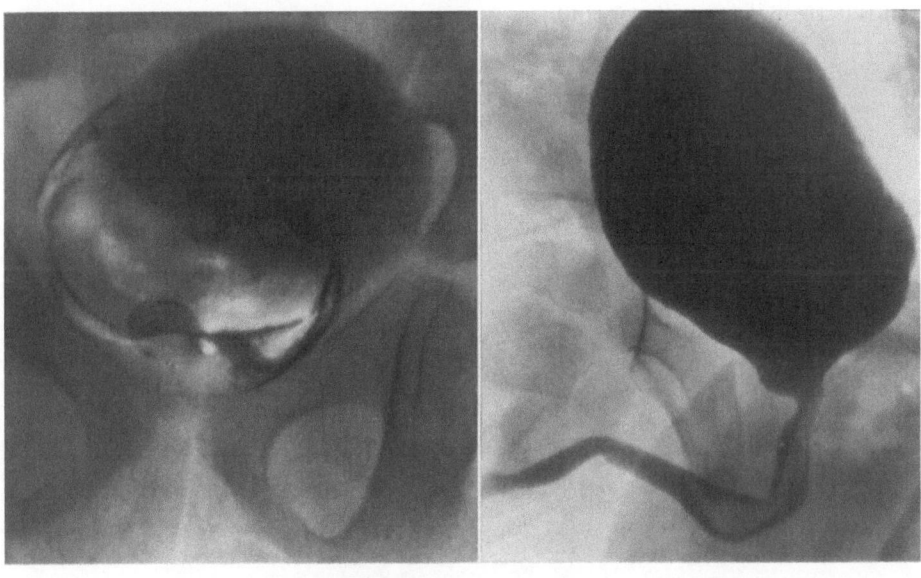

a   b

Fig. 444. Boy with benign polyp in urethra originating at colliculus. Polyp has long stalk making possible localization of polyp at retrograde filling a) in base of bladder and at micturition, b) in posterior part of pars pendula

6. Stone and foreign bodies

In cases of the passage of stone after an attack of renal colic, the stone may be arrested in the urethra for a certain period of time. Therefore, when stone is sought, the penis should be included in the examination of the male patient after such an attack, particularly upon checking after the disappearance of a previously seen stone.

Stone may be lodged or formed in the cavity found after prostatectomy. A urethral diverticulum may also contain stone.

Calcification may occur in desquamated tissue in connection with an operative procedure on the urethra, or on a suture after such a procedure.

Foreign bodies in the urethra are not uncommon in children and in certain psychotic patients. They may calcify completely or partly. They are usually easily detectable, even if not calcified, at plain films or at urethrocystography.

IV. Cystoureteric Reflux

The distal parts of the ureter consist of a paravesical part 2 to 3 cm long, with longitudinal muscle fibers; an intramural part 9 mm in length, also with longitudinal muscles surrounded by bladder muscles; and a submucous part 7 mm in length. The longitudinal muscles in the latter part deviate partly into the trigon, partly downward to the bladder outlet (GREGOIRE and DEBLED, 1971). In addition, muscle fibers from the bladder form the Waldeyers sheath around the distal part of the ureter for a distance of 1 to 3 cm.

This intricate muscle system with the corresponding nerve monitoring regulates urinary flow in the direction ureter to bladder, but blocks retrograde flow. Because of this regulatory mechanism, no reflux of contrast medium occurs to the ureters during urethro-cystography. A slight transitory reflux has been noted very occasionally, however, during cystography in children with no demonstrable urologic disease. Thus IANNACCONE and PANZIRONI (1955) found transitory regurgitation into a ureter in one out of 50 cases. IANNOCCONE later performed cystography periodically in infants and in only one case found a small transitory reflux (1966).

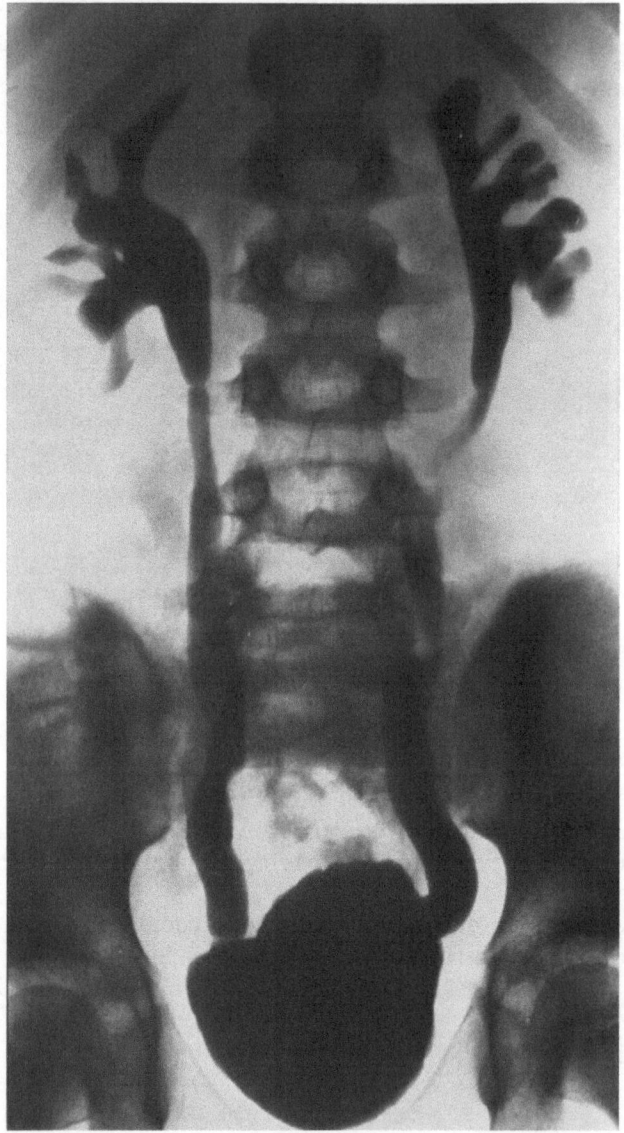

Fig. 445. Cystoureteric reflux during urethrocystography into both ureters, which are moderately dilated, up into pelvis of both kidneys with marked pyelonephritic changes and shrinkage

Reflux is common under pathologic conditions. Thus in children with obstruction to bladder drainage, with urethral valves, for example, a marked incompetence of one or both ureteral orifices is present, with dilatation of ureters and kidney pelves. In many other instances reflux is seen. GRAF et al. (1964) reviewed roentgenologic findings in 50 patients with spina bifida and myelomeningocele and found progressive renal damage occuring over a period of years. Ureteral reflux, demonstrated by delayed cystography, was present in more than half of the patients, in six of which the bladder was apparently normal. Twenty-three patients had dilated kidney pelves. Associated lower tract damage was present in the great majority of these patients.

DAMANSKI (1965), in 455 paraplegics studied by cystography, found reflux in one-fourth of the patients, with a higher incidence in upper motorneurone lesions than in lower.

Reflux causes damage in two ways: back pressure can cause severe damage to kidney function and reflux incurs spread of infection. KJELLBERG et al. (1957) found reflux in 34%

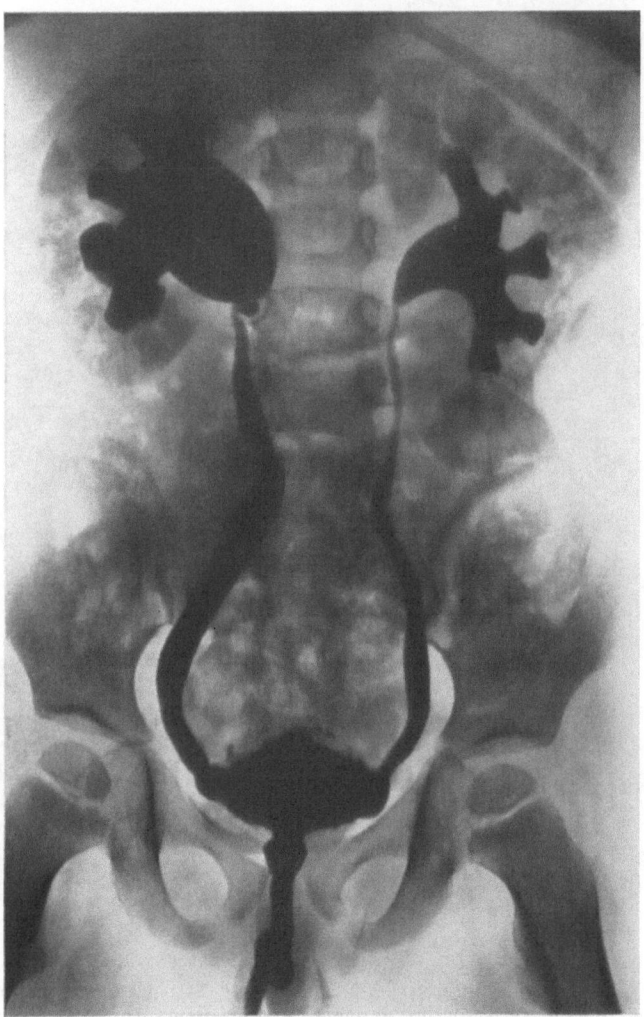

Fig. 446. Cystoureteric reflux. Injection of contrast medium during cystography with a pressure of 75 cm water. Marked reflux to both ureters and kidney pelves with dilatation on right side. Reflux continues up into renal tubuli

of children with recurrent urinary infection. The importance of reflux in pyelonephritis from both of the above-mentioned points of view has been stressed by HINMAN and HUTCH (1962) and by HODSON (1967), for example. The latter author believes that reflux provides the answer regarding the pathway of infection in the vast majority of cases of pyelonephritis and that it also provides a ready-made mechanism by which infection maintains itself (see Fig. 445).

STEPHENS and LENAGHAN (1963), however studied 34 patients with vesico-ureteric reflux for a period of up to ten years and found no infection or change in kidney function.

SUNDIN and FRITJOFSSON (1965) found three patients to have sterile urine and normal renal function one to 11 years after the first detection of reflux.

The reflux may be very marked and continue from the kidney pelvis into the tubules (Fig. 446).

A marked dilatation can be seen not infrequently of the kidney pelvis and the ureter on one or both sides in connection with cystoureteric reflux, where, during urography, no dilatation was seen (Fig. 447).

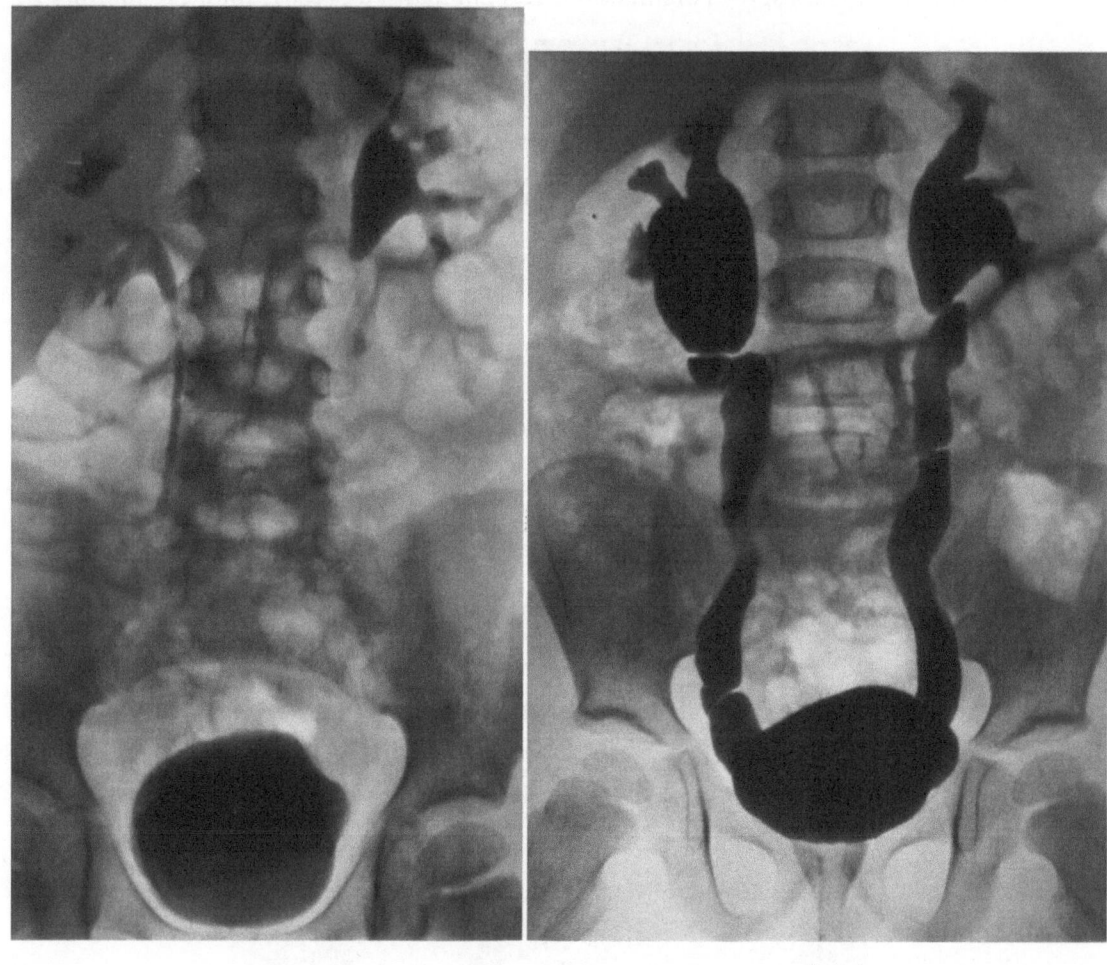

a   b

Fig. 447. a) Urography in patient with persistent urinary infection. Ordinary excretion. Marked plasticity especially of right kidney pelvis. b) Cystoureteric reflux in connection with cystography. Marked reflux to ureters and kidney pelves with marked dilatation as compared with conditions during urography

During urethrocystography reflux may occur into a ureter with an ectopic orifice in the urethra (Fig. 448).

Reflux may be iatrogenic, caused by surgical procedures. Thus extraction of a ureteric stone or meatotomy of the ureteric orifice to remove stone may occasionally cause reflux. GREGERSEN and BUUS (1971) found cysto-ureteric reflux in three patients out of 24 in whom meatotomy was performed. The reflux gave rise to symptoms of urinary tract infection in one patient, in whom the reflux improved after the infection had been treated.

Several surgical methods have been designed to arrest reflux. In this connection it should be pointed out that the clinical differentiation between primary and secondary reflux cannot be made roentgenologically. The latter type of reflux is supposed to be due entirely to infection, for example, and therefore in several instances a long period of anti-infectious treatment is recommended before surgical therapy is contemplated.

The reflux phenomenon may be rapid and transitory during cystography. The cysto-graphic examination should therefore be made under fluoroscopic control, when reflux

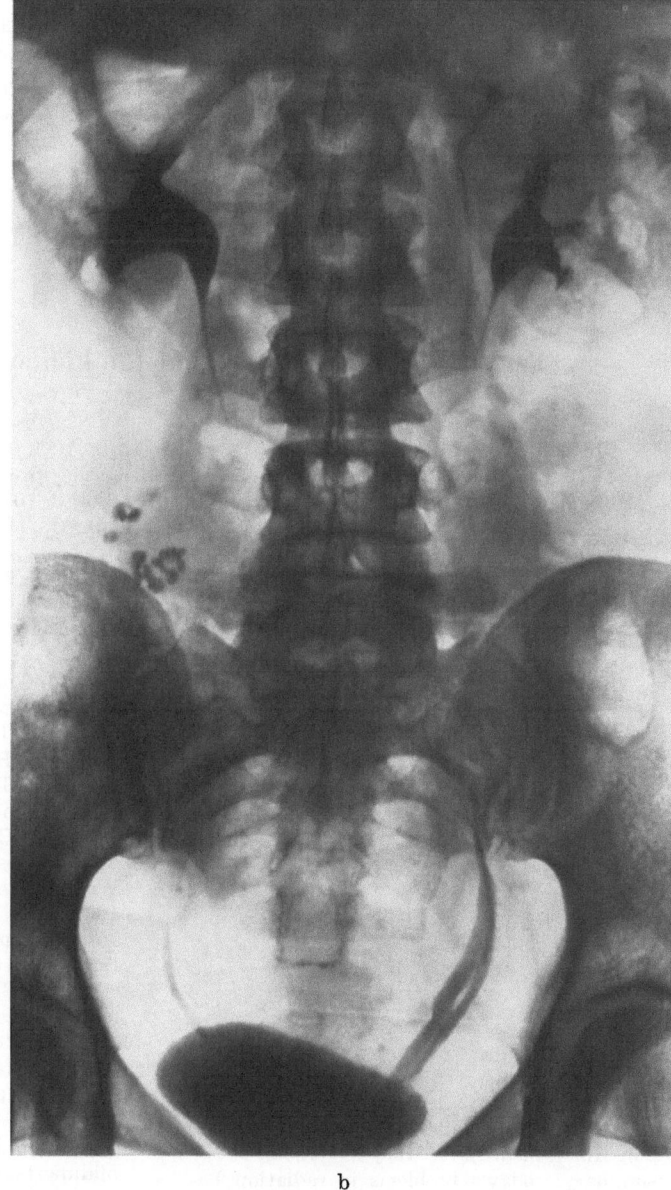
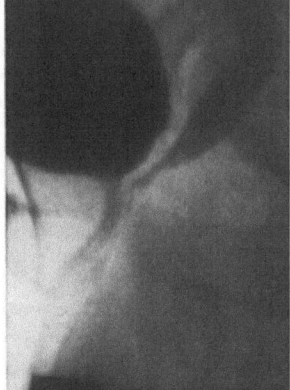

a   b

Fig. 448. Reflux from proximal part of urethra into ureter to cranial kidney pelvis in double kidney with ectopic orifice in proximal part of urethra a), urography b)

is usually easily seen. The examination should include films of the ureter and kidney pelves, with the patient in supine position, at least at the end of the examination, in order to determine if reflux of contrast medium has occurred. It must be stressed, however, that even in the presence of reflux seen and documented during fluoroscopy, the kidney pelves and the ureters may be completely empty at the end of the examination.

It must be stressed further that a normal appearance of the kidney pelves and ureters at urography does not exclude the presence of cysto-ureteral reflux. It is occasionally surprising to observe how in such a case a marked reflux may occur at cystography, with demonstration of widening of the proximal urinary pathways. Cystography should therefore be performed in each case where reflux could be a factor in the pathophysiology of a clinical situation. It should be pointed out here that in connection with surgical correction of the ureteric ostium because of vesico-ureteric reflux, the operative procedure may cause temporary, complete, or incomplete block of urine flow through the ureteric orifice. This causes stasis in the homolateral kidney. It is a good rule to check post-operative conditions by *urography* shortly after operation in this, as in all other operative procedures on the ureter.

References

Part I: Roentgen diagnosis of the kidney and the ureter

B. Examination Fundamentale

II. Radiation protection

ARDRAN, G. M., CROOKS, H. E., KEMP, F. H., OLIVER, R.: Radiation dose to staff in medical x-ray departments. Brit. J. Radiol. **30**, 600 (1957).

— KEMP, F. H.: Protection of the male gonads in diagnostic procedures. Brit. J. Radiol. **30**, 280 (1957).
Reduction of radiation doses administered during chest radiography. Tubercle (Lond.) **38**, 403 (1957).

BAKER, W. J., PORTNEY, F. R., FIRFER, R.: A study of x-ray hazards. Urol. Int. (Basel) **1**, 135 (1955).

— A study of x-ray hazards of retrograde urography. J. Urol. (Baltimore) **74**, 174 (1955).

BÖÖK, Jan A.: Joniserande strålning och genetisk morbiditet. Sv. Läk.-Tidn. (Stockholm) **54**, 517 (1957).

BRAESTRUP, C. B.: Past and present radiation exposure to radiologists from the point of view of life expectancy. Amer. J Roentgenol. **78**, 988 (1957).

CARLSSON, C.: Integral absorbed doses in roentgen diagnostics, a theoretical analysis and clinical application. Acta Universitatis Lundensis, Sectio II (1964).

CHAMBERLAIN, R. H.: Radiation protection comes of age. J. Amer. Med. Assoc. **153**, 488 (1953).

— A summary: today's problems in radiation hazards and what is being done to control them. Amer. J. Roentgenol. **78**, 1000 (1957).

COOLEY, R. N., BEENTJES, L. B.: Weighted gonadal diagnostic roentgen-ray doses in a teaching hospital with comments on x-ray dosages to the general population of the U.S. Amer. J. Roentgenol. **92**, 404 (1964).

DEUEL, H. J. jr., CHENG, A. L. S. KRYDER, G. D., BINGEMANN, M. E.: Protective effect against X-irradiation of methyl linoleate in the rat. Science **117**, 254–255 (1953).

DEUEL, H. J. jr., Exposure of man to ionizing radiation arising from medical procedures. Phys. in Med. Biol. **2**, 107–151 (1957).

FAILLA, G., McCLEMENT, P.: The shortening of life by chronic whole-body irradiation. Amer. J. Roentgenol. **78**, 946 (1957).

GLASS, B.: The genetic basis for the limitation of radiation exposure. Amer. J. Roentgenol. **78**, 955 (1957).

HAMMER-JACOBSEN, E.: Genetically significant radiation doses in diagnostic radiology. Acta radiol. Suppl. **222** (1963).

HOLTHUSEN, H., LEETZ, H.-K., LEPPIN, W.: Die genetische Belastung der Bevölkerung einer Großstadt (Hamburg) durch medizinische Strahlenanwendung. Heft 21 Strahlenschutz, Schriftenreihe des Bundesministers für Atomkernenergie und Wasserwirtschaft. München: Gersbach & Sohn 1961.

— International Commission for Radiation Protection, Bulletin Nr. 2 (1959.

KAPLAN, H. S.: An evaluation of the somatic and genetic hazards of the medical uses of radiation. Amer. J. Roentgenol. **80**, 696 (1958).

KAUDE, J., CARLSSON, C., SPANNE, P.: Patientendosis und Strahlenbelastung des Röntgenpersonals bei angiographischen Untersuchungen. In: Angiographie und ihre Fortschritte, Arbeits und Fortbildungstagung, Baden-Baden (1970). Stuttgart: Georg Thieme Verlag 1972.

KOCKUM, J., LIDÉN, K., NORMAN, O.: Radiation hazards attending use of transportable image intensifier. Acta radiol. (Stockh.) **46**, 369 (1958).

LARSSON, L.-E.: Radiation doses to patients and personnel in modern roentgen diagnostic work. Acta radiol. (Stockh.) **46**, 680 (1956).

— Radiation doses to the gonads of patients in Swedish roentgen diagnostics. Acta radiol. (Stockh.) Suppl. **157** (1958).

LAUGHLIN, J. S., MEURK, M. L., PULLMANN, I., SHERMAN, R. S.: Bone, skin, and gonadal doses in routine diagnostic procedures. Amer. J. Roentgenol. **78** (1957).

LINDELL, B., DOBSON, R. L.: Ionizing radiation and health. World Health Organiz. Public Health Papers Nr. **6** (1961).

NORWOOD, W. D.: Common sense approach to the problem of genetic hazard due to diagnostic radiology. J. Amer. med. Ass. **167**, 1928 (1958).

— The determination of injury from the internally deposited radioisotope plutonium. J. occupat. Med. **1**, 269 (1959).

— HEALY, J. W., DONALDSON, E. E., ROESCH, C. W., KIRKLIN, C.W.: The gonadal radiation dose received by the people of a small American city due to the diagnostic use of roentgen rays. Amer. J. Roentgenol. **82**, 1081 (1959).

RUSSELL, L. B., RUSSELL, W. L.: Radiation hazards to embryo and fetus. Radiology **58**, 369 (1952)

SPIEGLER, G. KEANE, B. E,: Scatter doses received on the lower extremities of the diagnostic radiologist. Brit. J. Radiol. **28**, 140 (1955).

STANFORD, R. W., VANCE, J.: Quantity of radiation received by reproductive organs of patients during routine diagnostic X-ray examinations. Brit. J. Radiol. **28**, 266 (1955).

STIEVE, F. E.: Untersuchungen über Maßnahmen zur Reduzierung der Strahlenbelastung der männlichen Keimdrüsen bei röntgendiagnostischen Maßnahmen in deren Umgebung. Fortschr. Röntgenstr. **90**, 373 (1959).

STONE, R. S.: COMMON sense in radiation protection applied to clinical practice. Amer. J. Roentgenol. **78**, 993 (1957).

SVAHN, G., CARLSSON, C. SPANNE, P.: Radiation doses in angiographic procedures. Paper presented at 31st Congress, Scandinavian Soc. for Med. Radiol. Reykjavik, 1971.

SWENSON, P. C.: The radiation hazards of diagnostic procedures. Radiology **63**, 876 (1954).

TAYLOR, L. S.: Practical suggestions for reducing radiation exposure in diagnostic examinations. Amer. J. Roentgenol. **78**, 983 (1957).

WARREN, S.: Longevity and causes of death from irradiation in physicians. J. Amer. med. Ass. **162**, 464 (1956).

WOERT jr., I. VAN, KEARNEY, P, I., KILICOZLU, I., ROACH, J. F.: Radiation hazards of intravenous pyelography. J. Amer. med. Ass. **166**, 1826 (1958).

WORLD HEALTH ORGANIZATION: Technical Report Series. Nr. **248** (1962) Radiation hazards in perspective: Third report of the Expert Comm. on Radiation.

— Nr. **306** (1965) Public health and the medical use of ionizing radiation: Fifth report of the WHO Expert Comm. on Radiation.

— WHO Public health Papers Nr. **6** (1961) Ionizing radiation and health (LINDELL, B., DOBSON, R. L.).

— WHO report on Conference on the public health aspects of protection against ionizing radiation (Düsseldorf 1962). (Distributed by WHO Regional Office. Copenhagen).

— WHO report on European seminar on public health aspects of the medical uses of ionizing radiation (Lund 1965). (Distributed by WHO Regional Office, Copenhagen).

III. Preparation of the Patient

BERG, O. C., ALLEN, D. H.: Use of carbonated beverage as an aid in pediatric excretory urography. J. Urol. **67**, 393 (1952).

BERG, V., DUFRESNE, M.: Excretory urography in the pediatric patient with the aid of carbonated beverage. Harper Hosp. Bull. **14**, 122 (1956).

COLLINS, E. N., ROOT, J. C.: Elimination of confusing gas shadows during cholecystography by use of pitressin. J. Amer. Med. Ass. **107**, 32 (1936).

DUNBAR, J. S., MacEWAN, D. W., HEBERT, F.: The value of dehydration in intravenous pyelography — an experimental study. Amer. J. Roentgenol. **84**, 813 (1960).

GÖTHLIN, J.: Vasopressin as an aid in eliminating intestinal gas before roentgen examination of the abdomen. Acta radiol. **12**, 100 (1972).

GYLLENSWÄRD, Å., LODIN, H., MYKLAND, O.: Prevention of undue intestinal gas in abdominal radiography in infants. Acta radiol. **39**, 6 (1953).

HEGEDÜS, V.: Röntgenförberedelse med kontaktlaxativ och diet. Läkartidningen (Stockh.) **68**, 4365 (1971).

JUTRAS, A., CANTERO, A.: Le Pitressin, hormone antipneumatosigne son emploi dans le radiodiagnostique abdominal. J. Radiol. et Electrol. **20**, 443 (1936).

KOSENOW, W.: Verbesserung der Säuglings- und Kleinkinder-Urographie durch gleichzeitige Flüssigkeits- und Luftfüllung des Magens. Fortschr. Röntgenstr. **83**, 396 (1955).

— Einfache Methode zur Verbesserung der Ausscheidungsurogramme bei Säuglingen und Kleinkindern. Mschr. Kinderheilk. **103**, 407 (1955).

LILJA, B., WAHREN, H.: On meteorism in pyelography. Acta radiol. **15**, 41 (1934).

MAGNUSSON, W.: On meteorism in pyelography and on the passage of gas through the small intestine. Acta radiol. **12**, 552 (1931).

MURPHY, T. E.: Effective evacuation of the bowel preparatory to urologic radiography. J. Urol. **86**, 659 (1961).

RAMBO, O., ZBORALSKE, F. F., JARROS, P. RIEGELMAN, S., MARGULIS, A.: Toxic studies on tannic acid administered by enema, I. II. III. Amer. J. Reontgenol. **96**, 488 (1966).

SCHEIBEL, O.: Concerning pitressin in roentgen examination of the abdomen as an agent for reducing shadows caused by intestinal gas. Acta radiol. **XVII**, 511 (1936).

SLANINA, J.: The value of hydrogen peroxide and tannic acid in cleansing enema. Radiol. clin. (Basel) **27**, 197 (1958).

STEINERT, R.: Effect of enemata on contrast excretion in urography. Acta radiol. **38**, 30 (1952).

WYATT, G. M.: Excretory urography for children. Radiology **36**, 664 (1941).

C. Examination Methods

I. Plain radiography

ALBRICHT, F., BAIRD, P. C., COPE, O., BLOOMBERG, E.: Studies on the physiology of the parathyorid glands. Amer. J. Med. Sci. **187**, 49 (1934).
— REIFENSTEIN, jr. E. C.: The parathyroid glands and metabolic bone disease. Baltimore 1948.

ANDERSEN, P. E.: Pneumoretroperitoneum in suprarenal disease. Acta radiol. **43**, 289 (1955).

ÅKERLUND, Å.: Über die Technik bei Röntgenuntersuchung der freigelegten Niere. Acta chir. scand. **79**, 553 (1937).

ARONS, W. L., CHRISTENSEN, W. R., SOSMAN, M. C.: Nephrocalcinosis visible by x-ray associated with chronic glomerulonephritis. Ann. Intern. Med. **42**, 260 (1955).

ASK-UPMARK, E.: Über Röntgenuntersuchung der Nieren bei gewissen diagnostisch schwer zu deutenden Krankheitsfällen in der inneren Medizin. Acta med. scand. **96**, 390 (1938).

ASTRALDI, A., URIBURU, J. V. Jr.: Radiologia del rinon durante el acto operatorio. Rév. Med. Lat. Amer. **21**, 891 (1936).

BASKIN, A. M., HARVARD, B. M., JANZEN, A. H.: Sterile fluoroscopy: preliminary report of a new technique for localization of renal calculi. J. Urol. **78**, 821 (1957).

BAUER, H.: Beitrag zu den Nierenverkalkungen. Btsch. Z. Chir. **254**, 1 (1940).

BECKER, R.: Beitrag zur Verbesserung der röntgenologischen Nierendiagnostik. Münch. med. Wschr. **97**, 1104 (1955).

BEER, E.: Roentgenological control of exposed kidneys in operations for nephrolithiasis with the use of special intensifying cassette. J. Urol. **25**, 159 (1931).

BENJAMIN, E. W.: Notes on the technique of x-ray control in the operating room. J. Urol. **25**, 165 (1931).

BERNARDINI e, R. SALVATI: Retropneumoperitoneo, nuovo mezzo di indagine radiologica Gas.-intes. Med. Chir. **44**, 301 (1950).

BEZOLD, K., FEINDT, H. R., PRESSLER, K.: Der Röntgenbildverstärker in Routinebetrieb. Fortschr. Röntgenstr. **85**, 447 (1956).

BIBUS, B.: Die Pneumoradiographie des Nierenlagers. Wien. klin. Wschr. **52**, 256 (1939).

BLAND, A. B.: A simplified apparatus for presacral carbon dioxide injection. J. Urol. **79**, 171 (1958).

BODNER, H., HOWARD, A. H., KAPLAN, J. H.: Cinefluorography for the urologist. J. Urol. **79**, 356 (1958).

BONOMINI e BACCAGLINI: Pneumoretroperitoneo e pneumomediastino. L'enfisema diagnostico dei tessuti areolari profondi del tronco. Bologna: Capelli 1953.

BRODNY, M. L., CHAMBERLAIN, H. A.: A simple apparatus for pneumoadrenalography. J. Urol. **42**, 211 (1939).

BURNETT, C. H., COMMONS, R. R., ALBRIGHT, F., HOWARD, J. E.: Hypercalcemia without hypercalcuria or hypophosphatemia, calcinosis and renal insufficiency. New Engl. J. Med. **240**, 787 (1949).

BUSCHER, A. K.: Beitrag zur Röntgendiagnostik an der freigelegten Niere. Urologia (Treviso) **22**, 217 (1955).

CAHILL, G. F.: Air injections to demonstrate the adrenals by x-ray. J. Urol. **34**, 238 (1935).

CARELLI, M. H.: Sur le pneumopéritoine et sur une méthode personelle pour voir le rein sans pneumopéritoine. Bull. Soc. Med. Hop. Paris **45**, 1409 (1921).

COCCHI, U.: Retropneumoperitoneum und Pneumomediastinum. Stuttgart: Georg Thieme 1957. Fortschr. Röntgenstr. Erg.-Bd. **79**.

COONEY, J. D., AMELAR, R. D., ORRON, A.: Renal displacement and rotation during retroperitoneal pneumography. Arch. Surg. (Chicago) **70**, 405 (1955).

COPE, O., SCHATZKI, R.: Tumors of the adrenal glands. Arch. Intern. Med. **64**, 1222 (1939).

DODSON, A. I.: Urological surgery. London 1956.

DURANT. E. M., LONG, J., OPPENHEIMER, M. J.: Pulmonary (venous) air embolism. Amer. Heart J. **33**, 269 (1947).

EVANS, A. T.: Combined use of contrast media in retroperitoneal tumors. Critical evaluation. Arch. Surg. (Chicago) **70**, 191 (1955).

EVANS, J. A., POKER, N.: Newer roentgenographic techniques in the diagnosis of retroperitoneal tumors. J. Amer. Med. Ass. **161**, 1128 (1956).

FAGERBERG, S.: Pneumoretroperitoneum. Acta radiol. **37**, 519 (1952).

FONTAINE, R., WARTER, P., FRANK, P., STOLL G., RABER, R.: De l'intéret du rétropneumopéritoine pour le diagnostic des malformations et néoplasmes du rein. J. Radiol. Electrol. **36**, 708 (1955).

FRANCIOSI, A. U., GOVONI, A. F., PASQUINELLI, C. G.: Retroperitoneum associated with laminography. Amer. J. Roentgenol. **72**, 1034 (1954).

FUSI, G.: Considerazioni sull'iperparatiroidismo in nefropatic. Radiol. Med. (Torino) **40**, 551 (1954).

GANDINI, D., GIBBA, A.: Present trends in the diagnoses of surgical renal diseases by means of pneumoretroperitoneum combined with the usual radio-urological technique. Nunt. Radiol. **20**, 707 (1954).

GENNES, L. DE, MAY, J. P., SIMON, G.: Le rétropneumoperitoine (Nouveau procedé d'exploration radiologique de l'abdomen.) Presse méd. **21**, 351 (1950).

GIRAUD, G., BETOULIERES, P., LATOUR, H., PELISSIER M.: La neumostratigrafia. Arch. esp. Med. interna **2**, 79 (1956).

GIRAUD, M., BRET, P., KUENTZ, M., ANJOU, A.: Bilan de cent examens après pneumorétroperitoine. J. Radiol. Electrol. **35**, 838 (1954).

GLASMANN, I., SHAPIRO, R., ROBINSON, F.: Air embolism during presacral pneumography: a case report. J. Urol. **75**, 560 (1956).

HAMRE, L.: Fibrolipomatosis renis. Nord. med. **58**, 1769 (1957).

HARRIS, P., ZBORALSKE, F. F., RAMBO, O., MARGULIS, A., RIEGELMAN, S.: Toxicity studies on tannic acid administered by enema. II. The colonic absorption and intraperitoneal toxicity of tannic acid and its hydrolytic products in rats. Amer. J. Roentgenol. **96**, 498 (1966).

HARROW, B. R., SLOANE, J. A.: The dromedary or humped left kidney. Amer. J. Roentgenol. **88**, 144–152 (1962).

HAUBRICH, R.: Zwerchfellpathologie, Berlin-Heidelberg: Springer-Verlag 1957.

HEGEDÜS, V.: Röntgenförberedelse med ett kontaktlaxativ (Toilax) och diet. Läkartidn. (Stockholm) **68**, 4365 (1971).

HEIDENBLUT, A.: Röntgendiagnostik des verkalkten Renalisaneurysmas. Fortschr. Röntgenstr. **83**, 868 (1955).

HELLSTRÖM, J.: Clinical experience of twenty-one cases of hyperparathyroidism with special reference to the prognosis following parathyroidectomy. Acta chir. scand **100**, 391 (1950).

— Further observations regarding the prognosis and diagnosis in hyperparathyroidism. Acta chir. scand. **105**, 122 (1953).

— Primary hyperparathyroidism. Observations in a series of 50 cases. Acta endocr. (Copenhagen) **16**, 30 (1954).

— Calcification and calculus formation in a series of seventy cases of primary hyperparathyroidism. Brit. J. Urol. **27**, 387 (1955).

HEUSSER, H.: Röntgenuntersuchung der operativ freigelegten Niere. Schweiz. med. Wschr. **18**, 630 (1937).

HODSON, C. J.: Physiological changes in size of the human kidney. Clin. Radiol. **12**, 91 (1961).

— DREWE, J. A., KARN, M. N., KING, A.: Renal size in normal children. A radiographic study during life. Arch. Dis. Child. **37**, 616 (1962); abstract in: Yearbook of Radiol. 1963–64, 228.

HOPE, J. W., MICHIE, A. J.: Hydronephrosis following retrograde pyelography. Radiology **72**, 844 (1959).

IAVAZYAN, A. V.: Visualization of kidney anomalies by the aid of presacral pneumoretroperitoneum (Russian text). Vestn. Rentgenol. Radiol. **32**, 60 (1957).

ISAACS, I.: Medial ptosis of the kidney. Clinical Radiology **22**, 214 (1971).

KESHIN, J. G., JOFFE, A.: Varices of the upper urinary tract and their relationship to portal hypertension. J. Urol. **76**, 350 (1956).

KOCKUM, J., LIDÉN, K., NORMAN, O.: Radiation hazards attending use of transportable image intensifier. Acta radiol. **49**, 369 (1958).

KRETSCHMER, H. L.: Intravenous urography. Surg. Gynec. Obst. **51**, 404 (1930).

KÖHLER, H.: Indikationsgebiet der Pneumoradiographie. Dtsch. Ges. Urol. 1926, S. 119.

LALLI, A. F.: Renal enlargement. Radiology **84**, 688 (1965).

LANDES, R. R., RANSOM, C. L.: Presacral retroperitoneal pneumography utilizing carbon dioxide: further experiences and improved technique. J. Urol. **82**, 670 (1959).

LEVINE, B.: Use of helium in perirenal insufflation: preliminary reports. J. Urol. **67**, 390 (1952).

LEWIS, S., DOSS, R. D.: Calcified hydropyonephrosis. Radiology **70**, 866 (1958).

LILJA, B., WAHREN, H.: On meteorism in pyelography. Acta radiol. **15**, 41 (1934).

LUDIN, H.: Tomographische Bestimmung der Nierengröße. Fortschr. Röntgenstr. **96**, 215 (1961).

MACARINI, N., OLIVA, L.: Sur l'insufflation rétropéritonéale associée à la stratigraphie tridimensionell. J. belge Radiol. **34**, 281 (1951).

MAJELA, DE ABREU GUEDES, G.: Nossa experiencia com o retro-pneumoperitoneo. Rev. Brasil. Cir. **32**, 193 (1956).

MARTZ, H.: Renal calcification accompanying pyloric and high intestinal obstruction. Arch. Intern. Med. **65**, 375 (1940).

MAY, F.: Ein Beitrag zur Röntgenphotographie der freigelegten Niere. Z. Urol. **36**, 89 (1942).

— Meßergebnisse des osmotischen Druckes der zur Zeit gebräuchlichsten Kontrastmittel. Schering AB. (Berlin-West) 1957.

MENCHER, W. H.: Perirenal insufflation. J. Amer. Med. Ass. **109**, 1338 (1937).

MENEGHINI, C., DELL'ADAMI, G.: Die Insufflation des extraperitonealen Bindegewebes in der Röntgendiagnostik der oberen Harnorgane mit besonderer Berücksichtigung der Möglichkeiten der Stratigraphie. Fortschr. Röntgenstr. **76**, 181 (1952).

METZLER, R., HABIGHORST, L. V., DIETHELM, L.: Komplikationen des Retropneumoperitoneum unter Verwendung von Kohlendioxyd als Insufflationsgas. Der Radiologe **12**, 367 (1972).

MISHALANY, H. G., GILBERT, D. R.: Benign ossified lesion of kidney. J. Urol. **78**, 330 (1957).

MONTERO, J. J.: Aplasia renal y retropneumoperitoneo. Arch. Espan. Urol. **14**, 26 (1958).

MOOS, F. VON: Die Tomographie beim Pneumoretroperitoneum. Schw. med. Wschr. **82**, 629 (1952).

MOSCA, L. G.: El enfisema retroperitoneal: Su técnica sus indicaciones y resultados. Pren, méd. Argentina **38**, 1025 (1951).

MOSENTHAL, A.: Unsere Erfahrungen mit der „Pneumoradiographie des Nierenlagers" nach P. Rosenstein. Z. Urol. Chir. **12**, 303 (1923).

MUSCHAT, M., KOOPLE, L.: Parenchymal calculosis of the kidneys. J. Urol. **42**, 293 (1939).

NESBIT, R. M., CRENSHAW, W. B.: Aneurysm of the renal artery. J. Urol. **75**, 380 (1956).

NUGENT, C. A., STOWELL, W.: Localization of the kidney for renal biopsy. J. Urol. **82**, 193 (1959).

OPPENHEIMER, G. D.: Evaluation of roentgenography of surgically exposed kidney in treatment of renal calculi. J. Urol. **43**, 253 (1940).

PACCIARDI, A., MICHELASSI, P. L.: Diagnostic criteria for the evaluation of renal calcifications on routine roentgenograms. Ann. Radiol. Diagn. (Bologna) **31**, 30 (1958).

PFLAUMER, E.: Die Röntgenphotographie der freigelegten Niere bei der Steinoperation. Z. Urol. **29**, 225 (1935).

PALUBINSKAS, A. J., HODSON, C. J.: Transintervertebral retroperitoneal gas insufflation. Radiology **70**, 851 (1958).

PANICHI, S., BONECHI, I.: Determinazione radiologica delle dimensioni del rene, Valori normali. Minerva Med. (Torino) **49**, 3261 (1958).

— Determinazione radiologica del volume del rene nel soggetto normale. Minerva Med. **49/50**, 2015 (1959).

PÉLISSIER, M., LEVÈRE, F., BETRANDO, L., PÉLISSIER, J.: Effraction et passage de l'air dans la cavité péritonéale. J. Radiol. Électrol. **35**, 482 (1954).

PENDERGRASS, H. P., TRISTAN, T. A., BLAKEMORE, W. S., SELLERS, A. M., JANNETTA, P. J., MURPHY, J. J.: Roentgen technics in the diagnosis and localization of pheochromocytoma. Radiology 78, 725 (1962).

PETRÉN, T.: La situation des reins en hauteur chez l'enfant. Stockholm: Iduns Tryckeri AB, 1934.

POLVAR, G., BRAGGION, P.: Mobilita renale e pneumoaddome extraperitoneale. Minerva Urol. (Torino) 4, 221 (1952).

PORCHER, BONOMINI, OLIVA: L'insufflazione retroperitonealy in radiodiagnostica. Torino: Minerva Medica 1954.

PUIGVERT-GORRO, A., MOYA-PRATS: Les infiltration periviscerales en radiologie urinaire. J. Urol. méd. chir. 55, 63 (1949).

PUHL, H.: Röntgenuntersuchung freigelegter Nieren. Zbl. Chir. 63, 1035 (1936).

RAMBO, O., ZBORALSKE, F. F., JARROS, P., RIEGELMAN, S., MARGULIS, A.: Toxicity studies on tannic acid administered by enema. I. Effects of enema-administered tannic acid on the colon and lower abdomen of rats. Am. J. Roentgenol. 96, 488 (1966).

RANSOM, C. L., LANDES, R. R., McLELLAND, R.: Air embolism following retroperitoneal pneumography: a nation-wide survey. J. Urol. 76, 664 (1956).

RAWSON, A. J.: Distribution of the lymphatics of the human kidney as shown in a case of carcinomatous premeation. Arch. Path 47, 283 (1949).

REINHARDT, K.: Zur Technik des Retropneumoperitoneums. Dtsch. med. Wschr. 77, 804 (1952).

REISNER, K., VAN DE WEYER, K. H.: Die Leistungsfähigkeit der Nephrotomographie unter Kontrastmittelinfusion. Fortschr. Röntgenstr. 104, 305 (1966).

RÉNI-VÁMOS, F.: Das innere Lymphgefäßsystem der Organe. Budapest 1960.

RIEMENSCHNEIDER, P. A.: Multiple large aneurysms of the splenic artery. Amer. J. Roentgenol. 74, 872 (1955).

RITTER, A., ALLEMAN, R.: Diagnostische Ergebnisse der Pyelographie und Pneumoradiographie. Schweiz. med. Wschr. 53, 927 and 955 (1923).

RHODIN, J. A. G.: Structure of the kidney. In: Diseases of the kidney. Ed. by M. B. Strauss & L. G. Welt. Boston: Little, Brown & Co 1963. p. 1–29.

RONNEN, J. R.: The roentgen diagnosis of calcified aneurysms of the splenic and renal arteries. Acta radiol. 39, 385 (1953).

ROSENBERG, M. L.: Hypercalcuria and metabolic bone disease. Calif. Med. 81, 382 (1954).

ROSENSTEIN, P.: Die Pneumoradiographie des Nierenlagers. Z. Urol. 15, 447 (1921).

ROSSI, L.: Il retropneumoperitoneo. Ann. Radiol. Diagn. (Bologna) 23, 340 (1951).

RUIZ RIVAS, M.: Nueva tecnica de diagnostico radiografico aplicable a organos y estructuras retroperitoneales, mediastinicas y cervicales. Rev. Clin. Espan. 25, 206 (1947).

— Diagnostico radiologico. El neumorrinon. Tecnica original. Arch. Espan. Urol. 4, 228 (1948).

RUIZ RIVAS, M.: Roentgenological diagnosis. Generalized subserous emphysema through a single puncture. Amer. J. Roentgenol. 64, 723–734 (1950).

RUSS, F. H., GLENN, D. L. GIANTURCO, C.: Gas embolism during extraperitoneal insufflation. Radiology 61, 637 (1953).

SALVATI, R.: Utilità e indicazioni della insufflazione retroperitoneale nella pratica e nella radiodiagnostica urologica. Minerva urol. (Torino) 8, 201 (1956).

SCHORR, S., BIRNBAUM, D.: Raised position of the right kidney. Radiol. Clin. (Basel) 28, 102 (1959).

— AVIAD, I., BIRNBAUM, D., LOWENTHAL, M.: Pyelography as an aid for the diagnosis of liver cirrhosis. With a study of the normal position of the kidneys. Amer. J. Roentgenol. 88, 1142 (1962).

SCHULTE, E.: Gasembolie bei der extraperitonealen Pneumoradiographie. Fortschr. Röntgenstr. 91, 87 (1959).

SENGER, F. L., HORTON, G. R., BOTTONE, J. J., CHIN, H. Y. H., WILSON, M. C.: Perirenal air insufflation by the paracoccygeal retrorectal route. N. Y. St. J. Med. 53, 2823 (1953).

SINNER, W.: Die Bedeutung des Retropneumoperitoneums in der Nierendiagnostik. Z. Urol. 48, 564 (1955).

STEINBACH, H. L., LYON, R. P., SMITH, D. R., MILLER, E. R.: Extraperitoneal pneumography. Radiology 59, 167 (1952).

— MILLER, E. R., SMITH, D. R.: Extraperitoneal pneumography. Calif. Med. 75, 202 (1951).

— Extraperitoneal pneumography in diagnosis of retroperitoneal tumors. Arch. Surg. 70, 161 (1955).

SUTHERLAND, C. G.: Renal roentgenoscopy and roentgenography at the operating table. J. Urol. 33, 1 (1935).

SÖVÉNYI, E.: Unsere Erfahrungen mit der retroperitonealen Luftinsufflation (Retropneumoperitoneum). Radiol. Clin. (Basel), 28, 198 (1959).

ÜBELHÖR, R.: Die Röntgenaufnahme der freigelegten Niere. Z. urol. Chir. 41, 275–279 (1936).

DE WARDENER, H. E.: The kidney. London: Churchill 1958.

VESPIGNANI, L.: The roentgen reticular appearance of the perirenal fat tissue in extraperitoneal pneumoabdomen (retropneumoperitoneum) and tomography. Acta radiol. 36, 509 (1951).

— ZENNARO, R.: La stratigraphie en projection latérale du rein normal et pathologique avec le "pneumo-abdomen extra-péritonéal". J. Radiol. Électrol. 32, 720 (1951).

WALTER, R. C., GOODWIN, W. E.: Aortography and retroperitoneal oxygen in urologic diagnosis: a comparison of translumbar and percutaneous femoral methods of aortography. J. Urol. 70, 526 (1953).

— Aortography and pneumography in children. J. Urol. 77, 323 (1957).

WILHELM, S. F.: Gas insufflation through the lumbar and presacral routes. Surg. Gynec. Obst. 99, 319 (1954).

WOLF, G. L., WILSON, WM. J.: Renal silhouette size before and after vasodilators as an index of renal vascular stenosis. Invest. Radiol. 6, 366 (1971).

WOLKE, K.: Pyelogramm mit einem durch einen Nierenarterienzweig verursachten Füllungsdefekt (Pseudodefekt). Acta radiol. **17**, 566 (1936).

ZANCA, P., BARKER, K. G., PYE, T. H., FU, WHEI-RUNG, HAAG, EDMUND, L.: Ureteral jet stream phenomenon in adults. Amer. J. Roentgenol. **92**, 341 (1964).

ZBORALSKE, F. F., HARRIS, P., RIEGELMAN, S., RAMBO, O., MARGULIS, A.: Toxicity studies on tannic acid administered by enema. III. Studies on the retention of enemas in humans. IV. Review and conclusions. Amer. J. Roentgenol. **96**, 505 (1966).

II. Additional methods

2. Retroperitoneal pneumography

ANDERSEN, P. E.: Pneumoretroperitoneum in suprarenal disease. Acta radiol. **43**, 289 (1955).

BERNARDINI, SALVATI, R.: Retropneumoperitoneo, nuovo mezzo di indagine radiologica. Gaz. int. Med. Chir. **44**, 301 (1950).

BIBUS, B.: Die Pneumoradiographie des Nierenlagers. Wien klin. Wschr. **52**, 256 (1939).

BLAND, A. B.: A simplified apparatus for presacral carbon dioxide injection. J. Urol. **79**, 171 (1958).

BONOMINI, BACCAGLINI: Pneumoretroperitoneo e pneumomediastino. L'enfisema diagnostico dei tessuti adreolari profondi del tronco. Bologna: Cappelli 1953.

BRODNY, M. L., CHAMBERLIN, H. A.: A simple apparatus for pneumoadrenalography. J. Urol. **42**, 211 (1939).

CAHILL, G. F.: Air injections to demonstrate the adrenals by X-ray. J. Urol. **34**, 238 (1935).

CARELLI, M. H.: Sur le pneumopéritoine et sur une methode personelle pur voir le rein sans pneumopéritoine. Bull. Soc. méd. Hôp. Paris **45**, 1409 (1921).

COCCHI, U.: Retropneumoperitoneum und Pneumomediastinum. Stuttgart: Georg Thieme 1957.
— Fortschr. Röntgenstr. Erg.-Bd. **79**.

COONEY, J. D., AMELAR, R. D. ORRON, A.: Renal displacement and rotation during retroperitoneal pneumography. Arch. Surg. (Chicago) **70**, 405 (1955).

COPE, O., SCHATZKI, R.: Tumors of the adrenal glands. Arch. intern. Med. **64**, 1222 (1939).

DODSON, A. I.: Urological surgery. London 1956.

DURANT, E. M., LONG, J., OPPENHEIMER, M. J.: Pulmonary (venous) air embolism. Amer. Heart J. **33**, 269–281 (1947).

EVANS, A. T.: Combined use of contrast media in retroperitoneal tumors. Critical evaluation. Arch. Surg. (Chicago) **70**, 191 (1955).

EVANS, J. A., POKER, N.: Newer roentgenographic techniques in the diagnosis of retroperitoneal tumors. J. Amer. med. Ass. **161**, 1128 (1956).

FAGERBERG, S: Pneumoretroperitoneum. Acta radiol (Stockh.) **37**, 519 (1952).

FONTAINE, R., WARTER, P., FRANK, P., STOLL, G., RABER, R.: De l'intérêt du rétropneumopéritoine pour le diagnostic des malformations et néoplasmes du rein. J. Radiol. Électrol. **36**, 708 (1955).

FRANCIOSI, I. U., GOVONI, A. F., PASQUANELLI, C. G.: Retroperitoneum associated with laminography. Amer. J. Roentgenol. **72**, 1034 (1954).

GANDINI, D., GIBBA, A.: Present trends in the diagnoses of surgical renal diseases by means of pneumoretroperitoneum combined with the usual radiourological technique. Nunt. Radiol. **20**, 707 (1954).

GENNES, L. DE, MAY, J. P., SIMON, G.: Le rétropneumoperitoine (nouveau procedé d'exploration radiologique de l'abdomen). Presse méd. **21**, 351 (1950).

GIRAUD, G., BETOULIERES, P., LATOUR, H., PELISSIER, M.: La neumostratigrafia. Arch. esp. Med. interna **2**, 79–103 (1956).

GIRAUD, M., BRET, P., KUENTZ, M., ANJOU, A.: Bilan de cent examens après pneumorétropéritoine. J. Radiol. Électrol. **35**, 838 (1954).

GLASSMAN, I., SHAPIRO, R., ROBINSON, F.: Air embolism during presacral pneumography: a case report. J. Urol. (**75**, 569 (1956).

IAVAZYAN, A. V.: Visualization of kidney anomalies by the aid of presacral pneumoretroperitoneum (Russian text). Vestn. Rentgenol. Radiol. **32**, 60 (1957).

KÖHLER, H.: Indikationsgebiet der Pneumoradiographie. Dtsch. Ges. Urol. 1926, pg 119.

LANDES, R. R., RANSOM, C. L.: Presacral retroperitoneal pneumography utilizing carbon dioxide: further experiences and improved technique. J. Urol. **82**, 670 (1959).

LEVINE, B.: Use of helium in perirenal insufflation: preliminary reports. J. Urol. **67**, 390 (1952).

MACARINI, N., OLIVA, L.: Sur l'insufflation rétropéritonéale associée à la stratigraphie tridimensionell. J. Belge Radiol. **34**, 281 (1951).

MAJELA DE ABREU GUEDES, G.: Nossa experiencia com o retro-pneumoperitoneo. Rev. Bras. Cir. **32**, 193 (1956).

MENCHER, W. H.: Perirenal insufflation. J. Amer. med. Ass. **109**, 1338 (1937)

MENEGHINI, C., u. G. DELL'ADAMI: G. Die Insufflation des extraperitonealen Bindegewebes in der Röntgendiagnostik der oberen Harnorgane mit besonderer Berücksichtigung der Möglichkeiten der Stratigraphie. Fortschr. Röntgenstr. **76**, 181 (1952).

MONTERO, J. J.: Aplasia renal y retropneumoperitoneo. Arch, esp. Urol. **14**, 26 (1958).

MOOS, F. VON: Die Tomographie beim Pneumoretroperitoneum., Schweiz. med. Wschr. **82**, 629 (1952).

MOSCA, L. G.: El enfisema retroperitoneal: Su técnica, sus indiacciones y resultados. Pren. méd. Argent. **38**, 1025 (1951).

MOSENTHAL, A.: Unsere Erfahrungen mit der „Pneumoradiographie des Nierenlagers" nach P. Rosenstein. Z. urol. Chir. **12**, 303 (1923).

PALUBINSKAS, A. J., HODSON, C. J.: Transintervertebral retroperitoneal gas insufflation. Radiology **70**, 851 (1958).

POLVAR, G., BRAGGION, P.: Mobilità renale e pneumoaddome extraperitoneate. Minerva urol. (Torino) **4**, 221 (1952).

PORCHER, BONOMINI, OLIVA: L'insufflazione retroperitoneale in radiodiagnostica. Torino: Minerva Medica 1954.

PUIGVERT-GORRO, A., MOYA-PRATS: Les infiltrations periviscerales en radiologie urinaire. J. Urol. méd. chir. **55**, 63 (1949).

RANSOM, C. L., LANDES, R. R., McLELLAND, R.: Air embolism following retroperitoneal pneumography: a nation-wide survey. J. Urol. **76**, 664 (1956).

REINHARDT, K.: Zur Technik des Retropneumoperitoneums. Dtsch. med. Wschr. **77**, 804 (1952).

RITTER, A., ALLEMANN, R.: Diagnostische Ergebnisse der Pyelographie und Pneumoradiographie. Schweiz med. Wschr. **53**, 927–961 (1923).

ROSENSTEIN, P.: Die Pneumoradiographie des Nierenlagers. Z. Urol. **15**, 447 (1921).

ROSSI, L.: Il retropneumoperitoneo. Ann. Radiol. diagn. (Bologna) **23**, 340 (1951).

RUIZ RIVAS, M.: Nueva tecnica de diagnostico radiografico aplicable a organos y estructuras retroperitoneales, mediastinicas y cervicales. Rev. clin. esp. **25**, 206 (1947).

— Diagnostico radiologico. El neumorriñon. Tecnica original. Arch. esp. Urol. **4**, 228 (1948).

— Roentgenological diagnosis. Generalized subserous emphysema through a single puncture. Amer. J. Roentgenol. **64**, 723 (1950).

RUSS, F. H., GLENN, D. L., GIANTURCO, C.: Gas embolism during extraperitoneal insufflation. Radiology **61**, 637 (1953).

SALVATI, R.: Utilità e indicazioni della insufflazione retroperitoneale nella practica e nella radiodiagnostica urologica. Minerva urol. (Torino) **8**, 201 (1956).

SCHNUR, B. M., SAKSON, J. A.: Trans-sacral retroperitoneal pneumography. J. Urol. **94**, 701 (1965).

SCHULTE, E.: Gasembolie bei der extraperitonealen Pneumoradiographie. Fortschr. Röntgenstr. **91**, 87 (1959).

SENGER, F. L., HORTON, G. R., BOTTONE, J. J., CHIN, H. Y. H., WILSON, M. C.: Perirenal air insufflation by the paracoccygeal retro rectal route. N. Y. St. J. Med. **53**, 2823 (1953).

SINNER, W.: Die Bedeutung des Retropneumoperitoneums in der Nierendiagnostik. Z. Urol. **48**, 564 (1955).

SÖVÉNYI, E.: Unsere Erfahrungen mit der retroperitonealen Luftinsufflation (Retropneumoperitoneum). Radiol. clin. (Basel) **28**, 198 (1959).

STEINBACH, H. L., LYON, R. P., MILLER, E. R., SMITH, D. R.: Extraperitoneal pneumography. Calif. Med. **75**, 202 (1951).

— SMITH, D. R.: Extraperitoneal pneumography in diagnosis of retroperitoneal tumors. Arch. Surg. (Chicago) **70**, 161 (1955).

VESPIGNANI, L.: The roentgen reticular appearance of the perirenal fat tissue in extraperitoneal pneumoabdomen (retropneumo, peritoneum) and tomography. Acta radiol. **36**, 509 (1951).

— ZENNARO, R.: La stratigraphie en projection latérale du rein normal et pathologique avec le "pneumo-abdomen extra-péritoneál". J. Radiol. Électrol. **32**, 720 (1951).

WALTER, R. C., GOODWIN, W. E.: Aortography and retroperitoneal oxygen in urologic diagnosis: a comparison of translumbar and percutaneous femoral methods of aortography. J. Urol. **70**, 526 (1953).

WALTER, R. C.: Aortography and pneumography in children. J. Urol. **77**, 323 (1957).

WILHELM, S. F.: Gas insufflation through the lumbar and presacral routes. Surg. Gynec. Obstet. **99**, 319 (1954).

III. Pyelography and urography

ABRAMS, H. L.: Screening techniques in reno-vascular hypertension. Book of Abstracts. Xth int. congr. of radiol. Montreal 1962 (p. 231—232).

ALFERMANN, F.: Die Anwendung des Bewegungspyelogramms zur Differentialdiagnostik von Bauchtumoren. Bruns Beitr. klin. Chir. **180**, 199 (1950).

ALLEN, R. P.: Neuromuscular disorders of the urinary tract in children. Radiology **65**, 325 (1955).

ALWALL, N.: Aspiration biopsy of the kidney. Acta med scand. **143**, 430 (1952).

— ERLANSSON, P., TORNBERG, A.: The clinical course of renal failure occurring after intravenous urography and/or retrograde pyelography. Acta med. scand. **152**, 163 (1955).

ALYEA, E. P., HAINES, C. E.: Intradermal test for sensitivity to iodopyracet injection, or "diodrast". J. Amer. med. Ass. **135**, 25 (1947).

AMPLATZ, K.: Catheter embolization. Editorial in: Radiology **91**, 392 (1968).

AMUNDSEN, P.: Metrizoate sodium (Isopaque), a new contrast medium for angiography and urography. Evaluation, initial clinical testing and clinical experience. Farmakoterapi (Oslo) **18**, 3 (1962).

ANSELL, G.: Adverse reactions to contrast agents. Investigative Radiology **5**, 375 (1970).

ARENDT, J., ZGODA, A.: Heterotropic excretion of intravenously injected contrast media. Radiology **68**, 238 (1957).

ARNELL, S., LIDSTRÖM, F.: Myelography with skiodan (abrodil). Acta radiol. **12**, 287 (1931).

ARNER, B.: Personal communications 1959.

— Treatment of hypersensitiveness to iodized roentgen contrast media. Acta allerg. (Copenhagen) **15**, 432 (1960).

ASTRALDI, A., URIBURU jr., J. V.: Radiologia del rinon durante el acto operatorio. Rév. med. lat.-amer. **21**, 891 (1936).

ATKINS, H. L., HODES, J. PH.: The use of oral antihistamines in intravenous urography. Radiology **69**, 384 (1957).

BABAIANTZ, L., WIESER, C.: Un noveau produit de contraste triiodé pour l' urographie intraveineuse. Praxis **44**, 454 (1955).

BACKLUND, V.: Über die Technik der simultanen Telefilmplanigraphie. Acta radiol. Suppl. **137**, (1956).

BACON, R. D.: Respiration pyelography. Amer. J. Roentgenol. **44**, 71 (1940).

BARTLEY, O., BENGTSSON, U., STATTIN, S.: Urography in relation to renal function. Acta radiol. **7**, 289 (1968).

BARTELS, E. D., BRUN, C. C., GAMMELTOFT, A., GJORUP, P. A.: Acute anuria following intravenous pyelography in patient with myelomatosis. Acta med. scand. **150**, 297 (1954).

BAURYS, W.: Serious complications associated with the newer diagnostic methods in urology. J. Urol. **75**, 846 (1956).

BEALL, A. C., Jr., CRAWFORD, E. S., COUVES, C. M., DeBAKEY, M. E., MOYER, J. H.: Complication of aortography. Factors influencing renal function following aortography with 70 per cent Urokon. Surgery 43, 364 (1958).

BECKER, J. A., GREGOIRE, A., BERDON, W., SCHWARTZ, D.: Vicarious excretion of urographic media. Radiology 90, 243 (1968).

BELL, E. T.: Renal diseases. London: Henry Kimpton 1950.

BELL, J. C.: Intravenous urography. Urol. cutan rev. rr, 460 (1940).

BENNHOLD, H., OTT, H., WIECH, M.: Difference in binding ability of hepatotrophic and nephtrophic substance with serum proteins. Deutsche med. Wschr. 75, 11 (1950).

BERG, O. C., ALLEN, D. H.: Use of carbonated beverage as an aid in pediatric excretory urography. J. Urol. 67, 393 (1952).

BERG, V., DUFRIESNE, M.: Excretory urography in the pediatric patient with the aid of carbonated beverage. Harper Hosp. Bull 14, 122 (1956).

BERGER, H. U., KARGL, O.: Beitrag zur Ureterankompression bei der Urographie. Bruns' Beitr. klin. Chir. 190, 13 (1955).

BERGMAN, F., NORMAN, O., SJÖSTEDT, S.: Perjodal H., Viscous, a water-soluble contrast medium containing dextran. Acta radiol. 46, 587 (1956).

BERNAGEAU, J., BISMUTH, V., DESPREZ-CURLEY, J. P., BOURDON, R.: La lymphographie dans les chyluries. J. Radiol. et d'Electrol. 45, 529 (1964).

BERNSTEIN, E. F., EVANS, R. L., AVANT, R. F., TYBERG, J. V.: Experimental studies of ditriokon toxicity. Amer. J. Roentgenol. 86, 1138 (1961).

— GREENSPAN, R. H., LOKEN, M. K.: Intravenous aortography. A. M. A. Arch. Surg. 80, 71 (1960).

— PALMER, J. D., AABERG, T. A., DAVIS, R. L.: Studies of the toxicity of Hyapaque-90 per cent, following rapid intravenous injection. Radiology 76, 88 (1961).

BERRY, C. D., CROSS, R. R.: Use of bag ureteral catheters for nephrograms: obstructive nephrograms. J. Urol. 74, 683 (1955).

BEZOLD, K., FEINDT, H. R., PRESSLER, K.: Der Röntgenbildverstärker im Routinebetrieb. Fortschr. Röntgenstr. 85, 447 (1956).

BLOCK, J. B., GRAHAM, D. E., BURROWS, B. A.: Influence of protein binding on I¹³¹ diodrast excretion. J. Clin. Invest. 38, 988 (1959).

BLOMMERT, G., BERGRANDY, J., MOLHUYSEN, J. A., DE VRIES, L. A., BORST, J. G. G.: Diuretic effect of isotonis saline solution compared with that of water. Lancet 1951, 1011.

BLOOM, J., RICHARDSON, J. F.: The usefulness of a contrast medium containing an antibacterial agent (retrografin) for retrograde pyelography). J. Urol. 81, 332 (1959).

BØRDALEN, B., WANG, H., HOLTERMANN, H.: Osmotic properties of some contrast media. Investigative Radiology 5, 559 (1970).

BORGARD, W.: Beobachtungen und Untersuchungen bei Pyelitis. Z. Urol. 41, 217 (1948).

BOWEN, J. A., SHIFLETT, E. L.: Intravenous urography in the upright position. Radiology 36, 672 (1941).

BRAEDEL, H. U.: Die Zwei-Katheter-Methode der Nephrographie. Röntgenblätter 14, 33 (1961).

BRAASCH, W. F., EMMETT, J. L.: Excretory urography as a test of renal function. J. Urol. 35, 630 (1936).

— Clinical urography. Philadelphia & London: W. B. Saunders Company, 1951.

BRADLEY, S. E., BRADLEY, G. P.: The effect of increased intra-abdominal pressure of renal function in man. J. clin. Invest. 26, 1010 (1947).

BRASCHE, H.: Ein Beitrag zur Technik der Aortographie. Fortschr. Röntgenstr. 88, 669 (1958).

BRAUN, J. P., SCHNEIDER, L.: L'opacification corollaire de la vésicule d'une substance de contrast urinaire. J. Radiol. Électrol. 40, 481 (1959).

BREAM, CH. A.: The clinical use of pitressin in excretory urography. Amer. J. Roentgenol. 78, 343 (1957).

BREUER, F.: Zur Bedeutung des Veratmungspyelograms für die Erkennung paranephritischer Abszesse. Zbl. Chir. 64, 683 (1937).

BURROS, H. M., BORROMEO, V. H. J., SELIGSON, D.: Anuria following retrograde pyelography. Ann. intern. Med. 48, 674 (1958).

CAFFARATTI, A., MORELLI, A.: Diagnostic value of pneumo-uretero-pyelography in nephro-ureterolithiasis. Ann. radiol. diag. 31, 423 (1958).

CAMPBELL, M.: Clinical pediatric urology. Philadelphia and London: W. B. Saunders Company 1951.

CARLSON, H. E.: The proven ineffectiveness of the compression bag in intravenous pyelography. J. Urol. 56, 609 (1946).

CASEY, W. C., GOODWIN, W. E.: Percutaneous antegrade pyelography in hydronephrosis. J. Urol. 74, 164 (1955).

CASTELLI, W. A., HUELKE, D. F.: The intrarenal vascular distribution in the human kidney. J. Urol. 102, 12 (1969).

CATEL, W., GARSCHE, R.: Studien bei Kindern mit dem Bildwandler. 2. Bewegungs- und Entleerungsvorgänge im Bereich von Nierenkelchen und Nierenbecken. Fortschr. Röntgenstr. 86, 66 (1957).

CATTEL, W. R.: Excretory pathways for contrast media. Investigative Radiology 5, 473 (1970).

CHAMBERLAIN, G. W., IMBER, I.: Pyelography for the diagnosis of lesions of the body and tail of the pancreas. Radiology 63, 722 (1954).

CHAPLIN, H. Jr., CARLSSON, E.: Changes in human red blood cells during in vitro exposure to several roentgenologic contrast media. Amer. J. Roentgenol. 86, 1127 (1961).

CHESNEY, W., McEVAN, HOPE, J. O.: Studies of the tissue distribution and excretion of sodium diatrizoate in laboratory animals. Amer. J. Roentgenol. 78, 137 (1957).

CHIAUDANO, M.: Comportamento arteriografico del rene normale. Minerva chir. (Torino) 13, 1082 (1958).

CHOI, J. K., WIEDEMER, H. S.: Chyluria: lymphangiographic study and review of literature. J. Urol. 92, 723 (1964).

CHRISTIANSEN, H.: Some practical hints on the performance of urography on infants. Acta radiol. 26, 46 (1945).

Clark's applied pharmacology, VIII edit. Revised by A. WILSON & H. O. SCHILD: London: Churchill Ltd. 1952.

CICCANTELLI, M. J., GALLAGHER, W. B., SKEMP, F. C., DIETZ, P. C.: Fatal nephropathy and adrenal necrosis after translumbar aortography. New Engl. J. Med. **258**, 433 (1958).

CLERMONT, A.: La microangiographie: Etude technique et applications en pathologie rénale. Monografi — Université Claude Bernard, Lyon (Imprimierie des Beaux Arts. J. Tixier et Fils, Lyon) 1971.

CONWAY, G. F., BICKNELL, F. B.: Anuria following retrograde pyelography. J. Urol. **96**, 805 (1966).

COOK, F. E. Jr., FLAHERTY, R. A., WILLMARTH, C. L., LANGELIER, P. R.: Chylothorax: a complication of translumbar aortography. Radiology **75**, 251 (1960).

COOK, I. K., KEATS, T. E., SEALE, D. L.: Determination of the normal position of the upper urinary tract on the lateral abdominal urogram. Radiology **99**, 499 (1971).

COUNTS, R. W., MAGILL, B. G., SHERMAN, R. S.: Death from intra-abdominal hemorrhage simulating reaction to contrast medium. J. Amer. med. Ass. **165**, 1134 (1957).

CRANE, J. J.: Sudden death following intravenous administration of diodrast for intravenous urography. J. Urol. **42**, 745 (1939).

CREPEA, S. B., ALLANSON, J. C., DeLAMBRE, L.: Failure of antihistaminic drugs to inhibit diodrast reactions, N.Y. St. J. Med. **49**, 2556 (1949).

CWYNARSKI, M. T., SAXTON, H. M.: Urography in myelomatosis (Preliminary communication). Brit. Med. J. **1**, 457 (1969).

DACIE, J. E., FRY, I., KELSEY: A comparison of sodium and methylglucamine diatrizoate in clinical urography. Brit. J. Radiol. **44**, 51 (1971).

DARGENT, M., PAPILLOS, J. MONTBARBON, J. F., COSTAL, G.: Etude systématique de l'urographie pré- et post-opératoire chez des malades traitées par association radium-chirurgie pour cancer du col de l'utérus au stade de début. Lyon chir. **51**, 711 (1956).

— Etude urographique du cancer du col utérin traité par l'association radium-lymphadénectomie. J. Radiol. Electrol. **39**, 109 (1958).

DAVIDSON, A. J., BECKER, J., ROTHFIELD, N., UNGER, G., PLOCH, D.: An evaluation of the effect of high-dose urography on previously impaired renal and hepatic function in man. Radiology **97**, 249 (1970).

DAVIS, G. D., KINCAID, O. W., HUNT, J. C.: Roentgenologic evaluation of multiple renal arteries. Amer. J. Roentgenol. **90**, 583 (1963).

DAVIS, L. A.: Reactions following excretory pyelography in infants and children. Radiology **71**, 19 (1958).

— KEE-CHANG HUANG, PIRKEY, E. L.: Water-soluble, non-absorbable radiopaque mediums in gastrointestional examination. J. Amer. med. Ass. **160**, 373 (1956).

DAWSON, J., McCHESNEY, E., TELLER, F.: Excretion of metrizoate in man. Acta radiol. **7**, 502 (1968).

DENNEHY, P. J.: A method of excretory urography in children. S. Afr. med. J. **28**, 949 (1954).

DETAR, J. A., HARRIS, J. A.: Venous pooled nephrograms: technique and results. J. Urol. **72**, 979 (1954).

DICK, D. R., HERRMANN, R. W., FERGUSON, CH., HEBERT, C. L.: The use of short acting, muscle relaxant drug in diagnostic urography. A preliminary report. J. Urol. **72**, 1260 (1954).

DIHLMANN, W.: Vergleichende Untersuchungen über den Wert der intravenösen Kompressionsurographie. Fortschr. Röntgenstr. **89**, 104 (1958).

DITTMAR, F.: Reflektorische Skoliosen bei Erkrankungen der Harnwege. Dtsch. Arch. klin. Med. **184**, 249 (1939).

DOLL, E.: Ausscheidungsurographie mit Urografin in der Kinderheilkunde. Medizinische **38**, 1384 (1957).

DOROSHOW, L. W., HA YOUNG YOON, ROBBINS, M. A.: Intrathecal injection, an unusual complication of translumbar aortography: case report. J. Urol. **88**, 438 (1962).

DOYLE, O. W.: The use of chlortrimeton with miokon in intravenous urography. J. Urol. **81**, 573 (1959).

DUDZINSKI, P. J., PETRONE, A. F., PERSOFF, M., CALLAGHAN, E. E.: Acute renal failure following high dose excretory urography in dehydrated patients. J. Urol. **106**, 619 (1971).

DUNBAR, J. S., MacEVAN, D. W., HEBERT, F.: The value of dehydration in intravenous pyelography. An experimental study. Amer. J. Roentgenol. **84**, 813 (1960).

DURE-SMITH, P.: The dose of contrast medium in intravenous urography: A physiologic assessment. Amer. J. Roentgenol. **108**, 691 (1970).

— McARDLE, G. H.: Tomography during excretory urography. Technical aspects. Brit. J. Radiol. **45**, 896 (1972).

— SIMENHOFF, M., ZIMSKIND, P., KODROFF, M.: The bolus effect in excretory urography. Radiology **101**, 29 (1971).

DURIO, A., GRIO, A., MASTROBUONO, N., SCAGLIONE, G.: Osservazioni sull' impiego della jaluronidase nella tecnica urografica dell' infanzia. Aggiorn. pediat **6**, 191 (1955).

DÜX, A., THURN, P.: Zur Methodik der Nierenarteriographie. Fortschr. Röntgenstr. **98**, 659 (1963).

EBERL, J.: Die urinschichtung bei der intravenösen Pyelographie. Fortschr. Röntgenstr. **86**, 74 (1957).

EBBINGHAUS, K. D.: Ist die intravenöse Pyelographie bei Nierenschäden kontraindiziert? Ärztl. Wschr. **10**, 736 (1955).

— Die technische Durchführung der intravenösen Pyelographie. Ärztl. Wschr. **97** (1955).

EDGREN, J. U., KÖHLER, R.: Urographie mit schneller Injektion großer Kontrastmittelmengen oder als Infusionsurographie. Diagnostischer Wert und Komplikationsfrequenz. Fortschr. Röntgenstr. **117**, 434 (1972).

EDLING, N. P. G., EDVALL, C. A., HELANDER, C. G.: Correlation of urography and tests of renal function. Acta radiol. **54**, 433 (1960).

— — PERNOW, B.: Comparison of urography with selective clearance as tests of renal function. Acta radiol. **45**, 85 (1956).

EDLING, N. P. G., HELANDER, C. G.: Cholegraphy with depression of the renal excretion of the contrast medium. Acta radiol. **49**, 187 (1958).
— — RENCK, L.: The correlation between contrast excretion and arterial and intrapelvic pressures in urography. Acta radiol. **42**, 442 (1954).
— — SELDINGER, S. I.: The nephrographic effect in depressed tubular excretion of umbradil. Acta radiol. **48**, 1 (1957).
EDLUND, Y., ZETTERGREN, L.: Toxicity of the methylglucamine salt of tetraiodophtalic acid morpholide. Acta radiol. **55**, 413 (1961).
EISLER, F.: Neueste Fortschritte der röntgenologischen Steindiagnose. Referat 5. Tagg. der Dtsch. Ges. für Urologie 1921, Wien. Dtsch. med. Wschr. 1921, 1380.
EKELUND, L., OLIN, T.: Catheterization of arteries in rats. Investigative Radiology **5**, 69 (1970).
ENGELKAMP, H.: Anwendung der Hartstrahltechnik (200 kV) bei Untersuchungen mit negativen Kontrastmitteln. Fortschr. Röntgenstr. **93**, 230 (1960).
ENGELL, H. C., DREWSEN, E.: Udvaskningsurografi og kirurgisk behandling af renal iskaemi. Nord. Med. **7 III 79**, 308 (1968).
EPSTEIN, B. S.: Subcutaneous urography in infants. J. Amer. med. Ass. **164**, 39 (1957).
ERIKSON, U., GRÄNGSJÖ, G., ULFENDAHL, H. R., WOLGAST, M.: A roentgenological method for the determination of renal blood flow. A preliminary report. Excerpta Medica (Radiology) **20**, 468 (1966).
ETTINGER, A.: Layer formation in pyelography. Amer. J. Roentgenol. **49**, 783 (1943).
FEY, B., TRUCHOT, P.: L'urographie intra-veineuse. Paris: Masson & Cie. 1944.
— — NOIX, M.: Étude radiocinématographique de l'uretère normal et pathologique. J. Radiol. Électrol. **39**, 328 (1958).
FIGDOR, P. P.: Akute Nierenschäden nach Pyelographien. Z. Urol. **49**, 133 (1956).
FINBY, N., EVANS, J. A., STEINBERG, I.: Reactions from intravenous organic iodide compounds: Pretesting and prophylaxis. Radiology **71**, 15 (1958).
— POKER, N., EVANS, J. A.: Ninety procent hypaque for rapid intravenous roentgenography; preliminary report. Radiology **67**, 244 (1956).
FISCHER, H. W., DOUST, V. L.: Evaluation of the role of pretesting in the problems of serious reactions to urographic contrast media. Investigative Radiology **6**, 367 (1971).
— An evaluation of pretesting in the problem of serious and fatal reactions to excretory urography. Radiology **103**, 497 (1972).
— ROTHFIELD, N., CARR, J.: Optimum dose in excretory urography. Amer. J. Roentgenol. **113**, 423 (1971).
FLEISCHNER, F. G., BELLMAN, S., HENKEN, E. M.: Papillary opacification in excretory urography. Radiology **74**, 567 (1960).
FLOYD, E., GUY, J. C.: Translumbar percutaneous antegrade pyelography as an adjunct to urologic diagnosis. J. Med. Georgia **45**, 13 (1956).
FORD, W. H. Jr., PALUBINSKAS, A. J.: Renal extravasation during excretory urography using abdominal compression. J. Urol. **97**, 283 (1967).

FREI, A.: Ein neues Kontrastmittel zur intravenösen Urographie. Dtsch. Med. Wschr. **79**, 1636 (1954).
FRIEDENBERG, M. J., CARLIN, M. R.: The routine use of higher volumes of contrast material to improve intravenous urography. Radiology **83**, 405 (1964).
FRIESE-CHRISTIANSEN, A.: Urography on children after administration of the contrast substance by mouth. Acta radiol. **27**, 197 (1946).
FROMMHOLD, W., BRABAND, H.: Zwischenfälle bei Gallenblasenuntersuchungen mit Biografin und ihre Behandlung. Fortschr. Röntgenstr. **92**, 47 (1960).
FRY, I., KELSEY, CATTELL, W. R.: Excretion urography in advanced renal failure. Brit. J. Radiol. **44**, 198 (1971).
FUCHS, W. A.: Selektive renale Phlebographie. Schweiz. med. Wschr. **91**, 1507 (1961).
— Zur Technik der Nierenangiographie. Radiol. clin. **32**, 121 (1963).
GARRITANO, A. P., WOHL, G. T., KIRBY, CH. K., PIETROLUONGO, A. L.: The roentgenographic demonstration of an arteriovenous fistula of renal vessels. Amer. J. Roentgenol. **75**, 905 (1956).
GEREMIA, B., GAMBA, A.: Urografia discendente destra da pielografin ascendente sinistra. Acta chir. Ital. **14**, 141 (1958).
GETZOFF, P. L.: Use of antihistamine drug prophylaxis against diodrast reactions. J. Urol. **65**, 1139 (1951).
GIDLUND, A.: Development of apparatus and methods for roentgen studies in hemodynamics. Acta radiol. Suppl. **130**, (1956).
GILG, E.: The influence of diphenhydramine (Benadryl) on the side-effects of diodone in urography. Acta radiol. **39**, 299 (1953).
GILLENWATER, J. Y.: Reactions associated with excretory urography: Current concepts. J. Urol. **106**, 122 (1971).
GILLESPIE, J. B., MILLER, G. A., SCHLERETH, J.: Water intoxication following enemas for roentgenographic preparation. Amer. J. Roentgenol. **82**, 1067 (1959).
GOODWIN, W. E., CASEY, W. C., WOOLF, W.: Percutaneous trocar (needle) nephrostomy in hydronephrosis. J. Amer. med. Ass. **157**, 891 (1955).
GOODWIN, W., CASEY, W. C.: Percutaneous antegrade pyelography & translumbar needle nephrostomy in hydronephrosis. A.M.A. Archives of Surgery **72**, 357 (1956).
GOLLMAN, G.: Zur Vermeidung störender Luftblasen bei der retrograden Pyelographie. Fortschr. Röntgenstr. **84**, 487 (1956).
GRAYSON, T., MARGULIS, A. R., HEINBECKER, P., SALTZSTEIN, S. L.: Effects of intra-arterial injection of Miokon, Hypaque and Renografin in the small intestine of the dog. Radiology **77**, 776 (1961).
GREENWOOD, F. G.: Cineradiography in urinary tuberculosis. Brit. J. Radiol. **30**, 493 (1957).
GRIEVE, J., LOWE, K. G.: Anuria following retrograde pyelography. Brit. J. Urol. **27**, 63 (1955).
GYLLENSWÄRD, Å., LODIN, H., MYKLAND, O.: Prevention of undue intestinal gas in abdominal radiography in infants. Acta radiol. **39**, 6 (1953).
GÜNTHER, G. W.: Röntgenuroskopie. Stuttgart: Georg Thieme 1952.

HAJÓS, E.: Methodik des Röntgen schichtverfahrens in der Urologie. Fortschr. Röntgenstr. **91**, 366 (1959).

HAENISCH, F.: Die Röntgenuntersuchung des uropoetischen Systems. In GROEDEL: Lehrbuch und Atlas der Röntgendiagnostik. München 1938.

HAMM, F. C., WATERHOUSE, K., WEINBERG, S. R.: Dangers of excretory urography. J. Amer. Med. Ass. **172**, 542 (1960).

HANLEY, H. G.: Cineradiography of the urinary tract. Brit. med. J. **199** II, 22.

— The pelvi-ureteric junction: A cine-pyelography study. Brit. J. Urol. **31**, 377 (1959).

HARRIS, J. H., HARRIS Jr., J. H.: Infusion pyelography. Amer. J. Roentgenol. **92**, 1391 (1964).

HARROW, B. R.: Intravenous urography using mixtures of radiopaque agents. Radiologie **65**, 265 (1955).

HARTMAN, H. R., NEWCOMB, A. W., BARNES, A., LOWMAN, R. M.: Renal infarction following selective renal arteriography. Excerpta Medica **20**, 664 (1966).

HELETÄ, T., VIRTAMA, P.: Bradykinin in renal angiography of normotensive and hypertensive patients. Investigative Radiology **5**, 149 (1970).

HELLMER, H.: On the technique in urography and the roentgen picture in acute renal and ureteral stasis. Acta radiol. **16**, 51 (1935).

— Nephrography. Acta radiol. **23**, 233 (1942).

HELWIG, F. C., SCHUTZ, C. B., CURRY, O. E.: Water intoxication: report of fatal human case, with clinical, pathologic and experimental studies. J. Amer. Med. Ass. **104**, 1569 (1935).

HENSON, P. E. Jr., BOYARSKY, S.: Constant Infusion Excretory Urography. J. Urol. **95**, 814 (1966).

HERSKOVITS, E.: Mit Perabrodil gefüllte Gallenblase während einer Ausscheidungspyelographie. Röntgenpraxis **10**, 261 (1938).

HERZAN, F. A., O'BRIEN, F. W.: Acceleration of delayed excretory urograms. Amer. J. Roentgenol. **68**, 104 (1952).

HESS, E.: Respiration pyelography as an aid in diagnosis. J. Urol. **42**, 4, 381 (1939).

HICKEL, R., CORNET, P.: Essai sur la significantion et la valeur des images et des signes urographiques fonctionnels. J. Radiol. Électrol. **29**, (1948).

HILDRETH, E. A., PENDERGRASS, H. P., TONDREAU, R. L., RITCHIE, D. I.: Reactions associated with intravenous urography: Discussion of mechanisms and therapy. Radiology **74**, 246 (1960).

HILGENFELDT, O.: Das Veratmungspyelogram. Dtsch. Z. Chir. **247**, 411 (1936).

HOFFMAN, H. A., DE CARVALHO, M. P.: Retrograde pyelography and use of contrast media containing neomycin. J. Amer. Med. Ass. **172**, 236 (1960).

HOFFMAN, W. W., GRAYHACK, J. T.: The limitations of the intravenous pyelogram as a test of renal function. Surg. gynec. Obst. **110**, 503 (1960).

HOGEMAN, O.: Elevated nonprotein nitrogen and urography. Upsala Läk.-Fören (Sweden). Förh. **57**, 161 (1952).

HOL, R., SKJERVEN, O.: Spinal cord damage in abdominal aortography. Acta radiol. **42**, 276 (1954).

HOLLANDER Jr., W., WILLIAMS, T. F.: A comparison of the water diuresis produced by oral and by intravenous water loading in normal human subjects. J. Lab. clin. Med. **49**, 182 (1957).

HOLMAN, R. L.: Complete anuria due to blockage of renal tubules by protein casts in a case of multiple myeloma. Arch. Path. (Chicago) **27**, 748 (1939).

HOPE, J. W., CAMPOY, F.: The use of carbonated beverages in pediatric excretory urography. Radiology **64**, 66 (1955).

HOPPE, J. O.: Some pharmacological aspects of radiopaque compounds. Ann. N.Y. Acad. Sci. **78**, 727 (1959).

— Urographic x-ray contrast media. Continuation course in urologic radiology for radiologists. Minneapolis 1961. Class notes (page 79—90).

HOWARDS, S., HARRISON, J., HARTWELL: Retroperitoneal phlegmon: a fatal complication of retrograde pyelography. J. Urol. **109**, 92 (1973).

HUGER, W. E., MARGOLIS, G., GRIMSON, K. S.: Protective effect of intra-aortic injection of procaine against renal injuries produced in experimental aortography. Surgery **43**, 52 (1958).

HULTBORN, K. A.: Allergische Reaktionen bei Kontrastinjektionen für die Urographie. Acta radiol. **20**, 263 (1949).

HUNNER, G. L.: The fallacy of depending on x-rays in the diagnosis of certain important urological conditions. J. Urol. **42**, 720 (1939).

HUTTER, K.: Zur Röntgendarstellung der Nierenhohlräume nebst Bemerkungen über die Lagebeziehung des Nierenbeckens zum Musculus psoas. Z. urol. Chir. **30**, 256 (1930).

IDHBORN, H., BERG, N.: On the tolerance of the rabbit's kidney to contrast media in renal angiography. Acta radiol. **42**, 121 (1954).

IMBUR, D., BOURNE, R.: Iodide mumps following excretory urography. J. Urol. **108**, 629 (1972).

INMAN, G. K. E.: A comparison of urographic contrast media, with particular reference to the aetiology and prevention of certain side effects. Brit. J. Radiol. **25**, 625 (1952).

JENSEN, F.: Ny kompressionsmetode ved intravenøs urografi. Nord. med. **58**, 1771 (1957).

JOSEPHSON, B.: Examination of diodrast clearance and tubular excretory capacity in man by means of two single injections of diodrast (Umbradil). Acta med. scand. **128**, 515 (1947).

— The mechanism of the excretion of renal contrast substances. Acta radiol. **38**, 299 (1952).

JULIANI, G., GIBBA, A.: Note di semeiotica roentgenchimografica pielo-ureterale. Radiol. med. (Torino) **42**, 209 (1957).

JUNKER, H.: Durchleuchtung und Momentaufnahme von Nierenbecken und Ureter. Z. Urol. **30**, 231 (1936).

JUTRAS, A.: Roentgen diagnosis by remote control. Telefluoroscopy and cineradiography. Medica Mundi **4**, 77 (1958).

KÅGSTRÖM, E., LINDGREN, P., TÖRNELL, G.: Changes in cerebral circulation during carotid angiography with sodium acetrizoate (Triurol) and sodium diatrizoate (Hypaque). Acta radiol. **50**, 151 (1958).

KAUFMAN, S. A.: The acceleration of delayed excretory urograms with ingested ice water. J. Urol. **74**, 243 (1955).

KEATES, P. G.: Improving the intravenous pyelogram: an experimental study. Brit. J. Urol. **25**, 366 (1953).

KENAN, P. B., TINDAL, G. T., MARGOLIS, G., WOOD, R. S.: The prevention of experimental contrast medium injury to the nervous system. J. Neurosurg. **15**, 92 (1958).

KIIL, F.: The function of the ureter and renal pelvis. Philadelphia and London: W. B. Saunders Company 1957.

KILLMANN, S., GJØRUP, S., THAYSEN, J. H.: Fatal acute renal failure following intravenous pyelography in patient with multiple myeloma. Acta med. scand. **158**, 43 (1957).

KITABATAKE, T.: Solidography of kidney study on rotatography. 16 reports. Nagoya J. Med. Sci. **18**, 159 (1955).

KJELLBERG, S. R., RUDHE, U.: The fetal renal secretion and its significance in congenital deformities of the ureters and urethra. Acta radiol. **31**, 243 (1949).

KLAMI, P.: Retrograde pyelography with hydrogen peroxide in the contrast medium. Acta radiol. **42**, 181 (1954).

KNEISE, O., SCHOBER, K. L.: Die Röntgenuntersuchung der Harnorgane. Leipzig 1941.

KNOEFEL, P. K., HUANG, K. C.: The biochemorphology of renal tubular transport: Iodinated benzoic acids. J. Pharmacol. & Exp. Therap. **117**, 307 (1956).

— The nature of the toxic action of radiopaque diagnostic agents. Radiology **71**, 13 (1958).

KOCH, C. C., NØRGAARD, B. G.: Intravenous pyelography. An examination of certain technical problems and a new radiopaque substance. Nord. med. **54**, 1351 (1955).

KRETSCHMER, H. L.: Intravenous urography. Surg. Gynec. Obstet. **51**, 404 (1930).

KUTT, H., McDOWELL, F.: Effects of iodinized contrast media upon electrophoretic mobilities of blood proteins and lipoproteins. J. Lab. Clin. Med. **59**, 118 (1962).

LAME, E. L.: Vertebral osteomyelitis following operation on the urinary tract or sigmoid. The third lesion of an uncommon syndrome. Amer. J. Roentgenol. **75**, 938 (1956).

LANG, E. K.: A survey of the complications of percutaneous retrograde arteriography. Radiology **81**, 257 (1963).

— Complications of retrograde percutaneous arteriography. J. Urol. **90**, 604 (1963).

LAPIDES, J., BOBBIT, J. M.: Preoperative estimation of renal function. J. Amer. med. Ass. **166**, 866 (1958).

LASIO, E., ARRIGONI, G., CIVINO, A.: Indicazioni e limiti dell'aortografia addominale in urologia. Minerva chir. (Torino) **13**, 1096 (1958).

LASSER, E. C.: Basic mechanisms of contrast media reactions. Radiology **91**, 63 (1968).

— Metabolic basis of contrast material toxicity-status. Amer. J. Roentgenol. **113**, 415 (1971).

— FARR, R. S., FUJIMAGARI, T., TRIPP, W. N.: The significance of protein binding of contrast media in roentgen diagnosis. Amer. J. Roentgenol. **87**, 338 (1962).

LASSER, E. C., LANG, J.: Contrast:Protein Interactions. Investigative Radiology **5**, 446 (1970).

— — Physiologic significance of contrast-protein interactions. I. Study in vitro of some enzyme effects. Investigative Radiology **5**, 514 (1970).

— LEE, S. H., FISCHER, E., FISCHER, B.: Some further pertinent considerations regarding the comparative toxicity of contrast materials for the dog kidney. Radiology **78**, 240 (1962).

— WALTERS, A., REUTER, S., LANG, J.: Histamine release by contrast media (Work in progress.) Radiology **100**, 683 (1971).

LAUBSCHER, W. M. L., RAPER, F. P.: A report of a case of the injection of a massive dose of urografin into the renal artery. Brit. J. Urol. **32**, 160 (1960).

LAURELL, H.: On the differential diagnosis: pyonephrosis or retroperitoneal tumour. Acta radiol. **3**, 226 (1924).

LEIGHTON, R. S.: Nephrography. Radiology **53**, 540 (1949).

LEUCUTIA, T.: Multiple myeloma and intravenous pyelography. Amer. J. Roentgenol. **85**, 187 (1961).

LEVICK, R. K., MITCHELL, J.: A simplified method of subtraction and its application to renal arteriography. Brit. J. Radiol. **35**, 843 (1962).

LICHTENBERG, A. v: Grundsätzliches zur Ausscheidungsurographie auf Grundlage von 2000 Untersuchungen mit sieben Nierenkontrastmitteln. Verh. III Internat. Radiologenkongr. Paris 1931, (s. 931).

— Principles and new advances in excretion urography Brit. J. Radiol. **3**, 119 (1931).

— The principles of intravenous urography. J. Urol. **25**, 249 (1931).

— Grundlagen und Fortschritte der Ausscheidungsurographie. Langenbecks Arch. klin. Chir. **171**, 1 3 (1932).

LILJA, B., WAHREN, H.: On meteorism in pyelography. Acta radiol. **15**, 41 (1934).

LILIENFELD, R. M.: Absorption of Urokon from the G. I. tract. Acta radiol. **51**, 251 (1959).

— ROSS, C. A.: Observations on the absorption of Urokon from the pathologic gastro-intestinal tract. Amer. J. Roentgenol. **83**, 931 (1960).

LINDBOM, Å.: Miliary tuberculosis after retrograde pyelography. Acta radiol. **25**, 219 (1944).

LINDGREN, P., TÖRNELL, G.: Blood circulation during and after peripheral arteriography. Acta radiol. **49**, 425 (1958).

— Hemodynamic responses to contrast media. Investigative Radiology **5**, 424 (1960).

LITTLE, E. H., BERGERON, R. B., TUTTON, R. H.: Antihistamine in excretory urography. Journal Louisiana Med. Soc. **117/8**, 257 (1965).

LOONEY, W. B.: An investigation of the late clinical findings following thorotrast (thorium dioxide) administration. Amer. J. Roentgenol. **83**, 163 (1960).

LOWMAN, R. M., DE LUCA, J. T.: Nephrotomography: its role in routine urographic studies. J. Urol. **83**, 308 (1960).

— SHAPIRO, H., LIN, A., DAVIS, L., KORN, F. E., NEWMAN, H. R.: Preliminary clinical evaluation of hypaque in excretory urography. Surg. Gynec. Obstet. **101**, 1 (1955).

LUDIN, H.: Vergleichende Prüfung des Kompressionseffektes von Einzel- und Doppelballonkompressorien bei der Ausscheidungsurographie (intravenöse Pyelographie). Radiol. Clin. **30**, 96 (1961).

MADSEN, E.: Effectiveness of urologic contrast media. Comparison between diodone and triiodyl (sodium acetriozoate). Acta radiol. **47**, 192 (1957).

MAGNUSSON, W.: On meteorism in pyelography and on the passage of gas through the small intestine. Acta radiol. **12**, 552 (1931).

MALUF, N.S.R.: Role of roentgenology in the development of urology. Amer. J. Roentgenol. **75**, 847 (1956).

MANFREDI, D., BEGANI, R., FREZZA, L. G.: La roentgencineangiografia renale selettiva. Minerva chir. (Torino) **13**, 1100 (1958).

MANGELSDORFF, B.: Die Veratmungspyelographie und ihre Verwertbarkeit in der urologischen Diagnostik. Fortschr. Röntgenstr. **74**, 416 (1951).

MARION, G.: Traité d'urologie. T. **1-2**, Paris 1928.

MARTIN, E. C., CAMPBELL, J. H., PESQUIER, C. M.: Cystography in children. J. Urol. **75**, 151 (1956).

MARTIN, J. F., DEYTON, W. E., GLENN, J. F.: The minute sequence pyelogram. Amer. J. Roentgenol. **90**, 55 (1963).

MAXWELL, M. H.: Reversible renal hypertension: clinical characteristics and predictive tests. Amer. J. Cardiol. **9**, 126 (1962).

— Use of the rapid-sequence intravenous pyelogram in the diagnosis of renovascular hypertension. New Engl. J. Med. **270**, 213 (1964).

MAY, F., SCHILLER, M.: Urografin, ein neues Mittel zur Ausscheidungsurographie. Med. Klin. **49**, 1403 (1954).

MAY, R. E., BOGASH, M.: Lymphangiography as a diagnostic adjunct in urology. J. Urol. **87**, 208 (1962).

McCHESNEY, E. W., HOPPE, J. O.: Studies of the tissue distribution and excretion sodium diatrizoate in laboratory animals. Amer. J. Roentgenol. **78**, 137 (1957).

McCLENNAN, B., BECKER, J., BERDON, W.: Excretory urography. Choice of contrast material-experimental. Radiology **100**, 585 (1971).

— — Excretory urography. Choice of contrast material-clinical. Radiology **100**, 591 (1971).

McDONALD, H. P., UPCHURCH, W. E.: Twenty-five years of progress in intravenous urography. Amer. Surg **21**, 989 (1955).

McFARLANE, R. K.: Routine water diuresis in excretory urography. Brit. J. Radiol. **35**, 798 (1962).

METYX, R., HORNYCH, A., BURIANOVA, U. B.: Die Nierenfunktion nach abdomineller Aortographie mittels verschiedener trijodierter Kontrastmittel Fortschr. Röntgenstr. **115**, 201 (1971).

MEYER, E.: Kritische Besprechung der direkten Kontrastfüllung der Harnwege und Erfahrungen mit dem neuen Kontrastmittel Thorotrast. Z. Urol. **26**, 157 (1932).

MIGLIORINI, M.: Condizioni neccessario per una valutazione sommaria della funzionalità ranel in corso di urografia. Radiol. med. (Torino) **43**, 462 (1957).

MIGLIORINI, M., TODDE, I.: Sull'uso dell'E.D.T.A. di Pb come di contrasto in radiologia. Atti Acad. Fisiocr. Siena **3**, 279 (1956).

MÖCKEL, G.: Medikamentöse Ganglienblockade zur Verbesserung der Röntgendiagnostik der Harnwege. Dtsch. med. Wschr. **79**, 1169 (1954).

MOORE, TH. D., MAYER, R. F.: Hypaque: an improved medium for excretory urography. Sth. Med. J. (Bgham, Ala.) **48**, 135 (1955).

MOORE, T. D., SANDERS. N: Reaction to urographic agents with and without antihistamines. J. Urol. **70**, 538 (1953).

MORINO, F., SESIA, G., QUAGLIA, C.: Varietà anatomiche e anomalie delle arterie renali revelate in vivo dall'arteriografia selettiva. Minerva Urol. **11**, 1 (1959).

MORROW, I., AMPLATZ, K.: Embolic occlusion of the renal artery during arteriography. Excerpta Medica **20**, 664 (1966).

MURPHY, T. E.: Effective evacuation of the bowel preparatory to urologic radiography. J. Urol. **86**, 659 (1961).

MYERS, WITTEN: Acute failure after excretory urography in multiple myeloma. Amer. J. Roentgenol. **113**, 583 (1971).

MYHRE, J. R., BRODWALL, E. K., KNUTSEN, S. B.: Acute renal failure following intravenous pyelography in cases of myelomatosis. Acta med. scand. **156**, 263 (1956).

NALBANDIAN. R. M., RICE, W. T., NICKEL, W. O.: A new category of contrast meida: water-soluble radioqaque polyvalent chelates. Ann. N. Y. Acad. Sci. **78**, 779 (1959).

NARATH, P. A.: The hydromechanics of the calyx renalis. J. Urol. **43**, 145 (1940).

— Renal pelvis and ureter. New York: Grune & Stratton 1951.

— The physiology of the renal pelvis and the ureter. in M. F. CAMPBELL, Urology. Philadelphia: W. B. Saunders Company 1954.

NECKER, F., WIESER, v. W.: Die Fehldeutung der Ausscheidungssperre und andere Irrtümer bei der intravenösen Pyelographie sowie Bemerkungen zur Indikationsstellung und Untersuchungstechnik. Radiol. clin. (Basel) **9**, 105, 129 (1940).

NESBIT, R. M.: Experience with the avoidance of allergic reactions to pyelographic media by the use of antihistamine drugs. Ann. N. Y. Acad. Sci. **78**, 852 (1959).

— The incidence of severe reactions from present day urographic contrast material. J. Urol. **81**, 486 (1959).

— DOUGLAS, D. B.: The subcutaneous administration of diodrast for pyelograms in infants. J. Urol. **42**, 709 (1939).

NICOLAI, C. H.: Major reactions to intravenous urographic media. Arch. Surg. **73**, 285 (1956).

— Miokon, a new intravenous urographic medium. J. Urol. **75**, 758 (1956).

NICOLICH, G., CERRUTI, G. B.: La nostra experienza in angiografia renale e vesicale. Minerva chir (Torino) **13**, 1109 (1958).

NITSCH, K., ALLIES, F.: Kurze Hinweise zur i. v. Urographie bei Kindern. Z. Urol. **50**, 353 (1957).

NOGRADY, M., BERNADETTE, DUNBAR, SCOTT, J.: Delayed concentration and prolonged excretion of urographic contrast medium in the first month of life. Amer. J. Roentgenol. **104**, 289 (1968).

— DUNBAR, J. S., MACEWAN, D. W.: The effect of (voluntary) bladder distention on the intravenous pyelogram. An experimental study. Amer. J. Roentgenol. **90**, 37 (1963).

O'CONNOR, J. F., NEUHAUSER, E. B. D.: Total body opacification in conventional and high dose intravenous urography in infancy. Amer. J. Roentgenol. **90**, 63 (1963).

OLIN, T., REES, D. O.: Renal function at urography with compression. Acta Radiol. **14**, 613 (1973).

OLIVERO, S., F. MORINO, F., MARGAGLIA, F.: Comportamento delle curve glicemiche a seguito dell'arteriografia addominale selettiva. Minerva chir. (Torino) **13**, 1111 (1958).

OLSSON, O.: On hepatosplenography with "jodsol". Acta radiol. **22**, 749 (1941).

— Contrast media in diagnosis and the attendant risks. Acta radiol. **116**, 75 (1954).

— Excretion of sodium metrizoate through the liver during urography. Acta radiol. **11**, 85 (1971).

— LÖFGREN, O.: Hyaluronidase as a factor hastening the spread and absorption of water-soluble radiopaque substances deposited intracutaneously, subcutaneously or intramuscularly. Acta radiol. **31**, 250 (1949).

ORTIZ, F., WALZAK, M. P., MARSHALL, V. F.: Chyluria: lymphatic-urinary fistula demonstrated by lymphangiography. J. Urol. **91**, 608 (1964).

OWEN R. H. R.: The concentration of pyelographic contrast media. A radiographic method of estimation of renal function. Brit. J. Radiol. **33**, 368 (1960).

OWMAN, T.: Urografi vid njurinsufficiens. Der Radiologe **13**, 283 (1973).

PALUBINSKAS, A. J.: "Stretching" of the arteries in renal arteriography. Radiology **82**, 40 (1964).

PAUL, L. E., JUHL, J. H.: The essentials of roentgen interpretation. New York: Paul B. Hoeber 1959.

PAYNE, W. W., MORSE, W. H., RAINES, S. L.: A fatal reaction following injection of urographic medium: a case report. J. Urol. **76**, 661 (1956).

PENDERGRASS, H. P., HODES, J. PH., TONDREAU, R. L., POWELL, C. C., BURDICK, E. D.: Further consideration of deaths and unfavourable sequelae following the administration of contrast media in urography in the United States. Amer. J. Roentgenol. **74**, 262 (1955).

PENDERGRASS, H.P., TONDREAU, R. L., PENDERGRASS, E. P., RITCHIE, D. J., HILDRETH, E. A., ASKOVITZ, S. I.: Reactions associated with intravenous urography: Historical and statistical review. Radiology **71**, 1 (1958).

PEART, W. S., SUTTON, D.: Renal vein catheterization and venography. Lancet **2**, 817 (1958).

PERILLIE, P. E., CONN, H. O.: Acute renal failure after intravenous pyelography in plasma cell myeloma. J. Amer. med. Ass. **167**, 2186 (1958).

PETTINARI, V., SERVELLO, M.: L'indagine arteriografica e flebografica del rene. Minerva chir. (Torino) **13**, 1117 (1958).

PIEMONTE, M., MAGNO, L.: Sulla eliminazione renale dei mezzi di contrasto iodati. Radiol. med. (Torino) **44**, 225 (1958).

— MAGNO, L.: Di-iodinated or tri-iodinated urographic contrast media? Further research on the mechanism of renal elimination of the contrast media for urography. Radiol. med. **45**, 744 (1959).

PIERCE, W. V., MINER, W. R.: Benign tumors of the ureter, Sth. med. J. (Bgham, Ala) **45**, 485 (1952).

PIERSON, L. E., HONKE, E. M.: Respiration pyelography in the diagnosis of perinephric abscess. J. Urol. **47**, 580 (1942).

PINET, F., DUCASSOU, J., CHARLES, F., GUIONIE, R., CALLICE, P., PÉRÈS, G.: L'arteriographie sous-gang1ioplégique dans l'exploration de l'appareil urinaire de l'adulte. J. radiol. **42**, 756 (1962).

PIRONTI DI CAMPAGNA, G. M., SERENO, L.: Contributo sperimentale al problema dell'eliminazione urografica. Tubulo-nefrosi da tetrationato di sodio e glomerulonefrite sperimentale da normali proteine eterogenee. Nunt. radiol. (Firenze) **22**, 1 (1956).

PITTS, R. F.: Physiology of the kidney and body fluids. Chicago: Year Book Medical Publishers Inc. 1963.

PIZON, P.: Les accidents de l'urographie intraveineuse. Presse méd. **64**, 1107 (1956).

POPPEL, M. H., ZEITEL, B. E.: Roentgen manifestation of milk drinker's syndrome. Radiology **67**, 195 (1956).

PRATHER, G. C.: MEDIAL ptosis of the kidney. New Engl. J. Med. **238**, 253 (1948).

PRÉVOT, R.: Intravenöse gezielte Pyelographie. Fortschr. Röntgenstr. **59**, 52 (1939).

— BERNING, H.: Zur Röntgendiagnostik der Pyelonephritis. Fortschr. Röntgenstr. **73**, 482 (1950).

PUIGVERT, A.: Un caso de inhibicion renal prolongada Chirurg Ginec. Urol. **8**, 273 (1954).

PYTEL, A.: Percutaneous antegrade pyelography (Russian text). Vestn. Rentgenol. Radiol. **33**, 15 (1958).

RABAIOTTI, A. L., ROSSI, PREVEDI, G.: Arteriografia addominale e delle estremità. Ed. Minerva Med. (Torino), 1956.

RAPOPORT, S., BRODSKY, W. A., WEST, C. D., MACKLER, B.: Urinary flow and excretion of solutes during osmotic diuresis in hydropenic man. Amer. J. Physiol. **156**, 433 (1949).

RAVASINI: Studium der Nierenfunktion in der Nierenchirurgie. Z. Urol. Chir. **40**, 470 (1935).

REINHARDT, K.: Ein Fall von Gallenblasendarstellung nach Perabrodilinjektion. Radiol. clin. (Basel) **23**, 193 (1954).

REITAN, H.: Prinzipien und Erfahrungen betreffend die Urographie. Acta radiol. **18**, 578 (1937).

RETHELYI, J.: Über die heterotope Ausscheidung Urografin. Fortschr. Röntgenstr. **97**, 316 (1962).

RIBBING, S.: Une source d'erreurs négligée dans l'interprétation des pyélographies. Acta radiol. **14**, 545 (1933).

— Über das sog. „Psoasrandsymptom" bei Pyelographie. Z. Urol. **28**, 306 (1934).

RIBBING, S.: La stratification des liquides opaques dans l'urographie. Acta radiol. **16**, 716 (1935).

RICHES, E. W.: The present status of renal angiography. Brit. J. Surg. **42**, 462 (1954-55).

ROCKOFF, S. D., BRASCH, R., KUHN, C., CHRAPLYVY, M.: Contrast media as histamine liberators. I & II. Investigative Radiology **5**, 503 (1970).

ROLLINS, M., BONTE, F. J., ROSE, F. A., KEATING, D. R.: Clinical evaluation of a new compound for intravenous urography. Amer. J. Roentgenol. **73**, 771 (1955).

ROSE, D. K.: Early diagnosis of cancer of the kidney. Surg. Clin. N. Amer. **29**, 1483 (1949).

ROSS, J. A.: One thousand retrograde pyelograms with manometric pressure records. Brit. J. Urol. **31**, 133 (1959).

ROSSI, A.: Aortografia translombare o arteriografia renale selettiva? Rassegna clinico-scientifica **34**, (1958).

— Aortografia addominale translombare, o arteriografia renale selletiva? Minerva chir. (Torino) **13**, 1131 (1958).

ROTH, M., NICHOLSON, T. A.: Comparative study of five urographic contrast media. J. Urol. **77**, 670 (1957).

ROTH, R. B., KAMINSKY, A. F., HESS, E.: Bactericidal additive for pyelographic mediums. J. Urol. **74**, 563 (1955).

SALINGER, H., SAALBERG, F.: Pyeloscopy. Acta radiol. **27**, 617 (1946).

SALZMAN, E., WARDEN, M. R.: Telepaque opacification of radiolucent biliary calculi. The "rim sign". Radiology **71**, 85 (1958).

— WATKINS, D. H., RUNDLES, W. R.: Opasification of radiolucent biliary calculi. J. Amer. med. Ass. **167**, 1741 (1958).

SAMMONS, B. P., LUND, R. R., PISCHNOTTE, W. O., RICHARDSON, J. F.: Simplified phlebography of the inferior vena cava in urologic diagnosis. Radiology **72**, 222 (1959).

SANDERS jr., P. W.: Medial renal ptosis. J. Urol. **77**, 24 (1957).

SANDSTRÖM, C.: Contrast media for the kidneys, heart and vessels, and their toxicity. Acta radiol. **39**, 281 (1953).

SAPEIKA, N.: Lead EDTA complex: a water-soluble contrast medium. S. Afr. med. J. **28**, 759 (1954).

— Lead EDTA complex: further radiographic studies. S. Afr. med. J. **28**, 953 (1954).

SARRUBI, ZALDIVAR, D.: Radiologie des pyelitis et pyelonephrits. J. Urol. **62**, 372 (1956).

SAUPE, E.: Magen- und Dünndarmfüllung nach Injektion von Per-Abrodil zur Durchführung einer Ausscheidungsurographie. Fortschr. Röntgenstr. **65**, 143 (1942).

SAVINO, F. M.: A pyelographic test for renal fixity during respiration. Brit J. Urol. **19**, 29 (1947).

SCHEELE, K.: Die Radiographie der oberen Harnwege als diagnostisches Mittel bei Tumoren des Bauches. Ergebn. med. Strahlenforsch. **4**, 41 (1930).

SCHENKER, B.: Drip infusion pyelography Radiology **83**, 12 (1964).

— Further experience with drip infusion pyelography. Radiology **87**, 304 (1966).

SCHERMULY, W.: Die heterotope Ausscheidung von Nierenkontrastmittel. Fortschr. Röntgenstr. **89**, 220 (1958).

SCHIFFER, E.: Füllungsdefekt bei retrograder Pyelographie, vorgetäuscht durch einen Nierenkelchkrampf. Acta radiol. **17**, 93 (1936).

SCHIMMERL, G.: Infusionsurographie. Fortschr. Röntgenstr. **104**, 306 (1966).

SCHLOSSMANN, D.: Thrombogenecity of vascular catheters. Akad. avh. University of Gothenburg 1972.

SCHLUNGBAUM, W.: Verteilung, Ausscheidung und Resorption nierengängiger, mit J^{131} markierter Röntgenkontrastmittel. Fortschr. Röntgenstr. **96**, 795 (1962).

— BILLION, H.: Untersuchungen der Verteilung von radioaktiven Urografin im menschlichen Organismus. Klin. Wschr. **34**, 633 (1956).

SCHNEIDER, H. J., HELBIG, U. W.: Zur Frage der Nierenschädigung nach Ausscheidungsurographie. Z. Urol. **55**, 529 (1962).

SCHOEN, H.: Zur Darstellung von Gallensteinen nach intravenösen Urogramm. Fortschr. Röntgenstr. **72**, 738 (1949–50).

SCHOLTZ, A.: Kontrasterzeugende Magenfüllung im Laufe einer Ausscheidungspyelographie. Z. Urol. **35**, 209 (1941).

SCHWARZ, E.: Puncture of the thoracic lymph duct with chylothorax: a rare complication of aortography. Radiology **75**, 248 (1960).

SCHWARTZ, R. H., BERDON, W. E., WAGNER, B. S., BECKER, J., BAKER, D. H.: Tamm-Horsfall urinary mucoprotein precipitation by urographic contrast agents: in vitro studies. Amer. J. Roentgenol. **108**, 698 (1970).

SCHWARTZ, W. B., HURWIT, A., ETTINGER, A.: Intravenous urography in the patient with renal insufficiency. New Engl. J. Med. **269**, 277 (1963).

SECRÉTAN, M.: Les accidents au cours des urographies intraveineuses. Urol. int. (Basel) **2**, 81 (1955).

— Les accidents au cours urographies intraveineuses. J. Belge. Radiol. **39**, 76 (1956).

SEGALL, H.: Gallbladder visualization following the injection of diatrizoate. Amer. J. Roentgenol. **107**, 21 (1969).

SENDEL, A.: Infusionspyelographie. Fortschr. Röntgenstr. **103**, 725 (1965).

SERVADIO, C. A.: A modified technique for intravenous pyelography. Brit. J. Urol. **37**, 385 (1965).

SHAPIRO, J. H., JACOBSON, H. G.: Oral 76 per cent sodium and methylglucamine diatrizoate, a new contrast medium for the gastrointestinal tract. Ann. N. Y. Acad. Sci. **78**, 966 (1959).

SHAPIRO, R.: Chelation in contrast roentgenography with special reference to lead disodium EDTA. Amer. J. Roentgenol. **76**, 161 (1956).

SHEA, T. E., PFISTER, R., Opacification of the gallbladder by urographic contrast media. Amer. J. Roentgenol. **107**, 763 (1969).

SHERWOOD, T., STEVENSON, J. J.: Antegrade pyelography: a further look at an old technique. Brit. J. Radiol. **45**, 812, (1972).

SINGER, P. L.: The use of antispasmodic drugs as preparation for intravenous pyelography. J. Urol. **58**, 216 (1947).

SINGLETON, E. B., HARRISON, G. H.: Excretory pyelography in infants. Technique for intravenous injection. Amer. J. Roentgenol. **75**, 896 (1956).

SMITH, P. G., RUSH, T. W., EVANS, A. T.: An evaluation of translumbar arteriography. J. Urol. **65**, 911 (1951).

SOBIN, S. S., FRASHER, W. G., JACOBSON, G., VAN EECKHOVEN, F. A.: Nature of adverse reactions to radiopaque agents. J. Amer. med. Ass. **170**, 1546 (1959).

SOUTHWOOD, W. F. W., MARSHALL, V. F.: A clinical evaluation of nephrotomography. Brit. J. Urol. **30**, 127 (1958).

SOVAK, M., LYNCH, P., MYGIND, T.: Improved technique for production of particulate contrast medium. Investigative Radiology **5**, 566 (1970).

SPEICHER, M. E.: A report on hypaque, a new intravenous urographic medium. Series of 800 cases. Amer. J. Roentgenol. **75**, 865 (1956).

STAGE, P., BRIX, E., FOLKE, K., KARLE, A.: Urography in renal failure. Acta radiol. **11**, 337 (1971).

STEINBERG, I., FINBY, N., EVANS, J. A.: A safe and practical intravenous method for abdominal aortography, peripheral arteriography, and cerebral angiography. Amer. J. Roentgenol. **82**, 758 (1959).

STEINERT, R.: Effect of enemata on contrast excretion in urography. Acta radiol. **38**, 30 (1952).

— A compression apparatus for urography. Acta radiol. **38**, 212 (1952).

STEVENSON, J. J.: Experience with Isopaque in intravenous pyelography. Farmakoterapi (Oslo) **18**, 18 (1962).

STRAIN, W. H.: Chemical composition and names of some principal water-soluble and cholecystographic contrast media. Investigative Radiology **5**, 498 (1970).

STRANDNESS, Jr., D. E.: The unilateral nonfunctioning kidney. A. M. A. Arch. intern. med. **101**, 611 (1958).

STRAUSS, M. B., DAVIS, R. K., ROSENBAUM, J. D., ROSSMEISL, E. C.: "Water diuresis" produced during recumbency by the intravenous infusion of isotonic saline solution. J. clin. Invest. **30**, 862 (1951).

SUSSMAN, R. M., MILLER, J.: Iodide "Mumps" after intravenous urography. New Engl. J. Med. **255**, 433 (1956).

SWANSON, G. E.: Lymphangiography in chyluria. Radiology **81**, 473 (1963).

SWICK, M.: The discovery of intravenous urography: Historical and developmental aspects of the urographic media and their role in other diagnostic and therapeutic areas. Bull. N. Y. Acad. Med. **42**, 128 (1966).

SVOBODA, M.: Beitrag zur Problematik der intravenösen Urographie beim Myelom. Radiologica Diagnostica **3**, 353 (1967).

TAYLOR, D. A., MACKEN, K. L., FIORE, A. S.: Mannitol Pyelography: A simplification of the drip technic. Radiology **88**, 1117 (1967).

TEPLICK, J. G., YARROW, M. W.: Arterial infarction of the kidney. Ann. intern. Med. **42**, 1041 (1955).

THEANDER, G.: On the visualization of the renal pelves in cholegraphy. Acta radiol. **45**, 283 (1956).

THEANDER, G.: Precipitation of contrast medium in the gallbladder. Acta radiol. **44**, 467 (1955).

THESTRUP ANDERSEN, P.: On tomography as an adjunct to urography. Acta radiol. **30**, 255 (1948).

TILLE, D.: Nicht patologische Füllungseffekte des Nierenbeckens und der Nierenkelche, Dtsch. Med. Wschr. **85**, 1414, 1422 (1960).

— Nierenangiographie durch Aortographie oder selektive Katheterisierung? Fortschr. Röntgenstr. **94**, 777 (1961).

TILLOTSON, P. M., HALPERN, M.: Selective renal arteriography. Amer. J. Roentgenol. **90**, 124 (1963).

TONIOLO, G.: Considerazioni critiche sull'uso delle alte percentuali di jodio nell'urografia funzionale. Nunt. radiol. (Firenze) **20**, 495 (1954).

TRUCHOT, P., NOIX, M., FABRE, R.: Valeur diagnostique des modifications morphologiques de l'image rénale au cours des examens radiologiques. J. Radiol. Electrol. **38**, 1141 (1957).

TUCKER, A. S., DI BAGNO, G., Intravenous urography, a comparative study of neoiopax and urokon. Amer. J. Roentgenol. **75**, 855 (1956).

UEBERSAX, R., SARASIN, R., LERUDULIER, J.-L.: Comparaison des résultat obtenus par différentes métodes urographiques. Radiol. clin. **32**, 495 (1963).

UTZ, D. C., THOMPSON, G. J.: Evaluation of contrast media for excretory urography. Proc. Mayo Clin. **33**, 75 (1958).

VESEY, J., DOTTER, C. T., STEINBERG, I.: Nephrography: simplified technic. Radiology **55**, 827 (1950).

VESIN, S.: Der diagnostische Wert cholinergischer Stoffe in der pharmakodynamischen Renovasographie. Der Radiologe **12**, 379 (1972).

VESTERDAHL, J., TUDVAD, F.: Studies on the kidney function in premature and full-term infants by estimating the inulin and paraaminohippurate clearances. Acta paediat. **37**, 429 (1949).

VIAMONTE, Jr. M., MYERS, M. B., SOTO, M., KENYON, N. M., PARKS, R. E.: Lymphography: its role in detection and therapeutic evaluation of carcinoma and neoplastic conditions of the genitourinary tract. J. Urol. **87**, 85 (1962).

VIX, V. A.: Intravenous pyelography in multiple myeloma. A review of 52 studies in 40 patients. Radiology **87**, 896 (1966).

VOUDOIKIS, I. J., BOUCEK, R. J.: Intercalative renal arteriography. Radiology **79**, 82 (1962).

VUORINEN, P., PYYKÖNEN, L., ANTTILA, P.: A renal cortical index obtained from urography films. Brit. J. Radiol. **33**, 622 (1960).

WADSWORTH, G. E., UHLENHUTH, E.: The pelvic ureter in the male and female. J. Urol. **76**, 244 (1956).

WAGNER, Jr., F. B., PRICE, A. H., SWENSON, P. C.: Abdominal arteriography. Amer. J. Roentgenol. **58**, 591 (1947).

WALD, A. M.: Nephrography during routine excretory urography. J. Urol. **75**, 572 (1956).

WALL, B., ROSE, D. K.: The clinical intravenous nephrogram: preliminary report. J. Urol. **66**, 305 (1951).

WALLDÉN, L.: Administration of contrast medium in urography via the bone marrow. Acta radiol. **25**, 213 (1944).

WALLINGFORD, V. H.: General aspects of contrast media research. Ann. N.Y. Acad. Sci. **78**, 707 (1959).

WALTER, R. C., GOODWIN, W. E.: Aortography and retroperitoneal oxygen in urologic diagnosis: a comparison of translumbar and percutaneous femoral methods of aortography. J. Urol. **70**, 526 (1953).

WARDENER DE, H. E.: The kidney: An outline of normal and abnormal structure and function. London: J. & A. Churchill Ltd. 1960.

WARRES, H. L., KIND, A. C.: Hyalurinidase in intramuscular excretory urography. Radiology **63**, 730 (1955).

WECHSLER, H.: Further studies of reactions due to intravenous urography. J. Urol. **78**, 496 (1957).

WEENS, H. S., FLORENCE, T. J.: Nephrography. Amer. J. Roentgenol. **57**, 338 (1947).

— The diagnosis of hydronephrosis by percutaneous renal puncture. J. Urol. **72**, 589 (1954).

WEIGEN, J. F., THOMAS, S. F.: Reactions to intravenous organic iodine compounds and their immediate treatment. Radiology **71**, 21 (1958).

WEISER, M.: Strahlentod durch Thorotrast. Röntgenblätter **10**, 270 (1957).

WEISSLEDER, H., EMMERICH, J., SCHIRMEISTER, J.: Gefäßbedingte Kontrastmittelaussparungen im urographischen Bild. Fortschr. Röntgenstr. **97**, 703 (1962).

— SCHOOP, W., KLÖSS, J.: Akuter Femoralisverschluß als Komplikation bei einer Arteriographie. Fortschr. Röntgenstr. **98**, 288 (1963).

WENDTH, A. J.: Drip infusion pyelography. Amer. J. Roentgenol. **95**, 269 (1965).

WHITESEL, J. A.: Lymphography: its place in urology. J. Urol. **91**, 613 (1964).

WHITESIDE, C. G.: Advances in the radiology of the urinary tract. In: Modern trends in urology. Ed. by Riches, E. W. London 1953, p. 20.

WICKBOM, I.: The influence of the blood pressure in urographic examination. Acta radiol. **34**, 1 (1950).

— Pyelography after direct puncture of the renal pelvis. Acta radiol. **41**, 505 (1954).

WINDHOLZ, F.: The roentgen appearance of the central fat tissue of the kidney: its significance in urography. Radiology **56**, 202 (1951).

WINTER, C. C.: The value of chlor-trimeton in the prevention of immediate reactions to 70 per cent urokon. J. Urol. **74**, 416 (1955).

— A clinical study of a new renal function test: The radioactive diodrast renogram. J. Urol. **76**, 182 (1956).

— The excretory urogram as a kidney function test. J. Urol. **83**, 313 (1960).

WINZER, K., LANGECKER, H., JUNKMAN, K.: Zur Frage der Verträglichkeit von Nieren- und Gallenkontrastmitteln. Sonderdruck aus Ärztl. Wschr. 9, 950 (1954).

WITT, H., BÜRGER, H.: Der Wert der Diuresepyelographie: Eine kritische Stellungnahme. Fortschr. Röntgenstr. **105**, 819 (1966).

WOHL, G. T.: Verbetral metastasis in renal carcinoma. An anatomic correlation. Amer. J. Roentgenol. **75**, 930 (1956).

WOLKE, K.: Some experiments in rectal pyelography. Acta radiol. **12**, 497 (1931).

— Pyelogramm mit einem durch einen Nierenarterienzweig verursachten Füllungsdefekt (Pseudodefekt). Acta radiol. **17**, 566 (1936).

WOLPERT, S. M.: Variation in kidney length during the intravenous pyelogram. Brit. J. Radiol. **38**, 100 (1965).

WOODRUFF, M. W.: The five-minute intravenous pyelogram as a measure of renal function. Amer. J. Roentgenol. **82**, 847 (1959).

WRIGHT, F. W.: Intravenous hydrocortisone in the treatment of a severe urographic reaction. Brit. J. Radiol. **32**, 343 (1959).

WYATT, G. M.: Excretory urography for children. Radiology 36, 664 (1941).

YOFFEY, J. M., COURTICE, F. C.: Lymphatics, lymph and lymphoid tissue. London: Edward Arnold Ltd. 1956, p. 201.

YOUNGBLOOD, V. H., WILLIAMS, J. O., TUGGLE, A.: Reactions due to intravenous urokon. J. Urol. **75**, 1011 (1956).

ZACCONE, G., CONZI, L.: Urografia a deflusso ostacolato (Proposta di tecnica). La Radiologia Medica, Vol. XXXIV Settembre 1948, p. 548.

ZANCA, P., BARKER, K. G., PYE, T. H.: WHEI-RUNG FU, HAAG, E. L.: Ureteral jet stream phenomenon in adults. Amer. J. Roentgenol. **92**, 341 (1964).

ZEITEL, B. E., LENTINO, W., JACOBSON, H. G.: POPPEL, M. H.: Renografin. A new intravenous urographic medium. J. Urol. **76**, 461 (1956).

ZIEGLER, J.: Bedeutung und Technik der Ureterkompression bei der Ausscheidungspyelographie. Dtsch. med. Wschr. **56**, 1772 (1930).

ZINNER, G., GOTTLOB, R.: Die gefäß-schädigende Wirkung verschiedener Röntgenkontrastmittel, vergleichende Untersuchungen. Fortschr. Röntgenstr. **91**, 507 (1959).

ZOLLINGER, H. U.: Thorotrastschädigung der Nieren mit Hypertonie. Schweiz. Med. Wschr. **87**, 1089 (1957).

Examination methods

IV. Renal Angiography

ABESHOUSE, B. S.: Thrombosis and thrombophlebitis of the renal veins. Urol. cutan. Rev. **49**, 661 (1945).

— TIONGSON, A. T.: Paraplegia, a rare complication of translumbar aortography. J. Urol. **75**, 348 (1956).

ABRAMS, H. L.: The response of neoplastic renal vessels to epinephrine in man. Radiology **82**, 217 (1964).

AGNEW, C. H.: Renal angiography. J. Kansas Med. Soc. **61**, 142 (1960).

AGUZZI, A., MARLEY, A., CHIUPPA, S.: Valutazione critica delle technice di aortografia abdominale. Boll. Soc. med. chir. Pavia **68**, 1153 (1954).

AHLBÄCK, S.: The suprarenal glands in aortography. Acta radiol. **50**, 341 (1958).

AHLBERG, N. E., BARTLEY, O., CHIDEKEL, N., WAHL-QVIST, L.: Njurvenskommunikanter. Anatomi och röntgenologi. Nord. Med. **74**, 1033 (1965).

AJELLO, L., MELIS, M., BALDUZZI, G., BENEDETTI, G.: L'arteriografia renale in condizioni normali e pathologiche. Minerva chir. (Torino) **13**, 1000 (1958).

ALKEN, C.: La rénovasographie peropératoire. J. Urol. méd. chir. **57**, 623 (1951).

— Renovasographie bei Teilresektionen der Niere und ihre Bedeutung für die Diagnostik isolierter Prozesse am Nierenparenchym. Z. Urol. Sonderh. 1952, 121.

— SOMMER, F.: Die Renovasographie. Z. Urol. **43**, 420 (1950).

ALLEN, C. D.: Urological symptoms produced by abdominal aneurysms. Urol. cutan. Rev. **44**, 462 (1940).

AMBROSETTI, A., SESENNA, B.: Arteriographische Untersuchungen an der tuberkulösen Niere. Urol. int. (Basel) **1**, 152 (1955).

AMUNDSEN, P.: Metrizoate sodium (Isopaque), a new contrast medium for angiography and urography. Evaluation of initial clinical testing and clinical experience. Farmakoterapi (Oslo) **18**, 3 (1962).

ANTHONY Jr., J. E.: Complications of aortography. Arch. Surg. **76**, 28 (1958).

ANTONI, N., LINDGREN, E.: Steno's experiment in man as complication in lumbar aortography. Acta chir. scand. **98**, 230 (1949).

— Aortography. J. Amer. Med. Ass. **148**, 652 (1952).

ARNOLD, M. W., GOODWIN, W. E., COLSTON, J. A. C.: Renal infarction and its relation to hypertension. Urol. Surv. **1**, 191 (1951).

ATKINS, H. L., HODES, PH. J.: The use of oral antihistamines in intravenous urography. Radiology **69**, 384 (1957).

BARNES, B. A., SHAW, R. S., LEAF, A., LINTON, R. R.: Oliguria following diagnostic translumbar aortography: report of a case. New Engl. J. Med. **252**, 1113 (1955).

BARON, G. J., KOENEMANN, R. H.: Arteriovenous fistula of the renal vessels. A case report. Radiology **64**, 85 (1955).

BASU, S. P.: Angiographic studies on renal circulation with rauwolfia serpentina. Indian J. Radiol. **16**, 105 (1962).

BAURYS, W.: Serious complications associated with the newer diagnostic methods in urology. J. Urol. **75**, 846 (1956).

BAZY, L., HUGUIER, J., REBOUI, H., LAUBRY, P., AUBERT, J.: Sur quelques aspects technique de l'artériographie. Arch. Mal. Coeur **41**, 97 (1948).

BECKER, J. A., GREGOIRE, A., BERDON, W., SCHWARTZ, D.: Vicarious excretion of urographic media. Radiology **90**, 243 (1968).

— POLLACK, H.: Cinefluorographic studies of the normal upper urinary tract. Radiology **84**, 886 (1965).

BECKMAN, G. F.: Translumbar aortography, Transactions of southeastern section of the A.U.A. (p. 144) Apr. 1954.

BEGNER, J. A.: Aortography in renal artery aneurysm. J. Urol. **73**, 720 (1955).

BENNESS, G. T.: Urographic contrast agents. A comparison of sodium and methoglucamine salts. Clin. Radiol. **21**, 150 (1970).

BERG, N. O., IDHBORN, H., WENDEBERG, B.: Investigation of the tolerance of the rabbit's kidney to newer contrast media in renal angiography. Acta Radiol. **50**, 285 (1958).

BERG, O. C.: Acute renal failure following translumbar aortography. Sth. med. J. (Bgham, Ala.) **49**, 494 (1956).

BERGENDAHL, S.: Zur Frage der Hydronephrose bei Nierengefäßvarianten. Acta chir. scand. Suppl. **45** (1936).

BERGSTRAND, I., SØRENSEN, S. E.: Renal angiography during straining. Brit. J. Radiol. **38**, 288 (1965).

BERLINER, R. W.: Outline of renal physiology. In: Diseases of the Kidney. Editd by M. B. Strauss & L. G. Welt. Boston; Little, Brown & Co. 1963, p. 30.

BERRY, J. F., ROBBINS, J. J., PIRKEY, E. L.: Abdominal aortography. Arch. Surg. **70**, 173 (1955).

BERRY, N. E., WHITE, E. P., METCALFE, J. O.: Abdominal aortography in urology. Canad. Med. Ass. J. **66**, 215 (1952).

BIERMAN, H. R., MILLER, E. R., BYRON, R. L., DOD, K. S., KELLY, K. H., BLACK, D. H.: Intraarterial catheterization of viscera in man. Amer. J. Roentgenol. **66**, 555 (1951).

BILLING, L.: The roentgen diagnosis of polycystic kidneys. Acta Radiol. **41**, 305 (1954).

— LINDGREN, Å. G. H.: Die pathologisch-anatomische Unterlage der Geschwulstarteriographie. Acta Radiol. **25**, 625 (1944).

BOBLITT, D. E., FIGLEY, M. M., WOLFMAN Jr., E. F.: Roentgen signs of contrast material dissection of aortic wall in direct aortography. Amer. J. Roentgenol. **81**, 826 (1959).

BODFORSS, B., MUTH, T., OLIN, T.: Renal function judged with radioactive diodrast after selective renal angiography in dogs. Acta radiol. **2**, 449 (1964).

BOHNE, A. W., HENDERSON, G. L.: Intrarenal arteriovenous aneurysm: case report. J. Urol. **77**, 818 (1957).

BOIJSEN, E.: Angiographic studies of the anatomy of single and multiple renal arteries. Acta Radiol. Suppl. **183** (1959).

— KÖHLER, R.: Renal arteriovenous fistulae. Acta Radiol. **57**, 433 (1962).

— — Renal artery aneurysms. Acta Radiol. **1**, 1077 (1963).

BOLIN, H.: Contrast medium in kidney during angiography: A densitometric method for estimation of renal function. Acta Radiol. Suppl. **257** (1966).

BREAM, CH. A.: The clinical use of pitressin in excretory urography. Amer. J. Roentgenol. **78**, 343 (1957).

CAFFARATTI, E., MORELLI, A.: Sul valore diagnostico della pneumoureteropielografia nello studio radiologico di alcune forme di calcolosi reno-ureterale. Ann. Radiol. Diagn. **31**, 423 (1958).

CALDICOTT, W. J. H., HOLLENBERG, N. K., ABRAMS, H. L.: Characteristics of response of renal vascular bed to contrast media: evidence for vasoconstriction induced by Renin-Angiotensin system. Investig Radiol. **5**, 539 (1970).

CAMPBELL, J. E.: Uretal peristalsis in duplex collecting systems. Amer. J. Roentgenol. **99**, 577 (1967).

CATTELL, W. R.: Comparison of the renal excretion of hypaque 45% and 60%. Brit. J. Radiol. **43**, 309 (1970).

CEN, M., ROSENBUSCH, G.: Nierenangiographie mit Adrenalin (Möglichkeiten der Pharmakoangiographie). Fortschr. Röntgenstr. **109**, 702 (1968).

CHAMBERLAIN, M. J., SHERWOOD, T.: The extrarenal excretion of diatrizoate in renal failure. Brit. J. Radiol. **39**, 765 (1966).

CHAUVIN, E.: Sull'arteriografia renale. Minerva chir. (Torino) **13**, 1134 (1958).

CHIAUDANO, C.: Arteriografia renale. Torino 1955.

CHIAUDANO, M.: Aspetti arteriografici dei reni in condizioni patologiche. Minerva chir. (Torino) **13**, 1074 (1958).

— Comportamento arteriografico del rene normale. Minerva chir. (Torino) **13**, 1082 (1958).

CHRISTOPHE, L., HONORÉ, D.: L'arteriographie par injection et prises de clichés automatiques. J. Chir. (Paris) **63**, 5 (1947).

CHVOJKA, J., DOLÉZEL, J.: Der Pharmakotest bei der Angiographie der Niere. Der Radiologe (1972).

CLARK, C. G.: Unilateral renal injury due to translumbar aortography. Lancet **1**, 769 (1958).

COMAR, O. B., SAGGESE, V.: Studio roentgencinematografico della dinamica calico-pielica. Rass. Int. Clin. Ter. **41**, 291 (1961).

CONGER, K. B., REARDON, H., AREY, J.: Translumbar aortography followed by fatal renal failure and severe hemorrhagic diathesis. Arch. Surg. **74**, 287 (1957).

COOK, K. K., KEATS, T. E., SEALE, D. L.: Determination of the normal position of the upper urinary tract on the lateral abdominal urogram. Radiology **99**, 499 (1971).

CREEVY, C. D., PRICE, W. E.: Differentiation of renal cysts from neoplasms by abdominal aortography: Pitfalls. Radiology **64**, 831 (1955).

CUÉLLAR, J.: New technique of translumbar aortic catheterization. J. Urol. **75**, 169 (1956).

CWYNARSKI, M. T., SAXTON, H. M.: Urography in myelomatosis. (Preliminary communication). Brit. Med. J. 1, **457** (1969).

DACIE, J., E., FRY, I. KELSEY: A comparison of sodium and methyolglucamine diatrizoate in clinical urography. Brit. J. Radiol. **44**, 51 (1971).

DAUGHTRIDGE, T. G.: Mucosal folds in the upper urinary tract. Amer. J. Roentgenol. **107**, 743 (1969).

DANIEL, P. M., PRICHARD, M. M. L., WARD-Mc QUAID, J. N.: The renal circulation after temporary occlusion of the renal artery. Brit. J. Urol. **26**, 118 (1954),

DAVIDSON, A. J., BECKER, J., ROTHFIELD, N., UNGER, G., PLOCH, D.: An evaluation of the effect of high-dose urography on previously impaired renal and hepatic function in man. Radiology **97**, 249, (1970).

DAVIS, L. A.: Reactions following excretory pyelography in infants and children. Radiology **71**, 19 (1958).

DETAR, J. H., HARRIS, J. A.: Venous pooled nephrograms: technique and results. J. Urol. **72**, 979 (1954).

DETERLING, Jr., R. A.: Direct and retrograde aortography. Surgery **31**, 88 (1952).

DIHLMANN, W.: Vergleichende Untersuchungen über den Wert der intravenösen Kompressionsurographie. Fortschr. Röntgenstr. **89**, 104 (1958).

DOLL, E.: Ausscheidungsurographie mit Urografin in der Kinderheilkunde. Medizinische **38**, 1384 (1957).

DOSS, A. K.: Translumbar aortography: its diagnostic value in urology. J. Urol. **55**, 594 (1946).

— THOMAS, H. C., BOND, T. B.: Renal arteriography, its clinical value. Tex. St. J. Med. **38**, 277 (1953).

DOS SANTOS, J. C.: L'angiographie Rénale. In Xme Congrès de la Soc. Int. d'Urol., Athènes, 1955 (Vol. I, p. 229).

DOS SANTOS, R., LAMAS, A., CALDAS, J. P.: L'artériographie des membres, de l'aorte et de ses branches abdominales. Bull. Soc. Nat. Chir. **55**, 587 (1929).

DOYLE, O. W.: The use of chlor-trimeton with miokon in intravenous urography. J. Urol. **81**, 573 (1959).

DREVVATNE, T.: Videotape Recorder ved Selektive Angiografier. Presented at Scand. Soc. med. Radiol. Congress, Copenhagen 1968.

DUDZINSKI, P. J., PETRONE, A. F., PERSOFF, M., CALLAGHAN, E. E.: Acute renal failure following high dose excretory urography in dehydrated patients. J. Urol. **106**, 619 (1971).

DUNBAR, J. S., MacEWAN, D. W., HEBERT, F.: The value of dehydration in intravenous pyelography – An experimental study. Amer. J. Roentgenol. **84**, 813 (1960).

DUNN, J., BROWN, H.: Unilateral renal disease and hypertension. J. Amer. Med. Ass. **166**, 18 (1958).

DURE-SMITH, P.: The dose of contrast medium in intravenous urography: A physiologic assessment. Amer. J. Roentgenol. **108**, 691 (1970).

— McARDLE, G. H.: Tomography during excretory urography. Technical aspects. Brit. J. Radiol. **45**, 896 (1972).

— SIMENHOFF, M., ZIMSKIND, P., KODROFF, M.: The bolus effect in excretory urography. Radiology **101**, 29 (1971).

DÜX, A., THURN, P., KISSELER, B.: Der physiologische Entleerungsmechanismus der ableitenden Harnwege im Röntgenkinematogramm. Fortschr. Röntgenstr. **97**, 687 (1962).

EDGREN, J., KÖHLER, R.: Urographie mit schneller Injektion großer Kontrastmittelmengen oder als Infusionsurographie. Diagnostischer Wert und Komplikationsfrequenz. Fortschr. Röntgenstr. **117**, 434 (1972).

EDHOLM, P., SELDINGER, S. I.: Percutaneous catheterization of the renal artery. Acta Radiol. **45**, 15 (1956).

EDLING, N. P. G.: Röntgenuntersuchung der Harnorgane. I: Lehrbuch der Röntgendiagnostik von Schinz, Baensch, Friedl und Uehlinger. Stuttgart: Georg Thieme Verlag 1952.

— EDVALL, C. A., HELANDER, C. G.: Correlation of urography and tests of renal function. Acta Radiol. **54**, 433 (1960).

EDLING, N. P. G, EDVALL, C. A., HELANDER, C. G., PERNOW, B.: Comparison of urography with selective clearance as tests of renal function. Acta Radiol. 45, 85 (1956).
— HELANDER, C. G.: On renal damage due to aortography and its prevention by renal tests. Acta Radiol. 47, 473 (1957).
— — Nephrographic effect in renal angiography. Acta Radiol. 51, 17 (1959).
— — Angionephrographic effect in renal damage. Acta Radiol. 51, 241 (1959).
— — PERSSON, F., ÅSHEIM, Å.: Renal function after aortography with large contrast medium doses. Acta radiol. 50, 351 (1958).
— — — — Renal function after selective renal angiography. Acta Radiol. 51, 161 (1959).
— — SELDINGER, S. I.: The nephrographic effect in depressed tubular excretion of umbradil. Acta Radiol 48, 1 (1957).
EDSMAN, G.: Accessory vessels of the kidney and their diagnosis in hydronephrosis. Acta Radiol. 42, 26 (1954).
— Angionephrography and suprarenal angiography. Acta Radiol. Suppl. 155, (1957).
— Angionephrography in malignant renal tumours. Urol. int. (Basel) 6, 117 (1958).
EIE, H.: Antihistamine treatment of side effects caused by injection of contrast media in angiographies. Farmakoterapi, Hefte 2, 39 (1970).
EIKNER, W. C., BOBECK, CH.: Renal vein thrombosis. J. Urol. 75, 780 (1956).
EKELUND, L.: Pharmakoangiographie der Nieren. Der Radiol. 13, 279 (1973).
— GÖTHLIN, J., LUNDERQUIST, A.: Diagnostic improvement with angiotensin in renal angiography. Radiology 105, 33 (1972).
ENGELL, H. C., DREWSEN, E.: Udvaskningsurografi og kirurgisk behandling af renal iskaemi. Nord. Med. 7 III, 308 (1968).
EVANS, A. T.: Renal arteriography. Amer. J. Roentgenol. 72, 574 (1954).
EVANS, J. A., GOVONI, A. F.: Angionefrografia associata a stratigrafia. Radiol. med. (Torino) 41, 1120 (1955).
— DUBILIER jr., W., MONTEITH, J. C.: Nephrotomography. Amer. J. Roentgenol. 71, 213 (1954).
— MONTEITH, J. C., DUBILIER, jr., W.: Nephrotomography. Radiology 64, 655 (1955).
— POKER, N.: Newer roentgenographic techniques in the diagnosis of retroperitoneal tumors. J. Amer. Med. Ass. 161, 1128 (1956).
FABRE, P.: L'angiographie rénale. X. congrès de la soc. int. d'urol. Aten 1955 (p. 345).
FARIÑAS, P. L.: A new technique for the arteriographic examination of the abdominal aorta and its branches. Amer. J. Roentgenol. 46, 641 (1941).
FISCHER, H., ROTHFIELD, NEVILLE, CARR, J.: Optimum dose in excretory urography. Amer. J. Roentgenol. 113, 423 (1971).
— DOUST, V. L.: Evaluation of the role of pretesting in the problems of serious reactions to urographic contrast media. Invest. Radiol. 6, 367 (1971).
— An evaluation of pretesting in the problem of serious and fatal reactions to excretory urography. Radiology 103, 497 (1972).

FOLIN, J.: Angiography in renal tumors.: Its value in diagnosis and differential diagnosis as a complement to conventional methods. Acta Radiol. Suppl. 267, (1967).
— Complications of percutaneous femoral catheterization for renal angiography. Der Radiologe 8, 190 (1968).
FONTAINE, R., WARTER, P., BILGER, F., KIM, M., KIENY, R.: De l'intérèt de l'aortographie pour le diagnostic des affections rénales. J. Radiol. Électrol. 37, 733 (1957).
FORST, H.: Der aortographische Nachweis der einseitigen Nierenaplasie. Z. Urol. 50, 366 (1957).
FREED, T. A., NEAL, M. P., VINIK, M.: The effect of Bradykinin on renal arteriography. Amer. J. Roentgenol. 102, 776 (1968).
FRIEDENBERG, M. J., CARLIN, M. R.: The routine use of higher volumes of contrast material to improve intravenous urography. Radiology 83, 405 (1964).
FRIMANN-DAHL, J.: Radiological investigations of urogenital tuberculosis. Urol. Int. 1, 396 (1955).
— Selective angiography in renal tuberculosis. Acta Radiol. 49, 31 (1958).
— Normal variations of the left kidney. Acta Radiol. 55, 207 (1961).
FRY, E., KELSEY, I., CATTELL, W. R.: Excretion urography in advanced renal failure. Brit. J. Radiol. 44, 198 (1971).
GANSAU, H.: Cavographie. Fortschr. Röntgenstr. 84, 575 (1956).
GARRITANO, A. P., WOHL. G. T., KIRBY, C. K., PIETROLUONGO, A. L.: The roentgenographic demonstration of an arteriovenous fistula of renal vessels. Amer. J. Roentgenol. 75, 905 (1956).
GASPAR, M. R., SECREST, P. G.: Chylothorax as a complication of translumbar aortography. Arch. Surg. 75, 193 (1957).
GAYLIS, H., LAWS, J. W.: Dissection of aorta as complication of translumbar aortography. Brit. Med. J. 1956, 1141.
GESENIUS, H.: Die abdominale Aortographie. Fortschr. Röntgenstr. 76, 24 (1952).
GIDLUND, Å.: Development of apparatus and methods for roentgen studies in haemodynamics. Acta radiol. Suppl. 130, (1956).
GIOUSTREMES, V., BOYARSKY, S., NEWMAN, H. R.: Fatal air embolism following presacral air insufflation. J. Urol. 85, 381 (1961).
GOLLMAN, G.: Die gezielte Angiographie und ihre diagnostischen Möglichkeiten (Kathetermethode). Radiol. Austr. 9, 117 (1956).
— Eine Modifizierung der Seldingerschen Kathetermethode zur isolierten Kontrastfüllung der Aortenäste. Fortschr. Röntgenstr. 87, 211 (1957).
— Zur Technik der Angiographie mittels Katheter. Fortschr. Röntgenstr. 89, 281 (1958).
— Die isolierte Angiographie der Aortenäste mit perkutan eingeführten Katheter, ihre Indikation und Ergebnisse. Fortschr. Röntgenstr. 89, 383 (1958).
GOODWIN, W. E., SCARDINO, P. L., SCOTT, W. W.: Translumbar aortic puncture and retrograde catherization of the aorta in aortography and renal arteriography. Ann. Surg. 132, 944 (1950).

Gospodinow, G. I., Topalow, J. B.: Phlebographie der Nierenvene auf dem Wege der Vena spermatica sinistra. Fortschr. Röntgenstr. **91**, 664 (1959).

Göthlin, J.: Ureteral jets. Der Radiologe **4**, 398 (1964).

— Vasopressin as an aid in eliminating intestinal gas before roentgen examination of the abdomen. Acta radiol. **12**, 100 (1972).

Gottlob, R., Zinner, G., Goldschmidt, F.: Über die Testmethoden zur Feststellung der lokalen schädlichen Wirkung von Röntgenkontrastmitteln bei der Angiographie. Langenbecks Arch. klin. Chir. **285**, 591 (1957).

Grant, B. P., Wigh, R.: Urine radiography of excreted iodide. A new renal function test. J. Amer. Med. Ass. **174**, 1304 (1960).

Graves, F. T.: The anatomy of the intrarenal arteries in health and disease. Brit. J. Surg. **43**, 605 (1956).

Gregg, D. McC., Allcock, J. M., Berridge, F. R.: Percutaneous transfemoral selective renal arteriography (including cineradiology). Brit. J. Radiol. **30**, 423 (1957).

Gremmel, H.: Darstellung von Bewegungsvorgängen. c) Bewegungspyelogramm. Handb. d. med. Radiol. **Bd. III**, (1960).

Grossman, L. A., Kirtley, J. A.: Paraplegia after translumbar aortography. J. Amer. Med. Ass. **166**, 1035 (1958).

Hajós, E., Magasi, P.: Das Röntgenbild der operierten Niere. Fortschr. Röntgenstr. **94**, 208 (1961).

Hamm, F. C., Waterhouse, K., Weinberg, S. R.: Dangers of excretory urography. J. Amer. Med. Ass. **172**, 542 (1960).

Handbuch der Inneren Medizin: Nierenkrankheiten, Teil 1, 2 & 3. Berlin & Heidelberg: Springer-Verlag 1968.

Handel, J., Schwartz, S.: Value of the prone position for filling the obstructed ureter in the presence of hydronephrotis. Radiology **71**, 102 (1958).

Hanley, H. G.: Cineradiography of the urinary tract. Brit. Med. J. **II**, 22 (1955).

— The pelvi-ureteric junction: A cinepyelographic study. Brit. J. Urol. **31**, 377 (1959).

Hare, W. S. C.: Damage to the spinal cord during translumbar aortography. J. Fac. Radiol. (Lond.) **8**, 258 (1957).

Harris, J. H., Harris Jr., J. H.: Infusion pyelography. Amer. J. Roentgenol. **92**, 1391 (1964).

Harrison, C. V., Milne, M. D., Steiner, R. E.: Clinical aspects of renal vein thrombosis. Quart. J. Med. **25**, 285 (1956).

Harvard, M.: Renal angiography. J. Urol. **70**, 15 (1953).

Hauschild, W.: Peridurale Kontrastmittelinjektion bei der Aortographie. Fortschr. Röntgenstr. **88**, 154 (1958).

Helander, C. G.: Nephrographic effect and renal arteriographic damage. Acta Radiol. Suppl. **163** (1958).

— Lindbom, Å.: Roentgen examination of the inferior vena cava in retroperitoneal expanding process. Acta Radiol. **45**, 287 (1956).

Hellström, J.: Über die Varianten der Nierengefäße, Z. urol. Chir. **24**, 253 (1928).

Henson, P. E. Jr., Boyarsky, S.: Constant Infusion Excretory Urography. J. Urol. **95**, 814 (1966).

Hilal, S., Sadek, K.: Trends in preparation of new angiographic contrast media with special emphasis on polymeric derivatives. Invest. Radiol. **5**, 458 (1970).

Hildreth, E. A., Pendergrass, H. P., Tondreau, R. L., Ritchie, D. J.: Reactions associated with intravenous urography: discussion of mechanisms and therapy. Radiology **74**, 246 (1960).

Hodson, C. J.: The radiological contribution toward the diagnosis of chronic pyelonephritis. Radiology **88**, 857 (1967).

Hoffman, H. A., de Carvalho, M. P.: Retrograde pyelography and use of contrast media containing neomycin. J.A.M.A. **172**, 236 (1960).

Hoffman, W. W., Grayhack, J. T.: The limitations of the intravenous pyelogram as a test of renal function. Surg. Gynec Obst. **110**, 503 (1960).

Hol, R., Skjerven, O.: Spinal cord damage in abdominal aortography. Acta Radiol. **42**, 276 (1954).

Holm, O. F.: Registrering genom aortografi av lokala recidiv efter nefrectomi för hyperneform (renalt adenocarcinom). Svenska Läkartidn (Stockholm) **54**, 3388 (1957).

Hoppe, J. O.: Urographic X-ray contrast media. Continuation course in urologic radiology for radiologists. Minneapolis 1961, class notes Pages 79–90.

Hou-Jensen, H. M.: Die Verästelung der Arteria renalis in der Niere des Menschen. Berlin: Springer-Verlag 1929.

Howards, Stuart, Harrison, J.: Retroperitoneal phlegmon: a fatal complication of retrograde pyelography. J. Urol. **109**, 92 (1973).

Hughes, F., Barcta, A., Fiandra, O., Viola, J.: Angiografia renal por via femoral. An. Hosp. S. Cruz (Barcelona) **17**, 1 (1957).

— Aneurysm of the renal artery. Acta Radiol. **49**, 117 (1958).

Hutter, K.: Zur Röntgendarstellung von Beckengefäßen bei urologischen Fällen. Acta radiol. **16**, 94 (1935).

Idhborn, H.: Angiographical diagnosis of carotid body tumors. Acta Radiol. **35**, 115 (1951).

— Renal angiography in cases of delayed excretion in intravenous urography. Acta Radiol. **42**, 333 (1954).

Idhborn, H.: Renal angiography in experimental hydronephrosis. Acta Radiol. Suppl. **136** (1956).

— Berg, N.: On the tolerance of the rabbit's kidney to contrast media in renal angiography. Acta Radiol. **42**, 121 (1954).

— Sjöstedt, S.: Ectopic ureter not causing incontinence until adult life. Acta Obstet. Gynec. Scand. **33**, 457 (1954).

Imbur, D., Bourne, R.: Iodide mumps following excretory urography. J. Urol. **108**, 629 (1972).

Indovina, I.: La circolazione renale studiata mediante isotopi radioattivi. Minerva chir. (Torino) **13**, 1090 (1958).

Isaac, F., Brem, T. H., Temkin, E., Movius, H. J.: Congenital malformation of the renal artery, a cause of hypertension. Radiology **68**, 679 (1957).

ISAAC, F., SCHOEN, I., WALKER, P.: An unusual case of Lindau's disease. Cystic disease of the kidneys and pancreas with renal and cerebellar tumors. Amer. J. Roentgenol. 75, 912 (1956).

JAMES, L.R., MATOOLE, J. J., DAVIS, H. L., HODGSON, P. E.: Morphologic responses to renal arterial perfusion with hypaque. Amer. J. Roentgenol. 93, 916 (1965).

JONES, R. N., WOOD, F. G.: Renal arteriography. Practitioner 175, 293 (1955).

JÖNSSON, G., OLLE OLSSON: A case of renal extopia with malrotation and vascular anomalies causing renal pain. Acta chir. scand. 123, 447 (1962).

KAHN, P. C.: The Epinephrine effect in selective renal angiography. Radiology 85, 301 (1965).

KALMON, E. H., ALBERS, D. D., DUNN, J. H.: Ureteral jet phenomenon. Radiology 65, 933 (1955).

KANEKO, M., SASAKI, T.: Der Wert der Serien-Frühurogramme und des Manitt-Auswasch-Urographie-Testes in der renovasculären Hypertension. Der Radiologe 10, 100 (1970).

KAUFMAN, J. J., BURKE, D. E., GOODWIN, W. E.: Abdominal venography in urological diagnosis. J. Urol. 75, 160 (1956).

KENDALL, A. R.: Experience with antidiuretic hormone in excretory urography. J. Urol. 84, 577 (1960).

KILLEN, D. A., LANCE, E. M.: Experimental appraisal of agents employed as angiocardiographic and aortographic contrast media. II. Nephrotoxicity. Surgery 47, 260 (1960).

KINCAID, O. W.: Renal angiography. Chicago: Year Book Publ. 1966.

— DAVIS, O. G., HALLERMANN, F., HUNT, J.: Fibromuscular dysplasia of the renal arteries: arteriographic features, classification and observations on natural history of the disease. Amer. J. Roentgenol. 104, 271 (1968).

KJELDSBERG, C. R., HOLMAN, R. E.: Acute renal failure in multiple myeloma. J. Urol. 105, 21 (1971).

KJELLBERG, S. R.: Die Mischungs- und Strömungsverhältnisse von wasserlöslichen Kontrastmitteln bei Gefäß- und Herzuntersuchungen. Acta radiol. 24, 433 (1943).

KNOEFEL, P. K.: The nature of the toxic action of radiopaque diagnostic agents. Radiology 71, 13 (1958).

KÖHLER, R.: Incomplete angiogram in selective renal angiography. Acta radiol. 1, 1011 (1963).

KRÜCKENMEYER, K., LESSMANN, H., PUDWITZ, K.: Nierenkarzinom als Thorotrastschaden. Fortschr. Röntgenstr. 93, 313 (1960).

LANDELIUS, E.: Death following renal arteriography in a child. Acta chir. scand. 109, 469 (1955).

LANDMANN, J., GENTILE, A., RIBEIRO, R., BEDRAN, Y: Insufficiéncia renal aguda por pielografia intravenosa. Bol. Cent. Estudos Hosp. Servidores 10, 237 (1958).

LASIO, E., ARRIGONI, G., CIVINO, A.: L'aortografia addominale in chirurgia urologica. Arch. ital. Urol. 27, 424 (1954).

— Indicazioni e limiti dell'aortografia addominale in urologia. Minerva chir. (Torino) 13, 1096 (1958).

LASSER, E. C.: Basic mechanisms of contrast media reactions. Radiology 91, 63 (1968).

— FARR, R. S., FUJIMAGARI, T., TRIPP, W.: The significance of protein binding of contrast media in roentgen diagnosis. Amer. J. Roentgenol. 87, 338 (1962).

— LEE, S. H., FISCHER, E., FISCHER, B.: Some further considerations regarding the comparative toxicity of contrast material for the dog kidney. Radiology 78, 240 (1962).

LEGER, L., PROUX, C., DURANTEAU, M.: Phlébographie rénale et cave inférieure par injection intra-parenchymateuse. Presse méd. 65, 141 (1957).

LÉLEK, I.: Untersuchung der akuten Nierenschädigung nach der Aortographie: experimentelle Arbeit an Hunden. Fortschr. Röntgenstr. 114, 790 (1971).

— Der Einfluß der renalen Arteriographie auf die Nierenfunktion, selektive Katheterisierung und Injektion: Experimentelle Arbeit an Hunden Fortschr. Röntgenstr. 114, 26 (1971).

LENKO, J.: Zur Frage der Kompressionsaufnahme bei Ausscheidungsurographien. Urologia (Treviso) 31, 52 (1964).

LENTZEN, W., FRIK, W., SCHIFFER, A.: Zur Frage einer Überlegenheit der Infusionsurographie gegenüber der konventionellen Urographie. Fortschr. Röntgenstr. 113, 396 (1971).

LERICHE, R., BEACONSFIELD, P., BOELY, C.: Aortography: its interpretation and value: a report of 200 cases. Surg. Gynec. Obstet. 94, 83 (1952).

LEUCUTIA, T.: Multiple myeloma and intravenous pyelography. Amer. J. Roentgenol. 85, 187 (1961).

LIESE, G. J.: Angiotomography: a preliminary report. Radiology 75, 272 (1960).

LINDBLOM, K.: Percutaneous puncture of renal cysts and tumors. Acta radiol. 27, 66 (1946).

— Diagnostic kidney puncture in cysts and tumors. Amer. J. Roentgenol. 68, 209 (1952).

LINDBLOM, K., SELDINGER, S. I.: Renal angiography as compared with renal puncture in the diagnosis of cysts and tumours. X. Congrès de la Soc. Int. d'Urol., Athens 1955 (page 331).

LINDGREN, E.: Technique of abdominal aortography. Acta radiol. 39, 205 (1953).

LITTLE, E. H., BERGERON, R. B., TUTTON, R. H.: Antihistamine in excretory urography. J. Louisiana Med. Soc. 117/8, 257 (1965).

LJUNGGREN, E., EDSMAN, G.: Remarques sur l'ateriographie rénale. X. congrès de al soc. int. d'urol. Aten 1955 II, pp. 140–147.

LOCKHART, J., POLLERO, A., CORLERE, A., HÉCTOR, J.: La cavografia de los tumores del testiculo. Arch. esp. Urol. 12 (1956).

LODIN, H., THORÉN, L.: Renal function following aortography carried out under ganglionic block. Acta radiol. 43 (1955).

LÖFGREN, F.: Das topographische System der Malpighischen Pyramiden der Menschenniere. Lund: A. B. Gleerupska Univ.-bokhandeln 1949.

LÖFGREN, F. O.: Renal tumour not demonstrable by urography but shown by renal angiography. Acta radiol. 42, 300 (1954).

514 References: Part I

LOOSE, K. E.: The importance of serial aortography for demonstration of blood vessels in pelvis and kidney. Radiol. clin. (Basel) **23**, 325 (1954).

LOPATKIN, N. A.: Renal angiography and its diagnostic significance (Russian text). Vestn. Hir. **78**, 74 (1957).

MacDONALD, J. S., WALLACE, E. N.: Lymphangiography in tumours of the kidney, bladder and testicle. Brit. J. Radiol. **38**, 93 (1965).

MALAMENT, M., SCHWARTZ, B., NAGAMATSU, G. R.: Extrarenal calyces: their relationship to renal disease. Amer. J. Roentgenol. **86**, 823 (1961).

MALISHOFF, S., CERRUTI, M.: Aneurysm of the renal artery. J. Urol. **76**, 542 (1956).

MALUF, N. S. R.: Internal diameter of renal artery and renal function. Surg. Gynec. Obstet. **107**, 415 (1958).

— McCOY, C. B.: Translumbar aortography as a diagnostic procedure in urology. Amer. J. Roentgenol. **73**, 533 (1955).

MANFREDI, D., BEGANI, R., FREZZA, L. G.: La roentgencineangiografia renale selettiva. Minerva chir. (Torino) **13**, 1100 (1958).

MARGOLIS, G.: Pathogenesis of contrast media injury: insights provided by neurotoxicity studies. Investig. Radiol. **5**, 392 (1970).

— TARAZI, A. K., GRIMSOM, K. S.: Contrast medium injury to the spinal cord produced by aortography. J. Neurosurg. **13**, 349 (1956).

MAYALL, G. F.: Mucosal folds in the upper urinary tract in childhood. Brit. J. Radiol. **38**, 303 (1965).

McAFEE, J. G., WILLSON, J. K. V.: A review of the complications of translumbar aortography. Amer. J. Roentgenol. **75**, 956 (1956).

McCORMACK, J. G.: Paraplegia secondary to abdominal aortography. J. Amer. Med. Ass. **161**, 860 (1956).

McDONALD, D. F., KENNELLY, jr., J. M.: Intrarenal distribution of multiple renal arteries. J. Urol. **81**, 25 (1959).

McDOWELL, R. F. C., THOMPSON, I. D.: Inferior mesenteric artery occlusion following lumbar aortography. Brit. J. Radiol. **32**, 344 (1959).

McFARLANE, R. K.: Routine water diuresis in excretory urography. Brit. J. Radiol. **35**, 798 (1962).

McLELLAND, R.: Renal artery aneurysms. Amer. J. Roentgenol. **78**, 256 (1957).

MEANEY, T. F., BUONOCORE E.: Contractions of the renal arteries during arteriography. Radiology **86**, 1 (1966).

MELDOLESI, G.: Il quadro aniografico renale nel blocco degli ureteri. Minerva Chir. (Torino) **13**, 1104 (1958).

MENG, C.-H., ELKIN, M.: Venous impression on the calyceal system. Radiology **87**, 878 (1966).

MERSEREAU, W. A. Robertson H. R.: Observations on venous endothelial injury following injection of various radiographic contrast media in rat. J. Neurosurg. **18**, 289 (1961).

MESCHAN, I., SCHMID, H. E., WATTS, F. C., WITCOFSKI, R.: The utilization of radioactive iodinated hippuran for determination of renal clearance rates. Radiology **81**, 437 (1963).

MIGLIARDI, L.: Sull'angiografia renale. Minerva Chir. (Torino) **13**, 1135 (1958).

MILLER, A. L., BROWN, A. W., TOMSKEY, G. C.: Pelvic fused kidney. J. Urol. **75**, 17 (1956).

MORINO, F., TARQUINI, A.: Il contributo dell'arteriografia selettiva allo studio della patologia renale. Minerva Chir. (Torino) **13**, 1018 (1958).

MORRIS, S., LASSER, E., FISCHER, B., LEE, S., GRANKE, R.: A comparative experimental approach to contrast materials in renal angiography. Radiology **77**, 764 (1961).

MOSER, F., HARTWEG, H.: Die Bedeutung der Nebennierenrindenhormone für die Röntgendiagnostik. Röntgenblätter **14**, 193 (1961).

MOTTRAM, R., LYNCH, P.: Circulatory effects of repeated intra-arterial injections of Conray 60. Investig. radiol. **5**, 534 (1970).

MULHOLLAND, S. W.: Abdominal crises with urologic implications. J. Amer. Med. Ass. **166**, 455 (1958).

MULLER, H.: Arteriography by retrograde catheterization of the aorta in renal pathology. Arch. Chri. Neerl. **5**, 108 (1953).

MURPHY, J. J., MYINT, M. K., RATTNER, W. H., KLAUS, R., SHALLOW, J.: The lymphatic system of the kidney. J. Urol. **80**, 1 (1958).

MURPHY, T. E.: Effective evacuation of the bowel preparatory to urologic radiography. T. Urol. **86**, 659 (1961).

MURRAY, R., TRESIDDER, G.: Renal angiography. Brit. Med. Bull. **13**, 61 (1957).

MYERS, M., WITTEN, D.: Acute failure after excretory urography in multiple myeloma. Amer. J. Roentgenol. **113**, 583 (1971).

MYGIND, T., ØIGAARD, A., SOVAK, M., DORPH, S.: Particulate radiographic contrast material for quantitative representation of blood-flow patterns. Investig. Radiol. **5**, 548 (1970).

MYHRE, J.R.: Arteriovenous fistula of the renal vessels: a case report. Circulation **14**, 185 (1956).

— BRODWALL, E. K., KNUTSEN, S. B.: Acute renal failure following intravenous pyelography in cases of myelomatosis. Acta med. scand. **156**, 263 (1956).

MÜLLER, H.: Suphrenische Gasansammlung nach Retroperitoneum. Fortschr. Röntgenstr. **94**, 636 (1961).

NESBITT, T. E.: A criticism of renal angiography. Amer. J. Roentgenol. **73**, 574 (1955).

NICOLICH, G., CERRUTI, G. B.: La nostra esperienza in angiografia renale e vescicale. Minerva chir. (Torino) **13**, 1109 (1958).

NITSCH, K., ALLIES, F.: Kurze Hinweise zur i. v. Urographie bei Kindern. Zschr. Urol. **50**, 353 (1957).

NOGRADY, M. B., DUNBAR, J.: Delayed concentration and prolonged excretion of urographic contrast medium in the first month of life. Amer. J. Roentgenol. **104**, 289 (1968).

— DUNBAR, J., MacEWAN, D.: The effect of (voluntary) bladder distention on the intravenous pyelogram. An experimental study. Amer. J. Roentgenol. **90**, 37 (1963).

NORDMARK, B.: Double formations of the pelves of the kidneys and the ureters. Embryology, occurrence and clinical significance. Acta radiol. **30**, 267 (1948).

NOTTER, G., HELANDER, C. G.: Über den Wert der Cavographie bei Diagnose und Behandlung retroperitonealer Testistumormetastasen. Fortschr. Röntgenstr. **89**, 409 (1958).

NUNNO jr., R. DE: L'arteriografia strumentale selettiva del rene. Arch. ital. Urol. **29**, 159 (1956).

— Technique, indications et limites de l'artériographie sélective instrumentale du rein. Presse méd. **65**, 792 (1957).

— L'arteriografia selettiva strumentala del rene. Minerva chir. (Torino) **13**, 1014 (1958).

O'CONNOR, J. F., NEUHAUSER, E. B.: Total body opacification in conventional and high dose intravavenous urography in infancy. Amer. J. Roentgenol. **90**, 63 (1963).

ÖDMAN, P.: Percutaneous selective angiography of the main branches of the aorta. Acta radiol. **45**, 1 (1956).

— RANNINGER, K.: The location of the renal arteries. Amer. J. Roentgenol. **104**, 283 (1968).

OLHAGEN, B.: Hypernefromdiagnos vid negativ urografi. Svenska Läkare Tidning (Stockholm) **51**, 7 (1954).

OLIN, T.: Studies in angiographic technique. (H. Ohlsson Boktryckeri, Lund, Sweden. 1963).

OLIN, T., REES, D.: Renal function at urography with compression. Acta radiol. **14**, 6/3 (1963).

— REUTER, S.: A pharmacoangiographic method for improving nephrophlebography. Radiology **85**, 1036 (1965).

OLIVERO, S., MORINO, F., MARGAGLIA, F.: Comportamento delle curve glicemiche a seguito dell'arteriografia addominale selettiva. Minerva chir. (Torino) **13**, 1111 (1958).

OLSSON, OLLE: Renal angiography. X. congrès de la soc. int. d'urol. Athena 1955 (p. 298).

— Arteriografia renale per via transfemorale. Minerva chir. (Torino) **13**, 1041 (1958).
Renal angiography in the pre-diagnostic phase. IX. I. C. R. München 1959.

— Contrast media in diagnosis and the attendant risks. Acta radiol. Suppl. **116**, 75 (1954).

— Renal radiography. In: Diseases of the Kidney. Edited by M. B. Strauss & L. G. Welt. Boston: Little, Brown & Co. 1963.

— Renal angiography in vascular and inflammatory diseases of the kidney. Congressus Radiolog. Chechoslov. Karlovy Vary 1963.

— Angiography in kidney masses; coeliacography; renal angiography in kidney trauma; renal angiography in pyelonephritis. In: Progress in Angiography. Edited by Viamonte M. & R. E. Parks. Springfield, Illinois: Thomas & Co. 1964.

— Renale Angiographie-Renovasographie. In: Vorträge der Angiographietagung in Baden-Baden 1965. Stuttgart: Thieme Verlag, 1966.

— Angiography in pyelonephritis. In: XIV Kongreß der Intern'l Gesellschaft f. Urologie, München 1967 (Vol. I, page 423).

— JÖNSSON, G.: Roentgen examination of the kidney and the ureter. In: Handbuch der Urologie. Heidelberg: Springer Verlag 1962.

OLSSON, OLLE, WEILAND, P.-O.: Renal fibrolipomatosis. Acta radiol. **1**, 1061 (1963).

— WHOLEY, M.: Vascular abnormalities in gross anomalies of kidneys. Acta radiol. **2**, 420 (1964).

OWEN, R. H.: The concentration of pyelographic contrast media. Brit. J. Radiol. **33**, 368 (1960).

PEIRCE, C.: Arteriografia renale transfemorale. Minerva Chir. (Torino) **13**, 1045 (1958).

PEIRCE, E. C.: Percutaneous femoral artery aortography: its use in the evaluation of retroperitoneal masses. J. Int. Coll. Surg. **20**, 16 (1953).

— RAMEY, W. P.: Renal arteriography: report of a percutaneous method using the femoral artery approach and a disposable catheter. J. Urol. **69**, 578 (1953).

PENDERGRASS, H. P., TONDREAU, R. L., PENDERGRASS, E. P., RITCHIE, D. J., HILDRETH, E. A., ASKOVITZ, S. I.: Reactions associated with intravenous urography: historical and statistical review. Radiology **71**, 1 (1958).

PETTINARI, V., SERVELLO, M.: L'Indagine arteriografica e flebografica del rene. Minerva Chir. **13**, 1117 (1958).

PIEMONTE, M., MAGNO, L.: Di-iodinated or tri-iodinated urographic contrast media? Further research on the mechanism of renal elimination of the contrast media for urography. (In Italian). Radiol. Med. Milan **45**, 744 (1959).

PIRONTI, L., TARQUINI, A.: Alcuni casi di tumore primitivo del rene studiati can l'arteriografia renale selettiva. Minerva Chir. **13**, 1122 (1958).

PITTS, R. F.: Physiology of the kidney and body fluids. Chicago: Year Book Medical Publishers 1963.

POIRIER, P., CHARPY, A.: Traité d'anatomie humaine. Paris: Masson & Cie. 1923.

POST, H. W. A., SOUTHWOOD, W. F. W.: The technique and interpretation of nephrotomograms. Brit. J. Radiol. **32**, 734 (1959).

POTTS, I. F.: Translumbar aortography. Med. J. Austr. **1**, 173 (1954).

— Further experiences in aortography. Med. J. Austr. **1955 I**, 232.

POUTASSE, E. F.: Occlusion of renal artery as cause of hypertension. Circulation **13**, 37 (1956).

— Renal artery aneurysm: report of 12 cases, two treated by excision of the aneurysm and repair of renal artery. J. Urol. **77**, 697 (1957).

— DUSTAN, H. P.: Arteriosclerosis and renal hypertension. J. Amer. Med. Ass. **165**, 1521 (1957).

— HUMPHRIES, A. W., McCORMACK, L. J., CORCORAN, A. C.: Bilateral stenosis of renal arteries and hypertension: Treatment by arterial homografts. J. Amer. Med. Ass. **161**, 419 (1956).

PROVET, H., LORD, J. W., LISA, J. R.: Aneurysm of the renal artery. Amer. J. Roentgenol. **78**, 266 (1957).

PYRAH, L. N., COWIE, J. W.: Two unnsual aortograms. J. Fac. Radiol. (Lond.) **8**, 416 (1957).

RADNER, S.: Subclavian angiography by arterial catheterization. Acta radiol. **23**, 359 (1949).

RANDALL, A., CAMPBELL, E. W.: Anomalous relationship of the right ureter to the vena cava. J. Urol. **34**, 565 (1935).

REAGAN jr., G. W., CARROLL, G.: Arteriography as observed in 80 patients at St. Louis city hospital. J. Urol. **66**, 467 (1951).

REDMAN, H. C., OLIN, T., SALDEEN, T., REUTER, S. R.: Nephrotoxicity of some vasoactive drugs following selective intra-arterial injection. Investig. Radiol. **1**, 458 (1966).

RICHES, E. W.: The present status of renal angiography. Brit. J. Surg. **42**, 462 (1955).

— GRIFFITHS, I. H.: Renal angiography. X. congrès de la soc. int. d'urol. Aten 1955, p. 271.

RILEY, J. M., HANAFEE, W.: Transaxillary renal angiography. J. Urol. **92**, 148 (1964).

RITTER, J. S.: Aortography. J. Urol. 155 (1955).

ROBECCHI, M., MORINO, F., TARQUINI, A.: L'arteriografia renale selettiva per via omerale nella pratica urologica. Minerva med. (Torino) **47**, 1639 (1956).

ROBINSON, ALAN, S.: Acute pancreatitis following translumbar aortography: case report with autopsy findings seven weeks following aortogram. A.M.A. Arch. Surg. **72**, 290 (1956).

ROCKOFF, S. D., KUHN, C., CHRAPLYVY, M.: Contrast media as histamine liberators. IV. In vitro mast cell histamine release by methyl-glucamine salts. Investig. Radiol. **6**, 186 (1971).

ROSS, J. A.: One thousand retrograde pyelograms with manometric pressure records. Brit. J. Urol. **31**, 133 (1959).

ROSSI, A.: Aortografia addominale translombare, o arteriografia renale selettiva? Minerva chir. (Torino) **13**, 1131 (1958).

ROUX-BERGER, J. L., NAULLEAU, J., CONTIADÈS, X. J. Cortico-surrénalome malin. Aortographie. Exérèse. Guérison opératoire. Bull. Soc. nat. Chir. **60**, 791 (1934).

SAMUEL, E., DENNY, M.: An evaluation of the hazards of aortography. Arch. Surg. (Chicago) **76**, 542 (1958).

SANCHEZ, L. M., DOMZ, C. A.: Renal patterns in myeloma. Ann. Int. Med. **52**, 44 (1960).

SANTE, L. R.: Evaluation of aortography in abdominal diagnosis. Radiology **56**, 183 (1951).

SANTOS, J. C. DOS: L'angiographie rénale. X. congrès de la soc. int. d'urol. Aten 1955, p. 229.

— Phlébographie d'une veine cave inférieure suturée. J. Urol. méd. chir. **39**, 586 (1935).

— Technique de l'Aortographie. J. int. Chir. **2**, 609 (1937).

SCHIMATZEK, A.: Aortographie. Verh. ber. der Deutsch. Ges. f. Urologie, Leipzig 1958 (page 257).

SCHLUNGBAUM, W.: Verteilung, Ausscheidung u. Resorption nierengängiger mit J^131 markierter Röntgenkontrastmittel. Fortschr. Röntgenstr. **96**, 795 (1962).

SCHNEIDER, H. J., HELBIG, W.: Zur Frage der Nierenschädigung nach Ausscheidungsurographie. Z. Urol. **55**, 529 (1962).

SCHNUR, B. M., SAKSON, J. A.: Trans-sacral retroperitoneal pneumography. J. Urol. **94**, 701 (1965).

SCHULZE-BERGMAN, G.: Über das arterio-venöse Aneurysma der Niere. Z. Urol. **47**, 661 (1954).

SCHWARTZ, J. W., BORSKI, A. A., JAHNKE, E. J.: Renal arteriovenous fistula. Surgery **37**, 951 (1955).

SELDINGER, S. I.: Catheter replacement of the needle in percutaneous arteriography. Acta radiol. **39**, 368 (1953).

SIDD, J. J., DECTER, A.: Unilateral renal damage due to massive contrast dye injection with recovery. J. Urol. **97**, 30 (1967).

SIEMENSEN, H. C., AUGUSTIN, H. J.: Untersuchungen zur Pharmakokinetik eines hepatotropen und eines renotropen Röntgenkontrastmittels unter Hämodialyse. Fortschr. Röntgenstr. **116**, 799 (1972).

SILVIS, R. S., HUGHES, W. F., HOLMES, F. H.: Aneurysm of the renal artery. Amer. J. Surg. **91**, 339 (1956).

SKOP, V., TEICHMANN, V.: The aortographic picture in Grawitz tumours of the kidney. Csl. Roentgenol. **9**, 148 (1955).

SLOMINSKI-LAWS, M. D., KIEFER, J., VERMEULEN, C.: Arteriovenous aneurysm of the kidney: case report. J. Urol. **75**, 586 (1956).

SMITH, G. I., ERICKSON, V.: Intrarenal aneurysm of the renal artery: case report. J. Urol. **77**, 814 (1957).

SMITH, P. G.: A résumé of the experience of the making of 1500 renal angiograms. J. Urol. **70**, 328 (1953).

— RUSH, T. W., EVANS, A. T.: An evaluation of translumbar arteriography. J. Urol. **65**, 911 (1951).

— The technique of translumbar arteriography. J. Amer. Med. Ass. **148**, 255 (1952).

SMITHUIS, T.: The problem of renal segmentation in connection with the modes of ramification of the renal artery and the renal vein. Acta Chir. Neerl. **8**, 227 (1956).

SOMMER, F., SCHÖLZEL, P.: Beobachtung einer aszendierenden Aortenthrombose nach Aortographie. Fortschr. Röntgenstr. **86**, 609 (1957).

STEIN, H., HILGARTNER, M. W.: Alteration of coagulation mechanism of blood by contrast media. Amer. J. Roentgenol. **104**, 458 (1968).

STEINER, R. E.: Venography in relation to the kidney. Brit. Med. Bull. **13**, 64 (1957).

STIRLING, W. B.: Aortography: its application in urological and some other conditions. Edingurgh: E. & S. Livingstone Ltd. 1957.

SWART, B.: Die zonographische Darstellung der Nieren- und Gallenwege. Der Radiologe **6**, 15 (1966).

SWICK, M.: The discovery of intravenous urography: historical and developmental aspects of the urographic media and their role in other diagnostic and therapeutic areas. Bull. New York Acad. Med. **42**, 128 (1966).

SVOBODA, M.: Beitrag zur Problematik der intravenösen Urographie beim Myelom. Radiol. Diagnostica **3**, 353 (1967).

TARAZI, A. K., MARGOLIS, G., GRIMSON, K. S.: Spinal cord lesions produced by aortography in dogs. Arch. Surg. (Chicago) **72**, 38 (1956).

THOMSON, H. S., MARGOLIS, G., GRIMSON, K. S., TAYLOR, H. M.: Effects of intra-arterial injection of iodine contrast media on the kidney of the dog. Arch. Surg. (Chicago) **74**, 39 (1957).

TILLANDER, H.: Magnetic guidance of a catheter with articulated steel tip. Acta radiol. **35**, 62 (1951).

TILLE, D.: Zur Technik und Indikation der Aortographie insbesondere der Renovasographie. Z. Urol. **52**, 121 (1959).

— Non-pathological filling defects of the renal pelvis and calyces. Germ. Med. Monthly **6**, 12 (1961).

TRUC, E., PALEIRAC, R.: I difetti di diffusione gassosa retro-peritonealy fisiologici. Minerva Chir. (Torino) **13**, 1135 (1958).

TRUSS, F.: Beitrag zur Nephrographie. 75. Tagung der Deutsch. Ges. f. Chir., München 1958.

UNGEHEUSER, E.: Indikationen zur Aortographie. Med. Klin. **52**, 16 (1957).

VELZER, D. A. VAN, LANIER, R. R.: A simplified technic for nephrotomography. Radiology **70**, 77 (1958).

VESTBY, G. W.: Perkutan punksjön av nyrecyster. Nord. Med. **79**, 633 (1968).

VOGLER, E.: Die Aortographie in ihrer Anwendung zur Darstellung der Durchblutung innerer Organe. Radiol. Austr. **9**, 13 (1956).

— HERBST, R.: Angiographie der Nieren. Stuttgart: Georg Thieme (1958).

VOTH, H., FINKE, H.: Zum Röntgenbild der Nierennekrose. Fortschr. Röntgenstr. **87**, 266 (1957).

VUORINEN, P., WEGELIUS, U.: Changes of renal size after drinking and intravenous glucose infusion. Brit. J. Radiol. **38**, 673 (1965).

WAGNER, F. B. Jr.: Arteriography in renal diagnosis: preliminary report and critical evaluation. J. Urol. **56**, 625 (1946).

WAKIM, K. G.: Normal anatomy and physiology of the kidneys and the pelves. Continuation Course in Urol. Radiol. for Radiologists. Univ. of Minnesota, Minneapolis 1961 (Class notes, pages 187–192).

WALTER, R. C., GOODWIN, W. E.: Aortography and pneumography in children. J. Urol. **77**, 323 (1957).

DE WARDENER, H. E.: The kidney: an outline of normal and abnormal structure and function. London: J. & A. Churchill Ltd. 1960.

WEIGEN, J. F., THOMAS, S. F.: Reactions to intravenous organic iodine compounds and their immediate treatment. Radiology **71**, 21 (1958).

WEYDE, R.: Abdominal aortography in renal diseases. Brit. J. Urol **25**, 353 (1952).

— Die abdominale Aortographie, insbesondere bei Nierenkrankheiten. Radiol. Clin. (Basel) **23**, 313 (1954).

WEYENETH, R., LE RUDULIER, J. L.: Image radiologique bizarre au niveau du trajet de l'uretère lombaire droit. Radiol. Clin. **31**, 67 (1962).

WIDÉN, C. C.: Unilateral renal disease and hypertension: Use of the radioactive diodrast renogram as a screening test. J. Urol. **78**, 107 (1957).

WINDHOLZ, F.: The roentgen appearance of the central fat tissue of the kidney: its significance in urography. Radiology **56**, 202 (1951).

WINTER, C. C.: The excretory urogram as a kidney function test. J. Urol. **83**, 313 (1960).

WOODARD, J. R.: Vascular imprints on the upper ureter. J. Urol. **87**, 666 (1962).

WOODRUFF, M. W., MALVIN, R. L.: Localization of renal contrast media excretion by stop-flow analysis. J. Urol. **84**, 677 (1960).

WOODRUFF, J. H. Jr., OTTOMAN, R. E.: Radiologic diagnosis of renal tumours by renal angiography. J. Canad. Ass. Radiol. **7**, 54 (1956).

WYATT, G. M., FELSON, B.: Aortic thrombosis as a cause of hypertension: an arteriographic study. Radiology **69**, 676 (1957).

WYMAN, A. C., CIMMINO, C. V.: Fluoroscopic examination of the urinary tract. J. Urol. **83**, 501 (1960).

ZACCONE, G., CONZI, L.: Urografia a deflusso ostacolato (Proposta di tecnica). La Radiol. Medica **XXXIV**, 548 (1948).

ZANCA, P., BARKER, K. G., PYE, T. H., FU, W.-R., HAAG, E. L.: Ureteral jet stream phenomenon in adults. Amer. J. Roentgenol. **92**, 341 (1964).

ZHEUTLIN, N., HUGHES, D., O'LOUGHLIN, B. J.: Radiographic findings in renal vein thrombosis. Radiology **73**, 884 (1959).

D. Anomalis

ABOULKER, P., MOTZ, C.: Un cas d'uretère rétro-cave. J. Urol. méd. chir. **59**, 391 (1953).

ABRAMS, A., FINKLE, L. u. A. L.: Reversible suppressed function in unilateral renal malrotation. J. Amer. med. Ass. **163**, 641 (1957).

ABRAMS, H. L., KAPLAN, H. S.: Angiocardiographic interpretation in congenital heart disease. Springfield (Illinois): Chas. C. Thomas Company 1956 (page 14).

ALLANSMITH, R.: Ectopic ureter termination in seminal vesicle; unilateral polycystic kidney: report of a case and review of the literature. J. Urol. **80**, 425 (1958).

ANDERSON, G. W., RICE, G. G., HARRIS jr., B. A.: Pregnancy and labor complicated by pelvic ectopic kidney. J. Urol. **65**, 760 (1951).

ANDERSSON, J. C., ROBERTSON, A. S. C.: Solitary ectopic pelvis kidney, Brit. J. Urol. **24**, 207 (1952).

ANDRÉN, L., BJERSING, L., LAGERGREN, L.: Congenital aplasia of the abdominal muscles with urogenital malformations. Acta radiol. **2**, 298 (1964).

ANZ, A. H., CHAN, W. F.: Ectopic thoracic kidney. Jr. Urol. **108**: 2, 211 (1972).

ANSON, B. J., KURTH, L. E.: Common variations in the renal blood supply. Surg. Gynec. Obstet. **100**, 157 (1955).

ASHLEY, D. J., MOSTOFI, F. K.: Renal agenesis and dysgenesis. J. Urol. **83**, 211 (1960).

ASK-UPMARK, E.: Über juvenile maligne Nephrosklerose und ihr Verhältnis zu Störungen in der Nierenentwicklung. Acta Path. Microbiol. Scand. **6**, 383 (1929).

AXILROD, H. D.: Triplicate ureter. J. Urol. **72**, 799 (1954).

BACHMANN, D., HAASNER, E.: Renal arteriography with special reference to anomalies of the renal arteries. Fortschritte Röntgenstr. **103**: 1, 71 (1965).

BAGGENSTOSS, A. H.: Congenital anomalies of the kidney. Med. Clin. N. Amer. **35**, 987 (1951).

BANKER, R. J., CARD, W. H.: Calyceal diverticula. J. Urol. **72**, 773 (1954).

BARLOON, J. W., GOODWIN, W. E., VERMOOTEN, V.: Thoracic kidney. J. Urol. **78**, 356 (1957).

BARTLEY, O., CEDERBOM, G., HEGNELL, B.: Multicystic renal disease in an adult. Acta radiol. 6, 424 (1967).

BEGG, R. C.: Sextuplicitas renum: a case of six functioning kidneys and ureters in an adult female. J. Urol. 70, 686 (1953).

BENNETT, J. P.: Renal cysts communicating with the pelvis. Illinois med. 79, 232 (1941).

DE BERNARDI, E., SPAZIANTE, G.: Aspects angiographiques dans quelques malformations et ectopies du rein. J. Radiol. Électrol. 44, 37 (1963).

BIBUS, B.: Ein seltener Fall von Nierenmißbildung. Z. Urol. 47, 28 (1954).

BIE, K.: Ureteral duplications, ectopic ureter and ureterocele. J. Oslo City Hosp. 8, 201 (1958).

BOATMAN, D., CORNELL, S., KÖLLN, C.-P.: The arterial supply of horeshoe kidneys. Amer. Jr. of Roentgenol. 113: 3, 447 (1971).

— KÖLLN, C.-P., FLOCKS, R. H.: Congenital anomalies associated with horeshoe kidney. Jr. Urol. 107: 2, 205 (1972).

BOIJSEN, E.: Angiographic studies of the anatomy of single and multiple renal arteries. Acta radiol. Suppl. 183, 1959.

BOLADO, J. L.: Rinon en herradura. Arch. esp. Urol. 13, 220 (1957).

BORELL, U., FERNSTROM, I.: Congenital solitary pelvic kidney. A study of its blood supply by aortography. J. Urol. (Baltimore) 72, 618 (1954).

BRAASCH, W. F.: Anomalous renal rotation and associated anomalies. Trans. Amer. Ass. gen.-urin. Surg. 23, 1 (1930).

BRAIBANTI, T.: Considerazioni su un caso di dispasia cistica del rene. Ann. Radiol. diagn. (Bologna) 21, 412 (1949).

BREKKAN, E., MYRVOLD, H., SCHNÜRER, L.-B.: Kolonkancer som senkomplikation vid ureterosigmoideostomi. Nord. Medicin 11 (II): 85: 6, 189 (1971).

BROOMÉ, A.: Komplex urogenital missbildning. Nord. Med. 59, 51 (1958).

BRUNELLI, B., DARDARI, M.: Raro aspetto di cisti pielogenica. Nunt. radiol. (Firenze) 21, 33—39 (1955).

BULGRIN, J. G., HOLMES, F. H.: Eventration of the diaphragm with high renal ectopia. Radiology 64, 249 (1955).

BURKLAND, C. E.: Clinical considerations in aplasia, hypoplasia and atrophy of the kidney. J. Urol. (Baltimore) 71, 1 (1954).

BUTLER, T. J.: Solitary ectopic pelvic kidney. Brit. J. Surg. 38, 522 (1951).

CAMPBELL, M. F.: Urology I. Philadelphia and London: W. B. Saunders Company 1954.

— Renal ectopy. J. Urol. 24, 187 (1930).

— Anomalies of the kidney. In: Urology. Edited by M. F. Campbell. Philadelphia: W. B. Saunders Company 1963 (Vol. 2, page 1564).

CAMPOS FREIRE, G.: Uretère rétrocave et rein hypoplasique. J. Urol. méd. chir. 59, 868 (1953).

CATHRO, A. J. McG.: Section of the inferior vena cava for retrocaval ureter: A new method of treatment. J. Urol. 67, 464 (1952).

CAVINA-PRATESI, A., FIOCCHI, C. E.: Considerazioni su un caso di "ectopia renale alta." Ann. Radiol. Diagn. (Bologna) 35, 90 (1962).

CECCARELLI, F. E., BEACH, P. D.: Multiple urogenital anomalies: pronephric, mesonephric and metanephric kidney elements with persistent Müllerian duct in an adult male. J. Urol. 85, 31 (1961).

CHALKLEY, T. S., SUTTON, L. E.: Infected solitary cyst of the kidney in a child, with a review of the literature. J. Urol. 50, 414 (1943).

CHAUVIN, H. F.: Sur les images radiologiques d'uretère rétro-cave. J. Urol. méd chir. 60, 266 (1954).

CHEN, K.-C.: Lymphatic abnormalities in patients with chyluria. J. Urol. 106: 1, 111 (1971).

— CHWALLA (1935) cit. GILL (1952).

COPPRIDGE, W. M.: Bilateral pelvic kidneys. J. Urol. 32, 231 (1934).

COUVELAIRE, R.: Autre exemple d'uretère rétro-cave. J. Urol. méd. chir. 59, 65 (1953).

CREMIN, B. J.: The urinary tract anomalies associated with agenesis of the abdominal walls. Brit. Jr. Radiol. 44, 767 (1971).

CULVER, H.: Extravesical ureteral opening into the genital tract in a male. Trans. Amer. Ass. gen.-urin. Surg. 30, 295 (1937).

DALGAARD, O. Z.: Polycystic disease of the kidneys. In: Diseases of the kidney. Edited by M. B. Strauss & L. G. Welt. Boston: Little, Brown and Company 1963 (pg 912).

DALLA BERNARDINA, L., RIGOLI, E.: La cisti pielogenica. Quad. radiol. 23, 109 (1958).

DAMM, E.: Solitärcysten der Niere. Z. urol. Chir. 35, 102 (1932).

DAVIDSON, B.: Renal ectopia with abdominal and pelvic symptomatology. Urol. cutan. Rev. 42, 334 (1938).

DAY, R. V.: Ectopic opening of the ureter in the male with report of a case. J. Urol. (Baltimore) 11, 239 (1924).

DEÁK, J.: Eine seltene Nierenentwicklungsanomalie. Fortschr. Röntgenstr. 85, 250 (1956).

DEMOULIN, M., NICKELS, L.: Kelchzysten der Niere. Fortschr. Röntgenstr. 83, 208 (1955).

DERBES, V. J., DIAL, W. A.: Postcaval ureter. J. Urol. 36, 226 (1936).

DESGREZ, H., HEITZ, F., VASELLE, B., CORNU, J., BARROIS, J.: Étude radiologique des uretères ectopiques s'abouchant dans l'urèthre postérieur. Jr. Radiol. d'Electrol. 45, 308 (1964).

DORSEY, J. W.: Solitary hydrocalyx secondary to a dumbbell calculus. J. Urol. 62, 742 (1949).

DREYFUSS, W.: Anomaly simulating a retrocaval ureter. J. Urol. 82, 630—632 (1959).

DUFF, P. A.: Retrocaval ureter: Case report. J. Urol. 63, 496 (1950).

DUFOUR, A., SESBOÜÉ, P.: L'uretère rétrocave, J. Urol. méd. chir. 58, 433 (1952).

— Uretère rétrocave diagnostiqué avant l'opération et guéri par uréteroplastie. J. Urol. méd. chir. 58, 390 (1952).

ECKERBOM, H., LILIEQUIST, B.: Ectopic ureter. Acta radiol. 38, 420 (1952).

EDSMAN, G.: Angionephrography and suprarenal angiography. Acta radiol. Suppl. 155 (1957).

EKSTRÖM, T.: Renal hypoplasia. A clinical study of 179 cases. Acta chir. scand. Suppl. 203 (1955).

— NILSON, A. E.: Retrocaval ureter. Acta chir. scand. 118, 53—59 (1959).

EMMETT, J. L., ALVAREZ-IERENA, J. J., McDONALD, J. R.: Atrophic pyelonephritis versus congenital renal hypoplasia. J. Amer. med. Ass. **148**, 1470 (1952).

ENGEL, W. J.: Aberrant ureters ending blindly. J. Urol. **42**, 674 (1939).

— The late results of partial nephrectomy for calyectasis with stone. J. Urol. (Baltimore) **57**, 619 (1947).

— Ureteral ectopia opening into the seminal vesicle. J. Urol. (Baltimore) **60**, 46 (1948).

ERICKSEN, L. G.: Rupture of congenital solitary kidney. Report of a case in which the diagnosis was made during life. Amer. J. Roentgenol. **39** 731 (1938).

ESCH, W., HALBEIS, K.: Zu den Kelchzysten der Niere. Radiol. Austr. **10**, 65 (1958).

EVERS, E.: Zwei Fälle mit seltener Ureteranomalie (akzessorische Blindureter). Acta radiol. **25**, 121 (1944).

FALLENIUS, GÖSTA: Beitrag zur Röntgendiagnostik der Nierenektopie. Acta radiol. **23**, 455 (1942).

FELTON, L. M.: Should intravenous pyelography be a routine procedure for children with chryptorchism or hypospadias? J. Urol. **81**, 335 (1959).

FERGUSON, G., WARD-McQUAID, J. N.: Stones in pyelogenic cysts. Brit. J. Surg. **42**, 595 (1955).

FEY, B., GOUYGOU, TEINTURIER: Diverticules kystiques des calcis. J. Urol. méd. chir. **57**, 1 (1951).

FOROUGHI, E., TURNER, J. A.: Congenital ureteral valve. Jr. Urol. **81**, 272 (1959).

GILL, R. D.: Triplication of the ureter and renal pelvis. J. Urol. **68**, 140 (1952).

GLENN, J. F.: Fused pelvic kidney. J. Urol. **80**, 7 (1958).

GOLDSTEIN, A. E., HELLER, E.: Ectopic ureter opening into a seminal vesicle. J. Urol. **75**, 57 (1956).

GONDOS, B.: High ectopy of the left kidney. Amer. J. Roentgenol. **74**, 295 (1955).

— Rotation of the kidney around its transverse axis. Radiology **74**, 19 (1960).

— Rotation of the kidney around its longitudinal axis. Radiology **76**, 615 (1961).

GRAF, R. A., SMITH, J. H., FLOCKS, R. H., VAN EPPS, E. F.: Urinary tract changes associated with Spina Bifida and Myelomeningocele. Amer. Jr. Roentgenol. **92**, 255 (1964).

GRAVES, F. T.: The anatomy of the intrarenal arteries in health and disease. Brit. J. Surg. **43**, 605 (1956).

GRAVES, R. C., DAVIDOFF, L. M.: Anomalous relationship of the right ureter to the inferior vena cava. J. Urol. **8**, 75 (1922).

GRUBER, G.: Entwicklungsstörungen der Nieren und Harnleiter. In HENKE-LUBARSCH' Handbuch der speziellen pathologischen Anatomie und Histologie, Teil 4. Berlin 1925.

HAMILTON, G. R., PEYTON, A. B.: Ureter opening into seminal vesicle complicated by traumatic rupture of only functioning kidney. J. Urol. **64**, 731 (1950).

HARRIS, A.: Renal ectopia — special reference to crossed ectopia without fusion. J. Urol. **42**, 1051 (1939).

HARRISON, J. H., BOTSFORD, T. W.: Experiences in the management of congenital anomaly of the kidney in the army. J. Urol. **55**, 309 (1946).

HEIDENBLUT, A.: Das Kelchdivertikel der Niere. Fortschr. Röntgenstr. **84**, 230 (1956).

HELLMER, H.: Nephrography. Acta radiol. **23**, 233 (1942).

HELLSTRÖM, J.: Über die Varianten der Nierengefäße. Z. urol. Chir. **24**, 253 (1928).

HENNIG, O.: Überbleibsel von Urnierenanlagen. Z. Urol. **47**, 493 (1954).

HESLIN, J. E., MAMONAS, C.: Retrocaval ureter: a report of four cases and review of the literature. Jr. Urol. **65**, 212 (1951).

HILL, J. E., BUNTS, R. C.: Thoracic kidney: case reports. Jr. Urol. **84**, 460 (1960).

HOLM, H.: On pyelogenic renal cysts. Acta radiol. **29**, 87 (1948).

HÖSLI, P. O.: Anomalien der Harnwege im Kindesalter und ihre chirurgische Behandlung. Basel: S. Karger 1960.

HOU-JENSEN, H.: Die Verästelung der Arteria renalis in der Niere des Menschen. Z. anat. Entwickl.-Gesch. **91**. 1 (1930).

IDBOHRN, H., SJÖSTEDT, S.: Ectopic ureter not causing incontinence until adult life. Acta obstet. gynec. scand. **33**, 457 (1954),

ITIKAWA, T., TANIO, H.: Über den Ureterprolapsus und das angeborene Divertikel des Nierenkelchs. Z. Urol. **33**, 395 (1939).

JEFFERY, R. F.: Unusual origins of renal arteries. Radiology **102**: 2, 309 (1972).

JUCKER, C., PRATES, A. C., PRINI, G.: Radiological findings in cases of hypoplastic kidney. Quad. Radiol. **27**: 3, 271 (1962).

KANASAWA, M., MOLLER, J., GOOD, R. A., VERNIER, R. L.: Dwarfed kidneys in children: the classification, etiology and significance of bilateral small kidneys in eleven children. Amer. Jr. Dis. Childh. **109**: 2, 130 (1965).

KATZEN, P., TRACHTMAN, B.: Diagnosis of vaginal ectopic ureter by vaginogram. J. Urol. **72**, 808 (1954).

KISSELER, B., MERTEN, M., THURN, P.: Zur röntgenologischen Diagnose des Kelchdivertikels der Niere. Fortschr. Röntgenstr. **96**, 222 (1962).

KRETSCHMER, H. L.: Hernia of the kidney. J. Urol. **65**, 944 (1951).

KYAW, M. M., NEWMAN, H.: Renal pseudotumors due to ectopic accessory renal arteries: the angiographic diagnosis. Amer. J. Roentgenol. **113**: 3, 443 (1971).

LAIDIG, C. E., PIERCE jr., J. M.: Retrocaval ureter — unusual cause of ureteral obstruction. J. Amer. med. Ass. **171**, 2312 (1959).

LAU, F. T., HENLINE, R. B.: Ureteral anomalies. J. Amer. med. Ass. **96**, 587 (1931).

LAUGHLIN, V. C.: Retrocaval (circumcaval) ureter associated with solitary kidney. J. Urol. **71**, 195 (1954).

LEITER, E.: Horseshoe kidney: discordance in monozygotic twins. J. Urol. **108**: 5, 683 (1972).

LEWIS, S., DOSS, R.: Calcified hydropyonephrosis. Radiol. **70**, 866 (1958).

LIBSHILTZ, H., BEN-MENACHEM, Y., KURODA, K.: Unusual renal vascular supply. Brit. J. Radiol. **45**, 536 (1972).

LJUNGGREN, E.: Beitrag zur Röntgendiagnostik der Nierentuberkulose. Z. Urol. **36**, 155 (1942).

— EDSMAN, G.: Remarques sur l'arteriographie rénale. X. Congrès de la Soc. Int. d'Urol. Aten 1955 (page 140).

LÖFGREN, F. O.: Das topographische System der Malpighischen Pyramiden der Menschenniere. Lund: A. B. Gleerupska Univ.-bokhandel 1949.

MALEK, R., KELALIS, P., BURKE, E.: Ectopic kidney in children and frequency of association with other malformations. Mayo Clinic Proceedings **46**, 461 (1971).

— GREENE, L.: Urologic aspects of Hippel-Lindau syndrome. J. Urol. **106**:6, 800 (1971).

MALTER, U., STANLEY, R.: The intrathoracic kidney, with a view of the literature. J. Urol. **107**:4 (1972).

MAYER, R. F., MATHES, G. L.: Retrocaval ureter. Sth. Med. J. (Bgham, Alabama) **51**, 945 (1958).

McDONALD, D. F., KENNELLY, J. M. jr.: Intrarenal distribution of multiple renal arteries. J. Urol. **81**, 25 (1959).

McQUIGGAN, M. C., RATLIFF, R. K.: Infant survival in the absence of renal function. J. Urol. **91**, 206 (1964).

MEHL, R. L.: Retro-iliac artery ureter. J. Urol. **102**:1, 27 (1969).

MEISEL, H. J.: Ectopic ureter opening into a seminal vesicle. J. Urol **68**, 579 (1952).

MENVILLE, J. G.: Horseshoe kidney with unilateral reduplication of the pelvis and ureter and ureteral ectopia. J. Urol. **73**, 25 (1955).

MESSERSCHMIDT, O.: Betrag zur Röntgendiagnose der „Cystome des nephrogenen Gewebes". Fortschr. **79**, 529 (1953).

MILLER, A. L. Jr., BROWN, A. W., TOMSKEY, G. C.: Pelvic fused kidney. J. Urol. **75**, 17 (1956).

MILLER, E. V., TREMBLAY, R. E.: Symptomatic blindly ending bifid ureter. J. Urol. **92**, 109 (1964).

MOLINA, L. F., SABUCEDO, R. M.: The retrocaval ureter. Radiologia (Panama) **7**, 115 (1957).

MOORE, G. W., BUCHERT, W. I.: Unilateral multicystic kidney in an infant. J. Urol. **78**, 721 (1957).

MUANGMAN, V., UEHLING, D.: Hydronephrosis secondary to vaginal atresia. J. Urol. **106**:1, 140 (1971).

MULLEN, W. H. Jr., ENGEL, W. J.: Circumcaval ureter. Radiology **59**, 528 (1952).

MURPHY, F. J., MAU, W., ZELMAN, S.: Nephrogenic polycythemia. J. Urol. **91**:5, 474 (1964).

NATVIG, P.: Two cases of solitary renal cyst with communucation to the renal pelvis. Acta radiol. **22**, 732 (1941).

NIELSEN, P. B.: Retrocaval ureter. Acta radiol. **51**, 179 (1959).

NILSSON, J.: Ektopisk ureter. Nord. Med. **68**, 1132 (1962).

NORDMARK, B.: Double formations of the pelves of the kidneys and the ureters. Embryology, occurrence and clinical significance. Acta radiol. **30**, 267—278 (1948).

OCHSNER, H. C.: Cysts of the kidney. Amer. J. Roentgenol. **65**, 185 (1951).

ØDEGAARD, H.: Crossed renal ectopia. Acta radiol. **27**, 543 (1946).

OLSSON, OLLE: Anomalies. In: Diseases of the kidney. Edited by M. B. Strauss & L. G. Welt. Boston: Little, Brown & Co. 1971 (page 155).

— JÖNSSON, G.: A case of renal ectopia with malrotation and vascular anomalies causing renal pain. Acta chir. Scand. **123**, 447 (1962).

— WHOLEY, M.: Vascular abnormalities in gross anomalies of the kidneys. Acta radiol. **2**:5, 420 (1964).

ÖSTLING, K.: Röntgenologische und pathologisch-anatomische Veränderungen bei Erweiterungen einzelner Nierenkelche. Acta radiol. **15**, 28 (1934).

PARKER, R. W.: Absence of abdominal muscles in an infant. Lancet **1**, 1252 (1895).

PASQUIER, C. M., WOMACK, R. K.: Ectopic opening of ureter into seminal vesicle. J. Urol. **70**, 164 (1953).

PASSARO, E. Jr., SMITH, J. P.: Congenital ureteral valve in children: a case report. J. Urol. **84**, 290 (1960).

PERRIN (1927) cit. GILL (1952) (see above).

PETROVČIĆ, F., KRIVEC, O.: Triple ureter: with report of a case. Brit. J. Radiol. **28**, 627 (1955).

— MILIČ, N.: "Horseshoe" kidney with crossed ureter condition after right nephrectomy. Brit. J. Radiol. **29**, 114 (1956).

PICK, J. W., ANSON, B. J.: Retrocaval ureter; report of a case, with discussion of its clinical significance. J. Urol. **43**, 672 (1940).

PONTHUS, P., BOUSTANY, F. N.: Sur le diagnostic radiologique du rein en fer à cheval. Rev. méd. Moy. Or. **13**, 93—98 (1956).

POTTER, E. L.: Pathology of the fetus and the newborn. Year Book Publ. (Chicago) 1952.

POTTS, I. F.: Solitary ectopic pelvic kidney. Med. J. Aust. **2**, 498 (1953).

PRATHER, G. C.: Calyceal diverticulum. J. Urol. **45**, 55 (1941).

PRESMAN, D., RAYMOND, F.: A diagnostic method for retrocaval ureter. Amer. J. Surg. **92**, 628 (1956).

PURPON, I.: Crossed renal ectopy with solitary kidney: a review of the literature. J. Urol. **90**, 13 (1963).

RAMSEY, J., BLIZNAK, J.: Klippel-feil syndrome with renal agenesis and other anomalies. Amer. J. Roentgenol. **113**:3, 460 (1971).

RANDALL, A., CAMPBELL, E.: Anomalous relationship of the right ureter to the vena cava. I. Urol. **34**, 565 (1935).

RAYER, P. F.: Traité des maladies des reins. (Paris) **3**, 507 (1841).

RENERT, W., RUDIN, L. J., CASARELLA, W. J.: Renal vein thrombosis in carcinoma of the renal pelvis. Amer. J. Roentgenol. **114**:4, 735 (1972).

RENTERSKIÖLD, G., WILBRAND, H.: „Ask-Upmark-Niere". Fortschr. Röntgenstr. **115**:6, 752 (1971).

RIBA, L. W., SCHMIDLAPP, C. J., BOSWORTH, N. L.: Ectopic ureter draining into the seminal vesicle. J. Urol. **56**, 332 (1946).

ROBERTS, R. R.: Complete valve of the ureter: Congenital urethral valves. J. Urol. **76**, 62 (1956).

RÖHRIG, H.: Kongenitale thorakale Ektopie der rechten Niere. Fortschr. Röntgenstr. **89**, 371 (1958).

ROWLAND, H. S. Jr., BUNTS, R. C., IWANO, J. H.: Operative correction of retrocaval ureter: a report of four cases and review of the literature. J. Urol. **83**, 820 (1960).

RUDSTRÖM, P.: Ein Fall von Nierenzyste mit eigenartiger Konkrementbildung. Acta chir. scand. **85**, 501 (1941).

SANDEGÅRD, E.: The treatment of ureteral ectopia. Acta chir. scand. **115**, 149 (1958).

SCHORR, S., BIRNBAUM, D.: Raised position of the right kidney. Radiol. clin. (Basel) **28**, 102 (1959).

SCHWARTZ, A., FRÄNKEL, M.: High renal ectopia, detected on routine chest examination. Acta radiol. **37**, 583 (1952).

SCHWARTZ, J.: An unusual unilateral multicystic kidney in infant. J. Urol. **35**, 259–263 (1936).

SEITZMAN, D. M., PATTON, J. F. Ureteral ectopia: combined ureteral and vas deferens anamoly. J. Urol. **84**, 604 (1960).

SELDOWITSCH, J. B.: Über die Multiplicität der Nierenarterie und deren chirurgische Bedeutung. Langenbecks Arch. klin. Chir. **89**, 1071 (1909).

SERVANTIE, G.: Un cas d'uretère rétro-cave. J. Radiol. Électrol. **37**, 935 (1956).

SESBOÜÉ, P.: L'uretère retro-cave. Thèse, Paris 1952.

SHIH, H. E.: Postcaval ureter. J. Urol. **38**, 61 (1937).

SHOPFNER, C. E.: Abstract, Genitourinary Radiology postgraduate course, Albert Einstein College of Medicine, New York, 1969.

SKALLEBERG, L.: Ureteranomali. Nord. Med. **70**, 829 (1963).

SPANGLER, E. B.: Complete triplication of the ureter. Radiology **80**, 795 (1963).

SPENCE, H. M.: Congenital unilateral multicystic kidney: an entity to be distinguished from polycystic kidney disease and other cystic disorders. J. Urol. **74**, 693 (1955).

SPILLANE, R. J., PRATHER, G. C.: High renal ectopy: a case report. J. Urol. **62**, 441 (1949).

STAEHLER, W.: Klinik und Praxis der Urologie. Stuttgart: Georg Thieme 1959.

STEVENS, A. R.: Pelvic single kidneys. J. Urol. **37**, 610 (1937).

STITES, J. R., BOWEN, J. A.: Crossed ectopia of the kidney. J. Urol. **42**, 9 (1939).

STOKKE, D., ANDRESEN, P.: Klinefelters syndrom. Nord. Med. 18 XI, **86**:46, 1333 (1971).

TEICHERT, G.: Kelchdivertikel der Niere mit Konkrement. Fortschr. Röntgenstr. **84**, 761 (1956).

THOMAS, G. J., BARTON, J. C.: Ectopic pelvic kidney. J. Amer. med. Ass. **106**, 197 (1936).

THOMPSON, G. J., PACE, J. M.: Ectopic kidney. Surg. Gynec. Obstet. **64**, 935 (1937).

THORSÉN, G.: Pyelorenal cysts. Acta chir. scand. **94**, 476 (1949).

VELZER, D. A. VAN, BARRICK, C. W., JENKINSON, E. L.: Postcaval ureter. A case report. Amer. J. Roentgenol. **74**, 490 (1955).

VIALLA, M., BADOSA, J., ARLES, H.: L'angiographie rénale dans l'exploration des reins en fer à cheval. J. Radiol. Electrol **44**, 131 (1963).

VITKO, R., CASS, A., WINTER, R.: Anomalies of the genitourinary tract associated with congenital scoliosis and congenital kyphosis. J. Urol. **108**:4, 655 (1972).

WALL, B., WACHTER, H. E.: Congenital ureteral valve: its role as a primary obstructive lesion: classification of the literature and report of an authentic case. J. Urol. **68**, 684 (1952).

WARD, J. N., DRAPER, J. W., LAVENGOOD Jr., R. W.: A clinical review of polycystic kidney disease in 53 patients. J. Urol. **98**:1 (1967).

WATKINS, K. H., Cysts of kidney due to hydrocalycosis. Brit. J. Urol. **11**, 207 (1939).

WEISS, R. M., MALONEY Jr., P. K., BELAND, G. A.: Crossed ectopia of a solitary kidney. J. Urol. **94**, 320 (1965).

WILLIAMS, J. I., CARSON, R. B., WELLS, W. D.: Renal aplasia: a report of two cases. J. Urol. **79**, 6 (1958).

WILMER, H. A.: Unilateral fused kidney: Report of 5 cases and review of the literature. J. Urol. **40**, 551 (1938).

WOODSON, H. D., HERRING, A. L.: Ureteral ectopia. J. Urol. **80**, 311 (1958).

WYRENS, R. G.: Calyceal diverticula or pyelogenic cysts. J. Urol. **70**, 358 (1953).

YELSA, C., BURHENNE, H. J.: Triple ureters, a case report. Radiol. clinica et biologica. **35**:4, 233 (1966).

YOUNG, J. N.: Ureteral opening into the seminal vesicle: report on a case. Brit. J. Urol. **27**, 57 (1955).

YOW, R. M., BUNTS, R. C.: Calyceal diverticulum. J. Urol. **73**, 663 (1955).

E. Nephro- and Ureterolithiasis

ÅKERLUND, Å.: Ein typisches Röntgenbild bei Konkrementbildung in einer Ureterozele. Acta radiol. **16**, 39 (1935).

ALBRIGHT, F., BAIRD, P. C., COPE, O., BLOOMBERG, E.: Studies on the physiology of the parathyroid glands. Amer. J. Med. Sci. **187**, 49 (1934).

— DIENES, L., SULKOWITCH, H. W.: Pyelonephritis with nephrocalcinosis. J. Amer. Med. Ass. **110**, 357 (1938).

— CONSOLAZIO, W. V., COOMBS, F. S., SULKOWITCH, H. W., TALBOTT, J. H.: Metabolic studies and therapy in a case of nephrocalcinosis with rickets and dwarfism. Bull. Johns Hopkins Hosp. **66**, 7 (1940).

— REIFENSTEIN Jr., E. C.: The parathyroid glands and metabolic bone disease. Baltimore 1948.

ALLYN, R. E.: Uric acid calculi. J. Urol. **78**, 314 (1957).

ANTHONSEN, W., CHRISTOFFERSEN, C. J.: Nephrolithiasis. Nord. med. **8**, 1943 (1940).

ARNALDSSON, Ö., HOLMLUND, D.: Defects in urographic contrast medium above and below a ureteric calculus. Acta radiol. **11**, 26 (1971).

ARNESEN, A.: Der akute Nierensteinanfall. Z. urol. Chir. Gynäk. 45, 94 (1939).

ASK-UPMARK, E.: Über Röntgenuntersuchung der Nieren bei gewissen diagnostisch schwer zu deutenden Krankheitsfällen in der inneren Medizin. Acta med. scand. 96, 390 (1938).

BAINES, G. H., BARCLAY, J. A., COOKE, W. T.: Nephrocalcinosis associated with hyperchloraemia and low plasma-bicarbonate. Quart. J. Med. 14, 113 (1945).

BAKER, R., CONELLY, J. P.: Bilateral and recurrent renal calculi. J. Amer. Med. Ass. 160, 1106 (1956).

BATESON, E. M.: Nephrocalcinosis in children: Review of the literature and report of a case complicated by Wilms Tumor. Clin. radiol. 13/3, 231 (1962).

— CHANDLER, S.: Nephrocalcinosis in cretinism. Brit. J. Radiol. 38, 581 (1965).

BEARD, D. F., GOODYEAR, W. E.: Hyperparathyroidism and urolithiasis. J. Urol. (Baltimore) 65, 638 (1950).

BIE, K., KJELSTRUP, Y.: Urinveiskonkrementer hos småbarn. Nord. Med. 58, 1777 (1957).

BIRDSALL, J. C.: The incidence of urinary tract obstruction in renal calculus formation. J. Urol. 42, 917 (1939).

BOEMINGHAUS, H.: Über die Funktion der Niere bei akutem komplettem Ureterverschluß. Langenbecks Arch. klin. Chir. 171, 109 (1932).

— ZEISS, L.: Zur Erholungsfähigkeit mechanisch bedingter Stauungszustände im Nierenbecken-Harnleistersystem. Z. Urol. 29, 83 (1935).

BORGHI, M., CONFALONIERI, A., COLOMBI, M.: La nefrocalcinosi. Ann. Medicin, 3 113 (1959).

BOSTRÖM, H.: Cystinuri-frekvensen i Sverige. Opuscula Medica (Stockholm) 3, 370 (1958).

BOYCE, W. H., GARVEY, F. K.: The amount and nature of the organic matrix in urinary calculi: a review. J. Urol. 76, 213 (1956).

— POOL, C. S., MESCHAN, I., KING Jr., J. S.: Organic matrix of urinary calculi. Microradiographic comparison of crystalline structure with microscopic and histochemical studies. Acta radiol. 50, 543 (1958).

BRUNSCHWIG, A., BARBER, H., ROBERTS, S.: Return of renal function after varying periods of ureteral occlusion. J. Amer. Med. Ass. 188, 5 (1964).

BURKLAND, C. E.: Fracture of giant ureteral calculus. J. Urol. 69, 366 (1953).

BURNETT, C. H., COMMONS, R. R.. ALBRIGHT, F., HOWARD, J. E.: Hypercalcemia without hypercalcuria. New Engl. J. Med. 240, 787 (1949).

BUTLER, A. M., WILSON, J. L., FARBER, S.: Dehydration and acidosis with calcification at renal tubulus. J. Pediat. 8, 489 (1936).

CAMIEL, M. R.: Stone in the intramural bladder portion of the ureter. Urographic observations. Radiology 78, 959 (1962).

CANTAROW, A., SCHEPARTZ B.: Biochemistry, 2nd edit., p. 779. Philadelphia: W. B. Sauders Company 1957.

CARR, R. J.: A new theory on the formation of renal calculi. Brit. J. Urol. 26, 105 (1954).

CLAESSON, U.: Nephrolithiasis hos barn efter immobilisering för fraktur. Nord. Med. 58, 1772 (1957).

COHEN, M. E. L., COHEN, G. F., AHAD, V., KAYE, M.: Renal osteodystrophy in patients on chronic hemodialysis: a radiologic study. Clin. radiol. 21, 124 (1970).

COLIEZ, R.: La stase pyélo-calicienne artificielle dans le diagnostic radiologique des affections des reins. Gaz. méd. Fr. 50, 189 (1943).

— Les signes radiologiques de stase et de surpression urétéro-rénale cours de l'urographie intra veineuse. J. Radiol. Éléctrol. 28, 311 (1947).

COMARR, A. E.: A long-term survey of the incidence of renal calculosis in paraplegia. J. Urol. 74, 447 (1955).

COMAAR, A. E., KAWAICHI, G. K., BORS, E.: Renal calculosis of patients with traumatic cord lesions. J. Urol. 87, 647 (1962).

CONWELL, cit. E. J. McCaque (1937).

COUNCILL, W. A., COUNCILL Jr., W. A.: Spontaneous rupture of the renal parenchyma associated with renal lithiasis. J. Urol. 63, 441 (1950).

COWIE, T.: Nephrocalcinosis and renal calculi. Radiological studies in calculus formation. Brit. J. Radiol. 27, 210 (1954).

CRAVEN, J. D., LECKY, J. W.: The natural history of postobstructive renal atrophy shown by sequential urograms. Radiology 101, 555 (1971).

CRONQVIST, S.: Renal osteonephropathy. Acta radiol. 55, 17 (1961).

DAVIDSON, C. N., DENNIS, J. M., McNINCH, E. R., WILLSON, J., BROWN, W. H.: Nephrocalcinosis associated with sarcoidosis. Radiology 62, 203 (1954).

DAVIS, H.: Metabolic causes of renal stones in children. J. Amer. Med. Ass. 171, 2199 (1959).

DODSON, A. I.: Urological surgery. London 1956.

DOLL, S. G., BERGMAN, R. T., AFFELDT, J. E.: Urolithiasis in poliomyelitic patients, J. Urol. 80, 371 (1958).

DRACH, G. W., BOYCE, W. H.: Nephrocalcinosis as a source for renal stone nuclei. Observations on humans and squirrel monkeys and on hyperparathyroidism in the squirrel monkey. J. Urol. 107, 897 (1972).

DUNCAN, H., WAKIM, K. G., WARD, L. E.: Renal lesions resulting from induced hyperuicemia in animals. Proceed., Mayo Clinic 38, 411 (1963).

DUNN, H. G.: Oxalosis: Report of a case with review of the literature. Amer. J. Dis. Childh. 90, 58 (1955).

DWORETZKY, M.: Reversible metastatic calcification (milkdrinker's syndrome). J. Amer. Med. Ass. 155, 830 (1954).

EBSTEIN, W., NICOLAIER, A.: Über die Wirkung der Oxalsäure und einiger ihrer Derivate auf die Nieren. Virchows Arch. path. Anat. 148, 366 (1897).

EDLING, N. P. G.: Der Interureterwulst im Röntgenbild. Acta radiol. 22, 573 (1941).

ELLIOT, J. S., TODD, H. E., LEWIS, L.: Some aspects of calcium phosphate solubility. J. Urol. 85, 428 (1961).

— Spontaneous dissolution of renal calculi. J. Urol. 72, 331 (1954).

ENFEDJIEFF, M.: Detrusorspasmus bei tiefsitzenden Uretersteinen im Röntgenbild. Verhandlungsber. der Dtsch. Ges. für Urologie, S. 276, Leipzig 1958.

ENGEL, W. J.: Nephrocalcinosis. J. Amer. Med. Ass. 145, 288 (1951).

— Urinary calculi associated with nephrocalcinosis. J. Urol. 68, 105–116 (1952).

ENGFELDT, B., LAGERGREN, C.: Nephrocalcionsis. Acta chir. scand. 115, 46 (1958).

EZICKSON, W. J., J. B. Feldmann,: Signs of vitamin A deficiency in the eye correlated with urinary lithiasis. J. Amer. Med. Ass. 109, 1706 (1937).

FASSBENDER, C. W.: Über Nieren- und Harnleiterkonkremente bei Kleinstkindern. Fortschr. Röntgenstr. 85, 451 (1956).

FEINDT, W.: Röntgenologischer Nachweis eines partiellen Sekretionsausfalles der Niere bei Harnleiterkonkrement und gedoppelter Ureteranlage. Fortschr. Röntgenstr. 73, 62 (1950).

FELBER, E.: Asynchronous bilateral benign papilloma of the ureter with subsequent cancer of ureteral stump, bladder, and vagina. J. Med. Ass. Georgia 42, 198 (1953).

FRITJOFSSON, A.: Njurstenar och deras behandling. Nord. Med. 59, 733 (1958).

GAUJOUX, J.: Four cases of urolithiasis impossible to see on the X-ray picture. Écho méd. Cevennes 55, 1 (1954).

GOLDSTEIN, A. E., ABESHOUSE, B. S.: Calcification and ossification of the kidney. Radiology 30, 544 (1937).

GOODWIN, W. E., COCKETT, A. T. K.: Surgical treatment of multiple, recurrent, branched, renal (staghorn) calculi by pyelo-nephro-ileo-vesical anastomosis. J. Urol. 85, 214 (1961).

GORDONSON, J., SARGENT, E. N.: Nephrobroncholithiasis: report of a case secondary to renal lithiasis with a nephrobronchial fistula. Amer. J. Roentgenol. 110, 701 (1970).

GRAHAM, J. B.: Recovery of kidney after ureteral obstruction. J. Amer. Med. Ass. 181 993 (1962).

GRANOFF, M. A.: Migration of renal stones associated with pyonephrosis and perinephric abscess into lung. J. Urol. 42, 302 (1939).

GREENSPAN, E. M.: Hyperchloremic acidosis and nephrocalcinosis. Arch. intern. Med. 83, 271 (1949).

GÜRSEL, A. E.: Renal lithiasis invisible without opaque medium. J. Radiol. Électrol. 36, 360 (1955).

HAGGITT, R. C., PITCOCK, J. A.: Renal medullary calcifications: a light and electron microscopic study. J. Urol. 106, 342 (1971).

HAMMARSTEN, G.: Terapi-inducerade urinvägsstenar. Opusc. med. (Stockholm) 3, 19 (1958).

HAMRE, L.: Bilaterale ureterstener med uremi. Nord. med. 58, 1775 (1957).

HARRELL, G. T., FISCHER, S.: Blood chemical changes in Boeck's sarcoid with particular reference to protein, calcium and phosphatase values. J. Clin. Invest. 18, 687 (1939).

HARRISON, H. E., HARRISON, H. C.: The inhibition of urine citrate excretion and the production of renal calculosis in the rat by acetazolamide (diamox) administration. J. Clin. Invest. 34, 1662 (1955).

HELLMER, H.: On the technique in urography and the roentgen picture in acute renal and ureteral stasis. Acta radiol. 16, 51 (1935).

— Nephrography. Acta radiol. 23, 233 (1942).

HELLSTRÖM, J.: Röntgendiagnostikens begränsning och möjligheter vid njur-och uretärstenar. Nord. Med. 8, 1725 (1934).

— Njur- och uretärsten. Inledn. föredrag vid Nord. Kir. för. 20th meeting, Copenhagen 1935.

HERZAN, F. A., O'BRIEN, F. W.: Acceleration of delayed excretory urograms. Influence of ingested ice water on the kidney function. Amer. J. Roentgenol. 68, 104 (1952).

HESSÉN, I.: Njursten av kiselsyra efter silikat som antacidum. Nord. med. 69, 424 (1963).

HICKEL, R.: Figures urographiques particulières: les ombres precapillaires (ou images dites "en boules") et la néphrographie. J. Radiol. Electrol. 27, 509 (1946).

HIGGINS, C. C.: Nonopaque urinary tract calculi. J. Urol. 70, 857 (1953).

— MENDENHALL, E. E.: Factors associated with recurrent formation of renal lithiasis with report of new method for qualitative analysis of urinary calculi. J. Urol. 42, 436 (1939).

HOLMLUND, D.: Ureterstensjukdomen: mekanik och konservativ behandling. Läkartidningen (Stockholm) 66, 4629 (1969).

— Ureteral stones: an experimental and clinical study of the mechanism of the passage and arrest of ureteral stones. Scand. J. Urol. & Nephrol. Suppl. 1, 1968.

HOLST, S.: Silikatsten i urinveiene. Nord. med. 60, 1169 (1958).

HOWELL, R. D.: Milk of calcium renal stone. J. Urol. 82, 197 (1959).

HURXTHAL, L. M., O'SULLIVAN, J. B.: Cushing's syndrome: clinical differential diagnosis and complications. Ann. Int. Med. 51, 1 (1959).

IDBOHRN, H.: Renal angiography in experimental hydronephrosis. Acta radiol. Suppl. 136, 1956.

— MUREN, A.: Renal blood flow in experimental hydronephrosis. Acta physiol. scand. 38, 200 (1956).

KAUFMANN, S. A.: The acceleration of delayed excretory uorgrams with ingested ice water. J. Urol. 74, 243 (1955).

KEATING F. R., Jr.: Some metabolic aspects of urinary calculi. J. Urol. 79, 663 (1958).

KEYSER, L. D.: Newer concepts of stone in the urinary tract. J. Urol. 42, 420 (1939).

KIMBROUGH, J. C., DENSLOW, J. C.: Urinary tract calculi in recumbent patients. J. Urol. 61, 837 (1949)

KING, J. S. Jr.: Etiologic factors involved in urolithiasis: a review of recent research. J. Urol. 97, 583 (1967).

KIRSNER, J. B., PALMER, W. L., HUMPHREYS, E.: Morphologic changes in the human kidney following prolonged administration of alkali. Arch. Path. (Chicago) 35, 207 (1943).

KJELLBERG, S. R.: Fälle mit geschichteten und facettierten Nierensteinen. Acta radiol. 16, 571 (1935).

KNEISE, O., SCHOBER, K. L.: Die Röntgenuntersuchung der Harnorgane. Leipzig: Georg Thieme 1941.

KNUTH, D.: Die seitliche Röntgenaufnahme in der Nierensteindiagnostik und ihre Fehlerquellen. Röntgenpraxis 11, 679 (1939).

KREEL, L.: Radiological aspects of nephrocalcinosis. Clin. radiol. 13, 218 (1962).

LAGERGREN, C.: Biophysical investigations of urinary calculi. Acta radiol. Suppl. 133 (1956).

— ÖHRLING, H.: Urinary calculi composed of pure calcium phosphate. Acta chir. scand. 117, 335 (1959).

LEDOUX-LEBARD, G., LAURENT, Y.: Lithiase et urétérocèle. J. Radiol. Electrol. 45, 325 (1964).

LÖFGREN, S., SNELLMAN, B., LINDGREN, Å.: Renal complications in sarcoidosis. Acta med. scand. 159, 295 (1957).

MACKENZIE, A. R.: Acetazolamide-induced renal stone. J. Urol. 84, 453 (1960).

McCAQUE, E. J.: The incidence and prevention of renal and vesical calculi in the fracture and traumatic group. Amer. J. Surg. 38, 85 (1937).

McCREA, L.: Formation of uric acid calculi during chemotherapy for leukemia. J. Urol. 73, 29 (1955).

MADSEN, H.: The value of tomography for the demonstration of small intrarenal calcifications. Brit. J. Radiol. 45, 203 (1972).

MALM, O. J.: Urinkalkutskillelsen vid sengeleie og immobilisering. Nord. med. 47, 1280 (1963).

MEADS, A. M.: Fibrin calculi of the kidney. J. Urol. 42, 1157 (1939).

MELDOLESI, G.: Il quadro angiografico renale nel blocco degli ureteri. Minerva chir. (Torino) 13, 1104 (1958).

MILLER, J. M., FREEMAN, I., HEATH, W. H.: Calcinosis due to treatment of duodenal ulcer. J. Amer. med. Ass. 148, 198 (1952).

MOËLL, H.: Kidney size and its deviation from normal in acute renal failure. Acta radiol. Suppl. 206 (1961).

— Size of normal kidneys. Acta radiol. 46, 640 (1956).

— Gross bilateral renal cortical necrosis during long periods of oliguria-anuria. Acta radiol. 48, 355 (1957).

MOORE, C. A., DODSON, C. C.: Urinary tract calculi in children, renal and vesical calculi in an 8-month-old child. Amer. J. Dis. Child. 88, 743 (1954).

MORTENSEN, J. D., BAGGENSTOSS, A. H., POWER, M. H., PUGH, D. G.: Roentgenographic demonstration of histologically identifiable renal calcification. Radiology 62, 703 (1954).

— EMMETT, J. L.: Nephrocalcinosis: a collective and clinicopathologic study. J. Urol. (Baltimore) 71, 398 (1954).

— — BAGGENSTOSS, A. H.: Clinical aspects of nephrocalcinosis. Proc. Mayo Clin. 28, 305 (1953).

MULVANEY, W. P.: A new solvent for certain urinary calculi. J. Urol. 82, 546 (1959).

MURPHY, G. P., SCHIRMER, H. K.: Nephrocalcinosis, urolithiasis and renal insufficiency in sarcoidosis. J. Urol. 86, 702 (1961).

MUSCETTOLA, G.: Raro caso di pseudocalcolo transparente intraureteropelvico in uretero-pielografia. Radiol. med. (Torino) 26, 767 (1939).

NEUSTEIN, H. B., STEVENSON, S. S., KRAINER, L.: Oxalis with renal calcinosis due to calcium oxalate. J. Pediat. 47, 624 (1955).

NICE, C. M., MARGULIS, A. R., RIGLER, L. G.: Roentgen diagnosis of abdominal tumors in childhood. Springfield, Ill.: Ch. C. Thomas 1957.

OLSSON, OLLE: Renal colic in cases of tumor and tuberculosis of the kidney: roentgenologic views. J. Urol. 63, 118 (1949).

— Backflow in excretion urography during renal colic. In: Modern trends in diagnostic radiology. Ed. by J. W. McLaren, London: Butterworth 1953 (chap. 13).

— Stone. In: Diseases of the kidney. Ed. by M. B. Strauss & L. G. Welt. Boston: Little, Brown & Co. 1971.

OSTRY, H.: Nephrocalcinosis. Canad. Med. Ass. J. 65, 465 (1951).

PAPAIOANNOU, A. N., BRUNSCHWIG, A.: Return of function of a kidney not visualized on intravenous pyelogram for $1^1/_2$ years. Arch. of Surg. 90, 376 (1965).

PARSONS, J.: Magnesium dibasic phosphate identified as a crystalline component of a urinary calculus. J. Urol. 76, 228 (1956).

PERSKY, L., CHAMBERS, D., POTTS, A.: Calculus formation and ureteral colic following acetazolamide (diamox) therapy. J. Amer. Med. Ass. 161, 1625 (1956).

PHEMISTER, D. B.: Ossification in kidney stones attached to the renal pelvis. Ann. Surg. 78, 239 (1923).

PITTS, H. H. Jr., SCHULTE, J. W., SMITH, D. R.: Nephrocalcinosis in a father and three children. J. Urol. 73, 208 (1955).

PRIEN, E. L.: Studies in urolithiasis. II. Relationships between pathogenesis, structure and composition of calculi. J. Urol. 61, 821 (1949).

— Studies in urolithiasis. III. Physicochemical principles in stone formation and prevention. J. Urol. 73, 627 (1955).

— Chrystallographic analysis of urinary calculi: a 23-year survey study. J. Urol. 89, 917 (1963).

— FRONDEL, C.: Chrystallography of the urinary sediments with clinical and pathological observations in sulfonamide drug therapy. J. Urol. 46, 748 (1941).

— Studies in urolithiasis. I. The composition of urinary calculi. J. Urol. 57, 949 (1947).

RANDALL, A.: The initiating lesions of renal calculus. Surg. Gynec. Obstet. 64, 201 (1937).

RENANDER, A.: Spontane konkrementäre Nierenbeckenperforation. Acta radiol. 21, 343 (1940).

— The roentgen density of the cystine calculus. Diss. Stockholm 1941.

RICHARDSON, R. E.: Nephrocalcinosis with special reference to its occurrence in renal tubular acidosis. Clin. radiol. 13, 224 (1962).

RICKER, W., CLARK, M.: Sarcoidosis. Amer. J. Clin. Pathol. 19, 725 (1949).

RIES, S. W., MALAMENT, M.: Renacidin: a urinary calculi solvent. J. Urol. 87, 657 (1962).

RISHOLM, L.: Studies on renal colic and its treatment by posterior splanchnic block. Acta chir. scand. Suppl. **184**, (1954).

ROSENBAUM, D., COGGESHALL, W. LEVIN, R. T.: Chronic glomerulonephritis with severe renal tubular calcification. Amer. J. med. Sci. **221**, 319 (1951).

ROSENDAL, T.: Renal tuberculosis. Urol. Cutan. Rev. **52**, 340 (1948).

ROSENOW, E. C.: Renal calculi: a study of papillary calcification. J. Urol. **44**, 19 (1940).

ROSTAD, H.: Ureterstenssykdommen: et operasjonsmateriale. Nord. med. **19: XI**, 1488 (1970).

SANDEGÅRD, E.: Prognosis of stone in the ureter. Acta chir. scand. Suppl. **219** (1956).

SAUPE, E.: Röntgendiagramme von menschlichen Körpergeweben und Konkrementen. Fortschr. Röntgenstr. **44**, 204 (1931).

SCHÄFER, H.: Nephrokalzinose und Nierensteinbildung bei Hyperparathreoidismus. Fortschr. Röntgenstr. **96**, 787 (1962).

SCHIFFER, E.: Füllungsdefekt bei retrograder Pyelographie, vorgetäuscht durch einen Nierenkelchkrampf. Acta radiol. **17**, 93 (1936).

SCHNEIDER, P. W.: Beitrag zur Nephrokalzinose. Radiol. clin. (Basel) **28**, 34 (1959).

SCHÜPBACH, A., WERNLY, M.: Hyperkalzaemie und Organverkalkungen bei Boeckscher Krankheit. Acta med. scand. **115**, 401 (1943).

SEIFTER, J., TRATTNER, H. R.: Simplified qualitative analysis of urinary calculi by spot tests. J. Urol. **42**, 452 (1939).

SGALITZER, M.: Röntgenuntersuchung im Krankenzimmer. Wien. med. Wschr. **86**, 864 (1936).

SMITH, D. R., KOLB, F. O., HARPER, H. A.: The management of cystinuria and cystine-stone disease. J. Urol. **81**, 61 (1959).

SNOBL, O., SVORC, J., BIBELKOVÁ, M.: Die Markschwammniere im Kindesalter. Fortschr. Röntgenstr. **113**, 644 (1970).

STAHL, F.: Urolithiasis als Komplikation bei orthopädischen Erkrankungen. Acta chir. scand. **87**, 342 (1942).

STENSTRÖM, R.: Nefrokalcinos vid poliomyelit med andningsförlamning. Nord. Med. **55**, 647 (1956).

STOUT, H. A., AKIN, R. H., MORTON, E.: Nephrocalcinosis in routine necropsies; its relationship to stone formation. J. Urol. **74**, 8 (1955).

TOVBORG-JENSEN, A., THYGESEN, J. E.: Über die Phosphatkonkremente der Harnwege. Z. Urol. **32**, 659 (1938).

TWINEM, F. P.: The relation of renal stone formation and recurrence to calyceal pathology. J. Urol. **44**, 596 (1940).

VERMEULEN, C. W., LYON, E. S., ELLIS, J. E., BORDEN, T. A.: The renal papilla and calculogenesis. J. Urol. **97**, 573 (1967).

VERMOOTEN, V.: The incidence and significance of the deposition of calcium plaques in the renal papilla. J. Urol. **46**, 193 (1941).

WIDÉN, T.: Renal angiography during and after unilateral ureteric occlusion. Acta radiol. Suppl. **162** (1958).

WIESER, C., ISLER, U. M.: Viszerale Röntgenbefunde bei Osteomyelosklerose. Radiol. clin. (Basel) **26**, 329 (1957).

WILDBOLZ, E.: Klinik der Pyurie im Kindesalter. Schweiz. med. Wschr. **89**, 665 (1959).

WINER, J. H.: Practical value of analysis of urinary calculi. J. Amer. Med. Ass. **169**, 1715 (1959).

WULFF, H. B.: Om värdet ay urografi vid diagnostiken av njur- och uretärstensanfallet. Nord. Kir. För. Förhandl. Copenhagen 1935.

— Urography in 125 cases of acute renal and abdominal conditions. Acta radiol. **16**, 77 (1935).

— Die Zuverlässigkeit der Röntgendiagnostik — besonders hinsichtlich des Wertes der Urographie — und die Prognose bei Nieren- und Harnleitersteinen. Acta radiol. Suppl. **32** (1936).

— Über die sog. reflektorische Steinanurie. Lund 1941.

— Urinary excretion in acute unilateral renal and ureteral blocking. Lund: Håkan Ohlssons boktryckeri 1948.

YEAN-CHIN, T.: Application of infra-red spectroscopy to analysis of urinary calculi. J. Urol. **86**, 838 (1961).

ZOLLINGER, H. U., ROSENMUND, H.: Urämie bei endogen bedingter subakuter und chronischer Calciumoxalatniere. Schweiz. Med. Wschr. **82**, 1261 (1952).

F. Renal, pelvic and ureteric tumors

ABOULKER, P., CHOME, J., CORNET, P.: Documents pour l'étude de l'artériographie rénale. J. Urol. méd. chir. **61**, 218 (1955).

ABRAMS, H. L.: The response of neoplastic renal vessels to epinephrine in man. Radiology **82**, 217 (1964).

— OBREZ, I.: Epinephrine in the study of renal tumors. In: Angiography. Edited by H. L. ABRAMS. Vol. II, pages 831–854. Boston: Little, Brown & Co. 1971.

ACKERMANN, L. V.: Mucinous adenocarcinoma of the pelvis of the kidney. J. Urol. **55**, 36 (1946).

ADAMS, P. S., HUNT, H. B.: Differential diagnosis of Wilms' tumour assisted by intramuscular urography. J. Urol. **42**, 688 (1939).

ADELMAN, B. P.: Angiomyolipoma of the kidney. Amer. J. Roentgenol. **95**, 403 (1965).

ADOLFSSON, G.: Hypernephroma metastasis in the lung with no demonstrable primary tumor. J. Urol. **97**, 221 (1967).

AGERHOLM-CHRISTENSEN, J.: A case of adenosarcoma of the kidney (Wilms' mixed tumor). Acta radiol. **20**, 69 (1939).

AGNEW, C. H.: Metastatic malignant melanoma of the kidney simulating a primary neoplasm. A case report. Amer. J. Roentgenol. **80**, 813 (1958).

AHLBÄCK, S.: The suprarenal glands in aortography. Acta radiol. **50**, 341 (1958).

AHLSTRÖM, C. G., WELIN, S.: Zur Differentialdiagnostik der Ewingschen Sarkome. Acta radiol. **24**, 67 (1943).

AINSWORTH, W. L., VEST, S. A.: The differential diagnosis between renal tumors and cysts. J. Urol. **66**, 740 (1951).

ALBERS, D. D., KALMON, E. H., BACK, K. C.: Pheochromocytoma: Report of five cases, one a spontaneous cure. J. Urol. **78**, 301 (1957).

ALLEN, A. C.: The kidney. Medical and surgical diseases. New York: Grune & Stratton 1951 (p. 504).

ALLEN, T. D., RISK, W.: Renal angiomyolipoma. J. Urol. **94**, 203 (1965).

ALMGÅRD, L.-E., EDSMYR, F., FRANZÉN, S., HAVERLING, M., HENRIKSSON, L.-E. LAGERGREN, C., LJUNGQVIST, A., VON SCHREEB, T., STJERNSWÄRD, J., WADSTRÖM, L., VÁNKY, F.: Kliniskt experimentella studier av adenocarcinoma renis. Läkartidningen (Stockholm) **69**, 153 (1972).

ANGERVALL, L., BENGTSSON, U., ZETTERLUND, C. G., SZIGMOND. M.: Renal pelvic carcinoma in a Swedish district with abuse of a phenacetin-containing drug. Brit. J. Urol. **XLI:4** (1969).

ANGULO, R.: Recurrent, nonfunctioning tumor of adrenal capsule. J. Urol. **78**, 309 (1957).

ANNAMUNTHODO, H., HUTCHINGS, R. F.: Nephroblastoma (Wilms' Tumor): Case report. J. Urol. **78**, 197 (1957).

ARCADI, J. A.: Mucus-producing cystadenocarcinoma of renal pelvis and ureter: fourth reported case. A.M.A. Arch. Path. **61**, 264 (1956).

ARCOMANO, J. P., BARNETT, J. C., BOTTONE, J. J.: Spontaneous disappearance of pulmonary metastases following nephrectomy for hypernephroma. Amer. J. Surg. **96**, 703 (1958).

ARVIS, G., STEG, A.: Léiomyosarcome bilatéral du rein (à propos d'un cas). J. d'urologie et de néphrologie **77**, 272 (1971).

AUSTEN jr., G.: Calcification of renal tumors. Amer. J. Roentgenol. **49**, 580 (1943).

BAILEY, M. K., YOUNGBLOOD, V. H.: Bilateral renal hypernephroma: report of a case. J. Urol. **63**, 593 (1950).

BAKER, W. J., RAGINS, A. B.: Pararenal teratoma: case report. J. Urol. **63**, 982 (1950).

BARTLEY, O., Hypernephroma in a pelvic kidney demonstrated by angiography. Report of a case. Acta radiol. **48**, 175 (1957).

— HELANDER, C. G.: Angiography in spontaneously healed hypernephromas. Acta radiol. **57**, 417 (1962).

— HULTQUIST, G. T.: Spontaneous regression of hypernephromas. Acta path. mirobiol. scand. **27**, 448 (1950).

BAUER jr., F. C., MURRAY, D. E., HIRSCH, E. F.: Solitary adenoma of the kidney. J. Urol. **79**, 377 (1958).

BEATTIE, J. W.: Hypernephroma in seven-year-old white girl. J. Urol. **72**, 625 (1954).

BECK, R. E., HAMMOND, R. C.: Renal and osseus manifestation of tuberous sclerosis: case report. J. Urol. **77**, 578 (1957).

BECKER, J. A., FLEMING, R., KANTER, I., MELICOW, W.: Misleading appearances in renal angiography. Radiology **88**, 691 (1967).

BEER, E.: Some aspects of malignant tumors of the kidney. Surg. Gynec. Obstet. **65**, 433 (1937).

BELL, E. T.: A classification of renal tumors with observations on the frequency of the various types. J. Urol. **39**, 238 (1938).

BENGTSSON, U., ANGERVALL, L., EKMAN, H., LEHMANN, L.: Transitional cell tumors of the renal pelvis in analgesic abusers. Scand. J. Urol. Nephrol. **2**, 145 (1968).

BERGMAN, H., FRIEDENBERG, R. M., SAYEGH, V.: New roentgenologic signs of carcinoma of the ureter. Amer. J. Roentgenol. **86**, 707 (1961).

BESSE jr., B. E., LIEBERMANN, J. E., LUSTED, L. B.: Kidney size in acute leukemia. Amer. J. Roentgenol. **80**, 611 (1958).

BILLING, L., LINDGREN, Å. G. H.: Die pathologisch-anatomische Unterlage der Geschwulstarteriographie. Acta radiol. **25**, 625 (1944).

BLUTH, I., VITALE, P.: Right renal enlargements causing alterations in descending duodenum: radiographic demonstration. Radiology **76**, 777 (1961).

BOHNE, A. W., CHRISTENSON, W. W.: Clinical evaluation of a concentrated iodine preparation. Radiology **60**, 401 (1953).

BOIJSEN, E.: Angiographic diagnosis of ureteric carcinoma. Acta radiol. **57**, 172 (1962).

— FOLIN, J.: Angiography in the diagnosis of renal carcinoma. Der Radiologe **1**, 173 (1961).

— — Angiography in carcinoma of the renal pelvis. Acta radiol. **56**, 81 (1961).

BOLDUS, R., BROWN, R., CULP, D.: Fungus balls in the renal pelvis. Radiology **102**, 555 (1972).

BOSHAMMER: Das Pyelogramm bei Nierentumoren. Langenbecks Arch. klin. Chir. **175**, 238 (1933).

BOSNIAK, M. A.: Abstract, Postgraduate Course in Genitourinary Radiology, Albert Einstein College of Medicine, New York City, 1969: Metastatic tumors to the kidney.

— STERN, W., LOPEZ, F., TEHRANIAN, N., O'CONNOR, S. J.: Metastatic neoplasm to the kidney. Radiology **92**, 989 (1969).

— FAEGENBURG, D.: The thick-wall sign: an important finding in nephrotomography. Radiology **84**, 692 (1965).

BOTTING, A. J., HARRISON jr., E. G., BLACK, B. M.: Metastatic hypernephroma masquerading as a polypoid tumor of the gallbladder and review of metastatic tumors of the gallbladder. Proc. Mayo Clin. **38**, 225 (1963).

BRAASCH, W. F., HENDRICK, J. A.: Renal cysts, simple and otherwise. J. Urol. **51**, 1 (1944).

BRECKENRIDGE, R. L., LYNCH, P. V., HOLFELNER, E. D.: Fibrous polyp of ureter. J. Urol. **90**, 160 (1963).

BRINDLE, M. J.: Alternative vascular channels in renal carcinoma. Clin. Radiol. **XXIII**, 321 (1972).

BRODY, H., LIPSHUTZ, H.: Concomitant intrarenal and pararenal angiomyolipomas. J. Urol. **74**, 741 (1955).

BRØNDUM NIELSEN, J.: Sjaelden nyrebaekkentumor. Nord. Med. **58**, 1774 (1957).

BUKERT, S., GARBSCH, H., KIESSWETTER, H., MAYRHOFER, P., SAPIK, J.: Über zwei Fälle von Hypernephrom in Hufeisennieren. Fortschritte **115**, 186 (1971).

BULKLEY, G. J., DRINKER, H. R.: Malignant mesenchynoma of the kidney: case report. J. Urol. 77, 583 (1957).

BUMPUS, H. C.: The apparent disappearance of pulmonary metastasis in a case of hypernephroma following nephrectomy. J. Urol. 20, 185 (1928).

BURKLAND, C. E., LEADBETTER, W. F.: Pyelitis cystica associated with an hemophilus influenzae infection in the urine. J. Urol. 42, 14 (1939).

CALDERÓN, D. O., MUSA, H. E., OTERO, G. O.: Renal osteoma. J. Urol. 93, 350 (1965).

CAMPBELL, J. H., PASQUIER, C. M., MARTIN, E. C. ST., WORLEY, P. C.: Hypernephroma associated with polycythemia and eczematoid dermatitis. J. Urol. 79, 12 (1958).

CAMPBELL, M. F.: Bilateral embryonal adenomyosarcoma of the kidney (Wilms' tumor). J. Urol. 56, 567 (1948).

CAPEK, V., SVÁB, L.: Bedeutung der gezielten Angiographie bei der Differentialdiagnose von Geschwülsten und Zysten der Niere. Radiol. diagn. 2, 441 (1961).

CARNEVALL, G., CATANIA, V. C., DI PIETRO, S.: Contributo radio-chirurgico allo studio dei surreni mediante pneumoretroperitoneo. Ann. Radiol. diag. 30, 466 (1958).

CARSKY, E. W., PRIOR, J. T., MOORE, R., HAMEL, J.: Cholesteatoma of the kidney: radiographic findings. Radiology 78, 796 (1962).

CHIAUDANO, M.: Aspetti arteriografici dei reni in condizioni patologiche. Minerva chir. 13, 1074 (1958).

CHIDEKEL, N., OBRANT, O.: Hypernephroma metastases demonstrated by pelvic angiography. Acta chir. scand. 114, 46 (1957).

CHYNN, K. Y., EVANS, J. A.: Nephrotomography in the differentiation of renal cyst from neoplasm: a review of 500 cases. J. Urol. 83, 21 (1960).

CLARK, R. E., PALUBINSKAS, A. J.: The angiographic spectrum of renal hamartoma. Amer. J. Roentgenol. 114, 715 (1972).

— MOSS, A., LORIMIER, A., PALUBINSKAS: A.: Arteriography of Wilms' tumor. Amer. J. Roentgenol. 113, 476 (1971).

CLARKE, B. G., GOADE jr., W. J., RUDY, H. L.: ROCKWOOD, L.: Differential diagnosis between cancer and solitary serous cyst of the kidney. J. Urol. 75, 922 (1956).

COPE, J. R., ROYLANCE, J., GORDON, I. R. S.: The radiological features of Wilms' tumor. Clin. Radiol. XXIII, 331 (1972).

COUVELAIRE, R., AUVERT, J.: La phlébographie cave inférieure dans l'exploration des tumeurs du rein droit. J. Urol. méd. chir. 62, 21 (1956).

CREEVY, C. D., PRICE, W. E.: Differentiation of renal cysts from neoplasms by abdominal aortography: pitfalls. Radiology 64, 831 (1955).

CREMIN, B. J., KASCHULA, R. O. C.: Arteriography in Wilms' tumor — the results of 13 cases and comparison to renal dysplasia. Brit. J. Radiol. 45, 415 (1972).

DEES, J. E.: Prognosis of primary tumors of renal pelvis and ureter. J. Urol. 75, 419 (1956).

DEININGER, H. K., TRAPP, P.: Angiographische und nuklear-medizinische Befunde der Nieren beim Pringle-Syndrom (Adenoma sebaceum). Fortschr. Röntgenstr. 114, 782 (1971).

DEUTICKE, P.: Nierentumoren. Dtsch. Z. Chir. 231, 767 (1931).

DE WEERD, J. H.: Lipomatous retroperitoneal tumors: urographic findings. J. Urol. 71, 421 (1954).

— HAGEDORN, A. B.: Hypernephroma associated with polycythemia. J. Urol. 82, 29 (1959).

DUFF, P. A., GRANGER, W. H.: Diagnosis of involvement of inferior vena cava in renal neoplasms. J. Urol. 65, 368 (1951).

EARLY, R., BROWN, B., TERPLAN, K.: Fibroblastoma of renal parenchyma. J. Urol. 80, 417 (1958).

EDELSTEIN, J. M., MARCUS, S. M.: Primary benign neoplasm of the ureter. J. Urol. 60, 409 (1948).

EDSMYR, F.: Kliniskt experimentella studier av adenocarcinoma renis. Läkartidningen (Stockholm) 69, 154 (1972).

ELLNER, H. J., BERGMAN, H., ALFONSO, G.: Two cases of solitary giant tubular adenoma of the kidney simulating carcinoma of the renal parenchyma. J. Urol. 84, 706 (1960).

ENDTNER, B., WILDBOLZ, E.: Tumoren der abführenden Harnwege und des männlichen Genitale. In: Diagnostik der Geschwulstkrankheiten. Ed. H. BERTELHEIMER u. H. J. MAURER. Stuttgart: Georg Thieme Verlag 1962, page 285.

ENGEL, W. J.: The significance of renal displacement. J. Urol. 76, 478 (1956).

ERIKSON, S.: Ein Fall von Nierenbeckentumor mit ungewöhnlichem Röntgenbild. Radiol. clin. 11, 173 (1942).

ESCOVITZ, W., WHITE, S. G.: Extensive metastatic calcification in a case of malignant melanoma. Ann. West. Med. Surg. 4, 339 (1950).

ETTINGER, A., ELKIN, M.: Value of plain film in renal mass lesions (tumors and casts). Radiology 62, 372 (1954).

EVANS, A. T.: Combined use of contrast media in retroperitoneal lumbar arteriography for its recognition. Radiology 69, 657 (1957).

EVANS, J. A.: Nephrotomography in the investigation of renal masses. Radiology 69, 684 (1957).

— DUBLIER, W., MONTEITH, J. C.: Nephrotomography Amer. J. Roentgenol. 71, 213 (1954).

— POKER, N.: Newer roentgenographic techniques in the diagnosis of retroperitoneal tumors. J. Amer. med. Ass. 161, 1128 (1956).

FELBER, E.: Asynchronous bilateral benign papilloma of the ureter with subsequent cancer of ureteral stump, bladder, and vagina. J. med. Ass. Ga. 42, 198 (1953).

FELSON, B., MOSKOWITZ, M.: Renal pseudotumors: the regenerated nodule and other lumps, bumps, and dromedary humps. Amer. J. Roentgenol. 107, 720 (1969).

FERGUSON, CH., CAMERON, G., CARRON, J.: Hemangioma of the kidney: report of two cases: J. Urol. 74, 591 (1955).

FOLIN, J.: Röntgenleeraufnahmen und Urographie in der Diagnostik von Nierentumoren. Der Radiologe 1, 166 (1961).

FOSTER, D. G.: Large benign renal tumors. J. Urol. 76, 231 (1956).

GALATIUS-JENSEN, F., ROSTGAARD-CHRISTENSEN, E.: Zur Differentialdiagnose von Abdominaltumoren bei Kindern. Fortschr. Röntgenstr. **93**, 127 (1963).

GEBAUER, A., LISSNER, J.: Differentialdiagnose retroperitonealer Tumoren. Fortschr. Röntgenstr. **88**, 200 (1958).

GIBSON, T. E.: Lymphosarcoma of the kidney. J. Urol. **60**, 838 (1948).

— Interrelationship of renal cysts and tumors: report of three cases. J. Urol. **71**, 241 (1954).

GILLENWATER, J. Y., HOWARD, R. S., PAQUIN, A.: Bilateral primary carcinoma of the ureter. J. Amer. Med. Ass. **197**, 1040 (1966).

GIRAUD, M., BRET, P., KUENTZ, M., ANJOU, A., COSTAZ, G., CHOLLAT, L.: Étude radiologique et stratigraphique des tumeurs surrénaliennes. J. Radiol. Élect. **38**, 893 (1957).

GLAY, A.: Roentgen manifestations of Hodgkin's disease involving the urinary tract. Amer. J. Roentgenol. **84**, 227 (1960).

GLENN, J. F.: Primary ureteral carcinoma eight years in duration. J. Urol. **81**, 649 (1959).

GLOOR, H. U.: Über Verdrängungen der Niere bei Milztumor. Acta radiol. **15**, 476 (1934).

GONDOS, B.: Urographic studies in abdominal masses: the diagnostic value of kidney rotation. Radiology **78**, 180 (1962).

GONZALES-ANGULO, A., REYES, H. A.: Neurofibromatosis involving the lower urinary tract. J. Urol. **89**, 804 (1963).

GOODWIN, W. E., MOORE, E. V., PEIRCE, E. C.: Roentgenographic visualization of adrenal glands: use of aortography and/or retroperitoneal pneumography to visualize adrenal glands: combined adrenalography. J. Urol. **74**, 231 (1955).

GRACIA, V., BRADFIELD, E. O.: Simultaneous bilateral transitional cell carcinoma of the ureter: a case report. J. Urol. **79**, 925 (1958).

GRAUHAN: Die Tumorniere im Röntgenbild. Z. urol. Chir. **17**, 1 (1925).

GREEN-BERG, A. L.: Right solitary renal cyst, left renal calculus. J. Urol. **42**, 87 (1939).

GREENE, L. B., HAYLLAR, B. L., BOGASCH, M.: Epithelial tumors of the renal pelvis and ureter. J. Urol. **79**, 697 (1958).

GREGG, D.: Renal and suprarenal tumours in adults. Br. J. Radiol. **37**, 128 (1964).

GROSS, M., MINKOWITZ, S.: Ureteral metastasis from renal adeno-carcinoma. J. Urol. **106**, 23 (1971).

GROSSMAN, I. W., KOPILNICK, M. D.: Peripelvic renal fibroma: Radiological, pathological and ultrastructural study of a unique lesion. J. Urol. **105**, 174 (1971).

GROSSMAN, A., WILLIAMS, M. J.: Kaposi's sarcoma simulating renal carcinoma. J. Urol. **88**, 473 (1962).

GRUMSTEDT, B., WAHLQVIST, L.: Gradering av njurcarcinom med hjälp av preoperativ njurkärlsröntgen. Nord. Med. **74**, 1033 (1965).

HAJDU, S. I., FOOTE, F. W.: Angiomyolipoma of the kidney: Report of 27 cases and review of the literature. J. Urol. **102**, 396 (1969).

HALLAHAN, J. D.: Spontaneous remission of metastatic renal cell adenocarcinoma: a case report. J. Urol. **81**, 522 (1959).

HAMER, H. G., NILES-WISHARD jr., W. M.: Osteogenic sarcoma involving the right kidney. J. Urol. **60**, 10 (1948).

HAMM, F. C., LAVALLE, L. L.: Tumors of the ureter. J. Urol. **61**, 493 (1949).

HAMM, F. C., SCORDAMAGLIA, L. J.: A diagnostic aid for visualization of the left suprarenal space. J. Urol. **73**, 885 (1955).

HARBAUGH, J.: Botryoid sarcoma of the renal pelvis: a case report. J. Urol. **100**, 424 (1968).

HARRISON, F. G., WARRES, H. L., FUST, J. A.: Neuroblastoma involving the urinary tract. J. Urol. **63**, 598 (1950).

HARRISON III, R. H., DOUBLEDAY, L. C.: Roentgenological appearance of normal adrenal glands. J. Urol. **76**, 16 (1956).

HÄRTEL, M., WEHLIN, L., LIEDBERG, C. F.: Zur radiologischen Differentialdiagnose hypervaskularisierter Nierentumoren. Fortschritte **118**, 498 (1973).

HAUGE, B. N.: Pheochromocytoma. J. Oslo Cy Hosp. **6**, 135 (1956).

HEIDENBLUT, A.: Plattenepithelkarzinom des Nierenbeckens. Fortschr. Röntgenstr. **83**, 95 (1955).

HEMPSTEAD, R. H., DOCKERTY, M. B., PRIESTLEY, J. T., LOGAN, G. B.: Hypernephroma in children: report of two cases. J. Urol. **70**, 152 (1953).

HOLM, O. F.: Nachweis über die Ausbreitung von Rezidiven und lokalen Metastasen durch Aortographie bei einem Falle von operiertem Hypernephrom. Fortschr. Röntgenstr. **86**, 399 (1957).

— Registrering genom aortografi av lokala recidiv efter nefrectomi för hypernefrom (renalt adenocarcinom). Svenska Läk.-Tidn. (Stockholm) **54**, 3388 (1957).

HUFFMAN, W. L.: Echinococcus disease of kidney: report of a case. J. Urol. **78**, 17 (1957).

HULSE, C., PALIK, E. E.: Renal hamartoma. J. Urol. **66**, 506 (1951).

HULTENGREN, N., LAGERGREN, C., LJUNGQVIST, A.: Carcinoma of the renal pelvis in renal papillary necrosis. Acta chir. scand. **130**, 314 (1965).

IMMERGUT, S., COTTLER, Z. R.: Peripelvic lipoma. J. Urol. **67**, 50 (1952).

ISFORT, A., RINSCHE, K. G.: Das Hamartoma der Niere im Angiogram. Fortschr. Röntgenstr. **112**, 231 (1970).

ISRAEL, J.: Über Fieber bei malignen Nieren- und Nebennierengeschwülsten. Dtsch. med. Wschr. **37**, 57 (1911).

JANSSON, G.: Die Röntgendiagnose bei Nierenbeckenpapillom. Acta radiol. **16**, 354 (1935).

JOHNSSON, S.: A contribution to the diagnostics of nephromata. Acta radiol. Suppl. **60** (1946).

JOHNSSON, S. H., MARSHALL jr., M.: Primary kidney tumors of childhood. J. Urol. **74**, 707 (1955).

JÖRG, H.: Nierenhamartome bei tuberöser Sklerose. Fortschr. Röntgenstr. **114**, 381 (1971).

KAHN, P. C., WISE, H. M.: Simulation of renal tumor response to epinephrine by inflammatory disease. Radiology **89**, 1062 (1967).

— — The use of epinephrine in selective angiography of renal masses. J. Urol. **99**, 133 (1968).

KAISER, T., HODSON, J. M., SEIBEL, R. E., ALBEE, R. D., FARROW, F. C., McMAHON, J. J.: Evaluation of asymptomatic renal masses by selective renal angiography and percutaneous needle puncture: a preliminary report. J. Urol. **98**, 436 (1967).

KAUDE, J., CHANG, T. T.: Angiography in evaluation of tuberous sclerosis complex. Der Radiologe **10**, 105 (1970).

KEATS, T. E., SESHANARAYANA: K. N.: Angiomyolipoma of the kidney. Amer. J. Roentgenol. **104**, 332 (1968).

KEEN, M. R.: Primary ureteral tumors. J. Urol. **69**, 231 (1953).

KENDALL, A. R., LAKEY, W. H.: Sclerosing Hodgkin's disease vs. idiopathic retroperitoneal fibrosis. J. Urol. **86**, 217 (1961).

KESSEL, L.: Spontaneous disappearance of bilateral pulmonary metastases. J. Amer. med. Ass. **169**, 1737 (1959).

KHILNANI, M. T., WOLF, B. S.: Hamartolipoma of the kidney: clinical and roentgen features. Amer. J. Roentgenol. **86**, 830 (1961).

KHILNANI, M., ABRAMS, R., BERENBAUM, E. R.: Angiographic features of hamartoma of the kidney. Radiology **90**, 999 (1968).

KING, M. C., FRIEDENBERG, R. M., TENA, L. B.: Normal renal parenchyma simulating tumor. Radiology **91**, 217 (1968).

KNOX, J., SLESSOR, A.: Phaechromocytoma and neurofibromatosis. Lancet I, 790 (1955).

KÖHLER, R.: Correlation between vascular supply to the kidney and excretion as shown by urography in renal tumours. Radiol. Clin. **32**, 100 (1963).

KOST, L. V., LEBERMAN, P. R.: Metastatic carcinoma to the ureter: a case report. J. Urol. **93**, 367 (1965).

KUCERA, J., DVORACEK, C.: A contribution to the diagnosis of renal adenoma. Acta radiol. bohemosl. **8**, 163 (1954).

KUCHINSKY, G. A., MARINBAKH, E. B., BORISOV, V. I.: The significance of aortography in retroperitoneal metastases of hypernephroid carcinoma of the kidney following nephrectomy. Sovjet radiological journal (1969).

KURSH, E. D., PERSKY, L.: Selective renal arteriography in renal lymphoma. J. Urol. **105**, 772 (1971).

KVALE, W. F., ROTH, G. M.: Some aspects of pheochromocytoma. Circulation **21**, 161 (1960).

KYAW, M., KOEHLER, R.: Renal and perirenal lymphoma: Arteriographic findings. Radiology **93**, 1055 (1969).

LAGERGREN, C., LJUNGQVIST, A.: Radiography in the differential diagnosis between carcinoma of the kidney and of the renal pelvis. Scand. J. Urol. Nephrol. **3**, 111 (1969).

LALLI, A. F.: Lymphoma and the urinary tract. Radiology **93**, 1051 (1969).

LAMBETH, J. T., RANNIGER, K.: Angiographic demonstration of a benign tumor of the ureter. Radiology **91**, 929 (1968).

LANG, E. K.: Coexistence of cyst and tumor in the same kidney. Radiology **101**, 7 (1971).

— Arteriographic assessment and staging of renal-cell carcinoma: analysis of a series of 120 patients. Radiology **101**, 17 (1971).

LANG, E. K.: The accuracy of roentgenographic techniques in the diagnosis of renal mass lesions. Radiology **98**, 119 (1971).

LASSER, E. C., STAUBITZ, W. J.: Translumbar aortography in urologic diagnosis. J. Amer. med. Ass. **163**, 1325 (1957).

LATTIMER, J. K., MELICOW, M. M., USON, A. C., Wilms' tumor: a report of 71 cases. J. Urol. **80**. 401 (1958).

LAWS, J. W.: Radiology of the suprarenal glands: Brit. J. Radiol. **31**, 352 (1958).

LEBLANC, G. A.: Contralateral ureteral metastasis from renal adenocarcinoma. J. Urol. **86**, 316 (1961).

LEWIS, J. A., VIERALVES, G., LANDES, R. R., POWELL, L. W.: Malakoplakia of the renal pelvis, calyces and upper ureter: case report. J. Urol. **85**, 243 (1961).

LIEBERTHAL, F.: Multi-locular solitary cyst of the renal hilus. J. Urol. **42**, 321 (1939).

LINDBLOM, K.: Percutaneous puncture of renal cysts and tumors. Acta radiol. **27**, 66 (1946).

LINKE, C. A., ROSENTHAL, I., KIEFER, J. H.: Bilateral pheochromocytoma in a 12-year-old boy. J. Urol. **79**, 781 (1958).

LITZKY, G. M., SEIDEL, R. F., O'BRIEN, J. E.: Leiomyoma of the renal pelvis. J. Urol. **105**, 171 (1971).

LJUNGGREN, E.: Partial nephrectomy in renal tumor. Acta chir. scand. Suppl. **253** (1960).

— HOLM, S., KARTH, B., POMPEIUS, R.: Some aspects of renal tumors with special reference to spontaneous regression. J. Urol. **82**, 553 (1959).

LJUNGQVIST, A., LAGERGREN, C.: The arterial vasculature of renal adenocarcinomas. Acta pathol. microbiol. Scand. **67**, 55 (1966).

LOEB, M. J.: Solitary cysts of the kidney. An hypothesis of common pathogenesis of cysts. Report of three unusual cases. Urol. cutan. Rev. **48**, 105 (1944).

LÖHR, E., MELLIN, P., GÖBBELER, TH.: Über die Grenzen der angiographischen Diagnostik parenchymatöser Nierentumoren. Fortschr. Rontgenstr. **109**, 696 (1968).

LONG, W. W., LYNCH, K. M.: A case report. J. Urol. **106**, 177 (1971).

LOVE, L., FRANK, S. J.: Angiographic features of angiomyolipoma of the kidney. Amer. J. Roentgenol. **95**, 406 (1965).

LOWMAN, R. M., DAVIS, L.: The role of barium contrast studies in the diagnosis of retroperitoneal tumors. Radiology **69**, 641 (1957).

LOWSLEY, O.: Malignant cyst of the kidney. J. Urol. **74**, 586 (1955).

LUSTED, L. B., BESSE jr., B. E., FRITZ, R.: The intravenous urogram in acute leukemia. Amer. J. Roentgenol. **80**, 608 (1958).

MACLEAN, J. T., FOWLER, V. B.: Pathology of tumors of the renal pelvis and ureter. J. Urol. **75**, 384 (1956).

MACQUET, P., VANDENDORP, F., LEMAITRE, G., DU BOIS, R.: L'aortographie dans le diagnostic des tumeurs rénales. J. Radiol. Électrol. **38**, 221 (1957).

MAGEE, P. N., BARNES, J. M.: The experimental production of tumours in the rat. Acta Un. Int. Cancer **15**, 187 (1959).

MALUF, N. S. R., McCoy, C. B.: Translumbar aortography as a diagnostic procedure in urology. Amer. J. Roentgenol. **73**, 533 (1955).

MANN, L. T.: Spontaneous disappearance of pulmonary metastases after nephrectomy for hypernephroma. J. Urol. **59**, 564 (1948).

MASSON, G. M. C., CORCORAN, A. C., HUMPHREY, D. C.: Diagnostic procedures for pheochromocytoma. J. Amer. med. Ass. **165**, 1555 (1957).

McAFEE, J. G., BALLI, C. E.: Radiological diagnosis of diseases of adrenal origin. Amer. J. med. Sci. **232**, 572 (1956).

McCULLOUGH, D. L., SCOTT jr., R., SEYBOLD, H.: Renal angiomyolipoma (Hamartoma): Review of the literature and report of seven cases. J. Urol. **105**, 33 (1971).

McKAY, R. T.: Metastatic deposit from renal carcinoma presenting as an arteriovenous aneurysm, with angiographic demonstration. Brit. J. Radiol. **43**, 217 (1970).

MEANEY, T. F.: Errors in angiographic diagnosis of renal masses. Radiology **93**, 361 (1969).

MEISEL, H. J.: Bilateral polyadenomatous kidneys; adenomatosis of the kidneys simulating polycystic disease. J. Urol. **72**, 1140 (1954).

MENG, C. H., ELKIN, M.: Angiographic manifestations of Wilms' tumor. Amer. J. Roentgenol. **105**, 95 (1969).

MIMS, M. M.: Multiple acquired diverticulosis of the ureter. J. Urol. **84**, 297 (1960).

MOONEY, K.: Hamartoma of kidney. J. Urol. **73**, 951 (1955).

MURPHY, F. J., MAU, W., ZELMAN, S.: Nephrogenic polycythemia. J. Urol. **91**, 474 (1964).

MYERS, G. H., FEHRENBAKER, L. G., KELALIS, P.: Prognostic significance of renal vein invasion by hypernephroma. J. Urol. **100**, 420 (1968).

NAUMANN, H. N., SABATINI, S. A.: Cholesteatoma of kidney simulating squamous cell carcinoma. J. Urol. **69**, 467 (1953).

NICOL, M., STABERT, CH., GUERIN, G.: Néphro-épithélioma calcifié. J. Radiol. Électrol. **39**, 64 (1958).

NILSON, A. E.: Implantation metastasis in renal pelvis from primary tumours of bladder. Acta. chir. scand. **116**, 306 (1959).

NILSSON, S., ANGERVALL, L., BENGTSSON, U., GOTTFRIES, A., JOHANSSON, S., WAHLQVIST, L.: Multipel lokalisation av uroepiteliala tumörer. Nord. Med. **85**, 1156 (1971).

OCKULY, E. A., DOUGLASS, F. M.: Retroperitoneal perirenal lipomata. J. Urol. **37**, 619 (1937).

O'CONOR, V. J.: The diagnosis of tumors of the renal pelvis and ureter. J. Urol. **75**, 416 (1956).

— CANNON, A. H., LAIPPLY, TH. C., SOKOL, K., BARTH, E.: Renal tumors, a round table discussion. Radiology **58**, 830 (1952).

OLSSON, O.: Zur Röntgendiagnostik der Nierentumoren. Der Radiologe **1**, 163 (1961).

OWMAN, T.: Die Aniograpie des renalen Hamartoms (Angiomyolipom). Der Radiologe **13**, 287 (1973).

PALMISANO, P.: Renal hamartoma (angiomyolipoma). Its angiographic appearance and response to intraarterial epinephrine. Radiology **88**, 249 (1967).

DE LA PEÑA, A., USON, A. C., OLIVEROS, M.: Benign renal angiolipoma. Amer. J. Surg. **96**, 590 (1958).

PENNISI, A. A., RUSSI, S., BUNTS, R. C.: Multiple dissimilar tumors in one kidney. J. Urol. **78**, 205 (1957).

PERLMUTTER, A. D., RETIK, A. B., HARRISON, J. H.: Simultaneous bilateral carcinoma of the ureter present for five years before surgery. J. Urol. **93**, 582 (1965).

PEROU, M. L., GRAY, P. T.: Mesenchymal hamartomas of the kidney. J. Urol. **83**, 240 (1960).

PETERSON, C. C., JACKSON jr., H. J. MOORE, J. G.: A Re-evaluation of nephrotomography stressing limitations of the procedure. J. Urol. **98**, 721 (1967).

PFEIFFER, G. E., GANDIN, M. M.: Massive perirenal lipoma with report of a case. J. Urol. **56**, 12 (1946).

PHILLIPS, C. A. S., BAUMRUCKER, G.: Neurilemmoma (arising in the hilus of left kidney). J. Urol. **73**, 671 (1955).

PHILLIPS, T. L., CHIN, F. G., PALUBINSKAS, A. J.: Calcification in renal masses: an eleven-year survey. Radiology **80**, 786 (1963).

PICK, R., CASTELLINO, R., SELTZER, R.: Arteriographic findings in renal lymphoma. Amer. J. Roentgenol. **111**, 530 (1971).

PIRONTI, L., TARQUINI, A.: Alcuni casi di tumore primitivo del rene studiati con l'arteriografia renale selettiva. Minerva chir. **13**, 1122 (1958).

PISANO, D. J., ROSEN, R. H., RUBINSTEIN, B. M., JACOBSON, H. G.: The roentgen manifestations of carcinoma and cyst in the same kidney. Amer. J. Roentgenol. **80**, 603 (1958).

PLAUT, A.: Diffuses dickdarmähnliches Adenom des Nierenbeckens mit geschwulstartiger Wucherung von Gefäßmuskulatur. Z. urol. Chir. **26**, 562 (1929).

POOLE, C. A., VIAMONTE, M.: Unusual renal masses in the pediatric age group. Amer. J. Radiol. **109**, 368 (1970).

PORSTMANN, W., KUCHINSKY, G. A., TRAPEZNIKOVA, M. F.: Angiographic diagnosis of tumours of the kidneys and of their retroperitoneal metastases. Sovjet radiological journal (1969).

POST, H. W. A., SOUTHWOOD, W. F. W.: The technique and interpretation of nephrotomograms. Brit. J. Radiol. **32**, 734 (1959).

POUTASSE, E. F.: Value and limitation of roentgenographic diagnosis of adrenal disease. J. Urol. **73**, 891 (1955).

PRATHER, G. C.: Differential diagnosis between renal tumor and renal cyst. J. Urol. **64**, 193 (1950).

PROVET, H., LISA, J. R., TRINIDAD, S.: Tubular carcinoma of the kidney within a solitary cyst. J. Urol. **75**, 627 (1956).

PUIGVERT, A.: Polykystose rénale et cancer bilatéral. J. Urol. méd. chir. **64**, 30 (1958).

RABINOWITZ, J. G., KINKHABWALA, M., HIMMELFARB, E., ROBINSON, T., BECKER, J. A., BOSNIAK, M., MADAYAG, M.: Renal pelvic carcinoma: an angiographic reevaluation. Radiology **102**, 551 (1972).

RAGINS, A. B., ROLNICK, H. C.: Mucus producing adenocarcinoma of the renal pelvis. J. Urol. **63**, 66 (1950).

RANNIGER, K.: Selective renal arteriographic appearance of necrotic hypernephroma. Radiology 83, 405 (1964).

RATCLIFF, R. K., BAUM, W. C., BUTLER, W. J.: Bilateral primary carcinoma of the ureter, a case report. Cancer 2, 815 (1949).

REILLY, B. J., NEUHAUSER, E. B. D.: Renal tubular ectasia in cystic disease of the kidneys and liver. Amer. J. Roentgenol. 84, 546 (1960).

RICHES, E.: Tumours of the kidneys and suprarenals in adults. Brit. J. Radiol. 37, 124 (1964).

RICHES, E. W., GRIFFITHS, I. H., THACKRAY, A. C.: New growths of the kidney and ureter. Brit. J. Urol. 23, 297 (1951).

ROBECCHI, M., CHIAUDANO, G.: Diagnosi differenziale arteriografica fra cisti e tumori. Boll. soc. piemont. chir. 26, 275 (1956).

ROBSON, C. J.: Radical nephrectomy for renal cell carcinoma. J. Urol. 89, 37 (1963).

— CHURCHILL, B. M., ANDERSON, W. M.: The results of radical nephrectomy for renal cell carcinoma. J. Urol. 101, 297 (1969).

ROSS, L. S., BALTAXE, H.: The value of epinephrine in the diagnosis of epidermoid carcinoma of the kidney. Amer. J. Roentgenol. 112, 600 (1971).

ROY, J. B., WALTON, K. N.: Secondary tumors of the kidney. J. Urol. 103, 411 (1970).

RUDSTRÖM, P.: Ein Fall von Nierenzyste mit eigenartiger Konkrementbildung. Acta chir. scand. 85, 501 (1941).

RUSCHE, C.: Renal hamartoma (angiomyolipoma): report of three cases. J. Urol. 67, 823 (1952).

SALIK, J. O., ABESHOUSE, B. S.: Calcification, ossification and cartilage formation in the kidney. Amer. J. Radiol. 88, 125 (1962).

SALMON, R., KOEHLER, P. R.: Angiography in renal and perirenal inflammatory masses: report of three cases. Radiology 88, 9 (1967).

SALTZ, N. J., LUTTWAK, E. M., SCHWARTZ, A., GOLDBERG, G. M.: Danger of aortography in the localization of pheochromocytoma. Ann. Surg. 144, 118 (1956).

SALVIN, B. L., SCHLOSS, W. A.: Papillary adenocarcinoma of the kidney, with aortography resembling huge renal cyst. J. Urol. 72, 135 (1954).

SAMELLAS, W., MARKS, A. R.: Metastatic melanoma of the urinary tract. J. Urol. 85, 21 (1961).

SANDOMENICO, C., MANSI, M.: Contributo clinicoradiologico alla diagnosi dell'echinococcosi renale. Nunt. Radiol. 22, 270 (1956).

SANTOS, R. DOS: L'aortographie dans les tumeurs rénales et pararénales. Arch. Mal. Reins 8, 313 (1934).

SARGENT, J. W.: Ureteral metastasis from renal adenocarcinoma presenting a bizarre urogram. J. Urol. 83, 97 (1960).

SAVIGNAC, E. M.: Primary carcinoma of the ureter. Amer. J. Roentgenol. 74, 628 (1955).

SCHMITZ-DRÄGER, H. G.: Gleichzeitige Feststellung eines Hypernephroms und seiner Metastase durch retrograde Aortographie. Fortschr. Röntgenstr. 93, 382 (1960).

SCHOLL, A, J.: Peripelvic lymphatic cysts of the kidney. Report of two cases. J. Amer. Med. Ass. 136, 4 (1948).

SCHULTE, T. L., ÉMMETT, J. L.: Urography in the differential diagnosis of retroperitoneal tumors. J. Urol. 42, 215 (1939).

SCHWIEBINGER, G. W., HODGES, C. V.: Coexistence of renal tumor and solitary cyst of the kidney. A.M.A. Arch. Surg. 71, 115 (1955).

SCHRUGGS, C. D., AINSWORTH, T.: Renal cell carcinoma in children: a review of the literature and report of two cases. J. Urol. 86, 728 (1961).

SELTZER, R. A., WENLUND, D. E.: Renal lymphoma: arteriographic studies. Amer. J. Roentgenol. 101, 692 (1967).

SHELLEY, H. S.: Renal adenoma. Pyelograms showing the growth over a five year period. J. Urol. 69, 480 (1953).

SHERWOOD, T., STEVENSON, J. J.: The management of renal masses. Clin. Radiol. 22, 180 (1971).

SHIMKIN, P. M., BUCHIGANI, J. S., SOLOWAY, M. S.: Blood borne metastases to the kidney. An angiographic investigation of three vascular tumors. Acta radiol. 12, 387 (1972).

SHIVERS, T. C. H., DE, AXILROOD, H. D.: Solitary renal cysts. J. Urol. 69, 193 (1953).

— A clinical comparison between benign solitary cysts and malignant lesions of the renal parenchyma. J. Urol. 79, 363 (1958).

SIDAWAY, M. E.: Wilm's tumor in a horseshoe kidney. Brit. J. Radiol. 35, 431 (1962).

SIEGELMANN, S. S., HAYT, D., ANNES, G. P., GOODGOLD, M.: Angiography in carcinoma of the proximal ureter. Radiology 91, 925 (1968).

SIMRIL, W. A., ROSE, D. K.: Replacement lipomatosis and its simulation of renal tumors: A report of two cases. J. Urol. 63, 588 (1950).

SINCLAIR, D. J., RITCHIE, G. W.: Renal carcinoma diagnosed by cyst puncture: a case of mistaken identity. Brit. J. Radiol. 44, 885 (1971).

SMITH, B. A., WEBB, E. A., PRICE, W. M. E.: Retroperitoneal hypernephroid mesonephroma. J. Urol. 94, 616 (1965).

SOUTHWOOD, W. E. W., MARSHALL, V. F.: A clinical evaluation of nephrotomography. Brit. J. Urol. 30, 127 (1958).

SPENCE, H. M., BAIRD, S. S., WARE jr., E. W.: Cystic disorders of the kidney — Classification, diagnosis, treatment. J. Amer. Med. Ass. 163, 1466 (1957).

SPILLANE, R. J., SINGISER, J. A., PRATHER, G. C.: Fibromyxolipoma of the kidney. J. Urol. 68, 811 (1952).

STAHL, D. M.: Unusual primary hypernephroma (renal cell carcinoma) of the ureter in a child. J. Urol. 80, 176 (1958).

STEARNS, D. B., SHAPIRO, M. W., GORDON, S. K.: Reticulum cell sarcoma of the kidney. J. Urol. 81, 395 (1959).

STEINBACH, H. L., HINMAN jr., F., FORSHAM, P. H.: The diagnosis of adrenal neoplasms by contrast media. Radiology 69, 664 (1957).

SUKTHOMYA, C., LEVIN, B.: Pseudotumors of kidney secondary to anticoagulant therapy. Radiology 88, 701 (1967).

SUNDBERG, J.: Ein Fall von malignem Tumor in einer Beckenniere. Der Radiologie 12, 377 (1972).

Süsse, H. J., Radke, H.: Nachweis und Lokalisierung von Nebennierentumoren mittels Aortographie. Fortschr. Röntgenstr. **86**, 599 (1957).

Suzuki, H., Siminovitch, M.: Primary mucus-producing adenocarcinoma of the renal pelvis: report of a case. J. Urol. **93**, 562 (1965).

Taylor, J. S.: Carcinoma of the urinary tract and analgesic abuse. Med. J. Australia **1**, 407 (1972).

Taylor, J. N., Genters, K.: Renal angiomyolipoma and tuberous sclerosis. J. Urol. **79**, 865 (1958).

Taylor, W. N.: Tumors of the kidney pelvis. J. Urol. **82**, 452 (1959).

Teplick, J. G., Laress, M., Steinberg, S.: Echinococcosis of the kidney. J. Urol. **78**, 323 (1957).

Thompson, I. M.: Peripelvic lymphatic renal cysts. J. Urol. **78**, 343 (1957).

Twiss, A. C.: Cortical adenomas of arteriosclerotic kidneys. Illinois med. J. **95**, 311 (1949).

Uson, A. C., del Rosario, C., Melicow, M. M.: Wilms' tumor in association with cystic renal disease: report of two cases. J. Urol. **83**, 262 (1960).

— Melicow, M. M., Lattimer, J. K.: Is renal arteriography (aortography) a reliable test in the differential diagnosis between kidney cysts and neoplasms? J. Urol. **89**, 554 (1963).

Vermillion, C. D., Skinner, D. G., Pfister, R. C.: Bilateral renal cell carcinoma. J. Urol. **108**, 219 (1972).

Villaume, C.: Diffuse papillomatosis of the urinary tract. Acta radiol. **37**, 401 (1952).

Voegeli, E.: Hypovaskuläre Nierentumoren, Korrelation zwischen Histologie und Angiographie. Fortschr. Röntgenstr. **114**, 373 (1971).

Wahlqvist, L.: Factors of importance for primary surgical therapy in renal carcinoma-nephrectomy and kidney resection. Scand. J. Urol. Nephr. Suppl. **4** (1969).

Wallach, J. B., Sutton, A. P., Claman, M.: Hemangioma of the kidney. J. Urol. **81**, 515 (1959).

Watkins, J. P.: Wilms' tumor with ureteral metastases extending into the bladder. J. Urol. **77**, 593 (1957).

Watson, R. C., Fleming, R. J., Evans, J. A.: Arteriography in the diagnosis of renal carcinoma. Radiology **91**, 888 (1968).

Weaver, R. G., Carlquist, J. H.: Two rare tumors of the renal parenchyma. J. Urol. **77**, 351 (1957).

Weiss, M., Kröpelin, T., Oechslen, D.: (Schaukasten) Bilaterale Nierentumoren. Fortschr. Röntgenstr. **115**, 828 (1971).

Wesolowski, S.: Primary tumors of the ureter. J. Urol. **82**, 212 (1959).

Weyde, R.: Abdominal aortography in renal diseases. Brit. J. Radiol. **25**, 353 (1952).

Wharton, L.R.: Hypernephromas that are too early to diagnose. J. Urol. **42**, 713 (1939).

Whitlock, G. F., McDonald, J. R., Cook, E. N.: Primary carcinoma of the ureter.: a pathologic and prognostic study. J. Urol. **73**, 245 (1955).

Wiggli, U.: Doppelseitiges Nierenbeckencholesteatom. Fortschr. Röntgenstr. **114**, 388 (1971).

Witten, D. M., Greene, L. F., Emmett, J. L.: An evaluation of nephrotomography in urologic diagnosis. Amer. J. Roentgenol. **90**, 115 (1963).

Woodard, J. R., Levine, M. K.: Nephroblastoma (Wilms' tumor) and congenital aniridia. J. Urol. **101**, 140 (1969).

Woodruff, J. H., Chalek, C. C., Ottoman, R. E., Wilk, S. P.: The roentgen diagnosis of renal neoplasms. J. Urol. **75**, 615 (1956).

— Ottoman, R. E.: Radiologic diagnosis of renal tumours by renal angiography. J. Canad. Ass. Radiol. **7**, 54 (1956).

Woods, F. M., Melvin, P. D., Coplan, M. M., Raim, J. A.: Renal adenoma: two cases requiring surgical intervention. J. Urol. **85**, 17 (1961).

Ziter, F. M. H., Wieche, D. R., McAndrews, J. F.: Renal leiomyosarcoma: a case report with angiographic findings. J. Urol. **105**, 776 (1971).

G. Renal Cyst and polycystic disease

Ainsworth, W. L., Vest, S. A.: Differential diagnosis between renal tumors and cysts. J. Urol. **66**, 740 (1951).

Andresen, K.: Beitrag zur Röntgenologie der solitären Nierenzysten. Röntgenpraxis **8**, 505 (1936).

Ask-Upmark, K. E. F., Ingvar, D.: A follow-up examination of 138 cases of subarachnoid hemorrhage, Acta med. scand. **138**, 15 (1950).

Barnett, L. E.: Hydatid disease. Aust. N. Z. J. Surg. **12**, 240 (1943).

Bartley, O., Cederbom, G., Henell, B.: Multicystic renal disease in an adult. Acta radiol. **6: 5**, 424 (1967).

Baurys, W.: Echinococcus disease of the kidney. J. Urol. **411** (1952).

Beltran, J. C.: Congenital unilateral multicystic kidney in infancy. J. Urol. **81**, 602 (1959).

Berger, I. R., Gowart, G. T.: Renal echinococcus disease. Radiology **62**, 852 (1954).

Billing, L.: The roentgen examination of polycystic kidneys. Acta radiol. **41**, 305 (1954).

Boggs, L. K., Kimmelstiel, P.: Benign multilocular cystic nephroma: report of two cases of so-called multilocular cyst of the kidney. J. Urol. **76**, 530 (1956).

Borski, A. A., Kimbrough, J.: Bilateral carcinoma in polycystic renal disease — an unique case. J. Urol. **71**, 677 (1954).

Braasch, W. F., Emmett, J.: Clinical Urology. Philadelphia & London: W. B. Saunders Co. 1951.

Braedel, H. U.: Zur angiographischen Diagnose der solitären Nierencyste. Röntgenbl. **16**, 44 (1963).

Buchet, R., Leblanc, J.: Maladie polykystique du foie et des reins (à propos de deux cas).: aspect radiologique de problème. J. Radiol. Électrol. **43**, 12 (1962).

Buttarazzi, P. J., Poutasse, E. F., Devine jr., C. J., Fiveash jr., J., Devine, P. C.: Aspiration of renal cyst. J. Urol. **100**, 591 (1968).

Campbell, M. F.: Anomalies of the kidney. In: Urology. Philadelphia: W. B. Saunders Co. 1963 (Vol. 2, page 1654).

Cannon, A. H., Zanon jr., B., Karras, B. G.: Cystic calcification in the kidney. Amer. J. Roentgenol. **84**, 837 (1960).

CIMMINO, C. V.: Congenital unilateral multicystic disease of the kidney. Amer. J. Roentgenol. **92**, 281 (1964).

CLAESSEN, G.: The roentgen diagnosis of echinococcus tumors. Acta radiol. (Stockh.) Suppl. **6** (1928).

CLARKE, B. G., GOADE jr., W. J., RUDY, H. L., ROCKWOOD, L.: Differential diagnosis between cancer and solitary serous cyst of the kidney. J. Urol. (Baltimore) **75**, 922 (1956).

COPPRIDGE, A. J., RATLIFF, R. K.: Unilateral multicystic disease. J. Pediat. **53**, 330 (1958).

CRUMMY, A. B., MADSEN, P. O.: Parapelvic renal cyst: the peripheral fat sign. J. Urol. **96:4**, 436 (1966).

DALGAARD, O. Z.: Polycystic disease of the kidneys. In: Diseases of the kidney. Ed. by M. B. Strauss & L. G. Welt. Boston: Little, Brown and Company (1963, 1971).

DEAN, A. L.: Treatment of solitary cyst of the kidney by aspiration. Trans. Amer. Ass. gen.-urin. Surg. **32**, 91 (1939).

DEW, H. R.: Hydatid disease. Sidney: Australian medical publishing Co. 1928.

DE WEERD, J. H., SIMON, H. B.: Simple renal cysts in children: review of the literature and report of five cases. J. Urol. **75**, 912 (1956).

DOBBEN, G. D.: Benign adenomatous polycystic kidney tumor. Radiology **76**, 100 (1961).

DUBILIER, W., EVANS, J. A.: Peripelvic cysts of the kidney. Radiology **71**, 404 (1958).

ETTINGER, A., KAHN, P. C., WISE jr., H. M.: The importance of selective renal angiography in the diagnosis of polycystic disease. Jr. Urol. **102:2**, 156 (1969).

FAWCETT, A. W.: Case of congenital cystadenoma of the kidney. Brit. J. Surg. **20**, 678 (1933).

FETTER, T. R., YUNEN, J. R., BOGAEV, J. H.: Parapelvic renal cyst: report of three additional cases. J. Urol. **88**, 599 (1962).

FINE, M. G., BURNS, E.: Unilateral multicystic kidney: report of six cases and discussion of the literature. J. Urol. **81**, 42 (1959).

FISH, G. W.: Large solitary serous cysts of the kidney. J. Amer. Med. Assoc. **112**, 514 (1939).

FRAZIER, T. H.: Multilocular cysts of the kidney. J. Urol. **65**, 351 (1951).

FRIMANN-DAHL, J.: Radiology in renal cysts, particularly on the left side. Brit. J. Radiol. **37**, 146 (1964).

GHIGO, M., MAGRINI, M.: Aspetti radiografici della bilharziosi urinaria. Radiol. Med. **46**, 341 (1960).

GIBSON, T. E.: Multilocular cyst of the kidney: case report. J. Urol. **87**, 297 (1962).

GIRL, J., TUHY, J.: Schwierigkeiten der Diagnosestellung der solitären Nierencyste. Der Radiologe **11:6**, 219 (1971).

GOLDSTEIN, H. H., LIEBERMAN, M. L., OBESTER, G. E.: Echinococcic disease of the kidney: report of a case of unusual size. J. Urol. **81**, 596 (1959).

GORDON, I. R. S.: Renal puncture. J. Fac. Radiol. (Lond.) **9**, 108 (1958).

GÖTHLIN, J., OLIN, T.: Determination of renal blood flow in humans in connection with renal angio-graphy. Proceedings of 2nd Congr. European Ass. Radiol., Amsterdam, 1971 (page 182).

GRABSTAD, H.: Catheterization of renal cyst for diagnostic and therapeutic purposes. J. Urol. **71**, 28 (1954).

HARROW, B. R., SLOANE, J. A.: Polycystic renal disease with renal and splenic artery aneurysms. J. Urol. **84**, 447 (1960).

HECKEL, N. J., GOULD, H. V.: A report of a papillary cystadenoma of the kidney. J. Urol. **44**, 200 (1940).

HELLMER, H.: Beitrag zur Kenntnis des Röntgenbildes der Dermoidzyste. Acta radiol. XVIII: 1—2, **No. 101 — 102**, 81 (1937).

HUDSON, P. L.: Echinococcus disease. Sth. med. J. (Bgham, Ala.) **38**, 584 (1945).

HUFFMAN, W. L.: Echinococcus disease of kidney: report of a case. J. Urol. **78**, 17 (1957).

ISAAC, F., SCHOEN, I., WALKER, P.: An unusual case of Lindau's disease. Cystic disease of the kidneys and pancreas with renal and cerebellar tumors. Amer. J. Roentgenol. **75**, 912 (1956),

IVEMARK, B. I., LINDBLOM, K.: Arterial ruptures in the adult polycystic kidney. Acta chir. scand. **115**, 100 (1958).

von IWIG, J., THIEMANN, K. J.: Zur angiographischen Symptomatologie der extrarenalen parapelvinen Zyste. Fortschr. Röntgenstr. **109:2**, 247 (1968).

JOHNSSON, S.: A contribution to the diagnostics of nephromata: analysis of a roentgenological and patho-anatomical material. Acta radiol. Suppl. **60** (1946).

KHORSAND, D.: Carcinoma within solitary renal cysts. J. Urol. **93**, 440 (1965).

KRETSCHMER, H. L.: Echinococcus disease of kidney. Surg. Gynec. Obstet. **36**, 196 (1923).

KROPP, K. A., GRAYHACK, J. T., WENDEL, R. M., DAHL, D. S.: Morbidity and mortality of renal exploration for cyst. Surg. Gynec. Obstet. **125:4**, 803 (1967).

KYAW, M. M., NEWMAN, H.: Adult multicystic renal disease. Brit. J. Radiol. **44**, 881 (1971).

LAGEMAN, K., VÖLTER, D.: Der Hydrokalix: Pathogenese — Diagnostik — Therapie. Fortschr. Röntgenstr. **112:2**, 238 (1970).

LANG, E. K.: The differential diagnosis of renal cysts and tumors. Radiology **87**, 883 (1966).

LATHAM, W. J.: Hydatid disease. J. Fac. Radiol. (Lond.) **5**, 65 (1953).

LINDBLOM, K.: Diagnostic kidney puncture in cysts and tumors. Amer. J. Roentgenol. **68**, 209 (1952).

— Percutaneous puncture of renal cysts and tumors. Acta radiol. **XXVII**, 66 (1946).

LOWSLEY, O. S., CURTIS, M. S.: The surgical aspects of cystic disease of the kidney. J. Amer. Med. Assoc. **127**, 112 (1945).

MENASHE, V., SMITH, D. R.: Apparently unilateral polycystic kidney. A cause for abdominal calcific shadows. Amer. J. Dis. Childh. **94**, 313 (1957).

MISHALAN, H. G., GILBERT, D. R.: Benign ossified lesion of the kidney — report of a case resembling a hydatid cyst. J. Urol. **78**, 330 (1957).

MOORE, G. W., BUCHERT, W. I.: Unilateral multicystic kidney in an infant. J. Urol. **78**, 721 (1957).

MUIR, J. B. G.: Hydatid cyst of kidney. Aust. & N. Z. J. Surg. **17**, 305 (1948).

MURPHY, F. J., MAU, W., ZELMAN, S.: Nephrogenic polycythemia. J. Urol. **91**: 5, 474 (1964).

NATVIG, P.: Two cases of solitary renal cyst with communication to the renal pelvis. Acta radiol. **22**, 732 (1941).

OLIVERO, S.: Il problema diagnostico dei reni cistici con particolare riguardo alla semeiologia arteriografica. Minerva urol. (Torino) **11**, 31 (1959).

OLSSON, OLLE: Renal cyst. In: Diseases of the kidney. Edited by M. B. Strauss & L. G. Welt. Boston: Little, Brown & Co. 1971 (page 165).

— Renal tumor and cyst. In: Angiography. Edited by H. L. Abrams. Boston: Little, Brown & Co. 1971 (Chapter 49).

PARKKULAINEN, K. V., HJELT L., SIROLA, K.: Congenital multicystic dysplasia of the kidney. Acta chir. scand. Suppl. **244**, (1959).

PISANO, D. J., ROSEN, R. H., RUBINSTEIN, B. M., JACOBSSON, H. G.: The roentgen manifestations of carcinoma and cyst in the same kidney. Amer. J. Roentgenol. **80**, 603 (1958).

PUIGVERT, A.: Polykystose rénale et cancer bilatéral. J. Urol. méd. chir. **64**, 30 (1958).

RALL, J. E., ODELE, H. M.: Congenital polycystic disease of the kidney: review of the literature and data on 207 cases. Amer. J. Med. Sci. **218**, 399 (1949).

REAY, E. R., ROLLESTON, G. L.: Diagnosis of hydatid cyst of the kidney. J. Urol. **64**, 26 (1950).

ROLOFF, D. W., BAILLIE, E. E., WEAVER, D. K.: Macrobullous medullary polycystic kidney and cystic lung disease: report of rare association in a child. Amer. J. Dis. Childh. **121**, 318 (1971).

SALANO, P. B. E.: Consideraciones sobre 452 casos de quistes renales, revisados en el "Armed Forces Instit. of Pathology". Arch. Español. **13**, 299 (1957).

SCHIMATZEK, A.: Solitärzysten der Nieren im Aortogramm. Radiol. Austr. **11**, 149 (1961).

SHIVERS, C. H., DE T., AXILROD, H. D.: Solitary renal cysts. J. Urol. **69**, 193 (1953).

SNOW, W. T.: Urachal cyst with calculi. Amer. J. Roentgenol. **78**, 323 (1957).

SPENCE, H. M.: Congenital unilateral multicystic kidney: an entity to be distinguished from polycystic kidney disease and other cystic disorders. J. Urol. **74**, 693 (1955).

SPRING, M., GROSS, S. W.: Ruptured aneurysm of the circle of Willis associated with polycystic kidneys. Amer. Med. Assoc. Arch. Intern. Med. **102**, 806 (1958).

STAUBITZ, W. J., JEWETT, jr., T. C., PLETMAN, R. J.: Renal cystic disease in childhood. J. Urol. **90**, 8 (1963).

TEPLICK, J. G., LABESS, M., STEINBERG, S.: Echinococcosis of the kidney. J. Urol. **78**, 323 (1957).

VESTBY, G. W.: Perkutan punksjon av nyrecyster. Nord. Med. **78**, 633 (1968).

VIDAL, B., ENGLARO, G.: Sulla semeiologia radiologica del rene policistico. Radiol. med. (Torino) **43**, 647 (1957).

VOEGELI, E.: Die Pathogenese des Fibrolipomatose. Der Radiologe **11**, 209 (1971).

WARD, J. N., DRAPER, J. W., LAVENGOOD jr., R. W.: A clinical review of polycystic kidney disease in 53 patients. J. Urol. **98**, 1 (1967).

WHEELER, B. C.: Use of the aspirating needle in the diagnosis of solitary renal cysts. New Engl. J. Med. **226**, 55 (1952).

WHITE, E. W., BRAUNSTEIN, L.: Renal cystic disease. J. Urol. **71**, 17 (1954).

H. Renal tuberculosis

AMBROSETTI, A. SESANNA, R.: Arteriographische Untersuchungen an der tuberkulösen Niere. Urol. int. (Basel) **1**, 153 (1955).

BECKER, J. A., WEISS, R. M., LATTIMER, J. K.: Renal tuberculosis: the role of nephrotomography and angiography. J. Urol. **100**, 415 (1968).

BIONDETTI, P., MARANI, F.: Diagnosi differenziale arteriografica della tubercolosi renale. Minerva chir. (Torino) **13**, 1049 (1958).

CAVAZZANA, P., MENEGHINI, C.: Considerazoni sull'evoluzione radiologica e clinica della tubercolosi urinaria in soggetti trattati con streptomicina e chemioterapici antitubercolari. Radiol. med. (Torino) **42**, 977 (1956).

CHLAUDANO, C., GIONGO, V.: Trattamento chirurgico conservativo della tubercolosi urinaria. Minerva med. Saluzzo 1958.

CIBERT, J.: La tuberculose rénale. Paris 1946.

COOK, E. N., GREENE, L. F.: The use of streptomycin in the treatment of tuberculosis of the urinary tract. J. Urol. **60**, 187 (1948).

EITZEN, A. C.: Tuberculous contracted kidney: case report. J. Urol. **42**, 288 (1939).

ELKE, M., RUTISHAUSER, G., BAUMANN, J.: Vorschlag einer einfachen Stadieneinteilung der Nierentuberkulose auf Grund röntgenologischer und therapeutischer Gesichtspunkte. Der Urologe **6**, 40 (1967).

ERICSSON, N. O., LINDBOM, Å.: Intravenous urography in renal tuberculosis. Brit. J. Urol. **22**, 201 (1950).

FRANZAS, F.: Clarification of radiograms in renal tuberculosis. Acta chir. scand. **106**, 429 (1954).

FRIMANN-DAHL, J.: The radiological investigation of renal tuberculosis. The XXVII Meeting of the scand. surg. soc. in Oslo 1955, p. 22.

— Radiological investigations of urogenital tbc. Urol. intern. (Basel) **1**, 396 (1955).

— Selective angiography in renal tuberculosis. Acta radiol. **49**, 31 (1958).

FRITJOFSSON, Å., EDSMAN, G.: Angionephrography in renal tuberculosis. Acta chir. scand. **118**, 60 (1959).

GAY, R.: Focal exclusions in renal tuberculosis. Acta radiol. **32**, 129 (1949).

GIUSTRA, P., WATSON, R., SHULMAN, H.: Arteriographic findings in the various stages of renal tuberculosis. Radiology **100**, 597 (1971).

GREENWOOD, F. G.: Cineradiography in urinary tuberculosis. Brit. J. Radiol. **30**, 493 (1957).

HALKIER, E.: Behandling af nyretuberkulose med kemoterapeutica. Copenhagen: Arnold Busck 1956.

— MEYER, J.: Chemotherapy of renal tuberculosis. Dan. Med. Bull. **6**, 97 (1959).

HANLEY, H. G.: Cineradiography of the urinary tract. Brit. Med. J. II, 22 (1955).

HEINZE, H. G., KLEIN, U., SCHMIDT-MENDE, M.: Selektive Serien-Renovasographie zur Beurteilung von Morphologie und Therapie der Nierentuberkulose. Fortschr. Röntgenstr. 114, 758 (1971).

JACOBS, L. G.: Total tuberculosis calcification of a kidney and ureter. Amer. Rev. Tubercul. 71, 437 (1955).

KELALIS, P. P, GREENE, L. F., WEED, L. A.: Brucellosis of the urogenital tract: a mimic of tuberculosis. J. Urol. 88, 347 (1962).

LANE, T. J. D.: Some observations on renal tuberculosis. Brit. J. Urol. 27, 27 (1955).

LINDBOM, Å.: Fornix backflow in excretion urography. Acta radiol. 24, 411 (1943).

— Miliary tuberculosis after retrograde pyelografi. Acta radiol. 25, 219 (1944).

LINDÉN, K.: Prognostic and therapeutic aspects of urogenital tuberculosis. Acta chir. scand. Suppl. 153 (1950).

LJUNGGREN, E.: Zur Röntgendiagnostik der Nierentuberkulose. Z. Urol. 32, 40 (1938).

— Beitrag zur Röntgendiagnostik der Nierentuberkulose. Z. Urol. 36, 155 (1942).

— Le diagnostic précoce de la tuberculose rénale. Presse méd. 91, 2089 (1956).

MAY, F.: Zur Behandlung der Urogenitaltuberkulose. Wschr. Klinik u. Praxis 35, 1525 and 1563 (1959).

NESBIT, R. M., BOHNE, A. W.: A present-day rationale for the treatment of urinary tuberculosis. J. Amer. Med. Ass. 138, 937 (1948).

OBRANT, K. O. F.: Studier över urogenitaltuberkulosens behandling. Diss. Göteborg 1953.

OLSSON, OLLE: Die Urographie bei der Nierentuberkulose. Acta radiol. Suppl. 47 (1943).

— Über die Bedeutung der Verkalkungen in der Niere für die Röntgendiagnose der Nierentuberkulose. Z. f. Urol. Band XXXVIII: 9–10, 21 (1944).

— Röntgenuntersökningen i diagnostiken av urogenitaltuberkulosen. Nord. med. 29, 517 (1946).

— La urografia en la tuberculosis urinaria. Arch. Espan. de Urol. III: 1 (1946).

— Röntgenundersökning vid njurtuberkulos. Nord. med. 39, 1647 (1948).

— Renal angiography. X Congr. Soc. Int'l d'Urol., Aten 1955, I, 298.

— Tuberculosis. In: Diseases of the kidney. Ed. by M. B. Strauss & L. G. Welt. Boston: Little, Brown & Co. 1971. (page 166).

PUIGVERT, A.: La néphrectomie partielle pour tuberculose. Urol. int. (Basel) 1, 199 (1955).

RENANDER, A.: Röntgenbefunde bei Nierentuberkulose. Acta radiol. 20, 341 (1939).

RODRIQUEZ-LUCCA, B.: Renal tuberculosis simulating hypernephroma. J. Urol. 77, 589 (1957).

ROSENDAL, T.: Renal tuberculosis. Urol. cutan. Rev. 52, 340 (1948).

SENGER, F. L., BELL, A. L., WARRES, H. L., TIRMAN, W. S.: Fate of the ureteral stump after nephrectomy. Amer. J. Surg. 73, 69 (1947).

STEINERT, R.: Renal tuberculosis and roentgenologic examination. Acta radiol. Suppl. 53 (1943).

WESOLOWSKI, S.: Sténoses de l'uretère tuberculeux. III Symposium for the study of urogenital tuberculosis. Anacapri–San Michele 1959 (page 139).

WEYDE, R.: Abdominal aortography in renal diseases. Brit. J. Radiol. 25, 353 (1952).

I. Primary vascular lesions

ABESHOUSE, B. S.: Aneurysm of the renal artery: report of two cases and review of the literature. Urol. cutan. Rev. 55, 451 (1951).

ABRAMS, H. L., BAUM, S., STAMEY, T.: Renal venous washout time in renovascular hypertension. Radiology 83, 597 (1964).

— CORNELL, S. H.: Patterns of Collateral Flow in Renal Ischemia. Excerpta Medica 20, 1 (1966).

D'ABREU, F., STRICKLAND, B.: Developmental renal artery stenosis. Lancet II, 517 (1962).

ACKER, E. D., DOOLEY, J. V., HERMAN, W. F.: Multiple aneurysms of the right renal artery: a case report. J. Urol. 87, 759 (1962).

ALBERS, P., HABIGHORST, L. V., KÖSSLING, F. K.: Zur Diagnostik des arteriellen Kollateralkreislaufs der Niere, Fortschr. Röntgenstr. 105, 793 (1966).

ALFIDI, R. J., TARAR, R., FOSMOE, R., FERRARIO, C., BULTUCH, R., GIFFORD, R.: Renal-Splanchnic Steal and Hypertension. Radiology 102, 545 (1972).

AMPLATZ, K.: Assessment of curable renovascular hypertension by radiographic technics. Radiology 83, 816 (1964).

— Two radiographic tests for assessment of renovascular hypertension. Radiology 79, 807 (1962).

ANSAY, J., BUISSERET, J., MAHIEU, F.: L'artériographie rénale dans l'hypertension. J. Belge de radiol. 45, 15 (1962).

ASK-UPMARK, E.: Arteriell hypertension och sjukdomar i några artärprovinser med särskild hänsyn till deras kirurgiska tillgänglighet. Schola Postgraduata Medica 5, 2505 (1962).

ATKINSON, R. L.: Aneurysm of the renal artery. J. Urol. 72, 117 (1954).

BEGNER, J. A.: Aortography in renal artery aneurysm. J. Urol. 73, 720 (1955).

BERGENTZ, S. E., HOOD, B., KJELLBO, H.: Njurartärstenos. Sv. Läkartidn. (Stockholm) 67, 3383 (1970).

BJÖRK, L: Anomalous pulmonary venous drainage to below the diaphragm. Acta Radiol. 7, 231 (1968).

BLAKE, HEFFERNAN, McCANN: Renal arteriovenous fistula after percutaneous renal biopsy. Brit. M. J. 1, 1458 (1963).

BOHNE, A. W., HENDERSON, G. L.: Intrarenal arteriovenous aneurysm: case report. J. Urol. 77, 818 (1957).

BOIJSEN, E., JÖNSSON, G.: Renal arteriovenous aneurysm. To be published in Acta radiol.

— KÖHLER, R.: Renal artery aneurysms. Acta radiol. I, 1077 (1963).

— Renal arteriovenous fistulae. Acta radiol. 57, 433 (1962).

BOOKSTEIN, J. J.: Segmental renal artery stenosis in renovascular hypertension. Radiology 90, 1073 (1968).

BÖTTGER, E., REGULA, H., BURGHARD, A.: Angiographische Befunde vor und nach Streptokinasebehandlung bei Nierenarterienembolie. Fortschr. Röntgenstr. 115, 742 (1971).

BRAEDEL, H. U., HERAVI, P.: Tierexperimentelle Untersuchungen zur Nierenvenendarstellung mit nur gering nierengängigen Kontrastmitteln. Fortschr. Röntgenstr. 117, 270 (1972).

BRESCIA, M. J., CIMINO, J. E., APPEL, K., HURWICH, B. J.: Chronic hemodialysis using venipuncture and a surgically created arteriovenous fistula. New Engl. J. Med. 275, 1089 (1966).

BROLIN, I.: Renal artery changes in hypertension. Acta radiol. 6, 401 (1967).

— STENER, I.: Collaterals in obstruction of the renal artery. Acta radiol. IV, 449 (1966).

BROWN, J. J., OWEN, K., PEART, W. S., ROBERTSON, J. I. S., SUTTON, D.: The diagnosis and treatment of renal artery stenosis. Brit. Med. J. 2, 327 (1960).

BROY, H.: Die Querschnittslähmung, eine fatale angiographische Komplikation, Kasuistik und Übersicht. Fortschr. Röntgenstr. 114, 353 (1971).

VON BÜREN, W. W., BOURQUIN, J., STÄHLIN, G.: Verschluß einer Nierenarterie während der Angiographie. Fortschr. Röntgenstr. 114, 23 (1971).

CEDERMARK, J., LINDBLOM, K., HENSCHEN, F.: Om diagnosen av njurinfarkt, särskilt med hjälp av aortografi. Nord. Med. 10, 1793 (1941).

CEN, M. ROSENBUSCH, G.: Nierenangiographie mit Adrenalin (Möglichkeiten der Pharmakoangiographie). Fortschr. Röntgenstr. 109, 702 (1968).

CHAIT, A., STOANE, L., MOSKOWITZ, H., MELLINS, H.: Renal vein thrombosis. Radiology 90, 886 (1968).

CHISHOLM, G. D.: An arteriovenous fistula in a polycystic kidney: A cause of acute renal failure and hematuria. J. Urol. 96, 854 (1966).

CHOI, S., GATZEK, H., KENNY, G. M., MURPHY, G. P.: Techniques and results with arteriograms in human renal allotransplants. Amer. J. Roentgenol. 109, 155 (1970).

CHUTE, R., O'HARA, E. T., GOLDMAN, R. N., HOUGHTON, J. D., TOY, B. L.: The inferior vena cava as a good source of tissue for renal artery patch grafting for renal revascularization for hypertension. J. Urol. 89, 303 (1963).

CLARK, R., McNAMARA, T., PALUBINSKAS, A.: Intrarenal mycotic aneurysm detected angiographically. Brit. J. Radiol. 45, 66 (1972).

COCKETT, A. T. K., MAXWELL, M., KAUFMAN, J. J.: Delayed appearance time of intravenous urographic contrast media in renal ischemic hypertension. J. Urol. 87, 799 (1962).

CORDONNIER, J. J. Unilateral renal artery disease with hypertension. J. Urol. 82, 1 (1959).

CORNELL, S. H., KIRKENDALL, W. M., WALTER, M.: Neurofibromatosis of the renal artery: An unusual cause of hypertension. Radiology 88, 24 (1967).

CORREA, R. J., STEWART, B. H., BOBLITT, D. E.: Intravenous pyelography as a screening test in renal hypertension. Amer. J. Roentgenol. 88, 1135 (1962).

DAVIDSON, A. J., TALNER, L., DOWNS, W.: A study of the angiographic appearance of the kidney in an aging normotensive population. Radiology 92, 975 (1969).

DE CAMP, P. T., BIRCHALL, R.: Recognition and treatment of renal arterial stenosis associated with hypertension. Surgery 43, 134 (1958).

DEMING, C. L., HARVARD, B. M., GLENN, J. F.: Urological aspects of hypertension. J. Urol. 85, 859 (1961).

DEYTON, W. E., MARTIN, J. F., BOYCE, W. H., GLENN, J. F.: Differential renal function evaluation by minute sequence pyelography. J. Urol. 90, 611 (1963).

DON, C.: Unilateral manifestations of bilateral renal artery disease. Canad. M. A. J. 85, 1188 (1961).

— Asymmetry of the kidneys in disease of the main renal artery. J. Canad. Ass. Radiol. 12, 15 (1961).

DUSTAN, H. P., PAGE, I. H., POUTASSE, E. F.: Renal hypertension. New Engl. J. Med. 261, 647 (1959).

DÜX, A., THURN, P.: Das Aneurysma der Arteria renalis. Fortschr. Röntgenstr. 96, 471 (1962).

EFSEN, F., LORENZEN, U.: Nephroangiography in periarteritis nodosa: Report of a case. Acta radiol. 7, 225 (1968).

EIKNER, W. C., BOBECK, C. J.: Renal vein thrombosis. J. Urol. 75, 780 (1956).

EISEN, S., FRIEDENBERG, M. J., KLAHR, S.: Bilateral ureteral notching and selective renal phlebography in the nephrotic syndrome due to renal vein thrombosis. J. Urol. 93, 343 (1965).

EKELUND, L., GÖTHLIN, J., LINDHOLM, T., LINDSTEDT, E., MATTSSON, K.: Arteriovenous fistulas following renal biopsy with hypertension and hemodynamic changes: report of a case studied by dye-dilution technique. J. Urol. 108, 373 (1972).

EKESTRÖM, S., HANSSON, L. O.: Kirurgisk behandling av njurartärstenos. Sv. Läkartidn. (Stockholm) 58, 184 (1961).

ELKIN, M.: Renal vacular shunts. Clin. Radiol. XXII, 156 (1971).

— CHIEN-HSING, M.: Angiographic study of the effect of vasopressors — epinephrine and levarterenol — on renal vascularity. Amer. J. Roentgenol. 93, 904 (1965).

ELLIOT, J. A.: Post-nephrectomy arteriovenous fistula. J. Urol. 85, 426 (1961).

ENGEL, W. J. PAGE, I. H.: Hypertension due to renal compression resulting from subcapsular hematoma. J. Urol. 73, 735 (1955).

ESCAT, J., TON THAT, H., MERIEL, P., GOUZI, J.-L., LAZORTHES, F., CONTE, J., JUSKIEWENSKI, S., SUC, J.-M.: Fistule artérioveineuse chirurgicale destinée à la réalisation d'hemodialyses périodiques par ponction veineuse. Revue de Médicine de Toulouse III, 233 (1967).

ESCH, I., KRAMMER, J.: Vorgetäuschte Stenosen im Angiogramm der Nierenarterien. Fortschr. Röntgenstr. 115, 193 (1971).

FAHR, T. in HENKE, F., LUBARSCH, O.: Handbuch der spez. pathologischen Anatomie und Histologie. Berlin, Julius Springer 1925, 6, pt. 1, 438.

FAUST, H.: Diagnose und Verlauf intrarenaler arteriovenöser Fisteln: eigene Beobachtungen nach offener Nierenbiopsie. Fortschr. Röntgenstr. 109, 729 (1968).

FAURÉ, C., VERSPYCH, R., PARIENTY, R., SALOMON, A.: Les anévrysmes du pédicule rénal. J. Radiol. Electrol. **43**, 583 (1962).

FEINBERG, S. B., GOLDBERG, M. E.: Arteriovenous communication of the kidney in a patient with hypertension. Radiology **81**, 601 (1963).

FERNSTRÖM, I., LINDBLOM, K.: Selective renal biopsy using roentgen television control. J. Urol. **88**, 709 (1962).

FLEMING, R. J., STERN, L. Z.: Multiple intraparenchymal renal aneurysms in polyarteritis nodosa. Radiology **84**, 100 (1965).

FREED, T. A., HAGER, H., VINIK, M.: Effects of intra-arterial acetylcholine on renal arteriography in normal humans. Amer. J. Roentgenol. **104**, 312 (1968).

GARRITANO, A. P., WOHL, G. T., KIRBY, C. K., PIETROLUONGO, A. L.: The roentgenographic demonstration of an arteriovenous fistula of renal vessels. Amer. J. Roentgenol. **75**, 905 (1956).

GAROFALO, F. A., BACCARANI, C. P., SASDELLI, M.: L'angiografia nelle complicanze locali degli shunts arterio-venosi e delle fistole interne. Minerva urol. **22**, 61 (1970).

GARTI, I., SIRKEN, C., SALINGER, H.: Arterial hypertension and position of the kidneys – an angiographic study. Brit. J. Radiol. **44**, 682 (1971).

— SALINGER, H.: Arterial hypertension and position of the kidneys. Brit. J. Radiol. **42**, 21 (1969).

GARUSI, G. F.: Il circolo collaterale nelle stenosi ipertensive dell'arteria renal. Radiol. clin. biol. **34**, 1 (1965).

— Collateral circulation in hypertensive stenosis of the renal artery. Radiol. clin. biol. **34**, 1 (1965).

GERSTEN, B. E., STEGMAN, C. J., BOOKSTEIN, J. J.: Antegrade flow in extrarenal arteries arising distal to renal artery stenosis. Another aid in evaluating hemodynamic significance. Radiology **98**, 93 (1971).

GEYER, J. R., POUTASSE, E. F.: Incidence of multiple renal arteries on aortography. Report of a series of 400 patients, 381 of whom had arterial hypertension. J. Amer. Med. Ass. **182**, 120 (1962).

GILL, W., MEANEY, T.: Medial fibroplasia of the renal artery. Radiology **92**, 861 (1969).

GILL, W. B., COLE, A. T., WONG, R. J.: Renovascular hypertension developing as a complication of selective renal arteriography. J. Urol. **107**, 922 (1972).

GILLENWATER, J. Y., BURROS, H. M., NACKPHAIRAJJ, S.: Varicosities of the renal pelvis and ureter. J. Urol. **90**, 37 (1963).

GILSANZ, V., ESTRADA, V., MALILLOS, E., BARRIO, E.: Transparietal renal phlebography, in the nephrotic syndrome – Renal vein thrombosis: cause or complication of the nephrotic syndrome. Angiology **22**, 431 (1971).

GLAZIER, M., LOMBARDO, L. J.: Disease of renal artery. J. Urol. **81**, 27 (1959).

GOLDBLATT, H., LYNCH, J., HANZAL, R. F., SUMMERVILLE, W. W.: Studies on experimental hypertension. J. Exp. Med. **59**, 347 (1934).

GYEPES, M. T., KAUFMAN, D. B., McINTOSH, R. M.: Excretory urography following percutaneo usrenal biopsy in children and adolescents. Radiology **99**, 159 (1971).

HAAGE, H., REHM, A.: Zum Kollateralkreislauf der Niere. Fortschr. Röntgenstr. **100**, 736 (1964).

HABIGHORST, L. V., KÖSSLING, F. K., ALBERS, P.: Die perirenalen Arterien und der Kollateralkreislauf der Niere im postmortalen Angiogramm. Fortschr. Röntgenstr. **105**, 35 (1966).

HAIMOVICI, H., ZINICOLA, N.: Experimental renal artery stenosis: Diagnostic significance of arterial hemodynamics. J. Cardiovas. Surg. **3**, 259 (1962).

HALIKIOPOULOS, H. J., BALLOU, L., McDONALD, D. F. The excretory urogram and radiographic kidney size as screening devices in hypertension of unilateral renal origin. J. Urol. **88**, 456 (1962).

HALL, R., JENKINS, J. D.: Intravenous pyelography in acute idiopathic inferior vena caval thrombosis. Brit. J. Radiol. **43**, 781 (1970).

HALPERN, M., EVANS, J. A.: Coarctation of the renal artery with "notching" of the ureter. Amer. J. Roentgenol. **88**, 159 (1962).

— FINBY, N., EVANS, J. A.: Percutaneous transfemoral renal arteriography in hypertension. Radiology **77**, 25 (1961).

— Spontaneous closure of traumatic renal arteriovenous fistulas. Amer. J. Roentgenol. **107**, 730 (1969).

— Acute renal artery embolus. A concept of diagnosis and treatment. J. Urol. **98**, 552 (1967).

HARE, W. S., KINCAID-SMITH, P.: Dissecting aneurysm of the renal artery. Radiology **97**, 255 (1970).

HARRISON, E. G., HUNT, J. C., BERNATZ, P. E.: Morphology of fibromuscular dysplasia of the renal artery in renovascular hypertension. Amer. J. Med. **43**, 97 (1967).

HARROW, B. R., SLOANE, J. A.: Aneurysm of renal artery: report of five cases. J. Urol. **81**, 35 (1959).

HARTWICH, A.: Der Blutdruck bei experimenteller Urämie und partieller Nierenausscheidung. Z. ges. exp. Med. **69**, 462 (1930).

HEITZMAN, E. R., PERCHIK, L.: Radiography features of renal infarction. Radiology **76**, 39 (1961).

HILLMAN, W., ALLEN, J., KIGER, R., THOMAS, C.: Hemodynamic changes of arteriovenous fistula demonstrated by arteriography. Surgical Forum **X**, 476 (1959).

HOOD, B., KJELLBO, H., VIKGREN, P.: Njurartärstenos och hypertoni. Sv. Läkartidn. **58**, 173 (1961).

HORNER, B. A., HUNT, J., KINCAID, O. W., DE WEERD, J. H.: Perirenal hematoma secondary to intrarenal microaneurysm of periarteritis nodosa demonstrated radiographically, Mayo Clin. Proc. **41**, 169 (1966).

HOWARD, J. E., BERTHRONG, M., GOULD, D. M., YENDT, E. R.: Hypertension resulting from unilateral renal vascular disease and its relief by nephrectomy. Bull. Johns Hopkins Hosp. **94**, 51 (1954).

HUGHES, F., BARCIA, A., FIANDRA, O., VIOLA, J.: Aneurysm of the renal artery. Acta radiol. **49**, 117 (1958).

HUNT, J. C., HARRISON jr., E. G. KINCAID, O. W., BERNATZ, P. E., DAVIS, G. D.: Idiopathic fibrous and fibromuscular stenoses of the renal arteries associated with hypertension. Proc. Staff Meetings Mayo Clinic **37**, 181 (1962).

HUNTINGTON, S. S., McCLURE, C. F.: The development of the veins in the domestic cat. Anat. Rec. **20**, 1 (1920).

HURWICH, B. J.: Brachial arteriography of the surgically created radial arteriovenous fistula in patients undergoing chronic intermittent hemodialysis by venipuncture technique. Amer. J. Roentgenol. **104**, 394 (1968).

JANEWAY, T. C.: Note on the blood pressure changes following reduction of the renal arterial circulation. Proc. Soc. exp. Biol. & Med. **6**, 109 (1909).

JANOWER, M. L., WEBER, A. L.: Radiologic evaluation of acute renal infarction. Amer. J. Roentgenol. **95**, 309 (1965).

KAMMERER, V., DEININGER, H.-K., PIEPGRAS, U.: Passagerer vollständiger Verschluß einer Nierenhauptarterie im Verlauf einer Arteriographie. Fortschr. Röntgenstr. **114**, 843 (1971).

KARANI, S., MORRIS, L., RUSSELL, I.: Angioma of the renal artery causing hypertension. Clin. Radiol. **13**, 287 (1962).

KAUDE, J., LINDSTEDT, E.: Angiographic studies in patients with Cimino-Brescia fistulae. In: Studies in therapeutic arteriovenous fistulae. Scand. J. Urol. Nephrol. Suppl. **14**, 23 (1972).

KAUFMAN, J. J., MAXWELL, M. H.: Ureteral varices. Amer. J. Roentgenol. **92**, 346 (1964).

— SCHANCHE, A. F., MAXWELL, M. H.: Excretory urography in the diagnosis of renovascular hypertension: methods of enhancing its value. J. Urol. **89**, 498 (1963).

KERK, L., BUSCHMANN, O., WILLICH, E.: Die Renovasographie im Kindesalter, Fortschr. Röntgenstr. **103**, 675 (1965).

KEY, E., ÅKERLUND, Å.: Fall von verkalkten Aneurysma in der Arteria renalis. Fortschr. Röntgenstr. **25**, 551 (1917–1918).

KINCAID, O. W., DAVIS, G. D., HALLERMANN, F. J., HUNT, J. C.: Fibromuscular dysplasia of the renal arteries. Amer. J. Roentgenol. **104**, 271 (1968).

KÖHLER, R.: Incomplete angiogram in selective renal angiography. Acta radiol. **1**, 1011 (1963).

LANG, E. K.: Arteriographic diagnosis of renal infarcts. Radiology **88**, 1110 (1967).

LEADBETTER, W. F., BURKLAND, C. E.: Hypertension in unilateral renal disease. J. Urol. **39**, 611 (1938).

LECKY, J., CRAVEN, J.: A refinement of the analysis of the rapid sequence excretory urogram in hypertensive patients – volume difference. J. Urol. **108**, 840 (1972).

LEGER, L., GEORGE, L. A.: Thrombose de la veine rénale. Presse méd. **62**, 721 (1954).

LESTER, P. D., KOEHLER, P. R.: The renal angiographic changes in scleroderma. Radiology **99**, 516 (1971).

LIEDHOLM, K.: Total vänstersidig njurinfarkt hos hjärtfrisk pojke. Nord. Med. **23**, 1530 (1944).

LINDSTEDT, E.: Use of arteriovenous shunts (external and internal) for hemodialysis. Fourth International Congress of Nephrology – Stockholm 1969, vol. **3**, 188 (Karger, Basel/München/New York 1970).

LOVE, L., MONCADA, R., LESCHER, A. J.: Renal arteriovenous fistulae. Amer. J. Roentgenol. **95**, 364 (1965).

— BUSH, I. M.: Demonstration of renal collateral arterial supply. Amer. J. Roentgenol. **104**, 296 (1968).

LJUNGGREN, E., EDSMAN, G.: Remarques sur l'artériographie rénale. Dixième Congrès de la Soc. Int. d'Urol. Athènes 10–18 Avril 1955. Vol. II, p. 140. Athènes 1956.

LUNDSTRÖM, B.: Angiographic changes following percutaneous needle biopsy of the kidney. Akademisk avhandling. University of Umeå 1971.

MacDONALD, J. S., McMILLAN, J. A.: Fibromuscular hyperplasia of the renal arteries. Clin. Radiol. **XIV**, 392 (1963).

MARSHALL, W. H., CASTELLINO, R. A.: Hypertension produced by constricting capsular renal lesions ("Page" kidney). Radiology **101**, 561 (1971).

MATHÉ, C. P.: Aneurysm of renal artery causing hypertension: report of three cases. J. Urol. **82**, 412 (1959).

MAXWELL, M. H.: Reversible renal hypertension: clinical characteristics and predictive tests. Amer. J. Cardiol. **9**, 126 (1962).

— Use of the rapid sequence intravenous pyelogram in the diagnosis of renovascular hypertension. New Engl. J. Med. **270**, 213 (1964).

McCORMACK, L. J., POUTASSE, E. F., MEANEY, T. F., NOTO, T. J., DUSTAN, H. F.: Pathologic-arteriographic correlation of renal arterial disease. Amer. Heart J. **72**, 188 (1966).

McKIEL jr., C. F., GRAF, E. C., CALLAHAN, D. H.: Renal artery aneurysms: A report of 16 cases. J. Urol. **96**, 593 (1966).

McLELLAND, R.: Renal artery aneurysms. Amer. J. Roentgenol. **78**, 256 (1957).

MEANEY, T. F., DUSTAN, H. P., McCORMACK, L. J.: Natural history of renal arterial disease. Radiology **91**, 881 (1968).

MELLINS, H. Z.: Renal vein thrombosis. Genitourinary Radiology Postgraduate Course, New York City, May 1969.

MENG, C-H., ELKIN, M.: Immediate angiographic manifestations of iatrogenic renal injury due to percutaneous needle biopsy. Radiology **100**, 335 (1971).

MÉRIEL, P., GALINIER, F., MOREAU, G., BASTIDE, G., SUC, J.-M., BOUNHOURE, J.-P.: Deux nouveaux cas de thrombose veineuse rénale avec syndrome néphrotique: Intéret diagnostique de l'association de la cavographie à la ponction-biopsie rénale. Bull. Soc. Med. Hop. **75**, 109 (1959).

MILLER, G. E., DUSTAN, H. P., PAGE, I. H.: Renal lengths vs "split function tests" in evaluating arterial stenosis. Excerpta Medica **20**, 3115 (1966).

MOLDENHAUER, W.: Nierenarterienverkalkungen. Fortschr. Röntgenstr. **90**, 522 (1959).

MORROW, I., AMPLATZ, K.: Embolic occlusion of the renal artery during aortography. Radiology **86**, 57 (1966).

MUNGER, H. V.: Renal thrombosis. J. Urol. **71**, 144 (1954).

OCKER, jr., J. M., LEBMAN, T. H., MOORE, R. J., HODGES, C. V.: Experiences with differential function studies in renal vascular hypertension. J. Urol. 91, 639 (1964).

PAGE, I. H.: Production of persistent arterial hypertension by cellophane perinephritis. J. Amer. Med. Ass. 113, 2046 (1939).

PALMER, J. M., CONNOLLY, J. E.: Intrarenal arteriovenous fistula: Surgical excision under selective renal hypothermia with kidney survival. J. Urol. 96, 599 (1966).

PALUBINSKAS, A. J., PERLOFF, D., WYLIE, E. J.: Curable hypertension due to renal artery lesions. Radiol. clin. 33, 207 (1964).

— Roentgen diagnosis of fibromuscular hyperplasia of the renal arteries. Radiology 76, 634 (1961).

PAUL, R. E., ETTINGER, A., FAINSINGER, M. H., CALLOW, A. D., KAHN, P. C., INKER, L. H.: Angiographic visualization of renal collateral circulation as a mean of detecting and delineating renal ischemia. Radiology 84, 1013 (1965).

PERLOFF, D., SOKOLOW, M., WYLIE, E. J., SMITH, D. R., PALUBINSKAS, A. J.: Hypertension secondary to renal artery occlusive disease. Circulation 24, 1286 (1961).

POKIESER, H.: Röntgendiagnostische Aufgaben im Rahmen der Nierentransplantation (mit besonderer Berücksichtigung angiographischer Untersuchungen). Fortschr. Röntgenstr. 114, 1 (1971).

POUTASSE, E. E.: Renal artery aneurysm: report of 12 cases, two treated by excision of the aneurysm and repair of renal artery. J. Urol. 77, 697 (1957).

PROVET, H., LORD, J. W., LISA, J. R.: Aneurysm of the renal artery. Amer. J. Roentgenol. 78, 266 (1957).

QUINTON, W., DILLARD, D., SCRIBNER, H.: Cannulation of blood vessels for prolonged hemodialysis. Trans. Amer. Soc. artif. intern. organs 6, 104 (1960).

RATHE, J. C.: Differential "nephropacification": A screening procedure for unilateral renal artery occlusion. Radiology 76, 629 (1961).

RENCK, G.: Über das Renalisaneurysma, besonders vom röntgenologischen Gesichtspunkt. Acta radiol. 7, 309 (1926).

RILEY, J. M.: Renal arteriovenous fistula: a complication of percutaneous renal biopsy. J. Urol. 93, 333 (1965).

DEL RIO, G.: Trombosis de la vena renal. Progr. Pat. Clin. 7 (1960).

ROSENBERG, J. C., AZCARATE, J., PULTAVITUMA, A., SILVA, Y.: Gaining access to vessels for hemodialysis: Role of angiography. Angiology 23, 427 (1972).

ROTHFIELD, N. J. H.: Experimental fibromuscular arterial dysplasia. Radiology 93, 1291 (1969).

SCHÄFER, H.: Nierenverkalkungen. Fortschr. Röntgenstr. 91, 531 (1959).

SCHEIFLEY, C. H., DAUGHERTY, G. W., GREENE, L. F., PRIESTLEY, J. T.: Arteriovenous fistula of the kidney. Circulation 19, 662 (1959).

SCHOEN, D., PAPASSOTIRIUO, V.: Die Bedeutung der Röntgendiagnostik bei perirenalen Blutungen infolge von Gerinnungsstörungen. Fortschr. Röntgenstr. 115, 747 (1971).

SCHREIBER, M. H.: Angiographic demonstration of the causes of external arteriovenous haemodialysis shunt failure. Clin. Radiol. 22, 210 (1971).

SCHULTZE-BERGMANN, G.: Über das arteriovenöse Aneurysma der Niere. Z. Urol. 47, 661 (1954).

SCHWARTZ, J. W., BORSKI, A. A., JAHNKE, E. J.: Renal arteriovenous fistula. Surgery 37, 951 (1955).

SIENIEWICZ, D. J., MOORE, S., MOIR, F. D., McDADE, D. F.: Atheromatous emboli to the kidneys. Radiology 92, 1231 (1969).

SIEGELMAN, S., CAPLAN, L. H.: Acute segmental renal artery embolism.: A distinctive urographic and arteriographic complex. Radiology 88, 509 (1967).

— Renal artery emboli and renal infarction. Genitourinary Radiology Postgraduate Course, New York City, May 1969.

SIGGERS, R. L.: Differential renal function in Goldblatt type of hypertension. Acta radiol. 56, 94 (1961).

SLOMINSKI-LAWS, M. D., KIEFER, J. H., VERMEULEN, C. W.: Arteriovenous aneurysm of the kidney: case report. J. Urol. 75, 586 (1956).

SMITH, G. I., ERICKSON, V.: Intrarenal aneurysm of the renal artery: case report. J. Urol. 77, 814 (1957).

SPROUL, R. D., FRASER, R. G., MACKINNON, K. J.: Aneurysm of the renal artery. J. Canad. Ass. Radiol. 9, 45 (1958).

SQUIRE, L. F., SCHLEGEL, J. U.: Pyelography in renal disease with hypertension. Radiology 73, 849 (1959).

STEJSKAL, R. E., STAUB, E. V., LOKEN, M. K., AMPLATZ, K.: The value of the urea washout test in the assessment of curable renovascular hypertension. Amer. J. Roentgenol. 92, 1397 (1964).

STÖSSEL, H.-G., REICH, E.: Über das arteriovenöse Aneurysma der Niere. Fortschr. Röntgenstr. 114, 17 (1971).

TAYLOR, D. A., BOYES, T. D.: Filling of a varicose left ovarian vein following retrograde pyelography: a new cause of notching of the ureter. Brit. J. Radiol. 37, 625 (1964).

— A Symposium: Evaluation of diagnostic techniques in unilateral renovascular hypertension. Proc. Tel-Hashomer Hospital, Vol. II, No. 2 (1963).

TEPLICK, J. G., YARROW, M. W.: Arterial infarction of the kidney. Ann. intern. Med. 42, 1041 (1955).

THELEN, M., FROTSCHER, U., FROMMHOLD, H., KOZUSCHEK, W.: Angiographische Darstellung von arteriovenösen Shunts bei Dialyspatienten. Fortschr. Röntgenstr. 117, 438 (1972).

THOMAS, R. G., LEVIN, N. W.: Ureteric irregularity with renal artery obstruction. A new radiological sign. Brit. J. Radiol. 34, 438 (1961).

TURNER, A. F., JACOBSON, G.: Renal arteriovenous fistula following percutaneous renal biopsy. Radiology 85, 460 (1965).

TWIGG, H. L., PRADHAN, R., PERLOFF, J. K.: Arteriovenous fistula of the renal vessels. Amer. J. Roentgenol. 88, 1148 (1962).

VARELA, M. E.: Aneurisma arteriovenoso de los vasos renales y asistolia consecutiva. Rev. méd. lat. amer. **14**, 3244 (1928/29).

VELZER, D. A. VAN, BURGE, C. H., MORRIS jr., G. C.: Arteriosclerotic narrowing of renal arteries associated with hypertension. Amer. J. Roentgenol. **86**, 807 (1961).

WHITLEY, J., WITCOFSKY, R. L., QUINN, J. L., MESCHAN, I.: The radiologic diagnosis of renovascular hypertension. Radiology **78**, 414 (1962).

VIDAL, B., ENGLARO, G. C.: Sopra un non commune reperto radiografico: la calcificazione dell'arteria renale. Radiol. Med. (Torino) **46**, 282 (1960).

WÓJTOWICZ, J.: Relationship of the surface of the kidney to the size of the renal artery. Investigative Radiology **2**, 231 (1967).

WESTERBORN, A.: Embolie in der Arteria renalis. Z. Urol. **21**, 687 (1937).

YENDT, E. R., KERR, W. K., WILSON, D. R., JAWORSKI, Z. F.: The diagnosis and treatment of renal hypertension. Amer. J. Med. **28**, 169 (1960).

YOUNG jr., J. D., KISER, W. S.: Obstruction of the lower ureter by aberrant blood vessels. J. Urol. **94**, 101 (1965).

ZEITLER, E.: Angiographische Probleme zur Diagnostik und Therapie der renovasculären Hypertonie. Der Radiologe **11**, 43 (1971).

J. Injury to the kidneys and the urinary tract

ADAMS, P.: Traumatic rupture of the kidney. Amer. J. Surg. **61**, 316 (1943).

ANZILOTTI, A.: Late results of a severe injury of the kidney. Radiol. med. (Torino) **26**, 144 (1939).

BAICHWAL, K. S., WAUGH, D.: Traumatic renal artery thrombosis. J. Urol. **99**, 14 (1968).

BAIRD, H. H., JUSTIS, H. R.: Surgical injuries of the ureter and bladder. J. Amer. Med. Ass. **162**, 1357 (1956).

BANKS jr., R.: Spontaneous rupture of the kidney. South. Med. J. **47**, 1079 (1954).

BARETZ, L. H.: Rupture of the kidney following pyelography. J. Amer. Med. Ass. **106**, 980 (1936).

BECKLY, D. E., WATERS, E. A.: Avulsion of the pelviureteric junction — a rare consequence of non-penetrating trauma. Brit. J. Radiol. **45**, 423 (1972).

BRAEDEL, H. U., HERAVI, P., LÜBKE, P.: Funktionelle und morphologische Beobachtungen am Gegefäßsystem bei Nierenverletzungen: eine experimentelle Studie. Fortschr. Röntgenstr. **114**, 777 (1971).

CAPEK, V., FOJTIK, F.: The significance of selective renal angiography in injuries of the kidney in childhood. Amer. J. Roentgenol. **90**, 75 (1963).

CARLTON jr., C. E., SCOTT jr., R.: Penetrating renal injuries: an analysis of 100 cases. J. Urol. **84**, 599 (1960).

CASS, A., IRELAND, G.: Comparison of the conservative and surgical management of the more severe degrees of renal trauma in multiple injured patients. J. Urol. **109**, 8 (1973).

CIBERT, J. A. V., CAVAILHER, H.: Hématomes spontanés périrénaux. J. Urol. méd. chir. **50**, 65 (1942).

CLARKE, H.: Spontaneous rupture of the kidney pelvis. Brit. J. Urol. **27**, 162 (1955).

COLSTON, J. A. C., BAKER, W. W.: Late effects of various types of trauma to the kidney. Arch. Surg. (Chicago) **34**, 99 (1937).

DAVIES, J. A., TOMSKEY, G. C.: Shell fragment injuries of the kidney. J. Urol. **83**, 535 (1960).

DENIS et PLANCHAIS cit. M. F. LEGUEU: Rupture traumatique a une hydronéphrose. Bull. Soc. Chir. Paris **35**, 382 (1909).

DRUCKMANN, A., SCHORR, S.: Roentgenographic observation of perforation of the kidney following retrograde pyelography. J. Urol. **61**, 1028 (1949).

DUCHAMP, J., BARGY, P., TOUITOU, C., VAQUIER, P.: Considérations sur lévolution des signes radiologiques dans les contusions rénales chez l'enfant. J. Radiol. Électrol. **41**, 92 (1960).

EKMAN, H.: Displacement of the kidney consequent upon spontaneous perirenal hematoma. Acta chir. scand. **93**, 531 (1946).

ELKIN, M., MENG, C.-H., DE PAREDES, R. G.: Correlation of intravenous urography and renal angiography in kidney injury. Radiology **86**, 496 (1966).

ENGEL, W. J., PAGE, I. H.: Hypertension due to renal compression resulting from subcapsular hematoma. J. Urol. **73**, 735 (1955).

ETTINGER, A., PAUL, R. E.: The role of intravenous urography in ureteral fistulas: The value of delayed films. Radiology **79**, 285 (1962).

FORSYTHE, W. E., HUFFMAN, W. L., SCHILDT, P. J., PERSKY, L.: Spontaneous extravasation during urography. J. Urol. **80**, 393 (1958).

FRIEDENBERG, R. M., NEY, C., ELKIN, M.: Trauma to the ureter. Amer. J. Roentgenol. **90**, 28 (1963).

FROST, B.: Selektive renale Angiographie bei Nierenruptur. Fortschr. Röntgenstr. **96**, 260 (1962).

GOLDSTEIN, A. G., CONGER, K. B.: Perforation of the ureter during retrograde pyelography. J. Urol. **94**, 658 (1965).

GYEPES, M. T., KAUFAM, D. B., McINTOSH, R. M.: Excretory urography following percutaneous renal biopsy in children and adolescents. Radiology **99**, 159 (1971).

HALPERN, M.: Angiography in renal trauma. Surg. Clinics of N. Amer. **48**, 1221 (1968).

HAMMEL, H.: Subcutane Nierenverletzung und Ausscheidungsurographie. Z. urol. Chir. **41**, 502 (1936).

HAREIDE, I.: Über die Röntgenuntersuchung bei Nierenverletzungen unter besonderer Berücksichtigung der intravenösen Urographie. Acta radiol. **21**, 292 (1940).

HARROW, B. R., SLOANE, J. A.: Nontraumatic perirenal hemorrhages. Sth. Med. J. **57**, 363 (1964).

HÄRTEL, M., FUCHS, W. A., WICKY, B.: Röntgendiagnostik des Nierentrauma. Fortschr. Röntgenstr. **116**, 110 (1972).

HEMLEY, S. D., FINBY, N.: Renal trauma. Radiology **79**, 816 (1962).

HERMAN, J., MELLY, B.: Abrodillel végzett intravenás pyelographiáról. Orv. Hétil. **75**, 1—5 (1931). Ref. Z. Urol. **27**, 510 (1933).

HODGES, C. V., GILBERT, D. R., SCOTT, W. W.: Renal trauma; study of 71 cases. J. Urol. **66**, 627 (1951).

INCLÁN BOLADO, J. L., CORRAL CASTANEDO, J.: Fracturas de rinon. Estudio clinico. Arch. esp. Urol. **13**, 135 (1957).

JASIENSKI, G.: Sur un cas d'hématomie périrénal spontané chez un hémophile. J. Urol. méd. chir. **44**, 487 (1937).

JEPPESEN, F. B.: Spontaneous rupture of the kidney. J. Urol. **86**, 489 (1961).

JEVTICH, M. J., MONTERO, G.: Injuries to renal vessels by blunt trauma in children. J. Urol. **102**, 493 (1969).

JONES, R. F.: Surgical management of transcapsular rupture of the kidney: 24 cases. J. Urol. **74**, 721 (1955).

KAIJSER, R.: Über das sog. spontane perirenale Hämatom. Upsala Läk.-Fören. Förh. **44**, 283 (1938/39).

KEMM, N.: Rupture of the kidney: delayed symptoms; operation; recovery. Brit. med. J. **1923 II**, 1218.

KITTREDGE, W. E., CRAWLEY, J. R.: Surgical renal lesions associated with pregnancy. J. Amer. med. Ass. **162**, 1353 (1956).

KÖHLER, R.: Investigations on backflow in retrograde pyelography. Acta radiol. Suppl. **99** (1953).

KRAHN, H., AXENROD, H.: The management of severe renal lacerations. J. Urol. **109**, 11 (1973).

LAMESCH, A.: Die Bedeutung der Angiographie bei Nierenruptur. Langenbecks Arch. Klin. Chir. **305**, 168 (1964).

LANG, E. K., TRICHEL, B. E., TURNER, R. W., FONTENOT, R., REED, A., JOHNSON, B., MARTIN, E. C. ST. Arteriographic assessment of injury resulting from renal trauma: an analysis of 74 patients. J. Urol. **106**, 1 (1971).

— — — — JOHNSON, B., MARTIN, E. C. ST: Renal arteriography in the assessment of renal trauma. Radiology **98**, 103 (1971).

LARSEN, K. A., PEDERSEN, A.: Spontaneous rupture of the kidney pelvis. J. Oslo City Hosp. **5**, 121 (1955).

LEFKOVITS, A. M.: Fatal air embolism during presacral insufflation of air. J. Urol. **77**, 112 (1957).

LEVANT, B., FELDMAN, B.: Traumatic rupture of Wilms' tumor. J. Urol. **67**, 629 (1952).

LISKA, J. R.: Recognition and management of trauma to kidney. J. Urol. **78**, 525 (1957).

LJUNGGREN, E.: Die Bedeutung der Pyelographie bei subkutanen Nierenverletzungen. Z. Urol. **30**, 650 (1936).

LOCKARD, V. M.: Lesions of the upper gastro-intestinal tract in infants and children. Radiology **58**, 696 (1952).

LOPEZ, F.: Pelvicalyceal extravasations. Amer. J. Roentgenol. **112**, 593 (1971).

LOWSLEY, O. S., MENNING, J. H.: Treatment of the ruptured kidney. J. Urol. **45**, 253 (1941).

LUNDSTRÖM, B.: Angiographic changes following percutaneous needle biopsy of the kidney. Univ. of Umeå (Sweden) avhandling 1971.

LYNCH jr., K. M.: Management of the injured kidney: preliminary report. J. Urol. **60**, 371 (1948).

— Traumatic urinary injuries: pitfalls in diagnosis and treatment. J. Urol. **77**, 90 (1957).

— LARGE jr., H. L.: Post-traumatic ischemic infarction of the kidney due to arteriospasm. Sth. Med. J. (Birmingham, Alabama) **44**, 600 (1951).

MALCHIODI, C., REGGIANI, G., BERTI-RIBOLI, E. P., CERRUTI, G. B.: L'Angiographia nella diagnostica urologia. Ed. Minerva Medica (Torino) (1957).

MARQUARDT, H. D.: Zur Methodik der Röntgenuntersuchung der Harnorgane. Medizinische **8**, 316 (1958).

McKAY, H. W., BAIRD, H. H., LYNCH jr., K. M.: Management of the injured kidney. J. Amer. med. Ass. **141**, 575 (1949).

MENG, C., ELKIN, M.: Immediate angiographic manifestations of iatrogenic renal injury due to percutaneous needle biopsy. Radiology **100**, 335 (1971).

MERTZ, H. O.: Injury of the kidney in children. J. Urol. **69**, 39 (1953).

MILLER, J. A., CORDONNIER, J. J.: Spontaneous perirenal hematoma associated with hypertension. J. Urol. **62**, 13 (1949).

MORROW, J., MENDEZ, R.: Renal trauma. J. Urol. **104**, 649 (1970).

MUTZENBACH, P., MAURER, P.: Angiographische Differenzierung des akuten Nierentrauma. Fortschr. Röntgenstr. **3**, 374 (1969).

NATION, E. F., MASSEY, B. D.: Renal trauma: experience with 258 cases. J. Urol. **89**, 775 (1963).

NAVAS, J.: Contusion renal y litiasis. Arch. Español. Urol. **12**, 96 (1956).

NILSSON, J., SANDBERG, N.: Healing of kidney injuries. Acta chir. scand. **123**, 228 (1962).

O'CONOR, V. J.: Immediate management of the injured ureter. J. Amer. Med. Ass. **162**, 1201 (1956).

OLSSON, OLLE, LUNDERQUIST, A.: Angiography in renal trauma. Acta radiol. **1**, 1 (1963).

— Trauma. In: Diseases of the kidney. Ed. by M. B. Strauss & L. G. Welt. Boston: Little, Brown & Co. 1971 (page 174).

ORKIN, L. A.: Evaluation of the merits of cystoscopy and retrograde pyelography in the management of renal trauma. J. Urol. **63**, 9 (1950).

OSTRUM, B. J., SODER, P. D.: Periarteritis nodosa complicated by spontaneous perinephric hematoma. Amer. J. Roentgenol. **84**, 849 (1960).

OVERGAARD, K.: A case of internal uroplania. Acta radiol. **17**, 542 (1936).

PALAVATANA, C., GRAHAM, S. R., SILVERMAN, F. N.: Delayed sequels to renal injury in childhood. Amer. J. Roentgenol. **91**, 659 (1964).

POLLACK, H., POPKY, G.: Spontaneous subcapsular renal hemorrhage: its significance and roentgenographic diagnosis. J. Urol. **108**, 530 (1972).

PRIESTLEY, J. T., PILCHER, F.: Traumatic lesions of the kidney. Amer. J. Surg. **40**, 357 (1938).

RENANDER, A.: Another case of spontaneous rupture of the renal pelvis. Acta radiol. **22**, 422 (1941).

RITVO, M., STEARNS, D. B.: Roentgendiagnosis of contusions of the kidney. J. Amer. med. Ass. **109**, 1101 (1937).

ROSS jr., R., ACKERMAN, E., PIERCE jr., J. M.: Traumatic subintimal hemorrhage of the renal artery. J. Urol. **104**, 11 (1970).

SARGENT, J. C., MARQUARDT, C. R.: Renal injuries. J. Urol. **63**, 1 (1950).

SCHOEN, D., PAPASSOTIRIOU, P.: Die Bedeutung der Röntgendiagnostik bei perirenalen Blutungen infolge von Gerinnungsstörungen. Fortschr. Röntgenstr. **115**, 747 (1971).

SCOTT jr., R., CARLTON, C. E., ASHMORE, A. J., DUKE, H. H.: Initial management of non-penetrating renal injuries: clinical review of 111 cases. J. Urol. **90**, 535 (1963).

— CARLTON jr., C. E., GOLDMAN, M.: Penetrating injuries of the kidney: an analysis of 181 patients. J. Urol. **101**, 247 (1969).

SIMON, O.: Das Hämatom des Nierenlagers im Röntgenbild. Fortschr. Röntgenstr. **59**, 178 (1939).

STAEHLER, W.: Klinik und Praxis der Urologie. Stuttgart: Georg Thieme 1959.

STEINBOCK, A.: Intravenous urography and retrograde pyelography in subcutaneous injuries of kidney. Ann. Chir. Gynaec. Fenn. **37**, Suppl. 4 (1948).

STRNAD, F.: Nierenperforation und pyelovenöser Reflux. Fortschr. Röntgenstr. **53**, 175 (1936).

TRUETA, J., BARCLAY, A. E., DANIEL, P. M., FRANKLIN, K. J., PRICHARD, M. M. L.: Studies of the renal circulation. Oxford: Blackwell scientific publications 1947.

USON, A. C., KNAPPENBERGER, S. T., MELICOW, M. M.: Nontraumatic perirenal hematomas: a report based on 7 cases. J. Urol. **81**, 388 (1959).

VANDENDORP, F., LEMAITRE, G., DU BOIS, R.: L'Angiographie dans les contusions du rein. J. Radiol. Electrol. **46**, 344 (1965).

VOEGELI, E., SAXER, R.: Nierenhämatome bei Antikoagulantientherapie. Fortschr. Röntgenstr. **117**, 187 (1972).

VOGLER, E., BERGMANN, M.: Angiographie bei stumpfen Nierentraumen. Fortschr. Röntgenstr. **98**, 675 (1963).

WALKER, J. A.: Injuries of the ureter due to external violence. J. Urol. **102**, 410 (1969).

WATNICK, M., SPINDOLA-FRANCO, H., ABRAMS, H. L.: Small hypernephroma with subcapsular hematoma and renal infarction. J. Urol. **108**, 534 (1972).

WILLIAMS, R. D., ZOLLINGER, R. M.: Diagnostic and prognostic factors in abdominal trauma. Amer. J. Surg. **97**, 575 (1959).

WOODRUFF jr., J. H., COCKETT, R. T. K., CANNON, R., SWANSON, L. E.: Radiologic aspects of renal trauma with the emphasis on arteriography and renal isotope scanning. J. Urol. **97**, 184 (1967).

— OTTOMAN, R. E., SIMONTON, J. H., AVERBROOK, B. D.: The radiologic differential diagnosis of abdominal trauma. Radiology **72**, 641 (1959).

YDÉN, S.: Cyst rupture in 6 cases of polycystic renal disease. Acta radiol. **42**, 17 (1954).

K. Dilatation of the urinary tract

ALLEN, R. P., CONDON, V. R., COLLINS, R. E.: Multilocular cystic hydronephrosis secondary to congenital (ureteropelvic junction) obstruction. Radiology **80**, 203 (1963).

ANDERSON, J. C.: Hydronephrosis and hydrocalycosis. In: E. W. RICHES: Modern Trends in Urology (page 96). London: Butterworth & Co. (1953).

BAKER, E. C., LEWIS jr., J. S.: Comparison of the urinary tract in pregnancy and pelvic tumors. J. Amer. med. Ass. **104**, 812 (1935).

BAUER, K. M.: Das Rücklaufzystogramm. Medizinische **1**, 47 (1957).

BENJAMIN, J. A., BETHEIL, J. J., EMMEL, V. M., RAMSEY, G. H., WATSON, J. S.: Observations on ureteral obstruction and contractility in man and dog. J. Urol. **75**, 25 (1956).

BERGENDAL, S.: Zur Frage der Hydronephrose bei Nierengefäßvarianten. Acta chir. scand. Suppl. **45** (1936).

BISCHOFF, P.: Mißbildungen und Entleerungsstörungen der oberen Harnwege im Kindesalter. Verhandlungsber. der Dtsch. Ges. für Urologie, S. 29. Leipzig 1958.

BLIGH, A. S.: Pyelographic changes in pregnancy. Brit. J. Radiol. **30**, 489 (1957).

BOHNE, A. W., URWILLER, R. D., PANTOS, T. G.: Routine intravenous urograms prior to prostatectomy. J. Urol. **86**, 171 (1961).

BOIJSEN, E.: Angiographic studies of the anatomy of single and multiple renal arteries. Acta radiol. Suppl. **183** (1959).

BRAASCH, W. F., EMMETT, J. L.: Excretory urography as a test of renal function. J. Urol. **35**, 630 (1936).

— Clinical Urology. Philadelphia & London: W. B. Saunders Co. 1951.

— MUSSEY, R. D.: Complications in the urinary tract during pregnancy. Minn. Med. **28**, 543 (1945).

BUCHMANN, E.: Ureterstenosierung und Hydronephrosenbildung durch Krebsinfiltration und Strahleninduration des Parametriums beim Collumcarcinom. Strahlentherapie **99**, 20 (1956).

CAMPBELL, M.: Clinical pediatric urology. Philadelphia and London: W. B. Saunders Co. 1951.

CASEY, W. C., GOODWIN, W. E.: Percutaneous antegrade pyelography and hydronephrosis. J. Urol. **74**, 164 (1955).

CERNY, J., SCOTT, T.: Non-idiopathic retroperitoneal fibrosis. J. Urol. **105**: 1, 49 (1971).

CONTIADES, X.-J.: A propos de l'origine hormonale de la stase urinaire gravidique. 37. Congr. franc. d'Urol. Paris 1937, p. 473.

COVINGTON jr., T., REESER, W.: Hydronephrosis associated with overhydration. J. Urol. **63**, 438 (1950).

CRABTREE, E. G., PRATHER, G. C., PRIEN, E. L.: End-results of urinary tract infections associated with pregnancy. Amer. J. Obstet. Gynec **34**, 405 (1937).

CRUVEILHIER: Zit. F. HOFF, Der Schwangerschaftsureter. Beilageheft zu Z. Geburtsh. Gynäk. **125** (1945).

CUKIER, D. S., EPSTEIN, B. S.: The reversal of hydronephrosis due to extrinsic ureteral pressure from pelvic masses in women. Radiology **78**, 68 (1962).

ECKERBOM, H., LILIEQUIST, B.: Ectopic ureter. Acta radiol. **38**, 420 (1952).

EDELBROCK, H. H.: Ureterovesical obstruction in children. J. Urol. **74**, 492 (1955).

EDSMAN, G.: Accessory vessels of the kidney and their diagnosis in hydronephrosis. Acta radiol. **42**, 26 (1954).

ERICSSON, N. O.: Ectopic ureterocele in infants and children. Acta chir. scand. Suppl. **197** (1954).

FALK, D.: Intermittent obstruction at the ureteropelvic juncture. J. Urol. **79**, 16 (1958).

FETTER, T. R., WARREN, K. C.: Congenital urinary tract obstructions in children. J. Urol. (Baltimore) **75**, 173 (1956).

FINLAY jr., A. M.: Importance of the postvoiding film in pediatric excretory urography. Tex. St. J. Med. **53**, 781 (1957).

FRIEDBERG, V.: Njure och graviditet. Med. documentation CIBA-GEIGY (Basel) 1963.

GIBSON, TH. E.: Hydronephrosis: diagnosis and treatment of ureteropelvic obstructions. J. Urol. **75**, 1 (1956).

GOLDMAN, H. J., GLICKMAN, S. I.: Ureteral obstruction in regional ileitis. J. Urol. **88**, 616 (1962).

GOODWIN, W. E., CASEY, W. C., WOOLF, W.: Percutaneous trocar (needle) nephrostomy in hydronephrosis. Jr. Amer. Med. Assoc. **157**, 891 (1955).

— — Percutaneous antegrade pyelography and translumbar needle nephrostomy in hydronephrosis. Amer. Med. Assoc. Archives of Surgery **72**, 357 (1956).

GOVAN, D. E.: Experimental hydronephrosis. J. Urol. **85**, 432 (1961).

GRAF, R. A., SMITH, J. H., FLOCKS, R. H., VAN EPPS, E. V.: Urinary tract changes associated with spina bifida and myelomeningocele. Amer. J. Roentgenol. **92**, 255 (1964).

GRAHAM, J. B.: Recovery of kidney after ureteral obstruction. J. Amer. Med. Ass. **181**: 11, 993 (1962).

GREENE, L. F., PRIESTLEY, J. T., SIMON, H. B., HEMPSTEAD, R. H.: Obstruction of the lower third of the ureter by anomalous blood vessels. J. Urol. **71**, 544 (1954).

GUYER, P. B., DELANY, D.: Urinary tract dilatation and oral contraceptives. Brit. Med. J. **4**, 588 (1970).

HANDEL, J., SCHWARTZ, S.: Value of the prone position for filling the obstructed ureter in the presence of hydronephrosis. Radiology **71**, 102 (1958).

HARTMANN, G.: Ein Beitrag zur Angiographie der sog. einseitigen funktionslosen Niere. Z. Urol. **52**, 161 (1959).

— Die Bedeutung der Angiographie für Diagnostik und Therapie der sogenannten funktionslosen Niere. Münch. med. Wschr. **101**, 1264 (1959).

HERMANN, J. V., KRAUS, A. F.: Zur Indikationsstellung der Prostatektomie auf Grund der Ausscheidungsurographie. Z. urol. Chir. **41**, 441 (1936).

HOFF, F.: Der Schwangerschaftsureter. Ein experimenteller Beitrag zum Nachweis seiner Entstehung. Beilageheft Z. Geburtsh. **125** (1945).

HOLDER, E.: Die mechanische Hydronephrose und ihre Fähigkeit zur Rückbildung im Experiment. Ergebn. Chir. Orthop. **40**, 266 (1956).

HUTTER, K.: Zur Röntgendarstellung von Beckengefäßen bei urologischen Fällen. Acta radiol. **16**, 94 (1935).

IDBOHRN, H., MUREN, A.: Renal blood flow in experimental hydronephrosis. Acta physiol. scand. **38**, 200 (1956).

— SJÖSTEDT, S.: Ectopic ureter not causing incontinence until adult life. Acta obstet. gynec. scand. **33**, 457 (1954).

KEATES, P. G.: Physical, physiological and hormonal aspects of hydronephrosis. J. Fac. Radiol. (Lond.) **6**, 123 (1954).

JEWELL, J. H., BUCHERT, W. I.: Unilateral hereditary hydronephrosis: a report of four cases in three consecutive generations. J. Urol. **88**, 129 (1962).

KAUPPILA, A., PIETILÄ, K., KONTTURI, M.: Simultaneous uterine phlebography and retrograde pyelography: a method for investigating ureteric dilatation following pregnancy. Brit. J. of Radiol. **45**: 535, 496 (1972).

KENDALL, A. R., KARAFIN, L.: Intermittent hydronephrosis: hydration pyelography. J. Urol. **98**: 6, 653 (1967).

KJELLBERG, S. R., ERICSSON, N. O., RUDHE, U.: The lower urinary tract in childhood. Stockholm: Almqvist & Wiksell 1957.

KRETSCHMER, H. L., SQUIRE, F. H.: The incidence and extent of hydronephrosis in prostatic obstruction. J. Urol. **60**, 1 (1948).

LICH jr., R.: The obstructed ureteropelvic junction. Radiology **68**, 337 (1957).

— BARNES, M. L.: A clinicopathologic study of ureteropelvic obstructions. J. Urol. **77**, 382 (1957).

— MAURER, J. E., BARNES, M. L.: Pyelectasis. J. Urol. **75**, 12 (1956).

LIEDBERG, N.: Die Urographie als Untersuchungsmethode vor der Prostatektomie. Lund: Håkan Ohlssons förlag 1941.

LINDBLOM, K.: Roentgenographic studies of hydronephrosis due to obstruction at the ureteropelvic junction. Acta radiol. **32**, 113 (1949).

MALUF, N. S. R.: A method for relief of upper ureteral obstruction within bifurcation of renal artrey. J. Urol. **75**, 229 (1956).

MARCEL, J.-E., MONIN, G.: Complications urinaires hautes après curie et roentgenthérapie pour cancer du col utérin. J. Urol. méd. chir. **61**, 249 (1955).

MARSHALL, S., LYON, R., MINKLER, D.: Ureteral dilatation following use of oral contraceptives. J. Amer. Med. Assoc. **198**, 782 (1966).

MARTIN, C. L.: Ureteral obstruction in stage III cancer of the cervix relieved by low intensity radium needle implantation. Amer. J. Roentgenol. **85**, 479 (1961).

MELNICK, G., BRANWIT, D.: Bilateral ovarian vein syndrome. Amer. J. Roentgenol. **113**: 3, 509 (1971).

MINDER, J.: Über den diagnostischen und klinischen Wert der Ausscheidungspyelographie. Z. ur. Chir. Gynäk. **42**, 312 (1936).

MONCADA, R., WANG, J. J., LOVE, L., BUSH, I.: Neonatal ascites associated with urinary outlet obstruction (urine ascites). Radiology **90**, 1165 (1968).

MUANGMAN, V., UEHLING, D.: Hydronephrosis secondary to vaginal atresia. J. Urol. **106**, 140 (1971).

NESBIT, R. M.: Diagnosis of intermittent hydronephrosis: importance of pyelography during episodes of pain. J. Urol. **75**, 767 (1956).

NEUHAUSER, E. B. D., O'CONNOR, J. F.: Total body opacification in conventional and high dose intravenous urography in infants. Book of Abstracts, Xth Int'l Congr. Radiol. Montreal 1962 (page 320).

NILSSON, J.: Ektopisk ureter. Nord. med. **68**, 1132 (1962).

O'CONNOR, V. J.: Diagnosis and treatment of hydronephrosis. Trans. Amer. Ass. gen.-urin. Surg. **46**, 103 (1954).

OLSSON, OLLE: Angiography as a test of renal function. Continuation course in urologic radiology for radiologists. Univ. of Minnesota (Minneapolis), 1961. Class notes pages 336–339.

— Postpartum persistence of slight, right-sided dilatation of the renal pelvis and the ureter. Indian J. Radiol. 1 (1956).

— Urinary tract dilatation. In: Diseases of the kidney. Edited by M. B. Strauss & L. G. Welt. Boston: Little, Brown & Co. 1971 (page 169).

ORMOND, J. K.: Idiopathic retroperitoneal fibrosis: a discussion of the etiology J. Urol. 94, 385 (1965).

ÖSTLING, K.: Röntgenologische und pathologisch-anatomische Veränderungen bei Erweiterungen einzelner Nierenkelche. Acta radiol. 15, 28 (1934).

— The genesis of hydronephrosis. Acta chir. scand. Suppl. 72 (1942).

PELLEGRINO, A., GIUDICELLI, P.: L'urographie intra-veineuse dans la bilharziose urinaire. J. Radiol. Electrol. 39, 599 (1958).

PERSKY, L., BONTE, F. J., AUSTEN, G.: Mechanisms of hydronephrosis: radioautographic backflow patterns. J. Urol. 75, 190 (1956).

PETKOVIĆ, S.: Versuche zur Behandlung des Mega-ureters. Verhandlungsber. der Dtsch. Ges. für Urologie, S. 69, Leipzig 1958.

PONTI, C. DE, POGGI, U.: Rilievi clinico-radiologici sui vasi anomali renali. Nunt. radiol. (Firenze) 23, 702 (1957).

PUGI, U., JACOBI, H.: Über „fixierte" Schwangerschaftsatonie des Ureters. Z. urol. Chir. 35, 384 (1932).

RABINOWITZ, J. G., PRESENT, D. H., BANKS, P. A., JANOWITZ, H. D.: The roentgenographic features of ureteral obstruction secondary to granulomatous disease of the bowel. Clin. radiol. 22: 2, 205 (1971).

RENERT, W. A., BERDON, W., BAKER, D., ROSE, J.: Obstructive urologic malformations of the fetus and infant-relation to neonatal pneumomediastinum and pneumothorax (airblock). Radiology 105: 1, 97 (1972).

ROBERTSON, H. E.: Hydronephrosis and pyelitis of pregnancy. Philadelphia & London: W. B. Saunders Co. (1944).

ROLLESTON, G. L., REAY, E. R.: The pelvi-ureteric junction. Brit. J. Radiol. 30, 617 (1957).

ROMINGER, C. J., FLANDREAU, R. H., McGINNIS, F. T., SCHNALL, C.: Ureteral obstruction from regional enteritis. Amer. J. Roentgenol. 86, 114 (1961).

ROONEY, D. R.: Post-voiding films as an aid to opacifying the obstructed ureter. J. Urol. 84, 300 (1960).

ROSE, R. S., SMITH, J. P.: Hydronephrosis in infants with meningomyelocele: its early recognition. J. Urol. 90, 129 (1963).

SCHEWE, E. J., SALA, J. M.: Bilateral ureteral obstruction complicating the treatment of carcinoma of the cervix. Amer. J. Roentgenol. 81, 125 (1959).

SCORER, C. G., FINLAY, H. V. L.: Massive unilateral hydronephrosis in early infancy. Brit. J. Surg. 49, 144 (1961).

SENG, M. I.: Dilatation of the ureters and renal pelvis in pregnancy. J. Urol. 21, 475 (1929).

SHARP, R. F.: Hydronephrosis: development of present concept of management. J. Urol. 85, 206 (1961).

SIEGELMAN, S., BOSNIAK, M. A.: Renal arteriography in hydronephrosis, its value in diagnosis and management. Radiology 85: 4, 609 (1965).

SPJUT, H. J., NICOLAI, C. H.: The nonvisualizing kidney: a pathologic study of 83 nephrectomy specimens. J. Urol. 85, 115 (1961).

STIRLING, W. C.: Massive hydronephrosis complicated by hydro-ureter. J. Urol. 42, 520 (1939).

SWYNGEDAUW, J., WEMEAU, L., FLEURY, M., HÉRENT, J.: Les complications urinaires du traitement radio-thérapique du cancer du col utérin. J. Radiol. Electrol. 39, 618 (1958).

TRAUT, H. F., McLANE, C. M., KUDER, A.: Physiologic changes in the ureter associated with pregnancy. Surg. Gynec. Obstet. 64, 51 (1937).

TROELL, A.: Intravenöse Pyelographie zur Prüfung der Nierenfunktion bei Prostatikern. Chirurg 7, 513 (1935).

USON, A. C., JOHNSON, D. W., LATTIMER, J. K., MELICOW, M. M.: A classification of the urographic patterns in children with congenital bladder neck obstruction. Amer. J. Roentgenol. 80, 590 (1958).

WAGENEN, G. VAN, JENKINS, R. H.: An experimental examination of factors causing ureteral dilatation of pregnancy. J. Urol. 42, 1010 (1939).

WALL, B., WACHTER, H. E.: Congenital ureteral valve: its role as a primary obstructive lesion: classification of the literature and report of an authentic case. J. Urol. 68, 684 (1952).

WIDÉN, T.: Renal angiography during and after unilateral ureteric occlusion. Acta radiol. Suppl. 162 (1958).

WILHELM, G.: Beitrag zur Röntgendiagnostik der Hydronephrose durch Lagewechsel beim i.v. Pyelogramm. Fortschr. Röntgenstr. 84, 628 (1956).

— X-rays during pregnancy. J. Amer. Med. Assoc. 153, 218 (1953).

WOLFROMM, M. G.: Conclusions du forum. Sur le rein silencieux en urographie. 48 Congr. Français d'Urologie, Paris 1954 (pages 201–220).

YOUNG jr., J. D., KISER, W. S.: Obstruction of the lower ureter by aberrant blood vessels. J. Urol. 94, 101 (1965).

ZIMSKIND, P. D., FETTER, T. R., LEWIS, P. L.: Recovery from prolonged experimental ureteral occlusion: a radiologic study. J. Urol. 88, 731 (1962).

L. Generalized diseases of the renal parenchyma

ABESHOUSE, B. S., SALIK, J. O.: Pyelographic diagnosis of lesions of the renal papillae and calyces in cases of hematuria. Amer. J. Roentgenol. 80, 569 (1958).

ALEXANDER, J. C.: Pneumopyonephrosis in diabetes mellitus. J. Urol. 45, 570 (1941).

ALKEN, C. E.: Die Papillennekrose. Z. Urol. 32, 433 (1938).

ALLEN, A. C.: The kidney. In: Medical and surgical diseases. New York: Grune & Stratton 1951 (page 504).

ALWALL, N., NORVITT, L., STEINS, A. M.: On the artifical kidney. VII. Clinical experiences of dialytic treatment of uremia. Acta med. scand. 132, 587 (1949).

AMAR, A. D.: Simple ureterocele at the distal end of a blind-ending ureter. J. Urol. 106, 423 (1971).

ANHALT, M., CAWOOD, C. D., SCOTT, R.: Xanthogranulomatous pyelonephritis: a comprehensive review with report of four additional cases. J. Urol. 105, 10 (1971).

ATALA, A., ZAHER, M. F.: Biharzial calcification of the renal capsule: a case report. J. Urol. 101, 125 (1969).

AVNET, N. L., ROBERTS, T. W., GOLDBERG, H. R.: Tumefactive xanthogranulomatous pyelonephritis. Amer. J. Roentgenol. 90, 89 (1963).

AXELSON, U.: Papillitis necroticans renalis och hemolytisk anemi hos fenazonmissbrukare. Nord. Med. 59, 903 (1958).

BABICS, A.: Acute renal insufficiency of subrenal origin: results of the use of the artifical kidney. Soc. int. d'Urol. XIII Congr., London 1964 (page 280).

BARDEN, R. P.: Reflections of disease in the pulmonary medulla. Radiol. 75, 454 (1960).

BARTLEY, O., BENGTSSON, U., STATTIN, S.: Urography in relation to renal function. Acta radiol. 7, 289 (1968).

BASS, H. E., GREENBERG, D., SINGER, E., MILLER, M. A.: Pulmonary changes in uremia. J. Amer. Med. Ass. 148, 724 (1952).

BECK, R. E., HAMMOND, R. C.: Renal and osseous manifestation of tuberous sclerosis: a case report. J. Urol. 77, 578 (1957).

BELL, E. T.: Renal diseases. Philadelphia: Lea & Febiger 1950 (p. 295).

BENNETT, W. H.: Malakoplakia of the urinary tract. Urol. 70, 84 (1913).

BESEMANN, E. F.: Renal leukoplakia. Radiology 88, 872 (1967).

BOIJSEN, E: Angiographic studies of the anatomy of single and multiple renal arteries. Acta radiol. Suppl. 183, 1959.

BORGSTRÖM, K.-E., ISING, U., LINDER, E., LUNDERQUIST, A.: Experimental pulmonary edema. Acta radiol. 54, 97 (1960).

BRAASCH, W. F., EMMETT, J.: Clinical Urology. Philadelphia & London: W. B. Saunders Co. 1951.

— MERRICKS, J. W.: Clinical and radiological data associated with congenital and acquired single kidney. Surg. Gynec. Obstet. 67, 281 (1938).

BRANNAN, H. M., McCAUGHEY, W. T. E., GOOD, C. A.: The roentgenographic appearance of pulmonary hemorrhage associated with glomerulonephritis. Amer. J. Roentgenol. 90, 83 (1963).

BROOKFIELD, R. W., RUBIN, E. L., ALEXANDER, M. K.: Osteosclerosis in renal failure. J. Fac. Radiol. (Lond.) 7, 102 (1955).

BRUN, C.: Acute anuria. Diss. Copenhagen: Ejnar Munksgaard 1954.

BÜCHELER, E., THURN, P.: Lipomatosis renalis. Fortschr. Röntgenstr. 104, 320 (1966).

BYROM, F. B., PRATT, O. E.: Oxytocin and renal cortical necrosis. Lancet I, 753 (1959).

CARSKY, E. W., PRIOR, J. T., MOORE, R., HAMEL, J.: Cholesteatoma of the kidney: radiographic findings. Radiology 78, 796 (1962).

CHEN, P., LEBOWITZ, R.,, LEWICKI, A.: Spontaneous hematoma of the esophagus: a complication of uremia. Radiology 100, 281 (1971).

CHRISTOFFERSEN, J. C., ANDERSEN, K.: Renal papillary necrosis. Acta radiol. 45, 27 (1956).

VON CHUDACEK, Z.: Zum Röntgenbild der Periarteriitis nodosa der Niere. Fortschr. Röntgenstr. 105, 49 (1966).

CIAMPELLI, L.: Su due casi die sclerolipomatosi perirenal con spostamento anteriore della pelvi ed uretere associata a calcolosi ureterale. Radiol. Med. (Torino) 49, 988 (1963).

CLARK, R. E., MINAGI, H., PALUBINSKAS, A.: Renal candidiasis. Radiology 101, 567 (1971).

COHEN, M. E. L., COHEN, G. F., AHAD, V., KAYE, M.: Renal osteodystrophy in patients on chronic hemodialysis: a radiologic study. Clin. radiol. 21, 124 (1970).

COLIEZ, R. T.: La Nécrose papillaire du rein. J. Radiol. Electrol. 43, 361 (1962).

COWAN, D. E., DILLON jr., J. R., TALBOT, B. S., BRIDGE, R. A. C.: Renal moniliasis: a case report and discussion. J. Urol. 88, 594 (1962).

CRAMER, G. G., FUGELSTAD, J. R.: Cortical calcification in renal cortical necrosis. Amer. J. Roentgenol. 95, 344 (1965).

CRAWFORD, T., DENT, C. Lucas, P., MARTIN, N., NASSIM, J.: Osteosclerosis associated with chronic renal failure. Lancet II, 981 (1954).

CRONQVIST, S.: Renal osteonephropathy. Acta radiol. 55, 17 (1961).

CZEKALA, Z.: Periarteriitis nodosa der Nieren im Renovasogramm. Fortschr. Röntgenstr. III, 393 (1969).

DAVEY, P. W., HAMILTON, J. D., STEELE, H. D.: Radiation injury of kidney. Canadian Med. Ass. J. 67, 648 (1952).

DEJDAR, R.: Die chronische Pyelonephritis in röntgenographischer Darstellung. Fortschr. Röntgenstr. 90, 196 (1959).

— Zur Frage der Stenosen und Strikturen an den Kelchhälsen bei der chronischen Pyelonephritis. Fortschr. Röntgenstr. 92, 187 (1960).

— PRAT, V.: Das Röntgenbild der Nieren und der Harnwege bei der chronischen Pyelonephritis. Z. Urol. 51, 1 (1958).

DE PASS, S. W., STEIN, J., POPPER, M. H., JACOBSON, H. G.: Pulmonary congestion edema in uremia. J. Amer. med. Ass. 162, 5 (1956).

DIAZ-RIVERA, R. S., MILLER, A J.: Periarteritis nodosa: a clinico-pathological analysis of seven cases. Ann. intern. Med. 24, 420 (1946).

DOW, J. D.: Radiological findings in Bright's disease. Guy's Hosp. Rep. 107, 454 (1958).

EDMONDSON, H. A., MARTIN, H. E., EVANS, E.: Necrosis of renal papillae and acute pyelonephritis in diabetes mellitus. A.M.A. Arch. intern. Med. 79, 148 (1947).

EDVALL, C. A.: Unilateral renal function in chronic pyelonephritis and renal papillary necrosis. Acta chir. scand. **115**, 11 (1958).

EDWARDS, J. E.: Pathology of pyelitis and pyelonephritis. Continuation course in urologic radiology for radiologists, University of Minnesota, Minneapolis 1961 (Class notes, p. 273).

EKELUND, L., KAUDE, J., LINDHOLM, T.: Angiography in glomerular disease: a correlation with clinical findings and the stage of the disease. Amer. J. Roentgenol. To be published.

ELLEGAST, H., JESSERER, H.: Der röntgenologische Aspekt der renalen Osteopathie. Fortschr. Röntgenstr. **89**, 450 (1958).

ENGFELDT, B., LAGERGREN, C.: Nephrocalcinosis. Acta chir. scand. **115**, 46 (1958).

ESKELUND, V.: Necrosis of the renal papillae following retrograde pyelography. Acta radiol. **26**, 548 (1945).

EVANS, J. A., MONTEITH, J. C.: Nephrotomography. Amer. J. Roentgenol. **71**, 213 (1954).

— Ross, W. D.: Renal papillary necrosis. Radiology **66**, 502 (1956).

FAEGENBURG, D., BOSNIAK, M., EVANS, J. A.: Renal sinus lipomatosis. its demonstation by nephrotomography. Radiology **83**, 987 (1964).

FOORD, R. D., NABORRO, J. D., RICHES, E. W.: Diabetic pneumaturia. Brit. med. J. **I**, 433 (1956).

FRIEDENBERG, M. J., SPJUT, H. J.: Xanthogranulomatous pyelonephritis. Amer. J. Roentgenol. **90**, 97 (1963).

— EISEN, S., KISSANE, J.: Renal angiography in pyelonephritis, glomerulonephritis and arteriolar nephrosclerosis. Amer. J. Roentgenol. **95**, 349 (1965).

FREI, A.: Zur Röntgendiagnose der chronischen Pyelonephritis. Verhandl. der Dtsch. Ges. f. Urologie, Leipzig 1958 (S. 201).

FRIEDRICH, N.: Über Necrose der Nierenpapillen bei Hydronephrose. Archiv. f. pathol. Anatomie u. Physiologie u. kl. Medizin (Berlin), Band 69-XVIII, 308 (1877).

FRUMKIN, J.: Replacement lipomatosis of the kidney. J. Urol. **58**, 100 (1947).

FULTON, R. E., WITTEN, D. M., WAGONER, R. D.: Amer. J. Roentgenol. **106**, 623 (1969).

GARRETT, R. A., NORRIS, M. S., VELLIOS, F.: Renal papillary necrosis: a clinicopathologic study. J. Urol. **72**, 609 (1954).

GAUSTAD, V., HERTZBERG, J.: Acute necrosis of the renal papillae in pyelonephritis, particularly diabetes. Acta med. scand. **136**, 331 (1950).

GIBSON, T. E., BARETA, J., LAKE, G. C.: Malacoplakia: report of a case involving the bladder and one kidney and ureter. Urol. internat. **1**, 5 (1955).

GIFFORD, R. W., McCORMACK, L. J., PONTASSE, E. F.: The atrophic kidney: its role in hypertension. Mayo Clinic Proceedings, **40**: 11 (1965).

GILBERT, L. W., McDONALD, J. R.: Primary amyloidosis of the renal pelvis and ureter: report of one case. J. Urol. **68**, 137 (1952).

GILDENHORN, H. L.: Renal replacement lipomatosis. J. Amer. Med. Ass. **181**, 994 (1962).

GINGELL, J. C., ROYLANCE, J., DAVIES, E. R., PENRY, J. B.: Xanthogranulomatous pyelonephritis. Brit. J. Radiol. **46**, 99 (1973).

GLAY, A., RONA, G.: The pulmonary-renal syndrome of Goodpasture: case report. Radiology **83**, 314 (1964).

GONDOS, B.: Foreign body in the left kidney and ureter. J. Urol. **73**, 35 (1955).

— Ureteral manifestations in chronic pyelonephritis. Amer. J. Roentgenol. **92**, 329 (1964).

GORMSEN, H., HILDEN, T., IVERSEN, P., RAASCHOU, F.: Nyrebiopsi ved glomerulonefritis og nefrotisk syndrom. Nord. Med. **54**, 1341 (1955).

GROSSMAN, B. J.: Radiation nephritis. J. Pediatr. **47**, 424 (1955).

GROSSMAN, H., DISCHE, M., WINCHESTER, P., CANALE, V.: Renal enlargement in thalassemia major. Radiology **100**, 645 (1971).

GÜNTHER, G. W.: Die Papillennekrosen der Niere bei Diabetes. Münchener medizin. Wochenschr. **43**, 1695 (1937).

— Die Mark- und Papillennekrosen der Niere, Pyelonephritis und Diabetes. Z. Urol. **41**, 310 (1948).

HAARSTAD, J.: Papillitis necroticans renalis. Nord. Med. **58**, 1759 (1957).

HABIGHORST, P., ALBERS, P., KÖSSLING, F.: Zur Differentialdiagnose von Schrumpfnieren — postmortale arteriographische Untersuchungen. Fortschr. Röntgenstr. **112**, 309 (1970).

HAMM, F. C., DE VEER, J. A.: Fatty replacement following renal atrophy or destruction. J. Urol. **41**, 850 (1939).

HAMRE, L.: Fibrolipomatosis renis. Nord. Med. **58**, 1769 (1957).

HANLEY, H. G.: The post-operative results of nephrectomy. Brit. J. Surg. **27**, 533 (1940).

HARRISON, J. H.: Renal surgery for renal failure. Soc. int. d'Urol. XIII Congr., London 1964, 310.

— BAILEY, O. T.: The significance of necrotizing pyelonephritis in diabetes mellitus. J. Amer. Med. Ass. **118**, 15 (1942).

HARROW, B. R.: Early forms of renal papillary necrosis. Amer. J. Roentgenol. **95**, 335 (1965).

— Renal papillary necrosis: a critique of pathogenesis. J. Urol. **97**, 203 (1967).

HEGEDÜS, V., FAARUP, P.: Cortical volume of the normal human kidney: correlated angiographic and morphologic investigations. Acta radiol. **12**, 481 (1972).

— RAVNSKOV, U.: Cortical volume in apparently normal kidneys. Scand. J. Urol. & Nephrol. **6**, 159 (1972).

HEIDENBLUT, A.: Beitrag zur Röntgendiagnostik entzündlicher Schleimhauterkrankungen von Nierenbecken und Ureter. Fortschr. Röntgenstr. **92**, 658 (1960).

— Obliterierende Pyelonephritis. Fortschr. Röntgenstr. **92**, 183 (1960).

— Die Mark- und Papillennekrosen der Niere. Fortschr. Röntgenstr. **97**, 331 (1962).

HERRNHEISER, G.: Zur Röntgendiagnostik des Lungenödems. Fortschr. Röntgenstr. **89**, 125 (1958).

HILLENBRAND, H., FORST, J.: Renovasographie der chronischen Pyelonephritis. Verhandl. d. Dtsch. Ges. f. Urologie (Leipzig 1958).

HINMAN, F., HUTCH, J. A.: Atrophic pyelonephritis from ureteral reflux without obstructive signs ("Reflux pyelonephritis"). J. Urol. **87**, 230 (1962).

HIPONA, F., PARK, W.: Calcific renal cortical necrosis. J. Urol. **97**, 961 (1967).

HODSON, C. J.: The radiological contribution toward the diagnosis of chronic pyelonephritis. Radiology **88**, 857 (1967).

— Abstract, Postgraduate course in genitourinary radiology, Albert Einstein College of Medicine, New York, 1969.

HODSON, C. J., EDWARDS, D.: Chronic pyelonephritis and vesico-ureteric reflux. Clin. Rad. **XI**, 219 (1960).

HORNYKIEWYTSCH, T.: Röntgenologische Symptomatologie der Pyelonephritis. Radiolog. Austriaca Band **XIII**, 215 (1963).

HUGHES, B., GISLASON, G. J.: Osteonephropathy: a report of two cases. J. Urol. **55**, 330 (1946).

HULTENGREN, N.: Renal papillary necrosis. Acta chir. scand. **115**, 89 (1958).

— Renal papillary necrosis. Acta chir. scand. Suppl. **277** (1961).

HYAMS, J. A., KENYON, H. R.: Localized obliterating pyelonephritis. J. Urol. **46**, 380 (1941).

IDBOHRN, H.: Renal angiography in experimental hydronephrosis. Acta radiol. Suppl. **136** (1956).

IDBOHRN, H.: FAYERS, C. M.: Peripelvic reflux simulating a tumor of the renal pelvis. Urologia Int. (Basel), **197** (1957).

IMMERGUT, S., COTTLER, Z. R.: Peripelvic lipoma. J. Urol. **67**, 50 (1952).

JAMES, W. B.: Urological manifestations in schistosoma haematobium infestation. Brit. J. Radiol. **36**, 40 (1963).

JESSERER, H.: Röntgenveränderungen am Skelett als Folge von Nierenerkrankungen. Fortschr. Röntgenstr. **84**, 452 (1956).

JOHNSTON, D. H.: Repeated bouts of renal papillary necrosis diagnosed by examination of voided tissue. Arch. Intern. Med. **90**, 711 (1952).

JOHNSON, C., GRAHAM, C. B., CURTIS, F. K.: Roentgenographic manifestations of chronic renal disease treated by periodic hemodialysis. Amer. J. Roentgenol. **101**, 915 (1967).

JUCKER, C., PRATES, A. C., PRINI, G.: Rilievi radiologici in alcuni casi di rene ipoplasico. Quad. Radiol. **27**, 271 (1962).

KAUDE, J., CHANG, T. T.: Angiography in evaluation of tuberous sclerosis complex. Der Radiologe **10 : 3**, 105 (1970).

KEUHNELIAN, J. G., BARTONE, F., MARSHALL, V. F.: Practical considerations from autopsies on azotemic patients. J. Urol. **91**, 467 (1964).

KING, A. Y., SCHNEIDER, H. J., KING, L. R.: Roentgen appearance of small bowel during longterm hemodialysis for chronic renal disease. Radiology **99**, 331 (1971).

KNAPP, R., HOLLENBERG, N. K., BUSCH, G. J., ABRAMS, H. L.: Prolonged unilateral acute renal failure induced by intra-arterial Norepinephrine infusion in the dog. Investigative Radiology **B-II:3**, 164 (1972).

KNUTSSEN, A., JENNINGS, E. R., BRINES, O. A., AXELROD, A.: Renal papillary necrosis. Amer. J. Clin. Pathol. **22**, 327 (1952).

KUTZMANN, A. A.: Replacement lipomatosis of the kidney. Surg. Gynec. Obstet. **52**, 690 (1931).

KÖHLER, R.: Pyelo-ureteritis cystica. Acta radiol. **IV:2**, 123 (1966).

KRETSCHMER, H. L., PIERSON, L. E.: Fibrolipomatosis of the kidney: report of a case. Illinois Med. J. **61**, 336 (1932).

KROKOWSKI, E., KOLLWITZ, A. A.: Röntgenologische Lokalisation zur perkutanen Punktionsbiopsie der Nieren. Fortschr. Röntgenstr. **93**, 613 (1960).

LALLI, A. F., LAPIDES, J.: Osteosclerosis occurring in renal disease. Amer. J. Roentgenol. **93**, 924 (1965).

LARSSON, L. E., LINDQVIST, B., MORTENSSON, W.: Goodpasture's syndrome: a distinct clinicopathological entity or a postmortal retrospective diagnosis indicating malignant glomerulonephritis with pulmonary hemorrhage. To be published.

LEVITT, W. M., ORAM, S.: Irradiation-induced malignant hypertension cured by nephrectomy. Brit. Med. J. **2**, 910 (1956).

LINDHOLM, T.: On renal papillary necrosis with special reference to the diagnostic importance of papillary fragments in the urine, therapy (i.a. artificial kidney) and prognosis. Acta med. scand. **167**, 319 (1960).

LINDVALL, N.: Renal papillary necrosis. Acta radiol. Suppl. **192** (1960).

LJUNGQVIST, A., UNGE, G., LAGERGREN, C., NOTTER, G.: The intrarenal vascular alterations in radiation nephritis and their relationship to the development of hypertension. Acta path. microbiol. scand. Sect. A: **79**, 629 (1971).

LUSTED, L. B., STEINBACH, H. L., KLATTE, E.: Papillary calcification in necrotizing renal papillitis. Amer. J. Roentgenol. **78**, 1049 (1957).

MACDONALD, D. F., FAAGAN, C. J.: Fungus balls in the urinary bladder: case report. Radiology **104**, 734 (1972).

MACGIBBON, B. H., LOUGHRIDGE, L. W., HOURIHANE, D. O.'B., BOYD, D. W.: Auto-immune haemolytic anaemia with acute renal failure due to phenacetin and p-aminosalicylic acid. Lancet **I**, 7 (1960).

MAIER, K. J., BRADEN, E. S., BURKHEAD, H. C.: Renal papillary necrosis. Radiology **75**, 254 (1960).

MCALISTER, W. H., NEDELMAN, S. H.: The roentgen manifestations of bilateral renal cortical necrosis. Amer. J. Roentgenol. **86**, 129 (1961).

MCLACHLAN, M. S. F., WALLACE, D. M., SENEVIRATNE, C.: Pulmonary calcification in renal failure: report of three cases. Brit. J. Radiol. **41**, 99 (1968).

MANDEL, E. E.: Renal medullary necrosis. Amer. J. Med. **13**, 322 (1952).

— POPPER, H.: Experimental medullary necrosis of the kidney. A. M. A. Arch. Pathol. **52**, 1 (1951).

MARTINI, F.: Malattia di Besnier-Boeck-Schaumann in rene anomalo. Nunt. Radiol. **21**, 461 (1955).

MELCHIOR, J., MEBUST, W., VALK, W.: Ureteral colic from a fungus ball: unusual presentation of systemic aspergillosis. J. Urol. **108**, 698 (1972).

MILLARD, G.: Renal siderosis. Radiology **79**, 290 (1962).

MITCHELL jr., R. E., TITTLE, C. R., BOCKUS, H. L.: Nephrocalcinosis in patient with duodenal ulcer disease. Report of a case associated with parathyroid adenoma. Gastroenterology 30, 943 (1956).

MOËLL, H.: Gross bilateral renal cortical necrosis during long periods of oliguria-anuria. Acta radiol. 48, 355 (1957).

— Kidney size and its deviation from normal in acute renal failure. Acta radiol. Suppl. 206 (1961).

MOOLTEN, S. E., SMITH, I. B.: Fatal nephritis in chronic phenacetin poisoning. Amer. J. Med. 28, 127 (1960).

MOREAU, R., DEUIL, R., CROSNIER, J., BIATRIX, C., THIBAULT, P.: Nécrose papillaire rénale au cours du diabète. Presse méd. 62, 599 (1954).

MUIRHEAD, E. E., VANATTA, J., GROLLMAN, A.: Papillary necrosis of the kidney. J. Amer. Med. Ass. 142, 627 (1950).

MUNK, J., HAHN, E.: The radiological differentiation of the small kidney in hypertension of renal origin. Clin. Radiol. 13, 265 (1962).

NOURSE, M. H.: Pyelonephritis and the urologist. J. Urol. 85, 211 (1961).

NOYES, W. E., PALUBINSKAS, A.: Squamous metaplasia of the renal pelvis. Radiology 89, 292 (1967).

ODERR, C. P., PIZZOLATO, P., ZISKIND, J.: Emphysema studied by microradiology. Radiology 71, 236 (1958).

OLAFSSON, O., GUDMUNDSSON, K. R., BREKKAN, A.: Migraine, gastritis and renal papillary necrosis: a syndrome in chronic non-obstructive pyelonephritis. Acta med. scand. 179, 121 (1966).

OLSSON, OLLE: Spontanes Gaspyelogramm. Acta radiol. 20, 578 (1939).

— Renal fibrolipomatosis. Continuation course in urologic radiology for radiologists. University of Minnesota, Minneapolis, 1961 (Class notes, p.218).

— Roentgen examination of the kidney and the ureter. In: Handbuch der Urologie/Encyclopedia of Urology. Heidelberg: Springer-Verlag 1962 (p. 320).

OLSSON, OLLE, WEILAND, P.-O.: Renal fibrolipomatosis. Acta radiol. 1, 1061 (1963).

O'MALLEY, A. F., CHUTE, R., HOUGHTON, J. D.: Renal papillary necrosis. J. Urol. 86, 7 (1961).

OPIT, L. J., PROUDMAN, W. D., BONNIN, N. J.: Renal papillary necrosis. Brit. J. Surg. 50, 375 (1963).

OTTOMAN, R. E., WOODRUFF, J. H., WILK, S., ISAAC, F.: The roentgen aspects of necrotizing renal papillitis. Radiology 67, 157 (1956).

PALUBINSKAS, A. J.: Abstract, Postgraduate Course in Genitourinary Radiology, Albert Einstein College of Medicine, New York, 1969.

PAPILLON, J., PINET, F., BOUVET, R., PINET, A., CHASSARD, J. L.: A propos de deux cas de manifestations urinaires de la maladie de Hodgkin. J. Radiol. Electrol. 38, 974 (1957).

PAWLOWSKI, J. M.: Peripelvic urine granuloma. Amer. J. Clin. Pathol. 34, 64 (1960).

PEACOCK, A. H., BALLE, A.: Renal lipomatosis. Ann. Surg. 103, 395 (1936).

PILLAY, V. K. G., ROBBINS, P. C., SCHWARTZ, F. D., KARK, R. M.: Acute renal failure following intravenous urography in patients with long-standing diabetes mellitus and azotemia. Radiology 95, 633 (1970).

PLATT, R., DAVISON, J.: Clinical and pathological study of renal disease: diseases other than nephritis. Quart. J. Med. 19, 33 (1950).

PRAETORIUS, G.: Papillitis necroticans bei schwerer chronischer Pyelonephritis. Z. Urol. 31, 298 (1937).

PRÉVOT, R., BERNING, H.: Zur Röntgendiagnostik der Pyelonephritis. Fortschr. Röntgenstr. 73, 482 (1950).

PRIESTLEY, J. B.: Renal lipomatosis or fatty replacement of destroyed renal cortex. J. Urol. 40, 269 (1938).

PURPON, I., TAMAYO, R. P.: Malacoplakia of the kidney. J. Urol. 84, 231 (1960).

PYRAH, L. N.: Medullary sponge kidney. J. Urol. 95:3, 274 (1966).

RAKOVEC, S.: Hypertension due to vascular changes in chronic unilateral pyelonephritis. Urol. Int. (Basel) 6, 127 (1958).

REDD, B. L.: Radiation nephritis. Amer. J. Roentgenol. 83, 88 (1960).

REFVEM, O.: Lower nephron nephrosis-akut nyresvikt. Nord Med. 54, 1337 (1955).

ROBBINS, E. D., ANGRIST, A.: Necrosis of renal papillae. Ann. Intern. Med. 31, 773 (1949).

ROBBINS, S. L., MALLORY, G. K., KINNEY, T. D.: Necrotizing renal papillitis: a form of acute pyelonephritis. New Engl. J. Med. 235, 885 (1946).

ROJAS, A. G.: Insuficiencia renal aspectos fisiologicos. Soc. Int. d'Urol. XIII Congr. (Lond.) 1964, p. 249.

ROSENHEIM, M. L.: The syndromes of Bright's disease. Guy's Hosp. Reports 108, 403 (1959).

ROSENTHAL, L., LAGERGREN, C., OLHAGEN, B.: A clinical and roentgenological follow-up study of patients with uro-arthritis or pelvospondylitis. Acta rheum. scand. 17, 3 (1971).

ROTH, L. J., DAVIDSON, H. B.: Fibrous and fatty replacement of renal parenchyma. J. Amer. Med. Ass. III, 233 (1938).

ROUBIER, C., PLAUCHU, M.: Sur certains aspects radiographiques de l'oedème pulmonaire chez les cardia-rénaux azotémiques. Arch. méd.-chir. Appar. resp. 3, 189 (1934).

RUDEBECK, J.: Clinical and prognostic aspects of acute glomerulonephritis. Acta med. Scand. Suppl. 173 (1946).

RUTNER, A. B., SMITH, D. R.: Renal papillary necrosis. J. Urol. 85, 462 (1961).

SARGENT, J. C., SARGENT, J. W.: Unilateral renal papillary necrosis. J. Urol. 73, 757 (1955).

SARRUBI, Z.: Radiologie des pyélites et pyélonéphritis. J. Urol. méd. chir. 62, 372 (1956).

SCHROEDER, E.: Kliniske studier over nyrefunktionen hos nephrectomerede. Diss. Copenhagen: Ejnar Munksgaard 1944.

SCOTT, E., SCOTT jr., W. F.: A fatal case of malakoplakia of the urinary tract. J. Urol. 79, 52 (1958).

SHAPIRO, J. H., RAMSAY, C. G., JACOBSON, H. G., BOTSTEIN, C. C., ALLEN, L. B.: Renal involvement in lymphomas and leukemias in adults. Amer. J. Roentgenol. 88, 928 (1962).

SHEEHAN, H. L.: Medullary necrosis of the kidneys. Lancet II, 187 (1937).

SHEEHAN, H. L., MOORE, H. C.: Renal cortical necrosis of the kidney of concealed accidental haemorrhage. Oxford: Blackwell Scientific Publ. 1952.

SIEGEL, R. R.: The basis of pulmonary disease resolution after nephrectomy in Goodpasture's syndrome. Amer. J. Med. Sci. **259**, 201 (1970).

SIMON, H. B., BENNETT, W. A., EMMETT, J. L.: Renal papillary necrosis: a clinicopathologic study of 42 cases. J. Urol. **77**, 557 (1957).

SIMRIL, W. A., ROSE, D. K.: Replacement lipomatosis and its simulation of renal tumors: a report of two cases. J. Urol. **63**, 588 (1950).

SLIPYAN, A., BARLAND, S.: Renal papillary necrosis: case report. J. Urol. **68**, 430 (1952).

SOBBE, A., WESSEL, W., BITTSCHEIDT, H., VAHLEN, SIECK,W.: Angiographische, mikroangiographische, histologische und röntgenmorphometrische Untersuchungen an menschlichen Nieren nach entzündlichen und degenerativen Erkrankungen. Fortschr. **115**, 755 (1971).

SPÜHLER, O.: Probleme der interstitiellen Nephritis. Schweiz. med. Wschr. **83**, 145 (1953).

— ZOLLINGER, H. U.: Die chronisch-interstitielle Nephritis. Z. klin. Med. **151**, 1 (1953).

STANBURY, S. W.: Azotaemic renal osteodystrophy. Brit. med. Bull. **13**, 57 (1957).

STEINBACH, H. L., NOETZLI, M.: Roentgen appearance of the skeleton in osteomalacia and rickets. Amer. J. Roentgenol. **91**, 955 (1964).

STEPHENS, F. D., LENAGHAN, D.: The anatomical basis and dynamics of vesicoureteral reflux. J. Urol. **87**, 669 (1962).

— Aetiology of vesicoureteric reflux. J. Coll. Radiol. Aust. **7**, 23 (1963).

STERNBY, N. H.: Studies in enlargement of leukaemic kidneys. Acta haemat. (Basel) **14**, 453 (1955).

SUNDIN, T., FRITJOFSSON, A.: Njurfunktionsstudier vid vesicoureteral reflux. Nord. med. **73**, 620 (1965).

SWARTZ, D.: Renal papillary necrosis. J. Urol. **71**, 385 (1954).

TALLQVIST, G., PASTERNACK, A.: Njurarnas patologiska anatomi vid kollagensjukdomar. Nord. med. **26**, 833 (1968).

TARDOS, R.: Étude radiologique des lésions urétérales et rénales de la bilharziose urinaire. J. Radiol. Electrol. **44**, 187 (1963).

TESSLER, A. N., HOTCHKISS, R. S.: Renal cortical necrosis. J. Urol. **85**, 471 (1961).

THELEN, A.: Papillitis necroticans bei chronischer Pyelonephritis. Z. Urol. **40**, 67 (1947).

THORSÉN, G.: Pyelorenal cysts. Acta chir. scand. **98**, 476 (1949).

THURN, P., BÜCHELER, E.: Radiological visualization and assessment of the small kidney. Fortschr. Röntgenstr. **100**, 496 (1964).

TRINKLE, J. K., KISER, W. S.: Acute renal failure: diagnostics of etiology by radioisotope renography. J. Urol. **91**, 199 (1964).

TRUCKENBRODT, H.: Zur Diagnose der Nierenleukämie im Ausscheidungsurogramm. Der Radiologe **11**, 310 (1971).

TUCKER, A. S., NEWMAN, A. J., PERSKY, L.: The kidney in childhood leukemia. Radiology **78**, 407 (1962).

ÜBELHÖR, R., FIGDOR, P. P.: Betrachtungen über die Erholungsfähigkeit der Niere nach Anurie. Soc. Int. d'Urol. XIII Congr. London 1964, p. 287.

VALVASSORI, G. E., PIERCE, R. H.: Osteosclerosis in chronic uremia. Radiology **82**, 385 (1964).

VANDENDORP, F., WEMEAU, L., LEMAITRE, G., GRIGNON, M.: Signes radiologiques de la nécrose papillaire du rein (à propos de 12 observations personnelles). Ann. de radiologie **6**, 543 (1963).

VIX, V. A.: Urographic demonstration of renal medullary necrosis in hemoglobin SA and SC disease. Radiology **85**, 320 (1965).

VOEGELI, E.: Die Pathogenese des Fibrolipomatose. Der Radiologe **11**, 209 (1971).

VOLHARD, F., FAHR, T.: Die Brightsche Nierenkrankheit. Klinik, Pathologie u. Atlas. Berlin: Springer-Verlag 1914.

WALL, B.: Pyelographic changes in necrotizing renal papillitis. J. Urol. **72**, 1 (1954).

WELCH, N., PRATHER, G.: Pneumonephrosis: a complication of necrotizing pyelonephritis. J. Urol. **61**, 712 (1949).

WHITEHOUSE, F. W., ROOT, H. F.: Necrotizing renal papillitis and diabetes mellitus. J. Amer. Ass. **162**, 444 (1956).

WIESEL, B. H., McMANUS, J. F. A.: Necrotizing renal papillitis. Sth. med. J. (Birmingham, Alabama) **43**, 403 (1950).

WULFF, H.: Die Zuverlässigkeit der Röntgendiagnostik — besonders hinsichtlich des Wertes der Urographie — und die Prognose bei Nieren- und Harnleitersteinen. Acta radiol. Suppl. XXXII (1936).

ZETTERGREN, L.: Uremic lung. Acta Soc. Med. Upsalien (Uppsala) **60**, 161 (1955).

ZOLLINGER, H. U.: Problèmes des néphritis et néphroses. J. Urol. méd. chir. **61**, 581 (1955).

— Chronische interstitielle Nephritis bei Abusus von phenacetinhaltigen Analgetica, Saridon usw. Schweiz. med. Wschr. **85**, 746 (1955).

— Die Pathologie der chronischen Pyelonephritis. Verhandl. der Dtsch. Ges. f. Urologie (Leipzig) 1958 (S. 165).

ZUELZER, W. W., PALMER, H. D., NEWTON, W. A.: Unusual glomerulonephritis in young children, probably radiation nephritis. Amer. J. Pathol. **26**, 1019 (1950)

8. Papillary necrosis

ABESHOUSE, B. S., SALIK, J. O.: Pyelographic diagnosis of lesions of the renal papillae and calyces in cases of hematuria. Amer. J. Roentgenol. **80**, 569 (1958).

ALKEN, C. E.: Die Papillennekrose. Z. Urol. **32**, 433 (1938).

AXELSSON, U.: Papillitis necroticans renalis och hemolystik anemi hos fenazonmissbrukare. Nord. Med. **59**, 903 (1958).

CHRISTOFFERSEN, J. C., ANDERSEN, K.: Renal papillary necrosis. Acta radiol. **45**, 27 (1956).

EDMONDSON, H. A., MARTIN, H. E., EVANS, E.: Necrosis of renal papillae and acute pyelonephritis in diabetes mellitus. A.M.A. Arch. intern. Med. **79**, 148 (1947).

EDVALL, C. A.: Unilateral renal function in chronic pyelonephritis and renal papillary necrosis. Acta chir. scand. **115**, 11 (1958).

ESKELUND,V.:Necrosis of the renal papillae following retrograde pyelography. Acta radiol. **26**, 548 (1945).

EVANS, J. A., ROSS, W. D.: Renal papillary necrosis. Radiology **66**, 502 (1956).

FOORD, R. D., NABORRO, J. D. N., RICHES, E. W.: Diabetic pneumaturia. Brit. med. J. **1956 I**, 433.

FRIEDREICH, N.: Über Necrose der Nierenpapillen bei Hydronephrose. Archiv f. pathol. Anatomie u. Physiologie u. f. klin. Med. (Berlin), Band 69, XVIII, 308 (1877).

GARRETT, R. A., NORRIS, M. S., VELLIOS, F.: Renal papillary necrosia: a clinicopathologic study. J. Urol. **72**, 609 (1954).

GAUSTAD, V., HERTZBERG, J.: Acute necrosis of the renal papillae in pyelonephritis, particularly diabetes. Acta med. scand. **136**, 331 (1950).

GÜNTHER, G. W.: Die Papillennekrose der Niere bei Diabetes. Münch. med. Wschr. **84**, 1695 (1937).

— Die Mark- und Papillennekrosen der Niere, Pyelonephritis und Diabetes. Z. Urol. **41**, 310 (1948).

HARRISON, J. H., BAILEY, O. T.: The significance of necrotizing pyelonephritis in diabetes mellitus. J. Amer. med. Ass. **118**, 15 (1942).

HEIDENBLUT, A.: Die Mark- und Papillennekrosen der Niere. Fortschr. Röntgenstr. **97**, 331 (1962).

HULTENGREN, N.: Renal papillary necrosis. Acta Chir. Scand. Suppl. **277** (1961).

HYAMS, J. A., KENYON, H. R.: Localized obliterating pyelonephritis. J. Urol. **46**, 380 (1941).

JOHNSTON, D. H.: Repeated bouts of renal papillary necrosis diagnosed by examination of voided tissue. Arch. Intern. Med. **90**, 711 (1952).

KNUTSEN, A., JENNINGS, E. R., BRINES, O. A., AXELROD, A.: Renal papillary necrosis. Amer. J. Clin. Pathol. **22**, 327 (1952).

LINDHOLM, T.: On renal papillary necrosis with special reference to the diagnostic importance of papillary fragments in the urine, therapy (i.a. artificial kidney) and prognosis. Acta Med. Scand. **167**, 319 (1960).

LINDVALL, N.: Renal papillary necrosis. Acta radiol. Suppl. **192** (1960).

LUSTED, L. B., STEINBACH, H. L., KLATTE, E.: Papillary calcification in necrotizing renal papillities. Amer. J. Roentgenol. **78**, 1049 (1957).

MAIER, K. J., BRADEM, E. S., BURKHEAD, H. C.: Renal papillary necrosis. Radiology **75**, 254 (1960).

MANDEL, E. E.: Renal medullary necrosis. Amer. J. Med. **13**, 322 (1952).

— POPPER, H.: Experimental medullary necrosis of the kidney. Amer. Med. Ass. Arch. Pathol. **52**, 1 (1951).

MELLGREN, J., REDELL, G.: Zur Pathologie und Klinik der Papillitis necroticans renalis. Acta chir. scand. **84**, 439 (1941).

MOREAU, R., DEUIL, R., CROSNIER, J., BIATRIX, C., THIBAULT, P.: Nécrose papillaire rénale au cours du diabète. Presse méd. **62**, 599 (1954).

MUIRHEAD, E. E., VANATTA, J., GROLLMAN: Papillary necrosis of the kidney. J. Amer. Med. Ass. **142**, 627 (1950).

OLSSON, OLLE: Spontanes Gaspyelogramm. Acta radiol. **20**, 578 (1939).

— Renal papillary necrosis. Continuation course in urologic radiology for radiologists. Univ. of Minnesota, Minneapolis 1961 (Class notes, page 292).

O'MALLEY, A., CHUTE, A. R., HOUGHTON, J.: Renal papillary necrosis. J. Urol. **86**, 7 (1961).

OPIT, L. J., PROUDMAN, W. D., BONNIN, N. J.: Renal papillary necrosis. Brit. J. Surg. **50**, 375 (1963).

OTTOMAN, R. E., WOODRUFF, J. H., WILK, S., ISAAC, F.: The roentgen aspects of necrotizing renal papillitis. Radiology **67**, 157 (1956).

PRAETORIUS, G.: Papillitis necroticans bei schwerer chronischer Pyelonephritis. Z. Urol. **31**, 298 (1937).

PRÉVOT, R., BERNING, H.: Zur Röntgendiagnostik der Pyelonephritis. Fortschr. Röntgenstr. **73**, 482 (1950).

ROBBINS, E. D., ANGRIST, A.: Necrosis of renal papillae. Ann. Intern. Med. **31**, 773 (1949).

ROBBINS, S. L., MALLORY, G. K., KINNEY, T. D.: Necrotizing renal papillitis: a form of acute pyelonephritis. New Engl. J. Med. **235**, 885 (1946).

RUTNER, A. B., SMITH, D. R.: Renal papillary necrosis. J. Urol. **85**, 462 (1961).

SARGENT, J. C., SARGENT, J. W.: Unilateral renal papillary necrosis. J. Urol. **73**, 757 (1955).

SHEEHAN, H. L.: Medullary necrosis of the kidneys. Lancet **II**, 187 (1937).

SIMON, H. B. W., BENNETT, A., EMMETT, J. L.: Renal papillary necrosis: a clinicopathologic study of 42 cases. J. Urol. **77**, 557 (1957).

SLIPYAN, A., BARLAND, S.: Renal papillary necrosis: case report. J. Urol. **68**, 430 (1952).

SPÜHLER, O.: Probleme der interstitiellen Nephritis. Schweiz. med. Wschr. **83**, 145 (1953).

— ZOLLINGER, H. U.: Die chronisch-interstitielle Nephritis. Z. klin. Med. **151**, 1 (1953).

SWARTZ, D.: Renal papillary necrosis. J. Urol. **71**, 385 (1954).

THELEN, A.: Papillitis necroticans bei chronischer Pyelonephritis. Z. Urol. **40**, 67 (1947).

THORSÉN, G.: Pyelorenal cysts. Acta chir. scand. **98**, 476 (1949).

VANDENDORP, F., WEMEAU, L., LEMAITRE, G., GRIGNON, M.: Signes radiologiques de la nécrose papillaire du rein (à propos de 12 observations personnelles). Ann. de radiol. **6**, 543 (1963).

VIX, V. A.: Urographic demonstration of renal medullary necrosis in hemoglobin SA and SC disease. Radiology **85**, 320 (1965).

WALL, B.: Pyelographic changes in necrotizing renal papillitis. J. Urol. **72**, 1 (1954).

WELCH, N. M., PRATHER, G. C.: Pneumonephrosis: a complication of necrotizing pyelonephritis. J. Urol. **61**, 712 (1949).

WHITEHOUSE, F. W., ROOT, H. F.: Necrotizing renal papillitis and diabetes mellitus. J. Amer. Med. Ass. **162**, 444 (1956).

WIESEL, B. H., McMANUS, J. F. A.: Necrotizing renal papillitis. Sth. Med. J. (Birmingham, Alabama) **43**, 403 (1950).

ZOLLINGER, H. U.: Problèmes des néphritis et néphroses. J. Urol. méd. chir. **61**, 581 (1955).

M. Perinephritis, renal abscess and carbuncle

ALKEN, C. E.: Perinephritische Eiterungen mit seltenem Verlauf. Z. Urol. **31**, 772 (1937).

ATCHESON, D. W.: Perinephric abscess with a review of 117 cases. J. Urol. **46**, 201 (1941).

BALL, W. G.: Renal carbuncle. Brit. J. Urol. **6**, 248 (1934).

BANGERTER, J.: Über einen Fall von Nierenkarbunkel mit multiplen Rindabszessen in der anderen Niere, Schweiz. med. Wschr. **67**, 310 (1937).

BARON, E., ARDUINO, L. J.: Primary renal actinomycosis. J. Urol. **62**, 410 (1949).

BEER, E.: Roentgenographic evidence of perinephritic abscess. J. Amer. Med. Ass. **90**, 1375 (1928).

BERGSTRAND, H.: Über die Nierenveränderungen bei tödlicher Sulfathiazolschädigung. Acta med. scand. **118**, 97 (1944).

BRAMAN, R., CROSS jr., R. R.: Perinephric abscess producing a pneumonephrogram. J. Urol. **75**, 194 (1956).

CAMPBELL, M. F.: Urology I. Philadelphia & London: W. B. SAUNDRES Co. 1954.

— Renal ectopy. J. Urol. **24**, 187 (1930).

CAPLAN, L. H., SIEGELMAN, S., BOSNIAK, M. A.: Angiography in inflammatory space-occupying lesions of the kidney. Radiology **88**, 14 (1967).

DAVIDSON, B.: Solitary cortical abscess (carbuncle) of the kidney in a child simulating tumor. Urol. cutan. Rev. **40**, 260 (1936).

DEUTICKE, P.: Die Bedeutung der Pyelographie für die Diagnose des paranephritischen Abszesses. Zbl. Chir. **67**, 2214 (1940).

— Über die pyelographische Befunde bei Entzündungen des Nierenlagers. Z. Urol. **34**, 89 (1940).

DROSCHL, H.: Klinischer Beitrag zur Diagnose des Nierenkarbunkels. Zbl. Chir. **64**, 1209 (1937).

EMMETT, J. L., PRIESTLEY, J. T.: Solitary renal abscess (carbuncle): report of case. Proc. Mayo Clin. **11**, 764 (1936).

FECI, L.: Contributo radiologico alla diagnosi degli ascessi perirenal.. Arch. ital. Urol. **4**, 503 (1927).

FOULDS, G. S.: Diagnosis of perinephric abscess. J. Urol. **42**, 1 (1939).

FRIEDMAN, L. J.: Roentgen signs of perinephritic abscess. Med. J. Rec. **127**, 648 (1928).

FRIMANN-DAHL, J.: Rontgenundersøkelser ved akutte abdominalsykdommer. Oslo: Johan Grundt Tanum 1942.

GARDINI, G. F.: Contributo allo studio del forunculo renale. Arch. ital. Urol. **11**, 504 (1934).

GOLDSTEIN, A. E., MARCUS, O.: Roentgenological diagnosis of perinephritic abscess and perinephritis. Amer. J. Roentgenol. **40**, 371 (1938).

GRAVES, C. G., PARKINS, L. E.: Carbuncle of the kidney. J. Urol. **35**,1 (1936).

GUSZICH, A.: Zur Frage der Diagnostik des Nierenkarbunkels. Z. urol. Chir. **40**, 449 (1935).

HENCZ, L.: Späteres Schicksal eines Patienten mit operiertem Nierenkarbunkel. Z. urol. Chir. Gynäk. **43**, 186 (1937).

HJORT, E.: Om nyreabscess og nyrekarbunkel. Med. rev. Bergen **54**, 376 (1937).

HUNTER, A. W.: Gumma of kidney. J. Urol. (Baltimore) **42**, 1176 (1939).

ILLYÉS, G. DE: Suppurations of the renal parenchyma. Brit. J. Urol. **9**, 101 (1937).

INGRISH, G. A.: Carbuncle of the kidney: report of ten cases. J. Urol. **42**, 326 (1939).

JAMES, T. G. I.: A case of carbuncle of the kidney. Brit. J. Urol. **6**, 156 (1934).

KICKHAM, C. J. E., COLPOYS jr., F. L.: Periureteral fascitis. J. Amer. med. Ass. **171**, 2202 (1959).

LAURELL, H.: Ein Beitrag zur Röntgendiagnostik der Peri- bzw. der Paranephritis. Upsala Läk.-Fören, Förh. **26**, XXXVIII (1920/21).

LAZARUS, J. A.: Carbuncle of the kidney. Amer. J. Surg. **25**, 155 (1934).

LEAKE, R., WAYMAN, T. B.: Retroperitoneal encysted hematomas. J. Urol. **68**, 69 (1952).

LIPSETT, PH.: Roentgen-ray observations in acute perinephritic abscess. J. Amer. med. Ass. **90**, 1374 (1928).

LJUNGGREN, E.: Beitrag zur Röntgendiagnostik der Nierenkarbunkel. Z. urol. Chir. **31**, 258 (1931).

McNULTY, P. H.: Carbuncle of the kidney: review of the literature, discussion of unilateral localized lesions of the kidney and report of a case. J. Urol. **35**, 15 (1936).

MENVILLE, J. G.: The lateral pyelogram as a diagnostic aid in perinephritic abscess. J. Amer. med. Ass. **111**, 231 (1938).

MILLER, R. H.: Diagnosis of perinephric abscess. Ann. Surg. **106**, 756 (1937).

MITCHELL, G. A. G.: The spread of retroperitoneal effusions arising in the renal regions. Brit. med. J. 1134 (1939).

MOORE, T. D.: Renal carbuncle. J. Amer. med. Ass. **96**, 754 (1931).

MORALES, O.: A case of roentgenologically observed perirenal oedema after therapy with sulphanilamide preparations. Acta radiol. **26**, 334 (1945).

NESBIT, R. M., DICK, V. S.: Pulmonary complications of acute renal and perirenal suppuration. Amer. J. Roentgenol. **44**, 161 (1940).

O'CONOR, V.: Carbuncle of the kidney. J. Urol. **30**, 1 (1933).

ÖSTERLIND, S.: Über Pyelonephritis xanthomatosa. Acta chir. scand. **90**, 369 (1944).

ÖVERGAARD, K.: A case of paranephritic abscess with characteristic pyelogram. Acta radiol. **23**, 180 (1942).

PARKS, R. E.: The radiographic diagnosis of perinephric abscess. J. Urol. **64**, 555 (1950).

PORTER, R., WRIGHT, F. W.: Intracapsular perinephric gas-forming infection in a patient with diabetic coma. Brit. J. Radiol. **34**, 201 (1961).

PREHN, D. T.: A pyelographic sign in the diagnosis of perinephric abscess. J. Urol. **55**, 8 (1946).

PYTEL, A.: Unilateral chronic pyelonephritis and hypertension (Russian text). Urologia 1959.

RAASCHOU, F.: Studies of chronic pyelonephritis with special reference to kidney function. Copenhagen: Munksgaard 1948.

RÉVÉSZ, V.: Die direkte Röntgendiagnostik der peri- und paranephritischen Eiterungen und die Röntgenuntersuchung der chronischen Perinephritis. Fortschr. Röntgenstr. **34**, 48 (1926).

RIGLER, L. G., MANSON, M. H.: Perinephritic abscess. Amer. J. Surg. **13**, 459 (1931).

RIPPY, E. L.: Review of local cases of perinephritic abscess. Year Book of Urol. 1938 (page 208).

SCHULTZ jr., E. H., KLORFEIN, E. H.: Emphysematous pyelonephritis. J. Urol. **87**, 762 (1962).

SHANE, J. H., HARRIS, M.: Roentgenologic diagnosis of perinephritic abscess. J. Urol. **32**, 19 (1934).

SKARBY, H.-G.: Beiträge zur Diagnostik der Paranephritiden. Acta radiol. Suppl. **62** (1946).

SPENCE, H. M., JOHNSTON, L. W.: Renal carbuncle: case report and comparative review. Ann. Surg. **109**, 99 (1939).

STITES, J. R., BOWEN, J. A.: Diagnostic difficulties in perinephritic abscess. Sth. Med. J. (Birmingham, Alabama) **30**, 1062 (1937).

SZACSVAY, S. v.: Ein Beitrag zur Diagnose und Therapie des Nierenkarbunkels. Z. Urol. Chir. **40**, 70 (1935).

TAYLOR, W. N.: Carbuncle of the kidney. Amer. J. Surg. **22**, 550 (1933).

TURMAN, A. RUTHERFORD, C.: Emphysematous pyelonephritis with perinephric gas. J. Urol. **105**, 165 (1971).

VANDENDORP, F. G., LEMAITRE, G., REMY, J.: La radiologie des pyélonéphritis chroniques. Ann. de radiol. **5**, 77 (1962).

VOEGELI, E.: Diagnose von Abscessen im Bereiche der Nieren durch renale Angiographie und direkte Punktion. Der Radiologe **10**, 87 (1970).

— Die Pathogenese der Fibrolipomatose. Der Radiologe **11**, 209 (1971).

VRIES, G. H. DE: Angiogramm eines Nierenkarbunkels. Fortschr. Röntgenstr. **90**, 640 (1959).

WEINTRAUB, H. D., RALI, K. L., THOMPSON, I. M., ROSS, G.: Pararenal pseudocysts. Amer. J. Roentgenol. **92**, 286 (1964).

WELIN, S.: Über die Röntgendiagnostik der Paranephritis. Fortschr. Röntgenstr. **67**, 162 (1943).

WOODRUFF, S. R., GROSSMAN, S. L.: Renal carbuncle. Urol. Cutan. Rev. **40**, 240 (1936).

N. Gas in the urinary tract and fistula formation

BLOOM, B.: Spontaneous renoduodenal fistulas. J. Urol. **72**, 1153 (1954).

BOIJSEN, E., LEWIS-JOHNSSON, J.: Emphysematous cystitis. Acta radiol. **41**, 269 (1954).

BRAMAN, R., GROSS jr., R. R.: Perinephric abscess producing a pneumonephrogram. J. Urol. **75**, 194 (1956).

HARROW, B. R., SLOANE, J. A.: Ureteritis emphysematosa; spontaneous ureteral pneumogram; renal and perirenal emphysema. J. Urol. **89**, 43 (1963).

NARINS, L., SEGAL, H.: Spontaneous passage of a dendritic renal calculus by rectum. J. Urol. **82**, 274 (1959).

NOGUEIRA, T.: Zeitschr. f. Urol. BAND **29**, 275 (1935).

NORTH, J., LIVINGSTON, S., LOVELL, B.: Spontaneous renoduodenal fistula. Surgery **39**, 683 (1956).

OLSSON, OLLE: Spontanes gaspyelogramm. Acta radiol. **XX: 118**, 578 (1939).

— Diskussionsinlägg till B. Löfgren: Resultat av uretär-transplantation enligt Nesbit. Nord. med. **48**, 1467 (1952).

— Gas in the urinary pathways. In: Diseases of the kidney. Edited by B. M. Strauss & L. G. Welt. Boston: Little, Brown & Co. 1971 (page 180).

RATLIFF, R., BARNES, A.: Acquired renocolic fistula: report of two cases. J. Urol. **42**, 311 (1939).

ROST, G., KNOUF, C., FERGUSON, P., McCRARY, A.: Acquired renocolic fistula in remaining functioning kidney with recovery: case report. J. Urol. **75**, 787 (1956).

Schultz, E., KLORFEIN, E.: Emphysematous pyelonephritis. J. Urol. **87**, 762 (1962).

TURMAN, A., RUTHERFORD, C.: Emphysematous pyelonephritis with perinephric gas. J. Urol. **105**, 165 (1971).

VUORINEN, P., VIIKARI, S.: Ein Fall von chronischem spontanem Gaspyelogramm. Fortschr. Röntgenstr. **90**, 519 (1959).

WEISER, A.: Über einen Fall von Gasgangrän der Harnblase. Z. urol. Chir. Gynäk. **28**, 113 (1929).

O. Medullary sponge kidney

ABESHOUSE, B. S., ABESHOUSE, G. A.: Sponge kidney: a review of the literature and a report of five cases. J. Urol. **84**, 252 (1960).

ALKEN, C. E., SOMMER, F., KLING, F.: Renovasographie vor Teilresektion der Niere bei Markcystensteinbildung im oberen Pol. Z. Urol. **44**, 569 (1951).

ANTOINE, B., ANAGNOSTOPOULOS, T., WATCHI, J. M., PARIENTY, R.: L'ectasie canaliculaire précalicielle. J. Radiol. **45**, 663 (1964).

ARDUINO, L. J.: A case of pyelitis and cystitis cystica. J. Urol. **55**, 149 (1946).

BALESTRA, G., DELPINO, B.: In tema di rene a spugna e di nefrocalcinosi. Radiol. med. (Torino) **42**, 745 (1956).

BARATA, L. S.: Un caso de rim esponja. Urologia (P. Alegre) **1**, 40 (1951).

BEITZKE, H.: Über Zysten im Nierenmark. Charité-Ann. **32**, 285 (1908).

BRAIBANTI, T.: Considerazioni au di un caso di displasia cistica del rene. Ann. Radiol. diagn. (Bologna) **21**, 412 (1949).

BRUNI, P.: Rene a spugna associato a cistopatia cistica. Urologia (Treviso) **21**, 148 (1954).

BUTLER, A. M., WILSON, J. L., FARBER, S.: Dehydration and acidosis with calcification at renal tubules. J. Pediat. **8**, 489 (1936).

CACCHI, R.: La malattia cistica delle piramidi renali o „Rene a spugna". Relazione ufficiale al XXX. Congr. della Soc. Italiana di Urologia, Napoli **1** (1957). Cremona 1957.

— RICCI, V.: Sur une rare maladie kystique multiple des pyramides rénales le „rein en éponge". J. Urol. méd. chir. **55**, 497 (1949).

CARINATI, A.: In tema di displasie cistiche renali con particulare riguardo ad un caso di „rene a spugna". Radiol. **12**, 79 (1956).

CETNAROWICZ, H., CZECHOWSKA, Z., KOPEĆ, M., ZABOKRZYCKI, J.: Cystic disease of renal pyramids. Pol. Przegl. radiol. **22**, 233 (1958).

CIRLA, A., GALDINI, S.: Contributo allo studio del rene a spugna. Radiol. med. (Torino) **42**, 605 (1956).

CLAUS, H. G.: Die Schwammniere. Fortschr. Röntgenstr. **99**, 298 (1963).

DAMMERMANN, H. J.: Urologentreffen Düsseldorf 1948. Zit. GÜNTHER 1950.
— Markcystenniere unter dem Bild einer Solitärcyste. Z. Urol. 44, 230 (1951).
DARGET, R., BALLANGER, R.: Sur un cas de rein „en éponge". J. Urol. méd. chir. 69, 713 (1954).
DELL'ADAMI, G., MENEGHINI, C.: Il „rene a spugna": la prima osservazione in consanguinei. Arch. Ital. Urol. 27, 81 (1954).
DELMAS, J., RACHOU, R., PHILIPPON, J., BENEJAM, J.: Reins „en éponge". J. Radiol. Électrol. 39, 844 (1958).
DELZOTTO, L., TURCHETTO, P.: Il rene a spugna: contributo casistico. Urologia (Treviso) 22, 240 (1955).
DENSTAD, T.: Medullary sponge kidney. J. Oslo City Hosp. 9, 201 (1959).
DI SIENO, A., GUARESCHI, B.: Il quadro radiologico del rene a spugna midollare. Radiol. clin. (Basel) 25, 80 (1956).
— Il rene a spugna midollare con calcolosi multipla endocavitaria ed i suoi possibile rapporti con la nefrocalcinosi. Radiol. med. (Torino) 42, 167 (1956).
EKSTRÖM, T., ENGFELDT, B., LAGERGREN, C., LINDVALL, N.: Medullary sponge kidney. Stockholm: Almqvist & Wiksell 1959.
EVANS, J. A.: Medullary sponge kidney. Amer. J. Roentgenol. 86, 119 (1961)
FIUMICELLI, A., SAMMARCO, G., VERDECCHIA, G. C.: Rene a spugna midollare e nefrocalcinosi: diagnosi differenziale. Radiol. med. (Torino) 42, 1018 (1956).
FONTOURA, MADUREIRA, H.: Doenca quistica das piramides renais (Rim em esponja). J. Soc. Ci. Med. Lisboa 117, 6 (1943).
GAYET, R.: DEUX cas de maladie kystique des pyramides rénales ou rein en éponge. Actes du 44. Congr. Français d'urologie, p. 473. Paris: G. Doin & Cie. 1950.
— Discussion in HICKEL, R: Un cas de "rein en éponge". J. Urol. méd. chir. 59, 409 (1953).
GIANNONI, R., VIDAL, B., ENGLARO, L.: Contributo alla casistica del rene a spugna. Urologia (Treviso) 23, 625 (1956).
GIBBA, A., GANDINI, D.: Contributo casistico alla studio del rene a spugna. Urologia (Treviso) 21, 596 (1954).
GIORDANO, G.: Rene a spugna (caso con ipertensione a crisi). Nunt. Radiol. 22, 380 (1956).
GRANBERG, P.-O., LAGERGREN, C., THEVE, N. O.: Renal function studies in medullary sponge kidney. Scand. J. Urol. & Nephrol. 5, 177 (1971).
GÜNTHER, G. W.: Die Markcysten der Niere. Z. Urol. 43, 29 (1950).
HICKEL, R.: Un cas de „rein en éponge". J. Urol. méd. chir. 59, 408 (1953).
HOGNESS, J. R., BURNELL, J. M.: Medullary, cysts of kidneys. Arch. intern. Med. 93, 355 (1954).
IBACH, H. A., LAPSEN, L. L.: Roentgen manifestations of multiple cysts of the renal medulla. Radiol. 75, 363 (1960).
JOSSERAND, P., ANNINO, R., MUGNIERY, L., ROUVÉS, L., MERLE, H.: Le rein en éponge. Pédiatrie 7, 31 (1952).

KERR, D. N. S., WARRICK, C. K., HART-MERCER, J.: A lesion resembling medullary sponge kidney in patients with congenital hepatic fibrosis. Clin. radiol. 13, 85 (1962).
LAGERGREN, C., LINDVALL, N.: Medullary sponge kidney and polycystic diseases of the kidney: distinct entities. Amer. J. Roentgenol. 88, 153 (1962).
LENARDUZZI, G.: Reporte pielografico poco commune (dilatazione delle vie urinarie intrarenali). Radiol. med. (Torino) 26, 346 (1939).
— Sul rene a spugna. Radiol. med. (Torino) 35, 992 (1949).
— La forma circoscritta di rene a spugna. Radiol. med. (Torino) 37, 776 (1951).
— Evoluzione del rene a spugna. Radio. med. (Torino) 38, 57 (1952).
— Rene a spugna parcellare. Radiol. med. (Torino) 38, 1084 (1952).
LHEZ, A.: Le rein en éponge. J. Urol. méd. chir. 60, 575–588 (1954).
LINDVALL, N.: Roentgenologic diagnosis of medullary sponge kidney. Acta radiol. 51, 193 (1959).
MARINI, A.: Il rene a spugna. Boll. Soc. med.-chir. Cremona 11, 65 (1957).
MASETTO, I., BRAGGION, P.: Rene a spugna. Nunt. Radiol. 22, 47 (1956).
MATHIS, R. I., BERRI, G.: Rinen en exponja. Rev. argent. Urol. 24, 283 (1955).
MULVANEY, W. P., COLLINS, W. T.: Cystic disease of the renal pyramids. J. Urol. 75, 776 (1956).
MURPHY, W. K., PALUBINSKAS, A. J., SMITH, D. R.: Sponge kidney: a report of seven cases. J. Urol. 85, 866 (1961).
NEUHAUS, W.: Multiple Zysten der Tubuli recti. Fortschr. Röntgenstr. 84, 108 (1956).
NEVEU, J.: Un cas de „maladie kystique multiple des pyramides rénales". J. Urol. méd. chir. 56, 564 (1950).
PALUBINSKAS, A. J.: Medullary sponge kidney. Radiology 76, 911 (1961).
— Abstract, Postgraduate Course in Genito-urinary Radiology. New York: Albert Einstein College of Medicine 1969.
PANSADORO, V.: Su un caso di malattia cistica multipla delle piramidi renali o rene a spugna. Quad. Urol. 1, 125 (1952).
PELOT, G.: Discussione a HICKEL: Un cas de „rein en éponge". J. Urol. méd. chir. 59, 410 (1953).
— Discussione a LHEZ: le rein en éponge. J. Urol. méd. chir. 60, 587 (1954).
PENNISI, S. A., BUNTS, R. C.: Sponge kidney. J. Urol. 84, 246 (1960).
PETKOVIC, S.: Contribution à l'étude de la maladie kystique des pyramides rénales. J. Urol. méd. chir. 58, 425 (1952).
POLITANO, V. A.: Pyelorenal backflow: clinical significance and interpretation. J. Urol. 78, 1 (1957).
POWELL, R. E.: An unusual congenital deformity of the kidney. Canad. med. Ass. J. 60, 48 (1949).
PYRAH, L. N.: Medullary sponge kidney. J. Urol. 95, 274 (1966).

QUINARD, J., MARTIN, J., MOINE, D.: A propos de deux de spongiose rénale. J. Radiol. **43**, 235 (1962).

— MAUDUIT, A., ZUMBIEHL, J., SARIS, A., TOURETTE, G.: Cinq nouveaux cas de spongiose rénale. J. Radiol. d'Électrol. **45**, 267 (1964).

REBOUL, G., PÉLISSIER, M., BELTRANDO, L.: A propos d'un cas de rein en éponge. J. Radiol. Électrol. **39**, 795 (1958).

REILLY, B. J., NEUHAUSER, E. B. D.: Renal tubular ectasia in cystic disease of the kidneys and liver. Amer. J. Roentgenol. **84**, 546 (1960).

REBOUL, G., PÉLESSIER, M., BELTRANDO, L.: A propos d'un cas de rein en éponge. J. Radiol. Électrol. **39**, 795 (1958).

RONCORONI, L.: Le calcificazioni della loggia renale nelle formazioni cistiche e nel tumori. Radiol. med. (Torino) **42**, 953 (1956).

RUBIN, E. L., ROSS, J. C., TURNER, D. P. B.: Cystic disease of the renal pyramids ("sponge kidney"). J. Fac. Radiol. (Lond.) **10**, 134 (1959).

SECREST, P. G., KENDIG, T. A.: Medullary sponge kidney. Radiology **76**, 920 (1961).

SMITH, C. H., GRAHAM, J. B.: Congenital medullary cysts of the kidneys with severe refractory anemia. Amer. J. Dis. Child. **69**, 369 (1945).

TOTI, A., DELL'ADAMI, G.: Contributo alla conoscenza della dilatazione cistica delle vie urinarie prepelviche (rene a spugna). Atti Accad. Sci. Ferrara **27**, 2 (1948/49).

VERMOOTEN, V.: Congenital cystic dilatation of renal collecting tubules: New disease entity. Yale J. Biol. Med. **23**, 450 (1950/51).

VESPIGNANI, L.: Sull'associazione delle varie forme della malattia cistica renale Radiator. Radiobiol. Fis. med. **5**, 483 (1951).

— Rene a spugna. Ann. Radiol. diagn. (Bologna) **31**, 276 (1958).

ZAFFAGNINI, B., MACCHITELLA, A.: Rene a spugna. Acta chir. ital. **10**, 513 (1954).

P. The backflow phenomenon

ABESHOUSE, B. S.: Pyelographic injection of perirenal lymphatics. Amer. J. Surg. **25**, 427 (1934).

AHLGREN, P.: Renal uroplani-pyelosinøs refluks. Nordisk Medicin **13**, IV, 469 (1967).

AHLSTRÖM, C. G.: Experimentelle Untersuchung über die pyelovenöse Refluxe. Acta chir. scand. **75**, 162 (1934).

AUVERT, J. (Rapporteur): Les reflux à partir du bassinet (Refluxt pyélo-rénal). Ass. Française d'Urologie 51. session Paris, 7 au 12 octobre 1957. Rapport et informations.

BAUER, D.: Pyelorenal backflow. Amer. J. Roentgenol. **78**, 296 (1957).

BITSCHAI, J.: Demonstrationen zum Kapitel der Nierenchirurgie. Z. Urol. **21**, 891 (1927).

BOSSI, R., VIVIANI, G.: Considerazion radiologiche sui reflussi renali. Arch. Ital. Urol. **35**, 66 (1962).

BOYARSKY, S., TAYLOR, A., BAYLIN, G.: Extravasation in excretory urography. Urol. int. (Basel) **1**, 191 (1955).

BRIJS, A.: Extravasate bei intravenöser Urographie. Fortschr. Röntgenstr. **103**: 3, 375 (1968).

CEDERLUND, H.: Beitrag zur Frage des pyelovenösen Rückflusses. Acta radiol. **23**, 34 (1942).

CHEN, K.-C.: Lymphatic abnormalities in patients with chyluria. J. Urol. **106**: 1, 111 (1971).

FAJERS, C. M., IDBOHRN, H.: Peripelvic reflux simulating a tumour of the renal pelvis. Urologia Int. (Basel), **197** (1957).

FINE, M. G., VERMOOTEN, V.: Spontaneous extravasation associated with excretory urography. J. Urol. **84**, 409 (1960).

FLEISCHNER, F. G., BELLMAN, S., HENKEN, E. M.: Papillary opacification in excretory urography. Radiol. **74**, 567 (1960).

FORD jr., W. H., PALUBINSKAS, A. J.: Renal extravasation during excretory urography using abdominal compression. J. Urol. **97**: 6, 283 (1967).

FORSYTHE, W. E., HUFFMAN, W. L., SCHILDT, P. J., PERSKY, L.: Spontaneous extravasation during urography. J. Urol. **80**, 393 (1958).

FUCHS, F.: Untersuchungen über die innere Topographie der Niere. Z. urol. Chir. **18**, 164 (1925).

— Pyelovenous backflow in the human kidney. J. Urol. **23**, 181 (1930).

— Zur Frage der pyelographisch sichtbaren Nierenbeckenextravasate. Z. urol. Chir. **30**, 392 (1930).

— Die Hydromechanik der Niere. Z. urol. Chir. **33**, 1 (1931).

— Die physiologische Rolle des Fornixapparates. Z. urol. Chir. **42**, 80 (1936).

GIGON, A.: Quelques résultats expérimentaux et remarques concernant le métabolisme et spécialiment le diabète. Paris 1856. See: Acta med. scand. Suppl. **312**, 154, 481 (1956). in: BING, R.: Bull. Schweiz. Akad. Med. Wissensch. **12**: 91 (1956).

GREEN, N., FINGERHUT, A. G., FRENCH, S.: Mechanism of renovascular backflow. Radiol. **92**: 3, 531 (1969).

HAMPERL, H.: Vävnadsreaktion ("främmandekroppsreaktion") mot slem och urin. Nord. Medicin **41**, 66 (1949).

— DALLENBACH, F. D.: The extravasation and precipitation of urine in the hilus of the kidneys. J. of Mount Sinai Hosp. **24**, 929 (1957).

HARDY, E. G.: Spontaneous rupture of the renal pelvis from calculous obstruction of the ureter. Brit. J. Surg. **47**, 205 (1959).

HARROW, B. R.: Unusual renal peripelvic extravasation requiring operative drainage. J. Urol. **102**: 5, 564 (1969).

— Spontaneous urinary extravasation associated with renal colic causing a perinephric abscess. Amer. J. Roentgen. **98**: 1, 47 (1966).

— SLOANE, J. A.: Pyelorenal extravasation during excretory urography. J. Urol. **86**: 6, 995 (1961).

HAZMIN, M., PERSKY, L., STRORAASLI, J. P.: Backflow patterns in experimental chronic hydronephrosis. J. Urol. **84**, 10 (1960).

HENDRIOCK, A.: Intravenöse Urographie und pelvirenaler Übertritt. Zbl. Chir. **61**, 1822 (1934).

HERRNHEISER, G., STRNAD, F.: Die Perforationen des Nierenbeckens und des Harnleisters im Pyelogramm. Erg. Med. Strf. **7**, 259 (1936).

HINKEL, C. L.: Opacification of the renal pyramids in intravenous urography. Amer. J. Roentgenol. **78**, 317 (1957).

HINMAN, F.: Peripelvic extravasation during intravenous urography: evidence for an additional route for backflow after ureteral obstrution. J. Urol. **85**: 3, 385 (1961).

— LEE-BROWN, R. K.: Pyleovenous back flow. J. Amer. med. Ass. **82**, 607 (1924).

ILLYÉS, G. v.: Frühzeitige Feststellung einer kleinen Nierengeschwulst mittels pyelovenösen Refluxes. Z. urol. Chir. **34**, 186 (1932).

KÖHLER, R.: Investigations on backflow in retrograde pyelography. Acta radiol. Suppl. **99** (1953).

LAMMERS, H. J., SMITHUIS, TH., LOHMAN, A.: De pyelo-veneuze reflux. Ned. T. Geneesk. **99**, 3237 (1955).

LINDBOM, Å.: Fornix backflow in excretion urography. Acta radiol. **24**, 411 (1943).

— Miliary tuberculosis after retrograde pyelography. Acta radiol. **25**, 219 (1944).

LOEPER, J., MICHEL, J. R., EMERIT, J., SINGIER, J. R., FOUCHER, M., ZEILLER, B., CHASSAING, P.: Extravasation d'urine démontrée par urographie intraveineuse au cours d'une crise de colique néphrétique. J. Radiol. Électrol. **50**: 5, 293 (1969).

MARQUARDT, H., HEMMATI, A, KRÜGER, J.: Fornixrupturen bei der Ausscheidungsurographie. Fortschr. Röntgenstr. **115**: 2, 233 (1971).

MAYER, H.: Über einen Fall von ureterovenösem Reflux bei retrograder Pyelographie. Fortschr. Röntgenstr. **90**, 263 (1959).

McFARLANE, D. R.: Findings on excretory urography closely following extravasation of contrast material from the pelvic ureter. Amer. J. Roentgenol. **95**: 2, 424 (1965).

MEUSER, H.: Über Hypernephrome. Z. Urol. **37**, 251 (1943).

MINDER, J.: Experimentelle und klinische Beiträge zur Frage des pyelovenösen Refluxes und seine klinische Bedeutung. Z. urol. Chir. **30**, 404 (1930).

NARATH, P. A.: Extrarenal extravasation observed in the course of intravenous urography. J. Urol. **39**, 65 (1938).

OLIVIER, A.: Les aspects radiologiques des hémato-lymphochyluries filariennes. J. Radiol. Electrol. **38**, 286 (1957).

OLSSON, OLLE: Die Urographie bei der Nierentuberkulose, Acta radiol. Suppl. **XLVII** (1943).

— Studies on backflow in excretion urography. Acta radiol. Suppl. **70** (1948).

— Backflow in excretion urography during renal colic. In: Modern Trends in Diagnostic Radiology (Ed. by J. W. McLAREN). London: Butterworth & Co. (1953).

— In: Diseases of the kidney. Edited by M. B. Strauss & L. G. Welt. Boston: Little, Brown & Co. 1971.

OLSSON, OLLE: In: Angiography. Edited by H. L. Abrams. Boston: Little, Brown & Co. 1971.

— Frequency of backflow in acute renal colic. Acta radiol. **12**: 4, 469 (1972).

ORKIN, L. A.: Spontaneous or nontraumatic extravasation from the ureter. J. Urol. **67**, 272 (1952).

OSSINSKAYA, V. V.: Refluxes. Vestn. Rentgenol. Radiol. **16**, 25 (1936).

PERSKY, L., JOELSON, J. J.: Spontaneous rupture of renal pelvis secondary to a small ureteral calculus. J. Urol. **72**, 141 (1954).

— STORAASLI, J. P., AUSTEN, G.: Mechanisms of hydronephrosis: Newer investigative techniques. J. Urol. **73**, 740 (1955).

POLITANO, V. A.: Pyelorenal backflow. J. Urol. **78**, 1 (1957).

PYTEL, A.: A propos de la pathogénèse et du traitement des soi-disant hémorragies rénales essentielles. Acta urol. belg. **24**, 211 (1956).

— Über den Fornix-Venenkanal als Ursache gewisser Nierenblutungen. Urologia (Treviso) **25** (1958).

PYTEL, A: Über die Bedeutung der pyelorenalen Refluxe bei der Metastasierung der Nierentumoren. Ztschr. Urol. **53**, 133 (1960).

QUACK, G.: Pyelorenaler Reflux bei der Ausscheidungsurographie. Fortschr. Röntgenstr. **91**, 411 (1959).

RENANDER, A.: Röntgenbefunde bei Nierentuberkulose. Acta radiol. **20**, 341 (1939).

RABINOWITZ, J. G., RHONA, R. J.: WOLF, B. S.: Benign peripelvic extravasation associated with renal colic. Radiology **86**: 2, 220 (1966).

RISHOLM, L.: Studies on renal colic and its treatment by posterior splanchnic block. Acta chir. scand. Suppl. 184 (1954) (pp. 1–64).

— ÖBRINK, K. J.: Pyelorenal backflow in man. Acta chir. scand. **115**, 144 (1958).

ROLNICK, H. C., SINGER, P. L.: Effects of overdistention of the renal pelvis and ureter: a study on pyelovenous backflow. J. Urol. **57**, 834 (1947).

ROSS, J. A.: One thousand retrograde pyelograms with manometric pressure records. Brit. J. Urol. **31**, 133 (1959).

SAULS, C. L., NESBIT, R. M.: Pararenal pseudocysts: a report of four cases. J. Urol. **87**, 288 (1962).

SCHUBERTH, O.: Eine Komplikation bei Pyelographierung. Zbl. ges. Chir. Grenzgeb. **60**, 1825 (1933).

SENGPIEL, G. W.: Renal backflow in excretory urography. Amer. J. Roentgenol. **78**, 289 (1957).

SOARES DE GOUVÊA, G.: Spontaneous reflux during excretory urography. Rev. bras. Cir. **22**, 307 (1951).

STAUBESAND, J.: Beobachtungen an Korrosionspräparaten menschlicher Nierenbecken. Fortschr. Röntgenstr. **85**, 33 (1956).

STEINERT, R.: Renal tuberculosis and roentgenologic examination. Acta radiol. Suppl. **53** (1943).

SVOBODA, M.: Thorotrast residue in the kidneys thirteen years after retrograde pyelography. Zbl. Chir. **79**, 1930 (1954).

VOEGELI, E.: Die Pathogenese des Fibrolipomatose. Der Radiologe II, 209 (1971).

WEINER, M. E., ALCORN, F. S., JENKINSON, E. L.:
Subcapsular rupture of the kidney during intravenous urography. Radiology **69**, 853 (1957).

Q. Renal transplantation

ALFIDI, R. J., MEANEY, T. F., BUONOCORE, E.,
NAKAMOTO, S.: Evaluation of renal homotrans-
plantation by selective angiography. Radiology
87, 1099 (1966).
ALFIDI, R. J., MAGNUSSON, M.: Arteriography during
perfusion preservation of kidneys. Amer. J. Roent-
genol. **114**, 690 (1972).
BRÜCKE, P., POLIESER, H., PIZA, F., ZAUNBAUER, W.:
Angiographische Untersuchungen vor und nach
Nierentransplantation. In: Angiographie und ihre
Leistungen. Ed. by K. E. Loose. Stuttgart: Georg
Thieme Verlag 1968 (page 162).
CALNE, R. Y., LAUGHRIDGE, L. W., MACGILLIVRAY,
J. B., ZILVA, J. F., LEVI, A. J.: Renal transplan-
tation in man: a report of five cases using cada-
veric donors. Brit. Med. J. **II**, 645 (1963).
CRUMMY, A. B., HIPONA, F. A.: The roentgen diagno-
sis of renal vein thrombosis: experimental aspects.
Amer. J. Roentgenol. **93**, 898 (1965).
FLETCHER, E. W. L., LECKY, J. W.: The radiological
demonstration of urological complications in renal
transplantation. Brit. J. Radiol. **42**, 886 (1969).
GOODMAN, N., DAVES, M. L., RIFKIND, D.: Pulmonary roentgen findings following renal transplan-
tations. Radiology **89**, 621 (1967).
HUME, D. M.: Kidney transplantation. In: Human
transplantation. Ed. by F. T. Rapaport & J.
Dausse. New York & London: Grune & Stratton
1968.
IMRAY, T., GEDGAUDAS, E.: Excretory urography in
the evaluation of renal transplants. Radiology
95, 653 (1970).
KAUDE, J., SLUSHER, D. H., PFAFF, W. W., HACKETT,
R. L.: Angiographic diagnosis of rejection and
tubular necrosis in human kidney allografts. Acta
radiol. **10**, 476 (1970).
KNUDSEN, D. F., DAVIDSON, A. J., KOUNTZ, S. L.,
COHN, R.: Serial angiography in canine renal
allografts. Transplantation **5**, 256 (1967).
KOEHLER, P. R., BOWLES, W. T., MCALÍSTER, W. H.:
Renal arteriography in experimental renal vein
occlusion. Radiology **86**, 851 (1966).
KOUNTZ, S. L., WILLIAMS, M. A., WILLIAMS, P. L.,
KAPROS, D. C., DEMPSTER, W. J.: Mechanism of
rejection of homotransplanted kidneys. Nature
199, 257 (1963).
NAVANI, S., ATHANASOULIS, C., MONACO, A., CAVALLO,
T., LEWIS, E., HIPONA, F.: Renal homotransplan-
tation: spectrum of angiographic findings of the
kidney. Amer. J. Roentgenol. **113**, 433 (1971).
O'CONNOR, J. F., DEALY jr., J. B., LINDQUIST, R.,
COUCH, N. P.: Arterial lesions due to rejection in
human kidney allografts. Radiology **89**, 614 (1967).
OLIN, T., LINDSTEDT, E.: Angiografi vid njurtrans-
plantation på råtta. Nord. Med. **85**, 1164 (1971).
POKIESER, H.: Röntgendiagnostische Aufgaben im
Rahmen der Nierentransplantation (mit besonderer Berücksichtigung angiographischer Untersuchungen). Fortschr. Röntgenstr. **114**, 1 (1971).

PORTER, H. A., MARCHIORO, T. L., STARZL, T. E.:
Pathological changes in 37 human renal homo-
transplants treated with immunosuppressive drugs.
Brit. J. Urol. **37**, 250 (1965).
PROUT jr., G. R., HUME, D. M., LEE, H. M., WILLIAMS,
G. M.: Some urological aspects of 93 consecutive
renal homotransplants in modified recipients. J.
Urol. **97**, 409 (1967).
RAPHAEL, M. J., STEINER, R. E., SHACKMAN, R.,
WARE, R. G.: Postoperative angiography in renal
homotransplantation. Brit. J. Radiol. **42**, 873 (1969).
SAMUEL, E.: Radiology in the diagnosis of renal
• rejection. Clin. Radiol. **21**, 109 (1970).
STAPLE, T. W., DAVID, T. C.: Arteriography following
renal transplantation. Amer. J. Roentgenol. **101**,
669 (1967).
STARZL, T. E.: Experience in renal transplantation.
Philadelphia: W. B. Saunders Co. 1964.
— VANHOUTTE, J. J., BROWN, D. W., TAUBMAN,
J., STEARS, J. C., DAUES, M. L., HALGRIMSON,
C. G.: Radiology and organ transplantation. Ra-
diology **95**, 1 (1970).
VINIK, M., SMELLIE, W. A. B., FREED, T. A., HUME,
D. M., WEIDNER, W. A.: Angiographic evaluation
of the human homotransplant kidney. Radiology
92, 873 (1969).
WEIDNER, W., RILEY, J., HANAFFEE, W.: Angio-
graphic evaluation in renal transplantation. Ra-
diology **83**, 579 (1964).
WHITE jr., R., NAJARIAN, J., LOKEN, M., AMPLATZ,
K.: Arteriovenous complications associated with
renal transplantation. Radiology **102**, 29 (1972).

R. Miscellaneous changes particularly of the ureter

ABESHOUSE, B. S.: Primary benign and malignant
tumors of the ureter. A review of the literature
and report of one benign and twelve malignant
tumors. Amer. J. Surg. **91**, 237 (1956).
— TANKIN, L. H.: Leukoplakia of the renal pelvis
and the bladder. J. Urol. **76**, 330 (1956).
ÅKERLUND, Å.: Ein typisches Röntgenbild bei Konkrementbildung in einer Ureterozele. Acta radiol.
16, 39 (1935).
AKIMOTO, K.: Über amyloidartige Einweißnieder-
schläge im Nierenbecken. Beitr. path. Anat. **78**,
239 (1927).
ALTVATER, G.: Primäres Harnleiterkarzinom. Z. Urol.
49, 121 (1956).
AMSELEM, A.: Hidronefrosis bilateral gigante sin ob-
staculo sin organico aparente. Med. Españ. **23**, 230
(1950).
ANDREAS, B. F., OOSTING, M.: Primary amyloidosis
of the ureter. J. Urol. **79**, 929 (1958).
ARMSTRONG jr., C. P., HARLIN, H. C., FORT, C. A.:
Leukoplakia of the renal pelvis. J. Urol. **63**, 208
(1950).
ARNHOLDT, F.: Zur Diagnose der Leukoplakie des
Nierenbeckens. Z. urol. Chir. **44**, 292 (1939).
BARON, C.: Leukoplakia of the renal pelvis. J. Urol.
73, 941 (1955).
BATES, B. C.: Periureteritis obliterans: a case report
with a review of the literature. J. Urol. **82**, 58
(1959).

BENNETTS, F. A., CRANE, J. F., CRANE, J. J., GUMMESS, G. H., MILES, H. B.: Diseases of ureteral stump. J. Urol. **73**, 238 (1955).

BERMAN, M. H., COPELAND, H.: Filling defects of ureterogram caused by a varicose ureteral vein. J. Urol. **70**, 168 (1953).

BÉTOULIÈRES, P., JAUMES, F., COLIN, R.: Dilatation pseudokystique de l'uretère terminal. J. Radiol. Électrol. **40**, 582 (1959).

BIANCHI, E.: Roentgenologic findings in uretero-appendicular fistula. Radiol. med. (Milan) **42**, 286 (1956).

BORCH-MADSEN, P.: Primary benign tumour of the ureter. Nord. Med. **53**, 956 (1955).

BRADFIELD, E. O.: Bilateral ureteral obstruction due to envelopment and compression by an inflammatory retroperitoneal process. J. Urol. **69**, 769 (1953).

BRODNY, M. L., HERSHMAN, H.: Pedunculated hemangioma of the ureter. J. Urol. **71**, 539 (1954).

BURKLAND, C. E., LEADBETTER, W. F.: Pyelitis cystica associated with an hemophilus influenzae infection in the urine. J. Urol. **42**, 14 (1939).

CANIGIANI, T.: Ein Fall von cystischer Dilatation des vesicalen Ureterendes. Z. urol. Chir. **36**, 172 (1933).

CHINN, J., HORTON, R. K., RUSCHE, C.: Unilateral ureteral obstruction as sole manifestation of endometriosis. J. Urol. **77**, 144 (1957).

CHISHOLM, E. R., HUTCH, J. A.: BOLOMEY, A. A.: Bilateral uretral obstruction due to chronic inflammation of the fascia around the ureters. J. Urol. **72**, 812 (1954).

CIBERT, J., DURAND, L., RIVIÈRE, C.: Les compressions ureterales par sclerose du tissu cellulo-adipeux peri-ureteral "peri-ureteritis primitives". J. Urol. méd. chir. **62**, 705 (1956).

COMPERE, D. E., BEGLEY, G. F., ISAACKS, H. E., FRAZIER, T. H., DRYDEN, C. B.: Ureteral polyps. J. Urol. **79**, 209 (1958).

CRANE, J. F.: Ureteral involvement by aortic aneurysm. J. Urol. **79**, 403 (1958).

DAVIS, D. M., NEALON jr., TH. F.: Complete replacement of both ureters by an ileal loop. J. Urol. **78**, 748 (1957).

DAVISON, S.: Pyoureter seventeen years after nephrectomy. J. Amer. Med. Ass. **118**, 137 (1942).

DINEEN, J., ASCH, T., PEARCE, J.: Retroperitoneal fibrosis. Radiology **75**, 380 (1960).

DORST, J. D., CUSSEN, G. H., SILVERMAN, F. N.: Ureteroceles in children, with emphasis on the frequency of ectopic ureteroceles. Radiology **74**, 88 (1960).

DREYFUSS, W.: Anomaly simulating a retrocaval ureter. J. Urol. **82**, 630 (1959).

— GOODSITT, E.: Acute regional ureteritis. J. Urol. **79**, 202 (1958).

ELLEGAST, H., SCHIMATZEK, A.: Zur Differential-diagnose der Ureterstenosen. Radiol. Austr. **9**, 209 (1957).

ERICSSON, N. O.: Ectopic ureterocele in infants and children. Acta chir. scand. Suppl. **197** (1954).

EVERS, E.: Zwei Fälle mit seltener Ureteranomalie („Akzessorischer Blindureter"). Acta radiol. **25**, 121 (1944).

EWELL, G. H., BRUSKEWITZ, H. W.: Bilateral ureteral obstruction due to envelopment and compression by an inflammatory retroperitoneal process. Urol. cutan. Rev. **56**, 3 (1952).

FALK, C. C.: Leukoplakia of renal pelvis and ureter. J. Urol. **72**, 310 (1954).

FEY, B., TRUCHOT, P., NOIX, M.: Étude radiocinématographique de l'uretère normal et pathologique. J. Radiol. Électrol. **39**, 328 (1958).

FISHER, R. S., HOWARD, H. H.: Unusual ureterograms in a case of periarteritis nodosa. J. Urol. **60**, 398 (1948).

FRISCHKORN jr., H. B.: Roentgenographic behavior of the ureter. Amer. J. Roentgenol. **75**, 877 (1956).

GILBERT, L. W., McDONALD, J. R.: Primary amyloidosis of the renal pelvis and ureter: report of a case. J. Urol. **68**, 137 (1952).

GREENFIELD, M.: True prolapse of the ureter: case report and review of the literature. J. Urol. **75**, 223 (1956).

GUMMESS, G. H., CHARNOCK, D. A., RIDDELL, H. I., STEWART, C. M.: Ureteroceles in children. J. Urol. **74**, 331 (1955).

GUTIERREZ, R.: The modern surgical treatment of ureterocele. Surg. Gynec. Obstet. **68**, 611 (1939).

HACKETT, F.: Idiopathic retroperitoneal fibrosis — a condition involving the ureterus, the aorta and the inferior vena cava. Brit. J. Surg. **46**, 3 (1958).

HARLIN, H. C., HAMM, F. C.: Urologic disease resulting from nonspecific inflammatory conditions of the bowel. J. Urol. **68**, 383 (1952).

HEJTMANCIK, J. H., MAGID, M. A.: Bilateral periureteritis plastica. J. Urol. **76**, 57 (1956).

HELLSTRÖM, J.: Zur Kenntnis der isolierten Dilatation des pelvinen oder juxtavesikalen Harnleiterabschnittes. Acta radiol. **18**, 141 (1937).

HIGBEE, D. R., MILLETT, W. D.: Localized amyloidosis of the ureter: report of a case. J. Urol. **75**, 424 (1956).

HINKEL, C. L., MOLLER, G. A.: Multiple giant ureteral calculi. Amer. J. Roentgenol. **75**, 900 (1956).

HINMAN, F., JOHNSON, C. M., McCORKLE, J. H.: Pyelitis and ureteritis cystica. J. Urol. **35**, 174 (1936).

HOLLY, L. E., SUMCAD, B.: Diverticular ureteral changes. Amer. J. Roentgenol. **78**, 1053 (1957).

HOWARD, T. L.: Giant polyp of ureter. J. Urol. **79**, 397 (1958).

HUNNER, G. L.: Intussusception of the ureter due to a large papillomalike polypus. J. Urol. **40**, 752 (1938).

HUTCH, J. A., ATKINSON, R. C., LOQUVAM, G. S.: Perirenal (Gerota's) fascitis. J. Urol. **81**, 76 (1959).

IANNACCONE, G., MARSELLA, A.: Dilatations of the ureter: A casuistic contribution and critical review with particular regard to the problem of megaureter. Radiol. med. (Milan) **41**, 759 (1955).

— PANZIRONI, P. E.: Ureteral reflux in normal infants. Acta radiol. **44**, 451 (1955).

IOZZI, L., MURPHY, J. J.: Bilateral ureteral obstruction by retroperitoneal inflammation. J. Urol. **77**, 402 (1957).

IRELAND jr., E. F., CHUTE, R.: A case of triplicate-duplicate ureters. J. Urol. **74**, 342 (1955).

JACOBY, M.: Ureteritis cystica. Z. Urol. **23**, 722 (1929).

JEWETT, H. J., HARRIS, A. P.: Scrotal ureter: report of a case. J. Urol. 69, 184 (1953).

JOELSON, J. J.: Pyelitis, ureteritis and cystitis cystica. Arch. Surg. (Chicago) 18, 1570 (1929).

JULIANI, G., GIBBA, A.: Pyelo-ureteral roentgenkymography. Radiol. med. (Milan) 43, 209 (1957).

KAIRIS, Z.: Endometriose des Ureters. Verhandlungsber. der Dtsch. Ges. für Urologie, S. 271. Leipzig 1958.

KICKHAM, C. J. E., JAFFE, H. L.: The upper urinary tract in bladder tumors. J. Urol. 42, 131 (1939).

KINDALL, L.: Pyelitis cystica and ureteritis cystica. J. Urol. 29, 645 (1933).

KLINGER, M. E.: Bone formation in the ureter: a case report. J. Urol. 75, 793 (1956).

KNUTSSON, F.: The roentgen appearance in ureteritis cystica. Acta radiol. 16, 43 (1935).

LANDES, R. R., HOOKER, J. W.: Sclerosing lipogranuloma and peri-ureteral fibrosis following extravasation of urographic contrast media. J. Urol. 68, 403 (1952).

LEWIS, E. L., CLETSOWAY, R. W.: Megaloureter. J. Urol. 75, 643 (1956).

LINDBOM, Å.: Unusual ureteral obstruction by herniation of ureter into sciatic foramen. Acta radiol. 28, 225 (1947).

LIVERMORE, G. R.: Stone in the ureteral stump left when nephrectomy is done. J. Urol. 63, 786 (1950).

LOEF, J. A., CASELLA, P. A.: Squamous cell carcinoma occurring in the stump of a chronically infected ureter many years after nephrectomy. J. Urol. 67, 159 (1952).

LOITMAN, B. S., CHIAT, H.: Ureteritis cystica and pyelitis cystica. A review of cases and roentgenologic criteria. Radiology 68, 345 (1957).

LOW, H. T., COAKLEY, H. E.: Leukoplakia of the renal pelvis. J. Urol. 60, 712 (1948).

MAKAR, N.: The bilharzial ureter. Brit. J. Surg. 36, 148 (1948/49).

MAYERS, M. M.: Diverticulum of the ureter. J. Urol. 61, 344 (1949).

McCALL, I. W.: Case reports: an unusual manifestation of ureterocele. Brit. J. Radiol. 45, 218 (1972).

McGRAW, A. B., CULP, O. S.: Diverticulum of the ureter: report of another authentic case. J. Urol. 67, 262 (1952).

McNULTY, M.: Pyelo-ureteritis cystica. Brit. J. Radiol. 30, 648 (1957).

MILLARD, D. G., WYMAN, S. M.: Periureteric fibrosis: radiographic diagnosis. Radiology 72, 191 (1959).

MILLER, J. M., LIPIN, R. J., MEISEL, H. J., LONG, P. H.: Bilateral ureteral obstruction due to compression by chronic retroperitoneal inflammation. J. Urol. 68, 447 (1952).

MIRABILE, C. S., SPILLANE, R. J.: Bilateral ureteral compression with obstruction from a nonspecific retroperitoneal inflammatory process: case report. J. Urol. 73, 783 (1953).

MORLEY, H. V., SHUMAKER, E. J., GARDNER, L. W.: Intussusception of the ureter associated with a benign polyp. J. Urol. 67, 266 (1952).

MULVANEY, W. P.: Periureteritis obliterans: a retroperitoneal inflammatory disease. J. Urol. 79, 410 (1958).

NILSON, A. E.: Roentgen diagnosis of ureterocele and some impeding factors. Acta radiol. 52, 365 (1959).

NORING, O.: Nonspecific ureteritis elucidated by a case of primary ureteritis. J. Urol. 79, 701 (1958).

ORMOND, J. K.: Bilateral ureteral obstruction due to envelopment and compression by an inflammatory retroperitoneal process. J. Urol. 59, 1072 (1948).

PAULI, D. P., CAUSEY, J. C., HODGES, C. V.: Perinephritis plastica. J. Urol. 73, 212 (1955).

PETROVČIĆ, F., DUGAN, C.: Ureterocele. Report of an unusual case. Brit. J. Radiol. 28, 374 (1955).

POLITANO, V. A.: Leukoplakia of the renal pelvis and ureter. J. Urol. 75, 633 (1956).

PRÉVÔT, R., BERNING, H.: Zur Röntgendiagnostik der Pyelonephritis. Fortschr. Röntgenstr. 73, 482 (1950).

RAE, L. J.: Ectopic ureter in childhood. J. Fac. Radiol. (Lond.) 8, 402 (1957).

RANDALL, A.: Endometrioma of the ureter. J. Urol. 46, 419 (1941).

RAPER, F. P.: Bilateral, symmetrical, periureteric fibrosis. Proc. Roy. Soc. Med. 48, 736 (1955).

RATLIFF, R. K., CRENSHAW, W. B.: Ureteral obstruction from endometriosis. Surg. Gynec. Obstet. 100, 414 (1955).

RENNAES, S.: On double renal pelvis and ureteral calculus. Acta radiol. 31, 37 (1949).

RIESER, C.: A consideration of the ureteral stump subsequent to nephrectomy. J. Urol. 64, 275 (1950).

RIMONDINI, C.: Un caso di tumore primitivo dell'uretere destro. Considerazioni radiodiagnostiche e radioterapeutiche. Nunt. Radiol. 23, 596 (1957).

RÍOS, P.: Periureteritis primitiva unilateral. Arch. esp. Urol. 14, 97 (1958).

ROBBINS, J. J., LICH jr., R.: Metastatic carcinoma of the ureter. J. Urol. 75, 242 (1956).

ROBERTS, R. R.: Complete valve of the ureter: congenital urethral valves. J. Urol. 76, 62 (1956).

ROMANI, S., AMBROSETTI, A.: Le neoplasie dell'uretere. Riv. ital. Radiol. clin. 5, 121 (1955).

RONNEN, J. R. v., DORMAAR, H.: A case of pyelo-ureteritis cystica diagnosed by pyelography. Acta radiol. 34, 96 (1950).

ROSS, J. A.: Peri-ureteritis fibrosa, with notes on three cases. J. Fac. Radiol. 9, 142 (1958).

RUDHE, U.: A typical roentgen picture of very large ureteroceles. Acta radiol. 29, 396 (1948).

RUIU, A.: La pieloureterite cistica. Quad. Radiol. 23, 263 (1958).

SELMAN, J.: Ureterocele: roentgenologic diagnosis with report of an unusual case. Amer. J. Roentgenol. 80, 620 (1958).

SENGER, F. L., BELL, A. L. L., WARRES, H. L., TIRMAN, W. S.: Fate of the ureteral stump after nephrectomy. Amer. J. Surg. 73, 69 (1947).

— BOTTONE, J. J., KELLEHER, J. H.: Bilateral leukoplakia of the renal pelvis. J. Urol. 65, 528 (1951).

SHAHEEN, D. J., JOHNSTON, A.: Bilateral ureteral obstruction due to envelopment and compression by an inflammatory retroperitoneal process: report of two cases. J. Urol. 82, 51 (1959).

STAEHLER, W.: Klinik und Praxis der Urologie. Stuttgart: Georg Thieme Verlag 1959.

STUEBER jr., P. J.: Primary retroperitoneal inflammatory process with ureteral obstruction. J. Urol. 82, 41 (1959).

TALBOT, H. S., MAHONEY, E. M.: Obstruction of both ureters by retroperitoneal inflammation. J. Urol. 78, 738 (1957).

TAYLOR, J. A.: Primary carcinoma of the ureter. J. Urol. 65, 797 (1951).

TWINEM, F. P.: Primary tumors of the ureter. J. Amer. Med. Ass. 163, 808 (1957).

VELZER, D. A. VAN, BARRICK, C. W., JENKINSON, E. L.: Postcaval ureter. Amer. J. Roentgenol. 74, 490 (1955).

VEST, S. A., BARELARE jr., B.: Peri-ureteritis plastica: a report of four cases. J. Urol. 70, 38 (1953).

WADSWORTH, G. E., UHLENHUTH, E.: The pelvic ureter in the male and female. J. Urol. 76, 244 (1956).

WEAVER, R. G.: Ureteral regeneration: experimental and clinical, part III. J. Urol. 79, 31 (1958).

WELLENS, P.: La pyélo-urétérite (-cystite) kystique. J. belge Radiol. 41, 465 (1958).

WEMEAU, L., LEMAITRE, G., DEFRANCE, G.: Urétérocèle et prolapsus de l'urètre. J. Radiol. Électrol. 40, 275 (1959).

WILLIAMS, J. I., CARSON, R. B., WELLS, W. D.: Reflux ureteropyelograms in children. Sth. med. J. (Bgham., Ala.) 50, 845 (1957).

WILLICH, E.: Ureterostiumstenose-Ureterocele. Mschr. Kinderheilk. 105, 377 (1957).

WOOD, L. G., HOWE, G. E.: Primary tumors of the ureter: case reports. J. Urol. 79, 418 (1958).

ZERBINI, E.: Su di un caso di frattura dell'uretere. Nunt. Radiol. 22, 825 (1956).

Supplement to references

ASK-UPMARK, K. E. F., INGVAR, D.: A follow-up examination of 138 cases of subarachnoid hemorrhage. Acta med. scand. 138, 15 (1950).

DAVIDSON, C. N., DENNIS, J. M., McNINCH, E. R., WILLSON, J. K. V., BROWN, W. H.: Nephrocalcinosis associated with sarcoidosis. Radiology 62, 203 (1954).

HECHT, G.: Röntgenkontrastmittel. In: Handbuch der experimentellen Pharmakologie, Bd. 7, S. 79, Berlin: Springer 1938.

HIGGINS, C. C., HICKEN, N. F.: Perinephritic abscess. Ann. Surg. 96, 998 (1932).

IDBOHRN, H., NORGREN, A.: Personal communications. See: OLLE OLSSON, Renal angiography in the pre-diagnostic phase. IX. I. C. R. München 1959.

MATTSON, O.: Practical photographic problems in radiography. Acta radiol. Suppl. 120 (1955).

NOGUEIRA, A.: Spontane Gasfüllung der Harnwege. Z. Urol. 29, 275 (1935).

OLIN, T.: Personal communications. See: OLLE OLSSON, Renal angiography in the pre-diagnostic phase. IX. I. C. R. München 1959.

RISHOLM, L., ÖBRINK, K. J.: Pyelorenal backflow in man. Acta chir. scand. 115, 144 (1958).

SCHMERBER, F.: Les artères de la capsule graisseuse du rein. Int. Mschr. Anat. Physiol. 13, 269 (1896).

STAEHLER, W.: Klinik und Praxis der Urologie. Suttgart: Georg Thieme 1959.

STEINBOCK, A.: Intravenous urography and retrograde pyelography in subcutaneous injuries of kidney. Ann. Chir. Gynaec. Fenn. 37, Suppl. 4 (1948).

TROELL, A.: Intravenöse Pyelographie zur Prüfung der Nierenfunktion bei Prostatikern. Chirurg 7, 513 (1935).

VOGLER, E., HERBST, R.: Angiographie der Nieren. Stuttgart: Georg Thieme Verlag 1958.

Part II: Roentgen diagnosis of the distal part of the urinary tract

AAS, T. N., NILSON, A. E.: Ureterocele in adults. Clinical and roentgenographic follow up. Acta Chir. Scand. 116, 263 (1959).

ADLER, U., NICK, J.: Die Bedeutung der Tonometrie und Urethro-Cystographie bei der funktionellen Urininkontinenz. Gynaecologia (Basel) 146, 283 (1958).

ALONSO, A.: Un nuevo modelo de uretrógrafo. Rev. argent. Urol. 10, 348 (1941).

ALVAREZ IERENA, J. J.: La uretro-cistografia. Pren. méd. mex. 11, 72 (1946).

AMAR, A. D.: Vesicoureteral reflux causing improved visualization on the delayed excretory urogram. Radiology 101, 1 (1971).

AMSELEM, A., PALOMEQUE, L.: Accidentes vasculares de la uretrocistografia. Clin. y Lab. 49, 426 (1950).

ANDERSON, H. E.: Diagnosis of placenta praevia by use of cystogram. Urol. cutan. Rev. 42, 577 (1938).

ANDERSEN, P. E.: Calcification of the Vasa deferentia. Acta radiol. 34, 89 (1950).

ARANALDE BLANNO, J.: Estudio radiologico de la vena cava inferior como medio diagnostico en urologia. Tesis México 1953.

ARENAS, N., FOIX, A.: Importancia de la cistouretrografia en el tratamiento de la incontinencia de orina de esfuerzo. Sem. méd. (B. Aires) 106, 160 (1955).

ARRIGONI, G., LOVATI, G.: Studio uretrocistografico del collo vesicale dopo prostatectomia ipogastrica e perineale. Arch. Ital. Urol. **22**, 190 (1947).

ASTRALDI, A., LANARI, E. L.: Radiographic diagnosis of malignancy of bladder tumors – personal method. Urol. cutan. Rev. **37**, 222 (1933).

ASTRALDI, J.: Sur nue radiolgraphie de la vésicule séminale. Bull. Soc. franc. Urol. 1952, pp. 6–8.

BACH, H.: Ventil-polyp udgået fra prostata. Ugeskr. Laeg. **120**, 495 (1958).

BAENSCH, W.: Zur Technik der Harnröhrenfüllung. Warnung vor öligen Kontrastmitteln. Röntgenpraxis **8**, 316 (1936).

BALL, H., PELZ, H.: Tödlicher Zwischenfall bei der Urethrographie mit Bariumsulfat. Z. Urol. **46**, 539 (1953).

BALL, T. L., DOUGLAS, R. G.: Topographic urethrography in "continent" and "incontinent" women. Trans. New Engl. obstet. gynec. Soc. **4**, 65 (1950).

BALLENGER, E. G., ELDER, O. F., McDONALD, H. P.: Collapsed bladder skiodan cystograms. Sth. med. J. (Bgham, Ala.) **27**, 938 (1934).

BANDTLOW, K.: Urethrozystographie. Röntgenblätter **21**, 434 (1968).

— Urethrozystographie. Helvetia Chirurgica Acta **37**, 443 (1970).

BARRINGTON, F. J. F.: The diagnosis of stone in the urinary tract. II. Bladder and urethra. Med. Wld (Lond.) **74**, 515 (1951).

BÁRSONY, T., KOPPENSTEIN, E.: New method for roentgenoscopy. Orv. Hetil. **76**, 989 (1932).

— POLLÁK, E.: Intravenöse Urozystographie. Röntgenpraxis **4**, 956 (1932).

BARTLEY, O., HELANDER, C. G.: Double-contrast cystography in tumors of the urinary bladder. Acta radiol. **54**, 161 (1960).

— ECKERBOM, H.: Perivesical insufflation of gas for determination of bladder wall thickness in tumors of the bladder. Acta radiol. **54**, 241 (1960).

BAUER, K. M.: Seltene Erkrankungen der Samenblasen. Z. Urol. **49**, 287 (1956).

— Die Klinik der Samenblasenerkrankungen. Med. Klin. **55**, 529 (1960).

BAUMGART, R.: Diagnosestellung eines Blasenkarzinoms durch intravenöses Pyelogramm bei Unmöglichkeit der Cystoskopie wegen starker Hämaturie. Z. Urol. **47**, 382 (1954).

BEARD, D. E., GOODYEAR, W. E., WEENS, H. S.: Radiologic diagnosis of the lower urinary tract. Springfield/Ill.: Thomas 1952; Oxford: Blackwell 1952; Toronto: Ryerson 1952.

BEGG, R. C.: The verumontanum in urinary and sexual disorders. Brit. J. Urol. **1**, 237 (1929).

BELFIELD, W. T.: Vasotomy-radiography of the seminal duct. J. Amer. med. Ass. **61**, 1867 (1913).

— ROLNICK, H.: Roentgenography and therapy with iodized oils. J. Amer. pred. Ass. **86**, 1831 (1926).

BELL, J. C., HEUBLEIN, G. W., HAMMER, H. J.: Roentgen examination with special reference to methods and findings. Amer. J. Roentgenol. **53**, 527 (1945).

BENEVENTI, F. A., MARSHALL, V. F.: Some studies of urinary incontinence in men. J. Urol. **75**, 273 (1956).

BENJAMIN, J. A., JOINT, F. T., RAMSAY, G. H., WATSON, J. S., WEINBERG, S., SCOTT, W. W.: Cinefluorographic studies of bladder and urethral function. Trans. Amer. Ass. gen.-urin. Surg. **46**, 43 (1954).

— J. Urol. **73**, 525 (1955).

BENTZEN, N.: Urethrographic studies of prostatic tuberculosis. Thesis Copenhagen 1960.

BERLIN, L., WALDMAN I., WHITE, F. H., McLAIN, C. R., JR.: Endometriosis of the ureter. Amer. J. Roentgenol. **92**, 351 (1964).

BERNARDI, R., CHOIZZI, J. C.: Anestesia retroprostático-vesical; su visualización, radiográfica. Rev. argent. Urol. **17**, 431 (1948).

BERRI, H. D.: La importancia de la radiologia en las fistulas uretrales. Sem. méd. (B. Aires) **1**, 480 (1933).

BERTI-RIBOLI, E. P., CERRUTI, G. B., MALCHIODI, C., REGGIANI, G.: Studio angiografico dei tumori vesicali. Minerva pediat. (Torino) **9**, 11 (1957).

BEZZI, E., ROSSI, L., MACALUSO, G., RABAIOTTI, A.: Aspetti arteriografici della patologia prostatica. Minerva chir. (Torino) **12**, 867 (1957).

BIANCHINI, A.: Su di un caso di calcificazione quasi totale della vie deferenziali. Arch. Radiol. (Napoli) **6**, 228 (1930).

BIBUS, B.: Röntgenurologische Veränderungen bei Inguinalhernien. Fortschr. Röntgenstr. **94**, 633 (1961).

— Bladder tumors A. symposium. Philadelphia: J. B. Lippincott Co., 1957.

BLANC, H., NEGRO, M.: La cystographie; étude radiologique de la vessie normale et pathologique. Paris: Masson & Cie. 1926.

BLUM, E.: Renseignements fournis par l'urographie et la prostatographie dans les maladies de la prostate. Strasbourg méd. **10**, 423 (1959).

— SICHEL, D.: La radiographie de la prostate; technique, résultats, indications. Acta urol. belg. **25**, 381 (1957).

— — WOLFF, R., WAGNER, J. P.: L'exploration radiologique du prostatique; valeur comparée de l'urographie intraveineuse et de la prostatographie. J. Urol. méd. chir. **63**, 308 (1957).

BOBBIO, A., BEZZI, E., ROSSI, L.: Pelvic angiography in diseases of the prostatic gland. Amer. J. Roentgenol. **82**, 784 (1959).

BOEMINGHAUS, H. W.: Urologische Diagnostik und Therapie für Ärzte und Studierende. 2. erw. Aufl. Jena: Gustav Fischer 1931.

— Urologie. Operative Therapie, Klinik, Indikation. 2. Aufl. München: Werk-Verlag 1954.

— BALDUS, U.: Zur Physiologie der Samenblasen und der Spermien. Z. Urol. **28**, 433 (1934).

— — ZEISS, L.: Erkrankungen der Harnwege im Röntgenbild. Leipzig: Johann Ambrosius Barth 1933.

BOEVÉ, H. J.: Pyelography and cystography in children. Ned. T. Geneesk **16**, 690 (1929–1930).

BOHNERT, W. W.: Ureteral sciatic hernias: Case report of an infant with bilateral ureteral herniation into the sciatic foramina. J. Urol. **106**, 142 (1971).

BOIJSEN, E., LEWIS-JONSSON, J.: Emphysematous cystitis. Acta radiol. **45**, 269 (1954).

BOONE, A. W.: Cystourethrograms before prostatectomy. J. Urol. **67**, 358 (1952).

BOSCH SOLA, P.: Diverticulosis y diverticulitis vesical. Exploración roentgenólogica. Clin. y Lab. **20**, 217 (1932).

BOULLAND, G.: Rétention vésicale chez les prostatiques par le cysto-radiographie de profil. Paris: Le Grand 1928.

BOWEN, D. R., HEIMAN, L.: Combined roentgenoscopic and roentgenographic cystoscopic table. Amer. J. Roentgenol. **23**, 85 (1930).

BOYCE, W., HARRIS, H. J. A., VEST, S. A.: The dorsal cystogram or "squat shot": a technique for roentgenography of posterior bladder and pelvic ureters. J. Urol. **70**, 969 (1953).

BOYD, R. W.: Pneumocystogram. Canad. med. Ass. J. **43**, 221 (1940).

BRAASCH, W. F., EMMETT, J. L.: Clinical urography. Philadelphia: Lea & Febiger 1951.

BRAILSFORD, J. F., DONOVAN, H., MUCKLOW, E. H.: A simple estimation of residual urine in cases of prostatic disease following the ingestion of hippuran by mouth. Brit. J. Radiol. **27**, 183 (1954).

BRANDSTETTER, F.: Prüfungsverfahren zur Objektivierung der funktionellen Harninkontinenz unter besonderer Berücksichtigung der Urethrozystographie. Zbl. Gynäk. **77**, 1269 (1955).

BRELLAND, P. M.: Relationship of bladder shadow to bladder volume on excretion urography. J. Fac. Radiol. (Lond.) **9**, 152 (1958).

BRINEY, A. K., HODES, P. J.: Urinary incontinence in women: roentgen manifestations. Radiology **58**, 109 (1952).

BROCK, D. R.: Ureteral obstruction from endometriosis. J. Urol. **83**, 100 (1960).

BRODNY, M. L.: New instrument for urethrography in male. J. Urol. **46**, 350 (1941).

— Urethrography: its value in the study of male fertility and sterility. Fertil. and Steril. **4**, 386 (1953).

— ROBINS, S. A.: Enuresis; use of cystography in diagnosis. J. Amer. med. Ass. **126**, 1000 (1944).

— Use of new viscous water-miscible contrast medium rayopake (iodine preparation) for cysto-urethrography. J. Urol. **58**, 182 (1947).

— Value of roentgenography of male urethra following infection. Amer. J. Syph. **32**, 272 (1948).

— Urethrocystography in male child. J. Amer. med. Ass. **137**, 1511 (1948).

— Morbidity after prostatectomy: an urethrocystography study. J. int. Coll. Surg. **14**, 143 (1950).

— Urethrocystographic study; a guide for selective prostatectomy. J. int. Coll. Surg. **21**, 351 (1954).

— Urethrocystographic classification of prostatism. Schweiz. med. Wschr. **86**, Suppl. 541 (1956).

BROWNING, W. H., REED, D. C., O'DONNELL, H.: Delayed cystography: a valuable diagnostic tool. J. Kans. med. Soc. **60**, 22 (1959).

BRUNI, P.: Angioma dell'uretra e reflusso uretrovenoso. G. ital. Chir. **4**, 515 (1948).

BRYNDORF, J., CHRISTENSEN, E. R., SANDØE, E.: Suprapubic micturition cystography with constant filling in children. Acta radiol. **54**, 204 (1960).

BUCHMANN, E.: Röntgenologisch diagnostizierte Blasenruptur. Fortschr. Röntgenstr. **82**, 823 (1955).

BUDIN, E., EICHWALD, M.: Achalasia of the ureter. Radiology **75**, 757 (1960).

BUGYI, B.: Urethrography with umbradil viscous U preparation. Mag. Sebész. **10**, 375 (1957).

BUNGE, R. G.: Further observations with delayed cystograms. J. Urol. **71**, 427 (1954).

BURSTEIN, H. J.: Cystography as aid in urologic diagnoses. Illinois med. J. **64**, 344 (1933).

BUSCH, F. M., WEIBEL, D. C., MORRIS, W. E., POHL, C. E.: Congenital ureteral valve. J. Urol. **90**, 43 (1963).

BUTLER W. W. S., JR., PETERSON, C. H.: Roentgen ray study of prostatic urethra with special reference to resection. Sth. med. J. (Bgham, Ala) **27**, 690 (1934): also Virginia med. Monthly **61**, 276 (1934).

BUTTEN, F., SULLIVAN, J. R., BIRNBAUM, W. D.: Radiographic evidence indispensable aid in diagnosis of intraperitoneal rupture. West. J. Surg. **43**, 410 (1935).

CAMERINI, R., ZAFFAGNINI V., LOLLI, G.: Tomography as a research means of bladder walls. Radiol. clin. (Basel) **22**, 421 (1953).

CAMPBELL, M. F.: Cystography in infancy and childhood. Amer. J. Dis. Child. **39**, 386 (1930).

CANCRINI, A., NAPOLITANO, A.: Il pneumoperitoneo pelvico associato alla cistografia gassosa nello studio delle neoplasie vesicali. Ann. Ital. Chir. **36**, 365 (1959).

CAPORALE, L.: Manuale di urologia. Torino: Minerva medica 1952.

CARLSSON, E., GARSTEN, P.: Compression of the common iliac vessels by dilatation of the bladder: Report of a case. Acta radiol. **53**, 449 (1960).

CARNEIRO MONTEIRO, J.: Da uretrografia no homem e suas vantagens no diagnostico das afeccoes uretrais. Rev. Radiol. clin. **2**, 580 (1933).

CARRAL, P. E.: L'uretrografia negli ipospadici operati associando i procedimenti di plastica dell'Ombrédanne e del Leveuf. Arch. ital. Chir. **79**, 505 (1955).

CARTELLI, N.: Es suficiente la radiografia simple para asegurar una litiasis vesical. Sem. méd. (B. Aires) **1**, 1460 (1940).

— COMOTTO, C., BERRI, H. D.: Gran reflujo uretro venoso por uretrografia. Rev. argent. Urol. **15**, 59 (1946).

CARVALHO, M. A.: Study of 111 cystograms for diagnosis of placenta previa. Amer. J. Obstet. Gynec. **39**, 306 (1940).

CASTELLANOS, A., PEREIRAS, R.: La cistografia en el niño. Arch. Med. infant. **9**, 160 (1940).

CELLA, C.: Ricerche anatomoradiografiche sull'ampolla deferenziale dell'uomo nelle varie età. Ann. Radiol. diagn. (Bologna) **24**, 3 (1952).

CERNY, J., SCOTT, T.: Non-idiopathic retroperitoneal fibrosis. J. Urol. **105**, 49 (1971).

CHANDRACHUD, S.: Carcinoma in a urinary bladder diverticulum. Amer. J. Roentgenol. **75**, 925 (1956).

CHARBONNEAU, J.: Du diagnostic des tumeurs de la vessie par la cystographie. J. Hotel-Dieu Montréal **14**, 357 (1945).

CHARNOCK, D. A., RIDDELL, H. I., LOMBARDO, L. J., Jr.: Retroperitoneal fibrosis producing ureteral obstruction. J. Urol. **85**, 251 (1961).

CHAUVIN, H. F., ORSINI, A.: Rétrécissement du col vésical après prostatectomie. Présentation de radiographie. J. Urol. méd. chir. **57**, 739 (1951).

CHAVIGNY, C. L.: Beaded chain and catheter for cystograms. Obstet. and Gynec. **10**, 296 (1957).

CHEVASSU, M.: L'uréthrographie dans la tuberculose génitale male. Bull. Soc. franc. Urol. 274 (1936).

— Étude uréthrographique des cavités de prostatectomie sus-pubienne. Bull. Soc. franc. Urol. 109 (1937).

— L'uréthrographie à la diodone visqueuse. J. Urol. méd. chir. **58**, 149 (1952).

— MOREL, E.: L'exploration radiographique de l'urètre et de la prostate. Strasbourg méd. **95**, 101 (1935).

CHRISTIAN, E., CONSTANTINESCU, N. N.: Urethrography. Rev. rom. Urol. **2**, 112 (1935).

CIBERT, J., CAVAILER, H.: L'exploration radiographique chez les prostatiques. J. Urol. méd. chir. **52**, 35 (1944).

CIVINO, A, LOVATI, G.: Controllo clinico-radiologico di un gruppo di prostatectomizzati secondo il metodo di Hryntschak. Osped. maggiore **44**, 558 (1956).

COE, F. O., ARTHUR, P. S.: New medium (visco-rayopake, iodine preparation) for cystourethrography. Amer. J. Roentgenol. **56**, 361 (1946).

COLBY, F. H.: Early carcinoma of the prostate; diagnosis and treatment. J. Mich. med. Soc. **54**, 463 (1953).

— SUBY, H. I.: Casto-urethrograms: roentgen visualization of urethra, bladder and prostate. New Engl. J. Med. **223**, 85 (1940).

COLOMÉ BOUZA, A.: La cistografia en la práctica urológica. Vida nueva **53**, 17 (1944).

COMARR, A. E.: Position of the patient for roentgenologic interpretation of prostatogram. Amer. J. Roentgenol. **75**, 893 (1956).

— DODENHOFF, L.: A safe, simple method of performing urethrograms. J. Urol. **70**, 980 (1953).

CONRADT, J.: Les suites opératoires locales de la prostatectomic suspubienne étudiées par l'urethrographie. J. belge Urol. **11**, 21 (1938).

COOK, E. N.: Diverticulum of the female urethra: Problems in diagnosis and treatment. Surg. Gynec. Obstet. **99**, 273 (1954).

COTTALORDA, J. RUFF, H., SAVELLI, J.: Résultats uréthrographiques de l'opération de Millin. Marseille chir. **8**, 5 (1956).

COUVELAIRE, R.: Pathologie de l'appareil urinaire et de l'appareil génital masculin. Nouveau précis de pathologie chirurgicale, tome VI/I. Paris: Masson & Cie. 1949.

— FORET, J.: Sur la signification de l'asymétrie urographique des images urétéro-pyélo-calicielles du prostatique. J. Urol. méd. chir. **59**, 17 (1953).

CRABTREE, E. G.: Venous invasion due to urethrograms made with lipiodol (iodized oil). Trans. Amer. Ass. Gen.-Urin. Surg. **38**, 19 (1947); J. Urol. **57**, 380 (1947).

— BRODNEY, M. L.: Estimate of value of urethrogram and cystogram in diagnosis of prostatic obstruction J. Urol. **29**, 235 (1933).

CRABTREE, E. G., FORET, J., KONTOFF, H. A., MUELLNER, S. R.: Roentgenologic diagnosis of urologic and gynecologic diseases of the female bladder. J. Urol. **35**, 52 (1936).

CREEVY, C. D.: The Atonic distal ureteral segment (ureteral achalasia). J. Urol. **97**, 457 (1967).

CHRISTENSEN, E. R.: Cystography with controlled filling pressure in children. Acta radiol. **52**, 426 (1959).

CROOKS, M. L.: Roentgen examination of the urinary tract in children. X-Ray Techn. **23**, 24 (1951).

CRUZ, M.: Über dynamische Störungen der Urethra posterior und ihre Untersuchung mit Hilfe der Urethrographie. Z. Urol. **28**, 675 (1934).

CULP, O. S.: Ureteral diverticula: Classification of the literature and report of an authentic case. J. Urol. **58**, 309 (1947).

CURRARINO, G.: Narrowings of the male urethra caused by contractions or spasm of the bulbocavernosus muscle: cysto-urethrographic observations. Amer. J. Roentgenol. **108**, 641 (1970).

DAMANSKI, M., KERR, A. S.: The value of cysto-urethrography in paraplegia. Brit. J. Surg. **44**, 398 (1957).

— Vesicoureteric reflux in paraplegia. Brit. J. Surg. **52**, 168 (1965).

DAMM, E.: Die funktionelle Cysturethrographie. Z. Urol. **42**, 68 (1949).

DA MOTTA PACHECO, A. A.: Diagnóstico radiológico do adenoma da próstata. S. Paulo méd. **2**, 360 (1944).

— DE CASTRO, J. M., JANY, J., TUFF, H.: Cineuretrocistografia indirecta. Arch. bras. Urol. **4**, 7 (1946).

— DO ROSARIO, O. L.: A imagem do veru-montanum na uretrografia. An. Paul. Med. Cir. **42**, 293 (1941).

DANCKWARDT-LILIESTRÖM, G., FALKMER, S., RYBERG, C. H., STENPORT, G.: Idiopatisk retroperitoneal fibros. Nord. Med. **71**, 357 (1964).

DANNENBERG, M., BEILLY, J. S., BRODNEY, M. B., STORCH C.: Cystographic studies in placenta praevia. Amer. J. Roentgenol. **64**, 53 (1950).

DARGET, R.: L'exploration par l'air du rein et de la vessie. Bull. Soc. Chir. Bordeaux et Sud-Ouest 1932, 69.

— Nuove ricerche radiografiche in urologia. Minerva chir. (Torino) **10**, 367 (1955).

DEAN, A. L.: Carcinoma of the male and female urethra; pathology and diagnosis. J. Urol. **75**, 505 (1956).

— LATTIMER, J. K., McCOY, C. B.: The standardized Columbia University cystogram. J. Urol. **78**, 662 (1957).

DE AZEVEDO, G. V., CABELO CAMPOS, J. M.: Da uretrografia na mulher e seu valor pratico. Rev. Ass. Paul. Med. **1**, 400 (1932).

DE FIGUEIREDO, A.: Uretroscopia e uretrografia. Med. Chirurg. Farm. 1942, pp. 789–829.

DE LAMBERT, B. M., GREENSLADE, N. F.: Cystourethrography in the male. Med. J. Australia **41**, 159 (1954).

DE LA PENA, A., DE LA PENA, E.: Diverticular or cavitary chronic prostatitis. J. Urol. **55**, 273 (1946).

DELPORTE, T. V.: La uretrografia. Su importancia en urologia. Rev. méd. Rosario **33**, 165 (1943).

DENCK, H., HOHENFELLNER, R.: Über die chronische. unspezifische Prostatitis. Klin. Med. (Wien) 13, 245 (1958).

DESY, J.: L'uréthro-cystographie et ses déductions cliniques. Rev. méd. Liège 4, 491 (1949).

DI GRAETA, S., ORRENTINO, F.: La policistografia: metodologia ed indicazioni. Rif. med. 73, 1224 (1959).

DILLON, J. R.: Excretory cystograms after voiding. Calif. Med. 67, 17 (1947).

DINEEN, J., ASCH, T., PEARCE, J. M.: Retroperitoneal fibrosis. Radiology 75, 380 (1960).

DIONISI, H., FERNIOT, A.: La cistografia en el prolapso genital. Bol. Soc. Cir. Córdoba 8, 275 (1947).

DOLAN, P. A., KIRKPATRICK, W. E.: Multiple ureteral diverticula. J. Urol. 83, 570 (1960).

DOTTA, J. S., DELPORTE, T. V.: El reflujo venoso en la uretrografia. Rev. argent. Urol. 13, 133 (1944).

DOYLE, F. H.: Cystography in bladder tumours. A technique using "Steripaque" and carbon dioxide. Brit. J. Radiol. 34, 205 (1961).

DRAHOVSKY, V., KLIMES, M., DÉMANT, F., TISCHLER, P. V.: Enuresis bei Kindern und ihre Beziehung zu den Krankheiten der Harnwege. Proceedings of the 1st Czechoslovak-Swedish-Finnish Urological Symposium — Bratislava, May 1969. Publ. Osveta, Martin, Prague 1970.

DRAPER, J. W., SICELUFF, J. G.: Excretory cysto-urethrograms. J. Urol. 53, 539 (1945).

DUCLUZAUN, J. Q.: A propos des remainements radiographiques du bassin chez les cancéren prostatiques. Thèse Paris 1952.

DUFOUR, A.: Réflexions sur l'exploration radiologique de la vessie. Sem. Hop. Paris 33, 4324 (1957).

EDLING, N. P. G.: Urethrocystography in the male with special regard to micturition. Acta radiol. Suppl. 58, 1 (1945).

— On the roentgen aspect of prostatic cancer by urethrocystography. Acta radiol. 29, 461 (1948).

— On the roentgen aspect of prostatic atrophy. Acta radiol. 31, 145 (1949).

— Radiologic aspect of utriculus prostaticus during urethrocystography. Acta radiol 32, 28 (1949).

— Die Darstellung der Harnröhre und der Harnblase mittels wasserlöslicher Kontrastmittel. Fortschr. Rötgenstr. 72, 18 (1950).

— Roentgendiagnostik der Harnorgane. In SCHINZ, BAENSCH, FRIEDL u. UEHLINGER, Lehrbuch der Röntgendiagnostik, 5. Aufl. Bd. 7/8. Stuttgart: Georg Thieme 1952.

— The roentgen diagnosis of the diseases of the prostate. J. Urol. 67, 197 (1952).

— The radiologic appearances of diverticula of the male cavernous urethra. Acta radiol 40, 1 (1953).

EDSMAN, G.: Roentgenologic changes in the urinary bladder and the distal portion of the ureters in spermatocystitis. Acta radiol. 29, 371 (1948).

EDWARDS, D.: Cineradiography of the congenital neurogenic bladder. Proc. Roy. Soc. Med. 49, 898 (1956).

— Cineradiology of congenital bladderneck obstruction and the megaureter. Brit. J. Urol. 29, 410 (1957).

EISENLOHR, W.: Cit. in ORTMAYER, M.: Cystitis emphysematosa. J. Urol. 60, 757 (1948).

EISLER, F.: Röntgenuntersuchung der Harnblase, Rötgenpraxis 6, 204 (1934).

EKELUND, L., GÖTHLIN, J., HENRIKSON, H.: Angiography in dibuthylnitrosamine-induced rat bladder tumours. Acta path. microbiol. scand. Section A. 80, 691 (1972).

EKMAN, H.: Views on the value of urethrocystography in determining indications for surgery in prostatic hypertrophy. Acta chir. scand. 115, 18 (1958).

— Late results of prostatectomy for benign prostatic hyperplasia. A clinical study based on 370 cases. Acta chir. scand. Suppl. 250, pp. 1–140 (1959).

ENGEL, W. J.: Ureteral ectopia opening into the seminal vesicle. J. Urol. 60, 46 (1948).

Intravenous urography in the study of vesical neck obstructions. Amer. J. Roentgenol. 62, 661 (1949).

ENGELS, E. P.: Sigmoid colon and urinary bladder in high fixation: roentgen changes simulating pelvic ulcer. Radiology 72, 419 (1959).

FAZEKAS, I. G.: Plötzlicher Tod infolge des durch die Harnröhrenperforationen in den Blutkreislauf gelangten Röntgenbreies (Bariumsulfatschock). Z. Urol. 47, 673 (1954); Orv. Hetil. 95, 669 (1954).

FERDINAND, L.: Technic of urethrography. Rozhl. Chir. 35, 24 (1956).

FERNICOLA, A. R.: Extra-urethral confines of urethrographic contrast medium. J. Urol. 66, 132 (1951).

FERULANO, O., NAPOLI, D.: La proiczione assiale dorso-perineale nella indagine costigrafica. Arch. Radiol. (Napoli) 30, 225 (1955).

FEY, B., STOBBAERTS, P., TRUCHOT, P., WOLFROMM, G.: Exploration radiologique de l'appareil urinaire inférieur (vessie, urètre, prostate). Avec la collaboration de L. SABADINI et al. Paris: Masson & Cie. 1949.

FICHARDT, T.: Screening urethrocystography of adult Bantu males under manometric control; normal and pathological findings. Brit. J. Radiol. 32, 120 (1959).

FILHO MATTOSO, S.: El empleo del doble contraste en uretrografia. Arch. Esp. Urol. 5, 330 (1949).

FINKELSTEIN, S. I.: Axial roentgen projections in urology. Urologija, 24, 50 (1959).

FIRSTATER, M.: Cistografia de eliminación y uretro-prostatografia. Rev. argent. Urol. 22, 151 (1953).

FITZPATRICK, R. J., ORR, L. M.: Pelvio-prostatic venography: preliminary report. J. Urol. 68, 647 (1952).

FLECKER, H.: Position of urinary bladder. Med. J. Australia 2, 823 (1934).

FLOCKS, R. H.: The roentgen visualization of the posterior urethra. J. Urol. 30, 711 (1933).

FOCHEM, K., PALMRICH, A. H.: Zur zystographischen Symptomatik der relativen Harninkontinenz. Zbl. Gynäk. 76, 1741 (1954).

— Ein Fall einer Verkalkung einer Niere und des Ureters. Fortschr. Röntgenstr. 96, 570 (1962).

FORBES, K. A., CORDONNIER, J. J.: Circulatory collapse following combined use of rayopake and air for urethrocystography. J. Urol. 70, 975 (1953).

FRAIN-BELL, L., GRIEVE, J.: The micturating cysto-urethrogram in relation to function after prostatectomy. Brit. J. Urol. 29, 15 (1937).

FRANCKE, P., JR., LANE, J. W.: Cystitis emphysematosa, case report. Amer. J. Roentgenol. **75**, 921 (1956).

FRANKSSON, C., LINDBLOM, K.: Roentgenographic signs of tumor infiltration of the wall of the urinary bladder. Acta radiol. **37**, 1 (1952).

— — WHITEHOUSE, W.: The reliability of roentgen signs of varying degrees of malignancy of bladder tumors. Acta radiol. **45**, 266 (1956).

FRANZ, R.: Die Bedeutung der Cystographie für die Wahl der Therapie bei Harninkontinenz. Wien. klin. Wschr. **68**, 2170 (1956).

FRIEDENBERG, R. M., NEY, C.: Extravasation near the ureterovesical junction. Amer. J. Roentgenol. **90**, 72 (1963).

FRIEDHOFF, E.: Die intravenöse Urographie bei der Blasenhalsgeschwulst. Langenbecks Arch. klin. Chir. **274**, 132 (1953).

FRIEDMAN, P. S., SOLIS-COHEN, L., JOFFE, S. M.: Urethral calculus, its roentgen evaluation. Radiology **62**, 248 (1954).

FRÜHWALD, R.: Ein Urethrogramm bei Balanitis xerotica obliterans. Z. Haut- u. Geschl.-Kr. **24**, 157 (1958).

FULTON, H.: Delayed cystography in children. Amer. J. Roentgenol. **78**, 486 (1957).

GANDINI, D., GIBBA, A.: Modoficazione alla tecnica della cistografia combinata. Ann. Radiol. diagn. (Bologna) **26**, 64 (1953).

GARCIA, A. E., CASAL, J.: El diagnóstico uretrográfico de la enfermedad del cuello vesical. Rev. Méd. Hosp. Esp. (B. Aires) **23**, 83 (1953).

— — El diagnóstico uretrográfico de la enfermedad del cuello vesical. Rev. argent. Urol. **23**, 49 (1954).

— — ROCCHI, A.: El reflujo uretro-venoso como accidente de la uretrografia. Rev. argent. Urol. **15**, 423 (1946).

GAUDIN, H.: Roentgen examination of male urethra. N. Z. Med. J. **45**, 376 (1946).

— Fatal embolism following urethrography. J. Urol. **62**, 375 (1949).

GAUTIER, E. L.: Urologie. 4 etic. Rev. corr. et mise à jour par J. L. GAILLARD, Paris: Malonie 1954.

GÉRARD, P. L., DUFOUR, A., HELENON, C.: Intérét de l'exopneumopéritoine dans l'étude des tumeurs de la vesic. J. Radiol. Électrol. **40**, 341 (1959).

GHORAB, M. M. A.: Ureteritis calcinosa: complication of bilharzial ureteritis and its relation to primary ureteric stone formation. Brit. J. Urol. **34**, 33 (1962).

GIBBA, A., GANDINI, D.: Su di una recente modalita di tecnica cistografia combinata. Arch. ital. Urol. **25**, 245 (1951/52).

GIBSON, T. E.: Tumors of the seminal vesicla. Urology **2**, 1170 (1954).

— BARETA, J., LAKE, G. C.: Malacoplakia: report of a case involving the bladder and one kidney and ureter. Urologia internat. **1**, 5 (1955).

GIERTZ, G., LINDBLOM, K.: Urethro-cystographic studies of nervous disturbances of the urinary bladder and the urethra: a preliminary report. Acta radiol. **36**, 205 (1951).

GIROTTO, A.: Pneumourethrography in diagnosis of foreign bodies of male urethra. Ann. Ital. Chir. **21**, 651 (1942).

GIULIANI, L., PISANI, E.: L'intestino nella chirurgia plastica e sostitutiva della vesceca: Valutazione cistomanometrica e cestografica dei risultati. Arch. ital. Urol. **32**, 165 (1959).

GÖTZEN, F. J.: Über eine cystographische Besonderheit bei nerval gestörter Harnblase. Z. Urol. **49**, 340 (1956).

GOLDBERG, V. V.: X-Ray diagnosis of cancer of the prostate. Urologija **3**, 24 (1955).

GOLDMAN, H. J., GLICKMAN, S. I.: Ureteral obstruction in regional ileitis. J. Urol. **88**, 616 (1962).

GOODYEAR, W. E., BEARD, D. E., WEENS, H. S.: Urethrography: diagnostic acid in diseases of lower urinary tract. Sth. Med. J. (Bgham, Ala) **41**, 487 (1948).

GOUVÉA, G. S.: Iconografia urológica; bexiga. Rev. bras. Cir. **31**, 526 (1956).

GRAAS, G. MILLER, H.: Eine neue Methode zur Darstellung der Blase und ihrer pathologischen Inhalte. Fortschr. Röntgenstr. **87**, 218 (1957).

GRAJEWSKI, L. W., HOFFMAN, R. F.: Conditions of male and female urethra as demonstrated by cystourethrography. Alex. Blain Hosp. Bull. **5**, 87 (1946).

GRANBERG, P. O., SVARTHOLM, F.: Urethral diverticula in the female with special reference to the roentgenographic diagnosis and the result of surgery. Acta chir. scand. **115**, 78 (1958).

GRASHEY, R.: Atlas des chirurgisch-pathologischen Röntgenbildes. Lehmanns medizinische Atlas 3. Aufl. Bd. VI. München: J. F. Lehmann 1931.

GREGERSEN, E., BUUS, J. G.: Vesiko-ureteral refluks efter spaltning af ureterostiet. Nord. Med. **85**, 654 (1971).

GRENADINNIK, J. S.: Cystography in nocturnal incontinence. Vestn. Rentgenol. Radiol. **31**, 54 (1956).

GRIESBACH, W. A., WATERHOUSE, R. K., MELLINS, H. Z.: Voiding cystourethrography in the diagnosis of congenital posterior urethral valves. Amer. J. Roentgenol. **82**, 521 (1959).

GRIMALDI, A., ERASO, A. R.: Impregnación persistente del medio de contraste urografico: pielografia retrograde y eretrografia. Rev. argent. Urol. **24**, 680 (1955).

GUDBJERG, C. E., HANSEN, L. K., HASNER, E.: Micturition cysto-urethrography: automatic serial technique. Acta radiol **50**, 310 (1958).

GUICHARD, R., DUVERGEY, H.: L'Urethrographie. Paris: Masson & Cie. 1948.

GULLMO, Å.: A simple instrument for urethrocystography and fistulography in adults and children. Acta radiol. **45**, 473 (1956).

— SUNDBERG, J.: A method for roentgen examination of the posterior urethra, prostatic ducts and utricle (utriculography). Acta radiol. **48**, 241 (1957).

GÜNTHER, G. W.: Röntgenuroskopie: Nierenbecken und -kelche, Harnleiter, Blase, Harnröhre. Stuttgart: Georg Thieme 1952; New York: Grune & Stratton 1952.

HAAS, L., FILLENZ, K.: Contribution au radiodiagnostik de la prostate. J. Radiol. Electrol. **22**, 103 (1938).

HACKETT, F.: Idiopathic retroperitoneal fibrosis: A condition involving the ureters, the aorta and the inferior vena cava. Brit. J. Surg. **46**, 3 (1958).

HACKWORTH, L. E.: Urethrography in infants and children, J. Urol. **60**, 947 (1948).

HAGEMANN, E.: Eine rationelle Methode zur Röntgenuntersuchung der Harnblase. Dtsch. Gesundh.-Wes. **12**, 846 (1957).

HAHN, H.: Ligatur beider Aa. Hypogastricae und ihrer Zweige in der Therapie des fortgeschrittenen Prostatakrebses. Proceedings of the 1st Czechoslovak-Swedish-Finnish Urological Symposium-Bratislava, May 28–31, 1969. Prague: Osveta, Martin 1970.

HAJOS, E.: Methodik des Röntgenschichtverfahrens in der Urologie. Fortschr. Röntgenstr. **91**, 366 (1959).

HALLGREN, B.: Enuresis. Köpenhamn: Munksgaard 1957.

HALUZA, O.: Zur Ätiologie des vesikorenalen refluxes. Proceedings of the 1st Czechoslovak-Swedish-Finnish Urological Symposium — Bratislava, May 28–31, 1969. Prague: Osveta, Martin 1970.

HANAFEE, W. N., TURNER, R. D.: Some uses of cinefluorography in urologic diagnostic problems. Radiology **73**, 733 (1959).

HARDER, E.: The micturition cystourethrography in children. Radiography **21**, 255 (1955).

HARLIN, H.: Seminal vesiculitis. J. Amer. Med. Ass. **143**, 880 (1950).

HARTL, H.: Die Ergebnisse der Urethrographie bei der Frau. Fortschr. Röntgenstr. **82**, 680 (1955).

HARTUNG, W., FLOCKS, R. H.: Diverticulum of the bladder: method of roentgen examination and roentgen and clinical findings in 200 cases. Radiology **41**, 363 (1943).

HEDERRA, R.: Cistografia con doble medio de contraste. Arch. Soc. Ciru. Hosp. **13**, 210 (1943).

HEGEDÜS, V., OKMIAN, L.: Congenital posterior urethral polyp. Zeitschrift für Kinderchirurgie und Grenzgebiete **1:4**, 458 (1972).

HEIDENBLUT, A.: Beitrag zur Röntgendiagnostik entzündlicher Schleimhauterkrankungen von Nierenbecken und Ureter. Fortschr. Röntgenstr. **92**, 658 (1960).

HEIKEL, P. E., PARKKULAINEN, K. V.: A comparison between the results obtained by urography and mictiocystography in pediatric urological disease. Acta paediat. **48**, Suppl. 118, pp. 149–150 (1959).

— — The value of mictiocystourethrography in pediatric urological diagnosis. Ann. Med. Intern. Fenn. **48**, Suppl. **128**, 25 (1959).

HELLMER, H.: Beitrag zu Kenntnis des Röntgenbildes der Dermoidzyste. Acta radiol. **18**, 81 (1937).

HENLINE, R. B.: Prostatitis and seminal vesiculitis: acute and chronic. J. Amer. Med. Ass. **123**, 608 (1943).

HENNIG, O.: Die röntgenologische Darstellung der Prostatikerblase mit Bariumaufschwemmung und Luft am liegenden und stehenden Kranken; ein wirtschaftliches Verfahren. Langenbecks Arch. klin. Chir. **275**, 418 (1953).

HERBUT, P. A.: Urological pathology. Philadelphia: Lea & Febiger 1952.

HERMAN, L.: The practice of urology. Philadelphia and London: W. B. Saunders Co. 1943.

HEWETT, A. L., HEADSTREAM, J. W.: Pericystitis plastica. J. Urol. **83**, 103 (1960).

HICKEL, R.: Technique et résultats de l'exploration radiologique de la vessie. Sem. Hôp. Paris **33** 4311 (1957).

HIETALA, S. O.: Arteriografiska studier av urinblåsan före och efter strålbehandling av urinblåsecancer. Paper presented at Scand. Soc. Med. Radiol., Reykjavik, June 1971.

HINMAN, F., Jr., MILLER, G. M., MICKEL, E., MILLER, E. R.: Vesical physiology demonstrated by cineradiography and serial roentgenography: preliminary report. Radiology **62** , 713 (1954).

— — — STEINBACH, H. L., MILLER, E. R.: Normal micturition: certain details as shown by serial cystograms. Calif. Med. **82**, 6 (1955).

HOCK, E.: Diverticula of the prostate. J. Urol. **56**, 353 (1946).

HODGKINSON, C. P., DOUB, H. P.: Roentgen study of urethrovesical relationships in female urinary stress incontience. Radiology **61**, 335 (1953).

— — KELLY, W. T.: Urethrocystograms: metallic bead chain technique. Clin. Abst. **1**, 668 (1958).

HODSON, J. C., EDWARDS, D.: Chronic pyelonephritis and vesico-ureteric reflux. Clin. Radiol. **11**, 219 (1960).

HOFFMAN, W. W., TRIPPEL, O. H.: Retroperitoneal fibrosis: etiologic considerations. J. Urol. **86**, 222 (1961).

HOLDER, E.: Die Harnröhrenstriktur im Röntgenbild. Langenbecks Arch. klin. Chir. **272**, 224 (1952).

HOLM, O. F.: On the diagnosis of rupture of the urinary bladder. Acta radiol. **24**, 198 (1943).

HOPE, J. W., JAMESON, P. J., MICHIE, A. J.: Diagnosis of anterior urethral valve by voiding urethrography: report of two cases. Radiology **74**, 798 (1960).

HOWARD, F. S.: Hypospadias with enlargement of the prostatic utricle. Surg. Gynec. Obstet. **86**, 307 (1948).

HUDSON, E.: Urethro-cystography. Radiography **23**, 316 (1957).

HUGGINS, C.: The prostatic secretion. Harvey Lect. **92**, 148 (1946).

— BEAF, R. S.: Course of prostatic ducts and anatomy, chemical and X-ray diffraction analysis of calculi. J. Urol. **51**, 37 (1944).

— WEBSTER, W.: Duality of human prostate in response to estrogen. J. Urol. **59**, 258 (1948).

HULSE, C. A.: Radiographic procedures in urology. X-Ray Techn. **21**, 348 (1950).

HULTBORN, K. A., MORALES, O., ROMANUS, R.: The so-called shelf tumour of the rectum. Acta radiol. Suppl. **124**, pp. 1–46 (1955).

IANNACCONE, G.: Ureteral reflux in normal infants. Ann. Radiol. **9**, 31 (1966).

ICHIKAWA, T.: Über unsere Methode der Prostatographie. Z. Urol. **48**, 114 (1955).

INCLÁN BOLADO, J. L.: Algunas consideraciones sobre la vesiculografia. Arch. Esp. Urol. **12**, 26 (1956).

IVERSEN, O. H., NIELSEN, O. V.: Inkarcereret prolaps af ureterocele hos en voksen. Nord. Med. **69**, 512 (1963).

JAKHNICH, I. M.: Metodicheskie ukaraniia k provedeniiu rentgenologiche skogo issledovaniia nochevykh organov. Moskva: Medgiz 1957.

JAMES, W. B.: Urological manifestations in schistosoma haematobium infestation. Brit. J. Radiol. **36**, 40 (1963).

JENSEN, V.: A simple device for urethrocystography. Acta radiol. **45**, 403 (1956).

JOMAIN, J.: Prévention des embolies huileuses au cours de l'urethrographie par l'emploi d'un moyen de contraste hydrosoluble en solution visqueuse. J. Urol. Méd. Chir. **58**, 134 (1952).

JONES, R. F.: Symposium on prostatic cancer. V. Conclusion. J. Nat. Med. Ass. (N. Y.) **47**, 157 (1955).

JOHNSON, H. W., ANKENMAN, G. J.: Bilateral ureteral primary amyloidosis. J. Urol. **92**, 275 (1964).

JORUP, S., KJELLBERG, S. R.: Congenital valvular formations in the urethra. Acta radiol. **30**, 197 (1948).

JOUBERT, J. D.: Kistografie en urethragrafie. S. Afr. Med. J. **32**, 748 (1958).

JULES, R.: L'information déférento-vésiculographique dans le diagnostic de la tuberculose génitale profondo et dans celui du cancer de la prostate. Thèse Lille 1958.

JULIANI, G., GIBBA, A.: Quadri deferento-vesiculografici negzi adenomi e nei carcinomi della prostata. Nunt. radiol. (Firenze) **21**, 165 (1955).

KADRNKA, S. et, PONCET,: J. Vessie géante par cancer papillaire. Contribution à la cysto-radiographie de l'épithélioma. Rev. méd. Suisse rom. **54**, 789 (1934).

KAISER, R.: Selten lange Verweildauer des Kontrastmittels nach urethro-venösem Übertritt bei der Urethrographie. Chirurg II, 61 (1939).

KANAUKA, V.: Roentgen diagnosis of male urethra. Medicina (Kaunas) **16**, 487 (1935).

KATZ-GALATZI, T.: Le reflux uréthro-veineux et les dangers de l'emploi des huiles dans l'uréthre. J. Urol. Med. Chir. **44**, 300 (1937).

KAUFMANN, J. J., RUSSEL, M.: Cystourethrography, clinical experience with the newer contrast media. Amer. J. Roentgenol. **75**, 884 (1956).

KAUFMAN, P., IKLÉ, A.: Beitrag zur Beurteilung der relativen Urininkontinenz mit der lateralen Zystourethrographie. Geburtsh. u. Frauenheilk. **16**, 29 (1956).

KELLER, J.: Urologie. Ein Leitfaden für den Urologen und den urologisch interessierten Praktiker, 2. neubearb. Aufl. Dresden u. Leipzig: Theodor Steinkopff 1958.

KERR, H. D., GILLIES, C. L.: The urinary tract. A handbook of roentgen diagnosis. Chicago: Year Book Publ. 1944.

KIMBROUGH, J. C.: Symposium on prostatic cancer. II. Importance of early detection. J. Nat. Med. Ass. (N. Y.) **47**, 149 (1955).

KING, J., ROSENBAUM, H.: Calcification of the vasa deferentia in nondiabetics. Radiology **100**, 603 (1971).

KINGREEN, O.: Röntgendiagnostik des Chirurgen, 4. überarb. Aufl. Leipzig: Johann Ambrosius Barth 1958.

KJELLBERG, S. R., ERICSSON, N. O., RUDHE, U.: The lower urinary tract in childhood: some correlated clinical and roentgenologic observations. Chicago: Year Book Publ. 1957.

KJELLMAN, L.: A new instrument for urethrocystography. Acta radiol. **38**, 440 (1952).

KLIKA, M.: Die neueren Ansichten über die Anatomie und das Adenom der Prostata und ihre praktische Ausnützung. Urol. int. (Basel) **6**, 232 (1958).

KNEISE, O., SCHOBER, K. L.: Die Röntgenuntersuchung der Harnorgane, 4. Aufl. Leipzig: Georg Thieme 1952.

KNUTSSON, F.: On the technique of urethrography. Acta radiol. **10**, 437 (1929).

KORABEL'NIKOV, I. D.: Contrast cystography in diagnosis of retroperitoneal hematomas. Vestn. Rentgenol. Radiol. **2**, 91 (1955).

KORIN, D. L.: Cystography method in diagnosis of injuries of the bladder. Chirurgica 64, 1952.

KOTAY, P., SZERÉMY, L.: Nos expériencens sur l'examen combiné röntgen de la vessie. Acta Urol. Belg. **3**, 46 (1949).

KRAATZ, H.: Der Einfluß der vaginalen Radikaloperation auf die Harnblase. Ein Versuch, die postoperativen urologischen Komplikationen nach funktionellen Gesichtspunkten unter Zuhilfenahme der Zystoradiographie zu klären. Z. Geburtsh. Gynäk. **123**, 1 (1941).

— Die Bedeutung der Cystoradiographie für die gynäkologische Urologie. Zbl. Gynäk. **65**, 793 (1941).

KÜSS, R., NOIX: Étude radiocinématographique de la miction des vessies iléales. J. Urol. méd. chir. **62**, 519 (1956).

LAGERGREN, C.: Biophysical investigations of urinary calculi: an x-ray chrystallographic and microradiographic study. Acta radiol. Suppl. 133 (1956).

LANGE, J.: La tomographie dans les tumeurs de la vessie. J. Urol. méd. chir. **60**, 158 (1954).

LANGREDER, W., BRANDSTETTER, F.: Grundlagen zur röntgenologischen Inkontinenzdiagnostik. Arch. Gynäk. **188**, 344 (1957).

LASIO, E.: I tumori maligna della vesica. Milano: Delfino 1950.

— ARRIGONI, G., GVINO, A.: L'aortografia addominale in chirurgica urologica. Minerva Urol. (Torino) **7**, 8 (1955).

LEMAITRE, G., DEFRANCE, G., DUPUIS, C.: Radiologie des valvules urétrales du nourrisson et de l'enfant. J. Radiol. Électrol. **39**, 436 (1958).

LESPINASSE, V. D.: Urethrograms of male urethra. Quart. Bull. Northw. Univ. Med. Sch. **19**, 208 (1945).

LESTER, P., KYAW, M.: Ureteral diverticulosis. Radiology **106**, 77 (1973).

LEVI, L.: Sull'uretrografia nelle affezioni blenorragiche. G. ital. Derm. Sif. **71**, 1353 (1930).

— Sopra due casi di „falsa strada", accertati mediante l'uretrografia. Arch. ital· Derm. **7**, 501 (1931).

LEVINE, M. H., CROSBIE, S.: The value of a routine abdominal film. J. Amer. Med. Ass. **156**, 220 (1954).

LEVY, C. S.: Value of cystogram in cases of very large prostatic hypertrophies. Urol. Cutan. Rev. **44**, 644 (1940).

Lewis, L. G.: Symposium on prostatic cancer. III. Surgical approach for diagnosis and treatment. J. Nat. Med. Ass. (N.Y.) **47**, 152 (1955).

Liang, D. S.: Hemangioma of the bladder. J. Urol. **79**, 956 (1958).

Liess, G., Berwing, K.: Fehlermöglichkeiten bei der röntgenologischen Darstellung der Prostatahypertrophie mit Hilfe der Abrodilpfütze nach Kneise-Schober. Z. Urol. **48**, 240 (1955).

Lievre, J. A.: Le diagnostic des métastases osseuses du cancer de la prostate et de l'osteite fibreuse. Presse méd. **60**, 85 (1952).

Linbbom, Å.: Unusual ureteral obstruction by herniation of ureter into sciatic foramen. Acta radiol. **28**, 225 (1947).

Lloyd, F. A., Cottrell, T. L.: Diatrizoale sodium. Ann. N.Y. Acad. Sci. **78**, 987 (1959).

Loughnane, F. McG.: Examination of the male urethra. In: H. P. Whinsbury-White: Textbook of genito-urinary surgery (p. 374). Baltimore: Williams & Wilkins Co. 1948.

Lowsley, O. S., Kirwin, T. J.: Clinical urology, 2. edit, I–II. Baltimore: Williams & Wilkins Co. 1944.

Lund, C. J., Benjamin, J. A., Tristan, T. A., Fullerton, R. E., Ramsey, G. H., Watson, J. S.: Cinefluorographic studies of the bladder and urethra in women. I. Urethrovesical relationships in voluntary and involuntary urination. Amer. J. Obstet. Gynec. **74**, 896 (1957).

— Fullerton, R. E., Tristan, T. A.: Cinefluorographic studies of the bladder and urethra in women. II. Stress incontinence. Amer. J. Obstet. Gynec. **78**, 706 (1959).

Lund, H. G., Zingale, F. G., O'Dowd, J. A.: Cystitis emphysematosa. J. Urol. **42**, 684 (1939).

MacLaren, J. W.: Modern trends in diagnostic radiology. London: Butterworths 1970.

MacQuet, P., Lemaitre, G.: La cystographie à la flaque dans les tumeurs vésicales. J. Radiol. Électrol. **34**, 418 (1953).

Mándi, J., Tompa, G.: Pelvic venography in prostate surgery. Orv. Hetil. **97**, 1169 (1956).

Marchand, J. H., Barag, N., Clement, G., Le Vizon, L., Grimberg, M.: Contribution à l'étude radiologique de la prostate. J. Radiol. Électrol. **38**, 838 (1957).

— Le Vizon, C., Grimberg, B., Pinsky-Moore: Étude d'un rétrécissement urétral par le double procédé de l'urographie veineuse et de l'urétro-cystographie rétrograde. J. Radiol. Électrol. **38**, 1146 (1957).

— — — Traité d'urologie. Paris: Masson & Cie. (1940).

Markman, B. J.: Two mechanical devices for reducing risk of radiation exposure during certain types of roentgen examinations. Acta radiol. **27**, 388 (1946).

Marks, J. H., Ham, D. P.: Calcification of vas deferens. Amer. J. Roentgenol. **47**, 859 (1942).

Marshall, V. F.: Diagnosis of genito-urinary neoplasms. New York: Amer. Cancer Soc. 1949.

— Textbook of urology. London: Harper 1956.

Martinelli, V., Micieli G., Saracca, L.: Quadri deferentovesiculografici nella ipertrophia prostatica. Ann. Ital. Chir. **37**, 34 (1960).

Martinet, R.: La uretrografia retrograda. Arch. Esp. Urol. **4**, 318 (1948).

Martin-Luque, T.: La radiographie de la miction dans les affections prostato-urétrales. J. Urol. Med. Chir. **28**, 237 (1929).

Mason, J. T., Crenshaw, W. B.: Rectal obstruction by carcinoma of the prostate. Amer. J. Surg. **96**, 319 (1958).

Mathey-Cornat, R., Duvergey, H.: Sur l'exploration urétrographique des cancer de la prostate. J. Radiol. Électrol. **25**, 199 (1942/43).

Mayne, G. O.: Urethrography in urethral stricture. Brit. J. Vener. Dis. **32**, 119 (1956).

Mazurek, L. J.: Radiodiagnostyka kliniczna chorob narzada moczowego. Warszawa: Panstwowy Zaktad Wydawn. Lekarskich 1957.

McCall, I. W.: Case reports: An unusual manifestation of ureterocele. Brit. J. Radiol. **45**, 218 (1972).

McDonald, D. F., Fagan, C. J.: Fungus balls in the urinary bladder. Amer. J. Roentgenol. **114**, 753 (1972).

McDonald, H. P., Upchurch, W. E., Artime, M. E.: Visualization of vesical masses by excretory urography. Amer. Practit. **10**, 2140 (1959).

McDowell. J. F.: Cystographic diagnosis of placenta praevia. Amer. J. Obstet. Gynec. **33**, 436 (1937).

McIver, J.: Use of cystogram in diagnosing placenta praevia. Tex. St. J. Med. **32**, 471 (1936).

McKenna, C. M., Kiefer, J. H.: Congenital enlargement of the prostatic utricle with inclusion of the ejaculatory ducts and seminal vesicles. Trans. Amer. Ass. Gen.-Urin. Surg. **32**, 305 (1939).

Mellinger, G. T., Klatte, P. B.: Neocystoscopy and neocystography. Proc. North cent. Sect. Amer. Urol. Ass. 1957, 144; J. Urol. **79**, 459 (1958).

Mentha, C.: L'examen radiologique de la vessie (stéréo-pneumo-iodocystographie). J. Urol. méd. chir. **53**, 89 (1946/47).

Merricks, J. W.: The modern conception of the diagnosis and treatment of infections of the seminal vesicles with roentgenologic visualization of these organs by catheterization of the ejaculatory ducts. Int. Clin. **2**, 193 (1940).

Middlemiss, J. H.: Radiology in diseases of the prostate. J. Fac. Radiol. (Lond.) **4**, 115 (1952).

Miller, A.: Radiology in diseases of the prostate. J. Fac. Radiol. (Lond.) **4**, 125 (1952).

Mitty, H.: Roentgen features of reflux into the prostate, seminal vesicles, and vasa deferentia. Amer. J. Roentgenol. **112**, 603 (1971).

— Modern Trends in Urology, edit. by E. W. Riches. London: Butterworth & Co. 1953.

Montenegro, N.: Cálculos vesicales invisibles a la radiografía. Rev. argent. Urol. **9**, 531 (1940).

Morales, O., Romanus, R.: Urethrography in the male with a highly viscous, water soluble contrast medium, umbradilviscous U. Acta radiol. Suppl. 95 (1952).

— — Urethrography in the male: delimitation of the anterior and posterior urethra, the pars diaphragmatica, the pars nuda and the presence of a musculus compressor nudae. Acta radiol. **39**, 453 (1953).

— — Urethrography in the male: the boundaries of the different urethral parts and detail studies of the urethral mucous membrane and its motility. J. Urol.**73**, 162 (1955).

— — Manliga urethras funktion normalt och vid striktur samt indikationer för strikturbehandling. Nord Med. **52**, 1179 (1954).

MORALES, O., NILSSON, S., ROMANUS, R.: Urethrographic studies on the posterior urethra. I. Motility of the prostatic urethra. Acta radiol. **2**, 81 (1964).

— — — Urethrographic studies of the posterior urethra. II. Emptying of the prostatic urethra. Acta radiol. **2**, 305 (1964).

MOREAU, M. H., MOREAU, J. E.: Contribución a la técnica de la uretrografia; pinza para uretrografia. Radiologia (B. Aires) **8**, 174 (1945), also Rev. Asoc. Med. Argent. **60**, 818 (1946), and Pren. Méd. Argent. **33**, 2041 (1946).

MORTENSEN, H.: Use of cystourethrogram in diagnosis of various conditions in lower portion of urinary tract. Med. J. Aust. **1**, 157 (1942).

MUELLNER, S. R., FLEISCHNER, F. G.: Normal and abnormal micturition: study of bladder behavior by means of fluoroscopy. J. Urol. **61**, 233 (1949).

MUND, E.: Zur Kontrastdarstellung der männlichen Harnröhre. Dtsch. med. J. **7**, 126 (1956).

MUNOZ, H. D.: Uretrografia. Tesis, Universidad Buenos Aires. Buenos Aires: S. A. Casa Jacobo Penser 1942.

MUSIANI, A.: Aspects cystoscopiques et cystographiques de la rétraction inflammatoire de l'urétère. J. Urol. Méd.. Chir. **57**, 11 (1951).

MYGIND, H. B.: Urogenital tuberkulose hos manden; undersøgelse med vesikulografi og urethrografi; foreløbig meddelelse. Ugeskr. Laeg. **121**, 449 (1959).

— Urogenital tuberculosis in the human male. Vesiculographic and urethrographic studies. Dan. Med. Bull. **7**, 13 (1960).

NAVARRETE, E.: A propósito de un signo radiológico que presenta la cistografia en la mujer. Rev. méd. Peru. **19**, 459 (1946).

NEGRO, M.: La cistografia combinata idrobarina, olio gomenolato, aria. Minerva Urol. (Torino) **5**, 179 (1953).

NESBIT, R. M.: Problems in urological diagnosis. Series 1. Ann Arbor, Mich.: Edwards Bros. 1948.

NEY, C., DUFF, J.: Cysto-urethrography: Its role in diagnosis of neurogenic bladder. J. Urol. **63**, 640 (1950).

NILSEN, P. A.: Cystourethrography in stress incontinence. Acta obstet. gynec. scand. **37**, 269 (1958).

NILSSON, A. E.: The palpability of infiltrative bladder tumours: a diagnostic comparison with roentgenographic findings. Acta chir. scand. **115**, 132 (1958).

— Roentgen diagnosis of ureterocele and some impeding factors. Acta radiol. **52**, 365 (1959).

NILSSON, J.: Ektopisk ureter. Nord. Med. **68**, 1132 (1962).

— Angiography in tumours of the urinary bladder. Acta radiol. Suppl. 263, 1967.

NOIX, M.: La miction fractionnée dans les grands reflux cysto-urétéro-pyéliques. J. Radiol. Électrol. **45**, 335 (1964).

NÖLTING, D. E., CASO, R., STRATICO, J. R.: Contribución al diagnóstico radiológico de la placenta previa por medio de la cistografia. Bol. Inst. Matern. (B. Aires) **11**, 261 (1942).

NÖLTING, D. E., CASO, R., STRATICO, J. R.: Contribución al diagnóstico radiológico de la placenta previa por medio de la cistografia: a propósito de su utilización en el diagnóstico diferencial de 40 observaciones de hemorragias genitales del último trimestre del embarazo. Pren. Méd. Argent. **30**, 368 (1944).

NORDENSTRÖM, B. E. W.: A method of topographic urethrocystography in women. Acta radiol. **37**, 503 (1952).

— Some observations on the shape and course of the female urethra during miction. Acta radiol. **38**, 125 (1952).

— Roentgenologic demonstration during micturition of pathologic changes in the female urethra. Acta radiol. **38**, 264 (1952).

NOTTER, G., HELANDER, C. G.: Über den Wert der Cavographie bei Diagnose und Behandlung retroperitonealer Testistumormetastasen. Fortschr. Röntgenstr. **89**, 409 (1958).

OLIVIER, C., FELLUS, P.: Diagnostic cystographique d'un hématome pelvien sous-peritonéal. Presse Méd. **61**, 1243 (1953).

OLSSON, OLLE: Cystography with graduated compression. Acta radiol. **29**, 429 (1948).

OLSSON, T.: Ein Fall mit inkompletter Doppelurethra. Der Radiologe **3**, 427 (1963).

OLTRAMARE, J. H., MARTINET, R.: De l'uréthrographie. Schweiz. med. Wschr. **68**, 12 (1938).

OPPENHEIMER, G. D., GOLDMAN, H.: Periureteral fibrosis: an unusual complication of renal biopsy. J. Urol. **88**, 611 (1962).

ORANTES SUAREZ, A.: Radiografia clinica de la uretra. Rev. Urol. (Méx.) **2**, 322 (1944); Rev. méd. Hosp. Gen. (Méx). **6**, 111 (1944).

ORAVISTO, K. J., SCHAUMAN, S.: Urethrocystography in the differential diagnosis of cancer of the prostate. Duodecim (Helsinki) **71**, 395 (1955).

— — Urethrocystography in the differential diagnosis of prostatic cancer. J. Urol. **75**, 995 (1956).

ORMOND, J. K.: Idiopathic retroperitoneal fibrosis: a discussion of the etiology. J. Urol. **94**, 385 (1965).

OSADCHUK, V. I.: Experiences in the roentgenological investigation of seminal vesicles. Urologija **25**, 35 (1960).

PAALANEN H.: Malignant prostate. Ann. Chir. Gynaec. Fenn. **45**, Suppl. 10 (1956).

PABST, R.: Untersuchungen über Bau und Funktion des menschlichen Samenleiters. Z. Anat. Entwickl.-Gesch. **129**, 154 (1969).

PALM, L.: Bladder function in women with diseases of the lower urinary tract. Copenhagen: Munksgaard 1971.

PALMER, B. M.: Study of air cystograms in prostatic hypertrophy. Urol. Cutan. Rev. **44**, 795 (1940).

PANZIRONI, P. E., IANNACCONE, G.: La vesica urinaria nel lattante; studio anatomo-radiologico. Radiol. Med. (Torino) **40**, 1109 (1954).

PARONYAN, R. L.: Air embolism during cystography. Nov. Hir. Arch. **44**, 321 (1939).

PASSARO, E. P., JR., ROSE, R. S., TAYLOR, J. N.: Periureteric fibrosis: A review of the literature and presentation of two cases. J. Urol. **85**, 506 (1961).

PAZOUREK, J.: New experience with needle biopsy in diagnosis of carcinoma of the prostate. Proceedings of the 1st Czechoslovak-Swedish-Finnish Urological Symposium-Bratislava, May 28–31, 1969. Prague: Osveta, Martin 1970.

PEKAROVIC, E.: Intravesical obstruction in myelomeningocele. Proceedings of the 1st Czechoslovak-Swedish-Finnish Urological Symposium — Bratislava, May 28–31, 1969. Prague: Osveta, Martin 1970.

PEREIRA, A.: Roentgen diagnosis of diseases of neck of bladder. Amer. J. Roentge nol. **56**, 489 (1946).

— Information derived from examination of neck of bladder and of prostatic urethra. J. Urol. **57**, 1054 (1947).

PETKOVIĆ, S.: Die Bedeutung der Malignität von Blasentumoren. Z. Urol. **46**, 511 (1953).

PFEIFER, K.: Eine rationelle Methode zur Röntgenuntersuchung der Harnblase. Dtsch. Gesundh.-Wes. **12**, 809 (1957).

PFEIFER, W.: Grundlagen der funktionellen urologischen Röntgendiagnostik. Stuttgart: Georg Thieme 1949.

PFISTER, R. C., McLAUGHLIN, A. P., LEADBETTER, W. F.: Radiological evaluation of primary megaloureter. Radiology **99**, 503 (1971).

PINCELLI, C., PROSPERI, F.: L'indagine pneumocisto-stratografica associata a retropneumoperitoneo nello studio delle neoplasie vescicali. Minerva urol. (Torino) **11**, 215 (1959).

PONS, H., DENARD, Y., MOREAU, Y.: Un signe radiologique du diabète: la calcification des canaux déférents. J. Radiol. Électrol. **38**, 237 (1957).

POTSAID, M. S., ROBBINS, L. L.: Diprotrizoate sodium. Ann. N. Y. Acad. Sci. **78**, 993 (1959).

PRATHER, G. C., PETROFF, B.: Spinal cord injuries: urethrographic study of bladder neck. J. Urol. **57**, 274 (1947).

QUACKELS, R.: Propos sur la spermato-cystographie. Acta urol. belg. **25**, 413 (1957).

QUINN, W. P.: Radiologic methods in diagnosis and treatment of carcinoma of the prostate and urinary bladder. J. Nat. Cancer Inst. **20**, 109 (1958).

RANK, W. B., MELLINGER, G. T., SPIRO, E.: Ureteral diverticula: etiologic considerations. J. Urol. **83**, 566 (1960).

RATING, B.: Zur Darstellung von Urethravarizen. Fortschr. Röntgenstr. **63**, 214 (1941).

RAVICH, A., KATZEN, P.: Cystitis emphysematosa. J. Amer. Med. Ass. **98**, 1256 (1932).

REBAUDI, L., MOREAU, Y. M.: Radiografia de próstata. Rev. argent. Urol. **27**, 40 (1958).

RENANDER, A.: Roentgenologic differentiation of vesical uroliths. Acta radiol. **26**, 320 (1945).

REYGAERTS, J.: Aspects de la cystographie après opération de Michon et leur signification. Brux.-méd. **37**, 1483 (1957).

RIBA, L. W.: Carcinoma of the female urethra. Quart. Bull. Northw. Univ. Med. Sch. **28**, 347 (1954).

RIBA, L. W., SCHMIDLAPP, C. J., BOSWORTH, N. L.: Ectopic ureter draining into the seminal vesicle. J. Urol. **56**, 332 (1946).

RICHARDS, C. E.: Visco-rayopake (iodine preparation) in cystography. J. Urol. **58**, 185 (1947).

RITTER, J. S., RATTNER, I. N.: Umbrathor (thorium dioxide preparation) in urography. Amer. J. Roentgenol. **28**, 629 (1932).

ROBERTS, H.: Cystourethrography in Women. Brit. J. Radiol. **25**, 253 (1952).

ROBERTS, M. S., LATTIMER, J. K.: Advantages of floating lipiodol as further test for voiding efficiency. J. Pediat. **54**, 68 (1959).

ROBERTSON, J. P., HEADSTREAM, J. W.: The use of the cystogram and urethrogram in the diagnosis and management of rupture of the urethra and bladder. Sth. Med. J. (Bhgam, Ala) **44**, 895 (1951).

ROBLES FONTAN, W.: Diagnostico de las neoplasmas genito-urinarias. Thesis Mexico 1955.

ROLLESTONE, G. L.: Lower urinary tract disorders in children. J. Coll. Radiol. Aust. **4**, 15 (1960).

ROLNICK, D., CROSS, R. R., JR., LLOYD. F. A.: Urethrograms in the diagnosis and management of benign prostatic hypertrophy. J. Int. Coll. Surg. **31**, 683 (1959).

ROMANUS, R.: Pelvo-spondylitis ossificans in the male (Ankylosing spondylitis, Morbus Bechterew-Marie-Strümpell) and genito-urinary infection. Acta med. scand. Suppl. **280**, 1 (1953).

— YDÉN, S.: Pelvo-spondylitis ossificans. Rheumatoid or ankylosing spondylitis. Copenhagen: Munksgaard 1955.

ROSENTHAL, L., LAGERGREN, C., OLHAGEN, B.: A clinical and roentgenological follow-up study of patients with uro-arthritis or pelvospondylitis. Acta Rheum. Scand. **17**, 3 (1971).

ROTHFELD, S. H., EPSTEIN, B. S.: The size of the bladder in intravenous urography and retrograde cystography: a potential source of diagnostic error in children. J. Urol. **78**, 817 (1957).

RUBI, R. A., GOLGARECENA, J. A.: Uretrografias con un nuevo medio de contraste: umbradil U. Rev. Argent. Urol. **21**, 205 (1953).

RUBIN, A., SNOBL, O.: Cystoradiography in infants and in elder children. Pediat. Listy 8, 144 (1953).

RUCKENSTEINER, E.: Die Urethro-zystographie. Wien. med. Wschr. **109**, 168 (1959).

SABADINI, L.: L'importance des renseignements fournis par l'urétrographie préopératoire, et résultats de l'urétrectomie et de la réfection immédiate de l'urétre au cours des phlegmons diffus du périne. Mém. Acad. Chir. **74**, 515 (1948).

— Utilité des uréthro-cystographies immédiates post traumatique pour le diagnostic des ruptures de la véssie. Presse méd. **56**, 231 (1948).

SALA, S. L., BERGDOLT, E. G.: El diagnóstico radiólogico de la placenta previa por medico de la cistografia. Bol. Soc. Obstet. Ginec. B. Aires **19**, 131 (1940).

— — Nuevas experiencias sobre el diagnóstico de la placenta previa por medio de la cistografia. An bras. Ginec. **12**, 123 (1941).

— — Nuevas experiencias sobre el diagnóstico de la placenta previa por medico de la cistografia. Arch. Clin. obstet. ginec. „Canton" (B. Aires) **1**, 164 (1942).

SALGADO, C., ROCHA, A. H.: A cistografia no diagnóstico da placenta prévia. Rev. paul. Med. **24**, 319 (1944).

SANCHEZ, SALVADOR, A., La cistografia lacunar en el prostatismo; su valor en el diagnóstico del carcinoma de prostata. Arch. Esp. Urol. **12**, 49 (1956).

SANTE, L. R.: Manual of roentgenological technique, 14 ed. Ann. Arbor: Edwards 1947.

SCARCELLO, N. S., KUMAR, S.: Multiple ureteral diverticula. J. Urol. **106**, 36 (1971).

SCHAEFER, O.: Die Bedeutung der urologischen Röntgenuntersuchung für die Frauenheilkunde. Thèsis Würzburg 1956.

SCHEELE, K.: Gefahren der Urethrographie. Z. Urol. **48**, 141 (1955).

SCHIAPPA-PIETRA, T.: Ventajas a inconvencientes de las preparaciones de contraste para uso uretrografico. Rev. argent. Urol. **12**, 15 (1943).

SCHIFFER, E.: Urologiai röntgendiagnostica. Budapest: Tuodományos Könyvkiadó 1950.

SCHINZ, H. R., BAENSCH, W. E., FRIEDL, E., UEHLINGER, E.: Roentgen-diagnostics. Vol. 4: Gastrointestinal tract, gynecology, urology. Cumulative index. English transl. arr. and edit. by JAMES T. CASE. 1st Amer. ed. (based on 5th German ed.). New York: Grune & Stratton 1954.

SCHMITT, G., KAUFMANN, H., SCHEIDT, J.: Röntgendiagnostische Befunde und Strahlentherapie des primären Ureterkarzinoms. Fortschr. Röntgenstr. **115**, 780 (1971).

SCHOBER, K. L.: Die Abrodilpfütze nach Kneise-Schober und ihre Bedeutung für die Diagnose der Prostatahypertrophie. Z. Urol. **34**, 139 (1940).

SCHREYER, H.: Zur physiologie der Miktion, eine röntgenkinematographische Studie. Röntgenblätter **24**, 145 (1971).

SCHULTHEIS, T.: Zur Deutung des Kontrastbildes der Harnblase bei Ausscheidungsurographie. Langenbecks Arch. klin. Chir. **262**, 586 (1950).

SCHULZE-MANITIUS, H.: Wie entwickelte sich die Photographie und Kinematographie des Blaseninneren? Z. Urol. **52**, 376 (1959).

SCHUMANN, E.: Klärung eines jahrzentelangen Harnröhrenleidens durch Urethrocystographie. Z. Urol. **46**, 703 (1953).

SÉDAL, P., COTTALORDA, M.: Les complications urinaires de l'hysterectomie: étude radio-clinique. Marseille chir. **9**, 17 (1957).

SHAINUCK, L. I., HANO, J. E.: Bilateral ureteral obstruction following sulfamethoxazole. J. Urol. **98**, 466 (1967).

SHEA, J. D., SCHWARTZ, J. W.: Calcification of the seminal vesicles; case report. J. Urol. **58**, 132 (1947).

SHICK, J. E., SHEA, J. J.: Pyeloureteritis cystica. Radiology **74**, 468 (1960).

SHOPFNER, C. E.: Clinical evaluation of cystourethrographic contrast media. Radiology **88**, 491 (1967).

— Vesicoureteral reflux. Radiology **95**, 637 (1970).

— Cystourethrography. In: Medical Radiography and Photography (Eastman Kodak Company, Rochester, New York), Vol. 47, 1971.

— — HUTCH, J. A.: The normal urethrogram. Radiol. Clinics of North America **6**, 165 (1968).

SICHEL, D., BLUM, E.: Radiographie et tomographie de la prostate. J. Radiol. Électrol. **39**, 487 (1958).

SICHEL, D., BLUM, E, WALTER, J. P., WOLFF, R.: Étude radiographique et tomographique de l'hypertrophie et du cancer de la prostate. J. Radiol. Électrol. **39**, 321 (1958).

SIVAK, G. C.: Pheochromocytoma of bladder. J. Urol. **86**, 568 (1961).

SMITH, W. H.: The reliability of excretion urography in the diagnosis of bladder tumours. J. Fac. Radiol. (Lond.) **6**, 48 (1954).

SMYRNIOTIS, P. C.: Vingt-quatre années de radiodiagnostic de la bilharziose en Égypte. J. Radiol. Électrol. **30**, 514 (1949).

SQUIRE, F. H., KRETSCHMER, H. L.: Limitations of roentgen rays in diagnosis of bladder stone. J. Amer. Med. Ass. **145**, 81 (1951).

SRIVASTAVA, S. P.: Prostatic calculi. J. Indiana Med. Ass. 25, 404 (1955).

STAEHLER, W.: Die Behandlung der männlichen Adnexitis. Z. Urol. **38**, 72 (1944).

— Die Samenblase im Röntgenbild. Z. Urol. **38**, 93 (1944).

— Die Diagnose des Prostataabszesses im Röntgenbild. Z. Urol. **40**, 161 (1947).

— Die Diagnose der inneren männlichen Genitaltuberkulose im Röntgenbild. Helv. chir. Acta **15**, 476 (1948).

— Über die Röntgendiagnostik der entzündlichen Erkrankungen der inneren männlichen Genitalorgane. Fortschr. Röntgenstr. **72**, 202 (1949/50).

— Klinik und Praxis der Urologie. Stuttgart: Georg Thieme 1959.

STÄHLI, G.: Anwendung und Leistungsfähigkeit des Röntgenbildes bei der Untersuchung der Harnorgane. Med. Welt **20**, 927 (1951).

— Eine einfache Urethrographiemethode beim Manne mit gutem Strahlenschutz. Helv. chir. Acta **22**, 96 (1953).

STEGEMANN, W.: Cystourethrograms: use, technic and advantages, especially before prostatectomy. J. Urol. **46**, 549 (1941).

STENSTRÖM, B.: Das Röntgenbild der Prostatatuberkulose. Acta radiol. **20**, 303 (1939).

STENSTRÖM, R., ELO, J.: Nephrobarinosis after urethrocystography of micturition in children, J. Urol. **77**, 51 (1971).

STEPHENS, F. D.: Urethral obstruction in childhood: the use of urethrography in diagnosis. Aust.-N. Z. J. Surg. **25**, 89 (1955).

STEWART, C. M.: Delayed cystograms. J. Urol. **70**, 588 (1953), also Trans. West. Sect. Amer. Urol. **20**, 18 (1953).

— Delayed cystography. Bull. Moore-White Med. Fdn. **5**, 49 (1954).

STILSON, W. L., DEEB, P. H.: Unusual problems in urologic radiology. Urol. Cutan. Rev. **54**, 325 (1950).

ST. MARTIN, E. C., CAMPBELL, J. H., PESQUIER, C. M.: Cystography in children. Trans. South East. Sect. Amer. Urol. Ass. **19**, 86 (1955); J. Urol. **75**, 151 (1956).

STOBBAERTS, F.: L'urétrocystographie mictionnelle à double contraste. Procès-verb. Congr. franc. Urol. **40**, 264 (1946).

STOLZ, J. L., FOGEL, J.: The chain cystourethrogram. Radiology **103**, 204 (1972).

STRAUSS, B.: Roentgen demonstration of the perivesical spaces. J. Urol. 46, 520 (1941).

STROM, G. W., COOK, E. N.: Excretory cystogram as an aid in diagnosis. Proc. Mayo Clin. 17, 170 (1942).

SUGIURA, H., HASEGAWA, S.: Clinical evaluation of transrectal prostatography. Amer. J. Roentgenol. 111, 157 (1971).

TALANCÓN, G., ENGELKING LOPEZ, R.: Estenosis en longitud total de la uretra. Reflujo uretro-venose durante uretrografia. Rev. Urol. (Méx.) 6, 374 (1948).

TAUBER, A.: A new catheter for urethrography. J. Urol. 81, 700 (1959).

TAVOLARO, M.: Expermatocistografia por via retrógrada. Med. Cirurg. Pharm. 115, 1943.

TELTSCHER, E.: Große Cyste am Blasenhals. Z. Urol. 44, 172 (1951).

TEMELIESCO, J.: La cystopolygraphie. J. Urol. Méd. Chir. 62, 482 (1956).

TESCHENDORF, W.: Lehrbuch der röntgenologischen Differentialdiagnostik, 2. Aufl. (p. 533). Stuttgart: Georg Thieme 1950.

TEXTER, J. H., ENGEL, R. M.: Anterior urethral valve as cause for urinary obstruction: a case report. J. Urol. 107, 316 (1972).

THOMPSON, G. J., KELALIS, P. P.: Ureterocele: clinical appraisal of 176 cases. J. Urol. 91, 488 (1964).

THORNBURY, J. R.: The roentgen diagnosis of ureterocele in children. Amer. J. Roentgenol. 90, 15 (1963).

TRATTNER, H. R.: Introduction of solution into tubulo-alveolar system (by catheterization): a new method useful in diagnosis and therapy. J. Urol. 48, 710 (1942).

TREUTLER, H.: Beitrag zur Röntgendiagnostik des männlichen Chorionepithelioms. Fortschr. Röntgenstr. 82, 338 (1955).

TRUC, E., GUILLAUME, P., CANDON, J., PÉLISSIER, M., LEENHARDT, P.: Les tumeurs de la vessie; leur exploration par le double contraste et la péripneumocystographie. J. Radiol. Électrol. 35, 278 (1954).

— MARCHAL, PALEIRAC, R.: Le pneumo-exopéritoine par voie sus-pubienne; nouvelle technique d'insufflation. Semeilogie, radiologique de l'espace sous péritoneal abdomino-pelvien. J. Urol. méd. chir. 57, 125 (1951).

— PALEIRAC, R., GUILLAUME, P., BONNET, Y., CANDON, J.: L'impiego della parietografia vesicale nell'esplorazione della vesica. Minerva Urol. (Torino) 7, 26 (1955).

TRUCCHI, O.: L'associazione del pneumo-peritoneo pelvico e della pneumocistografia nell'esame radiologico della parete della vescia urinaria con particolare riguardo alla recerca delle neoplasie. Radiol. med. (Torino) 44, 421 (1958).

TURANO, L.: Diagnostica radiologica dell'apparato uropoietico, edit. 2. Roma: Soc. ed. Universo (Tip. S. GUISEPPE) 1948.

TWIGG, H. L.: Periureteral fibrosis. Amer. J. Roentgenol. 84, 876 (1960).

TZSCHIRNTSCH, K.: Die anamnestisch verheimlichte Lues im urologischen Röntgebild. Z. Urol. 44, 479 (1951).

ÜBELHÖR, R.: Urologie. Therapie und Praxis H. 11. Wien u. Innsbruck: Urban & Schwarzenberg 1958.

UHLÍR, K.: Tuberculosis of seminal vesicles: vesiculography. Acta Urol. Belg. 25, 53 (1957).

UNNÉRUS, C.-E., EISTOLA, P., KROKFORS, G.: Urethrocystography – Method and diagnostic aspects. Acta Obstet. Gynec. Scand. 64, Fasc. 2 (1965).

USON, A. C.: A classification of ureteroceles in children. J. Urol. 85, 732 (1961).

— JOHNSON, D. W., LATTIMER, J. K., MELICOW, M. M.: A classification of the urographic patterns in children with congenital bladder neck obstruction. Amer. J. Roentgenol. 80, 590 (1958).

VALLIER, G. R. M.: Possibilité de mettre en évidence par l'urographie intra-veineuse le contour intra-vésical des lobes prostatiques sans manœuvre instrumentale. Thèse, Paris: Clermont-Ferraud 1950.

VAQUIER, P. M.: La technique actuelle du radio diagnostic des affections urinaires. Thèse, Paris 1949.

VERNET, GIL, S. La tuberculose génitale masculine. Acta Urol. Bélg. 27, 264 (1959).

VERRIERE, P., NOOEL, H., NOVEL, R., BURLET, P.: Présentation d'un nouvel uréthrographie. J. Urol. Méd. Chir. 62, 700 (1956).

VESTBY, G. W.: Vasoseminal vesiculography in hypertrophy and carcinoma of the prostate with special reference to the ejaculatory ducts. Oslo: Oslo Univ. Press 1960.

— Vasoseminal vesiculography in hypertrophy and carcino ma of the prostate. Acta radiol. 50, 273 (1958).

VIEHWEGER, G.: Zur Kontrastdarstellung der Harnröhre. Ärztl. Wschr. 7, 318 (1952).

VILLELA ITIBERE, D., DE SOUZA ARANHA, E. W., MELLONE, O.: Refluxo uretrovenose na urethrografia. Rev. Méd. Brasil. 12, 187 (1942).

WALDRON, E. A.: Urethrocystography. J. Fac. Radiol. (Lond.) 4, 54 (1952).

WANGERMEZ, C., BONJEAN, P.: Appareil destiné à l'urétrographie rétrograde ches la femme. J. Radiol. Électrol. 49, 206 (1959).

WATSON, J. D., OCHSNER, S. F.: Compression of bladder due to "Rheumatoid" cysts of hip joint. Amer. J. Roentgenol. 99, 695 (1967).

WEBBER, M. M., KAUFMAN, J. J.: Multiple ureteral diverticula. Amer. J. Roentgenol. 90, 26 (1963).

WEBER, B., WEBER, A.: Urethrographie mit blutverträglichen viskösen Kontrastmitteln. Z. Urol. 49, 79 (1956).

WEBER, A. L., PFISTER, R. C., JAMES, A. E., HENDREN, W. H.: Megaureter in infants and children: roentgenologic, clinical and surgical aspects. Amer. J. Roentgenol. 112, 170 (1971).

WELFLING, J., POYAUD, P.: Utilisation d'un appareil à hystérographie pour l'uréthrographie rétrograde chez l'homme. J. Urol. méd. chir. 56, 492 (1959).

WELKENHUYZEN, P. VAN: Les modifications radiologiques des voies séminales par les lésions de la prostate. Acta urol. belg. 25, 34 (1957).

— Remarques sur l'interprétation des vésiculographies en cas de lésions de la prostate. Acta Urol. Belg. 26, 38 (1958).

WEMEAU, L., LEMAITRE, G., DEFRANCE, G.: Urétérocele et prolapsus de l'urètre. J. Radiol. Électrol. **40**, 275 (1959).

WENIG, H.: Eine vereinfachte Methode der funktionellen röntgenologischen Sphinkterometrie. Zbl. Gynäk. **80**, 1906 (1958).

WESSON, M. B., RUGGLES, H. E.: Urological roentgenology: A manual for students and practitioners. 3. edit. Philadelphia: Lea and Febiger 1950.

WHINSBURY-WHITE, H. P.: Textbook of genito-urinary surgery. Baltimore: Williams & Wilkins 1948.

WILLICH, E.: Röntgendiagnostik der Harntraktanomalien im frühen Kindesalter. Mschr. Kinderheilk. **107**, 474 (1959).

WINTER, C. C.: The problem of rectal involvement by prostatic cancer. Surg. Gynec. Obstet. **105**, 136 (1957).

WINTERBERGER, A., JENNINGS, E., MURPHY, G.: Arteriography in metastatic tumors of the bladder. J. Urol. **108**, 577 (1972).

WOLFROMM, G., DULAC, G., GILSON, M.: Sur trois méthodes de cystographie: la „flaque", la „flocculation", la „réplétion". J. Urol. Méd. Chir. **52**, 175 (1944/45).

— — GILSON, M.: De quelques perfectionnements dans la cystographie par la méthode la „flaque" (Kneise et Schobert). J. Urol. Méd. Chir. **53**, 332 (1946/47).

— ROUFLÉ-NADAUD, M.: Diverticule de la vessie étude grace au perfectionnement apporté par M. J. JOMAIN à la méthode de la flaque (Abrodil-pfütze) de Kneise et Schobert. J. Urol. Méd. Chir. **63**, 801 (1957).

WOLFROMM, G., SORIN, A.: La cystographie par la méthode de précipitation de Stobbaerts. J. Urol. Méd. Chir. **53**, 33 (1946/47).

WRIGHT, F. W., SANDERS, R. C.: Is retroperitoneal fibrosis a self-limiting disease? Brit. J. Radiol. **44**, 511 (1971).

WUGMEISTER, I.: Die röntgenographische Darstellung divertikulärer Gebilde der hinteren Harnröhre. Röntgenpraxis **8**, 313 (1936).

YALOWITZ, P. A., KELALIS, P. P.: Primary amyloidosis of the ureter: report of a case. J. Urol. **96**, 668 (1966).

YOUNG, B. W,, ANDERSON, W. L., KING, G. G.: Radiographic estimation of residual urine in children. J. Urol. **75**, 263 (1956).

YOUSSEF, A. F., MAHFOUZ, M. M.: Sphincteromethrography, a new technique for studying the physiology and pathology of urinary continence in the female. J. Obstet. Gynaec. Brit. Emp. **63**, 10 (1956).

ZAK, K.: Cystographic evaluation of surgical results in urinary incontinence in women. Csl. Gynaek. **19**, 178 (1955).

ZEMAN, E.: Pelveovenographie; ein neues diagnostisches Hilfsmittel bei den Blasentumoren. Z. Urol. **48**, 129 (1955).

ZIMMER, W.: Innendrüsenkarzinome der Prostata. Wien. med. Wschr. **108**, 1039 (1958).

ZOEDLER, D.: Beitrag zur Endometriose der Harnblase. Z. Urol. **50**, 243 (1957).

Namenverzeichnis — Author Index

Die *kursiv* gesetzten Zahlen beziehen sich auf die Literatur.

Page numbers in *italics* refer to the references.

Charnock, D. A., Riddell, H. I., Lombardo, L. L. *561*

Charnock, D. A., s. Gummess, G. H. *558*

Charpy, A., s. Poirier, P. 73, *515*

Chassaing, P., s. Loeper, J. *555*

Chassard, J. L., s. Papillon, J. *548*

Chauvin, E. *510*

Chauvin, H. F. *518*

Chauvin, H. F., Orsini, A. *562*

Chavigny, C. L. *562*

Chen, K.-C. 402, *518, 554*

Chen, K. C., Chwalla *518*

Chen, P., Lebowitz, R., Lewicki, A. *545*

Cheng, A. L. S., s. Deuel, H. J. jr. *492*

Chesney, W., McEvan, Hope, J. O. *499*

Chevassu, M. *562*

Chevassu, M., Morel, E. *562*

Chiat, H., s. Loitman, B. S. *558*

Chiaudano, C. 75, *510*

Chiaudano, C., Giongo, V. *534*

Chiaudano, G., s. Robecchi, M. *531*

Chiaudano, M. *499, 510, 527*

Chidekel, N., Obrant, O. *527*

Chidekel, N., s. Ahlberg, N. E. *509*

Chien-Hsing, M., s. Elkin, M. *536*

Chin, F. G., s. Phillips, T. L. *530*

Chin, H. Y. H., s. Senger, F. L. 19, *496, 498*

Chinn, J., Horton, R. K., Rusche, C. *557*

Chio, Kohler 199

Chisholm, E. R., Hutch, J. A., Bolomey, A. A. *557*

Chisholm, G. D. 273, *536*

Chiuppa, S., s. Aguzzi, A. *508*

Choi, J. K., Wiedemer, H. S. *499*

Choi, S., Gatzek, H., Kenny, G. M., Murphy, G. P. *536*

Choizzi, J. C., s. Bernardi, R. *560*

Chollat, L., s. Giraud, M. *528*

Chome, J., s. Aboulker, P. *525*

Chraplyvy, M., s. Rockoff, S. D. 57, *506, 516*

Christensen, E. R. *562*

Christensen, E. R., s. Bryndorf, J. 444, *561*

Christensen, W. R., s. Arons, W. L. *494*

Christeson, W. W., s. Bohne, A. W. *526*

Christian, E., Constantinescu, N. N. *562*

Christiansen, H. *499, 500*

Christoffersen, J. C., Andersen, K. *545, 550*

Christoffersen, C. J., s. Anthonsen, W. *521*

Christophe, L., Honoré, D. 68, *510*

von Chudacek, Z. *545*

Churchill, B. M., s. Robson, C. J. *531*

Chute, R., O'Hara, E. T., Goldman, R. N., Houghton, J. D., Toy, B. L. *536*

Chute, R., s. Ireland, Jr., E. F. *558*

Chute, R., s. O'Malley, A. F. *548, 550*

Chvojka, J., Dolézel, J. 83, *510*

Chwalla 89

Chwalla, s. Chen, K.-C. *518*

Chynn, K. Y., Evans, J. A. *527*

Ciampelli, L. *545*

Cibert, J. 250, 259, *534*

Cibert, J., Durand, L., Rivière, C. *557*

Cibert, J. A. V., Cavailher, H. *540, 562*

Ciccantelli, M. J., Gallagher, W. B., Skemp., F. C., Dietz, P. C. *500*

Cieviewich 262

Cimino, J. E., s. Brescia, M. J. 276, *536*

Cimmino, C. V. *533*

Cimmino, C. V., s. Wyman, A. C. *517*

Cirla, A., Galdini, S. *553*

Civino, A., Lovati, G. *562*

Civino, A., s. Lasio, E. *503, 513*

Claessen, G. *533*

Claesson, U. *522*

Claman, M., s. Wallach, J. B. 204, *532*

Clark, C. G. *510*

Clark, M., s. Ricker, W. *524*

Clark, M., s. Ries, S. W. *525*

Clark, R. E., McNamara, T., Palubinskas, A. 268, *536*

Clark, R. E., Minagi, H., Palubinskas, A. 378, *545*

Clark, R. E., Moss, A., Lorimier, A., Palubinskas, A. *527*

Clark, R. E., Palubinskas, A. J. *527*

Clarke, B. G., Goade, Jr., W. J., Rudy, H. L., Rockwood, L. *527, 533*

Clarke, H. *540*

Claus, H. G. *553*

Clement, G., s. Marchand, J. H. *567*

Clermont, A. *500*

Cletsoway, R. W., s. Lewis, E. L. *558*

Coakley, H. E., s. Low, H. T. *558*

Cocchi, U. 18, 179, *494, 497*

Cockett, A. T. K., Maxwell, M., Kaufman, J. J. *536*

Cockett, A. T. K., s. Goodwin, W. E. *523*

Cockett, A. T. K., s. Woodruff, Jr., J. H. *542*

Coe, F. O., Arthur, P. S. *562*

Coggeshall, W., s. Ries, S. W. 174, *525*

Cohen, G. F., s. Cohen, M. E. L. 176, *522, 545*

Cohen, M. E. L., Cohen, G. F., Ahad, V., Kaye, M. 176, *522, 545*

Cohn, R., s. Knudsen, D. F. 415, *556*

Cokier, Epstein **332**

Colby, F. H. *562*

Colby, F. H., Suby, H. I. *562*

Cole, A. T., s. Gill, W. B. *537*

Coliez, R. T. *522, 545*

Colin, R., s. Bétouliéres, P. 421, *557*

Collins, E. N., Root, J. C. 7, *493*

Collins, R. E., s. Allen, R. P. 318, *542*

Collins, W. T., s. Mulvaney, W. P. *554*

Colombi, M., s. Borghi, M. *522*

Colomé Bouza, A. *562*

Colpoys, Jr., F. L., s. Kickham, C. J. E. *551*

Colston, J. A. C., Baker, W. W. 303, *540*

Colston, J. A. C., s. Arnold, M. W. *509*

Comar, O. B., Saggese, V. *510*

Comarr, A. E. 127, *522, 562*

Comarr, A. E., Dodenhoff, L. *562*

Comarr, A. E., Kawaichi, G. K., Bors, E. 127, *522*

Commons, R. R., s. Burnett, C. H. 128, *494, 522*

Comotto, C., s. Cartelli, N. *561*

Compere, D. E., Begley, G. F., Isaacks, H. E., Frazier, T. H., Dryden, C. B. *577*

Condon, V. R., s. Allen, R. P. 318, *542*

Conelly, J. P., s. Baker, R. *522*

Confalonieri, A., s. Borghi, M. *522*

Conger, K. B., Reardon, H., Arey, J. 71, 73, *510*

Conger, K. B., s. Goldstein, A. G. *541*

Conn, H. O., s. Perillie, P. E. 55, *505*

Connolly, J. E., s. Palmer, J. M. *539*

Conradt, J. *562*

Consolazio, W. V., s. Albright, F. 174, *521*

Constantinescu, N. N., s. Christian, E. *562*

Conte, J., s. Escat, J. *536*

Constiades, X.-J. 336, *543*

Constiadès, X. J., s. Roux-Berger, J. L. *516*

Sachverzeichnis

Bei gleicher Schreibweise in beiden Sprachen sind die Stichwörter nur einmal aufgeführt

Subject Index

Where Englisch and German spelling of a word is identical, the German version is omited